P9-AOY-446

Comprehensive Psychiatric Nursing

COMPREHENSIVE PSYCHIATRIC NURSING

THIRD EDITION

Judith Haber, R.N., Ph.D., C.S.
College of Mount Saint Vincent
Riverdale, New York

Pamela Price Hoskins, R.N., Ph.D.
Anna Vaughn School of Nursing, Oral Roberts University
Tulsa, Oklahoma

Anita M. Leach, R.N., M.A., C.S.
State University of New York at Stony Brook
Stony Brook, New York

Barbara Flynn Sideleau, R.N., Ed.D.
School of Nursing, Fairfield University
Fairfield, Connecticut

McGRAW-HILL BOOK COMPANY

New York St. Louis San Francisco Auckland Bogotá Hamburg Johannesburg London
Madrid Mexico Milan Montreal New Delhi Panama Paris São Paulo Singapore
Sydney Tokyo Toronto

TO OUR SIGNIFICANT OTHERS

COMPREHENSIVE PSYCHIATRIC NURSING

Copyright © 1987, 1982, 1978 by McGraw-Hill, Inc.
All rights reserved.
Printed in the United States of America. Except as permitted under the United States Copyright Act of 1976, no part of this publication may be reproduced or distributed in any form or by any means, or stored in a data base or retrieval system, without the prior written permission of the publisher.

1 2 3 4 5 6 7 8 9 0 VNHVNH 8 9 4 3 2 1 0 9 8 7

ISBN 0-07-025415-X

This book was set in Zapf Book Light by Monotype Composition Company, Inc. The editors were Sally J. Barhydt and Susan Gamer; the designer was Joan Greenfield; the production supervisor was Joe Campanella. The drawings were done by Wellington Studios Ltd. Von Hoffman Press, Inc., was printer and binder.

Library of Congress Cataloging-in-Publication Data

Comprehensive psychiatric nursing.

Includes bibliographies and index.
1. Psychiatric nursing. 2. Nurse and patient.
I. Harber, Judith. [DNLM: 1. Psychiatric Nursing.
WY 160 C737]
RC440.C58 1987 610.73'68 86-18551
ISBN 0-07-025415-X

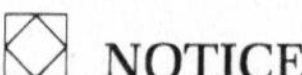

NOTICE

A new medical and nursing research and clinical experience broaden our knowledge, changes in treatment and drug therapy are required. The editors and the publisher of this work have made every effort to ensure that the drug dosage schedules herein are accurate and in accord with the standards accepted at the time of publication. Readers are advised, however, to check the product information sheet included in the package of each drug they plan to administer to be certain that changes have not been made in the recommended dose or in the contraindications for administration. This recommendation is of particular importance in regard to new or infrequently used drugs.

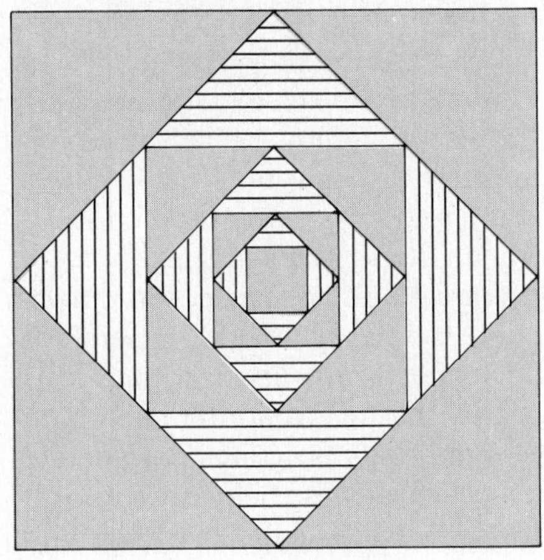

About the Authors

Judith Haber is an associate professor and coordinator of academic affairs in the Division of Nursing, College of Mount Saint Vincent, Riverdale, New York. Dr. Haber has worked with baccalaureate and associate degree nursing students for over 15 years. She holds a B.S., cum laude, in nursing from Adelphi University and an M.A. in adult psychiatric nursing and a Ph.D. from New York University. She is also certified as a clinical specialist in adult psychiatric nursing and has earned a Certificate of Advanced Achievement in Family Therapy from the Center for Family Learning.

Her psychiatric nursing experience includes a specialty in working with the chronically mentally ill in both residential and community settings. She also has extensive experience as a family therapist and maintains a private practive in family therapy. Her current clinical and research interests are focused on family therapy, in which she specializes in working with families who have marital conflict or dysfunctional adolescents or young adults, as well as families with physical health problems. She also has extensive clinical experience related to women's issues.

Dr. Haber has contributed numerous articles to professional journals, is a coauthor of a textbook on nursing research, and is a member of the editorial board of *Issues in Mental Health Nursing*. She is active nationally as both a speaker and a consultant to professional groups.

Pamela Price Hoskins received a B.S.N. from the University of Oklahoma and an M.A. in psychiatric–mental health nursing and a Ph.D. in nursing science, both from New York University. Her nursing practice has included pediatrics, work with clients with burns and disfiguring facial surgery, and operating room and postanesthesia recovery, as well as inpatient, outpatient, and community mental health nursing.

Dr. Hoskins has also taught in hospital school, associate degree, baccalaureate, and masters programs in nursing. She is especially interested in validating the efficacy of nursing theory being tested in practice settings that implement a specific theoretical model. Her desire to see clients healed has culminated in bringing together a strong belief in a healing, loving Savior and a nursing practice grounded in the theory of "nursing for the whole person." She speaks extensively and has provided leadership in several nursing organizations. Her current research project is "Factors That Maintain Discharged Psychiatric Patients in the Community."

The opportunity to join the editorial group of *Comprehensive Psychiatric Nursing*, third edition, has complemented the various avenues through which Dr. Hoskins has sought to serve the nursing profession. She is a tenured professor at Oral Roberts University Anna Vaughn School of Nursing, Tulsa, Oklahoma.

Anita M. Leach is Assistant Professor in the Department of Family and Community Nursing at the State University of New York at Stony Brook, where she is involved in teaching and research development in psychiatric nursing and family theory. She received a B.S. in Education from Brentwood College, New York; a diploma in nursing from St. Clare's Hospital School of Nursing; and an M.A. in Psychiatric Mental Health Nursing from New York University. She expects to complete her doctoral work in counseling at St. John's University, New York, in the spring of 1987.

Ms. Leach received her training in family therapy at the Center for Family Learning in New Rochelle and is certified as a Marriage and Family Counselor by the Board of Certified Counselors and as an Advanced Clinical Specialist in Adult Psychiatric Nursing by the ANA. Her career has included administrative positions in nursing and hospital administration, private practice, and consultation to geropsychiatric programs. Her research interests include ethics, the aging family, and the pastoral and spiritual care of clients. She is happily married to Robert Joseph McMahon.

Barbara Flynn Sideleau is an associate professor of nursing who has worked with undergraduate students for 20 years. She received a diploma in nursing from St. Vincent's School of Nursing, Bridgeport, Connecticut; a B.S.N. from the University of Bridgeport; an M.S.N. from Yale University; and an Ed.D. from Teachers College, Columbia University. She is on the faculty at Fairfield University, maintains a private practice in family counseling, and consults with corporations on stress management.

Her career in education has focused on curriculum development. She has conducted numerous professional workshops for practitioners that focus on health-promotive nursing. In addition, she has been involved in community programs designed to increase parents' effectiveness, help parents understand and deal with adolescents' drug use, and facilitate communication between adolescents and their parents.

She is interested in the mental health issues of families, particularly those with adolescents and those disrupted by divorce or death. She has been involved in research on the influence of birth order and disruption of family integrity on mental health. She is currently conducting research related to the nursing care of people with Alzheimer's disease.

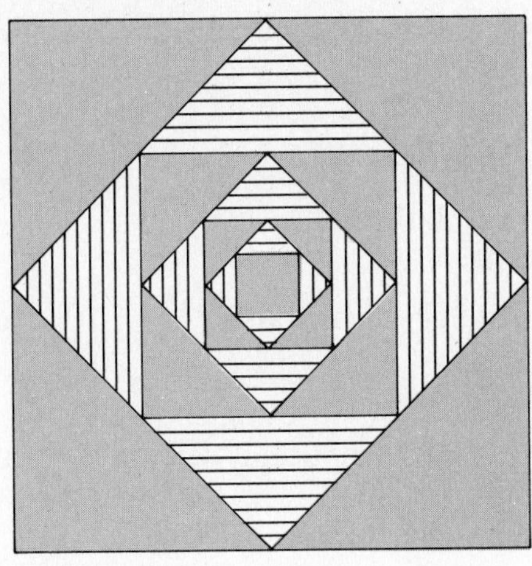

Contents

APPENDIXES

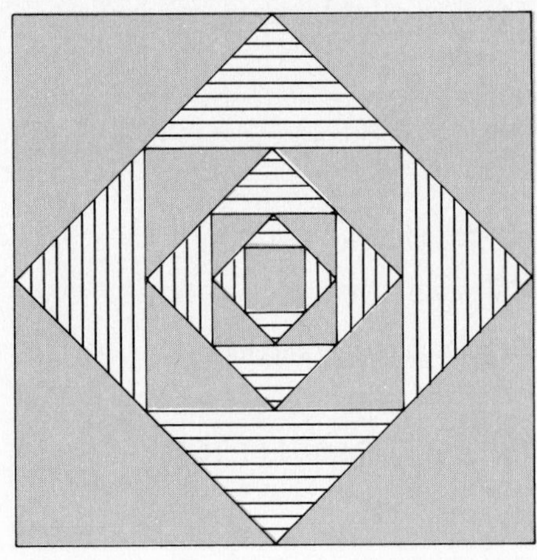

List of Contributors

Judith Ackerhalt, R.N., M.S.
Assistant Professor
Marion Buckley School of Nursing
Adelphi University
Garden City, New York

Ann Bello, R.N., M.A.
Associate Professor
Department of Nursing
Norwalk Community College
Norwalk, Connecticut

Lynn Bernstein, R.N., Ph.D.
Director
Sarasota Counseling and Psychotherapy Center
Sarasota, Florida
Private Practice, Licenced Nurse Psychologist

Judith Gregorie D'Afflitti, R.N., M.S.N., C.S.
Clinical Manager
Harvard Community Health Plan
Wellesley, Massachusetts

Joy Feldman, R.N., M.A.
Clinical Assistant Professor
School of Nursing
State University of New York at Buffalo
Buffalo, New York

Hope Fox, R.N., M.A., A.C.M.F.C.
Codirector
South Shore Mental Health Services
Wantaugh, New York
Trustee and Instructor
South Shore Institute for Mental Health
Wantaugh, New York

Karen Davis Frank, R.N., M.A.
Psychiatric Nurse Coordinator
Englewood Hospital
Englewood, New Jersey

Mary Giuffra, R.N., Ph.D., C.S.
Professor and Director
Department of Nursing
College of Mount Saint Vincent
Riverdale, New York

Judith Haber, R.N., Ph.D., C.S.
Associate Professor
Coordinator of Academic Affairs
Department of Nursing
College of Mount Saint Vincent
Riverdale, New York
Private Practice, Family Therapy

Pamela Price Hoskins, R.N., Ph.D.
Professor
Anna Vaughn School of Nursing
Oral Roberts University
Tulsa, Oklahoma

Sandra Jaffe-Johnson, R.N., Ed.D., C.S., C.A.C.
Clinical Associate Professor
School of Nursing
State University of New York at Stony Brook
Stony Brook, New York
Private Practice, Individual Psychotherapy

Suzanne Sayle Jimerson, R.N., M.S., C.S.
Assistant Professor
School of Nursing
University of Maryland
Bethesda, Maryland

Eugenia McAuliffe Kelly, R.N., M.A.
Director of Psychiatric Nursing
Coney Island Hospital
Brooklyn, New York

Norine J. Kerr, R.N., M.N.
Clinical Nurse Consultant
Western Missouri Mental Health Center
Kansas City, Missouri

Judith Belliveau Krauss, R.N., M.S.N.
Dean and Professor
School of Nursing
Yale University
New Haven, Connecticut

Anita M. Leach, R.N., M.A., C.S.
Assistant Professor
School of Nursing
State University of New York at Stony Brook
Stony Brook, New York
Private Practice, Marriage and Family Therapy

Suzanne Lego, R.N., Ph.D., C.S.
Private Practice
New York, New York; Demarest, New Jersey

Elise Lev, R.N., Ed.D.
Assistant Professor
College of New Rochelle
New Rochelle, New York

Nada Light, R.N., M.A.
Adjunct Faculty
Department of Nursing
Greater Hartford Community College
Hartford, Connecticut

Doris Troth Sommerfield Lippman, R.N., Ed.D.
Associate Professor
School of Nursing
Fairfield University
Fairfield, Connecticut

Lenora McClean, R.N., Ed.D.
Dean and Professor
School of Nursing
State University of New York at Stony Brook
Stony Brook, New York

Fern Mims, R.N., Ed.D.
Professor
School of Nursing
University of Wisconsin at Madison
Madison, Wisconsin

Thomas Francis Nolan, R.N., Ph.D.
Professor
Department of Nursing
Sonoma State University
Rohnert Park, California

Jane Norbeck, R.N., D.N.Sc., F.A.A.N.
Associate Professor
School of Nursing
University of California at San Francisco
San Francisco, California

Alice Marie Obrig, R.N., M.S., M.P.H.
Assistant Professor
School of Nursing
Fairfield University
Fairfield, Connecticut
Certified Nurse-Midwife

Luc Reginald Pelletier, R.N., M.S.N., C.S.
Assistant Clinical Professor
and Clinical Applications Analyst
University of California at Los Angeles
Los Angeles, California

Patricia Pothier, R.N. M.S., F.A.A.N.
Professor
School of Nursing
University of California at San Francisco
San Francisco, California

Victoria Schoolcraft, R.N., M.S.N.
Associate Professor and Assistant Director
of the Baccalaureate Program
College of Nursing
University of Oklahoma
Oklahoma City, Oklahoma

Barbara Flynn Sideleau, R.N., Ed.D.
Associate Professor
School of Nursing
Fairfield University
Fairfield, Connecticut
Private Practice, Individual and Family Therapy

Marie Cella Smith, R.N., M.A.
Private Practice
Nanuet, New York

Laura Coble Zamora, R.N., M.A.
Assistant Professor
College of Nursing
State University of New York at Downstate
Medical Center
Brooklyn, New York

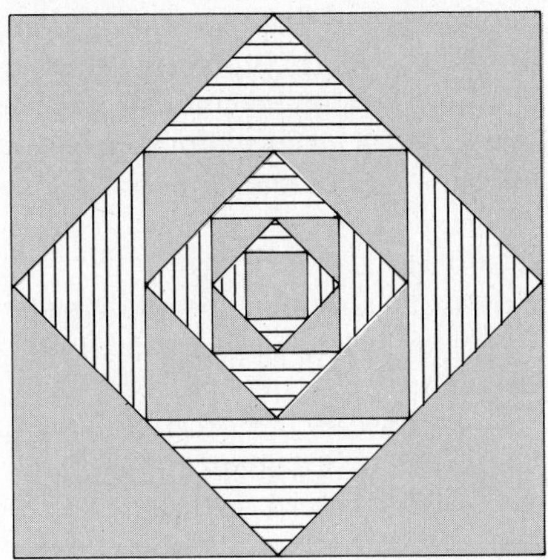

Preface

The publication of the third edition of *Comprehensive Psychiatric Nursing* marks the culmination of a decade of change and development in the text as well as evolution in the professional practice of psychiatric–mental health nursing.

In 1978 *Comprehensive Psychiatric Nursing* was a trailblazer among textbooks in the field. It was the first comprehensive psychiatric–mental health nursing textbook to use a holistic framework that addressed the four primary domains of nursing: *client, nursing, health,* and *environment.* It was the first psychiatric–mental health nursing textbook designed for use in an integrated curriculum. From its inception, the textbook has encompassed clients of all ages who are experiencing threats to mental health from a variety of sources and interacting environments including the family, the settings where nursing care is delivered, and the relevant influential societal context. It was also the first textbook to apply the nursing process to psychiatric–mental health phenomena. The conception of the original project by Anita M. Leach was based on the belief that nurses provide esential therapeutic experiences through their relationships with clients and that nurses must engage in an ongoing process of increasing their self-awareness if they are to maximize their therapeutic use of self with clients. Emphasis has been placed on the person-environment interactions that occur in relation to mental health and illness. The relevance of the textbook's approach to psychiatric–mental health nursing care and the wide acceptance of the text are evidence of its contribution to the nursing profession.

The second edition of the text, published in 1982, expanded and strengthened the focus on the client, nursing, health, and the environment, particularly the family, as operationalized through the nursing process and the nurse's therapeutic use of self.

The third edition of *Comprehensive Psychiatric Nursing* represents another milestone in the development and articulation of psychiatric–mental health nursing theory and practice. This edition further emphasizes the four domains—client, nursing, health, and environment—and strengthens the overall conceptual framework. Each domain is defined, and these definitions influence how the nursing process is applied in the text. The evolution of the application of the nursing process, evident in this edition, is reflected in the refinement and clarification of the components, particularly with regard to nursing diagnoses, outcome criteria, and the evaluation process. The commitment to the need for self-awareness, the nurse's therapeutic use of self, the importance of the family, and the significance of the interactional nature of human phenomena are retained and integrated. In addition, the editors emphasize and integrate current nursing research findings throughout the text. To facilitate the collaborative interdisciplinary nature of psychiatric–mental health nursing, DSM III nomenclature has been included in relevant chapters.

Several new chapters have been included in the third edition, and content from the second edition has been reorganized, expanded, and updated. The editors have developed brief introductory chapters for each of the seven parts of the text to highlight the implementation of the conceptual framework.

These chapters introduce the reader to the definition of the significant concept addressed within the chapters that follow. In this edition, separate chapters address the sociocultural issues related to psychiatric–mental health nursing, the history of psychiatric and mental health care, and the inpatient and outpatient contexts of care. In addition, chapters focus on what it means to become a client needing psychiatric care; on behavioral and cognitive approaches to care; and on problems of the elderly, the chronically mentally ill, and borderline clients. The chapters on holistic health concepts, legal and ethical issues, family theory, alternative and somatic therapies, patterns of depression, patterns of dysfunction in adolescence, and patterns of abuse have been expanded and extensively revised in this edition.

The third edition is organized into seven parts. Part One introduces and describes the conceptual framework in Chapter 1. Parts Two through Seven each begin with an introductory chapter that defines the domain (person or client; nursing; health; or environment) discussed in that part.

Part Two (Chapters 2 through 6) develops the concept of the *person*. In the introductory chapter, the editors define *person* as a living and developing being with physical, mental, and spiritual dimensions who functions in identifiable patterns with the environment to achieve a chosen life purpose. Self-awareness, concepts related to an understanding of the person as all one is and can become, and biopsychosocial developmental issues are discussed.

Part Three (Chapters 7 through 14) elaborates on the concept of *nursing*. The introductory chapter defines *nursing* as a goal-directed process that promotes synchronous patterns of interaction between person and environment. The historical development of mental health care and psychiatric–mental health nursing, the role of the nurse, the legal and ethical issues related to psychiatric–mental health nursing, and the nursing process are presented. Communication theory, the therapeutic nurse-client relationship, and the nursing process, which comprise the essence of nursing care, are also included in Part Three.

Part Four (Chapters 15 through 26) introduces the concept of environment from the perspective of becoming a client and participating in a therapeutic mental health context. In the introductory chapter, *environment* is defined as the relevant systems and processes external to and in interaction with the person, family, or community. The process of becoming a client in the mental health care system, the elements of inpatient and outpatient contexts of care, and the therapies used by nurses in these settings are examined.

Parts Five and Six discuss the concept of *health*. In this textbook, *health* is defined as a synchronous pattern of interaction in a person-environment system. Parts Five and Six each have an additional introductory chapter which defines the particular dysynchronous health pattern (psychosocial or biopsychosocial) that is the focus of the chapters in each part. Part Five (Chapters 27 through 39) deals specifically with dysynchronous *psychosocial* patterns of health that are manifested as overt and avoidant anxiety, borderline behavior, violence, substance abuse, depression, elation, self-destructiveness, dysfunctional reality orientation, sexual dysfunction, and patterns of dysfunction in adolescence. Part Six (Chapters 40 through 45) describes *biopsychosocial* patterns of health. The biopsychosocial dimensions of grappling with illness, stress-related illness, disability and chronic physical illness, organic mental disorders, and the dying process are presented.

In Part Seven (Chapters 46 through 54), the environment is addressed from a community perspective which includes descriptions of special groups of clients and their mental health problems. In the introductory chapter, *community* is defined as a group of people with common characteristics, location, or interests who live together within a larger society. Separate chapters are devoted to promotion of mental health in childbearing and child-rearing families; high-risk families; the maintenance and restoration of mental health in child-rearing families; the rehabilitation of mental health in children; problems of abusive families; rape; the chronic mentally ill; and the mental health issues of the elderly.

With this third edition, the editors have developed two supplements to facilitate a more effective teaching-learning process. A student activity manual provides instructors with chapter outlines and chapter-specific experiential learning exercises that are the original work of the editors and contributors. These exercises are designed to enhance the student's affective learning and creativity. They also provide students with opportunities to apply concepts presented in the correlated textbook chapters.

A computerized test bank, available as a printed manual and on a disk, was also developed for faculty use in evaluating learning or in helping students develop test-taking skills. Test bank questions include items on the theory base of practice and the application of the nursing process to psychiatric–mental health nursing.

The third edition of *Comprehensive Psychiatric Nursing* includes the contributions of many colleagues who helped make the first and second editions possible and the contributions of several new authors whose expertise broadens the scope of this edition. The value and quality of the project have been increased by the talents of the diverse individuals in nursing education and practice who have participated with us in this effort. In particular, the contribution of Sylvia Schudy to the first and second editions as an editor, author, and supportive person is gratefully acknowledged. The addition to the editorial board of Pamela Price Hoskins enhanced the development and implementation of the project. Her expertise and her commitment have been valuable contributions to the editorial board.

Acknowledgements

We wish to acknowledge the loving support, nurturance, patience, understanding, and forbearance of the many persons who helped us through the months of preparation of the third edition.

A special note of thanks is due to our families: Lenny, Laurie, and Andrew Haber; Mark and Whitney Price Hoskins; the Leaches and R. J. McMahon; and Bob, Greg, Michelle, Brian, Robert, and Katie Sideleau.

We are grateful for the encouragement and support of friends and colleagues whose names are too numerous to mention. A project of this size would not have been possible without our energetic and faithful secretaries: Sandra Csuka, Sylvia Robart, Diane Speiss, and Betty Vinci. McGraw-Hill editors have been tireless facilitators of our efforts. We are most grateful to Sally Barhydt, the editor of both the first and the third editions, for her support and guidance; and to Susan Gamer, whose attention to detail produced a more readable text.

Judith Haber
Pamela Price Hoskins
Anita M. Leach
Barbara Flynn Sideleau

Comprehensive Psychiatric Nursing

PART ONE
Conceptual Framework

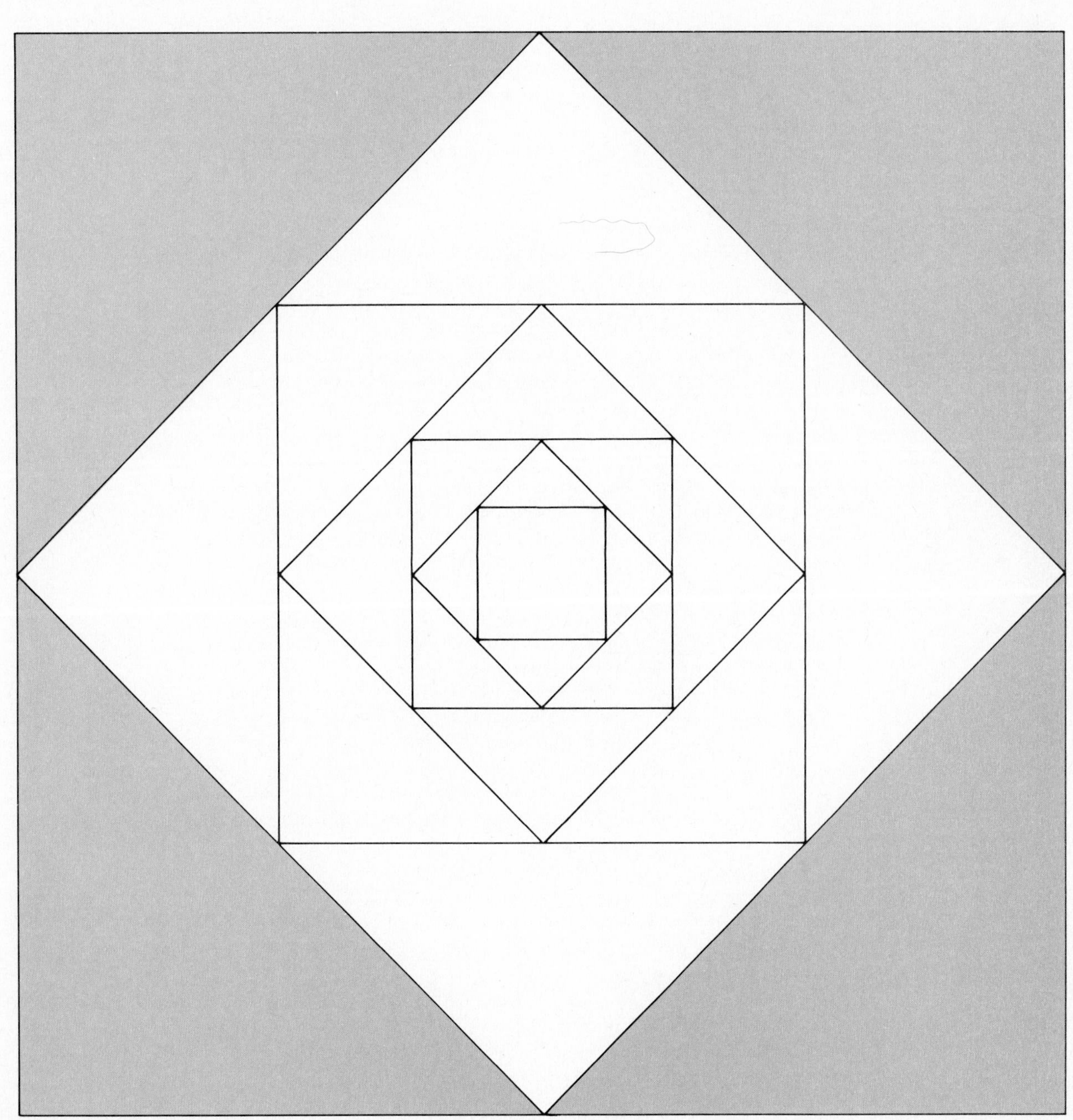

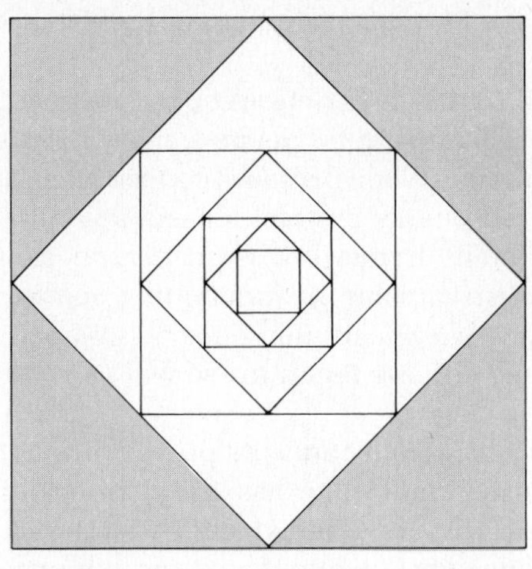

CHAPTER 1

Conceptual Framework for Psychiatric–Mental Health Nursing

Judith Haber

Pamela Price Hoskins

Anita M. Leach

Barbara Flynn Sideleau

LEARNING OBJECTIVES

After studying this chapter, the student should be able to:

1. Describe the conceptual framework of this book.
2. Define the terms *person, environment, health,* and *nursing,* as they are developed in this book.
3. Provide examples of how the conceptual framework is useful in nursing.
4. Recognize how a conceptual framework can be applied to nursing diagnoses, client outcomes, and nursing interventions in psychiatric–mental health care.
5. Recognize how a conceptual framework provides freedom.

What do nurses who work with psychiatric patients do? What kinds of tools do they use? Where do they work? What are the special challenges of working with psychiatric patients? Are there also special rewards? Why do nurses choose to work with psychiatric patients in the hospital or community? How does knowledge about mental health assist nurses in other areas of practice?

These and similar questions may be answered by means of a conceptual framework. The purpose of this chapter is to introduce and explore the conceptual framework of *Comprehensive Psychiatric Nursing.* Definitions, descriptions, and examples of the concepts are presented, and the influence of the concepts is specified.

Knowledge basic to nursing can be organized around four fundamental concepts: *person, environment, health,* and *nursing* itself. These four concepts are developed throughout the nursing curriculum. At the end of a nursing program, a student is expected to have a very complex understanding of each and to know how they are related to one another. That understanding is called the *knowledge base* of nursing.

STAGES OF THEORY DEVELOPMENT

Before an explanation of reality actually becomes a theory, it must pass through four developmental stages: (1) concept, (2) conceptual framework, (3) theoretical framework, (4) theory.

Stage 1: Concept

A *concept* is an abstract idea originating in or referring to the real world. A concept is intangible; it cannot be weighed or seen. But it does emerge from thought about tangible or observable phenomena. For instance, although the concept of *self* cannot be weighed or seen, it consists of specific observable elements that can be measured: self-concept, self-identity, self-image, self-esteem, moral image, and body boundary.

Stage 2: Conceptual Framework

Concepts are particularly useful when they can be related to one another. Relationships among concepts are called a *conceptual framework.* A conceptual framework is somewhat analagous to the framework of a building, which tells us a good deal about the shape of the building even before the rest of it is in place.[1]

Conceptual frameworks determine the approach to the four basic concepts: person, environment, health, and nursing. When *person* is conceptualized as an organized energy system, for example, that is a very different framework from *person* as a biological system capable of functioning socially. Here, the framework can influence assessment, goals, and interventions that a nurse will use with a client.

The four fundamental concepts provide nursing with its identity, knowledge base, and priorities. How the concepts are defined and operationalized—the framework—differentiates various nursing programs from each other. If, for instance, a biological framework is used—that is, if *person* is defined as a biological system—a nursing curriculum will probably emphasize biological systems (respiration, circulation, and so on). If a spiritual framework is used, *person* will be defined as a spiritual entity, and the curriculum will probably emphasize how the human spirit is reflected in behavior.

What one *does* in nursing emerges from what one *knows* and thus from a conceptual framework. Graduates from different programs may approach clients, and the art and science of nursing, in very different ways. The same four concepts are developed in every nursing program, but the frameworks—definitions, descriptions, operationalizations, and interrelationships—differ.

Stage 3: Theoretical Framework

The next stage of development is the *theoretical framework.* At this level, relationships among concepts are stated and interrelated very specifically. If a conceptual framework is like the framework of a building, a theoretical framework might be seen as a complete set of specifications, a sort of blueprint. The relationships detailed in a theoretical framework have been tested in research and found useful in practice. Elisabeth Kübler-Ross's work on death and dying is an example of a theoretical framework.

Stage 4: Theory

A theory can be considered the most advanced stage of knowledge. It is like a completed building—

the theoretical framework plus everything else. In nursing, when a conceptualization has reached the stage of theory, predictions can be made about the effectiveness of a given intervention for a specific client with a specific set of behaviors. Today there are in nursing a multitude of conceptual frameworks, several theoretical frameworks, and a few theories.

PURPOSE OF THE CONCEPTUAL FRAMEWORK

One purpose of the conceptual framework in this book is to provide a complex understanding of the four fundamental concepts; each chapter will build on the definitions and descriptions provided in this opening chapter. A second purpose is to provide a specific understanding of these concepts in the context of psychiatric–mental health nursing.

The following example shows how important a conceptual framework can be in nursing. One definition of *person* includes self-determination—the ability to set goals and behave rationally. If this framework is used, alcoholics might be seen as disgusting because they simply fail to exercise willpower. A nurse who was operating within such a framework might avoid an alcoholic client, or express anger toward such a client. A very different definition of *person* includes unconscious forces over which people have no control. Within this framework, alcohol abuse would be seen as a symptom of unresolved unconscious conflicts; alcoholics would be considered victims of unconscious, uncontrollable forces. A nurse working within this framework might ignore alcohol abuse as such regard it as merely a symptom, and help alcoholic clients to make their conflicts conscious. The action a nurse takes, then, can be derived from a conceptual framework.

CONCEPTS FOR COMPREHENSIVE PSYCHIATRIC NURSING

Below, the four fundamental concepts—person, environment, health, and nursing—are defined, described, and interrelated. These concepts will be explored throughout *Comprehensive Psychiatric Nursing*. How they are developed and interrelated is illustrative of systems theory.[2]

Person

A *person* is defined as a living being with physical, mental, and spiritual dimensions, who functions in identifiable patterns with the environment to achieve a chosen life purpose.

The *physical dimension* is the body—anatomy and physiology. The *mental dimension* is the ability to think and feel. The *spiritual dimension* is the ability to dream, to be aware of mortality, to relate to and commit oneself to God or to some being or essence greater than oneself. Although these three dimensions are defined separately, they are really inseparable within the person.

The person functions, or behaves, in *identifiable patterns with the environment.* People knowingly participate in the patterning of their lives. The patterns a person establishes with the environment are interactive and observable over time. Behavioral patterns are useful to the person because they are reliable ways to interact with the environment in different situations. Such patterns are learned and repeated until they become automatic. They are unique to each person and are a part of personal identity. For instance, a parent can come into the kitchen and find the cabinet door open, drops of grape juice on the floor and counter, and the jar on the counter next to a half-empty glass. The parent will think, "Janet must be home," because even though Janet is not visible, Janet's behavior pattern is.

Behavior patterns exist for a purpose; they are methods of interacting with the environment, developed to *achieve a chosen life purpose.* Purposes are chosen early in life, always as an outgrowth of interaction with the environment. Life purposes are sometimes chosen "because of" the environment and sometimes "in spite of" it. They may be realistic, ridiculous, visionary, ordinary, or tragic. Sometimes they are given to, and accepted by, children: "You'll be president someday, Gail." Sometimes they are formed because of attitudes of significant others: "Look at the shoulders on that kid," Jeff heard his father say, and so Jeff decided to be a model. Sad or tragic purposes can emerge from interactions such as these: "You'll kill your mother someday, son." "You'll never do anything with your life, Gina." "Your uncle was a drunk, and you're just like him." "Someday the police will come and take you away." The point is that human beings have a unique characteristic: we need a meaningful, purposeful life. Behavior patterns are ways to fulfill purposes.

Elements of the person include self, self-image, self-concept, self-esteem, self-awareness, body image, and identity. Each of these aspects has a physical, mental, and spiritual component. Identity, for instance, includes a system of beliefs about body, mind, and spirit; ideas about how one should and should not interact with others and the environment; and beliefs about what one will accomplish in life. For example, when a little girl was asked, "Who are you?" she answered, "I am Whitney. I am this tall (patting herself on the head), my eyes are blue, and God made me just right. I know my ABCs and numbers, and when I grow up, I'm going to drive to mommy's work to see her students." One can sense an identity beginning to emerge; here is someone who is growing, who is "just right," and who will someday be autonomous and will interact with others as her mother does. Her identity is not completely formed, but even at 3 years of age, she is exhibiting important aspects of being a person. (The aspects of *person* are developed in Chapter 3.)

Environment

Environment is defined as relevant systems and processes external to and in interaction with the client. Theoretically, environment is the universe: everything and everyone external to the client. Practically, of course, the universe is too vast to deal with. In nursing, as attempts are made to understand and intervene in clients' interactions with the environment, nurses and clients must determine which external systems and processes are relevant. Thus only the systems and processes considered relevant for a client are defined as the client's environment. The nurse, clearly, is part of the environment of the client.

Systems are defined as organized structures that influence and are influenced by the client. Systems include the family and the neighborhood in which one lives or works. They may also include school, church, unemployment office, parole department, public assistance office, visiting nurse, or child protection unit. Organizations such as Bible study classes, Parents Without Partners, Alcoholics Anonymous, parent effectiveness training groups, and state nurses' associations may also be systems.

Processes are defined as organized, purposeful patterns or operations. They include the dynamics of the person, family, group, and community. Processes that are especially relevant to mental health are satisfaction of needs, growth, and development.

Aspects of the environment include the family, the health care system, nursing, and resources relevant to the pursuit of life goals. For example:

> When Peggy was discharged from the psychiatric unit, there were several relevant systems and processes to be considered. Her family wanted her to come home and resume her role as wife and mother but were afraid that she would become suicidal again. She was discharged, given an antidepressant, and assigned to an outpatient therapy group. Peggy's primary nurse had worked with her to construct a plan that would help her stay out of the hospital, develop a better self-image, and eventually go to college (she wanted to be a meteorologist). The relevant systems in Peggy's environment were the family, the health care system, and the therapy group. The relevant processes were growing children, family dynamics, and personal growth.

Health

Health is defined as a synchronous pattern of interaction in the person-environment system. A synchronous pattern is a maximum level of wellness, which is different for each person. The pattern of interaction between person and environment determines health status. Patterns of interaction that are harmonious, synchronous, or congruent are healthy; patterns that are dissonant, dysynchronous, or incongruent are not healthy. The patterns of interaction are reflected in the functioning of the client. The nurse assesses patterns of interaction on a continuum ranging from severe dysfunction to maximum function. A nursing diagnosis is a summary of such an assessment. Health is one dynamic aspect of a client (whether person, family, or community).

Here is an example of the way health is determined by a pattern of interaction with the environment:

> Harold had just started a new business and was under tremendous pressure to get it established. He began gaining weight as the pressure increased. His clothes were too tight, he began to have obsessive thoughts about food, and he became a compulsive eater. His cholesterol level and blood pressure shot up, and he

became depressed and discouraged. His business began to founder. He then focused on his wife as the source of his stress. This allowed him to exert some control over his eating and thinking, so that his business began to pick up; but his marriage began to founder. The family began therapy, and the nurse counselor assisted the family members to take responsibility, each for his or her own stress. Harold stopped making his wife a scapegoat; but he developed premature ventricular contractions (PVCs). When a thorough cardiac evaluation uncovered no pathology, Harold and his wife made an effort to clarify their life purposes and recommit themselves to their marriage vows. Harold lost 80 pounds, developed a stronger sense of self-worth, and eventually established a financial base for his business, which succeeded.

Nursing

Nursing is defined as a goal-directed process that promotes synchronous patterns of interaction between client and environment. The term *synchronous patterns of interaction* is synonymous with *health* or *high-level wellness;* therefore, nursing is a goal-directed process that promotes health.

The *goals of nursing* as a profession are promotion, maintenance, restoration, and rehabilitation of health.

- *Promotion of health* is defined as nursing activities that facilitate more synchronous patterns of interaction.
- *Maintenance of health* is defined as nursing activities that continue or preserve the current health status.
- *Restoration of health* is defined as nursing activities that facilitate the return of health status to previous levels.
- *Rehabilitation of health* is defined as nursing activities that break into established dysfunctional patterns to facilitate the establishment of more functional patterns.

In any one client, some patterns should be promoted, some patterns should be maintained, and some patterns should be restored. In the chronically ill client, there are dysfunctional patterns that need to be rehabilitated. Table 1-1 gives examples of the goals of nursing. (Parts Five through Seven of this book develop the goals of nursing.)

Interventions in nursing are categorized as supportive-educative, partly compensatory, or wholly compensatory.[3] *Supportive-educative interventions* are used in situations where clients are able or should learn to care for themselves but need assistance, such as support, guidance, provision of a developmental environment, or teaching. For example:

John and Mary were referred to a clinical nurse specialist by a child abuse prevention center. The nurse determined that neither parent had an accurate perception of their 3-year-old son's developmental needs and abilities. The supportive-educative intervention used was teaching and demonstrating discipline techniques appropriate for a 3-year-old.

Partly compensatory interventions are used in situations where both client and nurse provide care. Their use varies with the client's limitations,

Table 1-1 Examples of the Goals of Nursing

Promotion	Maintenance	Restoration	Rehabilitation
Encourage concepts of right and wrong in a 7-year-old.	Help a recently raped woman to come to terms with her concepts of right and wrong in light of her experience.	Encourage forgiveness in a young man who has been physically handicapped through child abuse.	Assist a woman who has been incarcerated for 16 felonies to develop a sense of right and wrong.
Suggest the use of problem solving and values clarification to a couple deciding whether or not to have a baby.	Assist a family whose baby was stillborn to grieve appropriately.	Assist a man who has experienced a series of business failures to remold and reestablish abilities to solve problems and set priorities.	Help a man unemployed for 6 years to volunteer to work in the mail room of the community mental health center.
Assist a paraplegic mother of a 2-week-old in using nurturing skills.	Assist a family in promoting circulation for a terminally ill family member dying at home.	Teach range-of-motion exercises to a woman with dependent edema following a radical mastectomy.	Encourage the acquisition of cooking skills by a 32-year-old paraplegic man with 3 dependent children.

the knowledge and skill required, and the client's readiness to perform or to learn the needed activities. For example:

When the physician made rounds, Jay became confused and anxious and couldn't think of the questions he wanted to ask about his illness. The nurse role-played with Jay, helped him to write his questions, and stayed with him, prompting him to deal assertively with the physician. Once or twice the nurse asked a question for Jay. These partly compensatory interventions were performed by both Jay and the nurse, acting as a team to achieve the goals of gaining information and developing communication skills.

Wholly compensatory interventions are used in situations where the clients have no active role; the nurse provides all required care, compensates for the clients' inability to care for themselves, and supports them in the recipient role. For example:

Mary, 20 years old, was admitted to the intensive psychiatric unit in a totally regressed state. She maintained a fetal position, was incontinent, and was not eating or drinking. Mary's primary nurse took care of her totally, bathing, feeding, rocking, changing, talking to, and nurturing her. These wholly compensatory interventions were replaced with partly compensatory interventions as Mary began to respond.

A general example of nursing may be useful at this point:

Susan is an 18-year-old first-semester college student, away from home for the first time in her life. She is seen in the college clinic for severe constipation. The nurse assesses Susan's patterns of interaction with her environment and discovers that her bowels are not the only aspect of her life at a standstill. Susan feels confused and disoriented, can't think, feels unable to make even minor decisions, has not made any friends in her dormitory, and has lost her roommate (who dropped out after the first week of classes). She feels depressed and defeated but can't decide if she should go home. The nurse determines that although Susan has feelings of worthlessness and futility, she has not thought about suicide.

The nurse establishes with Susan the goal of getting her life moving again. Susan and the nurse work out a long-range plan aimed at eating well, establishing regular hygiene and health habits, making friends, and doing well in college. This week Susan will eat every meal with someone; she will not eat alone. She will choose high-fiber foods with lots of protein and will stay away from sugars and empty starches. When she returns to see the nurse the next week, work will begin on other objectives. These interventions are supportive-educative and partly compensatory.

RELEVANCE OF THE CONCEPTUAL FRAMEWORK

The conceptual framework interrelates the four basic concepts—person, environment, health, nursing. Each is a system in itself as well as a subsystem in the larger system which they form together. Nursing and health are relevant to person and environment; nursing is an essential part of the development of health in society and in individuals. None of these elements is static: health and the capacity for health are always developing and changing, as are the person and the environmental challenges that influence health. In other words, the person-environment-health-nursing system is dynamic, usually changing in the direction of more complexity and greater differentiation. A framework helps us to make sense of it. (Parts Two, Three, and Four are presented within this context.)

A conceptual framework is also practical; it can be used by the nurse to organize thinking about and planning for care of clients. Nurses can respond to clients spontaneously, using the self as a therapeutic tool, when observations are guided by a conceptual framework. A framework can free nurses from prescribed rules and allow them to think conceptually about interactions with clients. For instance, a traditional rule has been that nurses should refuse gifts from clients or their families. Two examples illustrate the importance of thinking through situations within a conceptual framework rather than relying on rules.

Tracy, diagnosed with anorexia nervosa, is a painfully thin 19-year-old whose father is an international financier. Her mother died when Tracy was 10 years old, and Tracy has taken over the wife's role in the family, including business entertaining. Tracy is extremely competitive and jealous of women in her father's life. You and Tracy work well together, and she is making progress. Her father, who is grateful for her improvement, brings you a silk scarf from his latest trip to France. Do you accept this gift?

Megan, a 17-year-old suffering from psychotic depression, mutilates her legs and arms with anything she can find whenever she can manage to be alone.

(One night she makes superficial cuts on her legs with a broken bottle.) She feels worthless and is certain that she has nothing to give to any relationship. Eventually, Megan begins to trust you and can sit near you in silence for about 10 minutes or more before becoming uncomfortable. One day she brings you a scrap of construction paper, on which she has drawn a tiny spring flower just poking its head above ground. She says, "Here," and stretches her hand toward you, holding the picture. Do you accept this gift?

A conceptual framework provides a structure within which to choose among alternatives, to formulate responses, to use the self therapeutically, to be a unique person interacting in an affirming way with another unique person. This is much better than following a set of rules, in any situation.

IMPLEMENTING THE CONCEPTUAL FRAMEWORK

The conceptual framework is the unifying theme of this book; it provides the elements needed for consistent development of knowledge in psychiatric–mental health nursing. It will be useful in the nursing process because it structures what is known about psychiatric–mental health nursing.

Assessment

A nurse's conceptual framework determines how a client is seen. The client is a whole, irreducible, person, whose identity and direction in life are expressed in three dimensions: mind, body, and spirit. Nurses see the client as needing fulfillment and purpose in life and therefore assess and minister to the client physically, mentally, and spiritually. To ignore any dimension of the person is to denigrate and dehumanize clients. A nurse must develop the ability to assess body, mind, and spirit and to discern life purposes. The nurse must be able to recognize relevant patterns of interaction between the client and the environment and determine relevant systems and processes in the client's environment.

Nursing Diagnosis

Much work has been done on the necessity, relevance, and form of nursing diagnosis; but most proposed taxonomies are based on divergent concepts, defined in different ways. The format for nursing diagnosis used in this book is based on *consistent* definitions and descriptions of nursing concepts. Patterns of interaction are emphasized, since nurses diagnose health status; and *health status* is defined as a pattern of interaction between client and environment. (At times, only a description of the client's pattern will be given; this is necessary when it is not clear what factors in the environment are part of the interaction. In such areas, exploratory research is needed.)

Among the health disciplines, the focus on patterns of interaction is unique to nursing. Besides being practical, it is also politically useful: it helps nurses communicate to other disciplines, to the consumer, and to government agencies what nurses do.

Goals for Nurses

The conceptual framework sets four goals for nurses: promotion, maintenance, restoration, and rehabilitation of synchronous patterns of interaction. Nursing takes place not within the person but in the interaction of the person with the environment. This makes nursing immediate and practical, visible to the client and in the environment. Nurses are concerned with life and living, here and now, day after day.

Client Outcomes

In addition, the conceptual framework provides parameters for appropriate outcomes. The desired general outcome is synchronous patterns of interaction, or functional behaviors. Clients participate in determining, and often do determine, the specific outcomes they are willing to pay for. Vague statements about enhancing self-worth and clarifying identity are much less significant in deciding what nursing is worth than specific statements of measurable outcomes, such as these: "Completes three job interviews, including appropriate completion of applications"; "good hygiene practices"; "appropriate choice of clothing"; "keeps appointments on time"; "good evaluation of the interview process by the employer."

Nursing Interventions

The conceptual framework provides a structure within which nursing interventions can be developed. In this conceptual framework, interventions are aimed at altering the interaction between client and environment. Defining *person* as body, mind, and spirit makes a broad spectrum of appropriate interventions possible. For instance, helping a client to clarify a life purpose is an intervention that makes sense only in a framework that mentions life purpose.

Evaluation

The evaluation phase of the nursing process has several purposes. It is, of course, an opportunity to evaluate the appropriateness and effectiveness of client outcomes and interventions; but it is also an excellent opportunity to build and test theories.

The various phases of the nursing process can also be parts of the process of developing theory. Nursing diagnoses are hypotheses about reality, and client outcomes specify what should happen if nursing interventions are appropriate. When enough successful interventions bring about similar outcomes, an excellent basis will have been provided for a theory and for more rigorous research.

Theories can also be tested through the nursing process. If a client's pattern of interaction is, in the nurse's judgment, best explained by a particular theory, then the interventions will reflect that theoretical understanding. If in fact the interventions prove valuable and help the client alter the pattern of interaction, then the theory has been supported. If, however, the interventions do not help, or even seem to make the situation worse, the theory is not supported. As a care plan is evaluated, the nurse thinks about where things went wrong. The nurse may decide that the theory, though it should have facilitated understanding, did not describe reality for a particular client and therefore is in need of modification.

SUMMARY

The conceptual framework is a way to organize the knowledge base of nursing. It describes who the client is, what assessment should include, what client outcomes are appropriate, what interventions are appropriate, and what form of evaluation should be included. In other words, the conceptual framework gives nursing its identity and defines its nature.

The four stages of theory development are concept, conceptual framework, theoretical framework, and theory. The unifying theme of *Comprehensive Psychiatric Nursing* is at the second level; it is a conceptual framework. It consists of four concepts. *Person* is defined as a living being with physical, mental, and spiritual dimensions, who functions in identifiable patterns with the environment to achieve a chosen life purpose. *Environment* is defined as relevant systems and processes external to and in interaction with the client. *Health* is defined as a synchronous pattern of interaction in the person-environment system; a synchronous pattern is the maximum level of wellness. *Nursing* is defined as a goal-directed process that promotes synchronous patterns of interaction between client and environment.

The conceptual framework is relevant for two reasons: (1) it helps organize all the knowledge the nurse must have to be a competent practitioner; (2) it helps the nurse to work effectively and efficiently.

The conceptual framework influences the implementation of each phase of the nursing process. In *assessment,* the conceptual framework determines how the client is perceived and what information needs to be collected. In *nursing diagnosis,* the conceptual framework determines what a diagnosis should consist of and how it should be stated. In *nursing goals* and *client outcomes,* the conceptual framework establishes the kinds of results which a nurse can help bring about. The conceptual framework determines what *interventions* a nurse can use; what one does comes from what one knows. A nurse can use an intervention only if the knowledge base is strong enough to support its use. *Evaluation* may contribute to building and testing theories, and this can help nursing to mature as a profession.

REFERENCES

1. The analogy was developed by Joann P. Wessman at the First Annual Conference on Nursing for the Whole Person, Oral Roberts University, Anna Vaughn School of Nursing, August 1982.

2. Ludwig Von Bertalanffy, *Robots, Men, and Minds*, Braziller, New York, 1967.
3. Dorothea Orem, *Nursing: Concepts of Practice*, 2d ed., McGraw-Hill, New York, 1980.

BIBLIOGRAPHY

Peggy L. Chinn, ed., *Advances in Nursing Theory Development*, Aspen Systems, Rockville, Md., 1982.

Peggy Chinn and Maeona K. Jacobs, *Theory and Nursing: A Systematic Approach*, Mosby, St. Louis, 1983.

Jacqueline Fawcett, *Analysis and Evaluation of Conceptual Models of Nursing*, Davis, Philadelphia, 1983.

Joyce Fitzpatrick and Ann Whall, *Conceptual Models of Nursing and Analysis Evaluation: Applications*, Brady, Bowie, Md., 1983.

Julia George, *Nursing Theories: The Base for Professional Nursing Practice*, Prentice-Hall. Englewood Cliffs, N.J., 1985.

Hesook S. Kim, *The Nature of Theoretical Thinking in Nursing*, Appleton-Century-Crofts, New York, 1983.

Catherine Norris, *Concept Clarification in Nursing*, Aspen, Rockville, Md., 1982.

Joan P. Riehl, and Sr. Callista Roy, *Conceptual Models for Nursing Practice*, Appleton-Century-Crofts, New York, 1980.

Martha E. Rogers, *Introduction to the Theoretical Basis of Nursing*, Davis, Philadelphia, 1970.

Callista Roy, *Introduction to Nursing: An Adaptation Model*, Prentice-Hall, Englewood Cliffs, N.J., 1976.

Barbara Stevens, *Nursing Theory: Analysis, Application, Evaluation*. Little, Brown, Boston, 1984.

Janice A. Thibodeau, *Nursing Models, Analysis, and Evaluation*. Brooks-Cole, Monterey, Calif., 1982.

PART TWO
The Person

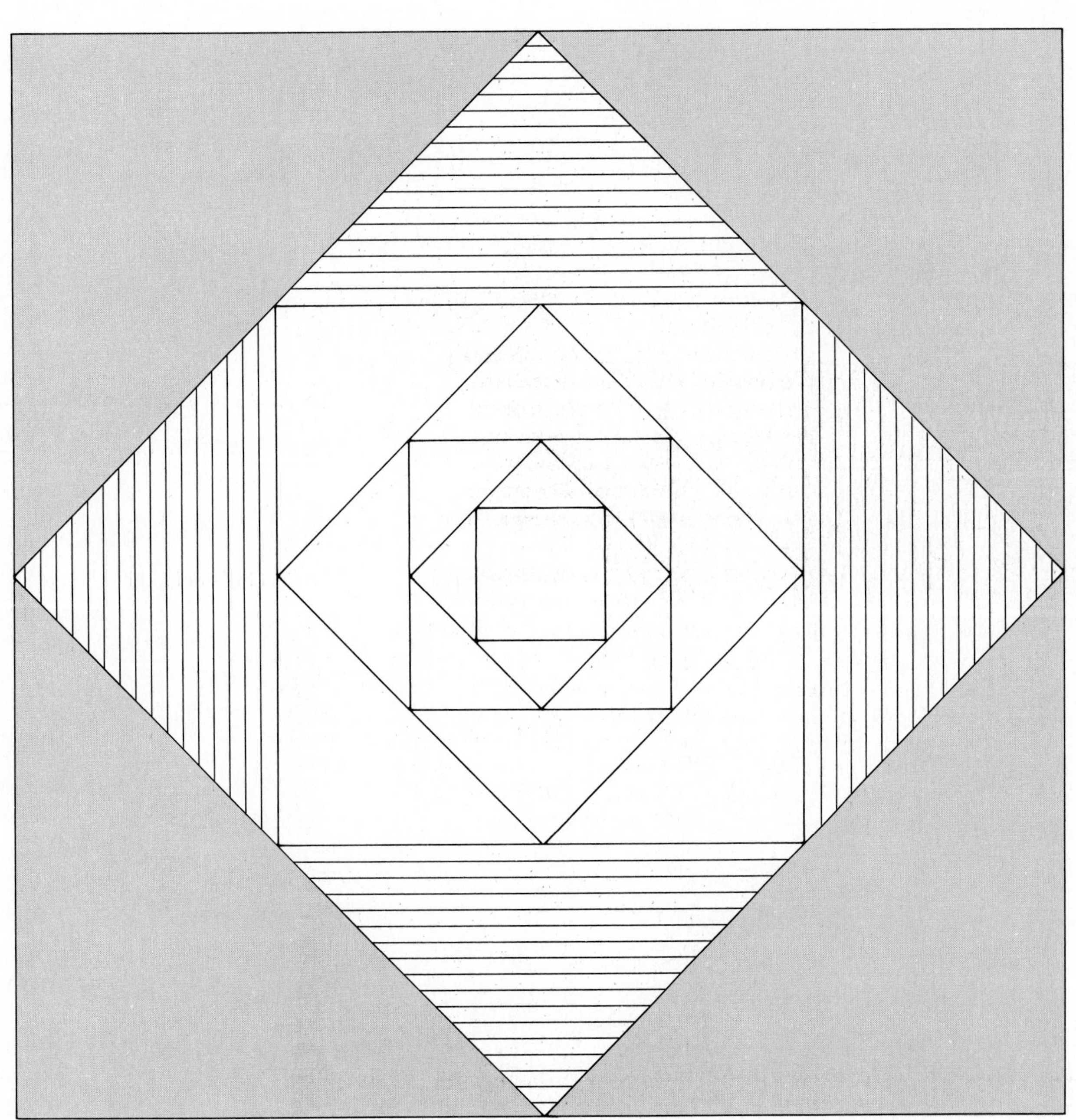

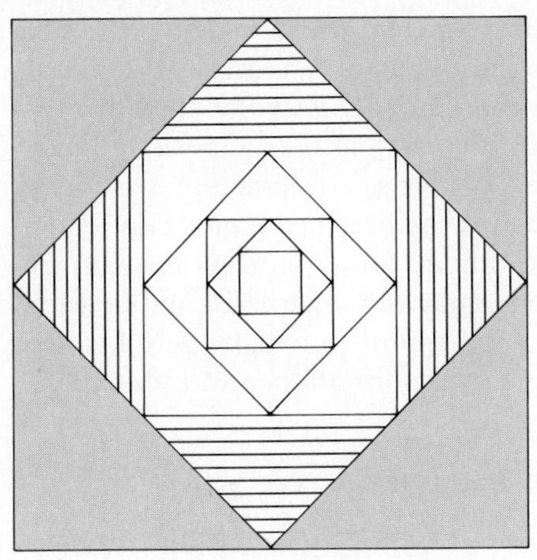

CHAPTER 2
Defining the Person

Judith Haber
Pamela Price Hoskins
Anita M. Leach
Barbara Flynn Sideleau

LEARNING OBJECTIVES

After studying this chapter, the student should be able to:

1. Elaborate on the definition of *person.*
2. Relate the definition of *person* to the concepts of holistic health, self-awareness, developmental processes, and sociocultural influences.

The purpose of this chapter is to expand on the definition of *person* and to provide a conceptual framework for the subjects covered in Part Two. The dimensions of person, patterns of interaction, and chosen life purposes will be explored. A rationale will be provided for relating the person to holistic health, self-awareness, developmental processes, and sociocultural issues.

THE CONCEPT OF PERSON

Person is defined as a living being with physical, mental, and spiritual dimensions who functions in identifiable patterns with the environment to achieve a chosen life purpose. Examining three aspects of the person will clarify this definition: (1) dimensions of the person, (2) identifiable patterns of interaction with the environment, and (3) chosen life purpose.

Dimensions of the Person

A person is defined as having three dimensions: physical, mental, and spiritual. These dimensions reflect the capacity for self-identity: recognizing oneself as separate and unique and being able and willing to regulate one's human functions and interact constructively with others. That is, the capacity for self-identity involves all three dimensions.

From the standpoint of mental health, the physical dimension of the person involves body image—a mental picture of one's own body. The mental dimension involves self-concept—a cognitive representation of everything one perceives oneself to be. The spiritual dimension involves self-esteem—the regard with which one holds oneself. Self-esteem reflects what one believes about one's own existence and nature.

Identity, then, consists of body image, self-concept, and self-esteem. It is, clearly, developed through perception of physical, mental, spiritual, and environmental input. But a person's ability to synthesize an almost infinite number of messages into patterned representations of self-identity is not so clear and may indeed be as mysterious as creation itself.

Identifiable Patterns of Interaction with the Environment

Only a few of a person's interactions with the environment become patterns. Patterns of interaction are identifiable, rhythmic, measurable, stable over time, and describable. (To give a very simple example, children can predict what their parents will say when they ask for their allowance before "payday.") Such patterns of interaction are part of a person's gestalt: a reciprocal, ongoing connection with the environment. How patterns develop depends upon personal and environmental boundaries, that is, on the extent to which there is a free exchange of energy, information, and influence.

Chosen Life Purpose

The need for a purpose in life seems to be a uniquely human characteristic. This need and the capacity of exercising free will combine so that each person actively chooses a purpose. The quality of the choice is an important focus for nurses working with clients with mental or emotional problems. A life purpose is an integrative spiritual function that gives life its meaning.

RATIONALE FOR THE ORGANIZATION OF PART TWO

There are four chapters in Part Two. Each of them contributes to the understanding of the concept *person*.

In Chapter 3, "Holistic Health Concepts," the theme of personal wholeness is developed. Variations in wholeness over the life span influence health status.

Chapter 4, "Self-Awareness," emphasizes the importance of understanding all that one is and can become. The person's influence on the environment and connectedness with it—particularly with regard to a therapeutic nursing role—are explored.

Chapter 5, "Developmental Processes," delineates biopsychosocial growth and the developmental cycle common to all human beings, considering similarities among individuals but also emphasizing the uniqueness of each person. The impact of developmental issues on mental health is illustrated.

Chapter 6, "Sociocultural Issues," explores the context within which the person is socialized. Sociocultural background influences definitions of health and illness; perception of diagnoses, treatments, and outcomes; and choices concerning participation in the pursuit of health.

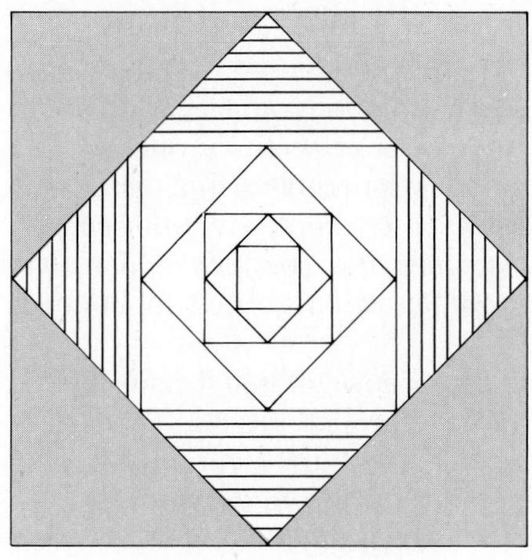

CHAPTER 3
Holistic Health Concepts

Judith Haber
Pamela Price Hoskins
Anita Leach
Barbara Flynn Sideleau

LEARNING OBJECTIVES

After studying this chapter, the student should be able to:

1. Relate self-concept, identity, moral image, self-esteem, and body image to the concept of self.
2. Relate the four-dimensional model of the self to the assessment of the person.
3. Define the five modes of perceiving.
4. Discuss the developmental and integrative needs for sensory input.
5. Discuss the impact of sensory-input disturbances.
6. Relate theory about rhythms to health and dysfunction.
7. Relate patterns of tiredness to sleep.
8. Relate dreaming and daydreaming to the capacity to function.
9. Describe the concept of space and its relationship to communication.
10. Discuss the concept of time and its influences on perception.
11. Determine the significance of emotions in personal integration and expression.
12. Define and give examples of selected emotions.
13. Analyze the sources and functions of anxiety.
14. Describe the effect of levels of anxiety on the ability to perceive and learn.
15. Discuss the dynamics of grieving.
16. Understand the existential significance of loneliness.
17. Discuss the relevance to nursing of the concepts explored in this chapter.

Nursing is developing both an identity within the health care system and a science upon which to base its practice. Knowledge about interactions between the person and the environment, and the effects of these interactions upon health, is derived from certain concepts and theories which must be systematically developed and tested through nursing research.

Nursing has evolved from a traditional focus on disease toward a focus on health. The nursing model has a holistic orientation to the client and to the delivery of health care. Mind, body, and spirit are perceived as inseparable and interactive; the person is perceived as interacting with and influencing the environment.

Using the nursing model as a framework, the nursing profession bases its practices on concepts and theories that classify and describe human phenomena. The concepts and theories that make up its knowledge base serve the profession by guiding:

1. The assessment process
2. Organization and classification of facts about the client in interaction with the environment, thus providing an understanding of the client, existing problems, and influencing factors
3. Conceptualization of the client's problem and formulation of nursing diagnoses
4. Collaboration with the client in establishing goals that become outcome criteria used to evaluate nursing care
5. Selection of interventions and evaluation of their effectiveness

The purpose of this chapter is to describe dimensions of the person in interaction with the environment that are relevant to the delivery of nursing care for promotion, maintenance, restoration, and rehabilitation of health. The concepts and theories to be examined include the self, sensory patterns, rhythm patterns, spatial and temporal patterns, emotional patterns, and stress. The examination of each of the concepts addresses a basic aspect of the person-environment interaction as it relates to health and to nursing.

The authors gratefully acknowledge the contribution of Roberta F. Mattheis in the original development of this chapter.

THE SELF

The *self* is the body, the body image, and certain nonbodily parts.[1] It is a concept of oneself as a whole person, distinct from other people or objects in the environment. To conceptualize the self, it is necessary to recognize the complex dimensions that interact to produce an integrated, functioning individual.

Development of a sense of self begins before birth and continues throughout life. It involves maturation, interaction with the environment, psychosexual development, and ego development. An infant does not recognize any difference between external stimuli and internal states, and probably has little sense of differences between internal states themselves. For example, hunger and anxiety experienced simultaneously are perceived as one sensation, and the infant does not perceive any outside source that would relieve this state of tension. As a person matures physiologically and psychologically and interacts with significant others, the self is differentiated from the environment. The person is able to recognize and label experiences and identify to varying degrees whether a source of tension is located in the environment or within the self. The person comes to perceive the self, the "I," as separate and worthwhile. Separation and self-differentiation are lifelong processes. Dimensions that contribute to an understanding of self include self-concept, identity, moral image, self-esteem, and body image.

Self-Concept

Self-concept is the synthesis of perceptions, feelings, and beliefs about oneself, and it includes characteristics, personality traits, and evaluations of the worth of these traits. Development of self-concept is a process which utilizes self-system, personification, self-feelings, and self-awareness.

Development of the self-concept has three components:

1. Actual responses of others toward the person
2. Perceived responses of others toward the person
3. Internalization by the person of these perceived responses

A sense of being separate and unique and having a personal boundary is fundamental to this process.

Development of a sense of separateness leads to an intrapsychic representation of the self as distinguished from a representation of the environment.[2]

The quality and nature of parental nurturing profoundly influence children's development, the clarity of children's personal boundaries, and their self-concepts. Siblings, grandparents, and other members of the extended family also influence children's lives and self-perceptions. As children grow older, teachers, school principals, and peers also interact with and influence them, affecting the development of self-concept through their perceptions and definitions of what these children should be. These perceptions and definitions are communicated verbally and nonverbally to children through social interaction. Children are motivated to acquire information about themselves that will maintain, validate, or enhance the self; they therefore actively seek those who will provide them with data.

Sullivan's theory about the self-system provides further understanding of the development of self-concept. According to Sullivan, the self develops in relation to social norms and behavior patterns. Significant others serve as intermediaries between the person and the culture.[3]

Sullivan hypothesized that during infancy a set of response patterns develops through interactions with significant others, and a composite of these response patterns becomes the self-system. The function of the response patterns is to avoid or minimize anxiety. In time, these behaviors form a habitual pattern of avoidance, which is resistant to change and may or may not promote growth. The self-system provides meaning to what is experienced and done, and it enables people to function more or less effectively in their sociocultural world.

Since the self-system is organized to avoid anxiety, others' perceptions will be internalized and accepted as belonging to the self if they support avoidance. Thus a child begins to "own" other people's definitions, evaluations, and judgments of the self—that is, begins to believe responses from significant people in the environment. It is important to note that children internalize, not other people's actual responses, but their own perceptions of these responses. Both the child's perceptions and (in this qualified sense) the perceptions of significant others mediate and thereby modify available data. Any limitation on, interference with, or distortion of the reception, processing, or integration of sensory data will produce misperception.

During the final phase of developing a self-system, the child creates a self that is congruent with the definitions, judgments, and evaluations made by significant others. Through this process, one may reject one's own self-perception in favor of the perceptions of others, even when these are incongruent with the self-perception.[3]

Sullivan's theory of *personification* also adds to an understanding of the self-concept. *Personification* is a symbolic conception of the other and of the self as "good" or "bad." Among the significant personifications that develop in infancy are "good mother" and "bad mother," and personifications of self as "good me," "bad me," and "not me." The "good mother" personification results from interactions with a nurturing parent that give satisfaction and reduce anxiety. The personification of the "bad mother" results from experiences that leave needs unmet and produce anxiety.[3]

Over time, the child begins to respond to the mother in terms of the way the mother is personified. Sullivan proposes that the child, through repeated interactions with the mother, develops responses that reflect "good me," "bad me," and "not me" personifications. The "good me" is a pattern of recurrent self-referent responses (perceptions, images, recollections, thoughts) that are learned in satisfying interactions with the mother. A "good me" conception of self contributes to positive self-regard. The "bad me" conception of self is a recurrent pattern of negative self-referent responses learned in relationship situations characterized by anxiety. A "bad me" conception of self contributes to negative self-regard. The "not me" conception is a constellation of self-referent responses that remains undifferentiated because it relates to experiences involving extreme tension, intense anxiety, horror, and loathing. Semantic perceptions become associated with the "good me" and the "bad me" perceptions and thus become invested with language. The "not me" continues to operate at an imagined and nonverbalized level. The "not me" reflects an overwhelming and intolerable level of anxiety.

With the development of self-concept comes the development of *self-feelings*. Self-feelings form the nucleus of self-regard. These feelings may be either positive or negative. Positive feelings are derived from praise, recognition, love, and acceptance by significant others. Negative feelings result from criticism or being labeled *bad, lazy, worthless,* or *useless* and from perceptions of rejection.[3]

One dimension of the self-concept is *self-awareness,* the recognition of one's own existence and uniqueness and of other's evaluations of the self. Self-awareness includes recognition of:

- One's own behavior and its impact on others
- Feelings toward the self, others, and situations
- Factors that influence perceptions, thoughts, feelings, and behavior, including past perceptions, experiences, and relationships
- One's own needs and wishes
- How one's efforts to fulfill needs and wishes affect others
- How one participates with others in a situation

Self-knowledge that increases self-awareness begins with ongoing self-assessment. It requires willingness to examine one's own perceptions, thoughts, feelings, and behaviors. It also requires an effort to understand and accept one's personal development and the familial, societal, and circumstantial influences that have affected it.

The self-concept established during the formative years is stable and consistent, but it is subject to some modification as the social environment changes. Others' perceptions of oneself, idealized conceptions of what one should be, and personal conceptions of what is desirable or useful are assessed and compared. Development of self-concept is a lifelong process of comparing, assessing, reinterpreting, and internalizing perceived appraisals.

Identity

Identity, which is a part of the self, is an awareness of being a person separate and distinct from all others. It is based on the integration of the body image. Both ego and superego functions are involved in giving the person a sense of identity. Identity is a product of continually changing psychological, social, spiritual, and physical processes throughout the life span. Developmental and interacting environmental factors make it necessary to revise one's sense of identity continually.

Social identity is the integrated self, developed through social labeling processes which classify the person within society. This identity is made up of demographic classifications such as sex, age, race, ethnicity, legal status, family status (for example, son, wife, or grandchild), occupational status, socioeconomic status, educational status, and group membership status.

The elements of social identity are not simply classifications. They have an evaluative dimension that conveys worth, importance, and desirability. Society determines these judgments, but even though they are external to the self, they affect personal judgment—that is, what social identity means to self and self-concept.[4]

Classifications having to do with conformity and nonconformity to societal norms are also evaluations that contribute to one's identity. For example, *alcoholic, insane,* and *criminal* are societal labels that not only classify people but also define negative identities. Even when people are classified as ex-alcoholics, ex-mental patients, or ex-convicts, there is still an associated social stigma. *Philanthropist* and *pillar of society* also classify and define people, but these labels convey positive social identities.

A social identity, including its evaluative dimension, is more than an accumulation of labels.[5] The labels are interconnected and form a holistic, integrated structure within which the self is organized. Some elements are central or pivotal and significantly influence how the self is perceived and valued; other elements are peripheral and less influential.

According to Fogarty,[5] self-identity has nine elements: (1) spiritual self, (2) values, (3) abstract thinking, (4) concrete thinking, (5) feelings, (6) emotions, (7) physical self, (8) imagination (fantasy), and (9) craziness (the irrational). Each of these elements interacts with the others.

People have varying degrees of awareness about each of the elements of identity; this seems to reflect each person's internal and external contexts. In most contexts, parts of the self remain relatively intact and in force; however, different situational contexts elicit and require responses from different aspects of the self. The parts of self that constitute the "I" are different with friends, family, colleagues, and authority figures. With each of these people in different contexts, awareness of self in relation to each element also varies.

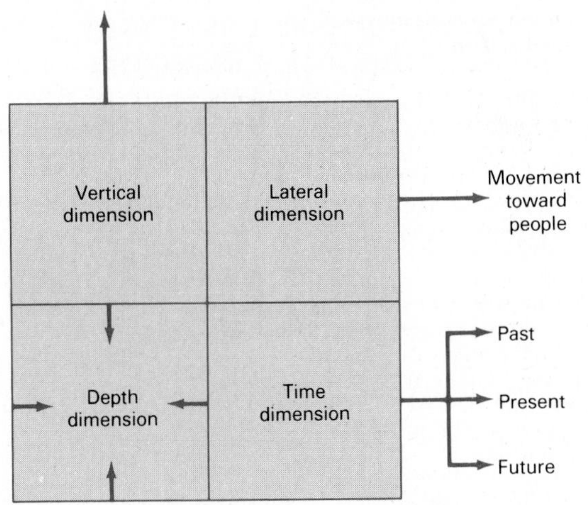

Figure 3-1 The four-dimensional self.

(SOURCE: From T. F. Fogarty, "System Concepts and the Dimensions of Self," in P. Guerin, ed., *Family Therapy: Theory and Practice*, Gardner, New York, 1976, pp. 144–153. Used with permission.)

Fogarty constructs a four-dimensional model of self; it is presented in Figure 3-1. The four elements of self, represented by quadrants in the model, are (1) time, (2) lateral dimension, (3) vertical dimension, (4) depth dimension. Each quadrant represents 25 percent of the person when the self is in a state of equilibrium.

The *time dimension* involves movement (since movement takes time) and has three aspects or orientations: past, present, and future. Maintaining balance among these time orientations allows a person to learn from past experiences and recall positive and pleasurable experiences that enhance the self in the present, to function effectively in the present, to anticipate the future, and to use the present to prepare for the future.

The *lateral dimension* is characterized by movement toward people, feelings of closeness and connectedness, and involvement with others.

The *vertical dimension* is characterized by movement toward objects. (For example, time, energy, and interest are invested in daily living activities, hobbies, and sports.)

The *depth dimension* does not involve movement. It is composed of spiritual elements, abstract and concrete thinking, feelings that one is aware of, unconscious emotional processes, imagination, and one's physical dimensions. It represents capacity rather than actuality. Fogarty's four-dimensional model is further delineated in Table 3-1; examples are given.

Self-Image and Moral Image

Self-image, which develops through self-perceptions, has two components: an "idealized" image and a "committed" image. Both are imaginative visions of the desired self. The committed image is more realistic; the idealized image is a glorified vision that is unrealistic and unattainable.[6] In conjunction with a desired self-image, people also hold a *moral image*—what they perceive and feel they should be. This moral image is learned through relationships with others. It encompasses standards that guide decisions and behaviors, and it has three aspects: conscience, role demands, and idiosyncratic self-demands.[6]

Ethical standards—definitions of right and wrong—are governed by the *conscience*. Interactions with parents, teachers, and religious instructors contribute to the development of the conscience. For example, a child learns from parents, teachers, and religious instructors that taking what belongs to another is stealing, which is morally wrong.

Role demands communicate standards for behavior. These standards not only specify acceptable and unacceptable behavior, but also require people to act responsibly and hold them accountable for their actions. For example, role prescriptions for students require them to make efforts to learn assignments, listen attentively to the teacher, prepare for classes and exams, and submit written assignments when they are due and in the required format.

Idiosyncratic self-demands have to do with personal feelings and beliefs about what is owed to oneself and others.[6] An example of self-demands is the belief of some nurses that they should never feel angry, disgusted, or hopeless about their clients, and that clients should comply with their recommendations.

Self-Esteem

Self-esteem is the internal image of oneself formed by the interaction of bodily experiences with influential variables in the environment at a particular

Table 3-1 Fogarty's Four-Dimensional Self

Dimension	Example
Time	
When orientation to the past is dominant, the person may spend time ruminating about past mistakes and regrets or reminiscing about the "good old days"; the person is "stuck" in the past, and is less able to cope with the present, and to anticipate and plan for the future.	Depressed and disengaged elderly people are often overinvolved with the past, and consequently they are unable to function effectively in the present.
When orientation to the present is dominant, the person may fail to learn from past experiences. Examinations of past experiences that could contribute to self-awareness are unavailable because only the present occupies interest. Since these people live for the moment, the future is out of awareness. Such people become vulnerable to crises because they fail to anticipate problems and take action to prevent them or lessen their impact.	Substance abusers organiz their lives around drugs and are overconcerned with immediate gratification; they are overinvolved in the "here and now" to the exclusion of interest in the past and future.
When orientation to the future is dominant, the person may be impatient, impulsive, and dissatisfied or feel caught in the present. Rather than attending to the present and resolving existing problems, these people focus on unrealistic future hopes, expectations, and dreams. Because they ignore the present and fail to use the past, they are ill prepared for the future; in time, the future becomes an unsatisfactory present.	The dreamer lives for fantasies of future successes, but lacks the self-discipline and self-responsibility in the "here and now" and the awareness of past patterns of ineffective coping that could facilitate the realization of dreams.
Lateral	
When imbalance occurs in this dimension, the person invests a disproportionate amount of energy and activity either in the pursuit of or involvement with others or in withdrawal from interpersonal relationships and connectedness. When the imbalance involves excessive concern with relations with others, it occurs at the expense of the other dimensions.	The person has little tolerance for solitude and is vulnerable to episodes of acute loneliness. The excessive need for involvement with others may lead to intrusiveness in the lives of others.
Vertical	
When imbalance occurs in this dimension, the person's attention is disproportionately focused on an object or activity; interpersonal relationships are limited, superficial, or conflicted. Introspection and self-awareness also may be limited.	Television or golf addicts, workaholics, alcoholics, and drug addicts organize their lives around watching programs, getting on the course, putting in overtime, or getting a drink or a drug. When this dimension is restricted in a person, he or she has little interest in solitary activities or self-amusement.
Depth	
When this dimension is the primary focus, the person withdraws into the self. Consequently, reality-based feedback is diminished. The inner reality dominates at the expense of the outer reality. Self-awareness is limited because the intellectual process of seeking new factual information and the emotional process of experiencing life events are impaired.	The lonely, isolated older person who ruminates about physical complaints and bodily functions such as eating, sleeping, and elimination of waste products exemplifies this inward focus. People who have hallucinations and delusions have an exaggerated withdrawal from reality. A classic example of people who have withdrawn from reality are those who keep learning about themselves but do not change.

SOURCE: T. F. Fogarty, "System Concepts and the Dimensions of Self," in P. Guerin, ed., *Family Therapy: Theory and Practice*, Gardner Press, New York, 1976, pp. 144–153.

stage in the life span. Self-esteem has an evaluative dimension; it can be either positive or negative. Positive self-esteem requires self-acceptance and a healthy attitude toward one's worth and limitations. One must recognize and accept each quality as being a part of self.

Interactions with others, particularly during childhood, contribute to self-esteem. Self-perceptions and attitudes that develop through these interactions generate feelings toward the self, such as pride, shame, respect, love, and hate. These self-perceptions and the evaluation one makes of one's identity influence the perception of self-worth. Additional factors include one's own and others' recognition of personal achievements; accomplishment of goals; increasing personal power and influence over events and people; a sense of personal acceptance; being valued and cared about; and acting in ways that are consistent with personal beliefs.[7]

People need positive self-esteem. They need to feel that they are worthy, competent, and loved. Positive feelings about oneself facilitate involvement in relationships with others, motivation, achievement, and a sense of personal worth and power.

Body Image

The *body image* is a mental representation of one's body derived from internal sensations, emotions, fantasies, posture, and experience of and with outside objects and people. It is an internal evaluative representation of one's body that is largely determined by how one thinks one looks to others. It includes a spatial idea of one's own body which changes according to the sensory information received from one's body and the environment.

Body Image Development

The development of the mental picture that constitutes body image is a process that evolves through the multiple interaction of maturation, sociocultural influences, family relationships, perceptions of significant others, peers' attitudes, topological bodily experiences, behavioral bodily experiences, and innermost somatic bodily experiences. Bower[1] proposes the nursing model for body image presented in Figure 3-2. This model is based on a holistic view of the person in continual interaction with environmental influences.

Innermost somatic bodily experiences derived from biological processes such as endocrine and metabolic changes are subtle influences in the development of the core of the body image. Maturational changes that produce these experiences include the hormonal shifts that occur during toddlerhood, adolescence, and middle age, as well as other significant maturational biological changes. Physiological responses to fear and anxiety also contribute to this core body image.

Behavioral bodily experiences come from data acquired and processed by the perceptual system. Movement, vision, hearing, and thinking contribute to the development of the body image. Personality

Figure 3-2 Nursing model of body image.

(SOURCE: From F. L. Bower, ed., *Normal Development of Body Image,* Wiley, New York, 1977. Used with permission.)

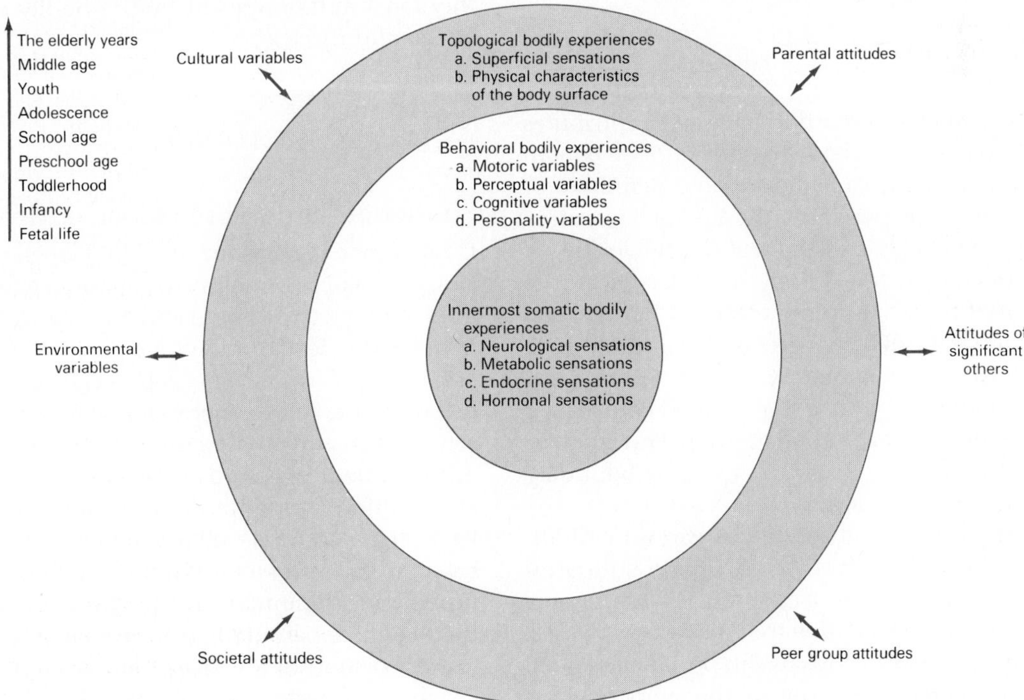

characteristics such as aggressiveness and passiveness mediate experiences and thereby also influence body image.

Topological bodily experiences are those that emanate from the surface of the body. Pain, pressure sensations, hearing, vision, and taste are examples of these experiences. A person's perception and experience in relation to the boundary that separates the body from the environment help to define the body.

Sensory stimulation that contributes to both behavioral and topological experiences significantly influences body image. Somatosensory stimulation and the integrity of the perceptual systems are of critical importance in the development of the body image, particularly during infancy. Newborns and older infants perceive and respond to sensory stimulation in a diffuse, undifferentiated manner. The interaction between neurological, maturational, and sensory stimulation contribute to (1) the definition of body boundaries, (2) the discriminations in relation to the location and quality of the stimulus, and (3) the feelings evoked. Rocking, patting, stroking, bathing, and other playing and care-giving activities provide this stimulation. Since the initial experience of one's body mediates future body and life experiences, the quality and sensitivity of early playing and care giving are vital to the development of a positive body image.

Body Boundary

The interaction of sensory stimulation that produces sensations on the body surface contributes to the development of body boundary. *Body boundary* is a mental idea related to how definitely or indefinitely one experiences the line of separation between one's body and the rest of the world.[1]

As a person matures, body boundary becomes demarcated more and more clearly. Changes that occur across the life span require continual revisions of the body boundary. Adolescence, pregnancy, middle age, and old age are accompanied by alterations in body configuration and appearance that require a revision of the body boundary as well as the self-concept.

Definitiveness of body boundary varies in adults. Women tend to have less well-defined boundaries than men. Sociocultural factors also influence the way in which people define their body boundaries. Whether a person develops health problems related to internal body organs or to the body surface appears to be related to the definitiveness of body boundary. People with a less distinct boundary seem to be more vulnerable to gastrointestinal symptoms such as diarrhea or stomach cramps, and those with a more defined body boundary appear to be susceptible to skin rashes and musculoskeletal symptoms such as joint and muscle pains.[1]

Body Image Integration

The interpersonal interactions that influence the development of self-concept play an equally significant role in the development of body image. Like self-concept, body image needs continual revision across the life span because of maturational and situational changes.

A wide variety of socioenvironmental factors influence the development of the body image. The family mediates cultural attitudes; and in our society communications media also have a direct impact on people and their perceptions about themselves. Interactions with parents, family members, and significant others influence body image much as they influence the self-concept.

A person's body and body image and intangibles such as mind, soul, and spirit interact and contribute to the holistic person. The intangibles make each person unique, so that personality transcends the constraints imposed by the bodily alterations of age and disease.

RELEVANCE TO NURSING

Promotion and Maintenance of Health

Development and integration of the many dimensions of self are concerns of nursing. Nurses using interventions to promote and maintain health must address the development of a positive self-concept and identity, a realistic self-image, a useful and helpful moral image, increasing self-awareness, high self-esteem, and an integrated and acceptable body image in their clients. The changes that occur with growth, development, and pregnancy, and the related needs to revise self-concept and body image, have to be assessed. When actual or potential problems are identified, nurses can collaborate with the clients experiencing the problems to facilitate the integration of a revised self-concept and body image.

Restoration of Health

Nurses also need to help clients whose self-concept and body image have been disturbed by illness, trauma, and surgery. Scars and mutilation (such as amputations, neurological deficits, and radical neck resections),[8] drastic weight loss or gain, and hair loss and changes in skin tone, color, and texture associated with cancer and its therapies all cause major alterations in self-image and body image which may also be distressing.

Rehabilitation of Health

Many chronic illnesses cause changes in appearance. These illnesses may also produce changes that are not as visible but are equally threatening to self-concept and body image. When people recognize a gradual loss of mental faculties, stamina, motor coordination, and well-being, their concept of who they are and how they are perceived by others is also altered. People requiring long-term hemodialysis must deal with such changes as well as the disfiguring shunt and the disruption in body boundaries that occur with connection to a dialysis machine.

Psychiatric illnesses characterized by disordered thinking, perceiving, feeling, or behaving often contribute to distorted self-image and body perceptions. Body boundaries may be ill-defined, or energy may be overinvested in protecting the self from imagined ill will. Nursing interventions can help clients experiencing such symptoms to reestablish personal boundaries, integrate the self, and feel safer in the hospital and at home.

Nurses have a responsibility to promote a healthy self-image and body image in clients of all ages and to help those whose self-image and body image have been altered by illness, surgery, or therapy to integrate and accept the changes. Nursing interventions that help clients ventilate their feelings about the changes, recognize their strengths, and minimize their limitations facilitate this process of integration and acceptance.

SENSORY STIMULATION

Human beings are in constant interaction with their environment, exchanging a wide variety of sensory information. This exchange enables them to maintain contact with their environment and their own bodies. Without the information gained from continuous interaction, integration of the self would not occur, and people would be unable to manipulate the environment to satisfy basic needs.

Information processing is the interaction between sensory stimuli and the functioning of the person. The central nervous system (CNS) is the matrix in which this information processing occurs. Sensory stimuli are the input, and the CNS is the "computer" which processes information that maintains the person's internal and relational functioning.[9] Behavior reflects both the quantity and the quality of sensory stimuli and the effectiveness of the information processing. Integration and utilization of sensory stimulation are necessary for the person to function effectively.

Perception is a significant variable in sensory stimulation. All senses are selectively receptive to environmental changes. Perception includes the physical, physiological, and psychological recognition of stimuli by sensory systems. It involves not only the selection and organization but also the interpretation of incoming stimuli. When the information-processing system is functioning properly, incoming information is evaluated, relevant data are sent on to the appropriate location in the brain, and irrelevant or excessive information is screened out or discarded.

Perception and Sensory Input*

Traditionally, sensory reception has been associated with the five senses. Bartley however, points out that to speak of only five senses is incorrect. He proposes that there are five *modes of perceiving*: (1) basic orienting system, (2) haptic system, (3) savor system, (4) auditory system, and (5) visual system.[10]

Basic Orienting System

The *basic orienting system* interacts with the other four perceptual systems to provide a frame of reference. The vestibular mechanism in the inner ear plays an important part in physical orientation. It reacts to forces of acceleration and indicates the direction of gravity and the beginnings and endings of body movement. The basic orienting system is composed of six interacting subsystems that

* From R. Mattheis, "Holistic Health Concepts," in the second edition of this book.

perform functional and exploratory activities: postural, orienting-exploratory, locomotor, appetitive, expressive, and semantic.[10]

POSTURAL SUBSYSTEM. The postural subsystem is used to relate to the forces (mechanical and gravitational) that influence body position. The ability to move and to remain in stationary positions requires data about where the body is located in space and where all parts are when one moves. The postural subsystem includes receptors for this data, information-processing capabilities, and feedback mechanisms that produce revisions and adjustments.

ORIENTING-EXPLORATORY SUBSYSTEM. The orienting-exploratory subsystem, which is also a part of the basic orienting system, moves body parts (such as the head, mouth, and limbs) to gain information about the environment. This subsystem provides data about the size, shape, consistency, and surface characteristics of objects such as their smoothness, lumpiness, squareness, or roundness.

LOCOMOTOR SUBSYSTEM. The locomotor subsystem is the mechanism by which activities of approach, avoidance, and transportation are performed. This system allows a person to move around in the environment and to adjust bodily position.

APPETITIVE SUBSYSTEM. The appetitive subsystem is involved with the interaction between the person and the environment. This subsystem is concerned with activities such as eating, breathing, eliminating, and sexual performance. The senses of hunger, satiation, need for oxygen, and sexual attraction and satisfaction are recognized by this system.

EXPRESSIVE SUBSYSTEM. The expressive subsystem mediates gestures, facial expressions, vocalizations, and activities conveying attitudes and feelings.

SEMANTIC SUBSYSTEM. The semantic subsystem, which sends and interprets all types of movements and activities, is an important dimension of the interactive processes with other systems. This subsystem is involved in the labeling and categorizing of sensory experiences. Without language to interpret sensory stimuli, the stimuli would remain diffuse and meaningless; conceptualization and abstract thinking about the sensory input would not be possible. Language contributes to understanding, and understanding is the first step toward purposeful interaction with the external environment to satisfy needs.

Haptic System

The second mode of perception proposed by Bartley, the *haptic system*, uses receptors in the skin, muscles, and joints to acquire information (sensations) about objects in the environment and about people's own external body configurations. Part of the process of getting to know one's body involves the reception and integration of data acquired through touching.

Savor System

The *savor system*, the third mode of perception, is used to detect and appreciate materials that enter the nose or mouth and to discriminate among them. Nasal receptors provide the odor or fragrance sensations of which smell is made up. Receptors in the mouth interpret sensations that produce taste. Receptors in the nose and mouth for touch, temperature, and pain provide further information about whether materials are hot or cold, hard or soft, or lumpy or smooth.

Auditory System

The *auditory system*, the fourth mode of perception, is involved with receiving and interpreting minute vibrations. Information about the nature and direction of the sound waves and their patterns is received through the ear. The semantic system interacts to give meaning to communication.

Visual System

The *visual system*, the fifth mode of perception, registers light wave (photic radiation) patterns. This information interacts with data from other systems, such as the orienting-exploratory and semantic systems, to interpret the picture formed by the light waves. The eye is the primary location of receptors for this system. When visual receptors are impaired, as in blindness, the haptic, auditory, and basic orienting systems play major roles in providing information that can be used to imagine an object in the environment.

Verdicality

Another dimension of perception and sensory stimulation is that of *verdicality*, or *truth telling*, which has to do with the accuracy of interpretation of perceptions. Illusions provide an example of the influence of verdicality on the interpretation of raw sensory data. The visual system processes raw sensory data provided by light waves. With an illusion, the raw sensory data are misperceived. The visual experience is real, since a real object in the environment is perceived. However, the data received—or the uses of the data—provide a mental picture of the object that is not accurate. If interpretation of a set of conditions (such as the lighting) is combined with data from another sensory system (such as the haptic system), the original misperception is then revised. In most instances, the revision better approximates the reality of the object. For example, a sphere suspended in the distance may be misperceived as a flat, two-dimensional circle because of body position and light reflection. This misperception can be corrected by moving the body position (using the locomotor system) and examining this apparent circle from a new angle while touching it (using the haptic system), which would result in the correct perception of a sphere.

Developmental Need for Sensory Input

Sensory stimulation has been associated with a person's development potential. Infants and children need stimulation to grow and develop physically, mentally, and spiritually. Research in learning of infants suggests that early stimulation is important for a person's future learning capacity. To maintain optimal health, people of all ages need sensory stimulation.

People vary in their need for sensory stimulation, and each person has a unique pattern of preferred sensory modes. Developmental, personal, and situational factors influence people's perception of, utilization of, and response to sensory stimulation. At various points across the life span there are theoretical ranges for optimal sensory stimulation—that is, for stimulation conducive to healthy functioning.

Touch

Touch is an important source of sensory input, primarily experienced through the skin. Montague[11] describes the skin as "a cloak that covers the body." It is the most sensitive of the body organs, the first medium of communication, and an efficient form of protection. Haptic system receptors are the primary mechanisms for acquiring information related to touch. Sensory input from cutaneous stimulation plays a direct role in the development of self-concept and an indirect role in behavior that reflects self-perception. The relationship between sensations produced by different types of cutaneous stimulation and human behavior is reflected in such common expressions as "She rubs me the wrong way," "He is a soft touch," and "She gets under my skin."

PHYSIOLOGICAL THEORY. Sensory and motor integrity are maintained by continuous stimulation of the skin. The brain must receive sensory feedback in order to maintain overall physical, psychological, and social functioning. Cutaneous stimulation provides sensory data which contribute to CNS integration and control over bodily functioning. This sensory input is required for accurate interpretation or verification of data from the other perceptual systems. Tactile information is used to define self-concept, body boundary, and body image.[11]

TACTILE STIMULATION. Studies seem to support the belief that infant monkeys and infant humans in all cultures show attachment to and dependence on the care-giving parent. Warmth, pleasure, comfort, contentment, satisfaction of needs, and care are all significant in relationships. Studies of monkeys reared in either total or partial social isolation, which involved deprivation of body contact, showed that the earlier and greater the isolation, the greater the behavioral deficits.

In humans, touching has two components: (1) sensations produced by stimulation of the haptic system receptors; and (2) an associated affect, that is, an emotion. Initially, parents' contacts with an infant are exploratory in nature. Fingertips are used and holding is perfunctory. Gradually, parents use the whole hand to maximize contact. Stroking and patting produce greater cutaneous stimulation. Holding patterns, such as cuddling, caressing, and rocking, appear when the nurturing one is comfortable. Rhythmic tactile stimulation of the infant is more likely to occur at this time. If the nurturing one is anxious, rejects the care-giving role, or finds this role to be unsatisfying, there may be no rhythmic tactile stimulation of the infant, or it may be inconsistent or harsh.

Montague speaks of the soothing effects of rhythm combined with tactile stimulation. Combined stimulation of the haptic and basic orienting systems enhances the integration of sensorimotor functions, and thus promotes growth and development. This need for patterned cutaneous stimulation and stimulation of the basic orienting system is lifelong: people of all ages need tactile stimulation—not only the physical sensation, but the emotional dimension as well.

Self-image and body image develop with cutaneous stimulation and the resulting sensations and affects. Adequate parenting, which involves complex cutaneous stimulation, activates the tactile response systems of the infant. Thus, these early life experiences prepare for later adequate functioning in all situations involving tactility.

USING TOUCH TO COMMUNICATE. Touch is also a means of communicating and relating that continues beyond the parent-child relationship. Handshakes, hugging, shoving, and hitting communicate feelings and help to define relationships between people. Early experiences influence uses of and responses to touch. Cultural proscriptions specify when not to touch, whom one cannot touch, how others can and cannot be touched, and how one responds to the touching behavior of others.

Touch may be comforting and supportive in one context and threatening in another. In spite of the human need for touching sensations and the related pleasurable affects, there are situations in which touching is inappropriate or stressful and produces intense discomfort or fear.

The skin is not only a receiving and mediating organ; it also transmits messages. The temperature of the skin can communicate information. Perspiration, goosebumps, rashes, and hives notify the external world that a person is warm, cold, or disturbed.

Sensory-Input Disturbances

When the intensity, quantity, or appropriateness of sensory stimuli exceeds the upper limit of one's ability to process the incoming information, *sensory overload* is experienced. When the stimuli fail to meet required needs, there is *sensory deprivation.*

Manifestations of sensory overload approximate those of sensory deprivation. Whether sensory input and variability are characterized by overload or deprivation, the person experiencing such sensations tends to manifest confusion, a sense of social isolation, anxiety and tension, inability to concentrate or organize thoughts, and increased suggestibility. When people experience deprivation, they may also experience vivid sensory imagery. The most common visual imagery is hallucinations involving delusions. There may be body illusions, somatic complaints, and intense subjective feelings.

Effects of brainwashing and solitary confinement on prisoners of war, hostages, and newly recruited cult members show how sensory overstimulation and understimulation have been used to alter perception, information processing, and behavior. Deprivation or intensification of unpatterned light, sound, and social interaction is destructive and disorienting.[12]

Sensory Deprivation

Sensory deprivation is a reduction or a loss of sensory stimulation, an interference with information processing, or both. Sensory deprivation at any age results in deterioration of nervous system integrity and psychosocial functioning.

Vulnerability to sensory deprivation increases when there is impairment of receptors, information-processing capabilities, or environmental sources of raw sensory data. Birth defects, trauma, or disease may produce dysfunction or loss in receptors. Impaired capacity to perceive raw data from any or several perceptual systems creates a situation that may result in deprivation. Because of the interactive characteristics of perceptual systems and the human potential for adjustment, people may compensate for the loss of sensory data input from one system by increasing the capabilities of other systems. In some instances, the capacities of all systems for reception and information processing may be adequate, but the environment fails to produce the needed raw sensory data. There may be few or no opportunities for social interaction.

Whether sensory deprivation is perceived to be stressful or capable of producing psychological dysfunction is in part culturally determined. In far eastern cultures, solitude is used in conjunction with various types of mental and physical exercises to induce desired altered states of consciousness. North American Indian tribes have used solitary time in the forest to seek communion with the spirits and thus obtain mystical power.[13] Social isolation and the sensory deprivation associated with it are likely to be viewed as stressful in our society. However, seclusion has been used effectively to control the behavior of psychiatric clients by decreasing environmental stimuli. It has also been used with anorectic clients as part of a behavior modification approach designed to alter eating patterns.[13]

Universally, isolation disrupts usual ways of coping and produces special kinds of psychological processes. Hallucinations and vivid dreams, unusual states of excitement and arousal, and great openness to experience commonly occur during periods of prolonged isolation. Returning to the normal social environment restores the ability to cope, but prolonged isolation may contribute to development and reinforcement of behaviors that might be considered bizarre in one society and religious experiences in another.[13]

People who make an optimal adjustment to isolation and sensory deprivation seem to be able to relax and enjoy the fantasies and other "primary process" material experienced. Whether a person uses solitude constructively or destructively is in part determined by expectations and cultural influences. Yogis and the American Indians who use solitude constructively are fulfilling societal roles. They have chosen their situation and perceive it as desirable; thus, they interpret what happens to them as nonthreatening. Hallucinatory visions, voices, and vivid dreams are perceived as spiritual experiences. In western society, such experiences could be viewed as evidence of mental illness. If isolation is to be used as a therapeutic intervention, the client must perceive, choose, and use it in the same way as the yogi or the Indian, and society must approve.

Sensory Overload

Sensory overload can be as destructive as sensory deprivation. *Sensory overload* involves multisensory experiences, usually dangerous and intense bombardments by sensory stimuli. *Sensory overload* is therefore characterized by excessive or inappropriate stimulation.

Overstimulation, or "flooding," of a young child may be the result of parental neglect. Children who live in a chaotic or violent household may be exposed to inappropriate and excessive sensory stimuli. Failure of the parents to provide times, places, and an atmosphere for adequate rest and uninterrupted sleep overtaxes the child's ability to receive and process sensations. Sexual stimulation of children, or any number of other situations in which there are failures to define and respect boundaries among family members or between the family and society, increases the risk of sensory overstimulation and consequent overload.

People are usually protected from sensory overload by a *stimulus barrier.* However, if the stimulus barrier is disrupted by faulty management of a child's environment and impaired relationships with parenting figures, or if an adult is overwhelmed by multiple or overintense sensations, overstimulation will result. For the child, defects in the maturing ego are an inevitable consequence.[12] In the adult, dysfunctional coping occurs.

Theoretical Frameworks for Sensory Disturbance

Psychological and physiological theories about the phenomenon of sensory deprivation are two of the most popular. Table 3-2 (page 30) lists the differences between the two explanations of sensory disturbance. The holistic view of the person implies that both of these theoretical frameworks contribute to the understanding of how sensory input is managed.

RELEVANCE TO NURSING

Sensory stimulation is a significant concept in nursing practice because of its role in the development of the self and in client-environment interactions. Each person has developed an optimal level of sensory stimulation. A wide variety of clients are vulnerable to distortion or overload of sensory input or to sensory deprivation.

Promotion and Maintenance of Health

The management of sensory stimulation is vitally important to the health and well-being of children. As they grow and develop, demands are placed on their physical, mental, spiritual, and social capacities. Thus, the range of sensory stimuli that facilitate

Table 3-2 Theories of Sensory Disturbance

	Psychological Theory	Physiological Theory	Cognitive Theory
Cause of sensory disturbance	Suppression of secondary mental processes related to logical thinking, delay of gratification, and regulation of instinctual demands; emergence of primary mental processes related to disorganized irrational thinking and immediate gratification of instinctual demands	Meaningless environmental input promotes an increased prominence of and attention to various internal stimuli, rehearsals of memory, heightened body image awareness with somatic illusions that are hallucinatory in character, and inner ear noise. In the absence of environmental stimuli, repressed material tends to become conscious	Sensory stimuli is absent, decreased, distorted, or in unmanageable quantities →impairment of cognitive organization of person-environment interaction→distortion of reality.
Influential factor in managing sensory input	Ego strength	A constant stream of meaningful environmental stimuli mediated through the ascending reticular activating system in the brain	Information-processing activities

optimal functioning varies according to developmental demands. Motor, intellectual, spiritual, and social development depend on appropriate and adequate sensory stimulation.

Because cutaneous stimulation is necessary for optimal growth and development, nurses, as promoters of health, should help parents use touch to enhance children's development. Even infants in neonatal intensive care units need human touching to facilitate maturation and healthy functioning. Interventions that reduce parental anxiety about care-giving activities such as bathing and feeding may help parents provide their infants with meaningful, nurturing touching. Parents' misconceptions about "spoiling" a child may interfere with the holding, stroking, and rocking needed by infants. Parents who themselves have been emotionally deprived or harshly treated may have less capacity for, or knowledge about, touching their infants. The nurse who nurtures, supports, and serves as a role model may help these parents acquire the capacity to use touch in a nurturing way.

Childbirth is usually characterized by varying degrees and periods of discomfort. Touch can be a useful intervention in relieving discomfort and helping the woman to cope effectively while participating maximally in the process of birth. Effleurage (gentle upward and outward stroking of the abdomen during a contraction) and massaging the lower back may be sources of comfort. The nurse may massage the woman's lower back area or show the expectant father how to do this.

Socially dysfunctional families need help in recognizing their offspring's needs and capacities for sensory stimulation. Nurses who work with parents in clinics or at home help these parents provide sensory input that facilitates their children's growth and development. Neglect can be a significant source of sensory deprivation, and inappropriate sexual stimulation and abuse a source of sensory overload.

Nurses may need to teach families about the selection of age-appropriate toys, games, and reading materials that can provide opportunities that enhance motor, social, and intellectual stimulation. In some instances parents may also need to learn how to spend quality time with their children that will enhance satisfaction of needs for love and belonging, self-esteem, recognition, and socialization. Violent, chaotic, and interpersonally dysfunctional family life may generate sensory stimulation that overwhelms or baffles the child's information-processing capacity. Defensive maneuvers may help the child to screen out unmanageable stimuli temporarily, but when these strategies are employed for extended periods of time, the child will develop operating styles that impair growth and development. For example, physically and sexually abused children and children who are exposed to distorted communication may retreat from social relationships into a world of fantasy. These children might exclude reality or become antisocial and insensitive or perhaps cruel toward others.

Clients with visual and auditory impairments need to be identified and helped to compensate for the absent or diminished sensory stimuli. Without intervention, these people are at risk of social isolation and increased sensory deprivation.

The elderly often have difficulties caused by sensory impairment. Chapter 54 explores nursing implications for this group of clients.

Impairment of taste may in later life lead to a loss of appetite and decreased intake of food. When this occurs, the person may not receive the nutrients needed to maintain health. Nursing interventions for such a client may involve seeking consultation with a nutritionist as well as helping to select and prepare food that maximizes available satisfactions.

Presbycusis, age-associated hearing loss, may be a significant factor in sensory deprivation. A hearing loss may interfere with the capacity to participate in meaningful social interactions. Consequently people with hearing loss withdraw socially, and this aggravates their social isolation and sensory deprivation.

Early identification of sensory impairment in the elderly as well as in other age groups allows the nurse to identify strategies that will help the client enhance existing capacities and compensate for irrevocable losses. New opportunities for socialization and pleasure derived from such activities as eating, reading, or listening to music can often be provided if interventions result in the acquisition of hearing aids, transportation, or spices which enhance sensory perception.

Restoration of Health

The distress associated with physical illness and surgical intervention compounds the stress induced by hospitalization and separation from significant others. The discomfort can be alleviated and therapeutic rest promoted through the use of touch. Bed baths and back massages can be used by nurses to provide touching that enhances relaxation and promotes rest.

Painful procedures are made more distressing if clients become anxious, tense their muscles, or cause tissue damage by sudden movement. In addition to preparing the client for what can be expected and how to cope, in some instances it is also helpful if the nurse holds the client's hand. Sometimes instructing the client to squeeze the nurse's hand when discomfort is great helps the client to cope and feel supported.

Illness and hospitalization, particularly confinement to a special-care unit such as a coronary-care, intensive-care, or burn unit, increases vulnerability to distortion, overload, or deprivation of sensory input. Respirators, the burn bubble, body casts, hyperbaric chambers, and reverse isolation impair sensory stimulation. The loss of control of physical functions such as those associated with elimination, respiration, and ingestion of nutrients produces sensory problems. The life-sustaining technology found in special-care units, the client's physical status, and the required care-giving activities generate sensory input that can become a meaningless and unmanageable flood of stimuli.

Impaired perception, integration, and response to environmental stimuli have been implicated in many psychiatric illnesses. Anxiety can be disorganizing to psychological processes. It may be generated by a failure of defense mechanisms, impaired screening processes, deficient information processing (recognition of inappropriate or incompetent behavior), and deficient social interaction. Nurses have a significant role in helping people who are experiencing severe anxiety, anger, or depression by managing the environmental sensory stimuli so that the client may engage in therapy.

People who are experiencing acute and exaggerated disordered thinking, feeling, perceiving, and behaving may experience touch as anxiety- or fear-producing. Schizophrenics whose boundaries are ill defined and poorly organized may experience panic if touched. Unable to distinguish between where they end and the nurse begins, they may fear that physical contact will somehow cause incorporation with the nurse—a loss of self.

Touching psychiatric clients who have poor impulse control and periods of violent hostility characterized by aggressiveness and assaultiveness also may be problematic. Their acute emotional state or antisocial relational capacity may cause them to misperceive a touch intended to calm, pacify, or support. The result may be an assault on the one who is touching them.

Rehabilitation of Health

Neurological deficits caused by trauma, strokes, viruses, or degenerative diseases interfere with the reception and processing of sensory data. Clients with such deficits experience losses in various perceptual systems. Mobility, balance, language, and the ability to interpret stimuli may be lost. Nurses have an important role in helping these people grieve over the losses imposed by their physical problems, optimize the rehabilitation process, and compensate for the losses with alternative sensory stimulation.

Interventions in which nurses address clients' physical and psychological responses to illness and hospitalization and the environmental influences that affect clients can facilitate return to optimal health. Management of sensory stimulation is an important dimension of nursing practice.

RHYTHMS*

Rhythms are patterns of regularly recurring phenomena occurring within a person or between a person and the environment. Regularity has been associated with health and optimal functioning, whereas irregularity has been correlated with disordered life processes and dysfunction. Identification of rhythmic patterns enables predictions to be made and thus provides useful criteria in the assessment of well-being.

Descriptive Terms

Rhythms can be classified as either exogenous or endogenous. *Exogenous* refers to rhythms that are external to the person. Movement of the stars and planets, fluctuations in gravitational and magnetic forces, variations in the tides, and different intensities of light waves are examples of exogenous rhythms. *Endogenous* refers to internal biological rhythms, such as variations in biochemical processes, steroid and electrolyte levels, body temperature, heart and respiration rates, brain activities, hunger levels, and other complex internal biological processes. Electrocardiographs (ECGs), which measure heart rhythms, and electroencephalographs (EEGs), which measure brain wave patterns, provide a way to measure endogenous rhythms so as to assess health status.

Rhythms occur in cycles, which means that the phenomenon is a continual process that starts from a specific (sometimes arbitrarily specified) point and returns to it. A *period* is the time required to complete a cycle. *Periodicity* refers to the pattern of cycles. *Frequency* is the number of times a cycle is repeated in a given length of time. (For example, sleep frequency in adult humans is generally one period of sleep every 24 hours.) The *amplitude* of a rhythm is the amount or extent of change within a period. *Phase* refers to the time in which part of a cycle takes place; it is usually identified on a graph as either a peak or a trough, with reference to some external point such as clock time. *Phases* are the parameters of biological rhythm. Figure 3-3 illustrates the wave phenomenon of a rhythm.

Researchers have documented more than 100 physiological and performance variables that are longer or shorter than the 24-hour period.[14] The term *circadian* refers to daily rhythms of 24-hour periodicity. A precise solar day is 24.0 hours, and a precise lunar cycle is about 24.8 hours. Body temperature rhythm, which is established after about the third month of life, is an example of a circadian rhythm. With clocklike regularity, the body temperature rises and falls each 24-hour period. The period of highest temperature usually is the time of day of greatest alertness and productivity, and the period of lowest temperature *(nadir point)* is the time of day when there is a marked decrease in activity, alertness, and productivity. Circadian rhythms are believed to be intrinsic to every cell and to persist under constant conditions.

Figure 3-3 Wave phenomenon.

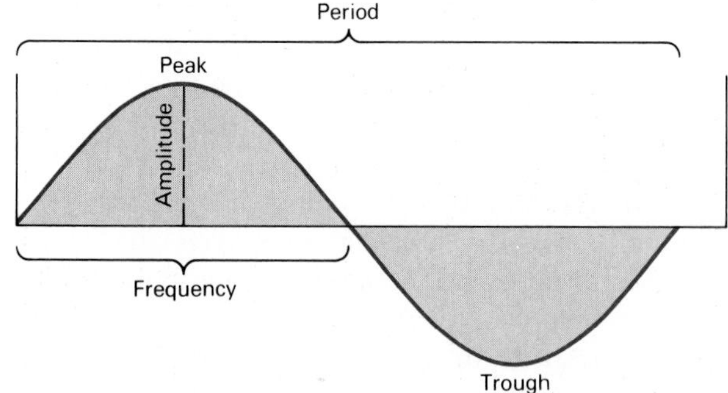

* From R. Mattheis, "Holistic Health Concepts," in the second edition of this book.

However, circadian biological rhythms are triggered by external cues such as light-darkness cycles, cosmic electromagnetic forces, and environmental social patterns; synchronization occurs through the hypothalamic-pituitary and adrenal steroid hormone system and social conditioning.

Rhythms of less than 24 hours are called *ultradian.* For instance, the 90-minute sleep-dream cycle is a basic rest-activity cycle (BRAC), which probably represents a fundamental periodicity in the activity of the CNS and occurs without relationship to the alternation of sleep and wakefulness. The BRAC lengthens from 50 to 60 minutes in infancy to 85 to 95 minutes in maturity. It has been suggested that these 90-minute cycles form a biological "tide" which is a part of lifelong alternation between charging and discharging of drive centers.[15]

Infradian rhythms are characterized by cycles longer than the circadian cycle. Examples are a 28-day menstrual cycle, the 17-ketosteroid 30-day rhythm, a seasonal thyroid production that helps to reduce body heat during the summer, variations in suicide rates peaking in May, deaths from arteriosclerosis in January, and the bipolar affective disorders that may have cycles of several years.

Development of Rhythms

The human infant is considered to have erratic biological rhythms, but data indicate that even the fetus has some intrinsic activity rhythms. The soothing rhythms of rocking and lullabies are now being related to intrauterine rhythmic experiences of the fetus. Montague points out that the fetal heart rate of 140 beats per minute is syncopated with the mother's heart rate of 70 beats per minute.[11] Since the fetus experiences this rhythmic environment, most children, not surprisingly, derive comfort from various rhythmic methods of rocking, head rolling, and, as their physiological development permits, dancing. Attempts to derive comfort from rocking and swaying movements are also easily observed among long-term residents of mental hospitals, retarded persons, and geriatric populations.

Only one circadian rhythm has been identified as being present at birth: electric skin resistance, which is higher in the morning and lower at night. But by the second or third week, urine flow is greater by day than by night, regardless of the amount of fluid intake. At 4 to 6 weeks, heart rate becomes circadian. Between 5 and 9 months, higher diurnal body temperatures are experienced, along with circadian periodicities in blood-sugar levels and urine constitutents.[16]

Environmental factors have been found to influence an infant's rhythmic functioning. A study of interactions among 3-month-old infants and their parents and strangers revealed that infants' heart rate rhythms are stronger and their behavior rhythms are more coherent with parents than with strangers.[17]

Many rhythms continue to stabilize throughout childhood, reaching the greatest level of stability as a person enters young adulthood. There is increasing evidence that some physiological rhythms may get out of phase as a person enters old age. The effect of social schedules on this dissociation has not been established, but certainly the circadian rhythms of old age more often resemble those of infancy than those of adulthood.

Rhythms and Functioning

In spite of the fact that biological periodicities play a major role in human functioning, we tend to remain unaware of them. People breathe, circulate blood, and experience brain, hormonal, biochemical, and temperature fluctuations without any consciousness of their rhythmic variations. Intervening stressors may contribute to dysynchronization and awareness of internal rhythms. People become aware of dysynchronization of internal rhythms when they recognize the symptoms of disrupted life processes.

Synchronization of Rhythms

Human functioning is a result of multiple, rhythmic interacting phenomena. Healthy people live in harmony internally (with synchronization of body rhythms) and with their environment. Physiological, psychological, cognitive, and social functioning occur in rhythmic, integrated patterns. Continual fluctuations in all human functions occur in a harmonious and predictable fashion. Sleeping, waking, eating, eliminating waste products, thinking, feeling, and relating to the environment occur with interactive periodicity.

Each person's inherited potentials, physical and social experiences, perception of events, and interactions with the environment influence the development of unique synchronous patterns. These rhythms and the development of the integrated patterns are probably synchronized through a variety of internal and external mechanisms.

One theory used to explain synchronization of rhythms states that a person is a kind of cosmic receiving station. Changes in a rhythmic geophysical environment, such as terrestrial magnetism, electric fields, background radiation, gravitation, and other signal sources, influence rhythmic human functioning.[18] Variations in the earth's magnetic field may form a spatial and temporal grid that influences the physiological rhythms of inherited human biological clocks. One study noted an association among solar flare activity (sun spots), geomagnetic disturbances, and increased aggressive behavior among hospitalized psychiatric clients.[18] After analyzing 6 years' worth of data, two geophysicists have concluded that there is a significant relationship between cardiac emergencies and geomagnetic activity.[18]

Developmental studies suggest that circadian rhythms may be acquired through interaction with both the social and the physical environment. Inherited propensities probably play a role in the synchronization of internal rhythms; however, environmental forces influence these rhythmic patterns and may interact with them so that there is synchrony with environmental periodicities. A 24-hour oscillator within living cells may help people survive by acting in tune with the environment.

Dysynchronization of Rhythms

Biological rhythms are remarkably stable; however, phase shifting and dysynchronization may be influenced by light-and-darkness cycles and stress, as well as by forces yet to be identified.

The pineal gland has been identified as a kind of biological clock. Melatonin, found in this gland, seems to influence pituitary function, which in turn influences other endocrine and nervous system functions. Melatonin production seems to be inhibited by light, and pineal gland function seems to be affected by exposure to light.[18]

The 24-hour rhythm of norepinephrine production also seems to be affected by light and darkness. Norepinephrine seems to influence pineal rhythms of melatonin and serotonin production, and thus indirectly to influence the pituitary, hypothalamus, and other glandular functions.[18]

Phase shifting, which also is often related to the light-darkness cycle, leads to decoupling of biochemical circadian hormone, electrolyte, neurohumoral, metabolite, and social rhythms. A shock-phase hypothesis of periodic health problems has been suggested. Stresses such as infection and emotional and physical trauma may upset the overall coordination of phase relations among the many internal biological rhythms. Such stresses may produce dysynchronization or phase shifting that influences the development of health problems.

The stresses associated with physical, psychological, and social traumas, as well as responses to stressors that occur at the same time each day, contribute to dysynchronization of rhythms and the development of symptomatic patterns. For example, if daily encounters with a supervisor or colleague are fraught with conflict or anxiety, the consequent emotional response may contribute to the development of an unconscious conditioned-response pattern. Such periodic stressful experiences are often easily remembered and are dysynchronizing within the context of the stressful experience.

The uncomfortable feelings and symptoms of an "anniversary" reaction to life-threatening or mutilative surgery or illness or the loss of a significant person through death or divorce represent an alteration in psychological and biological rhythms. For example, a person who experiences a depression on the anniversary of the death of a parent is symptomatic because of both the emotion and the physical memory of the loss.

Dysynchronization of body rhythms is reflected in disturbed patterns of body functions such as eating and sleeping, and in disrupted intrapersonal and interpersonal relationships. People's perceptions, environmental factors, traumatic events, chronic stresses, and conscious alterations in daily living patterns or lifestyles can produce a phase-shifting of rhythms. For example, sleep-wake cycles may be disturbed by a person consciously remaining awake, jet lag caused by changing time zones, anxiety generated by a perceived threat, or changes in the neuroendocrine system. Because body and social rhythms occur in an integrated pattern, a shift in one body rhythm influences the other interactive rhythms. For example, a reversal of the sleep-wake cycle influences eating, excretion of urine, and body temperature patterns. Interpersonal tension may disrupt eating and sleeping patterns and produce insomnia or binge eating.

Living arrangements, including the physical environment and people who share accommodations, may affect body rhythm. For example, one study found that women who spent 2 or more nights with men during a 40-day period exhibited a significantly higher rate of ovulation than those spending no nights or only one night with men.[19] When the unique rhythms of people within a family home or a group residence are incongruent, then tension and conflicting behaviors are likely to occur. (Some of this tension may also occur because individuals resist conforming to the rhythms of the group.) Research has shown that women who share a residence often develop synchronous menstrual cycles.[20] Thus, the effect of interpersonal influences on body rhythms extends beyond the obvious tension produced when "day people" and "night people" live together to more subtle influences on biological functioning.

Dysynchronization of biological rhythms is related to a loss of health and well-being. Disruption of sociobehavioral rhythms is related to both intrapersonal and interpersonal tension and conflict. High-energy people who have fast-paced behavioral and speech patterns and low-energy people who have slow-paced behavioral and speech patterns are apt to be in conflict in a work situation because of the discrepancy between their personal sociobehavioral rhythms.

Influence of Rhythms on Functioning

Research studies about rhythms are expanding the knowledge base which can be applied to health care. For instance, rhythmicity of biological, psychological, and social functions oscillates between minimum and maximum levels. Recognition of these cycles and their influence on people's overall capacity and ability to function effectively influences health care. Rhythmicity of biological, psychological, and social functions can affect people's interaction with the environment; use of nutrients, drugs, and resources; and vulnerability to stressors.[18]

Recent studies have indicated the importance of circadian rhythms in two significant areas of health care. There is increasing evidence that susceptibility to infection is greater during periods of isolation from environmental cues and during disruption of work-rest cycles. There is also significant variance in response to x-ray and chemical therapies at different points in the circadian cycle.[18]

Work Schedules

In our modern society, people are expected to perform at optimal levels at various hours of the day and night. Nurses and others who must work evening and night shifts must therefore phase-shift their biological, psychological, and social rhythms in order to function at a time when they would ordinarily be sleeping.

Switching from one work shift to another, particularly from day to night or vice versa, involves extensive phase shifting. During the process of phase shifting, efficiency levels are lower, alertness is decreased, and mistakes and misjudgments are more likely to occur. During the reversed work-rest cycle the quality of work, as well as the quality of sleep, is in question. Some investigators feel that sleep-deprivation problems should be a real concern during shift rotations, since a considerable length of time is required for phase shifting of the circadian rhythms.[21]

Studies have found an increased number of absences due to sicknesses, gastrointestinal and cardiovascular diseases, sleep disturbances, and fatigue among rotating shift workers. Shift workers also have exhibited a reluctance to consult a physician when they have symptoms of physical illness.[22] In a study of the effects of shift-rotation schedules on a group of policemen, sleep was reported to be longer and better with clockwise rotation of shifts (days-evenings-nights) than with counterclockwise rotation (nights-evenings-days). Systolic blood pressure and serum levels of triglycerides and glucose were also found to be lower after the clockwise rotation than after the counterclockwise rotation.[23] These findings indicate that clockwise rotation has a favorable effect on risk factors for ischemic heart disease and on impaired functioning. They further suggest the need to consider implementing a clockwise rotation for nurses in agencies where 24-hour care is provided.

A study of naval pilots revealed that the lowest accident or mishap rates are associated with flights that originate during the daytime, and the highest rates are associated with flights that originate during the evenings and nights. This finding suggests that dysynchronization of circadian rhythms, which would be more likely to occur during evening and night flights, increases the risk of errors that contribute to accidents.[24] If this is true for pilots, is it also true for nurses who work evening and night shifts?

One theory of the interaction between work and biorhythms proposes that the human race is still fundamentally operating as our earliest ancestors did in the climate of sub-Saharan Africa. Studies have documented the same daily rhythmic activity among people in various cultures and occupations all over the world. This is a bigeninous, or two-peaked, rhythm, with the late-morning peak more marked than the late-afternoon peak. This rhythm includes peak efficiency and productivity in the morning, regardless of when or whether the noon meal is taken. This high activity level is followed by a period of reduced activity in the afternoon when alertness is diminished. In tropical and nonindustrial societies there is a break from work during the afternoon; people nap, pursue less challenging and demanding activities, and sometimes socialize with their families. In the late afternoon there is a return to work, but the pace is slower than in the morning. In technological societies, this decrease in biorhythmic activity is ignored; one attributes the afternoon slump to the effect of lunch, despite the fact that the heavier evening meal in these societies is not followed by a dropoff in activity. In a study of accidents among woodworkers, the incidents of work-related injuries between 6 A.M. and noon, and 3 P.M. and 7 P.M., were found to be comparable, but a sharp increase occurred between noon and 3 P.M., the hours when alertness is diminished and activity is decreased.[14]

Nutrition and Metabolism

Biological rhythms influence nutrition and metabolism. Hormones such as insulin follow daily rhythms, as do blood glucose and amino acid levels. The body therefore uses carbohydrates, proteins, and fats in a rhythmic fashion. For example, proteins eaten at 8 A.M. rapidly raise amino acid levels in the blood, but at 8 P.M. the ingestion of the same proteins does not have the same effect. Foods may therefore be more efficiently utilized earlier rather than later in the day. Among diabetics, the dawn phenomenon, in which there is an abrupt fluctuation in plasma glucose and insulin requirements, has implications for programming open-loop insulin delivery systems.[25]

Hunger, which occurs in 90-minute cycles, and social patterns also influence eating patterns. Thus, a diet to treat undernutrition and overnutrition may prove to be more effective if it recognizes hunger, metabolic patterns, and social patterns.[18]

A study of newborn infants' sleep patterns and variations in diet, designed to affect the availability of Trp (the amino acid precursor of serotonin), suggests that diet may influence sleep patterns. Newborns who were fed Trp entered active sleep 14.1 minutes sooner and quiet sleep 20 minutes sooner than those fed Similac, and twice as soon as those fed Val (which competes with Trp for entry into the brain).[26] In another study, the investigators found that sleep deprivation and dysynchronization of the circadian rhythms were significantly correlated with reduced serum iron (Fe) levels.[27]

Diet and therapies altering sympathetic nervous system activity may influence sleep patterns. There is a need for greater understanding of the impact of dysynchronization and phase-shifting of rhythms on nutrition, and the implications of nutrition for the management of health problems.

Hormone Rhythmicity

Research has shown that manipulation of light-darkness cycles influences ovulation and the regularity of the menstrual cycle. The synodic month is 29 days, and the average menstrual cycle is 28 to 30 days. The movement of the sun and moon and light-darkness cycles may influence this biological function. Studies which employed indirect light during the nights of the fourteenth to fifteenth and sixteenth to seventeenth days of the menstrual cycle (counting the first day of menstruation) demonstrated that an irregular cycle that varied from 23 days to 48 days could be synchronized to a regular 29-day cycle. Premenstrual syndrome approximately parallels the lunar cycle, as do emotional cycles in men, although male cycles are more subtle. During the premenstrual syndrome, women experience more infections, higher rates of psychiatric admissions, higher accident and suicide rates, activation of chronic illnesses such as arthritis and ulcers, and notable changes in blood-sugar levels.

Men also show marked mood changes, with irritability, loss of energy, and depression occurring on a cyclic schedule.[18] Knowledge about environmental influences on human functioning contributes to the selection of interventions directed toward environmental manipulation which promote or restore health but are less intrusive.

Exercise also influences the menstrual cycle. Anovulatory cycles and oligomenorrhea are correlated with high levels of strenuous exercise. Since catecholamines and beta-endorphin are elevated after this type of exercise, they may interact with the endocrine system and suppress the release of luteinizing hormones at the hypothalamic-pituitary axis.[28]

Other studies of women's health have noted that in childbirth 60 percent of labor begins at night, with a peak occurring around 3 A.M. Research also shows that most stillbirths and births with fatal complications have occurred in the late afternoon.[29] Research also indicates that the 24-hour variation in birth incidence has an underlying endogenous circadian rhythmicity, possibly synchronized by the sun.[29] When labor is induced and there is delivery intervention, the rhythms of the work activity of hospital personnel are imposed. Whether this imposition of an exogenous rhythm on an endogenous rhythm is deleterious to the mother or fetus is not yet known.

The pineal gland influences the rate of sexual development indirectly, through the endocrine system. Knowledge about the relationship of light-darkness cycles on pineal development and function may be used in planning the environment for newborns. For example, the lighting pattern in hospital nurseries and intensive-care nurseries for premature infants may be physiologically important.

Menstrual irregularity influences conception, daily functioning, and perhaps overall health. For example, the frequency of occurrences of acute appendicitis in the luteal phase has been found to be more than twice that in the remaining half of the menstrual cycle, and a significant number of gangrenous, perforated appendices have been removed from women during the menstrual and follicular phases. These findings suggest that female sex hormones may play an important etiological role in acute appendicitis or influence the inflammatory process in the appendix.[30]

Medication and Rhythmicity

Research in chronopharmacology is contributing information regarding the timing of medications to ensure maximum therapeutic effect or minimal side effects. Blood levels of medications vary over a 24-hour period. For example, when the antidepressant amitriptyline is administered orally in the morning, its side effects—decreased salivation and sedation—are more marked than when the drug is administered in the evening. Since bioavailability of the drug does not differ between morning and evening, administering the drug in the evening is more desirable from the client's perspective.[31] Findings of current animal studies concerning changes in phase relations of circadian rhythms in cell proliferation may be applicable to the scheduling of chemotherapy and radiotherapy. Further research in this area will determine whether prescribed timing of these therapies will provide maximal effects upon the tumor with minimal undesirable side effects on vital physiological functions.[32]

RELEVANCE TO NURSING

Nurses have a significant responsibility to create a therapeutic climate for hospitalized clients and people who use clinics. Nurses need to be aware of the importance of rhythms and environmental influences in promoting health. Assessing environment and client will help the nurse to identify needs in both that must be satisfied through intervention in order for promotion, maintenance, restoration, and rehabilitation of health to occur.

It should also be pointed out that the effect of biorhythms can be important in the nurse's own work, especially when shifts are involved. Endogenous circadian rhythms, such as hormone production and temperature cycles, may take up to 3 weeks to change. Meanwhile, a nurse may be attempting to work with a body primed for sleep and to sleep with a body primed for work. The rate of readaptation at the end of a reversed cycle may also be a cause for concern, although that is generally much more rapid. The vulnerability associated with dysynchronization of body rhythms must be recognized before strategies can be identified that will lessen the impact of phase shifting. For example, many nurses have recognized that they perform their professional activities more safely when they work one shift for an extended period of time rather than several different shifts within the same week. Consequently, they have negotiated work contracts to avoid varied work schedules that would cause dysynchronization of their body rhythms. Theories and research findings have related biorhythmic patterns to accidents, and this has implications for nursing practice. If nurses want to give clients the best possible care, they must consider rhythmic functioning not only in planning care but also in determining their own effectiveness and safety as they provide it.

In people without overt emotional problems, changes in mood may be so gradual and moderate that they go unnoticed. Nevertheless, they influence decision making, family and work relationships, and job performance. If people become "tuned in" to their bodies and their feelings, and if they recognize rhythmic fluctuations, they can to some extent plan their lives to promote overall effectiveness and well-being. For example, there are "day people" and "night people." Some people function more alertly in the mornings and the early part of the day, whereas others are usually more attentive and physiologically active during the latter part of the day and the evening. These differences reflect the low and high periods of biological as well as social functioning. Nursing interventions that facilitate clients' well-being help them to recognize and predict rhythmic patterns, identify factors that influence the occurrence and severity of such patterns, and alter their own ways of coping.

As was noted earlier, rhythmic patterns in clients (for example, children's respiratory function) can be an important consideration in the timing of medication. Studies have found, for instance, that early-morning or midday doses of hormones have greater efficacy than similar doses later in the day.[18] If the administration of such medication is timed to maximize its effectiveness, a smaller dose can be used, which in turn lessens side effects. (Since hormone medication can retard growth, reducing the dose may be particularly desirable if the client is a child.) Immunity is also rhythmic to some extent. Future research in chronopharmacology may reveal that greater protection is afforded if immunization or chemotherapy that affects the immune system is administered at specific times. Thus nurses' responsibility for administering medications includes collaborating with physicians and clients. Identifying clients' rhythms, monitoring the efficacy of drugs, and timing the administration of drugs accordingly may enhance their therapeutic effect.[18]

Recent studies show a relationship among environmental light-darkness cycles, rhythmic hormonal functions, and the functional capacity of the nervous system and other body systems, on the one hand, and on the other the efficacy of treatments such as electroconvulsive therapy and responses to surgical intervention, as well as to drugs. Nurses need to keep up to date and to contribute to findings by applying research about biorhythms to the care of clients.

Since stress may cause a significant dysynchronization of biological rhythms, interventions must be directed toward repatterning dysynchronized rhythms in order to restore and promote health. Collaborative assessments with clients facilitate increased self-awareness and recognition of biological, psychological, and social rhythms. Biofeedback and related techniques for achieving self-regulation of unconscious body processes may contribute to this repatterning process.

The hospital itself may be a source of stress. Hospitals tend to maintain rigid schedules for clients with regard to care, meals, treatments, and so on. Clients incur stress in addition to their illnesses by having to adapt or phase-shift their own circadian rhythms to fit the hospital's schedule, often without having a wall clock or wristwatch.

Nurses play an important role in helping new parents recognize the importance of synchronizing rhythms between the parent and the child. Compatability of activity patterns in the parent-child relationship influences the child's well-being.

SLEEP*

Sleep is a regular, recurrent, easily reversible state characterized by relative quiescence and by a great increase in the threshold response to external stimuli relative to the waking state. It is basically a behavioral state of altered consciousness and an important biorhythmic human phenomenon. Sleep

* From R. Mattheis, "Holistic Health Concepts," in the second edition of this book.

has a restorative function that helps to maintain health. Disrupted sleep patterns and the biopsychosocial symptoms that occur as a result of sleep disturbances are examples of the impact of dysynchronization of body rhythms on well-being.

Tiredness

Tiredness precedes sleep. Two patterns of tiredness have been identified; these are compared in Table 3-3. Type 1 tiredness develops as a result of physical activity. Type 2 tiredness is related to mental or emotional fatigue and results in impaired cognitive functioning which in turn is reflected in difficulty in concentration, defective exclusion of extraneous stimuli, weakening of ego mechanisms, development of aggression, and impaired impulse control. The kind of sleep needed for each type of tiredness differs.[33]

Stages of Sleep

It is not possible to determine the exact onset of sleep, even with EEG monitoring. The essential difference between wakefulness and sleep is the loss of awareness. At the onset of sleep visual perception is lost and the eyes begin to drift slowly from side to side, either synchronously or asynchronously.[33] Sleep occurs in four stages. (This is a somewhat arbitrary division of a continuous process, although each stage is characterized by a distinct brain wave pattern). These stages are outlined in Table 3-4.

Table 3-3 Patterns of Tiredness

Type 1	Type 2
Product of physical exertion	Product of emotional stress and/or intellectual work involving new learning
Relaxed musculature, including the face and head	Muscle cramping; headache and eye strain
Relaxed feeling	Tense feeling
Falls asleep easily	Difficulty falling asleep
No mental or emotional symptoms	Irritability, discomfort, anger, anergia, inability to concentrate, loss of social adaptiveness, loss of superego functions

SOURCE: Adapted from E. L. Hartmann, "Psychology of Tiredness," in D. Goleman and R. J. Davidson, eds., *Consciousness: The Brain, States of Awareness, and Alternate Realities,* Irvington, New York, 1979.

Table 3-4 Stages and Characteristics of Sleep

Stage	Characteristics
1	This is the lightest stage of sleep and is characterized by dysynchronized brain wave activity. There is a feeling of floating or falling, which often terminates abruptly in a jerk that returns the person to wakefulness.
2	After a few seconds or minutes, stage 1 gives way to stage 2, which is characterized by a brain wave pattern that shows frequent spindle-shaped tracings and distinct spikes on EEG tracings.
3	Several minutes after stage 2 has begun, the brain waves change to the slow delta waves, which are a characteristic of stage 3.
4	After approximately 10 minutes, the delta waves become more dominant, which is characteristic of stage 4. Stage 4 lasts 30 to 40 minutes before the reascent through the stages of sleep begins.

As a person falls asleep, stage 1 is entered. Movement through the stages represents progressively deeper levels of anesthesia: it is most difficult to arouse a sleeper during stage 4. Sleepwalking (somnambulism), night terrors in children, and bedwetting begin to occur during this stage; however, actual micturition occurs during stage 1 or 2.[34]

Rapid-eye-movement (REM) *sleep,* which is also called *dysynchronized* (D) or *active sleep,* is both a period of emergence from stages 2, 3, and 4 and a separate stage of sleep. REM sleep is characterized by:

- Rapid conjugate eye movements
- Irregularity in pulse rate, respiratory rate, and blood pressure
- Full or partial penile erections
- Generalized muscular atony interrupted by sporadic movements in small muscle groups.

People have four or five such periods per sleep cycle. If awakened during one of these periods, they will report 60 to 90 percent of the time that they have been dreaming.[34]

Initially the body is immobile in REM sleep. Small, convulsive twitches of the face and fingertips develop. Snoring ceases, and breathing becomes irregular; this is rapidly followed by slow respirations and brief periods of apnea. Cerebral blood flow and brain temperature increase. The large muscles of the trunk appear completely paralyzed. Under the eyelids the eyes dart back and forth. Contraction, usually occurring during wakefulness as a response to various intensities and pitches of sound, appears in middle ear muscles.[34]

Nonrapid eye movement (NREM) *sleep,* which is also called *synchronized* (S) *sleep,* is quiet sleep. During a period of synchronized sleep, blood pressure, pulse, and respirations are relatively slow and steady, and the arousal threshold is much lower than during REM (or D) sleep.

Throughout the night, NREM (S) and REM (D) cycles alternate in 70- to 110-minute periods. In the early part of the sleep period, NREM dominates, particularly in stages 3 and 4. REM sleep becomes progressively longer during the latter part of the sleep period, and stage 2 represents the only NREM interruption.[34]

Functions of Sleep

REM (D) sleep may help to restore the ability to focus attention; maintain optimism, energy, and self-confidence; and interact effectively with the physical and social environment. This type of sleep seems to be needed more when a person has experienced stress or been involved in intense intellectual activity using new learning. It may help to consolidate learning and memory, and to integrate new concepts learned with conflicting beliefs and behaviors. Thus, REM (D) sleep is needed by people experiencing type 2 tiredness.[33]

NREM (S) sleep is the deepest and probably most intense part of sleep. It has a physically restorative function; physical restoration is especially needed after exercise or when catabolism has been increased. People experiencing type 1 tiredness benefit from NREM (S) sleep.[33]

Development of Sleep Rhythms

The duration of sleep is controlled by an endogenous circadian oscillatory system. Over a 24-hour period, sleep is controlled primarily by behavioral and environmental interactions. Social, occupational, and self-imposed pressures regulate the placement of sleep periods in a 24-hour time span.[33]

The distribution of the stages of sleep varies throughout the night. For instance, a typical sleep cycle begins with stage 1, progresses to stages 2, 3, and 4, returns to 3 and 2, and then (on an average of every 90 minutes) enters a D period. The cycle repeats itself but with a major variation in timing. In the early part of a sleep period, stage 4 predominates; in the last third of the period, stage 1 or D sleep prevails. It is postulated that this 90-minute cycle is a basic rest-activity cycle of the central nervous system, occurring straight through the 24-hour period as part of a circadian rhythm.[35]

The amount of time a person sleeps decreases across the life span. As people age, both S (NREM) and D (REM) sleep become, on the average, slightly shorter. A newborn usually sleeps 16 to 18 hours a day, and at least one-half of this time is in D sleep. Stage 4 sleep occurs most in infants and least in the elderly. A young adult usually sleeps 7 to 8 hours a day.[34]

The length and timing of sleep periods also change across the life span. Of the 16 hours of sleep required by newborns, up to 40 percent is in daytime naps. Naps usually stop by 5 years of age, and the total sleep requirement gradually decreases to the 8 hours per circadian cycle typical for adults. Disruption of sleep-wake patterns is normally a problem as a person ages.[36] Elderly people have the least total sleep time, although they often have daytime naps.

Dynamics of Sleep

The neural mechanisms that control sleep are not fully understood. However, the midline thalamus, the hypothalamus, and portions of the brain stem are known to play a part in sleep. The reticular activating system helps to maintain wakefulness and, with portions of the medulla, to initiate NREM (S) sleep. Neurons in the gigantocellular tegmental fields may play a part in initiating REM (D) sleep. Some researchers have proposed that chemical substances circulating in the blood, in the spinal fluid, or perhaps in both, may influence the sleep-wake cycle.[34]

The functions of sleep are not yet fully understood either. Hartmann hypothesizes that sleep may contribute to restoring the mechanisms of focused attention, and possibly of learning or memory, and preserving emotional integrity and social adaptation.[34]

Sleep Deprivation

Sleep deprivation is a stressful experience. During long periods of sleep deprivation, a person experiences a reduction in muscle tone and a fall in body temperature. Attention is impaired, and, as the person ages, the ability to mobilize decreases. The psychological disturbances that have been noted include illusions and sometimes visual and auditory hallucinations, disassociations, weakening defense mechanisms, and emerging primitive (usually repressed) thoughts. Subjects of sleep deprivation studies also exhibit increasing anger, irritability, and unfocused and antisocial behavior.[34]

Studies have found that people deprived of REM (D) sleep exhibit increased irritability and suspiciousness. If prolonged, sleep deprivation produces disturbances like those characterizing psychosis, including paranoid delusions, confused identity, and hallucinations. Deprivation of stage 4 sleep results in malaise, apathy, and depression. Recovery from sleep deprivation seems to occur more readily in young, healthy people.

Dreaming

A *dream* is a sequence of mental pictures, or images, that embodies the ideas or conceptions of the dreamer. A dream is not a consciously contrived waking fantasy, but an unconsciously fashioned expression of the mind in images.

Dreaming is both a psychological and a physical process. It helps to integrate emotionally significant events with existing memories. Severe depression is associated with disrupted sleep patterns characterized by rapid entry into intense dream sleep. It may be that the "overload" of emotions experienced in depression increases the need for and the intensity of dreaming.[37]

Dreams use symbols, or pictorial metaphors, to embody thoughts that are buried in the unconscious. Research suggests that the neural basis for dreams is located in the hippocampus. EEG findings indicate that bursts of rhythmic activity originate from this structure during dreaming periods. Motivational centers in the brain are activated during dreaming, and it is in these centers that the sensations of pleasure or punishment attached to certain situations, acts, or impulses may be based. This location of both pain and pleasure responses helps to explain the dichotomy between pleasant dreams and nightmares.[38]

A dream is the visual embodiment of conceptions—buried deep in the unconscious—of people, places, things, and situations. During sleep the "vigilance system" that ordinarily represses distracting, unwanted, or disturbing thoughts and impulses is not operative. Repressed material is therefore available and accessible for incorporation into dream activity.[38]

Jung proposed that dreams are more than repressed impulses. He suggested that they connect people to a "collective unconscious" of humanity. The common elements (archetypes) found in everyone's dreams, as well as in myths, reflect shared experiences, although they also have a unique dimension related to each person's life. Jung believed that through analysis of dreams, self-understanding and self-awareness can be developed.[39]

Interpretation of dreams, used in psychotherapy to facilitate the development of insight, was developed by Freud. The goal of such interpretation is to discover the meaning of a dream by translating its images into ideas. Ideas that can be used to increase self-knowledge and self-awareness include information about the self, others, the world, areas of conflict, and one's impulses (ways they are gratified, obstacles to their fulfillment, and penalties for breaking rules that control their satisfaction).[38]

Primitive societies use presleep instruction and early wakeful periods to advise people, particularly children, about how to reinterpret future dreams and benefit from orchestrated dream experiences. For example, children who have nightmares in which they are attacked by wild animals would be counseled to dream the next night that the animals are overcome and destroyed.[40] Current dream theory proposes that the mind uses dreams to heal psychological wounds.[39]

Daydreaming

Daydreams differ from nocturnal dreams in that they are fleeting fantasies or distracting images. Daydreams intrude suddenly into waking thoughts every day. Most of these daydreams take the form of fairly clear visual images. They occur primarily during private moments, just before bedtime, or during solitary travel.[41]

People who daydream withdraw part of their attention from the environment and screen out the surrounding stimuli. (A fixed steady stare at a particular spot allows the image to fade gradually away.) Exclusion of external stimuli makes it possible to focus greater attention on internal material.[41]

Most people enjoy their daydreams. Usually the content of daydreams involves plausible situations, but in some instances the content is wildly improbable. Some images involve violation of societal, family, or personal inhibitions; they range from the mundane to the bizarre. The peak period of daydreaming occurs during midadolescence and gradually declines, but some daydreaming persists into old age. During youth and young adulthood, daydreams tend to be future-oriented; as people grow older, daydreams tend to be past-oriented.[41] Seven categories of daydreaming patterns identified by Singer are described in Table 3-5.

Table 3-5 Daydreaming Patterns

Category	Content
General daydreaming	Varied content Interest in people rather than the environment
Self-recriminating daydreaming	Obsession with guilt and depression
Objective, controlled, thoughtful daydreaming	Reflective, scientific, and philosophical Curiosity about nature rather than people Masculine oriented Reflects emotional stability
Poorly controlled, kaleidoscopic daydreaming	Scattered thoughts Lack of systematic story lines Distractibility, boredom, and self-abasement
Autistic daydreaming	Content usually found in nocturnal dreaming Primary process material Poorly controlled quality of inner experiences
Neurotic, self-conscious daydreaming	Repetitive, egocentric, and body-centered fantasies
Enjoyable daydreaming	Enjoyable fantasies Use of fantasy for enjoyment and problem solving

SOURCE: J. L. Singer, "The Importance of Daydreaming," in D. Goleman and R. J. Davidson, eds., *Consciousness: The Brain, States of Awareness, and Alternate Realities,* Irvington, New York, 1979, pp. 53–57.

Daydreaming serves many functions. Research suggests that practiced daydreamers are able to work out fear or anger and alter moods rather than reduce drive energy. Among unpracticed daydreamers, daydreaming may increase anxiety; however, research evidence on this point is inconclusive. The functional role of daydreaming in relation to motivational or emotional processes needs to be examined further.

Daydreaming can be a source of pleasure and distraction during periods of solitude or in boring situations. However, when alertness and focused attention are needed to perform a complex task (such as operating machinery or a moving vehicle) daydreaming may be a dangerous distraction.

RELEVANCE TO NURSING

The specific relationship between sleep and mental health is not understood. Both external and internal factors influence restful sleep. Perception of the need for sleep may be a source of concern among some clients; a person who sleeps 6 hours a night, for instance, may believe that less than 8 hours of sleep is a symptom of insomnia. But some clients fail to recognize that they need more sleep than usual. For example, people often require more sleep when they are experiencing a change in occupation; increased mental activity, physical work, or exercise; an emotional upset; or stressful situations.

Nursing interventions may be needed to promote therapeutic rest and sleep in clients who are experiencing or convalescing from a medical problem or surgery. Additional sleep can conserve energy and mobilize the body's restorative capacities.[34]

Knowledge about the relationship between development and sleep patterns can be particularly useful to nurses working with elderly clients who express concern about their sleeping patterns, and to nurses working with mothers of newborns and infants. New parents need to know that neonates and some older infants usually wake every 3 to 4 hours and that as a child matures, this cycle will lengthen. The elderly often need to be reassured that less sleep, different patterns of sleeping, and short afternoon naps are common occurrences as one grows older.

Sleep disturbances (as was noted earlier) have been associated with depression. The early-morning awakening (EMA) and difficulty falling asleep (DFA) experienced by people with depression reflect dysynchronization of the sleep-wake cycle. Sleep patterns among depressed clients tend to shift quickly from stage to stage, and "phase advance"—a movement of REM sleep forward relative to the sleep-wake cycle as a whole—may account for some of the sleep abnormalities associated with depression: the greater the phase advance, the more severe the depression.[42] Tricyclic antidepressants seem to affect sleep patterns by increasing the amount of stage 4 sleep, slightly decreasing REM sleep, and lengthening the entire sleep cycle from about 90 to 120 minutes. Drugs such as phenelzine shorten the sleep cycle. Alcohol, amphetamines, and barbiturates also depress the REM cycle and affect the amount of dreaming that accompanies it. Significant improvement in depression occurs after REM deprivation.[33]

Sleep also can be important with regard to stress. Effective emotional interaction with the environment and positive moods affect the quality of REM sleep, and an increased quantity of this stage of sleep is needed during periods of stress.

Because promotion of restful sleep is an important nursing intervention, research is needed to discover nursing measures that increase synchrony of sleep patterns. Some people experience eight to ten sleep cycles per night, for example, instead of the usual four to five, with an accompanying disorganization in hormonal rhythms. These people may need nursing measures to promote restful sleep.

SPACE AND TIME

Space and time are inextricably linked, and life itself may be said to exist in a four-dimensional space-time matrix. However, for purposes of understanding space and time, each will be examined separately here.

Space

Space is notoriously difficult to define; but it may be described as distance extending without limit (or at least without boundaries) in all directions, or as that within which all material things are contained. The word *space* is also used to designate a specific area between or within things. Space is thus an aspect of the environment in which people interact. Properties and structures of environmental stimuli interact in space and influence people. Perceptions of space and distance are dynamic and vary according to the situation, past experiences, and expectations about the future. Culture, personal experiences, and personal needs further mediate these perceptions.

Physical properties of the spatial environment (such as heat, light, and sound) interact with physical, mental, and spiritual aspects of the person.

For example, the *thermal environment* (that is, air, temperature, wind velocity, and humidity), interacts with excess heat generated by a person's metabolic activity. Thyroid hormones influence the body's internal management of and sensitivity to environmental temperature.

The *acoustic environment*, which is not only a product of the sound directly generated by people and machines but a reflection of these sounds from surfaces in the environment, also interacts with people. Reverberation of sound is a function of amount and shape of space and absorptive properties of reflecting surfaces. Whether sound waves are widely scattered and rapidly absorbed by surfaces, or reverberated and intensified, influences perception and causes aural comfort or distress. Sound waves exert pressure on the auditory system. When the pressure increases beyond a certain point, it causes distress. Noise involves the interaction of both sound waves and unwanted auditory stimuli. Exposure to extreme levels of prolonged sound produces either immediate or eventual irreversible deafness. Up to a certain level, noise stimulates mental alertness; but excessive arousal can be followed by distortion and a loss of analytical and cognitive functioning. Individual differences in functioning of the auditory system influence sensitivity to auditory stimuli.

A person also interacts with the *visual environment*, which encompasses light, color, and texture, and thus an aesthetic dimension. Task performance and comfort are strongly influenced by the visual environment. Discomfort increases when light is glaring, flickering, or nonuniform. (Research indicates that in difficult visual conditions, the elderly have more problems performing tasks than the young.) An interesting aspect of the visual environment is windows. A window serves three purposes: (1) it provides contact with the outside world; (2) it admits daylight; and (3) it provides spatial and temporal variety, since the illumination it admits depends on external conditions. People prefer sunlight over artificial light (as long as there is no glare or overheating), even to the point of preferring a sunlit room with no view over a sunless room with a pleasant view.

Outer Space

Outer space (as opposed to inner space, which will be discussed later), may be defined as the area between objects. It can be described in terms of territoriality and distance zones.

TERRITORIALITY. *Territory* is a specific space limited or belonging to someone who defines its boundaries and predominates over it. *Territoriality* is behavior by which an organism characteristically lays claim to an area and defends it against members of its own species.

People are territorial. They evolve various symbols and structures (such as badges, laws, fences, hedges, walls, doors, and rooms) which serve as boundary markers for their territory. Both animals and people have critical distances or zones that, if violated, elicit defensive maneuvers. People define homes, workplaces, and areas of expertise as their territories, and they aggressively defend them when the critical zones are invaded.

Interpersonal distancing increases with age. The adolescent manifests a maturational need for four kinds of privacy: (1) freedom from unwanted intrusions; (2) freedom to determine times and places of communication with others; (3) time for solitude and seclusion; and (4) freedom to keep personal information from being known by others.[43] The elderly, however, begin to narrow the distance from others that was maintained during adulthood. This decrease in spatial requirements may be a result of three phenomena and perhaps others not yet identified. First, sensory perception becomes less acute with age; consequently, there is a need to maximize access to stimuli. Second, tactile stimuli exchanged between people may be perceived by the elderly as a way of enhancing communication and thus compensating for information that may be lost because of the decreased ability to receive other kinds of sensations. Third, although tactile stimulation is needed throughout life, it is often less available to the elderly; there may be a loss of intimate relationships that would provide such stimulation, such as death of a spouse or separation from offspring. Thus the elderly may tend to decrease their distance from others.[43]

DISTANCE ZONES. *Personal distance* is defined as the normal spacing maintained between members of a species. It is an "invisible bubble" that surrounds an animal or person. Social organization influences the size of these "bubbles." Dominant animals and high-status people tend to have larger personal distances than those lower in the social order.

Social distance is the situationally defined distance beyond the personal "bubble" that allows contact with others. Violation of personal and social distances elicits anxiety and defensiveness.

Hall[44] identified and described four distance zones based on observations of business and professional people who lived and worked in the northeastern seaboard of the United States: intimate, personal, social, and public. The characteristics of these four zones and the distances involved in them are presented in Table 3-6.

SPACE AND COMMUNICATION. Use of space is a form of communication. The way a person notifies others of the amount of personal space required and its boundaries is a message that conveys information and controls relationships. Expansion of personal space, permission to cross personal boundaries, and active or hostile defense of territory convey messages to others that influence relationships and interactions.[44] For example, the chair at the head of a rectangular table is usually selected by the leader of a group, not by any of the other members; a member who is allied with the leader tends to choose the chair on the leader's right.

Delineations of space requirements and activities that involve others' territorial and personal boundaries are influenced by the culture. Whether people allow others to enter their personal space to give comfort during periods of distress depends on what the society proscribes, on what imitative learning has occurred within the family, and per-

Table 3-6 Distance Zones

Zone	Distance	Communication	Social Use	Degree of Contact	Vision
Intimate space, close phase	Physical involvement	Whisper; most communication carried by other channels; telling a secret	Lovemaking; wrestling; comforting; protecting	Olfaction input increased; sensations of radiant heat increased	Sharp vision is blurred; images greatly enlarged
Intimate space, far phase	6–18 inches	Voice normal but at a low level or even whisper; confidential subject matter	Same as above; occurs in crowded public places but defensive devices are employed (e.g., immobility, rapid withdrawal if there is touching, muscle tension)	Body heat, odor, breath may be detected	Head is seen as enlarged in size; features distorted
Personal distance, close phase	$1\frac{1}{2}$–$2\frac{1}{2}$ feet	Soft voice; low volume; personal subject matter	Spousal; parent-child; sibling	Odors, body heat, and breath are less noticeable but can be detected	Noticeable feedback from muscles that control the eyes; three-dimensional quality to objects; surface textures are prominent and clearly differentiated
Personal distance, far phase	$2\frac{1}{2}$–4 feet	Subjects of personal interest and involvement; voice level moderate	Collaborative work relationship; some social situations	Outside easy touching distance; olfaction not noticeable; breath can sometimes be detected	Head size perceived as normal; facial details easily visible
Social distance, close phase	4–7 feet	Full voice	Impersonal business; some work relations	Not touching distance; odors and heat not usually perceived	Increased view of person; details clearly perceived
Social distance, far phase	7–12 feet	Full voice and noticeably louder and could be heard in an adjoining room	Business and social interactions of a formal nature	Odors and heat not perceived	View of whole person, but details less clearly visible; greater need for visual contact
Public distance, close phase	12–25 feet	Voice loud; formal style of interacting; careful choice of words and phrasing of sentences	Speaking to a group; recognizing someone in a crowd in a public place	Considerably minimized	At 16 feet body begins to lose roundness and appears flat; whole body can be seen
Public distance, far phase	25 feet or more	Voice amplified; communication shifts to gestures and body stance	Important public figures—a 30-foot distance	Precluded by physical distance	Whole person and setting are visible

SOURCE: Adapted from E. T. Hall, *The Silent Language*, Doubleday, New York, 1959; and *The Hidden Dimension*, Doubleday, New York, 1966.

haps on what professional training people have received with regard to supportive behavior.

Inner Space

Inner space is analogous to states of consciousness, or awareness. It involves knowing oneself as a thinking being: what one is doing and why, and what one is thinking, feeling, and sensing. It involves not only being self-aware—that is, being aware of being aware—but also knowing what is happening in the environment.

A MODEL FOR CONSCIOUSNESS. According to Tart, an ordinary state of consciousness is a very complex construction and serves as a tool for coping with the environment.[45] Current knowledge about consciousness is fragmented and incomplete.

Fishkin and Jones propose a model for consciousness which includes internal and external sensory data that supply the content for consciousness, attention control, and energy.[46] The phenomena that are potentially available to consciousness include:

- Perceptions of external events: sounds, light, messages from others, cutaneous stimulation, and heat or cold
- Perceptions of bodily events: posture, movement, and feelings
- Perceptions of brain-initiated events: imagery, dreams, visions, and hallucinations
- Verbal thinking: thoughts about what one might say (for example, descriptive and judgmental words like *ugly* and *beautiful*)
- Nonverbal thinking: notions or concepts that occur before expository words are selected
- Memories, some of which are more readily available than others
- Direct access to unconscious material under certain conditions
- Unspecified phenomena

Attention as such and the extent of attention determine what is present in consciousness. When attention is narrowly focused, the content available is also narrow.[46] Shifts in attention, and the rate of shifts, will affect what enters consciousness and how intense consciousness is. People develop various attention levels for various situations. For example, in a dangerous situation attention may be rigidly and narrowly focused on content that will ensure survival, whereas in benign situations attention may shift among various content areas.[46]

Energy for consciousness is supplied by the person and fluctuates in relation to the investments in attention, consciousness, and the sources of content. The greater the energy investment in one function, the less there is for the other functions.[46]

ORDINARY AND DISCRETE STATES OF CONSCIOUSNESS. A basic awareness of the physical environment, of the objects and people in it, and of its sounds, smells, and colors is an *ordinary state of consciousness.* It is volitional attention to things, to the actions of oneself and others, and to exchanges among people and between oneself and others. Within a person's normal range of consciousness, there are innumerable *discrete states of consciousness,* such as sleep, hypnosis, alcohol intoxication, meditation, fatigue, excitement, sexual arousal, rage, and fear. Each state of consciousness is unique as an experience and as a pattern of brain arousal.[45]

An ordinary state of consciousness is a construction of perceived reality that results in part through a socialization process. Thus, ordinary consciousness varies according to the cultural context. Potential for variations in consciousness exists within the person. The context facilitates development or repression of consciousness.

RELEVANCE TO NURSING

Internal physiological functioning and personal idiosyncrasies influence thermal preferences, such as what the room temperature will be. Since nurses are concerned with person-environment interactions, thermal preferences should be a consideration, as should theory about these interactions, in planning and delivering care. For example, research indicates that there is no difference between elderly and young persons' preference for environmental temperature or their thermal sensitivity. But the increased metabolic activity of an agitated hospitalized client and the vegetative immobility of a severely depressed client may require modification of the thermal environment. Failure to intervene in this respect would allow thermal stress to compound impaired functioning.

The acoustic environment is also a nursing concern. For example, some clients' capacity to manage environmentally generated aural stimulation is impaired. High levels of sound may be a source of stress that further disorganizes these clients and interferes with their ability to cope. Nurses need to be involved in creating environments that provide aural comfort. Curtains, carpets, and furnishings influence the reverberation and absorption of sound waves. The interaction between the environment of special-care units and clients' perceptions and comfort has been recognized. The noise level, rhythm of life-support systems and monitors, and the clients' perceptions of these stimuli must be considered in planning care and in selecting interventions.

The visual environment can become a stressor to both client and nurse, or it can be therapeutic. Decoration of clients' spaces within the hospital environment has a therapeutic dimension that nurses must influence on behalf of their clients. Soft lighting facilitates relaxation, but bright glare and flickering light increase tension and may impair functioning. Special-care units tend to have few or no windows. Clients therefore may not be able to tell if it is day or night, and they are deprived of daylight and subjected instead to continuous artificial light.

Territoriality influences relationships between nurses and their clients and colleagues. If its influences are understood and handled appropriately, these relationships can become collaborative, and outcomes can be both effective and satisfying.

A client's home or room in a treatment setting or long-term care setting often becomes that person's territory. Public health nurses on home visits and nurses in treatment or long-term care settings are intruding on people's territory. If the nurses recognize this intrusion and allow their clients to retain as much control as possible, the clients will feel more comfortable about their territorial boundaries.

Residential institutions and treatment facilities often have housekeeping policies that interfere with the development of territorial boundaries; without these boundaries, people may feel insecure or fail to develop a sense of belonging. Since people define their territory, they may feel that they have greater control over their lives and are more secure when they can choose whether their door is open or closed, hang their favorite pictures, arrange and decorate their room to suit their own tastes, and arrange personal items on dressers or nightstands.

Nurses also have professional territorial imperatives. Nurses' stations and nurses' lounges are often designated as their territory. Clients, visitors, and other staff members are often pointedly excluded from these spaces. When a designated nurses' lounge adjoins a nursing station, the territorial boundary becomes even more distinct and respected. Only nurses enter and sit down in this area; others (physicians, laboratory technicians, clients, and visitors) do not—they may stand at the door to talk to a nurse who is inside, but they do not cross the threshold without a specific invitation.

Doors, walls, glass panels, and waist-high partitions serve as boundaries for nurses' territories in health care settings. Doors, curtains, and furniture arrangements may define clients' territories.

In long-term treatment settings and residential settings, clients often define spaces outside their bedrooms as their territory. For example, in television or lounge areas a client may claim a particular chair. In a dining room, a particular table and seat at a table may also be claimed. If anyone else takes the "owned" chair or place at the table, that might be seen as an invasion, and the person who claimed it may defend it.

Nursing care usually requires the nurse to intrude into clients' intimate and personal spaces. The feelings generated in both nurse and client by such narrowing of personal space need to be recognized and dealt with if the care is to be effective. Defensive responses interfere with the nurse's capacity to be perceptive and helpful, and with the client's conservation of energy and ability to collaborate in problem solving and decision making.

The use of restraints with agitated clients involves physical invasion of intimate space and violation of body boundaries. Combativeness, disorganization, and aggressiveness when restraints are applied can be viewed as defenses against this invasion.

Nurses frequently care for clients whose inner space is in a state of upheaval. Levels of consciousness and overall functioning are an important concern with clients who are intoxicated, undergoing severe stress, or brain-damaged, and may determine when and how the nurse conveys information and describes expectations. Nurses need to recognize that information acquired during one state or level of consciousness may be recalled only partially, if at all, when there is a change to another level of consciousness. For example, clients who are intoxicated during their orientation to the hospital may remember very little of it when they become sober.

Time

Objective Time

Time may be considered in three ways: (1) as a continual flow; (2) as past, present, and future; and (3) as finite divisions, such as minutes, days, years, mornings, evenings, and nights.

A person's development of the concept of time is a gradual process.[47] Table 3-7 shows the development of the concept of time in young children. In young children, each day is its own universe and tomorrow is barely comprehensible.

Subjective Time

People develop an internal sense of time, which may or may not correspond with clock time. They respond to time structures that are often externally imposed. The clocks and calendars that govern lives in a highly technological society are designed for economic efficiency or convenience. These artificial measurements of time may not be based on any physiological clocks, and therefore they may violate basic physiological needs. The development of time sense is influenced by personal experiences within the family and society, and by physiochemical forces, conditioning, health problems, and use of drugs.

Table 3-7 Development of the Concept of Time in a Young Child

Age	Concept
18 months	Has little sense of time other than the present
2 years	Differentiates somewhat between simple time sequences in more or less the present
3 years	Understands the concepts of *bedtime* and *tomorrow* and that winter or a specific holiday happens every so often Has little sense of the duration of time such as an hour
4 years	Relates the sequence of events in a day to morning, afternoon, and evening Understands somewhat the cycles of the seasons Does not fully understand the idea of an hour's duration
5 years	Understands finer divisions of time, such as days and weeks

SOURCE: Adapted from D. P. Hymovich and R. W. Chamberlin, *Child and Family Development*, McGraw-Hill, New York, 1980.

FAMILY INFLUENCES. Children acquire time sense through family experiences that reflect cultural influences. Time sense and rhythm develop before language; thus, the learning is not overt and direct, but incidental and haphazard. Much of the learning of time sense probably comes from parents and role models. Daily living activities, such as eating, sleeping, and eliminating feces and urine, are made to conform to parents' work schedules, school schedules, and social demands rather than to the natural ebb and flow of internal rhythms. When eating and excretion are postponed time after time and when parents continually tell the child to "hurry up," he or she gradually becomes less sensitive to and less aware of internal rhythms.

CULTURAL INFLUENCES. Cultural attitudes affect the perception of time. Attitudes about time may also influence a society, but they are often unconscious and, therefore, unnoticed and unrecognized. For example, the Egyptians were preoccupied with the movements of the sun and the moon, and with an afterlife. These time orientations influenced their civilization, as their religious practices and the pyramids make clear. In an agrarian society, a calendar and the seasons are especially significant because they determine when crops are planted and harvested.[18]

The accelerating pace of technology in western society has resulted in an emphasis on efficiency and speed. A sense of urgency is pervasive. Phenomena as different as computers, rapid transit systems, microwave ovens, and fast-food chains all reflect a sense that time is scarce and valuable.

PHYSIOCHEMICAL INFLUENCES. The speed of transactions of neurons in the brain and body must be calibrated to the physical world and mediated by the way it is perceived. Thus, family and societal tempos influence an individual's physiochemical processes. The brain must respond at a certain rate to hear sounds of certain frequencies and to perceive light waves. The ability to perceive, integrate, and respond to moving phenomena is influenced by physiochemical processes that have, in turn, been modified by environmental influences.

As a person matures, the rate at which oxygen is consumed declines and metabolism slows. The higher metabolic rate of children suggests why time seems to move slowly for children, and the slower metabolic rate of adults suggests why time seems to pass more quickly for the elderly.

CONDITIONING INFLUENCES. When people awaken automatically at a preselected time, they may be responding to internal complex biological rhythms, or they may have programmed specific rhythms. Studies of animals suggest that time of day may become a conditioned stimulus.

Past events may "set" clocks in the nervous and endocrine systems as well as in other bodily systems. These past events may prove to be stressors that contribute to the development of health problems. In fact, symptoms may appear daily at the time when a trauma originally occurred, or annually on the date when it occurred. Apparently not only the mind but also the body can remember.

HEALTH PROBLEMS. People who suffer from psychoses experience various time distortions. The nervous system of depressed people tends to operate at an accelerated pace, which may explain why these clients often perceive clock time as much slower than real time. When people are physically ill, time distortion is common. If the metabolic rate and body temperature are elevated, 2 minutes of brain time can equal 1 minute of clock time. Brain time is moving faster than clock time, and the perception is that clock time is slow.[18]

INFLUENCES OF DRUGS. Drugs have been found to alter time sense. People under the influence of psychedelic drugs have felt that months of experience are compressed into a few hours. People under the influence of hallucinogenic and excitatory drugs such as LSD experience a sense of temporal contraction and spatial expansion—for example, they arrive early for appointments, and their signatures may be larger than usual. On the other hand, people under the influence of tranquilizers experience time expansion and space contraction. They will have a tendency to be late for appointments, and their signatures will appear cramped.[18]

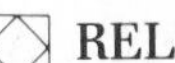

RELEVANCE TO NURSING

Because time is an abstract concept, its importance is often overlooked by nurses. When it is made operational, however, its significance in the caregiving process becomes obvious. When to give medications, perform treatments, teach clients and their families, and provide care and comfort should be part of any plan for meeting clients' needs.

Timing of Interventions

Institutions usually establish a fixed schedule for administering medications. For example, administrations of medications prescribed for three times a day (TID) in one institution may be scheduled for 7 A.M., 11 A.M., and 3 P.M., while in another institution they may be scheduled for 10 A.M., 2 P.M., and 6 P.M. Times for administering medicine may be influenced by nurses' shift schedules, or may be an arbitrary decision made by a hospital's administration. A more appropriate approach is to schedule interventions according to the client's biorhythm.

Research on biological rhythms has found that internal rhythms fluctuate within a 24-hour period, depending on whether the subjects are "day people" or "night people." Research has also shown that the time of day in which medication is administered influences its effectiveness and its side effects. For example, if the body's biological capacities are at a low ebb, drugs might be more potent than if capacities were high, but treatment would be less therapeutic.

Scheduling of surgical procedures and diagnostic tests also often fails to take clients' biological rhythms into consideration. A person who is at a low level of biological functioning may be at risk for an exaggerated response to anesthesia, or may be less able to respond to blood loss.

Clients may also be scheduled for various diagnostic tests and treatments with little regard for how the timing might influence the results or the client's toleration of the procedures. Research is needed to determine how timing effects results of diagnostic tests, efficacy of drug regimens, therapeutic effects of treatments, and toleration of surgical interventions. Hormones and other homeostatic physiological mechanisms fluctuate in a rhythmic way. Timing of the collection of blood and urine samples is important and influences the interpretation of findings from these diagnostic tests.[48]

Care and Comfort

Time is an important aspect of assessment. Determining when previous hospitalizations, health problems, symptoms, pain, and developmental milestones occurred provides significant information about a client. Also, people establish patterns for their daily activities. When nurses assess time schedules in relation to patterns of rising, sleeping, eating, and other activities, they are better able to provide individualized care and recognize deviations that may indicate problems. Some people are "morning people" who wake early and function optimally early in the day, and others are "night people" who sleep late and work best during the evening or night. When these people are hospitalized, institutional routines may be incongruent with their personal "timing." In the case of the "night person," nurses often in subtle ways enforce breakfast, bathing, ambulation in the early morning, and administration of bedtime medications hours before the client is ready. Nurses also may misinterpret a client's tendency to stay up late to watch television or read as an indication of sleep problems.

Clients who have elevated temperatures, are depressed, have certain health problems, or are receiving various medications may perceive clock time as being much longer than real time, because functioning of their nervous systems is accelerated. When these clients use the call light for a nurse, they will perceive the response as taking longer than usual. Knowing this, nurses need to respond more quickly when these clients make requests. Making these clients wait may escalate their fear, anxiety, and dependency, generate regression, and interfere with therapeutic rest.

A Sense of Urgency

Many clients, because of their physical condition, age, or situation, move slowly. Nurses on busy, short-staffed units are hurried and harried; their work load may demand careful planning and leave no room for unnecessary delays. Unfortunately, they may communicate this time pressure to clients. Clients who are fearful, anxious, or depressed will be reluctant to share their feelings with nurses who appear rushed or who complain about their overloaded work schedule. These clients may decide not to bother a nurse, and they may continue to live with their discomfort. Thus, sensitive, empathic care includes communicating the fact that time to talk is available. Repositioning and ambulating some clients may be time-consuming; however, if nurses communicate a sense of urgency, they may increase the clients' discomfort and anxiety.

Many people tend to slow their pace of living, their speech, and their performance of various activities as they grow older. Their stability may also be impaired by vision problems or changes in joint function, and they may prefer to walk more slowly. Nurses need to pace their speech and movements to be congruent with those of an elderly client.

Young children are not "clock watchers" and are easily distracted. By adult standards they often seem to dawdle when they dress or feed themselves. Physically and emotionally handicapped children may proceed at even a slower pace than well children. Nurses who wish to foster independence and competence in young clients need to recognize that a sense of urgency and impatience will interfere with this goal.

EMOTIONS

The words *feelings* and *emotions* tend to be used interchangeably, but they are separate and distinct concepts. *Feelings* are a background emotional coloring—a tone of pleasantness or unpleasantness in relation to something in the environment. They are transitory responses to sensations and perceptions. *Emotions* are attitudes toward a social environment which have a definite beginning and which run a characteristic course. They are defined affective inner experiences and attitudes toward persons and social situations. Anger, fear, joy, and disgust are examples of attitudinally derived emotions. They are inner experiences expressed through speech, posture, and symbolic gestures.[49]

A person's interpretation of a situation determines the emotion to be experienced and the expression of that emotion.[50] If an appraisal is inaccurate because it is based on false or irrational beliefs, or if it is derived from the past and based on unconscious material, the corresponding emotion may be inappropriate to the current situation.[49]

Emotions are influenced by culture. Culture prescribes emotions and emotional responses that conform to certain standards, limits types of responses and their expressions, and determines the appropriateness and acceptability of responses in specific situations.[50]

In addition to their cognitive and cultural aspects emotions also have a moral aspect. Many emotions are connected to, and may be congruent or in conflict with, moral principles; and emotions may be viewed as virtues (such as love, joy, and peace) or vices (such as envy, jealousy, and lust). Since emotions have a moral dimension, they may generate ethical issues. People are generally assumed to be responsible for their own emotions; but if a client chooses to maintain dysfunctional emotional patterns, is the nurse then responsible for attempting to alter them? For example, do nursing interventions that facilitate development of benevolence and the avoidance of another emotion, such as envy, present an ethical or moral dilemma?

Emotions and feelings are personal experiences which influence interactions with the environment. They have a biopsychosocial dimension. They reflect the holistic nature of the person. Some common emotions are defined, and examples of each are given, in Table 3-8. In this chapter, three emotions have been selected for examination and discussion: anxiety, grief, and loneliness. Each is a source of distress and may affect whether growth or dysfunction occurs in a nurse or a client.

Table 3-8 Definitions and Examples of Emotions

Emotion and Definition	Example
Anger: Burst of energy in reaction to an insult to one's sense of self, including one's values.	A well-meaning friend told Mary, "I think you choose men who turn out to be inconsiderate and unfeeling." Mary responded in anger, "That is not true, and you have no right to say such a thing."
Bitterness: A dispiriting emotion that pollutes and destroys everything it affects.	Bitterness first rose up in Michael when his father said Michael would never amount to anything. The bitterness distorted his relationships with other men, including his employer; people did not want to be Michael's friend because anything he did and said seemed poisoned.
Faith: Focus on things that are hoped for but have not yet become reality.	Debi and Michael's son didn't come home from school one day. He is now listed as a missing child. Debi and Michael believe that their son is alive and that he will be found and returned to them.
Fear: Respect for the power of another. Healthy fear allows constructive interaction with the powerful one; unhealthy fear compromises clear thinking, intelligent action, and assertive interaction.	Joann has recently begun to work in an intensive-care unit. The head nurse is a clinical nurse specialist with a master's degree who has an excellent professional reputation. Joann has a healthy fear of her new employer, and has developed an excellent working relationship with her.
Frustration: Buildup of energy which was to have been used to pursue a purpose or objective and which has been blocked.	Kevin had always wanted to be a professional baseball pitcher. He was ready to sign a contract with a professional team when he tore a shoulder ligament and dislocated his shoulder in an automobile accident. Kevin's nurse had difficulty communicating with him because he was hostile and sometimes emotionally explosive. Kevin was certain that he would never play baseball professionally, and he could not imagine what else he might do with his life.
Gentleness: Touching another, physically or emotionally, without invading that person's boundaries.	The clients at St. Alphonso Nursing Home love Joy, the RN in charge during the nights, because she is so gentle. You can overhear the clients talking about her. "She never startles me when she comes into the room." "When she rubs my back, all the tension pours out of me." "I feel that it's all right to be a little out of sorts; Joy gives me space, but doesn't let me stay off by myself."
Guilt: Sense of sin or wrongdoing against oneself or another.	While on a business trip, Mary met a very nice man and had sex with him. She felt guilty later, having broken faith with her husband and violated her own sense of right and wrong.

(Continued.)

Table 3-8 Continued

Emotion and Definition	Example	Emotion and Definition	Example
Helplessness: Inability to act effectively under compelling circumstances.	Nicole simply didn't know what to do to stop her friend and classmate, Anne, from abusing drugs. Both were juniors in the baccalaureate nursing program, studying hard, working part time, and concerned about their grades. Anne was taking "uppers" and "downers" in increasing quantities to handle the stress. Nicole had talked, warned, cajoled, and threatened, but Anne would not listen.	**Peace:** Prevailing calm that continues in spite of difficult circumstances.	Barbara was dying of cancer. She was surrounded by her children, and good friends came and went, bringing food and saying good-bye. Barbara had taken care of her business affairs, had reconciled all the loose ends of her life, had a strong belief in God, and felt ready to die. She was at peace with herself, her family, friends, and God.
Joy: Sense of fulfillment that strengthens and energizes.	Mark had successfully coached his wife through labor. The first moment he saw his baby daughter, he burst into tears and began laughing. "She's beautiful," he whispered as he held his daughter to his wife's breast to nurse.	**Rage:** Engulfing experience of destroying and being destroyed.	Missy had teased her brother Scott unmercifully about his new girlfriend, Kathy. He had determined he would not fight with Missy, but she knew all his vulnerable areas. He managed to get out of the room without fighting, but when he got to his bedroom, he was shaking with rage. He hit the wall with his fist and smashed through the plaster.
Love: Giving oneself to another unconditionally, without demanding anything in return.	The troop had been shelled by the enemy, and Jim couldn't find John in the scramble of the retreat. Though his life was in danger, Jim went back to find his friend.	**Temperance:** Disciplined balance of all aspects of one's person and lifestyle.	Marsha, committed to pursuing health as a personal goal, chose to maintain her weight, exercise daily, abstain from drugs and alcohol, and nurture her relationships with God, family, and friends.
Patience: Giving oneself and others the time, space, and nurturance needed for growth.	For 3 weeks Jason sat quietly next to Hannah for 5 minutes each shift. Gradually, Hannah became more comfortable. One day, Hannah spoke to Jason and said, "I thought you would go away. Why didn't you?"		

Anxiety*

Although anxiety is a universal experience and is characterized by uneasiness and tension, there is little agreement on what, exactly, constitutes anxiety and even less agreement on how it can be measured, explained, or predicted.

Anxiety is defined as apprehension which develops when there is a threat to some value considered essential to the personality.[51] It is an actual or symbolic signal of danger—to self-respect or to the respect of significant others, even if the others are only idealized figures from childhood.[52]

A person experiencing anxiety often is not aware of its causes. In fact, the person may not even recognize the anxiety or the role that it plays in influencing behavior.

The Experience of Anxiety

Anxiety, fear, excitement, tenseness, and stress appear to be a part of a broad attention-appraisal-response system. A threatening situation sets in motion a series of physiological mechanisms that produce physical manifestations (symptoms) and psychological states. Whether the source of the threat is a commonly recognized external danger or an event perceived as dangerous only by the person, the physiological changes that occur and the emotional state that is experienced are approximately the same. The cerebral cortex, the hypothalamus, and the endocrine, cardiovascular, and

* Portions of this section were taken from S.S. Jimerson, "Anxiety," in the second edition of this book.

autonomic nervous systems are activated. The fight-flight response that occurs is the same for fear and anxiety.

Physiological manifestations that occur with a temporary attack of *acute anxiety* or state anxiety, and a fear response include the following: palpitations, tremulousness, diaphoresis, hyperventilation causing paresthesias of the lips and fingers, carpopedal spasms, diarrhea, frequent urination, nausea, faintness, dizziness, dilation of the pupils, flushing of the skin, excessive facial and palmar sweating, shortness of breath, and tightness in the throat. Unpleasant subjective feelings associated with an anxiety-producing or fear-producing threat are helplessness, dread, apprehension, or a sense of impending disaster. People also experience a sense that sudden death, insanity, disorientation, or the urge to commit an aggressive or destructive act is imminently possible. Restlessness, lack of self-confidence, and difficulty in concentrating also occur.

In contrast, the person with *chronic anxiety*, which reflects a high level of trait anxiety (see Table 3-9), not only experiences unremitting episodes of acute anxiety that are frequent and prolonged, but also complains of insomnia, nightmares, back pain, headaches, and weakness.

Types of Anxiety

There are several types of anxiety: *trait, state, process, signal,* and *free-floating*. Table 3-9 gives the definition and an example of each.

Intensity of Anxiety

Anxiety can also be defined in terms of its intensity. Anxiety-producing experiences can range from mild disturbances to acute states of panic.[53] The ability to perceive, function, learn, solve problems, and make decisions becomes increasingly difficult as the degree of anxiety increases. Levels of anxiety and their influence on the person are presented in Table 3-10 (page 54).

Sources of Anxiety

There are various sources of anxiety. Genetic and biochemical factors, behavioral factors, and threats to biological integrity and self-concept have been associated with anxiety and anxiety-proneness.

Recent studies of twins provide direct support for the theory that there is a genetic predisposition to anxiety. Biochemical studies have found that people suffering from metabolic alkalosis may be prone to having anxiety attacks.

Behavioral and learning theorists propose a relationship between anxiety and physiological needs: anxiety generates a physiological state of arousal that demands resolution. Reinforcers condition the person to expect and respond to situational cues. The person learns which physiological, physical, emotional, and social responses can produce and increase anxiety and how to reduce or resolve anxiety.

A threat to biological integrity is some form of interference with the satisfaction of hunger, thirst,

Table 3-9 Types of Anxiety

Type	Definition	Example
Trait	Anxiety which exists as part of the personality over a long period of time; it can be measured.	A person becomes anxious in situations that do not make others anxious.
State	Anxiety elicited by stressful situations over which people feel no control; it can be measured.	A woman undergoes stress after receiving a call from the local hospital informing her that her husband has had a myocardial infarction.
Process	Anxiety in the form of a complex sequence of cognitive, affective, and behavioral patterns occurring in relation to some form of stress.	A student who has just been assigned to care for his first client becomes anxious when actually performing the research and formulating the care plan.
Signal	Anxiety elicited by an anticipated event similar to an earlier, unresolved, possibly forgotten traumatic event.	A mother becomes anxious at the thought of toilet-training her second child after having had a very difficult time toilet training her oldest child.
Free-floating	Anxiety which is ever-present and accompanied by feelings of dread; it is associated with ritualistic and avoidance behavior.	An adolescent girl constantly fears that she will be robbed while walking in public.

Table 3-10 Intensity of Anxiety, Associated Operations, and Learning Tasks

Intensity of Anxiety	Operations	Variations in the Form of Operation	Learning Tasks of the Anxious Person
Mild anxiety	Alertness	Noises seem louder. Restlessness. Irritability.	Recognition of anxiety as a warning sign that something is not going as expected. This can be done by: 1. Observing what goes on 2. Describing what was observed 3. Analyzing what was expected 4. Analyzing how expectations and results in the event differed 5. Formulating what can be done about the situation in terms of changing the situation or changing expectations 6. Validating with others
Moderate anxiety	Reduced ability to perceive and communicate; increased tension	Concentration on a problem. Someone talking may not be heard. Part of the room may not be noticed. Muscular tension, pounding heart, perspiration, gastric discomfort.	Recognition that in moderate and severe anxiety the focus is reduced and connections between details may not be seen; also that anxiety provides energy which can be reduced to mild anxiety and then used to find out what went wrong.
Severe anxiety	Only details are perceived; physical discomfort; emotional discomfort	Connections between details are not seen. Headaches, nausea, trembling, dizziness. Awe, dread, loathing, horror.	Moderate to severe anxiety may be reduced by: 1. Working at a simple, concrete task 2. Talking to someone who can listen 3. Playing a simple game 4. Walking 5. Crying
Panic	A perceived detail is elaborated and blown up.	Inability to communicate or function.	The person experiencing panic needs help in getting more comfortable. (In this stage learning cannot be expected to take place.)

SOURCE: Dorothea R. Hays, "Teaching a Concept of Anxiety to Patients," *Nursing Research*, vol. 10, Spring 1961, pp. 108–113.

warmth, or sexual needs. Threats to self-concept include actual or anticipated disapproval from a significant person; unfulfillment of one's own expectations; and insufficient respect and self-esteem.[54]

Fear and Anxiety

Theorists in the past have made a distinction between fear and anxiety, but such a distinction may be somewhat arbitrary in the light of recent psychophysiological research findings. *Fear* has been defined as a reaction to a known, specific danger that lies outside the person. In contrast, *anxiety* has been defined as a reaction to a perceived threat in which the real source of danger is unknown. Fear and anxiety tend to occur together, and in most instances they cannot be differentiated by the person who is experiencing the emotional state, by an objective observer, or by measurements of their physiological manifestations.

Anxiety and fear are now thought to form a continuum. Anxiety, at one end of the continuum, is a generalized, unfocused uncomfortable feeling of unknown origin; fear, at the other end, is a specific, focused feeling of known origin; and there are many gradations between them.

Functional Aspects of Anxiety

Anxiety is necessary for survival because it motivates people to make necessary changes in the environment. The major motivation created by anxiety is to rid the self of the discomfort associated with it—the queasy stomach, the jitteriness, the hollow feeling in the chest; and the feelings of threatened self-esteem, hopelessness, isolation, loneliness, insecurity, and overall lack of identity. Anxiety plays an important role in our daily experiences and in our ability to grow as individuals. Belief in one's ability to survive is strengthened and meaning is given to one's life when one succeeds in constructively overcoming anxiety-producing situations. Thus, a little anxiety is necessary and desirable. "Healthy anxiety" provides the energy needed to get on with life's tasks.

Defense Mechanisms

When anxiety is not "healthy" but is perceived as a threat, dysfunctional behavior may develop as people attempt to distance themselves from it through avoidance, denial, projection, and somatization. These mechanisms may work for a time. However, unwillingness to experience anxiety creates a situation somewhat like a pressure cooker with a clogged steam valve: sooner or later, the pressure will build up and steam will escape, even if it must do so in unusual ways or by exploding the top off the cooker. Anxiety that is not accepted can create a variety of dysfunctional symptoms ranging from minor physical problems to major psychotic illnesses or death. Figure 3-4 indicates functional and dysfunctional behaviors that are associated with anxiety.

Anxiety is the response of the ego to unconscious, threatening material that may emerge into consciousness. Because anxiety is such an unpleasant experience, people defend against it with several built-in mechanisms. The defense mechanisms outlined in Table 3-11 (page 56) keep threatening material repressed. Different defense mechanisms are used at various developmental stages, and different threats are experienced at each age.[55] Table 3-12 presents these.

RELEVANCE TO NURSING

The educational preparation of nurses is intellectually, physically, and emotionally demanding. Mastery of both the theoretical base for practice and the performance of the required technical skills is stressful and produces varying degrees of anxiety. Clinical application of what is learned is also stressful. The student must integrate, synthesize, and apply knowledge and skill to the care of people who often have complex, life-threatening health problems. The responsibility is often experienced as awesome. Errors may be perceived by the student and instructor as endangering a client's life and well-being.

In psychiatric settings, students may be confronted by clients who are out of control, and they may be disturbed when they encounter clients who resemble themselves or significant others. People who display these symptoms elicit fear and anxiety, particularly in novices.

People hospitalized for serious medical problems, surgery, or emotional disturbances are anxious and fearful. These feelings can easily be communicated to their families and care givers. The intimacy of the nurse-client relationship increases

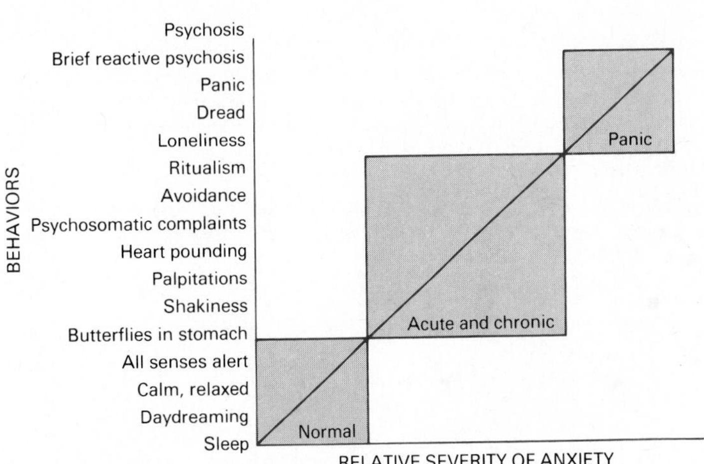

Figure 3-4 Functional and dysfunctional behaviors associated with anxiety.

Table 3-11 Ego Defense Mechanisms

Defense Mechanism	Example
Repression: A widely used unconscious mechanism. Painful experiences, disagreeable memories, unacceptable thoughts and impulses are barred from consciousness. Selfish, hostile, and sexual impulses are usually repressed. It takes a constant expenditure of energy to keep repressed material out of awareness. Consequently, less energy is available for constructive activity.	Mrs. S. does not remember having spent 6 months in a body cast at age 7. Mr. Z. does not remember having sexually exposed himself on a subway train.
Regression: The ego returns to an earlier stage of development in thought, feeling, or behavior. Regression is a normal component of our developmental sequence and appears transiently during times of stress when it is utilized as a retreat from anxiety and conflict. It becomes problematic when used as the primary defense, when the person fixates at an earlier level, or when the behavior immobilizes the person.	Mr. B., an adult, has temper tantrums (child behavior) when frustrated. Tim, a 4-year-old, is confronted with the birth of a new sister. He is toilet-trained and articulate but responds to the birth of the new baby by regressing to nighttime bed-wetting, daytime soiling, and baby talk. This stems from his effort to regain his old unchallenged position with his mother.
Identification: A person becomes like something or someone else in one or several aspects of thought or behavior. This contributes to ego development but does not replace the person's own ego. The personality consists of multiple identifications that have been tested for their ability to reduce anxiety.	Ms. Thomas, who is studying nursing, includes the assertiveness she admires in one of her nursing instructors.
Introjection: A form of identification which is a symbolic taking in or incorporation of a loved or hated object or person into the individual's own ego structure. Introjection is important in the development of the superego when the child incorporates the parents' instructions, rewards, and punishments.	Paul, a 5-year-old boy, tells his 2-year-old brother, "Look both ways when you cross the street." Paul has introjected the person who told him how to cross the street. Mr. K., a young man whose father has recently died, begins to talk and act like the father.
Reaction formation: Occurs when an individual consciously expresses feelings and wishes that are directly opposite to unconscious feelings and wishes.	Mr. J. has unconscious feelings of hate and anger toward his boss; he is excessively polite, believing he feels affection. Jane, a teenager, has an unconscious desire to be dependent and taken care of; this is masked by her excessively independent behavior.
Undoing: Closely related to reaction formation. A person negates an act by behavior which is the opposite of what was done before.	Ms. M. crosses her fingers while telling a lie. Peter, who just told his mother he hates her, now hugs and kisses her.
Isolation: The exclusion from awareness of the feelings connected to a thought, memory, or experience. The person remembers the experience or thought but does not reexperience the emotion that originally accompanied it.	Mrs. James, an obsessive client, relates her repeated thoughts of having thrown her baby out of the window. As the woman speaks, she conveys no affective response to the content of this frightening thought.
Displacement: The discharge of emotions, feelings, or ideas upon a subject other than the one to which the feelings rightly belong. This is a security operation in which the feelings are discharged away from the actual source of the emotion because it is not considered safe to express them directly.	Mrs. Green has had a difficult day at the office. A project she had worked hard on was rejected by her boss. When she comes home from work, she begins yelling at her husband and children, displacing onto her family the anger felt toward the boss.
Projection: The attribution of one's feelings, impulses, thoughts, and wishes to others or the environment in an effort to deny their existence in the self. Projection is used in a wide variety of normal situations. It is used excessively by clients with paranoid thought patterns.	David, a freshman, has failed an exam. He blames the instructor for having made a poor choice of questions on the exam. He projects his poor performance onto the instructor. Miss K., a suspicious client, projects hostile, aggressive feelings that are part of herself onto others when stating, "I can't eat; the food is poisoned," and "I can't go to sleep; they're just waiting to kill me." She really wishes to kill herself but has projected this wish onto others.

(Continued.)

Table 3-11 Continued

Defense Mechanism	Example
Rationalization: A coping mechanism that is universally employed. It is an attempt to make one's behavior appear to be the result of logical thinking rather than of unconscious impulses or desires. It is utilized when a person has a sense of guilt or uncertainty about something that has been done. It is a face-saving device that may or may not deal with the truth. It temporarily relieves anxiety.	Ms. S., a sophomore, fails a course and says the teacher was ineffective. Mr. W. has no friends; he says people do not appreciate his efforts at friendship. Miss B. says she wants to get married but has trouble dating. Every time she goes out with a man, she refuses a second date, saying, "He's not my intellectual equal." In doing this she is probably rationalizing deep fears of sexuality.
Denial: The total failure to acknowledge the existence of an affect, experience, idea, or memory. The person simply pretends that what is painful, anxiety-provoking, or threatening does not exist.	Mr. L., who has cancer, is told that he is terminally ill and has approximately 1 month to live. Later in the day, the nurse hears him talking to his travel agent. He is planning a trip to Europe next summer.
Substitution: The replacement of a highly valued, unacceptable object with a less valued one which is acceptable.	Mr. E. wants to marry Miss L., probably because she looks quite a bit like his mother.
Sublimation: Transformation of psychic energy associated with unwanted sexual or aggressive drives into socially acceptable pursuits. The activity or its object is changed, and the energy is discharged.	After Bobby's father forbade him to use the family car, Bobby spent 30 minutes punching a punching bag. Eleanor's boyfriend has left her to pursue a career as a rock musician. Now she spends much of her time writing love poems.

SOURCE: From P. P. Hoskins, "Theoretical Models," in the second edition of this book.

Table 3-12 Developmental Processes, Attendant Dangers, Fears, and Defenses

Developmental Stage	Danger Situations	Fears	Defenses
Oral: trust versus mistrust (birth to 2 years)	Satisfaction of basic physical and psychological needs Separation	Physiological distress Fear of losing a love object	Denial
Anal: autonomy versus shame and doubt (2–3½ years)	Separation Individuation	Fear of losing a love object	Introjection Displacement Substitution Reaction formation
Oedipal: initiative versus guilt (3½–6 years)	Establishing autonomy	Fear of body damage	
Latency: industry versus inferiority (6 years and older)	Development of superego	Fear of disapproval by superego	Undoing Isolation Sublimation Rationalization Dissociation

SOURCE: Adapted from L. B. Silver, "Recognition of Anxiety in Children and Adolescents," in W. E. Fann et al., *Phenomenology and Treatment of Anxiety*, S. P. Medical and Scientific Books, New York, 1979, pp. 104–105.

nurses' vulnerability to this anxiety. If nurses do not know how this anxiety is transmitted or what effects it can have on the therapeutic relationship, they may either unconsciously avoid anxious clients or introduce their own anxiety and thus aggravate the situation.

High levels of anxiety interfere with the nurse's sensitivity and proficiency in providing care. Nurses need to recognize and manage their own anxiety. Their personal growth and the quality of the care they provide depend in part on how effectively they manage their own anxiety.

Regression and increased dependency occur at high levels of anxiety and interfere with the ability to cope with stressful life events. To cope with stress, people need to engage in effective "worry work." For example, education is an important intervention that helps clients to manage anxiety related to childbirth, surgery, intrusive diagnostic procedures, and treatment regimens. Learning is enhanced when the client's anxiety is maintained at a mild level.

Nurses who work in primary health care settings and emergency rooms encounter clients in severe distress. Physical, psychological, and social assessment that provides opportunities for clients to describe their symptoms and life circumstances assist the nurse in recognizing and diagnosing acute anxiety. Health screening in primary care settings also needs to include the identification of covert anxiety that may be a contributing factor in the development of health problems.

Promotion and maintenance of health are primary concerns of nursing. Anticipatory guidance, education, and ventilation of feelings are significant ways nurses can help people prevent or manage problematic anxiety so that these goals can be achieved. From early childhood, developmental experiences influence people's general level of anxiety (trait anxiety) as well as their response to anxiety-producing situations (state anxiety); therefore, parent education and counseling are important nursing activities.

Chronic anxiety produces a variety of symptoms that interfere with personal relationships, work, and productivity, and may make it impossible to enjoy life. It is also a contributing factor in the development of health problems, absenteeism, and accident-proneness. Early identification and intervention promotes health and well-being.

Effective management of anxiety is an important nursing activity in promoting or restoring health, preventing disease, and facilitating a peaceful, dignified death. Nurses therefore need to develop and use interpersonal skills to help clients recognize their anxiety, maintain it at manageable levels, and use it to learn functional patterns or modify dysfunctional patterns.

Grief

Grief is a biopsychosocial response to the loss of a valued person, place, or thing—a love object. The value ascribed to the lost object is derived from what Freud called *cathecting*—the investment of emotional energy.[56] People invest emotional energy in other people (such as family members, friends, authority figures, and idols), roles, their own bodies, and places and things.

Significant others may contribute to satisfaction of needs, or they may represent an ideal; security, love, belonging, self-esteem, and recognition may be found in the relationship. If a significant person is lost, a mourning or grieving process is initiated.[56]

Energy may also be heavily invested in a role or career, which represents a considerable portion of one's identity and a major source of need satisfaction. The role or career becomes, in effect, a significant love object; and its loss evokes a grieving process. For example, an executive who is retired, a worker who is laid off, and a mother whose last child leaves home will each lose a role, a career, and a significant love object.[57]

One may also invest emotional energy in body parts and in one's appearance. The genitals, breasts, and limbs are (for obvious reasons) usually highly valued. Loss of an important body part through amputation, mutilative surgery, or disfigurement therefore elicits grief—mourning for the lost body part, the functions it performed, and the needs that were satisfied and the pleasures experienced when the body was intact.[57]

Places, and things—pets, a home or a neighborhood, cherished possessions—may also be highly valued or cathected. The death of a pet, a fire that destroys one's home, having to leave one's neighborhood, and even the loss of an heirloom can evoke grief.[57]

The devastating effects of loss are well known. For example, loss of a significant member creates a shock wave throughout an extended family and may produce illness in those who are especially vulnerable. There is even a correlation between a significant loss and sudden or premature death among the survivors.[58] Psychiatric illness has also been related to separation and loss. Stein and Susser, for instance, found that the percentage of bereaved spouses seeking psychiatric care for the first time is higher than would be expected.[59]

Loss of a spouse, particularly, seems to increase the risk of somatic, psychosomatic, and psychological illness, or even death, probably because of the emotional turmoil and social disruption associated with such a loss. The relationship between onset of illness and loss or separation has been studied by many researchers. In one study, 38 percent of the subjects—widows under age 60—reported a marked deterioration of health following the death of their husbands; and it has been found that widows in all age groups have a higher incidence of cancer than women who are married or single. A study of 150 women who applied for divorce reported that most had experienced a deterioration of health.[60]

Mourning

Mourning is the process of resolving grief. It occurs as a gradual process of "letting go" of the lost object, withdrawing emotional energy from it, and becoming able to invest energy in new relationships.

Upon experiencing a loss, a person immediately responds with shock and disbelief. This may be a transitory experience if the loss was anticipated. However, if the loss was unexpected, a longer time may be needed before the person develops awareness. Initially, the need to deny a loss is great. But denial is a primitive defense that cannot withstand reality very long; and as reality is recognized and accepted, there is a flood of conflicting feelings and emotions. At this point, symptoms of acute grief develop, and anger and resentment will be felt toward anyone who encourages acceptance of the loss. The emotional response is intense: reproaches, anger, and crying are characteristic. Other characteristics of this phase are yearning for and preoccupation with the lost object, a focus on situations associated with it, and a tendency to respond to any stimulus that suggests it.

During mourning, preoccupation with the lost object and memories of it may be particularly vivid. Rees[60] proposed that visual, auditory, and tactile hallucinations at this time can be considered normal. Guilt may also be felt over omissions that are perceived to have occurred. If the lost person had a terminal disease, the survivors may feel guilty for not having recognized the symptoms sooner and not having acted more assertively in seeking help. Even if a physician was consulted as soon as symptoms appeared, mourners may wonder whether they ignored or denied earlier evidence. Such guilt seems irrational to outsiders, but it is very real to the mourners, who will seek reassurance that they have not been neglectful or caused harm.

During the early stages of the grieving process, many people experience such intense and pervasive emotions that they become concerned for their own sanity. The acute symptoms of grief generally last from 4 to 8 weeks. However, new situations and anniversaries of the loss may reevoke such intense feelings that somatic symptoms reappear.[60] Yearning and protest tend to reach a peak during the second to fourth week and then gradually decrease.

According to Bowlby,[61] as the mourning process progresses, despair is felt. It is characterized by disorganization of the personality, apathy, aimlessness, and emotional pain, and it seems to be elicited by a gradual recognition of the reality of the loss. That is, when hope of reunion or recovery is surrendered, disorganization results. During this phase, restlessness, anxiety, depression, and symptoms of acute grief are common; and Parkes[62] has reported that panic is likely to be felt during the first month after a loss. Inability to accept reality may recur periodically. Some degree of toleration of all this disorganization and emotional pain is needed to bring about an eventual resolution of grief.[61]

After a period of time, detachment occurs. This is a phase of reorganization, withdrawing (decathecting), and investment of energy in new objects. Although a purpose in life and a future orientation may not return for a year (a fact which suggests that there is some lingering hope for reunion or recovery), thoughts about the lost object change gradually from a state of great intensity to one that is more balanced and allows other thoughts and interests.[61]

"Letting go" is a slow process of looking at and relinquishing one memory at a time. It requires an emotionally painful review of memories. In the beginning, the desire for reunion is acute and clearly recognized. But over time, if the process of "letting go" is proceeding, that desire diminishes. Emotional energy that is being decathected from the lost object can then be reinvested in new relationships.

"Quests"

During the phase of letting go, the desire for reunion and its accompanying fantasies become secretive "quests." Such a quest often remains unconscious, because it conflicts with what is known to be rational and true; it may be seen as disloyal and thus may jeopardize other relationships; and it may generate intolerable pain, loneliness, and longing. "Magical thinking" is an aspect of the quest; it reflects the regression that occurs with a significant loss. Quests can also be conscious, as in the case of adopted people seeking information about their biological parents.[63]

A quest is, in a sense, a precursor of grief. It helps to defend against the deeper emotion that comes with recognizing that a loss is final. But although it can be characterized by vitality and creativity, it may also be stagnatingly rigid and self-destructive. Expressions of the quest include searching; remembering and daydreaming; recreating painful feelings; using magical gestures and thoughts; feeling "presence"; using transitional objects; contemplating suicide, and denying the loss.[63]

SEARCHING. Unconscious searching takes many forms. Restless activity which may seem purposeless is an unconscious quest. In a young child, the search for the lost parent may be conscious and concrete; the child will actually look for the parent room by room. In an older child, the quest may be expressed unconsciously through stealing or other forbidden experiences. Older children and adolescents may turn to the external environment for instant gratification because dealing with their inner feelings is too painful. However, since a stolen object or forbidden experience fails to produce reunion, disillusionment sets in.[63]

In adults, motor restlessness and a frenetic search for something to do combined with an inability to initiate and maintain normal patterns of activity are characteristics of unconscious searching. Once the meaning of such behavior becomes conscious, it tends to lessen or stop, and the person is able to begin dealing with the loss and working it through.[63]

REMEMBERING AND DAYDREAMING. Remembering a lost person is a form of searching. It can occur as mental images of the lost person and shared experiences, or as recreations of bodily sensations. When children experience a loss before they have developed the capacity to hold on to and recall a mental image (object constancy) and the loss is a severe deprivation, then bodily sensations associated with it become the memory. For such children, remembering becomes an attempt to recreate physical sensations, even when they have grown up. For example, if the physical sensation associated with a loss is tactile, searching for the lost object will take the form of attempting to experience the tactile sensation again.

The developmental capacity to evoke a memory helps adults and children deal constructively with loss. Daydreams may be the first mental activity directed toward remembering.[63] The effective use of memories is enhanced when there is a sharing of recollections. Sharing with a custodial or surviving parent, or with other family members and friends, within a context in which the lost person has participated, evokes memories. Remembering can be conveyed by words, feelings, and descriptions of events and examined in a supportive relationship, thus helping to resolve the loss.[61]

RECREATION OF PAINFUL FEELINGS. Painful feelings associated with a loss may also be recreated as a way of searching for or getting in touch with the lost person. Children of divorced parents and those whose parents have died may use painful experiences as a form of quest. Children and adults often seek out situations and relationships that evoke painful feelings, unconsciously seeking a reunion with the lost person; but since a reunion is impossible, these situations and relationships are disappointing and regenerate feelings of rejection. If a loss occurs during childhood, the pattern of recreating the emotional pain associated with the loss may not emerge until young adulthood, when entering into relationships with others may have the unconscious purpose of recreating the lost relationship and its associated feelings. But the other person in these relationships is not the lost person; disappointment and frustration develop, the relationship is broken, and emotional pain is experienced again.

MAGICAL GESTURES AND THOUGHTS. Magical gestures and thoughts are forms of searching that involve some activity previously associated with the appearance of the lost person. These gestures and thoughts are used in the belief (conscious or unconscious) that they will produce a reunion.[61] (For example, a husband came home every evening while his wife was watching a certain television show. After his death, the wife insisted on watching the show every evening because she believed in some way that if she watched the show, the husband would return.) Magical activities inevitably lead to disappointment, of course. The growing capacity to deal with reality diminishes their perceived power and makes their repetition less and less likely.

"PRESENCE." The feeling that a lost person is present or seen in a crowd for a fleeting moment is commonly reported by people who are grieving. This phenomenon occurs more often when the lost person has died than when he or she is absent but still alive. Apparently, long-buried memories are revitalized after a loss; people in crowds become dreamlike figures that are neither hallucinations nor illusions but projections of memories.[61]

TRANSITIONAL OBJECTS. *Transitional objects* are things that form bridges between the self and the external world. A loss may lead to a "magical" dependence on some treasured object which has survived regardless of feelings, behaviors, or intentions toward it. Magical thinking is necessary for such an attachment to a transitional object.[61]

Following a significant loss, a person may become attached to an object or animal. The family pet or a good-luck charm may take on special significance. The presence of this object may be required at all times as a source of comfort and pleasure. The transitional object becomes part of the quest for reunion.[61]

SUICIDE. When attempts at reunion involve a renunciation of the self, an identification with the dead, lost person, or an internalization of hostility, the quest becomes self-destructive. The desire for reunion is reinforced by an unsatisfactory environment and by hopelessness. In such a situation there is a risk of suicide. A connection—conscious or unconscious—may be made between death and peaceful sleep, so that death comes to mean a merger or fusion—the wished-for reunion—with the lost person.[61]

In some instances, self-destructiveness is derived from a desire to be rid of a hated or devalued aspect of the lost person that has been incorporated into the self. An unsupportive environment or an identification with a hated aspect of a lost person increases the risk of suicide. Poorly developed self-boundaries also predispose people to self-destructive thoughts and behaviors.[61]

DENIAL. Outright denial of a loss occurs most frequently among young children. Older children, adolescents, and adults may protect the self from full recognition of a loss by screening the memory with stories involving wish fulfillment. These stories cover up painful reality.[63]

Children may be accused of lying when they use such stories to alter reality. Children whose parents are divorced and children who live with foster families may develop "dual truths" about their parents. Children who have lost a parent and experienced family disruption may lie to protect their inner selves and to handle contradictory knowledge about the lost parent.[64] Their lies cover up the truth and appear both to protect the child's inner integrity and to reproach the lost parent for being somehow untruthful.[63]

The mourning process, particularly in response to the loss of a significant other, extends for at least 1 year. This time frame provides the mourner with opportunities to experience the absence of the lost person during significant holidays, anniversaries, birthdays, and family gatherings. Each of these, as well as other events throughout the year, generates painful memories that must be reviewed before emotional investment can be withdrawn. As time passes, emotional pain decreases, even if only a little.

Sociocultural and Religious Influences on Grief

Grief and mourning are universal responses to loss and separation. Behavioral expressions of grief vary among cultures, but psychological reactions to loss are similar. Public tears, weeping, and wailing are culturally prescribed. Institutionalized mourning ceremonies also differ among societies, but these ceremonies always provide support to the survivors.

Roman Catholicism and Judaism have ceremonies that identify the relationship between the first year's anniversary of the loss and the end of the grieving process. Anniversary masses and the removal of the widow's veil are examples of social rituals and customs that help people to reflect on their losses and to redirect their energies toward the future.

Anticipatory Grief

Anticipatory grief is any grief which occurs before an actual loss. When there is a threat that a significant object will be lost, people frequently initiate the grieving process before the loss actually occurs. This anticipatory grief allows for a gradual recognition of the loss and resolution of the associated feelings. But problems arise when withdrawal and disengagement occur prematurely. Dying people will feel lonely and isolated if family members begin to withdraw and disengage psychologically from them. Clearly, such a situation will increase the emotional pain associated with imminent death. Moreover, anticipatory grieving may allow ambivalence to be expressed, so that hostile and destructive behavior toward the dying person may take place.

Anticipatory grief can facilitate the mourning process, but it does not always do so. People who have experienced anticipatory grief sometimes report that, in spite of it, they still find the loss to be a shock.

Delayed Mourning

When feelings about a lost person are strongly ambivalent, there may be no evidence of mourning at the time of the loss. If these feelings are unexpressed, they may cause physical and emotional distress and interpersonal dysfunction. Delayed mourning creates an additional problem in that, when grief is eventually expressed, it may puzzle others; consequently, support and understanding are not readily available. Moreover, when mourning begins months or years after a loss, mourners themselves may have no idea what is causing their overwhelming grief. For these people, healing begins as they search for the relationship between loss and grief.

RELEVANCE TO NURSING

Nurses continually encounter people who will experience or have experienced loss and separation. Knowledge about the grieving process and the importance of expressing feelings and reviewing memories can be used to help these people deal with loss effectively. Grief is the normal process of resolving the loss of a highly valued (cathected) object, place, or person.[57] It is the process of separation.

One of the more obvious separations in current American culture is divorce. Another important form of separation has to do with mobility. Even when a relocation is desired by all concerned, the separation process will occur. A change in jobs that does not require relocation still involves separation from colleagues, familiar responsibilities, and established routines. Urban renewal—the dissolution of "old" neighborhoods and dispersion of their residents throughout the city—involves separation and loss of familiar surroundings and familiar faces. Less obvious and obviously less disruptive separations are trading in an old car for a newer model (recalling memories of experiences in the old car), and discarding old clothing, memorabilia, or pieces of furniture.

Death, the ultimate separation, can be sudden and unexpected; such a death is often called *tragic* by survivors. Death can be predicted when there is a long serious illness or constant exposure to extreme danger, as in war. It can also be an accepted consequence of a long life, whether the lost object is a beloved family pet or an aged friend or relative.

With death, not only the survivors grieve. If the dying process occurs over time, the dying person must also separate from loved ones and from life itself. Thus, the dying person mourns the loss of self and relationships with friends and family. Nurses work with clients and families confronting such situations. Intervention can prevent misconceptions and the development of pathology among these people.

In medical or surgical treatment settings nurses often care for clients whose bodies have been mutilated by surgery or ravaged by disease. Grief is elicited by irrevocable changes in appearance, permanent loss of the perception of self as a healthy person, and diminished feelings of well-being. The loss of hair during chemotherapy, facial disfiguration, the amputation of a limb—all such experiences generate grief. Nursing interventions need to be directed toward helping these clients recognize and engage in "grief work."

Voluntary abortion, miscarriage, stillbirth, and birth of a defective child elicit varying degrees of grief. Nurses may help clients faced with such experiences, and their families, to resolve losses effectively and reinvest in the future.

When faced with an empty nest, the parents who have made a major commitment to child rearing grieve for their lost roles and the meaning of their lives. The maturation process involves many separations. For the child and the parents, gradual separation is a developmental task and is often symbolized by the child's graduation, moving out of the family home, first job, and marriage. The feelings of loss evoked by these separations result in a grieving process.

The hostility, ambivalence, guilt, and depression that accompany the loss of a significant love object may be pathogenic (capable of producing disease). Nurses have a significant role in helping people work through these feelings, avoid the problematic uses of repression and suppression of the associated feelings, and develop inner and family strengths through effective management of the grieving process.

Facilitation of the psychological processes required for resolution of the grieving process may be important in preventing the development of pathology. Encouraging the expression of feelings is an important aspect of the helping process. Empathic listening gives clients an opportunity to review memories, explore feelings, and let go of intense attachment to a lost object. Support groups whose members have experienced similar losses have been found helpful.

When families prevent expression of feelings and discussions about a lost object, early intervention is needed to help members work through the loss and become mutually supportive.

Early identification of delayed grieving and early intervention significantly influence the prevention of somatic, psychological, and social pathology. Helping people recognize their grieving process and accept as normal the feelings that are being experienced may be all that is needed.

The healthy resolution of grieving involves incorporating some aspect of the lost object into the ego structure of the griever. The intensity of grief is directly related to the intensity of attachment to the lost object. In due time, because of the working-through processes, emotional attachment to the lost object decreases, leaving usually pleasant, even idealized memories relatively free of the initial intense emotion. At this point, usually 6 to 12 months after the loss, the grieving process is completed and the regular patterns of living gradually resume.

One of the most helpful things one can do in preparation for dealing with loss of an object, and particularly death, is to be aware of one's own feelings. Religious beliefs, philosophical orientations, and childhood experiences all contribute to one's thinking about death. Being aware of those contributions and being comfortable with them is the best preparation for dealing with grief, either personally or professionally.

Loneliness

Despite its universality, loneliness and its accompanying moods, feelings, and experiences cannot be defined conceptually. *Loneliness* is a unique, pervasive human experience that has been described and observed in many ways. Descriptions of the experience of loneliness include emptiness, solitude, withdrawal, and pensiveness; loneliness has been compared to a creative force, a bottomless pit, calm seas, abandonment, death, and ultimate pain.

Many incongruent definitions of loneliness exist because there are actually four different states: aloneness, lonesomeness, loneliness, and pathological loneliness.

Aloneness is a state of social isolation which involves being physically apart from others by virtue of being an only, sole, or single person, or without company. One can be alone without being lonely, and lonely without being alone. It is well known that one can be lonely in the midst of a group of people; on the other hand, one can be alone on a mountain or a beach and not experience loneliness.

Lonesomeness, on the other hand, is a conscious recognition of aloneness and a simultaneous desire to be with others. It is expressed as an emotion, and people generally take steps to relieve it. For example, an elderly widower may experience lonesomeness following the death of his wife and plan to visit his grandchildren to help alleviate the emotion.

Loneliness is a restless search for connectedness with one's "center." It cannot really be understood abstractly but must be experienced. It has been called the *depth dimension* of the self; and Moustakas, among others, has suggested that it lies at the hub of life and cannot be avoided—it is part of the process of becoming a whole person.[65] The inevitable human search for the meaning of one's life, by necessity, leads a person to the existential, creative, and spiritual experience of loneliness. Loneliness can be a healthy, expansive experience that allows people to renew contact with themselves, feel their own apartness, and discover who they are and what their lives are really like. It is necessary for personal growth, self-discovery, formulation of values, and creativity. A sense of newness, even a new self, may emerge from loneliness. Solitude—spaces and times created so that loneliness can be experienced—can thus represent an opportunity to appreciate oneself, humanity, and the human condition.

Pathological loneliness, by contrast, is defined as social alienation and an inability to do anything while alone.[66] It has been described by Frieda Fromm-Reichman as a profound, nonconstructive, disintegrative experience which is symptomatic of, or leads to, a psychotic state. Pathological loneliness makes people emotionally paralyzed and helpless. Fromm-Reichman suggests that it is a form of anxiety which develops when there is a fundamental difference between what one is and what one pretends to be, or a gap between person and person. People who experience pathological loneliness are frightened by it, and tend to be secretive about it or to deny it. It is characterized by panic, a sense of unexplained threats, extreme restlessness, flight, and dissociation of memories, brought on by enforced isolation or voluntary isolation motivated by a desire to avoid the pain of rejection.[67] Sullivan proposes that it is an unconscious, exceedingly unpleasant drive which has to do with inadequate fulfillment of the need for human intimacy.[68] Pathological loneliness has been linked to several societal problems, and to illnesses such as schizophrenia, alcoholism, suicide, and depression. (Chapter 37 describes in detail the loneliness of people suffering from schizophrenia.)

RELEVANCE TO NURSING

Nurses are vulnerable to loneliness not only in themselves but also in their clients. In order for nurses to provide effective intervention for clients, they must look closely at their own experiences of loneliness, enter into them, and "own" them. The goal of such a subjective search is to become more comfortable with oneself and recognize solitude as dynamic and creative. Once nurses recognize what "triggers" loneliness for them, how they react to the experience, and how they can be comfortable with their own feelings about it, they are able to validate the experience empathically for clients.

The process of dealing with loneliness is facilitated by assessing one's own connections to others—family, friends, and society—and "tracking" the experience of loneliness in oneself and one's family. It is helpful to describe loneliness verbally, to form mental images of it, and to engage in solitary activities such as walking alone in a quiet place and writing in a journal. Spending time alone helps people discover themselves and others. A high level of self-differentiation and the ability to transform and transcend experiences can be achieved when people choose to enter into, rather than flee from, their loneliness.

STRESS

Stress is a paradoxical concept which may enable people to survive or may cause them to be disabled to the point of death. Stress has been defined in various ways and by different people; at present it is a major concept used in nursing, and it is being researched extensively in many other disciplines.

Stress is a state of imbalance within an organism, brought about by an actual or perceived disparity between environmental demands (stressors) and the organism's capacity to cope with them. It is manifested in a variety of physiological, emotional and behavioral response patterns.[69]

The Stress Syndrome

Selye defined stress as a rate of wear and tear in the body—a dynamic state which raises the body's resistance to threatening and dangerous agents. It is experienced as fatigue, uneasiness, or illness, and it is manifested by the general adaptation syndrome (GAS).[70] (See Table 3-13.) Selye's basic biochemical model of stress is based on the assumption that stress is a state manifested by a specific syndrome which consists of all the nonspecifically induced changes within a biological system.[70]

According to Selye, the response to stress—the GAS—has three stages. The first stage, an alarm reaction, is the direct effect of a stressor on the body. It is followed by the second stage, resistance, characterized by internal responses which in turn

Table 3-13 General Adaptation Syndrome (GAS)

Stage 1: Alarm Reaction
Weight loss
Enlargement of the adrenal cortex
Enlargement of lymph glands
Increase in hormone levels
Stage 2: Stage of Resistance (Adaptation)
Weight returns to normal
Adrenal cortex becomes smaller
Lymph glands return to normal
Hormone levels are constant
Stage 3: Stage of Exhaustion
Enlargement of adrenal glands
Adrenal-gland depletion
Weight loss
Enlargement of the lymph glands
Dysfunction of lymph system
Increase in hormone levels
Hormonal depletion

Table 3-14 Local Adaptation Syndrome (LAS)

Characteristics
Momentary vasoconstriction
Vasodilation with hyperemia (redness and heat)
Engorgement of the site
Leukocytes migrate to site
Capillary-wall permeability reduced
Leukocytes phagocytize foreign sustance and cellular debris
Leukocytes form a limiting circle around the site
A ring of fibrin is laid down around the site
Massive collection of leukocytes forms within ring
Bone marrow is stimulated to produce more leukocytes, particularly polymorphonuclear leukocytes

elicit defenses. If adaptation does not occur, a third stage, exhaustion, develops; in this third stage the internal responses stimulate "tissue surrender" by inhibiting defenses. The ability to resist and adapt depends upon the ability to reestablish a proper internal balance. Stages 1 and 2 of the GAS are experienced repeatedly throughout a lifetime. Thus for learning, growth, development, and survival itself, the ability to cope with stress is required. Stressful mental and physical activity, emotions, and relationships with others are unavoidable.

The local adaptation syndrome (LAS) is an inflammatory localized reaction to injury (see Table 3-14). It is an active defense reaction which very much resembles the GAS. An alarm signal caused by a stressor mobilizes defenses; this is followed by the stage of resistance. When exhaustion occurs, it is limited to the local area. However, several limited states of exhaustion may occur simultaneously in various parts of the body, and, if they are then extensive or intense enough, they can activate the GAS (Table 3-13).[70]

The stage of exhaustion in the GAS occurs when multiple severe stressors are affecting the body simultaneously or when a stressor is applied repeatedly or is overwhelmingly intense. When the resistance mechanisms are worn out, adaptation becomes impossible, and the body surrenders. Although the body is an open system capable of acquiring energy and information, its ability to exchange and utilize input is limited. According to Selye,[71] the ultimate consequence of unremitting stress is exhaustion; this indicates that adaptational energy is finite, although it is not yet measurable or operationally defined.

Exhaustion is reversible as long as it affects only parts of the body and as long as vigorous efforts are made to eliminate or mitigate the stressor. However, if all the body's defense systems are involved or if there are no respites, even brief ones, from stress, the body's capacity for defense will be exhausted, adaptational energy will be depleted, and survival will be uncertain.

Selye identified and described the GAS and LAS before production of endophorins in the brain had been discovered. These substances have morphine-like, painkilling, antistress properties, and, more important, they appear to play a role in transmitting alarm signals from the brain to the pituitary.[72]

Whereas Selye looked at the total phenomenon of stress, Lazarus[73] has examined a portion that he calls the *coping process.* He thinks that the visible reaction to a stressor is determined by the person's evaluation of it. A particular coping process selected may not be the best one for adapting to reality, but it is most appropriate for a person's *interpretation* of reality. Thus *perception* of a stressor and its effect is more significant than the stressor itself. A situation may provide an enjoyable challenge or even relief from boredom for one person, while it may be interpreted as threatening by another person. Even for one person, a situation may at one time be a pleasurable opportunity, but at another time it may become a threat (for example, when the person is already facing other difficulties).

Perceptions of stress are determined to a considerable extent by past experiences. Experience establishes a "history" of stressors and response patterns, so that when a new situation occurs, a person tends to react not to the present reality but to similar past experiences. (An example of this process may be found when a new mathematical concept is presented to a student who has a prodrome of an illness and therefore is unable to master it. When the concept is presented again, the student expects it to be difficult, even impossible, and experiences it as stress, even though the actual, original stressor—the illness—is no longer present.) The amazing variety of individual perceptions of stressors makes it generally impossible to establish a cause-and-effect relationship between a specific stressor and a physiological response or to predict what response a stressor will elicit.

Although much is unknown about stress, it can be said with certainty that some stress is necessary for living and adapting; the organism which no longer experiences stress is dead.

Physiological Responses to Stress

When people encounter stressors, the fight-flight response is activated: they either flee the situation or get ready for battle. Figure 3-5 illustrates the polarity of the responses as well as the behaviors and feelings which accompany both fight and flight.

Responses to stress include nervousness, inertia, insomnia, heart palpitations, trembling hands, sweating, headaches, dizziness, fainting, and nightmares. These symptoms, as well as psychopathology and organ and body-system dysfunction, develop as a consequence of stress and are mediated by the cerebral cortex, autonomic nervous system, endocrine system, and hypothalamus.*

Reactions to stressors begin with the perceptual system, which alerts the thalamocortical system and the central nervous system (CNS). The CNS can respond by initiating activity in any part of the body, since all vital organs are under its control.

* The student should consult a text on anatomy and physiology for information about the structure and function of these organs and systems.

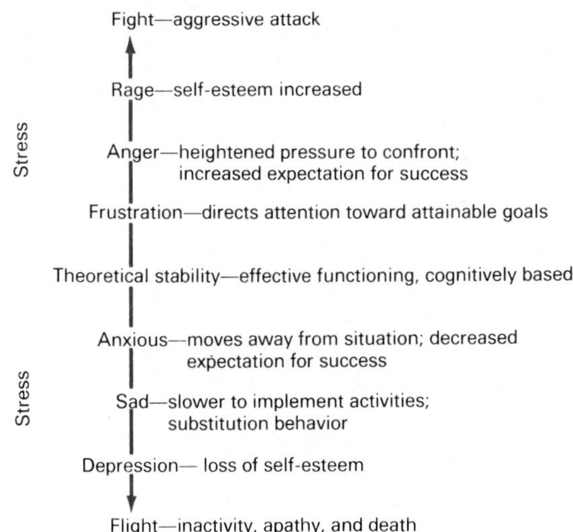

Figure 3-5 Fight-flight response to stress. Stress can elicit fight behavior (progressive confrontation) or flight behavior (progressive distancing from the source of stress).

There may be gross motor activity, which enables the person to run from the situation, as well as alterations in the functioning of the autonomic nervous system and in the activation of the endocrine system.

When a stressful event occurs, there are numerous biochemical and structural changes within the body. The carrier of signals that call for adaptation has yet to be identified; it may consist of metabolic by-products released during activity or trauma, or it may be depletion of a vital substance when a stress is experienced—that is, when a demand on the body is made. The alarm signal (whatever it is) disrupts homeostasis and excites the hypothalamus, which serves as a link between the brain and the endocrine system. Activation of the thalamocortical system generates signals that in turn activate neuroendocrine cells in the hypothalamus. The corticotrophic hormone-releasing factor also comes into play. The signal is relayed to the pituitary gland, causing the release of adrenocorticotrophic hormone (ACTH) into the general circulation. ACTH stimulates the adrenal cortex to secrete corticoids, specifically the glucocorticoids, cortisol and corticosterone. Hormones, such as the catecholamines, are also released; this is important for adaptation. Adrenaline is secreted; this supports the fight-flight response. Consequently, blood pressure and circulation to muscles increase; the central nervous system is stimulated; and blood coagulation is increased to prevent excess bleeding. Many other hormonal and chemical changes also occur during stress.[72] Tracing these stimuli and responses reveals the multiple ways in which stress affects organs and cells to produce symptomatic dysfunction.

Perception and Stress

Sensory stimuli—internal and external—are received through the perceptual system. The nervous system transmits stimuli to the cerebral cortex for interpretation. If a stimulus is found to be a threat, the stress syndrome is elicited; if a stimulus is interpreted as nonthreatening, the body's psychological and physiological defense mechanisms are not mobilized.

Any situation, thought, or agent which elicits fear, anger, anxiety, or elation is stressful. As was noted earlier, what makes a stimulus stressful is to a large extent a matter of how it is perceived. Two people in the same situation may perceive, and thus respond, differently because they perceive it differently. Perception is affected by inherited (genetic) traits, individual needs and aspirations, and earlier experiences (conditioning). Since each person is unique, what may be seen as a threat by one person is a challenge to another. Personality, structure, and ego integration affect perception of the degree of threat presented by a stressor and the number of stressors that can be managed at one time. Environmental support—"perceived security"—also affects the ability to deal with stress.

People react not only to the direct stressors, but also to threats and to symbols of the past. Each person perceives, interprets, and responds according to past experiences. For example, if a person has been rejected or treated harshly and unjustly by parental figures throughout childhood, confrontations with authority figures in adulthood will reactivate memories and elicit an expectation of similar treatment. Such a person will therefore approach authority figures with anxiety or hostility, which may be either overt or manifested by dysfunction in an organ or system.

Stressors

Stressors are agents, external events, or conditions that interact with and influence the person in such a way as to elicit the biopsychosocial stress-response syndrome. Stressors may be physical, emotional, cognitive, or spiritual. Sources of stress are found in both the external physical environment and society.

Physical Environment

The primary stressor encountered by organisms is in nature. The natural physical environment has several aspects which can act as stressors: heat, cold, humidity, geomagnetic forces, light, atmospheric electricity, pressure, and altitude. Overexposure to cold, for instance, may cause frostbite; and overexposure to heat may burn the skin. An inadequate supply of oxygen causes hypoxia; changes in atmospheric pressure can alter blood gases.

Technology also creates environmental stressors. Industrial pollution—noxious physical and chemical agents in the environment—includes high levels of dangerous gases, airborne particles, unwanted chemicals in water and food, and noise. All these are potential stressors, as are ionizing radiation, artificial lighting, radar screens, and computer cathode ray tubes.

Social Environment

The *social environment* encompasses interaction between individuals, between the individual and the family, and between the individual and society; all these interactions are potentially stressful.

PERSON-PERSON INTERACTIONS. As people interact with neighbors, friends, and coworkers, they encounter various situations in which their own beliefs, values, preferences, wishes, needs, and perceptions do not agree with other people's. In addition, when people work, live, or play in close proximity, idiosyncratic behaviors, mannerisms, and lifestyles can be abrasive and cause conflicts. Such conflicts can create acute stress or develop into chronically stressful patterns of interaction.

FAMILY-PERSON INTERACTIONS. Potential stressors in family-person interactions are generated by transitions in the family life cycle, by the family's adaptation to environmental demands, by situational crises, and by multigenerational conflicts. (See Table 3-15.)

Social support is an important resource for any family. Relatives and close friends can help a family

Table 3-15 Stressful Family-Person Patterns of Interaction

Stressful Patterns of Interaction	Helpful Responses
Family development Accession: changes in a family's structure through the addition of a member (birth, adoption, marriage) Separation: loss or departure of a member (child going to school, death, divorce, retirement)	Relinquish old patterns of interaction Acquire new behaviors Establish modified patterns of interaction
Individual growth and development	Revise old patterns of interaction Establish new patterns of interaction, as with adolescents or aging parents
Multigenerational problems Disruptions in the integrity of the family of origin Premature responsibilities	Create a functional family structure that does not duplicate the family of origin Mobilize the strengths and resources of all family members
Family resources Both parents working full time, balancing work and family demands and responsibilities Interactions among expectations: individual, spouse, society, employment Child care Decisions about allocation of time, energy, and other family resources Ethnic, sex, and racial discrimination	Mobilize the resources of all the family members and the resources of the family itself Develop strong support systems among friends and extended family Encourage societal supports Address societal issues which inhibit family health
Situational crises or catastrophes (natural disasters, rape, terrorism, etc.)	Help people express and work through feelings of hopelessness, grief, disruption, and destruction (individuals as well as family) Clearly identify and delineate stressors as they occur View stressors as family problems, not individuals' problems, that need mutually supportive, cohesive efforts Confront problems in an open, organized, solution-oriented way

survive a stressful event or period. Roles within the family need to be flexible. Highly empathic, open communication reinforces family cohesion and makes it possible to cope with stress more effectively. Avoidance patterns should be discouraged; approach patterns of support, problem solving, and decision making should be encouraged.[74]

PERSON-SOCIETY INTERACTIONS. Society itself is a potential stressor. One reason for this is that there are significant discrepancies between the real and the ideal in any society. For example, if the society emphasizes upward mobility, achievement, and success (the ideal) but provides very limited opportunities (the real), its members will experience this conflict as a source of stress.[75]

Social change is another source of stress. A transition from an agrarian to an industrial society, or—as is currently occurring in this country—from an industrial to an information society affects all spheres of life.[76] During such transitions, social institutions, norms, and beliefs are disrupted.[75] The environmental instability and unpredictability caused by such disruptions make members of the society feel insecure and confused. Rapid change challenges the ability of all members of society to cope. Dislocation, relocation, and perceived obsolescence of people, families, and communities are potential stressors.

Rapid development of high technology generates new economic entities that overshadow existing enterprises. Methods, skills, and entire industries may become obsolete. Industries rise and decline, or they are acquired by larger industries that either reorganize or dismantle them. Obviously, such changes are stressful in themselves, and they have the further effect of making the social environment seem threatening because it is so unstable.

Economic instability has implications for the society as a whole, for communities, and for individuals, particularly when social stratification is taken into account. Societies are stratified in many ways—by power, status, and money, for example.[71] People of low status are most likely to experience deprivation and disappointment when the economy is troubled; thus they are subject to intense, multiple stressors. Another source of stress is incongruence between economic position and other forms of social standing. People who have, for instance, more money than status or more status than money may experience an internalized conflict that becomes a stressor. If the economy fluctuates widely and frequently, potential stressors increase;[75] people's status, power, and economic resources may be lowered, affecting their lifestyle and self-esteem, or may be raised so rapidly that their personal values are in disarray.

A society's commitment to rights of working people, the young, the old, and the infirm is also important. If the society does little to prevent losses and uncertainty, a sense of hopelessness and futility will develop. Societies are human organizations, and like their individual members, they have moral obligations. When a society fails to uphold its moral principles, people within the society undergo serious stress.

RELEVANCE TO NURSING

Stress causes physical and emotional illness and social dysfunction. Therefore, management of stress is an integral part of the activities of nursing in maintaining, promoting, restoring, and rehabilitating health.

Outpatient services for family planning, maternity care, and well-child care are among the primary-care settings where nurses can facilitate stress management. Maternal stress affects not only the mother but the developing fetus as well. The expansion of families through procreation, adoption, and placement of foster children, and the contraction of families through death, divorce, and retirement, are inherently stressful. If these situations are mismanaged, family dynamics will become dysfunctional and adversely affect family members' ability to deal with either the present or the future.

Stressful situations develop in many homes, workplaces and schools. Public health nurses, occupational health nurses, and school nurses thus have opportunities to help clients recognize stress in their everyday lives. Awareness of stressors and of one's own responses to them is necessary for managing stress effectively.

Illness, surgery, and hospitalization are inherently stressful; almost everyone who undergoes these experiences is fearful and anxious. Nursing interventions can help clients manage, deal with these feelings effectively, control their fantasies, and improve their ability to cope. Nurses can also help clients engage in the necessary and manageable "worry work" that mobilizes physiological and emotional resources. Nurses also have a responsibility for lessening or resolving environmental and iatrogenic stress experienced by clients and their families.

Intensive-care and special-care units have clients whose medical or surgical problems are life-threatening. In such settings, both the clients' conditions and the environment tend to escalate stress. Nurses have a significant responsibility to modify these stressors and promote the well-being of clients and families.

In recent years, nurses have increasingly become aware of professional burnout—a progressive loss of idealism, energy, and purpose experienced by people in the helping professions as a result of work conditions. When burnout occurs, nurses' sensitivity and empathy are impaired, and they begin to experience the physical and psychological symptoms of stress. Thus, nurses must manage stress in both their personal and their professional lives. Their knowledge of organizational structures and functions and their own self-awareness will help them formulate strategies for this.

In every treatment setting and every nurse-client relationship, there are potential stressors. These stressors must be recognized before they can be managed. Nurses have a responsibility to identify stressors and to intervene appropriately. Stressors can promote growth if they are managed effectively; nurses therefore also have a responsibility to help clients use stressful events to learn how to cope with life.

Drug addiction, alcoholism, obesity, hypertension, dysfunction of various bodily systems (such as the respiratory and gastrointestinal systems), and frequent infections and colds are the result of stress mismanagement. Through education, clarification of values, and programs designed to foster a healthy lifestyle, nurses can facilitate effective stress management and promote health.

SUMMARY

The concepts in this chapter are part of the theoretical foundation of holistic nursing. People are the focus of nursing care. Each of the concepts examined here contributes to an understanding of the physical, mental, and spiritual aspects of the person, the person-environment interaction, and the relevance of this information to nursing practice. Self-concept, identity, moral image, body boundaries, self-esteem, and body image—and their relevance to health—have been explored. The effect of sensory stimuli upon effective functioning has been identified, as have the ways in which sensory stimuli are perceived. Disturbances of touch and sensory input have been related to health and dysfunction.

The rhythmical nature of human functioning has been explored. Particular attention has been given to sleep because of its significance in maintaining and restoring health. Both space and time, which help to conceptualize phenomena that influence the providers and consumers of health care and the sociocultural environment, have been examined.

Human emotion in general has been explored. Particular emphasis has been placed on anxiety, grief, and loneliness, which may be the most significant emotions in our time. Stress, a pervasive health problem, has also been examined, since it must be understood if it is to be dealt with adequately in a care-giving situation.

Each of these concepts has been defined and discussed, and its relevance to nursing has been identified. Examples have been used to illustrate the application of the concepts in the promotion, maintenance, restoration, and rehabilitation of health.

REFERENCES

1. F. L. Bower, ed., *Normal Development of Body Image*, Wiley, New York, 1977.
2. M. S. Mahler, F. Pine, and A. Bergman, *The Psychological Birth of the Human Infant*, Basic Books, New York, 1975.
3. H. S. Sullivan, *The Interpersonal Theory of Psychiatry*, Norton, New York, 1953.
4. M. R. Lyles et al., "Racial Identity and Self Esteem: Problems Peculiar to Biracial Children," *Journal of the American Academy of Child Psychiatry*, vol. 24, March 1985, pp. 150–153.
5. T. F. Fogarty, "System Concepts and the Dimensions of Self," in P. Guerin, ed., *Family Therapy: Theory and Practice*, Gardner, New York, 1976, pp. 144–153.
6. M. Rosenberg, *Conceiving the Self*, Basic Books, New York, 1979.
7. P. Bradshaw, *The Management of Self-Esteem*, Prentice-Hall, Englewood Cliffs, N. J., 1981.
8. F. L. Bower, *Distortions in Body Image in Illness and Disability*, Wiley, New York, 1977.
9. M. L. Kietzman et al., "Perception, Cognition and Attention," in A. M. Freedman, H. I. Kaplan, and B. J. Sadock, eds., *Comprehensive Textbook of Psychiatry*, 3d ed., Williams and Wilkins, Baltimore, 1980, pp. 334–371.
10. S. H. Bartley, "What Is Perception?" in D. Goleman and R. J. Davidson, eds., *Consciousness: The Brain, States of Awareness, and Alternate Realities*, Irvington, New York, 1979.
11. A. Montague, *Touching*, Columbia University Press, New York, 1971, pp. 1, 7.
12. P. Solomon and S. T. Kleeman, "Sensory Deprivation," in A. M. Freedman, H. I. Kaplan, and B. J. Sadock, eds., *Comprehensive Textbook of Psychiatry*, 3d ed., Williams and Wilkins, Baltimore, 1980, pp. 600–607.
13. P. Suedfeld, "Social Isolation: A Case for Interdisciplinary Research," in D. Goleman and R. J. Davidson, eds., *Consciousness: The Brain, States of Awareness, and Alternate Realities*, Irvington, New York, 1979, pp. 161–165.
14. M. J. Thompson and D. W. Harsha, "Our Rhythms Still Follow the African Sun," *Psychology Today*, vol. 18, January 1984, pp. 51–54.
15. A. Spielberger, *Biological Rhythms Research*, Elsevier, New York, 1965.
16. G. G. Luce et al., *Human and Animal Physiology*, Dover, New York, 1971.
17. M. W. Yogman, B. M. Lester, and J. Hoffman, "Behavioral Rhythmicity and Circadian Rhythmicity During Mother, Father, Stranger, Infant Social Interaction," *Pediatric Research*, vol. 17, no. 11, 1983, pp. 872–876.
18. *Biological Rhythms in Psychiatry and Medicine*, U.S. Department of Health, Education, and Welfare, National Institutes of Mental Health, Chevy Chase, Md., 1970.
19. J. L. Veith et al., "Exposure to Men Influences the Occurrence of Ovulation in Women," *Physiological Behavior*, vol. 31, no. 3, 1983, pp. 313–316.
20. D. C. Ziac, "Menstrual Synchrony in University Women," *American Journal of Physical Anthropology*, vol. 63, no. 2, 1984, p. 237.
21. W. P. Colguhoun, *Biological Rhythms and Human Performance*, Academic, London, 1971, p. 101.
22. M. Koller, "Health Risks Related to Shift Work: An Example of Time Contingent Effects of Long-Term Stress," *International Archives of Occupational and Environmental Health*, vol. 53, no. 1, 1984, pp. 59–76.
23. K. Orth-Gomer, "Intervention on Coronary Risk Factors by Adapting a Shift Work Schedule to Biologic Rhythmicity," *Psychosomatic Medicine*, vol. 45, no. 5, 1983, pp. 407–416.
24. M. S. Borowsky and R. Wall, "Naval Aviation Mishaps

and Fatigue," *Aviation, Space and Environmental Medicine*, vol. 54, no. 6, 1983, pp. 535–538.

25. G. B. Bolli and J. E. Gerich, "The Dawn Phenomenon: A Common Occurrence in Both Non-Insulin Dependent and Insulin Dependent Diabetes Mellitus," *New England Journal of Medicine*, vol. 310, no. 12, 1984, pp. 746–750.
26. M. W. Yogman and S. H. Zeisel, "Diet and Sleep Patterns in Newborn Infants," *New England Journal of Medicine*, vol. 309, no. 19, 1983, pp. 1147–1149.
27. E. Kuhn and V. Brodan, "Changes in the Circadian Rhythm of Serum Iron Induced by a 5-Day Sleep Deprivation," *European Journal of Applied Physiology, Occupational Physiology*, vol. 49, no. 2, 1984, pp. 215–222.
28. J. B. Russell, D. Mitchell, P. I. Musey, and D. C. Collins, "The Relationship of Exercise to Anovulatory Cycles in Female Athletes' Hormonal and Physical Characteristics," *Obstetrics and Gynecology*, vol. 63, no. 4, 1984, pp. 452–456.
29. E. Glattre and T. Bjerkedal, "The 24-Hour Rhythmicity of Birth: A Populational Study," *Acta Obstetric Gynecological Scandinavica*, vol. 62, no. 1, 1983, pp. 31–36.
30. E. Arnbjornsson, "Relationship Between the Removal of the Nonacute Appendix and the Menstrual Cycle," *Annals of Chir Gynaecology*, vol. 72, no. 6, 1984, pp. 329–331.
31. S. Nakano and L. E. Hollister, "Chrono Pharmacology of Amitriptyline," *Clinical Pharmacological Therapy*, vol. 33, no. 4, 1983, pp. 453–459.
32. D. J. Lakatua et al., "Change in Phase Relations of Circadian Rhythms in Cell Proliferation Induced by Time Limited Feeding in BALB-C X DBA-2 F-2 Mice Bearing a Transplantable Harding Paaey Tumor," *Cancer Research*, vol. 43, no. 9, 1983, pp. 4068–4072.
33. E. L. Hartmann, *The Functions of Sleep*, Yale University Press, New Haven, Conn., 1973, p. 30.
34. E. L. Hartmann, "Sleep," in A. M. Freedman, H. I. Kaplan, and B. J. Sadock, eds., *Textbook of Comprehensive Psychiatry*, 3d ed., Williams and Wilkins, Baltimore, 1980, pp. 2014–2029.
35. S. S. Campbell, "Duration and Placement of Sleep in a Disentrained Environment," *Psychophysiology*, vol. 21, no. 1, 1984, pp. 106–113.
36. C. F. Reynolds et al., "Electroencephalographic Sleep: Aging and Psychopathology New Data and State of the Art," *Biological Psychiatry*, vol. 18, no. 2, 1983, pp. 139–156.
37. "Coping with Dreams," *Science News*, vol. 123, 1983, p. 126.
38. C. Hall, "The Meaning of Dreams," in D. Goleman and R. J. Davidson, eds., *Consciousness: The Brain, States of Awareness, and Alternate Realities*, Irvington, New York, 1979.
39. A. Corrick, *The Human Brain: Mind and Matter*, Arco, New York, 1983.
40. M. C. Doyle, "Enhancing Dream Pleasure with Senoi Strategy," *Journal of Clinical Psychology*, vol. 40, no. 2, 1984, pp. 467–474.
41. J. L. Singer, "The Importance of Daydreaming," in D. Goleman and R. J. Davidson, eds., *Consciousness: The Brain, States of Awareness, and Alternate Realities*, Irvington, New York, 1979, pp. 53–57.
42. A. W. MacLean et al., "Rapid Eye Movement Latency and Depression Computer Simulations Based on the Results of Phase Delay of Sleep in Normal Subjects," *Psychiatry Research*, vol. 9, no. 1, 1983, pp. 69–80.
43. W. H. Ittelson, H. M. Proshansky, L. G. Rivlin, and H. Winkel, *An Introduction to Environmental Psychology*, Holt, Rinehart, and Winston, New York, 1974.
44. E. T. Hall, *The Hidden Dimension*, Doubleday, New York, 1966, pp. 7, 12, 109.
45. C. T. Tart, "Altered States of Consciousness: Putting the Pieces Together," in D. Goleman and R. J. Davidson, eds., *Consciousness: The Brain, States of Awareness, and Alternate Realities*, Irvington, New York, 1979, pp. 86, 87, 93.
46. S. M. Fishkin and B. M. Jones, "Drugs and Consciousness: An Attentional Model of Consciousness with Application to Drug-Related Altered States," in A. A. Sugarman and R. E. Tarter, eds., *Expanding Dimensions of Consciousness*, Springer, New York, 1978, pp. 273–292.
47. D. P. Hymovich and R. W. Chamberlin, *Child and Family Development*, McGraw-Hill, New York, 1980.
48. W. J. Bremmer, M. V. Vitiello, and P. N. Prinz, "Loss of Circadian Rhythmicity in Blood Testosterone Levels with Aging in Normal Men," *Journal of Clinical Endocrinology and Metabolism*, vol. 56, no. 6, 1983, pp. 1278–1281.
49. R. S. Peters, "The Education of the Emotions," in M. B. Arnold, ed., *Feelings and Emotions*, Academic, New York, 1970, pp. 187–203.
50. R. S. Lazarus, J. R. Averill, and E. M. Opton, Jr., "Toward a Cognitive Theory of Emotion," in M. B. Arnold, ed., *Feelings and Emotions*, Academic, New York, 1970, pp. 207–232.
51. Rollo May, *The Meaning of Anxiety*, Ronald, New York, 1950.
52. H. S. Sullivan, "The Psychiatric Interview," in M. S. Perry and M. L. Gawel, eds., *The Collected Works of Harry Stack Sullivan*, vol. 1, Norton, New York, 1953.
53. D. R. Hayes, "Teaching a Concept of Anxiety to Patients," *Nursing Research*, vol. 10, Spring 1961, pp. 108–113.
54. H. E. Peplau, "A Working Definition of Anxiety," in S. F. Burd and M. A. Marshall, eds., *Some Clinical Approaches to Psychiatric Nursing*, Macmillan, New York, 1963.

55. W. E. Fann et al., eds., *Phenomenology and Treatment of Anxiety*, S. P. Medical and Scientific Books, New York, 1979.
56. S. Freud and A. Freud, "Mourning and Melancholia," in J. Strachey, ed., *The Complete Psychological Works of Sigmund Freud*, Hogarth, London, 1966.
57. B. F. Sideleau, "Patient Response to Loss: An Exploratory Study," Yale University unpublished master's thesis, 1970.
58. D. C. Maddison and A. Viola, "The Health of Widows the Year Following Bereavement," *Journal of Psychosomatic Medical Research*, vol. 12, 1968, p. 297.
59. Z. Stein and M. Susser, "Widowhood and Mental Illness," *British Journal of Preventive and Social Medicine*, vol. 23, 1969, p. 106.
60. W. D. Rees, "The Bereaved and Their Hallucinations," in B. Schoenberg et al., eds., *Bereavement: Its Psychosocial Aspects*, Columbia University Press, New York, 1975.
61. J. Bowlby and C. M. Parkes, "Separation and Loss," in E. J. Anthony and C. Koupernik, eds., *International Yearbook for Child Psychiatry and Allied Disciplines: The Child and His Family*, vol. 1, Wiley, New York, 1970.
62. C. M. Parkes, "The First Year of Bereavement," *Psychiatry*, vol. 33, 1970, p. 344.
63. L. H. Tessman, *Children of Parting Parents*, Aronson, New York, 1978.
64. J. S. Wallerstein and J. B. Kelly, *Surviving the Breakup*, Basic Books, New York, 1980.
65. C. F. Moustakas, *Loneliness*, Prentice-Hall, Englewood Cliffs, N.J., 1963.
66. H. F. Peplau, "Loneliness," *American Journal of Nursing*, vol. 55, December 1955, pp. 1476–1481.
67. F. Fromm-Reichman, "Loneliness," *Psychiatry*, vol. 22, January 1959, pp. 1–15.
68. H. S. Sullivan, *The Interpersonal Theory of Psychiatry*, William Alanson White Psychiatric Foundation, ed., Norton, New York, 1953.
69. D. Stokols, "A Congruence Analysis of Human Stress," in I. G. Sarason and C. D. Spielberger, eds., *Stress and Anxiety*, vol. 6, Hemisphere, Washington, D.C., 1979.
70. H. Selye, *The Stress of Life*, McGraw-Hill, New York, 1956.
71. H. Selye, *Stress without Distress*, Lippincott, New York, 1974.
72. H. Selye, "History and Present Status of the Stress Concept," in L. Goldberger and S. Breznitz, eds., *Handbook of Stress*, Free Press, New York, 1982, pp. 7–17.
73. R. S. Lazarus, *Psychological Stress and the Coping Process*, McGraw-Hill, New York, 1966.
74. H. I. McCubbin, "Bridging Normative Stress and Catastrophic Family Stress," in H. I. McCubbin and C. R. Figley, eds., *Stress and the Family*, vol. 1, Brunner/Mazel, New York, 1983.
75. L. I. Pearlin, "The Social Contexts of Stress," in L. Goldberger and S. Breznitz, eds., *Handbook of Stress*, Free Press, New York, 1982, pp. 367–379.
76. J. Naisbitt, *Megatrends*, Warner, New York, 1984.

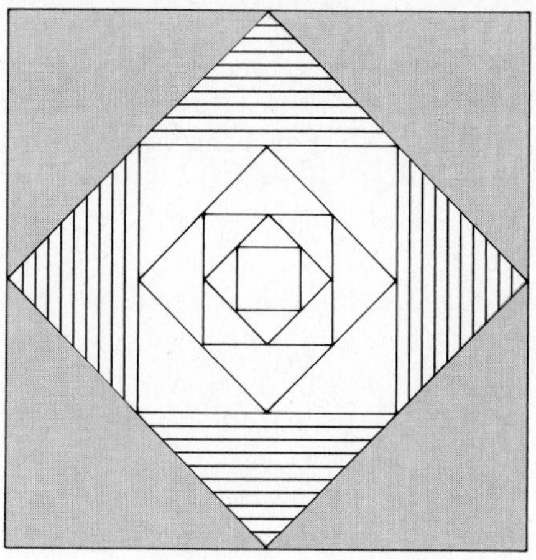

CHAPTER 4
Self-Awareness

Judith Haber
Pamela Price Hoskins
Anita M. Leach
Barbara Flynn Sideleau

LEARNING OBJECTIVES

After studying this chapter, the student should be able to:

1. Define *self-awareness*.
2. Discuss the reciprocal nature of the nurse-client relationship in relation to self-awareness.
3. Define the concept *self*.
4. Discuss the development of the self.
5. Discuss self-awareness from four perspectives:
   a. Cognitive
   b. Emotional
   c. Spiritual
   d. Physical
6. Describe the application of self-awareness to the nurse-client relationship.
7. Describe the problems that may emerge if thoughts, feelings, and values are not synchronous.
8. List self-assessment questions that can be used in developing self-awareness.
9. Describe the self-intervention process.

Nursing takes place in an interpersonal setting and has to do with relationships and interactions concerning the self, the self and others, and the environment. Feelings, thoughts, and behaviors continually emerge and change as a result of the dynamic, reciprocal interaction between nurses and clients.

Traditionally, the focus of the nurse-client relationship has been the client. The nurse has been identified as one who cares for, nurtures, and gives to clients; it is the client whose feelings, thoughts, and behaviors have been of paramount importance. More recently, however, the nurse-client relationship has been viewed as an interactive process in which the perceptions, feelings, and thoughts of both the client and the nurse are significant. Within such a relationship, the nurse and the client both have feelings and needs which are communicated verbally and nonverbally. The interaction process between the nurse and the client can thus be viewed as a two-way phenomenon in which the nurse affects the client and the client affects the nurse.[1,2] The perceptions, feelings, and thoughts that each brings to or experiences in the relationship will influence the nature and quality of the relationship. However, very often nurse and client are unaware of how and when these factors influence the process of the relationship.

Several examples illustrate this point:

> I can't get anywhere with this client. He seems to avoid me. I can't understand why. But then again, he is an alcoholic, and you can't do much with them anyway.

> I forgot to tell my client that we were leaving in 2 weeks. How could I have forgotten? I think that I have trouble saying good-bye, because partings have always been unpleasant for me.

> I feel so distant from my nurse. I feel as though we're on different wavelengths. I want to tell her about myself, but I'm not sure she'd listen or understand. When she has that frown on her face, I am afraid that she will judge me as I feel others do.

These examples reflect the fact that both nurses and clients bring a diversity of thoughts, feelings, behaviors, beliefs, and values to a therapeutic relationship. How do two people who are likely to be very different come together and interact so that one is assisted in gaining or regaining a sense of worth, energy, and direction?

Before nurses can help others, they must first come to know themselves, they must be able to answer the question, "Who am I?" They should be comfortable with themselves and capable of redirecting themselves. One becomes able to accomplish these tasks by achieving self-awareness.

Achieving self-awareness is a process of introspection in which a person—in this case, a nurse—examines and becomes sensitive to the cognitive, emotional, spiritual, and physical dimensions of self, including those that are not conscious. These dimensions include perceptions, feelings, thoughts, values, beliefs, and behavior, as well as stressors that affect them. Becoming aware of these forces through a process of introspection and self-assessment enables the nurse to engage in *self-intervention*, which is a process of understanding and modifying forces within the self that provoke anxiety and interfere with the nurse-client relationship. If nurses ask clients to examine their inner selves and modify dysfunctional patterns in their lives, must not nurses engage in a similar process? Reaching self-awareness increases self-understanding, self-acceptance, and options for action. Nurses who are self-aware will be better able to deal with their own anxiety, anger, sadness, and joy and thus to help clients with all kinds and degrees of problems. Self-awareness also tends to create a more harmonious relationship between mind, body, and spirit. If there is an unidentified problem in one of these three dimensions, the others will be affected as well; therefore, understanding and correcting a problem in one dimension will have a positive effect in others.

The purpose of this chapter is to explore the concept of self-awareness and how it affects nurse-client relationships. Strategies for coping with problems that arise in nurse-client interactions will also be presented. The goal is to improve nurses' therapeutic relationships with clients.

THE SELF

The self (which is discussed in some detail in Chapter 3) is a concept of one's own person as distinguished from other objects in the external world, as a separate, whole being. The self includes

The authors gratefully acknowledge the contribution of Sylvia M. Schudy in the original development of this chapter.

people's appraisals of themselves as well as the appraisals others make of them. It is never constant but is continually changing and emerging in new ways. It is influenced by interactions with others as well as by interaction with the environment; and it also influences the environment—that is, other persons, places, and things.

The appraisals of significant others and the way in which a person perceives them, relates to them, and incorporates them will influence the way in which they become part of the self. It is not uncommon for people to adopt qualities that have been repeatedly attributed to them. For example, when a girl is told that she is not bright and is criticized for her thoughts and opinions, it will probably not take long for her to think of herself in that way. This kind of message can evoke in her the very behaviors that people are ascribing to her. When this kind of input is consistent and sustained, it may become incorporated into her self-image and become a self-fulfilling prophecy. Initially she would be responding to critical external cues; later she would be responding to both external and internal cues as a negative self-view and dysfunctional behavior become established.

The self is not viewed solely in terms of appraisals by others. People do have the ability to bring their behavior under conscious control. They have the ability to communicate with themselves and evaluate discrepancies between their own views and the views of others. Consequently, they can modify their own behavior and guide their own actions.[3] The conclusions that they arrive at will influence the way they view themselves, others, and the environment. This will also play an important part in the way they interact with others. For example, the girl mentioned above who is repeatedly told that she is unintelligent may either incorporate that feedback into her self-image or evaluate it on the basis of what she knows about her own capabilities and discard all or part of it as untrue. The self-view that she develops will influence how she presents herself to and interacts with others. She may present herself as an intelligent, competent person; as a doubtful, semicompetent person; or as an unintelligent, incompetent person. She will participate in relationships in ways that reflect her self-perception.

A person's sense of self—an entity differentiated from the rest of the world—does not develop all at once. Nor does it ever stop developing. The self represents each person's unique pattern of values, attitudes, feelings, ideas, and needs.[4] This pattern results from a biological heredity, beliefs and values developed within a family and a culture, formal learning experiences, and interpersonal relationships. Together, these factors contribute to the formation of the self, the individual personality.

SELF-AWARENESS: A COGNITIVE PERSPECTIVE

The self is dynamic. It is partly conscious, partly unconscious; partly public, partly private. Some aspects of the self are known best by others; some aspects are known only by the self;[5] and some aspects remain largely undiscovered. Self-awareness will be influenced by the degree to which one has an accurate view of the different dimensions of self. Each person has the potential for expanding self-awareness by becoming more fully acquainted with each dimension.

The Johari window, illustrated in Figure 4-1, is a conceptual framework for the dimensions of self and their effect on self-awareness and interpersonal relationships. The self has four distinct components: (1) the public self, the self that is presented to and observed by others; (2) the semipublic self, the self as others perceive it, of which one may not be aware; (3) the private self, the self that is known only to oneself and not revealed to others; and (4) the inner self, the self that is unconscious and unknown even to the individual because its content is too anxiety-provoking to be consciously acknowledged.[5,6,7]

Figure 4-1 The self.
(SOURCE: From Joseph Luft, *Group Processes: An Introduction to Group Dynamics*, National Press Books, Palo Alto, Calif., 1970.)

	Known of self	Not known to self
Known to others	1 Public self	2 Semipublic self (blind area)
Not known to others	3 Private self	4 Inner self (area of unknown)

All four components represent the total self. Thus a change in the size of any area will mean that one or more of the other areas must increase or decrease so that the total remains the same. If the first area, the public self, is small, communication is poor; therefore the goal of this model is to enlarge area 1 and diminish one or more of the others.

Learning more about the self allows one to get in touch with its various dimensions. There are three steps in developing self-awareness cognitively:

1. Listening to yourself
2. Listening to others
3. Letting others listen to you

First, *listening to oneself* involves experiencing genuine emotions and identifying and accepting personal needs. It includes exploring one's own thoughts, feelings, memories, and impulses. It involves experiencing spirituality, as well as being responsive to one's body—experiencing freedom to move in an uninhibited, spontaneous way. In order to uncover these aspects of the self, the public and private selves (areas 1 and 3 of the Johari window) must be explored. For example, a nurse engaged in developing self-awareness might ask the questions shown in Table 4-1 to clarify and understand the uneasiness felt while working with a psychotic client.

Table 4-1

Questions	Answers
1. How do I feel now?	Tense.
2. What is the specific feeling I am experiencing?	Rejection, frustration, inadequacy.
3. What is making me feel this way? What happened to make this feeling arise?	The client told me that I'm a lousy therapist. He remains aloof and bizarre despite my efforts.
4. Is there anything about the way I'm feeling or behaving that may be contributing to the client's behavior?	Perhaps my frustration is being communicated to the client by my body language. I like to see results quickly. The client may sense my frustration and experience me as one more person he is unable to please. He gives up and withdraws rather than tell me what he is experiencing.

Second, by *listening to others*, people learn a lot about themselves. The feedback mechanism of communication opens up area 2 of the self—the semipublic self (see Figure 4-1)—and leads people to develop a greater awareness of themselves as others see them. Adequate knowledge of oneself is possible only through association with other people. As a person relates to others and receives feedback, the perception of self is expanded. This requires active listening as well as openness to the feedback that others provide.

When listening to others, people also learn a lot about the other person in an interaction. Good listeners tend to picture themselves in a situation similar to the one described by a speaker and usually compare their own feelings and responses with those of the other person. This inner activity stimulates greater insight into the self and an empathic understanding of others.

Third, *letting others listen to you* involves self-disclosure. Self-disclosure is a prerequisite for developing greater awareness of oneself; it is only as we reveal ourselves that we become more aware of our feelings, strengths, weaknesses, and areas of growth. This step involves taking risks because what is being disclosed usually belongs to area 3 in Figure 4-1, the private self, which a person avoids or hides from others. A high level of honesty about self and trust in others must be present for such sharing to occur, and it ultimately creates a feeling of greater closeness to people.[4,8]

As a person becomes more knowledgeable about and comfortable with areas 1, 2, and 3 in Figure 4-1, there is less need to be defensive about area 4, the inner self. Although area 4 never becomes completely accessible to consciousness, a person is able to get in touch with some of its anxiety-provoking aspects and work them through. Decreasing anxiety around sensitive "trigger" areas will free energy that can enable the person to perceive and respond to the needs of self and others more effectively.

SELF-AWARENESS: AN EMOTIONAL PERSPECTIVE

Understanding one's own feelings and developing empathy for the feelings of others will make efforts to communicate with others more effective.[9] Self-awareness and empathy are closely related.[2] The ability to understand one's own feelings, the feelings of others, and the way in which they affect one another is difficult to develop because each person is unique. For example:

> Joan, a student nurse, discovers that she is surprisingly intolerant when working with depressed clients. She complains that they seem to be "stuck in their own mud," are full of self-pity, are forever crying about their problems, but are unwilling to do anything to change their self-view or situation. She feels that they enjoy their depression and use it as a way of avoiding responsibility. She finds herself admonishing them to "get hold of themselves," "grow up," and "stop wallowing in self-pity." Joan has had many problems in her life but has rarely allowed herself to experience her own sadness. She humorously describes herself as an advocate of self-control and repression. Her discomfort with negative feelings interferes with her ability to empathize and effectively work with clients who communicate such feelings and are unable to control them.

All people have emotional "triggers," that is, particular feelings such as sadness, anger, fear, anxiety, guilt, and hurt derived from the totality of past experience, which may generate varying degrees of discomfort in the present. On a conscious, public level a feeling such as sadness may be experienced as annoyance, irritation, or anger. Such feelings, when encountered in others, may be responded to with irritation, sarcasm, or disdain. On a deeper, private level, sadness may be experienced as hurt, hopelessness, helplessness, or abandonment and may be too anxiety-provoking and painful to confront directly. On a still deeper level, feelings of profound despair, loneliness, or emptiness may exist but may remain unconscious because they are too painful and anxiety-provoking to be admitted to awareness.

In the example above, emotional triggers may explain Joan's response to depressed clients. The clients' sadness generates similar feelings in Joan, but she experiences and expresses them as annoyance and irritation. Her expressed, or surface, feelings mask the deeper feelings generated by her clients—feelings that are were too painful and anxiety-provoking for her to confront and deal with. In such cases it is difficult for nurses to distinguish their own feelings from those of clients—to know how much they are projecting their own feelings onto the clients, or to what extent the clients' feelings are entering the nurses' own emotional "reservoirs."[1,10]

The settings in which nurses work may also evoke emotional triggers of which the nurse is unaware and which can create problems and impede therapy.

The following example shows how a setting can be an emotional trigger.

> David had been working on a critical-care unit for 6 months. At his 6-month evaluation conference, his head nurse related to him that while his technical skills were satisfactory, he appeared tired, tense, and jumpy; that he had taken the maximum number of sick days possible; and that he seemed to spend time with clients only when they needed physical care. David said, "I feel very pressured by the responsibility of working on a critical-care unit. It seems like an unending struggle to stay ahead of death. I thought that working in critical care would give me a chance to give people the kind of care some of my own family didn't seem to get when they were in similar settings. But it's too much for me; too fast-paced, and every move is too crucial." The head nurse said, "I wonder how your own feelings about having been personally involved with your family when they were in critical-care units has influenced both your desire to work in this setting and your difficulties in fulfulling your responsibilities in a way that seems appropriate to you." David replied, "It's not the clients so much as the setting and what working in it represents to me. Perhaps it's my way of trying to rescue people, in a way that I couldn't with my own relatives. What bothers me, I think, is that I can't rescue everybody, not even in this highly sophisticated unit."

Whenever such a trigger exists, nurses should be able to identify it as well as understand its origin in their life experiences. It is only then that nurses are able to separate their feelings from that which is actually happening in the setting.

Feelings that go unrecognized are expressed indirectly through behavior. For example, unrecognized anger may be expressed as impatience or sarcasm which alienates other people, or as tension headaches or backaches. If a person is completely unaware of an underlying feeling, behavior may be its only manifestation.

In many life situations, and particularly in the nurse-client relationship, unconscious feelings present several problems. First, unrecognized feelings may be manifested as behaviors that are difficult to modify precisely because the underlying feeling is unknown. (For example, a person with underlying guilt may be a chronic worrier and apologizer.)

Second, when people do not recognize their feelings, they are likely to translate those feelings into self-protective behaviors rather than therapeutic ones. (For example, nurses may be anxious about their own mental health and consequently become very distant with and avoid clients who are actively psychotic.)

Third, when people have many feelings that go unrecognized, they may experience only a limited range of feelings; their felt emotions may be few and repetitive. This limits their objectivity and their ability to experience events: they will look for and perceive only what fits their limited range of feelings. For example:

> One nurse had a very hopeless outlook on life. This was reflected in the way she viewed the clients and her job. Regardless of how much clients' behavior improved, she would respond, "They're not really getting better; they're just playing the game to get discharged. They'll be back; nothing much ever really changes." This view made it difficult for her to recognize change in clients, to be supportive of their efforts to change, or to make them feel that she was behind them.

Fourth, when inner feelings go unrecognized, people are unlikely to recognize the same feelings in others; this makes it difficult for them to be empathic. (For instance, Joan, the student nurse in an earlier example, found it difficult to empathize with depressed clients because of her own unresolved feelings of sadness and loss. Joan's lack of awareness of these feelings contributed to the difficulties she was having with her clients.)

Fifth, when feelings go unrecognized, it is difficult to make appropriate decisions because the unrecognized feelings influence decisions in unknown ways. People may also have difficulty separating "shoulds" from the "wants." (For example, a nurse may say, "I *want* to spend time with that client today, but I *should* catch up on paperwork," not recognizing that because the client is withdrawn, the paperwork is the real "want"—a way to avoid rejection.)

Sensitivity to feelings—one's own and others'—can be learned and developed. It is important to recognize feelings because just as much as thoughts, they guide the way we view ourselves and others. Feelings are also instrumental in our view of reality. Becoming more aware of one's feelings includes acknowledgment of positive and negative feelings—both of which can interfere with relationships. Recognizing, acknowledging, and accepting feelings makes nurses less likely to misinterpret people and events, to distort the meaning of messages, to accept other people's ideas as their own, or to make poor decisions. Also, when one is aware of feelings, the feelings are available for modification. Finally, nurses who accept their own feelings can allow clients to have and express feelings too.[1,3,10]

SELF-AWARENESS: A SPIRITUAL PERSPECTIVE

Spirituality is another dimension of the self that nurses come to know, explore, and appreciate. It cannot be described in physical terms, and it is difficult (if not impossible) to measure, but it is reflected in a myriad of behaviors that are unique to each person. Spirituality may be expressed in basic beliefs—a philosophy of life.[11] A system of beliefs, then, is the beginning of a philosophical perspective. Many nurses have religious beliefs and incorporate them in their personal and professional lives. Others experience spirituality, not in a religious sense, but as ethics or as an approach to life or work, such as scientific method. It is from the spiritual part of the self that values, morals, and ethics are derived. The depth and nature of one's spirituality are often determined by significant personal experiences; people sometimes say that they have become aware of the essence of life through the beauty of a sunset, the aroma of a rose, or an act of giving. Such experiences create a sense of connection to life itself and, for some people, to something beyond life. Spirituality is that part of the self which asks questions about the importance, direction, and purpose of life.[11]

Values

Values are personal beliefs about, and attitudes toward, the truth, beauty, or worth of any thought, object, or behavior. They express, or articulate, the spiritual dimension of self-awareness.

Values provide individualized rules by which people live. They are inculcated by family, religious, and cultural teachings that are both overt and covert.

During childhood, people have *child values*—values they have incorporated as acceptable according to the significant authority figures in their lives, such as parents. In adulthood, people may either blindly retain these child values and continue to use them for decision making, or they may sort out and reevaluate child values. If child values are reevaluated, several results are possible. First, child values may, on examination, continue to be valid. They will then become *adult values* and be used to guide decisions. Second, some or all child values may no longer be valid. These may be refined or discarded and replaced by other values that more accurately represent new beliefs and attitudes. Third, both child and adult values may be periodically scrutinized, reassessed, and clarified in response to new experiences. For example, a child value or even an adult value regarding premarital sex may never need to be clarified until, say, one's best friend chooses to live with a lover before marriage. It is also possible to encounter a situation for which one has developed no "official" value and must suddenly formulate one, or a situation which requires that a vague value be clarified. For example:

> Before becoming a nurse, Mark had never thought much about euthanasia. After working on a critical-care unit for 1 year, he developed a very clear value about sustaining clients on life-support systems that guided his decision making.

Beliefs, Attitudes, and Opinions

Understanding the process of valuing means understanding how people come to hold certain beliefs and establish certain behavior patterns. Beliefs that are supported by available evidence are called *rational beliefs*. Beliefs that are adhered to without evidence are called *blind beliefs*. Beliefs that are adhered to despite contrary evidence are called *irrational beliefs*. Dogmatically held beliefs are both blind and irrational, and they are not based on personal experience.[12]

Nurses who adhere dogmatically to blind and irrational beliefs without engaging in a process of self-examination and self-assessment are likely to distort experience to fit their preconceptions. They tend to view people and situations in terms of preconceived notions, rather than as they actually exist. The outcome may be that the nurse operates and relates to people on the basis of stereotypes and myths. For example, a commonly held blind belief is that clients in psychiatric hospitals are violent and dangerous. Nurses who hold this belief will view all clients with whom they work as a threat. This will limit the nurses' ability to accurately view each client in terms of both good and bad qualities. It will also inhibit the nurses' ability to feel secure and work therapeutically with such clients.

Most people do not question beliefs that they hold strongly. They are also unlikely to welcome new information; if other information were allowed to seep in, they might be forced to find validity in other points of view and thus to question their own beliefs. Remaining ignorant of other points of view allows them to avoid change, of course, but it severely limits potential for personal growth and learning that could be derived from the unknown parts of the self.

When a feeling toward a person or a situation exists over time, it is called an *attitude*. When an attitude is coupled with an idea or a belief, it is called an *opinion*. An opinion involves both thoughts and feelings.[12] People feel most comfortable when their beliefs and attitudes are consistent with each other. In order to maintain consistency, they may distract their awareness from ideas that conflict with their beliefs or attitudes, repress a belief or attitude that is inconsistent with one that is more important, or distort their perceptions to fit existing attitudes or beliefs. For example, if nurses have an opinion that family planning is unacceptable, in teaching a postpartum couple, they may omit information about family planning.

Nurses need to be aware of their strongly held beliefs, attitudes, and opinions and how they influence actions and perceptions. To avoid self-deception, it is helpful to acknowledge where one is coming from and to become involved in the process of values clarification.

Values Clarification

Each person is continuously faced with situations which call for thoughts, opinions, decision making, and actions. Nurses are constantly faced with choices in both their personal and their professional lives. Ideally, their choices are based on the values they hold, but frequently they are not clear about what they value.[12]

People have two types of values, cognitive and active. *Cognitive values* are those that are verbally identified and ascribed to. *Active values* are those that people put effort into enacting.[13] The extent to which values are active is reflected in interests, preferences, decisions, and actions. For example:

> Mike has said that he values being honest and direct with clients about their progress. However, other staff members have observed that when clients approach him to talk about their progress, he says that he is too busy and will get to them later. The next day the client will say, "Hey, you never got back to me," and Mike will say, "In a few minutes." Apparently, although he pays lip service to honesty and directness, this nurse is operating on other values. In contrast, Allan works in a day hospital program for chronic psychotic clients. He said that he believes each client has a potential for health. No matter how many times clients have regressed or been rehospitalized, Allan remains interested, encouraging, and involved in helping them care for themselves and function in the community. Allan clearly puts his values into action.

Valuing, according to Raths,[13] is composed of three processes and seven subprocesses:

1. Prizing one's beliefs and behaviors
   a. Prizing and cherishing
   b. Publicly affirming, when appropriate
2. Choosing one's beliefs and behaviors
   a. Choosing from alternatives
   b. Choosing after consideration of consequences
   c. Choosing freely
3. Acting on one's beliefs
   a. Taking action
   b. Demonstrating a pattern of action that is consistent and repetitive

Valuing processes are not meant to instill any particular set of values. Rather, they are to be used in connection with beliefs and behavior patterns that are already formed or emerging.[1]

There are several ways in which people learn values. The process described above is an example of *values clarification*, that is, a systematic way of teaching the *process* of valuing rather than the *content* of a specific set of values. To accomplish this, teachers use strategies which help students become aware of their beliefs and values, choose among alternatives, consider the consequences of the various alternatives, and match their actions with their stated beliefs. Other ways in which people learn values are through moralizing, laissez-faire situations, and modeling. *Moralizing* is a direct, if somewhat subtle, method of inculcating one's own or desired values in another person. A *laissez-faire approach* leaves people alone to forge their own values. This may be a problem for young people, who tend to feel confused and to experience conflict if they are left totally on their own. *Modeling* transmits values by setting an example. Actions should match value statements if learning by example is to occur.[14]

Simon and others indicate that the small amount of research done so far shows the values clarification approach to be the most advantageous of the four ways of learning values. They indicate that people who engage in values clarification are less apathetic, less conforming, less contentious but more critical in their thinking, and more likely to follow through in their actions. This learning process should allow time for discussion and assessment of both comfortable and uncomfortable values.[14]

SELF-AWARENESS: A PHYSICAL PERSPECTIVE

In addition to its cognitive, emotional, and spiritual dimensions, self-awareness has a physical dimension. Physical processes communicate information about the body. Nurses (like other people) must attend to this information in order to maintain physical well-being.

Attending to aspects of the physical self involves knowing what one is like—"who one is"—physically. This includes being aware of what is "normal," or synchronous, with regard to different body rhythms. For example, nurses should be aware of the usual patterns of their sleep-wake cycles, including how many hours of sleep leave them feeling rested and vibrant as opposed to feeling fatigued and lethargic, and whether they are "day people" or "night people"—that is, whether their peak functioning occurs during the morning, the afternoon, the evening, or the night.[15] A nurse can use this information in selecting work hours that are congruent with optimal periods of wakefulness.

This information can also help nurses to understand their feelings of fatigue, lethargy, and irritability when the sleep-wake cycle and the work cycle do not mesh. The body's thermostat—that is, one's temperature—may also be rhythmical, fluctuating not only with the temperature of the external environment, but with the internal environment as well. For example, a person who is fatigued often feels chilled even if the weather is warm or the room is well heated. Similarly, a person who is anxious may feel hot, flushed, and diaphoretic even in cold weather or a chilly room. It is important for people to know what a comfortable body temperature feels like, so that "feeling cold" and "feeling hot" can be evaluated in terms of a norm. Another rhythmical phenomenon is the menstrual cycle; for women, the physical self varies with phases of the cycle. Women who experience premenstrual syndrome (PMS) should recognize that irritability, depression, or fatigue before the onset of menstruation often affect work performance. For a nurse, irritability caused by PMS may manifest itself in feelings of helplessness with clients or colleagues.

Nurses also need to be aware of their optimal body weight, one that is neither too high nor too low. A person who is too thin may be easily fatigued, anergic, or susceptible to infections. A person who is too heavy may feel "blobby," listless, and uncomfortably bloated. Both types of people may sense that they are not functioning optimally, may feel unattractive, and thus may be uncomfortable with the physical self.

All people, including nurses, must be receptive to internal and external clues—messages about levels of physical well-being. Fatigue, irritability, apathy, boredom, lack of emotional responsiveness, and reactions that seem out of proportion to what is happening are among the many clues to dysynchronization within the body.

For nurses, dysynchronization in one or more parameters of physical being may have a profound effect on work performance and relationships. For example:

> Andrea, a staff nurse on a surgical unit, rotated to all three shifts within any given month. She never felt that she had gotten enough sleep. She felt tired, drained, and listless. She found that she had difficulty concentrating on her work and completing her assignment and was losing patience with clients and colleagues alike. She also knew that she was not eating properly; her irregular sleep pattern had disrupted her eating pattern as well as her appetite. She was losing weight, too. Andrea was so fatigued that she had no interest in exercising or socializing. As she said to a colleague on the unit, "I feel awful; it's as if my body doesn't belong to me, and I know that I've been ignoring what it's been telling me."

Respect for one's physical being includes being sensitive to physical clues or signals. Providing for adequate rest, exercise, recreation, and a balanced diet keeps the body physically fit, restores and maintains energy, and enhances responsiveness and relatedness.

THERAPEUTIC USE OF SELF

The basic therapeutic tool used by the nurse is the self.[16] Therapeutic use of self requires that nurses be aware of and confront their thoughts, feelings, values, and actions. This is a prerequisite to developing understanding about how these factors affect the nurse-client relationship. Nurses must identify and understand their own feelings, values, thoughts, and actions so that they can separate those that belong to themselves from those that belong to clients.[1] Nurses who are able to do this will be able to distinguish between behaviors that are occurring in response to their own thoughts, values, and feelings and those that are occurring in response to what is going on with clients. This increases nurses' ability to accurately assess clients' needs and intervene appropriately.[17]

A balance between the nurse's thoughts, feelings, and values provides the context in which intervention based on clients' needs can occur. When thoughts, feelings, and values are not synchronous and the nurse is unaware of the discrepancy, several problems can emerge. First, the perceptual field will be distorted, inhibiting the nurse's ability to collect objective, verifiable data. Instead, the nurse may operate on the basis of expectations; preconceived beliefs, attitudes, or opinions; or projected feelings. Second, the lack of objective data may lead the nurse to make connections between ideas, events, and feelings that are not necessarily logical or valid. Third, the nurse may make assumptions which are erroneous. Fourth, decision making, intervention, and evaluation are impaired because they have been built on an inaccurate data base.[1,3,10]

An example of dysynchronization in thoughts, feelings, and values follows:

> A young nurse named Cindy was working on an inpatient unit of a psychiatric hospital. Jerry, aged 19, was a client on the unit. Overtly, he was a handsome, well-dressed, charming, intelligent, witty adolescent. He was "into" Zen and other mystical religions. In fact, he had spent some time in India studying with a guru. Cindy liked him and said to the rest of the staff, "He's not crazy; he's a free spirit, and he reminds me of my younger brother." At the same time, Jerry's impulsivity and destructiveness were driving the rest of the staff to distraction. Cindy was unable to assess his behavior accurately because her feelings were distorting her perceptual field. She was overidentifying with the client. The treatment plan consisted of setting limits and establishing consistency. Cindy did not agree with the rest of the staff, nor did she see the need for this approach. Thus, she sabotaged the treatment plan by not enforcing the limits agreed upon by the team.

SELF-ASSESSMENT

Nurses spend most of their time trying to help clients whose thoughts, feelings, and values are not working together in a synchronous way. Before nurses can do this with clients, they must be able to do it with themselves. A myriad of feelings are generated in the nurse-client relationship because it is a reciprocal process. Self-awareness is necessary to examine feelings and restore a sense of objectivity and empathy. Some self-assessment questions a nurse might ask in relation to the individual, the family, and the community appear in Table 4-2.

When feelings, thoughts, and behaviors are identified through self-assessment and synchronized through self-awareness, the nurse is able to perceive how these dimensions of self are influencing clients' behavior and care whether the client is an individual, a family, or a community. The acknowledged feelings may be unpleasant, but once understood, they pose less of a threat to the self than unacknowledged feelings do. When nurses have developed skill in listening to themselves and are ready to acknowledge and accept what they feel, they are ready to begin listening to clients and to hear what they are saying. They will then be better able to understand the dynamics of clients' behavior and

Table 4-2 Questions for Self-Assessment

Individual
1. Who is this client?
2. What does the client mean to me?
3. What are my feelings about this client, both positive and negative?
4. What problematic behaviors are being exhibited by the client?
5. What are my feelings about the client's behavior?
6. How do I handle those feelings?
7. What other situations have elicited the same feelings? How did I deal with the feelings in those situations?
8. What kinds of attitudes or opinions do I have about the client's behavior?
9. Where do these ideas, feelings, and values come from?
10. To what extent does the way I am feeling right now interfere with my ability to relate therapeutically to this client?
11. How am I feeling physically? Am I tired, restless, apathetic, and so on?
12. How do my perceptions compare with those of other team members?
13. Does this client remind me of significant others, and, if so, how?
14. Does the setting for care influence my ability to intervene effectively?
15. Is there anything I could have done differently to provide better care for this client?
Family
1. When am I uncomfortable with the client's family?
2. Are there people in the client's family who remind me of my own family?
3. With whom do I feel most uncomfortable in my family?
4. How do I view the family's participation in the client's problem?
5. Do I ally with either the client or the family around a particular issue?
6. Do I identify with the problems family members have in managing the client?
7. To what extent do I take on family roles that maintain dysfunctional behavior?
Community
1. What feelings are generated in me by this community?
2. What are the problematic issues in the community that I respond to?
3. Have I encountered such issues on other occasions?
4. How I have dealt with them?
5. How successful do I perceive myself to have been in dealing with them?
6. What about the present problem is interfering with my ability to deal with it effectively?

focus more on the *process* of interactions than the *content*.

In the therapeutic setting, nurses help clients to become aware of and to disclose feelings, desires, and thoughts. If these feelings are validated by another as being acceptable, clients feel that they are "OK," and this leads to greater self-acceptance. Self-acceptance leads to the ability to sort out feelings and thoughts and discover how they interact as well as to take risks in developing alternative behaviors that may be more satisfying.

Therapeutic "stalls" occur in the nurse-client relationship when expectations are not met and feelings are experienced which are not consciously acknowledged. Feelings that are not acknowledged cannot be analyzed and worked through; hence they lead to a vague sense of threat which gives rise to actual anxiety. Rising levels of anxiety further undermine awareness, leading to stereotyping and judgmental behavior, which interferes with the continuing therapeutic process. When this occurs, both nurse and client must return to the self-awareness process to identify feelings and determine what is causing the stall. Only when the relevant issues and feelings are resolved can the therapeutic process resume.

Nurses who value self-disclosure face a challenge in a society which says, "Mind your own business," and "Don't ask personal questions." However, self-awareness puts them in a much better position to empathize with clients and encourage self-disclosure. Students and beginning practitioners need to learn when and how to use selective self-disclosure in interactions with clients. Clients move toward wellness as they are helped to become aware and accepting of their real selves.[2]

The nurse-client interaction can be thought of as "pivoting" on six *core dimensions*: empathic understanding, concreteness, respect, genuineness, confrontation, and immediacy (see Chapters 12 and 13). All require self-awareness on the part of the nurse. Nurses' understanding of their clients is in large part a result of awareness of the feelings clients generate in them. Nurses' self-awareness facilitates the helping process, which moves the client toward health. Thus, the nurse is better able to assess the client's situation, understand the dynamics of the client's behavior, formulate nursing diagnoses and outcome criteria, and carry out nursing interventions in a more accurate, comprehensive way. The nurse then need not hide from feelings and thoughts but is free to delve into the self and explore the impact and purpose of clients' behavior; thus it becomes possible to formulate effective interventions.

SELF-INTERVENTION

Attaining self-awareness is a dynamic, ongoing process. Nurses strive to discover the forces within themselves that are influencing the nurse-client relationship. Once these thoughts, feelings, values, and behaviors have been discovered, nurses must examine the specific ways in which they positively or negatively affect relationships with clients. In addition, they must identify ways to modify such forces so that they can be more effective care givers. The combined process of discovery and change can be called *self-intervention*.

Nurses can engage in the self-intervention process in several different ways. First, they can use individual introspection to design change. However, since the perceptual field often has blind spots that limit the ability to see oneself and others clearly, that method has limitations, at least for beginners who may not have extensive self-understanding or experience with the self-awareness process. Second, they can use a supervisory relationship with a liaison nurse, a clinical specialist, or an instructor which is designed to monitor the nurse-client relationship, provide objective feedback regarding the process and content of the relationship, and provide an arena for identifying strategies for implementing and evaluating change.[18] Nurses may also use professional counseling to increase self-awareness and personal growth. Third, supervision by a peer group can provide a forum for case presentations and give objective feedback about problems experienced in the nurse-client relationship, as well as suggestions for change. Such supervision can be viewed as an opportunity for collaborative exchange which becomes a learning experience for everyone involved. Fourth, conferences of a nursing team or interdisciplinary team offer another opportunity to participate in collaborative learning experiences. Different team members working with the same client or group of clients take the opportunity to present their views of the client, their work with the client, and problems encountered. These conferences provide another forum for the exchange of thoughts, feelings, and potential strategies and provide feedback from a variety of sources. Each person's viewpoint may have something valuable to offer. Exchanging viewpoints provides data that can increase self-awareness.

Whichever method is used, nurses have to be active participants in the self-awareness process. If a nurse does not offer the data for examination, whether in a one-to-one relationship or a group, then nothing will be accomplished, regardless of the context.

Specific suggestions for self-intervention are given below.[1,3,10,19]

1. Use active listening skills to identify positive and negative patterns in interpersonal style. These data can also be identified by using process recordings, audiotapes, or videotapes.
2. Reflect on one's own past life in terms of the influences that have been instrumental in creating the person that exists today. Use a systematic review process; constructing a genogram (a family map) is one way of doing this (see Chapter 19). This enables the person to identify repetitive patterns, to appreciate significant actions, and to find meaning in data.
3. Identify how various past experiences and learning are influencing current relationships. This involves acknowledging both positive and negative thoughts, feelings, and values. All too often people have learned to block off their awareness and expression of certain feelings. Children have been taught in obvious and subtle ways that certain feelings (such as anger and sadness) and certain behaviors (such as assertiveness, rudeness, and selfishness) are unacceptable to significant others. In order to retain love and approval, they comply, not by eliminating a feeling or behavior, but rather by acting as if it did not exist. Nurses may receive similar messages from teachers or colleagues. They may perceive that it is not acceptable to find a client repulsive or to feel frustrated with, angry with, or hopeless about a client. Positive feelings such as attraction and love, can also interfere with interactions if they remain unrecognized.
4. Explore any conflict between feelings, thoughts, values, and behavior and the way in which it is manifested in nurse-client relationships. Nurses should also explore conflicts between theory and personal experience. Continuous expansion of one's knowledge base may provide a foundation for reorganizing perceptions and attitudes which in turn influence behavior. Continuing education may also provide a vehicle for accomplishing this.
5. Analyze clients' behavior that the nurse perceives to have precipitated problematic feelings or conflict. Doing this provides a way for the nurse to look at his or her own response. Through a process of analysis nurses may be able to differentiate between feelings, thoughts, values, and behavior that belong to the client and those that belong to the nurse. Aspects of self which have been projected onto another can then be clarified and redefined. This enables all participants to be clear on their parts in the process and facilitates constructive relationships. The nurse will be able to perceive both self and client in a more accurate way, draw unbiased impressions from the client based on behavioral observations, respond to clients' cues, and address clients' concerns.
6. Accept feelings, thoughts, and values for what they are. This makes nurses less vulnerable to other people's ideas about how they should feel. It enables them to separate their personal selves and experiences from those of others. Nurses, instead of feeling hurt or insulted when clients imply disapproval about what they feel, should realize that clients may merely disapprove of their feelings, not their treatment. When nurses accept in a more complete way their right to their own feelings, they can allow clients the right to have and express their own feelings as well.
7. Recognize mental, emotional, spiritual, and physical stress in the nurse's personal and professional life. Nurses whose lives are very stressful are vulnerable to personal and professional burnout. Nurses must maintain their well-being by taking care of themselves. They need to be assertive and have the ability to say "no" to excessive demands, and to set limits on their own behavior. For example, working too many hours or beyond one's level of skill may be stressful and thus indicate a need for self-intervention. Time reserved for rest, relaxation, soli-

tude, socialization, exercise, fun, and self-improvement is essential for renewing vitality and enthusiasm. Nurses who can take some time off return to work feeling refreshed and ready for involvement. This is obviously preferable to waiting until patience runs out and then breaking away inappropriately—becoming distant, aloof, or aggressive.

Self-intervention is essential for maintaining effective nurse-client relationships. Nurses are responsible for finding the most effective vehicles for this process.

SUMMARY

The nurse-client relationship is an interactive therapeutic encounter in which the perceptions, feelings, thoughts, beliefs, and values of both the client and the nurse are significant. Because each person brings different elements to the relationship, it is necessary to have a vehicle or method for coming together and interacting in a way that will help the client regain a sense of worth, energy, and direction.

Before nurses can help others, they must come to know themselves. In order to do this, they must develop *self-awareness* through a process of introspection in which they try to heighten their sensitivity to the cognitive, emotional, spiritual, and physical dimensions of self, including those that operate unconsciously. The outcome of this process is greater self-understanding, greater self-acceptance, and more options for action.

The self is a concept of one's own person as distinguished from others. It consists of one's own appraisals as well as the appraisals of others. Nurses can look at the self and develop self-awareness from cognitive, emotional, spiritual, and physical perspectives. From a cognitive perspective, the Johari window can be used to become more aware of aspects of the self (the public self, the semipublic self, the private self, and the inner self); and one can become more self-aware in three ways: by *listening to yourself; listening to others;* and *letting others listen to you.* From an emotional perspective, understanding one's own feelings and developing empathy will make efforts to communicate with others more effective. Awareness of one's own emotional "triggers," or sensitivities, is essential for understanding reactions to clients. From a spiritual perspective, nurses need to understand the beliefs and values that give meaning and purpose to their own lives as well as to the lives of others. Development and clarification of values are critical. From a physical perspective, self-awareness includes communication with one's body and awareness of information the body provides about physical well-being.

The basic therapeutic tool used by the nurse is the self. Therapeutic use of self requires that nurses be aware of and confront their own thoughts, feelings, values, beliefs, physicality, and actions. This is a prerequisite to developing an understanding of how these factors affect the nurse-client relationship. The therapeutic use of self in such a situation is based on a process of self-assessment and self-intervention.

REFERENCES

1. P. Seeger, "Self-Awareness and Nursing," *Journal of Psychiatric Nursing and Mental Health Services,* August 1979, pp. 24–26.
2. C. K. Gulino, "Entering the Mysterious Dimension of Others: An Existential Approach to Nursing Care," *Nursing Outlook,* no. 6, 1982, pp. 352–357.
3. J. Campbell, "The Relationship of Nursing and Self-Awareness," *Advances in Nursing Science,* 1980, pp. 15–24.
4. Gertrude Ujhely, *Determinants of the Nurse-Patient Relationship,* Springer, New York, 1968.
5. Joseph Luft, *Group Processes: An Introduction to Group Dynamics,* National Press Books, Palo Alto, Calif., 1970.
6. Leda Saulnier and Teresa Simard, *Personal Growth and Interpersonal Relations,* Prentice-Hall, Englewood Cliffs, N.J., 1973.
7. G. J. Chelhune et al., *Self-Disclosure: Origins, Patterns, and Implications of Openness in Interpersonal Relationships.* Jossey-Bass Publishers, Washington, D.C., 1979.
8. Sidney Jourard, *The Transparent Self,* Van Nostrand-Reinhold, New York, 1971.
9. E. LaMonica, "Construct Validity of An Empathy Instrument," *Research in Nursing and Health,* vol. 4, no. 4, 1981, pp. 389–400.
10. S. McGaran, "On Developing Empathy: Teaching Students Self-Awareness," *American Journal of Nursing,* vol. 78, no. 5, May 1978, pp. 859–861.
11. J. A. Shelly et al., *Spiritual Dimensions of Mental Health,* Inter Varsity, Downers Grove, Ill., 1983.

12. Diane B. Ustal, "Searching for Values," *Images*, vol. 9, no. 1, 1977, pp. 15–17.
13. L. Raths, H. Merril, and S. Simon, *Values and Teaching*, Merrill, Columbus, Ohio, 1966.
14. S. B. Simon, L. W. Howe, and H. Kirschenbaum, *Values Clarification: A Handbook of Practical Strategies for Teachers and Students*, Hart, New York, 1972.
15. C. N. Hoskins, "Chronobiology and Health," *Nursing Outlook*, vol. 29, no. 10, 1981, pp. 572–576.
16. Madeleine Clemence, Sr., "Existentialism: A Philosophy of Commitment," *American Journal of Nursing*, vol. 66, no. 3, March 1966, pp. 500–505.
17. Hildegard Peplau, *Interpersonal Relationships in Nursing*, Putnam, New York, 1952.
18. P. J. Karns and T. A. Schwab, "Therapeutic Communication and Clinical Instruction," *Nursing Outlook*, vol. 30, no. 1, 1982, pp. 39–43.
19. B. Talento and L. Crockett-McKeever, "Improving Interviewing Techniques," *Nursing Outlook*, vol. 31, no. 4, 1983, pp. 234–235.

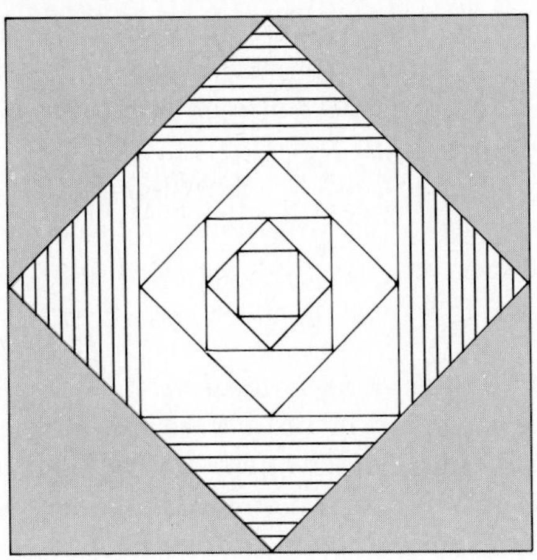

CHAPTER 5 Developmental Processes

Judith Haber

LEARNING OBJECTIVES

After studying this chapter, the student should be able to:

1. Discuss the systems properties of wholeness, interrelatedness, and complexity in the developmental process.
2. Compare and contrast the developmental theories of Freud, Erikson, Sullivan, Mahler, Piaget, Levinson, Lidz, Sheehy, Neugarten, and Havighurst.
3. Describe the significance of developmental processes to nursing practice.
4. Identify the phases of the life cycle.
5. Discuss physical, cognitive, psychosocial and spiritual development in each phase of the life cycle.
6. Define developmental stall.
7. Identify potential developmental stalls in each phase of the life cycle.
8. Using a developmental model, provide anticipatory guidance to individuals and families.

Development is a continuous evolutionary process that becomes increasingly complex and diverse and has no "final" stage. All aspects of human development are interrelated and integrated.

The systems properties of wholeness, interrelatedness, and complex interaction make it impossible to look at human development as a rigid sequence of events that occurs without fail at specific times and in specific ways for everyone.[1] Each person's development is a unique process that emerges out of continuous interaction with the environment. Because behavior is probabilistic and unique and cannot be predicted in an absolute way, developmental norms are relative, not absolute, and serve as tools for communication rather than as generalizations about people.[2] The complete study of the life cycle must take into account all of the physical, cognitive, psychosocial, and spiritual forces that combine to provide a unique matrix for the growth and development of each individual.

The human life cycle can be divided into nine phases: (1) infancy, (2) early childhood, (3) middle childhood, (4) late childhood, (5) adolescence, (6) young adulthood, (7) adulthood, (8) middle adulthood, and (9) late adulthood. The completion of each phase represents a turning point, or a transition to the next phase. Some disequilibrium is inherent in any transition, of course; in this context, disequilibrium can be seen as arising when developmental tasks of one phase[3] are challenged by the demands of the next. The person's sense of comfort and security is disrupted; thus insecurity and struggle may result.

Developmental turning points, and the disequilibrium associated with them, are often referred to as *maturational,* or *developmental, crises.* Each crisis represents a situation that has the potential for either positive resolution and human growth or negative resolution and developmental stall. The term *developmental stall* implies that, at some stage, developmental needs are unmet, issues are unresolved, and tasks are not mastered. As a result, movement to the next stage is inhibited, and, therefore, dysfunctional behavior patterns may emerge.

ORGANIZING THEORIES

Theoretical models of growth and development provide a framework for examining the life cycle. The theories of Freud, Sullivan, Erikson, Mahler, and Piaget (among others) have contributed to our understanding of human development. Each of these theorists described developmental processes, issues, and conflicts from a unique viewpoint.

Freud, a founder of the psychoanalytic school, described stages from birth through adolescence, focusing primarily on psychosexual development as well as aspects of consciousness and personality.[3]

Sullivan,[4] a founder of the interpersonal school, also described stages from birth through adolescence, but dealt only generally with adulthood. He was interested primarily in the interpersonal forces that contribute to development of the self.

Erikson,[5] a psychoanalyst who considered social forces as being essential to development, identified eight stages of development from birth through late adulthood; his is the most comprehensive schema of development throughout the life cycle. He dealt mainly with developmentally related psychosexual conflicts that result from personal and social experiences.

Mahler described a "separation-individuation" process that takes place, for the most part, during the first 3 years of life. It is out of this process that the sense of self as a separate being and autonomous ego functions emerge.[6,7]

Piaget discussed the processes of cognitive development from birth through adolescence.[8,9]

Other theorists, such as Lidz, Levinson, and Sheehy,[10–12] have focused on the developmental processes of youth through middle adulthood. Havighurst and Neugarten[13,14] described the developmental processes of late adulthood. (Their theories will be discussed in the appropriate developmental sections of this chapter.

Table 5-1 presents a comparative picture of the primary developmental focuses of these theorists and Freud, Erikson, Sullivan, Mahler, and Piaget.

Freud*

The major assumption of Freud's theoretical model is that all behavior is meaningful. Freud, a psychoanalyst, considered every thought, feeling, action, and dream to be an expression of a unique and important aspect of the person. He considered the primary motivation of behavior to be anxiety,

* Portions of this section from Pamela Price Hoskins, "Theoretical Models," in the second edition of this book.

which is an unconsciously motivated experience of tension or dread related to loss of self-image. Freud's theoretical model has two major parts: aspects of consciousness and aspects of personality.[3]

Aspects of Consciousness

Aspects of consciousness are the conscious, the preconscious, and the unconscious. The *conscious* includes all elements that are easily remembered. Elements that are somewhat difficult to remember but can be recalled with help are *preconscious*. *Unconscious* materials are thoughts, feelings, actions, experiences, and dreams that are not remembered, are very difficult to bring into consciousness, and are not recognized if one is told of them.

Aspects of Personality

Freud divided the personality into the id, the ego, and the superego. The *id* includes instinctive forces and is primarily unconscious. If uncontrolled by the ego, the superego, or both, the id would lead people to "kill, plunder, and destroy." The id's unconscious forces find expression through thoughts, feelings, and perceptions. Expressions of id would include, for instance, devouring several pounds of cotton candy at a country fair or having a temper tantrum after finding out about a low grade. The *ego* appraises the environment, assesses reality, stays in touch with bodily and environmental changes, and directs motor activity. The *superego* contains the rigid, absolute rules that direct thoughts, feelings, and actions. The term *conscience* is thought to be analogous to *superego*, but conscience is generally present in conscious awareness, whereas the superego includes unconscious as well as conscious material. The superego often directly opposes the id; the ego, with its reality orientation, maintains the balance between the id and the superego. *Ego strength* is the ability of the ego to maintain a sense of reality, to keep unconscious material buried, and to deal effectively with the forces of the id and superego. Whether a person exhibits neuroses or psychoses depends on ego strength. A person with a high degree of ego strength is better able to maintain a sense of reality even when experiencing severe anxiety.

Certain experiences, thoughts, and feelings generate tremendous anxiety; the ego defends against this anxiety by relegating these unacceptable experiences to the unconscious. The more energy is required to keep these experiences unconscious, the less is available for innovative, fulfilling experiences. When a person must avoid experiences that threaten to allow unconscious material to emerge, a neurotic personality configuration develops.

Stages of Development

Freud thought that sexual development was the basis of many unconscious conflicts and formulated a schema of sexual growth to clarify stages and emerging conflicts. Table 5-1 (pages 90–96) lists the time of development and the characteristics of each developmental stage. According to Freudian theory, if all stages of development are negotiated successfully, a person is emotionally mature. But difficulty in negotiating one of the stages also makes the next stage more difficult, and unresolved conflicts at any stage remain part of the personality. Such conflicts are often unconscious and thus must find expression through dreams or through inappropriate emotions or thoughts.[3]

RELEVANCE TO NURSING

Several of Freud's theoretical constructs can help nurses develop a perspective for understanding human behavior. First, Freud implies that behavior is never random or purposeless. For example, a woman's repeated pregnancies may be viewed as results of her unconscious wish to remain dependent, her unconscious need for love objects, or simply her conscious wish for a large family.

Second, the Freudian model of personality structure—id, ego, and superego—provides a useful framework for thinking about how the personality functions or dysfunctions. For example, a nurse who sees a toddler coloring on a wall with crayons would understand that although this behavior is unacceptable, it is natural at the child's stage of development because at this stage the ego and superego are only rudimentary. (The nurse would set limits on the child's behavior or redirect it.) On the other hand, if a 7-year-old did the same thing, a nurse would consider the child's ego and superego development inadequate; by age 7, a child should know that this is inappropriate.

Third, the Freudian schema for growth and development makes it clear that each phase of sexual growth and development involves specific experiences and conflicts; these must be success-

Table 5-1 Comparison of the Major Developmental Theorists

	Freud	Erikson	Sullivan	Mahler	Piaget	Levinson, Lidz, Sheehy	Neugarten	Havighurst
Stage	Oral	Infancy	Infancy	1. Symbiosis 2. Separation-individuation Phase 1: Differentiation Phase 2: Practicing	Sensorimotor			
Age	Birth to 18 months	Birth to 18 months	Birth to 18 months	1. Birth to 4–5 months 2. Phase 1: 4–5 months to 7–10 months Phase 2: 7–10 months to 16–18 months	Birth to 18 months			
Central task	Learning to deal with anxiety-producing experiences by using the mouth and tongue	Trust versus mistrust *Positive resolution:* Learning to trust others. Developing a sense of trust in self *Negative resolution:* Mistrust, withdrawal, estrangement	Learning to count on others to gratify wishes and needs	Development of a symbiotic bond with the nurturing figure. Increasing awareness of self as a separate person. Beginning imitative use of autonomous ego functions	Learning about self and the environment through sensorimotor exploration of objects and events and imitation			
Stage	Anal	Early childhood	Childhood	Separation-individuation Phase 3: Rapprochement Phase 4: Object constancy	Preoperational Preconceptual phase			
Age	18 months to 3 years	18 months to 3 years	18 months to 6 years	Phase 3: 16–18 to 25 months Phase 4: 25 to 36 months	2 to 4 years			

Central task	Learning muscle control, especially that involved with urination and defecation	Autonomy versus shame and doubt *Positive resolution:* Learning self-control and the extent to which the environment can be influenced by direct manipulation *Negative resolution:* Compulsive self-restraint or compliance; willfulness, defiance	Learning to accept interference with one's wishes in relative comfort, to delay gratification	Development of an acute awareness of self as a separate person. Resolution of separation anxiety; expanded use of autonomous ego functions such as memory, perception, and reality testing leads to internalization of mental images that results in object constancy	Learning to think in terms of mental images; development of expressive language and symbolic play
Stage	Phallic	Late childhood	Childhood (continued)		Preoperational Intuitive phase
Age	3 to 6 years	3 to 5 years	18 months to 6 years		4 to 7 years
Central task	Learning sexual identity and developing awareness of the genital area	Initiative versus guilt *Positive resolution:* Learning the extent to which assertiveness and purpose will influence the environment; beginning ability to evaluate one's own behavior *Negative resolution:* Lack of self-confidence, pessimism, fear of wrongdoing, overcontrol and overrestriction of own activities	Learning to accept interference with one's wishes in relative comfort, to delay gratification		Learning to separate disparate objects and events into a rudimentary classification system. Egocentric thought is reflected in persistent thought and animism. Expansion of expressive language

(Continued.)

Table 5-1 Continued

	Freud	Erikson	Sullivan	Mahler	Piaget	Levinson, Lidz, Sheehy	Neugarten	Havighurst
Stage	Latency	School age	Juvenile		Concrete operations			
Age	6 to 12 years	6 to 12 years	6 to 9 years		6–8 to 12 years			
Central task	Quiet stage during which sexual energy is repressed and sexual development lies dormant	Industry versus inferiority *Positive resolution:* Learning to use energies to create, develop, and manipulate. Development of a sense of competence *Negative resolution:* Disappointment in own abilities; loss of hope; sense of being mediocre, sense of inadequacy	Learning to form satisfactory relationships with peers		Learning to reason in a systematic way and apply rules to things that are seen and heard. Beginning of abstract thought and reversible operations			
Stage	Genital	Adolescence	Preadolescence Early adolescence Late adolescence		Formal operations			
Age	12 years to early adulthood	12 to 20 years	9 to 12 years 12 to 14 years 14 to 21 years		12 years through adulthood			
Central task	Developing sexual maturity and learning to form satisfactory relationships with the opposite sex	Identity versus role diffusion *Positive resolution:* Integration of life experiences into a coherent sense of self; plans for actualizing one's abilities *Negative resolution:* Doubt about sexual identity; inability to find an occupational identity; personality confusion	Learning to relate to a friend of the same sex. Learning to master independence and to establish satisfactory relationships with members of the opposite sex. Developing an enduring, intimate relationship with a member of the opposite sex		Learning to think using abstract, conceptual operations. Refinement of reasoning abilities leads to the capacity to visualize multiple logical relationships between classes or between and among several different properties			

Stage	Young adulthood	Young adulthood
Age	18 to 25 years	20 to 28 years
Central task	Intimacy versus isolation *Positive resolution:* Development of an intimate relationship with another person; commitment to work *Negative resolution:* Avoidance of intimacy, avoidance of relationship, career, or lifestyle commitments	Development of a life dream; development of an occupational choice which represents the selection of a way of life Decision making about marital, parenting, or relationship choices and options
Stage	Adulthood	Adulthood
Age	21 to 45 years	29 to 39 years
Central task	Generativity versus stagnation *Positive resolution:* Establishing a family and guiding the next generation. Expansion of creativity, productivity, and concern for others *Negative resolution:* Self-concern and self-indulgence, pseudointimacy, lack of interests and commitments	Extension or revision of work and relationship commitments Childbearing and childreaming Consolidation of self-identity

(Continued.)

Table 5-1 Continued

	Freud	Erikson	Sullivan	Mahler	Piaget	Levinson, Lidz, Sheehy	Neugarten	Havighurst
Stage		Maturity				Midlife transition	Midele age	Middle age
Age		45 years to death				39 to 42	40 to 49	40 to 49
Central task		Integrity versus despair *Positive resolution:* Acceptance of one's life as having been meaningful, fulfilling, and worthwhile. Extension of interests and relationships; providing a legacy for the next generation *Negative resolution:* Fear of death, sense of loss, lack of perceived meaning in one's life				Confronting the discrepancies between one's hopes and dreams of youth and what has actually been achieved. Realistic evaluation of values, future directions, and life as a whole. Adjustment to physiological changes, growing children, and relationship changes	Achieving adult responsibilities as parent, worker, and community member Seeing the environment as one that rewards risk taking and boldness Feeling that personal energy matches the energy of the outer world	Achieving adult, civic, and social responsibility Establishing and maintaining an economic standard of living Assisting teenagers to become responsible adults Developing leisure-time activities Relating to one's spouse as a person Accepting the physiological changes of middle age Adjusting to aging parents

Stage	Maturity	Middle age	Middle age	Middle age
Age	45 years to death	42 to 65–70 years	50 to 65–70 years	50 to 65–70 years
Central task	Integrity versus despair As above	Reintegration of self-identity Acceptance of aloneness and individuality. Extension of relationships Renewal and extension of secondary interests Launching of children and grandparenting Acceptance of physical manifestations of aging Redefined attitudes about money, religion, and death	As above as well as: Ability to redefine current emotional investments and capacity to invest meaningful emotion in new activities, relationships, and experiences Capacity to use, in the solutions to new problems, experience and prior mental sets as guidelines for flexible decision making Capacity to pursue a set of varied activities in life; to value one's self for more than one life role	As above as well as: Preparing for retirement Deriving satisfaction from increased availability of leisure time Developing interdependent relationships with grown offspring and other members of the younger generation, e.g., grandchildren

(Continued.)

Table 5-1 Continued

	Freud	Erikson	Sullivan	Mahler	Piaget	Levinson, Lidz, Sheehy	Neugarten	Havighurst
Stage		Maturity to old age					Late life	Later maturity
Age		45 years to death					65–70 years to death	65–70 years to death
Central task		Integrity versus despair As above					Capacity to feel whole, worthwhile, and happy because of one's social and mental powers, whether or not health is perfect; lack of preoccupation with health, physique, and body comfort Capacity to accept the death of the body as less important than knowing that a future has been built through children, other relationships, and community, contributions—a feeling of enduring significance—capacity to adjust to current life situations	Adjusting to decreased physical strength and health, to retirement and reduced income, and to death of a spouse Establishing a specific affiliation with one's age group Adjusting and adopting social roles in a flexible way Establishing satisfactory living arrangements

fully resolved if a person is to master succeeding stages and become mature. This idea is very important in nursing interventions with children and their families. For example, in order to avoid parents' forcing early toilet training or rigid bathroom schedules on their children, nurses can inform parents not only about body rhythms and myelinization of nerve tissues, but also about Freud's ideas on connections between excretion, sexuality, and developmental conflicts. Offering options for toilet training may decrease power struggles between children and parents, help children learn how to deal effectively with authority figures, and prevent experiences that can remain troublesome, though forgotten, in later life.

Erikson

Erik H. Erikson is a psychoanalyst who has added another dimension—society—to Freud's theories. He hypothesized that every person is a product not only of heredity and experience, but also of society. Thus all personal anxiety (for example) reflects social concerns. Erikson emphasized the ego and its development. He thought that the gradual stage-by-stage growth of ego identity, based on experiences of social health and cultural solidarity, culminates in a sense of humanity.[5]

Stages of Development

In addition to hereditary influences, Erikson postulated eight social developmental stages (these may be contrasted with Freud's five stages of sexual development). Erikson's developmental stages, time frames, and developmental tasks, with examples, are outlined in Table 5-1.

Erikson theorized that psychosocial development proceeds in a series of crises and that success or failure in negotiating one stage will influence the ability to deal with the next stage. Tasks are dealt with, however, not in an either-or manner but on a continuum. According to Erikson, the motivation for behavior is anxiety generated by failure to successfully negotiate stages of development.

RELEVANCE TO NURSING

Erikson's stages of social development are useful concepts for nurses working with children, adults, and their families. The idea that growth is a lifelong process is heartily embraced by nursing. When formulating intervention plans for clients, nurses also acknowledge the influence of society on health and behavior. (However, although Erikson saw sex roles as being based essentially on biology and heredity, nursing considers sex-role behavior to be culturally learned.) Like the psychotherapists who use Erikson's model, nurses can use his theory as a basis for therapeutic interventions.

Sullivan

Harry Stack Sullivan formulated a theory that major life events and sources of serious difficulty are the result of interpersonal relationships within a societal context. Sullivan saw human beings as gifted animals who must be socialized before they become able to live in a social organization. Sullivan's theory implies that anxiety is, in a sense, intolerable; he thought that learned ways of coping with anxiety can limit the capacity to have meaningful experiences later in life. The motivation for behavior, in Sullivan's view, is avoidance of anxiety and the satisfaction of needs.[4]

Stages of Development

Sullivan's behavioral theories centered on interpersonal growth and development (in contrast with Freud's emphasis on sexual development and Erikson's focus on social growth and development). Sullivan thought that biological changes determined the needs and growth; he saw biological changes and emerging capacities as *tools* and the direction of growth and development as *tasks.* His developmental schema appears in Table 5-1; it includes stages of development, developmental tools and tasks, and examples. Sullivan felt that if tasks at early stages are accomplished successfully, the cumulative result will be a person capable of fulfilling the tasks of late adolescence, of becoming interdependent, and of learning to form a durable sexual relationship with a chosen member of the opposite sex.

Modes of Perception

Sullivan called reality orientation the *syntaxic mode* of perception. This orientation occurs when perceptions form whole, logical, coherent pictures that can be validated by others. But the first kind of perceptual experience, which is characteristic of infancy, is the *prototaxic mode,* the sense of self and the universe as an undifferentiated whole; and in the *parataxic mode*—characteristic of childhood and juvenile periods—the undifferentiated whole is differentiated into parts that are momentary, illogical, and disconnected.

Self-System

Sullivan also focused on the self-system, which he considered to be an organization of experiences that exists to defend against anxiety and to satisfy needs. Aspects of the self-system are known as the "good me," the "bad me," and the "not me." Children learn behaviors that are approved of by parents and identify them as "good me." For example, children will identify cleanliness as a positive quality if it is regarded as "good" by parents, and they will incorporate cleanliness into their self-systems as "good me."

Behaviors that receive disapproval generate anxiety and are identified by children as "bad me." For example, an adult who as a child was punished for eating between meals may talk about the habit as being "bad."

Behaviors generating an extreme level of anxiety are denied and identified as "not me." For example, an adult who was strongly conditioned in childhood against showing hostility may say, "I never hate anybody; that's not me."

The self-system is dynamic, changeable, and positively directed; it must be reorganized if substantial change is to be effected.[4]

RELEVANCE TO NURSING

Nurses can use Sullivan's interpersonal theory of development and his view of self in different ways. First, his developmental schema provides another model for understanding developmental processes. The focus on development as an interplay of interpersonal forces is congruent with the nursing perspective that is operationalized throughout this text. Second, his view of self and person—as being more simply human than not—implies that people are more similar than different; this enables nurses to respond to people and their problems in a humanistic way.

Piaget

Piaget's theory is primarily concerned with *cognition,* the process of knowing and understanding. He was concerned with how we come to know what we know—with explaining how different methods of thinking develop in children and adolescents. The theory stresses both biological changes and maturation as determinants of cognitive development.

Piaget saw intellectual development as occurring in four stages: the *sensorimotor stage* (birth to 18 months), the *preoperational stage* (2 to 7 years), the *concrete-operations stage* (7 to 12 years), and the *formal-operations stage* (12 years to adulthood).[9] At the end of each stage, he believed, a person has attained "near equilibrium" in the assimilation and accommodation of environmental events; it is the remaining inconsistencies that serve to usher in a new phase of higher learning.[8,15] Each stage will be described in greater detail later in this chapter, in the section on cognitive development for each developmental period.

Four concepts—adaptation, assimilation, accommodation, and schema—will help the reader understand Piaget's theory. *Adaptation* refers to any interchange between a person and the environment. Adaptation results in a modification of the person that enhances the capacity for further interchange. It has two components, assimilation and accommodation.

Assimilation refers to the process of absorbing new information from the environment and using existing mental structures to deal with the information.[8,15] For example, an infant comes to know the environment through sensorimotor exploration. When a breast or bottle nipple that provides milk is repeatedly encountered, the infant will absorb the sensory perception of the nipple into the knowledge storehouse and use the stored perception as a reference point. When nipples are encountered and perceived in the future, the infant will know what is being presented.

Accommodation refers to the process of adjusting behavior to the requirements of an object or event that has just been assimilated. For example, neonates have a sucking reflex. They assimilate the perception of a nipple and then learn how to adjust their random sucking behavior so that they can effectively suck on a particular breast or bottle nipple. Accommodation, like assimilation, allows people to integrate new learning with old.

A *schema* is a mentally organized pattern of behavior.[8,15] For example, as infants physically explore the environment, they will initially accidentally touch objects and notice that they swing, bounce, tilt, or move in some other way. The infants may repeat the activity and find that the same thing happens. The actions that initiated the movement will be mentally organized into a structure that eventually will involve a purposeful series of behaviors that infants can initiate at will to achieve the same result. Stimuli are assimilated and accommodated into schemata that are revised, refined, and changed as new stimuli are encountered. For example, infants may initially have a set of mental operations that enables them to purposefully touch a ball. However, if an infant wants to pick the ball up in two hands, the touch schema must be revised to include touch and grasping patterns. A state of relative equilibrium is reached when there is a balance between assimilation and accommodation of environmental stimuli. For example, when an infant has a sharply defined schema about touching and grasping a ball and, therefore, can execute the behavior without thought, a state of relative equilibrium exists. If the infant now wants to rotate the ball and does not have an existing schema, the equilibrium is disrupted by this gap in knowledge, and the process of revision begins again.

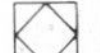 RELEVANCE TO NURSING

Piaget's theory is relevant to mental health nursing because it provides a framework that describes how people learn about and adapt to their world. It also provides a vehicle for assessing cognitive development so that deviations can be identified, realistic expectations can be formulated, and corrective experiences can be provided if necessary. This becomes particularly important for nurses who are involved in health teaching and must consider the client's level of cognitive functioning and understanding. For example, if a 9-year-old, newly diagnosed diabetic has to learn to self-administer insulin, it will be important for the nurse to know that a 9-year-old in the stage of concrete operations learns most effectively when presented with an abstract explanation plus an opportunity to see and manipulate objects that illustrate the concept. Nurses who provide parents with anticipatory guidance can also use Piaget's theory to suggest developmentally appropriate cognitive expectations, parent-child activities, play skills, games, and toys.

Mahler

Mahler's research provided a detailed theory about the separation-individuation process,[6,7] which takes place during the first 3 years of life. *Separation* involves the development of a mental picture of self as distinctly separate from other people. *Individuation* involves the development of autonomous ego functions that produce intrapsychic autonomy such as cognition, perception, memory, and reality testing. Both processes culminate in *object constancy*—the development of a whole, internalized image of the object that can be maintained, irrespective of either satisfying or unsatisfying experiences. An example of object constancy would be a 30-month-old child who is able to leave his or her mother for a period of time, become involved in current activities, later ask where mommy is, and become reabsorbed in the activity when mommy does not appear. This child is sustained by an internalized representation of mommy that exists whether mommy is present or absent.

In the separation-individuation process, a *symbiotic* stage precedes separation-individuation itself, which in turn has four subphases: *differentiation, practicing, rapprochement,* and *object constancy.* Both stages contribute to the formation of a separate sense of self and object constancy. The stages and subphases are summarized below[6,7] and will be discussed in more detail in the developmental sections later in the chapter.

Symbiotic Stage (Birth to 4 or 5 Months)

The initial part of the first stage consists of a normal *undifferentiated autistic experience.* The infant has relatively little awareness of external stimuli, does not view the self as separate from the mother, and experiences the world as an undifferentiated matrix without object-relatedness.

The latter part of the first stage involves a *symbiosis* between the infant and the mother, a psychic fusion of the two individuals. The "I" is still not differentiated from the "not I," and the infant is

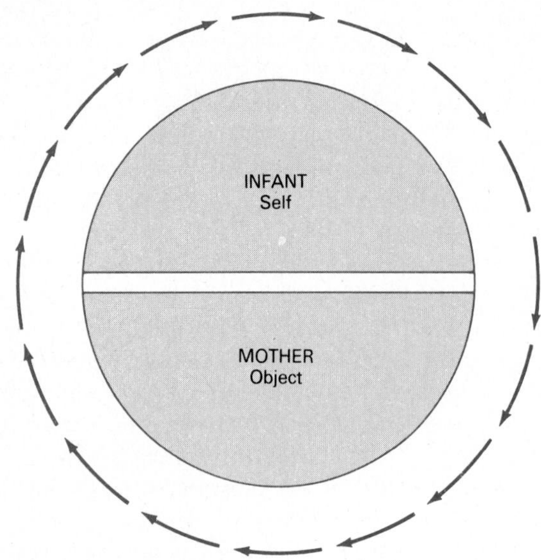

Figure 5-1 Symbiotic orbit.
The fused self-object immersed in a symbiotic stage of the separation-individuation process.

only beginning to sense the difference between inside and outside stimuli. There is dim awareness of objects outside the self that satisfy needs, but they become incorporated into the *symbiotic orbit*, a term which refers to the boundary between mother and infant that forms the totality of the infant's world. This notion is represented in Figure 5-1.

Separation-Individuation Stage (4 or 5 Months to 3 Years)

The second stage comprises four subphases: differentiation, practicing, rapprochement, and object constancy.

DIFFERENTIATION (4 OR 5 MONTHS TO 7 TO 10 MONTHS). In this stage the infant-mother symbiosis continues. The infant has become familiar with the mothering half of the symbiotic self, develops a specific bond with the mother, but begins to break away from the fusion, in a physical sense, by sitting and crawling. There is more awareness of and connectedness with objects outside the symbiotic orbit; the infant begins to discriminate between "mom" and "not mom." Anxiety may be experienced when the child is held by an unfamiliar person.

PRACTICING (7 TO 10 MONTHS TO 16 TO 18 MONTHS). In this stage there is greater awareness of a separate self as the infant becomes capable of independent locomotion. The child, intoxicated with independence, leaves the mother to explore and then returns for emotional "refueling" through physical contact. The beginning of individuation occurs as the infant increasingly masters cognitive functions. Sensory memory traces evolve into mental representations but these are derived from imitation of others and are not lasting. For example, a 1-year-old child may imitate the funny faces of mom or dad but be unable to duplicate them unless the parents repeat them. Mental images are also based on object representations: the child is able to "see" or experience only current behavior. For example, if the mother is nurturing and cuddly on a particular day, that is how she is perceived by the baby on that day, because the baby does not have the ability to synthesize into an integrated mental image the totality of behaviors displayed by the mother on all days.

RAPPROCHEMENT (16 TO 18 MONTHS TO 25 MONTHS). In this stage the child has an acute awareness of a separate self—so much so that a need for closeness with the mother reemerges as children recognize their own smallness, relative helplessness, and vulnerability. Individuation proceeds with the growth of cognitive abilities such as mental representation, symbolic play, and expressive language. This contributes to internalization of object representations. The child is able to create split representations: one image is the "good mother"; the other image is the "bad mother." These two conflicting images are not yet integrated realistically into one person, the "whole mother."

OBJECT CONSTANCY (25 TO 36 MONTHS). In this stage self-boundaries become relatively stable and firm. There is increased trust and confidence in self and others, so that the child is able to cope with being apart from the mother. Expanded cognitive functioning contributes this process in that the mother can now be replaced temporarily by a reliable internal image. Object constancy is achieved when the child resolves and combines the split images of "good mother" and "bad mother" into a unified whole. This unified whole object representation is internalized as an image that remains relatively stable regardless of instinctive needs or psychological discomfort.

The *mother-child relationship* is an integral part of the separation-individuation process. Nurturing behavior and the infant's receptivity to it, synchrony of rhythms and cues, and interaction patterns determine the quality of self-perceptions and object perceptions. Emotional availability and responsiveness seem to be key factors in facilitating the separation-individuation process.

The separation-individuation process sets the stage for relationships with other people and the environment in future life. If the needs at any particular stage or subphase are over- or undergratified, the child is at risk of getting "stuck" there and having difficulty moving on. For example, if the mother does not encourage the infant's attempts at separation and if the infant perceives separation as abandonment, the infant may remain symbiotically fused with the mother (because that is less anxiety-provoking) and may have difficulty throughout life establishing a sense of individuality. Failure to complete this process results in a child or adult who perceives self and others as confusing, strange, and unreliable and the world as unpredictable.

RELEVANCE TO NURSING

Nurses can use Mahler's theory as a developmental guide when providing anticipatory guidance to parents of young children. They can explain common behaviors at each stage of childhood and suggest appropriate parenting behaviors that will help children accomplish the tasks of each stage. Nurses can also use this theory to trace the origins of emotional problems such as pervasive developmental disorders, the borderline syndrome, schizophrenia, and adolescent adjustment reactions.

THE LIFE CYCLE

The theories of Freud, Erikson, Sullivan, Mahler, and Piaget (along with those of Levinson, Lidz, Sheehy, Neugarten, Havighurst, and others) provide an eclectic base from which nurses can conceptualize physical, cognitive, psychosocial, and spiritual development throughout the life cycle.

It is essential for nurses to have basic knowledge of developmental processes so that they can understand the feelings, thoughts, and actions of clients and families in all stages of the life cycle and provide anticipatory guidance.

In using these theories as a guide the student should remember that human development is a variable process, unique to each individual. Deviations from expected developmental norms are common, since growth and change do not proceed on a fixed timetable, and deviations do not necessarily indicate developmental problems—usually, they simply reflect a normal range of variation. Developmental deviations should be noted, however, because they are often an early warning of emerging problems. In such cases the individual, family, and environment must be thoroughly assessed.

Infancy (Birth to 18 Months)

Infancy is a period of rapid physical, cognitive, and psychosocial growth.[15] The central task of infancy is the development of trust in self and others.[4,5]

Physical Development in Infancy

In infancy physical development exceeds that in any other period in the postnatal life cycle. Infants triple their birth weight in the first year and increase their length by 50 percent.[16] Development proceeds in a cephalocaudal direction (from head to foot), in a proximal-distal direction (from the center outward), and from general to specific movements. *Cephalocaudal direction* is well-illustrated by the fact that oral functions related to sucking are highly developed in the newborn, whereas control of the anal sphincter does not occur until the second half of the first year of life. *Proximal-distal direction* is illustrated by the fact that the infant's perceptual apparatus is initially unable to detect objects outside the self and only gradually moves to perception of objects in the immediate environment and then to objects in the wider environment. *General-to-specific* development can be illustrated by grasping. Infants can crudely hold larger objects with both hands by about 4 months. They can hold smaller objects in one hand between thumb and forefinger (pincer grasp) by about 1 year of age.[17]

During infancy, the most important physical functions are the rhythmical integration of body processes such as sleeping, eating, elimination, sensory perceptions, and movement. Rhythmical body processes are initially erratic; stable, predictable patterns need to be developed through both internal regulatory mechanisms and interpersonal interactions. Internal regulatory mechanisms are the rhythms with which the infant experiences bodily needs. Initially, the needs do not necessarily occur in regular patterns; only gradually do they take on a predictable rhythm. As needs arise, tension is felt. The way the nurturing figure deals with these needs will either reduce tension or allow it to continue.[4,6]

For example, infants experience hunger-satiation cycles about every 3 to 4 hours, but not necessarily on a predictable schedule. How the nurturing figure meets this need establishes associations that will be connected with the feeding process in the future. The mother must be sensitive to clues that the infant is experiencing hunger and be flexible and available to provide both food and emotional warmth. The infant learns to correlate being hungry with the need to eat and the relief of hunger with ingesting food. The rhythm of this cycle becomes predictable to both mother and infant. They develop a set of cues for indicating need and responding to it.

Sleep-wake rhythms also vary greatly during the first year of life. Immediately after birth, infants spend most of their time sleeping. Their sleep-wake cycles, however, are short and unpredictable. Parents must be willing to modify their own cycles until the infant's cycle lengthens. From the beginning, infants may demonstrate distinct preferences with regard to sleeping and waking. Most infants move toward longer sleep-wake periods and sleep through the night by 4 to 7 months. But others prefer to sleep during the day and remain wakeful at night. Parents who are used to sleeping uninterruptedly at night may discover a mismatch between their rhythm and their infant's. This lack of synchrony can make it difficult for the parents to remain emotionally available to their child; they may find themselves increasingly fatigued and irritable. Over time, infants usually settle into a morning and afternoon nap and a full night of sleep. However variations do exist; families have to develop a match that accommodates both children's and parents' sleep-wake rhythms.

Cognitive Development in Infancy

Infants have the potential for cognitive development, but initially their intellectual capacities are completely undifferentiated and are essentially a matter of maturation. Cognitive development in infancy is perhaps best described in terms of Piaget's *sensorimotor period.* In this period, which lasts from birth to 2 years, the major mode of learning is motor activity and sensory impressions. There are six substages in the sensorimotor period: *reflex stage, primary circular reactions, secondary circular reactions, coordination of secondary schemas, tertiary circular reactions,* and *invention of new means through mental combinations.*[8,9] Five of the six substages are related to cognitive development. There is no overt end to one substage or beginning of the next; thus the associated behaviors can be observed over a wide age range. More important than *when* behaviors emerge is the fact that they develop *in sequence*. Table 5-2 lists the six substages of the sensorimotor period and observable behaviors associated with each.

Psychosocial Development in Infancy

DEVELOPMENT OF TRUST AND SENSE OF SELF. The psychosocial tasks of the first 18 months of life have to do primarily with the development of *trust*.[4,5] The infant does not view the self as an object separate from others or the environment. Mahler[6,7] states that the infant first views the self as an undifferentiated matrix, then as an object symbiotically fused with the nurturing figure, and only later, toward the end of the first year, as an emerging separate self.

The helplessness of infants forces them to trust that the nurturing figure will gratify basic physical and emotional needs. Predictability and continuity are internalized through the developing olfactory, visual, auditory, and tactile senses.

The symbiotic relationship with the mother is the foundation for the self-concept. The infant whose needs are met in a positive way will experience both the mother and the self—a fused part of the mother—as good. This is a basis for trust in self and others. As a result of varied interchanges between the nurturing person and the child, confidence is developed.[4,5]

In infancy, the mouth is the primary vehicle for communication and gratification. Consequently,

Table 5-2 Piaget's Sensorimotor Period

Substage	Learning	Observable Behaviors
Reflex stage, birth to 1 month	Learning takes place through naturally occurring reflexes	Rooting Sucking Swallowing Head turning Nonspecific smiling Grasping Startling
	Assimilates stimuli; learns to differentiate among stimuli and accommodate to them	At birth, the infant will suck whenever nonspecific stimuli are presented, as when the corner of the mouth is stroked with a finger. With repeated experience the infant learns to suck when the nipple is presented and will not be satisfied by a substitute.
Primary circular reactions, 1 to 2 or 3 months	Learning takes place through behavior that by chance leads to an interesting or advantageous result. The infant attempts to rediscover or reinstate the behavior through trial and error. If the behavior is rediscovered, it may be repeated and lead to habit formation. The infant pays more attention to outside stimuli.	Sucking on a specific object (thumb, pacifier, toy). Showing anticipatory behavior before routine procedures; for example, stops crying when placed by mother in a feeding position. Turning to look in the direction of a sound. Smiling at a familiar face. Visual tracking of people and objects.
Secondary circular reactions, 4 to 8–10 months	Learning begins to take place through intentional behaviors. Infants discover that they can alter stimuli themselves by motor effort and can make interesting events last. They begin to have a rudimentary object concept. If an object disappears, they will make an attempt to find it. Objects that are out of sight for a moderate period of time are lost.	By sitting, crawling, or transferring objects from hand to hand infants discover that they can do things (shake a rattle, move a mobile, push a ball). They put objects into and out of the mouth, play peekaboo, look in direction of mother's voice from another room, reach for a toy partially hidden by a diaper.
Coordination of sensory schemas, 8 to 12 months	Learning begins to take place in an organized, goal-directed way. The infant needs and uses more than one behavior to attain a goal. Expanded interaction with the environment has produced a sizable repertoire of schemas which pave the way for the development of coordinated schemas. Separate skills are put together to achieve a specific goal. The child can apply what has been learned to new situations.	Sit alone, crawl, stand, walk. Play with small objects using pincer movement of thumb and forefinger. Look for objects that have totally disappeared. Can combine picking up and rotating a toy to get it through the bars of the crib. Imitate actions of others such as making faces.
Tertiary circular reactions, 12 to 18 months	Learning occurs through incorporation of schema combinations and results of child experiments. Seeking out and exploring of new objects leads to new understanding of relationships. Object permanence increases as children search in new ways for vanished objects. They can figure out which objects belong and which do not belong in their world.	Independent locomotion. Explore closets, wastebaskets, and toy chests, manipulate knobs, switches, and dials. Stack blocks. Imitative play such as throwing a kiss, waving bye-bye, actively playing peekaboo. Beginning expressive language such as "mama" and "dada." Example: Buckled into a car seat, a child drops a toy and cannot retrieve it, then reaches for mother's hand and pushes it toward the object. This indicates that the infant knows where the object is and wants it returned.

(Continued.)

Table 5-2 Continued

Substage	Learning	Observable Behaviors
Invention of new means through mental combinations, 18 to 24 months	Learning occurs through formation of mental representations that become internal memory pictures of people and events. Children try to think about problems and develop solutions on a mental rather than on a physical level. Simple new forms of behavior are carried out without past trial-and-error steps. Object permanence has developed. The child no longer needs the physical object in order to remember it.	Example: A 20-month-old boy propels himself on a toy motorcycle. He catches a wheel on the edge of the carpet. He stands up to see what is obstructing his movement. He lifts the wheel over the carpet immediately and proceeds on his self-propelled ride. Also: Expansion of expressive language to phrases and sentences.

SOURCES: Developed from J. Piaget, *The Child's Conception of the World,* Littlefield, Adams, New York, 1963; J. Piaget, "The Stages of the Intellectual Development of the Child," *Bulletin of the Menninger Clinic,* vol. 26, no. 4103, 1962, pp. 120–132.

feeding becomes an important activity.[3] Prompt feedings accompanied by ample tactile stimulation increase the infant's confidence that needs will be met and that the environment can be trusted. Sporadic feedings and inconsistent feedings communicated by the mother will lead to uncertainty, anxiety, and mistrust. Then, the infant's anxiety will be manifested in behavior that may generate further inadequate or inconsistent nurturing patterns—thus a cycle of anxiety and mistrust of others and the environment is indicated. Maladaptive behavior patterns emerge quickly in an infant. A sequence of protest, crying, withdrawal, despair, and death can appear within 4 to 6 weeks of inadequate nurturing and stimulation.

A gradual decrease in symbiosis occurs toward the end of the first year of life as the infant begins to recognize self as a separate object. This coincides with an expanding awareness of objects and events outside the self, active exploration of the self and the environment, and increasingly sophisticated cognitive operations. An expanded awareness of self and the outer environment leads to exploration of self and others which includes tactile exploration of body parts; visual exploration of self and others by means of direct observations, mirrors, and reflections; and auditory exploration through listening and repetition of sounds that become increasingly purposeful. Exploration of the environment is accomplished by motor and sensory activity such as crawling, standing, walking, touching, and tasting.[6,7]

Parents' attitudes will, in part, determine the extent to which the child engages in exploratory behavior. Parents who understand that exploratory behavior is a vehicle for learning will encourage and facilitate it and will be less concerned about the domestic disarray that often results. For example, parents can provide age-appropriate toys that will facilitate this process and not forbid a child to play with more than one toy at a time. However, realistic limits and boundaries—based on safety, consideration for others, and the family's own needs—should begin to be established and consistently enforced. Children who feel free to explore within safe, secure boundaries and whose efforts are rewarded will develop self-confidence and enthusiasm about themselves and their environment.

If children leave this stage without having developed a strong sense of self and trust in others, they may encounter problems in later life: mistrust, superficial relationships, lack of self-confidence, dependency, and depression.[5]

Spiritual Development in Infancy

Pregnancy and the birth of a child often heighten parents' spiritual awareness—they have a stronger sense of the meaning and purpose of life and of connections between the generations and among all living things. When a new child is welcomed, the parents' spiritual well-being allows them to nurture the spiritual dimension in the child.

During infancy the basis for later spiritual development is established. Although babies are essentially amoral, early experiences within the family that involve development of trust are the seeds for spiritual growth later on.[18]

Early Childhood (18 Months to 3 Years)

In the transition from infancy to early childhood, children develop motor coordination and speech skills to such an extent that their parents and other adults view them as children rather than babies. Toddlers, as they are called at this stage, strive for a measure of self-reliance and independence as their sense of self develops.

Physical Development in Early Childhood

During early childhood, the rate of physical growth is slower than it was during infancy but proceeds at a continuous pace. Children gain approximately 4 pounds and grow about 2 to 3½ inches a year. The arms and legs grow fastest during childhood—more than the trunk. Growth of the head is much slower, mainly because the head circumference has already reached 68 percent of its adult size by age 2.[15]

Neuromuscular coordination improves as the nervous system matures and as muscles grow larger and increase in strength. Practice refines neuromuscular skills and improves the efficiency with which such skills are used. For example, by age 2, children walk upstairs holding onto someone's hand, a rail, or a wall and placing both feet on each step before proceeding to the next. By age 3, they alternate feet (one to a step) and do not hold on to anything. Neuromuscular coordination leads to gross and fine motor accomplishments. *Gross motor accomplishments* involve use of the large muscle groups such as the arms and legs. The 2- to 3-year-old is usually able to throw a ball overhand, pedal a tricycle, and jump in place. *Fine motor accomplishments* involve the use and coordination of small muscle groups such as the fingers. The 2- to 3-year-old is usually able to build an eight-block tower, copy a circle and imitate a vertical line, and string large beads.[15,16] Parents need to encourage physical activity that enhances the development of gross and fine motor skills.

Cognitive Development in Early Childhood

Cognitive development expands as the child enters Piaget's stage of *preoperational thought*, which lasts from about ages 2 to 7.[8,9] The *preconceptual phase* of this stage occurs from ages 2 to 4. Children are increasingly able to form mental images rather than assimilate and accommodate new phenomena only through exploration and manipulation. Exploration and manipulation remain an important part of learning, but thinking in terms of mental images now allows children to operate on a new level: they are no longer limited to present physical experiences but can transcend time and space by remembering and thinking about things in the past and things that are out of sight. Play becomes more symbolic, filled with fantasy figures and elements of "let's pretend."

Piaget gave specific names to the mental images that children use to represent objects or situations and the objects or situations themselves. The mental images (words, nonverbal symbols) are called *signifiers*. The objects or events to which they refer are called *significates*. In the dual process of assimilation and accommodation, young children apply signifiers to more and more diverse significates. Acquisition of expressive language in the form of words, phrases, and then sentences provides a way to share meanings that are mutually agreed upon. However, children are still often unable to phrase questions that would help clarify their thoughts.[8,9,17]

The ability to use mental images, although it begins in early childhood, will not be refined for several more years. For example, young children often have difficulty differentiating between the real and the unreal—for instance, between actual events and fantasies. Thus, witches, goblins, ghosts, and dreams seem very real. The concept of time also remains nebulous for young children, who have difficulty understanding the difference between yesterday, today, and tomorrow.

Psychosocial Development in Early Childhood

The psychosocial tasks of the second and third years of life revolve around the development of *autonomy*.[5] The child shifts from dependence on others and symbiotic relationships to a beginning of self-reliance and further separation-individuation.

DEVELOPMENT OF SELF. Mahler describes separation-individuation during toddlerhood as *rapprochement*.[6,7] In the second half of the second year of life, children become more and more aware of their physical separateness. The sense of clear boundaries between self and others expands as the child differentiates self from the mother.

The child pulls away from the mother so that a separate sense of self is experienced. This is pleasurable, but it is accompanied by separation anxiety and fear of loss of the mother. The child recognizes that the mothering figure is not an inevitable extension of self and develops a clearer sense of dependency. The wish to reunite with the mother conflicts with reluctance to be engulfed by her. The child wants to be separate but worries about being vulnerable and powerless. The toddler now seems to have a need for the mother to share in the acquisition of new skills and experience. The child "shadows" the mother, requesting her involvement, and then darts away, reclaiming independence. But as the children realize their power and ability to move away from the mother and satisfy needs independently, the conflict dissipates.[6,7] At this time the mother-child world expands to include the father as a separate love object.

At the same time as children develop a sense of separateness, they also develop *object constancy*. In the rapprochement phase, self and objects are initially seen as split representations: the child creates two mental images that exist separately. For example, one object image is the "good mother"; the other object image is the "bad mother." These two images are in conflict and are not yet resolved into one person, the "real mother." At the end of this phase (near age 3), the child resolves and combines the two object images into one person (the "real mother") and internalizes this cognitive and affective picture as a stable mental image. This is the beginning of object constancy. The same process occurs with self-representations. Object constancy provides stability and predictability for the child in all relationships.[6,7]

SOCIALIZATION. Children begin to learn socially acceptable behavior when they can forgo self-gratification to some extent and incorporate their parents' demands, which are representative of the larger society.[4,5] At this period, sexuality and gratification center on the anal zone of the body.[3] Issues of control—which can develop into a power struggle—have to do primarily with the child's need to coordinate "holding on" and "letting go." Toilet training is probably the most important example; it is accomplished only when the child complies with the parents' wishes in order to retain their approval and love and reduce anxiety to a minimum.[4,5] Children who are not expected to exercise control beyond their physical capacities will experience satisfaction over this achievement.

Children of this age also develop other means of self-regulation. They begin to learn rules of social behavior (how to act at the table; not to kick or bite) and guidelines for safety (not to touch dangerous objects). Realistic, consistent limits set by parents will support children's own efforts at self-control; if their developing autonomy is respected, they will come to feel that they can cope with difficulties. Basic concepts that help establish a balance between love and hate, cooperation and willingness, and self-expression and suppression are developed.

Failure to negotiate the tasks of this stage is manifested in feelings of shame and doubt, fear of self-disclosure, and ritualistic behavior.[5] In adulthood, lack of autonomy may persist and express itself as excessive need for control, order, and approval, overconforming behavior, and irrational rituals.

Spiritual Development in Early Childhood

In early childhood, the spiritual dimension begins to develop. The conflict between toddlers' increasing autonomy and their fear of separation from their parents is a crucial aspect of spiritual development.[17,18] If children learn that they are allowed to be themselves, they will develop faith in themselves as well as in others—including, perhaps, a supreme being. If children are given freedom within distinct, safe limits, they learn that the world is a safe, orderly, yet exciting place, and that other people are also reliable and safe. Such children begin to develop a sense that existence—their own, that of others, and that of the environment—has a meaning, purpose, and consistency. Within this context, toddlers learn to differentiate "good" from "bad"; to obey rules which are seen as coming from a higher authority; and to exercise rudimentary judgment and respect rituals which make them feel secure. Observing holiday traditions and saying bedtime and meal-time prayers are examples of ways in which spirituality can be introduced into a child's life. At this age, children have a boundless appreciation of the wonders of the world. It is delightful to observe a 2-year-old astounded by the magnificance of nature. (For example, during the autumn, one toddler said to her mother in a wondering voice, "Look, Mommy; how did all those leaves get painted?")

Middle Childhood (3 to 6 Years)

The transition from early to middle childhood involves consolidation of the sense of self as a separate person, the beginnings of sexual identity, and expansion of the social world.

Physical Development in Middle Childhood

Physical development continues at the slow, even rate of early childhood. Refinement of gross and fine motor skills continues as the nervous system matures and as physical activity provides opportunities for practice. Children in this age group can usually run with ease, hop on one foot, catch a bounced ball, and walk backward. They can draw crude figures, copy a square, and begin to write letters and numbers.[15,16] Parents need to provide age-appropriate activities that will enhance development.

Cognitive Development in Middle Childhood

At this age cognitive development continues in the preoperational stage; children make the transition to the *intuitive phase* of preoperational thinking.[8,9] *Intuitive* refers to the emerging ability of young children to separate disparate objects and events into some rudimentary classification. However, their classifications remain unsystematic and faulty by adult standards. For example:

> A boy of 4 was given 12 pieces of red-colored paper shaped in circles, squares, and rectangles and was asked to put them into groups that looked alike. the child returned 5 minutes later with all the shapes in one bag. When asked why he had not separated them into groups, he replied, "Oh, I did. They're all the same color, so I have one group." This made perfect sense to the child. The adult, thinking in a more sophisticated way, had expected the child to classify the objects by shape.

Thought during this phase is egocentric; that is, children view everything in relation to themselves. This makes it difficult for them to shift attention from one need, desire, or aspect of a problem to another and can make them appear single-minded, persistent, and stubborn. Egocentric thought is also exhibited in *animism*—attribution of life, consciousness, and will to physical objects. Pincushions feel the prick of a pin. Weeds hurt when they are pulled out of the ground. Clouds feel heavy when they are full of rain. The nature of the child's thinking also gives lifelike qualities to dreams, names, and events.

Expressive language becomes more sophisticated as two- and three-word phrases become sentences. Several ideas can be grouped in a sentence. Pronouns are used more, and vocabulary multiplies rapidly. Pronunciation of words becomes more precise, so that the child's speech is better understood by others.

Psychosocial Development in Middle Childhood

The psychosocial tasks of the third to sixth years of life revolve around the development of *identity* and *initiative*.

DEVELOPMENT OF RELATIONSHIPS. The separation process and the development of object constancy provide a sense of identity and expand the child's world. The child is able to define self and others as recognizably separate people.[6,7] The focus shifts from preoccupation with self and the mother to a wider circle of significant people including relatives, family friends, and peers. Children see themselves in an adult-dominated world and form attitudes toward authority. Issues of compliance and defiance are dealt with by role modeling and setting limits.

Relationships with peers take the form of "parallel play": children play together in a group, but each child usually focuses on a separate project. They come together only occasionally for cooperative activity. While children are playing separately, however, they are gaining the positive benefits from the presence of others: empathy and stimulation, for example. Children may turn from exclusive consideration of their own needs to consideration of the needs of others. They begin to appreciate the rights and feelings of other people. Social abilities develop as relationships expand and feedback is received about behavior from significant others. These abilities include leading, following, sharing, and competing.[15,19]

Having discovered the self as a separate person, children develop a sense of initiative and become curious about how much they can do, what they can become, and who else they can be. The child finds answers to these questions through observation, investigation, and play. Observation of diverse phenomena leads to many questions from the curious preschooler. "Why?" is the standard question as the child attempts to satisfy curiosity and deal with an expanding world. Exploration of self and the environment is vigorous and involves discovery of ways to undertake, plan, and carry out a task.[5] Rivalry is every-present because the child wants to succeed, win, and demonstrate superior ability. From this kind of successful exploratory activity the child begins to develop a feeling of being, to some extent, the master of his or her own fate. Play offers an opportunity for imagination and fantasy and for experiments with roles and interpersonal styles. (The child often plays "house," for instance, or dresses up and pretends to be another person.) Through play, then, a child gets a sense of what life is like for other people.

SEXUAL IDENTITY. During this period sexuality and gratification center on the genital area. Sexual identity and rivalry with the parent of the same sex for attention of the parent of the opposite sex becomes important. (The child may even express a desire to marry the parent of the opposite sex.) Children are preoccupied with sexual topics and body parts. They often react with surprise and shock to observation of genital differences between men and women. Girls often wonder why they do not have a penis and may begin to feel inferior because they are missing this body part.[5] Fantasies about reproduction abound. (For example, children commonly think that a person can become pregnant by swallowing a seed.)

Sexual identity is developed through identification with the parent of the same sex as infantile sexual striving toward the parent of the opposite sex is renounced. Children recognize that they cannot have the same kind of relationship with the parent of the opposite sex that mommy or daddy does. Fantasy, imagination, and preoccupation with the body result in normal guilt about dreams, wishes, and thoughts relating to self and parents.[4,5]

DEVELOPMENT OF INTERNAL CONTROLS. During this period a rudimentary sense of conscience develops as external prohibitions are internalized and incorporated as part of the self. Children begin to establish internal "barometers" of right and wrong and develop *signal anxiety*—anticipation of wrongdoing by connecting a wish with its consequence. The development of conscience also serves to control their initiative. Children not only fear the consequences of being caught in wrongdoing by their parents but also fear being tormented by their own self-accusations and prohibitions. The development of conscience is necessary for the formation of moral values. However, the child's conscience can be punitive and cruel. If children experience excessive guilt about their feelings, thoughts, or actions, they will deny their own wishes and curtail their activities. Children need to develop internal contacts that will control impulsive and aggressive behavior without becoming burdened by unrealistic self-restrictions that limit expansion of skill and energies.[5]

Children who are adjusting well will talk about the future and their possible roles in it. Children who have encountered developmental stalls, on the other hand, may feel that they have no right to dream. The secure child feels worthy and competent even though small.[20] Failure to successfully negotiate the issues of this developmental stage leads to psychosexual confusion, rigidity, and guilt, loss of initiative, and reluctance to explore new skills.

Spiritual Development in Middle Childhood

Spiritual development during middle childhood is directly related to the emergence of the superego. The 3-year-old begins to understand social requirements, norms, and expectations, and wants to conform to the family's norms rather than other people's. Differences between one's own family and other families are noted and remarked on. However, the child does not yet have a system for evaluating the "rightness" or "wrongness" of one family's norms in comparison with another's. The child is likely to blindly assert "My daddy does it best," regardless of what the father does or how he does it.[18]

Between ages 4 and 6, superego development is much more pronounced. Children begin to give evidence of a value system. Ideal traits, behaviors, and role models are incorporated by children so that they become inner standards and goals. These inner values provide direction for behavior and thus contribute to self-assurance and independence. From them, a system of "shoulds" evolves. Children need the opportunity to discuss values with parents and significant others. They want explanations about even the most fundamental philosophical and spiritual issues; they may ask, for instance, "Why are people mean to each other?" "Why do people get married?" "How do I know if I'm a good person?"

Children of this age think in concrete terms. When they imagine a spiritual being, such as God, they form animistic, literal images; they have difficulty separating God from parents and other authority figures. In drawings by preschoolers, for example, God wears pants and a shirt and eats with a fork; and many a young child has pointed to the family's minister or rabbi and said, "Look—there's God!" Children of this age believe that God is responsible for everything, yet "good" and "bad" continue to be what their parents approve of or forbid.[18]

Late Childhood (6 to 12 Years)

School-age children expand their mastery of the environment through industry and learning. Mastery of specific skills serves as a source of self-esteem. Children also expand their sense of self through new sources of identification as relationships with people outside the family develop.

Physical Development in Late Childhood

During late childhood, bodily proportions become more mature: the arms and legs grow longer, the abdomen flattens, the shoulders and trunk broaden, and facial proportions change. There is a distinct change in body image as children move from the toothless, babyish look of the 6-year-old to the lean, muscular preadolescent look of the 12-year-old. Growth is slower than it was in early childhood and slower than it will be in adolescence. Height increases at a rate of 2 to 3 inches in a year and weight gain varies from 3 to 6 pounds a year. Fat deposits are burned off and muscles grow stronger as children engage in physical activity. Gross motor coordination becomes increasingly refined as children ride bicycles and skateboards, swim, play baseball, run, climb, and jump. Fine motor coordination develops as children write, paint, model clay, weave, collect stamps, sew, take photographs, build models, and so on. Parents often describe their child as becoming physically competent during this period—youngsters who can really be a help in many situations.[15,19]

Cognitive Development in Late Childhood

During this stage cognitive development marks a transition from preoperational thought to *concrete operations*.[8,9] This period begins somewhere between ages 6 and 8, depending on the child. Concrete operations involve the ability to reason in a systematic way and to apply previously learned rules to new things and situations. That is, rules now help children understand and classify new phenomena. The rules constantly undergo revision. For example, a school-age child who sees a baby alone in a room will reason that a mother must be nearby because babies cannot take care of themselves. When a group of adults enters the room, the child will search out the most probable mother. If the mother does not go over to the baby and the father attends the baby instead, the child will have to revise the rule to include the fact that adults other than mothers also take care of babies.

Children who perform concrete operations can mentally reverse the operations—they can imagine how things were before the operations took place. This ability depends on a skill called *conservation*. Conservation is the ability to understand that a quantity does not change simply because the form it takes varies. For example, a child who can "conserve substance" realizes that a given amount of water does not change when it is poured from a short glass to a tall glass. This enables the child to view the same situation in a variety of ways. A child at this age is also able to classify phenomena according to similar attributes and order them serially by height, size, shape, and so on. The ability to synthesize diverse phenomena, formulate relationships, and speculate about causality provides a foundation for objectivity and problem solving, and these in turn lead to the beginning of abstract rather than rote learning—a capacity fundamental for the development of academic skills. However, most children still need to manipulate concrete objects to demonstrate logical abilities; they cannot deal with reversibility, classification, or rules in words alone.

Psychosocial Development in Late Childhood

The psychosocial tasks of the 6- to 12-year-old revolve around *industry* and *learning*.

SELF-CONCEPT. The child believes, "I am what I learn." Self-esteem is derived from accomplishment, and the child learns to win recognition by producing things. Children take pride in mastering tasks and feeling useful. They feel good about themselves when diligence produces a completed task. Positive appraisal from significant people such as parents, teachers, and friends reinforces their good feelings. While some feelings of inadequacy are bound to occur during late childhood, a sense of industry can be fostered by sensitive adults who counterbalance negative feedback with constructive criticism, suggestions, and praise.[5]

SEXUALITY. Theorists such as Freud and Erikson have stated that the school-age period is one of sexual latency; that is, sexual energy is sublimated into industry and learning.[3,4] However, current research indicates that for many children sexual curiosity actually increases. They tell each other the "facts of life" and share "dirty jokes," and many read anything related to sex that they can get their hands on.[15] Toward the end of late childhood sexual desires intensify, and there may be a reappearance of masturbation and sexual fantasy. Much of this sexual feeling is mixed with aggression and is sublimated into physical activity. However, changes in body image lead to intense preoccupation with appearance, especially if physical changes occur early. At this stage, sexuality is also a consolidation of "feeling male" or "feeling female" and thus sets the stage for puberty.

PEER RELATIONSHIPS. For children of school age, the peer group and the school become major influences on socialization, along with the family. As friends and "ego ideals," such as teachers, become the center of the child's universe, parents' influence decreases. Through cooperation, compromise, and collaboration, children take their place in their peer group, which is the core of their social life.[4,5] Friends are used as sounding boards, and the group becomes a testing ground for values and attitudes learned at home. In many cases the peer group can be more democratic than the home. Rules are not laid down by authority figures but are debated, with some of or all the group having a say in what they should be. Home values and attitudes may be strengthened or watered down.

During late childhood, friendships become more stable. Friends of the same sex are sought out, and "best friends" develop. Individual friendships provide opportunities for intimacy, sharing, and self-disclosure that may not have been experienced previously outside the family. Group relationships usually involve organized activities, such as scouting, sports, and community group projects, which provide a sense of belonging, teamwork, and cohesiveness. Other group activities such as secret societies, gangs, and team sports offer opportunities for playful aggression and acceptable sublimation of hostility.[4,5,15]

Failure to develop self-esteem and a sense of mastery at this stage may lead to feelings of inadequacy and inferiority which persist in later life. A child who has not developed a sense of initiative may be unprepared for school, or the school itself may fail to help the child develop necessary skills. The child may feel, "I'll never be good at anything," and may increasingly display reluctance to explore the environment and human relationships.[5]

Spiritual Development in Late Childhood

One of the crucial tasks of school-age children is moral development, which in this stage depends less on their automatic obedience to parents and more on their internal judgments. As the superego or conscience matures, children begin to discriminate between their own motives and motives derived from parents' demands. By late childhood, children can be expected to understand most of the things that family and society define as unacceptable, but they cannot always be expected to have control over their unacceptable urges. Nor can they always be expected to consider the rights and needs of others. To reach higher levels of moral judgment, children need experiences with choosing right and wrong and opportunities to reason out the whys and wherefores of their choices. Ultimately, they will be able to distinguish between right and wrong without external reminders.[21,22]

Thinking is still concrete in school-age children, but they begin to use abstract concepts to describe their religious and spiritual world. They start to develop an interest in the idea of a power greater than themselves or their parents. It is most common for this power to take the form of a God who is everywhere, creates happiness and sadness, and makes trees and flowers grow. As children progress through this stage, their ability to conceptualize increases and they also begin to think about how faith of one kind or another relates to life; they can discuss and explain what they believe. They may even begin to evaluate what they have been taught.[18]

Adolescence (12 to 18 Years)

This is a time of rapid growth (in fact, growth in this stage is equaled only in infancy and early childhood).[17,23] Physical, cognitive, and psychosocial changes occur simultaneously: nothing is the same; everything is changing at once. These changes do not always occur in a uniform, integrated way. There are delays in some areas, while overlapping and acceleration occur in others. However, the general magnitude of change in adolescence makes this stage a period of upheaval and turmoil for everyone. Issues of individuation and differentiation are of paramount importance for adolescents, as they prepare to assume adult identities.

Physical Development in Adolescence

The onset of *puberty* (changes accompanying the arrival of sexual maturity) varies from person to person. Puberty usually encompasses 1 to 2 years of rapid growth and development before a girl or boy becomes capable of reproducing children.[15,23] Sexual maturity is preceded by the development of secondary sex characteristics. In girls, as hormonal changes occur and estrogen is secreted, the breasts begin to enlarge, pubic and axillary hair appears, the hips widen, and menstruation begins. This process begins at about age 11, but time of onset can vary widely from age 9 to age 15. In boys, as behavioral changes occur and androgens are secreted, the penis, testes, and scrotum increase in size, pubic hair appears, the voice deepens as the shape of the larynx changes, the hips become slimmer, the body becomes more muscular, and the production and emission of sperm begin. Facial, body, and axillary hair appear as later physical changes. Puberty begins about 2 years later in boys than in girls, at about age 13. As with girls, the time of onset of this process can vary widely. In both sexes endocrine changes also include activation of the sweat and facial oil glands. The increased activity of these glands predisposes the adolescent to suffer from body odor, pimples, and blackheads, which constitute a disturbing alteration in body image.

Height and weight increase dramatically; full adult height and weight are attained during adolescence. Girls are initially taller than boys, but boys generally become taller in middle to late adolescence. The sudden and dramatic changes in body proportions often contribute to feelings of awkwardness, clumsiness, and self-consciousness. Teenagers may find that they have difficulty judging movements. For example, a boy may find that his big feet and longer legs are only two steps away from the snack table, rather than four, as they knock it over. Clumsiness probably results from failure to adapt quickly enough to changed body proportions; by the end of adolescence, the boy or girl has reached physical maturity and has had a chance to incorporate a new body image.[15,23]

Cognitive Development in Adolescence

The last stage of cognitive development occurs during adolescence. It is called the *formal-operations stage* and constitutes the highest level of intellectual functioning.[8,9] This stage provides the foundation for cognitive operations throughout adulthood. Formal operations involve abstract conceptual thought. The ability to reason becomes more complex as the adolescent is able to see multiple logical relationships between classes or between and among several different properties (such as height, weight, and density). This involves seeing all possible variations of a problem, separating all possible variables, and testing variables systematically. Such a process of deductive reasoning includes systematic analysis of real and hypothetical problems. (For example, in order to test teenagers' deductive reasoning, Piaget asked them to discover the right combination of chemical liquids to produce a yellow-colored liquid.[8])

Research indicates that the development of formal-operations skills may be, to some extent, a function of culture and education.[15] In areas where children begin school early and are given extensive instruction in written language, formal operations emerge slightly before the teenage years. Written language helps children go beyond concrete, here-and-now thinking. Children who read are helped to think about abstract as well as concrete possibilities. Nonreaders, poor readers, and people in cultures that do not use written language extensively may not reach the formal-operations stage at all.

Psychosocial Development in Adolescence

CONSOLIDATION OF SELF-CONCEPT. Psychologically, a sense of personal identity is being forged in adolescence. The adolescent asks, "Who am I?" "Where have I been?" "Where am I going?" "Who will I become?" Adolescence provides an opportunity to go through a second process of separation and individuation.[7]

Before identity can be consolidated, a stage of self-consciousness and disorganization must be endured. Teenagers experience ambivalent feelings as they engage in a process of rebellious experimentation and testing. Until a comfortable fit is achieved, they swing back and forth between independence and dependence. (For example, one minute they will be asking for help with homework, and the next minute they will accuse their parents of trying to run their lives.) Adolescents may defy parental authority, creating tension and conflict between parents and children. They may want to maintain a childlike role while they enjoy adult privileges. (For example, they may expect that someone will clean their room and prepare meals for them but, at the same time, feel that they should be able to use the family car and should have no curfew.) This conflict is accompanied by feelings of loneliness and confusion. The teenager must accept the finality of the end of childhood and the responsibilities of adulthood.

It is difficult for parents to know how to react to young people who are adults one minute and children the next. Parents need to strike a balance between freedom and realistic expectations. The process of separating from parents brings feelings of loss and emptiness that, although normal, are difficult for the adolescent to express and resolve. Such feelings, and denial of an unresolved emotional attachment, may in part account for the mood swings so characteristic of adolescence.

Adolescents begin to blend "wants" and "shoulds" of significant others with their own, but judgments by significant others still largely determine their sense of self-worth.[5] Sexuality must be dealt with and expressed in acceptable ways. This is a problem for the adolescent who is often overwhelmed by sexual feelings and has no outlet for them other than self-stimulation. The adolescent needs to know that these feelings are completely normal.

SOCIAL RELATIONSHIPS. Socially, adolescents are in role transition; they must form a concept of acceptable social roles through experimentation. Their inner lack of trust in themselves is manifested in conformity to a group. Cliques and gangs are often intolerant of those who do not belong. Rigid clothing styles, mannerisms, fetishes, and codes of behavior reflect a need to be accepted, wanted, and loved. If the adolescent experiences acceptance in a group, then individual heterosexual relationships will probably be sought. On the basis of these, a more or less enduring relationship with a member of the opposite sex may develop, and first love may be experienced.[4,20]

EDUCATIONAL AND CAREER CONCERNS. Contemplation of the future—"who I want to be and what I want to do"—begins in adolescence, and finding a career becomes a concern. The adolescent is continuously bombarded by questions about career plans. Uncertainty is compounded, since people of this age have not participated extensively in the world of work and have observed only fragments of work situations and job roles.[20] Consequently, they find it difficult to commit themselves to a full-time job or to identify career choices.

Failure to negotiate the tasks of this stage results in failure to consolidate an idea of "who I am," which leads to role confusion, deficits in assuming responsibility, a sense of inadequacy in controlling the self, and an inability to compete successfully.[5]

Spiritual Development in Adolescence

Adolescents strive to understand the meaning and purpose of life and to use this understanding in making present and future decisions. Their quest for understanding may involve questioning their parents' values and beliefs, rejecting formal religious beliefs and practices, comparing philosophical and religious beliefs of their friends, and examining their own beliefs. Perhaps the most common question posed by adolescents is, "What is life all about, anyway?" During adolescence life takes on a new note of seriousness; for perhaps the first time there is an awareness of mortality and of the need to find meaning within the context of mortality.[17,18,21]

A belief system is searched for that is congruent with the concept of self. Because this stage of development is pervaded with uncertainty, adolescents may hold contradictory beliefs or act in ways that are incongruent with their beliefs. For example, adolescents may espouse the belief that a person should be able to think and act in a unique way but may nevertheless make fun of anyone whose clothing, friends, social life, or goals do not conform to their own.

Beliefs develop by trial and error throughout life. Adolescents examine their parents' values and beliefs and may reject or modify them. They will, naturally, be confused when they find inconsistencies in the behavior of role models (for example, when an athletic coach preaches fairness on the playing field but then urges the team to win at any cost). Adolescents who consider loyalty, justice, and honesty important will be disillusioned when they discover that even those they admire make mistakes or act ruthlessly.

Adolescents will challenge, test, and perhaps even reject social, moral, and religious norms under which they have been reared. Attendance at a place of worship may diminish; interfaith dating may occur. Parents' commitment or lack of commitment to a religion may be questioned; religious practices may be seen as hypocrisy. At this time, beliefs of a peer group are often respected more than those of the family. But the belief system that people ultimately adopt as adults is usually more similar to than different from their parents', even if they have protested and rebelled during adolescence. By the time young people leave adolescence, they may have a system of beliefs to guide their thoughts, feelings, and actions. However, it is usually too early to know whether that will be the foundation of an adult belief system.[18]

Young Adulthood (18 to 25 Years)

Young adulthood is a time when men and women struggle with the urge to remain dependent and sheltered by others as opposed to the urge to prepare for and master the future.[5,10,12,24] Not everyone becomes independent at this point. Many people are not emotionally ready for independence and need to continue exploring the world and themselves. Others remain dependent because they have not completed their education or for financial reasons. However, most young adults do locate themselves in a peer group, a sex role, and an anticipated or actual occupation. They also develop an ideology or world view.

Physical and Cognitive Development in Young Adulthood

Young adulthood is essentially a period of psychosocial development. Physical development has been completed, except that males, more often than females, may continue to grow.[15] Cognitive development has been completed in terms of high-order cognitive operations. The young adult continues to refine and expand use of such operations.[8]

Psychosocial Development in Young Adulthood

Equipped with only a provisional sense of identity, the young adult is usually caught between wanting to prolong the irresponsibility of adolescence and wanting to assume adult commitments. Irresponsibility is more easily continued by those who do not begin to work, either because they remain in school or for other reasons. Some young adults want to make intelligent adult commitments, but they worry about making irrevocable decisions that will lock them into a permanent structure. Others want to forge new creative paths that will involve them in pursuits which are not accepted norms for adulthood. For example, some young people may join a commune or a religious cult, and some may pursue scholarly, political, artistic, or other nonmaterialistic interests. Others may choose more traditional paths, such as career, marriage and parenthood, or both, at this time.[12]

Young men at this time are likely to embark upon careers that will enable them to realize the occupational dreams of childhood. They may also formulate short- and long-term goals in traditional or nontraditional careers. In the past, women making the transition into adulthood usually focused on getting married and having a family. The expected role for women was primarily that of wife, mother, and homemaker. However, this traditional role has changed, and many new options now exist for women. Increasingly, young women are formulating the same kinds of occupational goals as men. Thus they, too, have short- and long-term career goals in traditional and nontraditional careers.

Although choosing a marriage partner and starting a family are major tasks of young adults, there is an increasing acceptance of diverse lifestyles that support a wide range of commitment and intimacy. Many young adults choose alternative options. Childless marriages, cohabitation (living together), and remaining single are becoming increasingly acceptable. For those who elect to marry, the motivation must be seriously examined. The marital relationship, at its best, represents true integration and leads to interdependence rather than dependence. Such "closeness without fusion" must be managed so that intimacy is possible but neither partner merges, loses, or gains self-identity at the expense of the other.[12]

To some people, young adulthood may appear to have been wasted if traditional or acceptable paths are not followed. One frequently hears family members say, when talking about a young adult, "When is he (or she) going to stop fooling around and get busy being a grown-up?" It is important to remember, however, that experimentation at this stage may be necessary. Some people need time to integrate identity, role, and separation issues to achieve a workable balance.[24]

Resolution of the problems of this stage occurs as young adults consider careers and establish personal and professional goals. People also locate themselves in social groups, intimate relationships, or both. Choices are made about lifestyles that involve varying levels of intimacy and commitment. Young adults are able to exercise increasing self-reliance in making choices, which at this point are not necessarily irrevocable. They arrive at a degree of personal uniqueness which shows itself in consistent ways of feeling and behaving.

Young adults who fail to achieve personal integration during this stage may have their options cut off too early. They may make decisions about work, marriage, and parenthood on the basis of values and wishes of others rather than their own. People who fail to develop some form of an intimate relationship at this stage risk isolation later in life—avoidance of close relationships or participation only in relationships that are short-lived, superficial, and stereotyped.[17]

Spiritual Development in Young Adulthood

Young adults continue to search for spiritual identity, sorting through the values and beliefs they learned as children and striving to arrive at a belief system of their own. Essentially, they ask, "What do *I* believe in?" and, "What do *I* see as the fundamental purpose of life?" Parents' values are discarded, modified, or adopted according to how well they "fit" with the young adult's own emerging beliefs. Spirituality is usually not a primary concern for young adults; there is too much else going on in their lives as they establish themselves in the adult world. However, societal or personal crises—such as war, natural disasters, traumatic accidents, or death of a significant other (such as a parent or friend)—may intensify the search for spiritual meaning. Young adults who marry and begin to raise a family during this period are likely to develop a spiritual identity that includes religious and moral values which they will pass on to the next generation.[25]

Adulthood (25 to 38 Years)

Adulthood is a time when men and women have a sense of personal integration and work toward taking their place in the world. Many decisions and commitments are made about career, marriage, parenthood, and community involvement. Activity is directed toward establishing what the adult wants to do and reaching these goals.[5,10,12]

Physical and Cognitive Development in Adulthood

The physical changes that occur in adulthood vary widely from person to person. Physical growth has ceased, and bodily integrity depends greatly on diet, exercise, rest, stress, genetic factors, and whether health problems or disabilities develop. The first physical signs of aging may appear in the late twenties and throughout the thirties. Skin begins to lose its resilience and elasticity, and wrinkles appear. This may be upsetting to men and women unless they feel that wrinkles add character to their appearance. Hair may grow more slowly, be lost, or turn grey. Genetic predisposition to baldness or early greying, nutritional factors, disease, drugs, and hormones may contribute to these changes.[15]

Cognitively, adulthood is a very productive stage. Brain weight and maturation of brain cells peak in the late twenties. Although a gradual shrinking process begins after that, cognitive functioning remains high throughout this period. Abstract thought is applied to a wide range of phenomena; inductive and deductive logic are used to solve problems and deal with human relationships.

Psychosocial Development in Adulthood

In adulthood, multiple role changes occur. Adults in their late twenties assume new roles as workers, lovers, spouses, parents, and participants in the community.

In the world of work, adults in their late twenties are busy setting goals, trying to bring about significant change, and seeking mentors who can guide them in their careers. Hope and energy abound, and demonstrating competence is of great importance. Some adults continue to explore and experiment with career options throughout the twenties. At this time, people begin to build a foundation for a safe future, but decisions are still not viewed as irrevocable.[12]

Other major choices are made at this time, if they have not been made before. Options for marriage and parenthood may be considered and implemented. Selection of a lover or spouse creates an opportunity for intimacy and consolidation of sexuality without loss of differentiation. Some people elect to remain unmarried. Others may enter into a significant, lasting relationship with another person without formal marriage. There are many reasons why a person may choose not to marry, if only for the time being. Perhaps the "formality" of marriage is frightening or unappealing. Perhaps there are financial obstacles. Commitment to career goals and the fear that marriage might inhibit career plans often lead one to choose not to marry or at least to postpone marriage until later in life, when some career success has been achieved. Those who choose to marry are confronted with a variety of relationship issues. For women, the question of combining marriage and career arises. Questions about having a family emerge. Some couples decide to have children immediately or shortly after marriage. When this decision is made, some women opt to interrupt their career for a number of years, while other women choose to return to work or to start working shortly after a baby is born. Some couples decide to postpone parenthood indefinitely. The decision the couple makes will result in role and identity shifts. A decision to postpone parenthood may imply that an occupational role or identity is paramount; a decision to have children or to stay home and nurture them may bring the parenting role and identity to the forefront. Conflict can occur when both marriage and career are desired. This requires role modification for both partners so that marriage, family, and careers can be successfully combined. (The dual-career family, an increasingly important phenomenon, is discussed in Chapter 47.)

Adults in their thirties are usually preoccupied with the question, "What do I want out of life now that I'm doing what I ought to do?" It is a time of greater introspection. There is often a feeling of restlessness and restriction accompanied by an urge to expand one's horizons. This is an outgrowth of commitments made during the early twenties. Important choices that start people on new roads may be made, and existing commitments may be altered or deepened. Career plans may be reviewed. Many people are eager to convert dreams of success into specific goals. Branching out into one's own business is not uncommon if working for an employer seems too constricted. People feel that they still have time to achieve, that things can still change. There is a sense of impatience, but not urgency.

The marriage relationship is examined by both partners, and qualities to be retained or discarded are evaluated. Men and women alike are making decisions regarding their lives. At this point, for example, many women want to expand their horizons if they have interrupted their career to raise children who are now in school. They have more free time, and the role of mother and wife is no longer sufficient. Such women have to make decisions regarding future directions. Often, previous career choices are no longer appropriate or desirable, and reentering the job market will require retraining or returning to school. Many women question their personal identity; they want to reject "shadow" roles—roles based on having a husband ("X's wife") or a child ("Y's mother"). However, they may not feel confident about leaving the home. Can they cope with the public world? What do they have to offer it?[12] Another problem such women may face is the attitude of their husbands. Many men are intent on pursuing their own career goals; they want to be free to do so without interference and thus may pay as little attention as possible to their marital and family responsibilities. They may want their wives to expand their horizons, but they do not want any sharing of marital chores that would facilitate their partners' plans.

Single men and women in their thirties may question earlier decisions about postponement of marriage and parenthood. They may have achieved their career goals and may now be ready to forgo a career or combine it with marriage and parenthood. Relationships may now seem more important than achievements. Single people may be ready for a change.

The sexual relationship is another area for renegotiation. At this time, women usually experience an increase in sexuality that may or may not be compatible with the sexual interests of their partners—men's sexuality tends to remain constant or decrease as a result of preoccupation with work or other tensions. However, increased self-confidence and openness in other areas of life can lead to an exploration of new levels of sexual satisfaction for both partners within the relationship. On the other hand, couples may begin to grow apart if they progress—intellectually, emotionally, sexually, and socially—at different rates. They may have different levels of personality development, values, and role expectations. Unless commitments are renegotiated, couples' relationships may dissipate to the point where they are no longer viable.

Spiritual Development in Adulthood

As people make the transition into adulthood, those who are functional adults experience spiritual "consolidation." That is, they have a clear concept of right and wrong, and they make moral, religious, and ethical decisions on the basis of a value system. Their life plans are usually also based on this fundamental spiritual core. Individual, family, societal, and (for some people) religious ethics operationalize the spiritual dimension. Energy is spent identifying and achieving goals congruent with a life plan.

Those who begin to question or reevaluate their chosen life plan at some point during this phase may also contemplate and reevaluate spiritual beliefs and values.

Middle Adulthood (38 to 65 or 70 Years)

Middle adulthood includes two phases, the *midlife crisis* and *restabilization*. The midlife crisis of the late thirties and early forties is a time of reevaluation for people at the midpoint of life. They ask, "Where have I been?" "What have I accomplished?" "How am I going to spend the future?" The period from the late thirties through the forties is a time when people must try to adjust to the gaps between what they wanted to accomplish, what they actually have accomplished, and what they still can accomplish before time runs out. People in their late thirties and forties may feel that this is their last chance and will, therefore, examine their inner selves. It is a time when one feels prompted to examine past accomplishments and renew previous commitments.

Men and women in their fifties and sixties who weather the midlife crisis restabilize in terms of identity and commitments. They feel a new freedom to be independent and follow their interests. They can enjoy the privileges of middle age without envying others. They have less fear of aging and death.

Physical and Cognitive Development in Middle Adulthood

During middle adulthood, there is a gradual slowing down of all physiological functions, and tissues have less capacity to regenerate. Degenerative changes such as arthritic joint disease may begin at this time. Other changes occur, such as wrinkling and sagging due to loss of tissue elasticity; balding and greying continue. Varying amounts of distress are experienced because of these changes.[15]

The outstanding physical changes during this period, in both men and women, have to do with the reproductive system. The reproductive organs begin to atrophy with advancing age. The end of the female reproductive cycle is relatively clearly marked by *menopause*, which occurs between the ages of 40 and 55. The male *climacteric* is gradual, and the point at which it is concluded is less obvious; whether it is a purely physical syndrome is uncertain at this time. Neither menopause nor the male climacteric need appreciably alter the sex drive. It may remain powerful throughout the life span.

Cognitive development does not advance. In fact, nerve impulses in the brain travel more slowly across neurons, causing a decrease in reaction time. However, in spite of these degenerative changes, most people retain full use of their intellectual abilities throughout the middle years. They continue to add new words to their vocabulary and organize and process new information. The degree to which intellectual functioning is maintained in the middle years appears to be a function of ongoing mental stimulation and variation in life experience.[15]

Psychosocial Development in Middle Adulthood

THE MIDLIFE CRISIS. The midlife crisis is a period of acute psychosocial discomfort experienced as men and women face the discrepancy between their youthful ambitions and their actual achievement. They may feel bored and dissatisfied with the way their life has developed; they may feel ambivalence and uncertainty about the future.

Multiple role changes occur. Children leave the home, and active parenting is completed. Thus some former meaningful roles are gone. Women in their forties whose lives have been bound up in motherhood and keeping house may feel that they have lost their purpose in life as their children become more independent. The "empty nest" syndrome stems from the sense of purposelessness many women experience at this time. As children are launched and allowed to lead their own lives, the woman's former identity no longer fits. She is confronted with the question, "Who am I?" and asks, "What is the purpose of the rest of my life?" Every woman needs to develop a sense of individual importance and a means of independent survival; otherwise, she will continue to depend on the well-being and largess of her husband and children for her identity.[26] Even women who have had careers and whose identities have not been as wrapped up in parenting experience a loss when their children are launched.

Men in middle life may feel that their opportunities for advancement are limited and that younger people with better knowledge and skills are crowding them out. They may have to give up the idealized self of the twenties and thirties for a more realistic one. Men also question what the purpose will be for the rest of their lives. They may have to give up early hopes and dreams and find value in what they have, in fact, accomplished.[11] Many men and women must confront the necessity of finding a new career, or the fact that they have become unemployable. Even people who have attained their goals need new ideas to renew their zeal.

The marital relationship also changes. Husbands and wives are alone together as they have not been in years. They may find that they no longer share interests or values or that they have gotten into the habit of communicating through their children. They may find that they need to renew their relationship and develop new interests which will enrich their lives. Role reversals occur. Adults become parents to their own parents as the parents age and become infirm. The last shreds of childhood dependence are severed. The adult realizes that "I am alone." This moment of self-confrontation is often terrifying.

In their middle years, men and, particularly, women who earlier elected not to marry and or become parents often have to confront the fact that they will not bear children. This awareness can lead to feelings of depression.

Physical changes occur which reflect changes in body image. There is a growing difference between the sexual capacity of men and women. Men find that they are unable to perform as frequently as in previous years; women, on the other hand, experience no loss of sexual ability and may actually feel increased desire owing to freedom from fear of pregnancy, freedom from the responsibilities of earlier years, and a positive redefinition of self, particularly if they return to work. However, menopause and the accompanying physiological changes may contribute to emotional disequilibrium and add to a woman's sense of loss and depression.[10]

The capacity for love and intimacy is not decreased for men or women, and sexuality in the middle years can be most fulfilling if creative approaches are taken to sexual activity. The general physical process of aging, however, confronts people with their own mortality. Illness and death among friends and relatives make it difficult to deny that endurance and physical capacity are decreasing. But in a youth-oriented culture, many people do try to hold on to a youthful self-concept. They look back at the past to evaluate whether they have had enough "kicks" and ask whether they want to pursue such youthful pleasures now. They may seek the exclusive company of people younger than themselves, have extramarital affairs with younger people, or maintain a frantic pace of life. They may dye their hair, have cosmetic surgery, or dress in a very youthful way. All these activities may be attempts to deny the aging process and to maintain a sense of vigor and self-esteem.

RESTABILIZATION. If the tasks of midlife crisis—self-confrontation and change—have been accomplished, men and women may find their fifties and sixties to be the most personally rewarding period of their lives. People come to terms with mortality and reconcile what is with what might have been.

Marriage, if it survives the midlife crisis, can provide opportunities for renewed intimacy, now that children no longer occupy so much of the partners' time.[12] Adults in the later middle years become concerned with *generativity*—establishing and guiding the next generation. Parents recognize their children as separate adults, not merely extensions of themselves.[25] They enjoy family events such as marriage of children and birth and growing up of grandchildren. People who have not married or had children of their own may expand and deepen relationships with nieces and nephews, younger colleagues, or students.

Although sexual activity may be less important, sexual relationships can remain satisfying if partners find mutually agreeable ways to stimulate and enjoy each other.

Involvement in community activities can provide an expanded network of social relationships at a time when friendship networks tend to contract because of geographic moves and death. Interests left dormant during earlier preoccupation with establishing a family, a career, or both can be redeveloped. Previous hobbies or interests can blossom and become very involving. (For example, a builder concentrated his interest and skill on building a sailboat, a hobby left untouched from his teenage years. A woman turned a lifetime love of shopping into a business when she started a local shopping service.)

The basic crisis of the middle years is one of introspection, self-confrontation, and renewal. The process of peeling away the layers is often painful because feelings which have been buried for years emerge. People are not sure they like what they see. However, this is a unique opportunity to put things together and come to accept oneself. At this stage, many people are no longer preoccupied with pleasing others. They make this a time to enrich their lives, do what they themselves want, and discover the unique answers they need.

If these issues are not confronted in middle adulthood, they crop up again in later years. Failure to negotiate these tasks and accept one's own finiteness results in denial, depression, psychosomatic symptoms, boredom, and stagnation.

Spiritual Development in Middle Adulthood

The middle years are a period of introspection and reassessment in the spiritual dimension as well as other dimensions of the self. People reevaluate their values and their philosophy of life. The resulting spiritual "position" often reflects accumulated wisdom and underlying beliefs that have evolved over many years. A renewed spiritual self is better able to cope with the challenges of the future.

As a result of their own reassessment, middle-aged people are often more flexible about accepting philosophical, moral, ethical, and religious differences among people; they accept the right of each person to choose a belief system. Within individual contexts, people may be able to renew their commitments to religious doctrines. Participation in church-affiliated activities often increases during the middle years. However, spiritual beliefs often extend beyond the confines of one's own religion. A sense of philanthropy may create a deep commitment to ecumenical religious and secular interests, and to the community.[12,17]

Accepting their own mortality leads middle-aged people to grapple with the need for transcendence—when they accept the inevitability of death, there may be a simultaneous need to believe in some form of immortality. But immortality need not be envisioned as personal survival. For some people it can take the form of accomplishments that will live on; and for some it is seen in terms of children, grandchildren, nieces, nephews, and other significant youngsters—links between generations. People place more and more importance on immortality as their own sense of vulnerability becomes acute and as their parents and peers grow infirm and die.[5]

This phase of life can be particularly meaningful for people who are able to reaffirm or renew the guiding principles of their spiritual dimension. They are then able to savor the riches of their life and philosophically accept the disappointments.

Late Adulthood (65 to 70 Years to Death)

No other developmental stage is so rigidly stereotyped as late adulthood. Except in cultures where the aged are revered, it is a stage that is synonymous with decline. This is particularly true in the United States; although older adults make up about 10 percent of the population, American culture places a high value on youth and tends to view old age as uniformly negative. Yet there is a great diversity in later maturity, just as there is in other stages of life. The way in which people experience late adulthood appears to be a function of a complex interrelationship of physical, cognitive, and psychosocial factors. Adjustment to late adulthood appears to be a direct consequence of ego development in earlier years. Most people who have demonstrated the ability to adapt to stress, change, and the social milieu over a lifetime have enough ego integrity and self-differentiation to cope with the stresses that confront them in late adulthood. Then they can consolidate, protect, and hold on to the sense of identity that has accrued over a lifetime and accept the life that has been lived as worthwhile.[10,27,28]

Physical and Cognitive Development in Late Adulthood

The physical appearance and cognitive functioning of people over 65 vary as much as those of people of earlier developmental stages. Chronological age cannot be used as a predictor of physical and cognitive decline.[29] The physical and cognitive aspects of aging are, to some degree, a result of changes in the ability of individual cells to perform specialized, integrated functions.[29] Once many cell types have undergone final developmental mitosis, the nuclear DNA is not replaced. Consequently, cell multiplication and tissue repair are reduced. But although change is inevitable, its rapidity and extent are highly correlated with the individual's investment or lack of investment in living.

PHYSICAL CHANGES. During the gradual onset of aging, the body experiences degeneration in structure and functions. Loss of bone density and mass (a condition known as *osteoporosis*) causes a compression of bones, especially in the vertebral area, so that there is a slight decrease in height. All bones break more easily and heal more slowly. A loss of cartilage makes painful joint complaints more common and decreases range of movement and mobility. A curved posture becomes increasingly common with age.

Visual acuity decreases beyond the sixties. Because of changes in the eye, older people accommodate more slowly to light and dark, color, and depth. Night driving may be more hazardous for this reason. Color and depth perception are also less accurate.

Hearing acuity decreases with age as the mean pure tone threshold at all sound frequencies increases in both sexes. Many older people, either unaware of or hesitant to admit a hearing loss, may pretend to understand messages that they do not hear completely. They may try to piece together what they did hear and fill in the blanks. As a result, they may receive the wrong message.

Taste buds and the sense of smell decrease with age; this contributes to a loss of appetite—and loss of appetite, in turn, may lead to an unbalanced diet and inadequate nutritional intake, especially if finances are limited or preparing food becomes difficult. The integrity of teeth depends on regular dental maintenance. Many people retain their own teeth; but others wear partial or full dentures.

Changes in skin and tissues are common. Pigment deposits in the skin may produce "age spots"; loss of elasticity produces wrinkles and jowls. The sebaceous glands slow down, and the skin may become dry and scaly. There is also a decrease in body hair and an increase in facial hair, owing to a decrease in hormone secretion.

Sexual activity usually diminishes markedly during this stage, more so in men than in women. In men the erectile capacity decreases, and ejaculation may or may not occur even if an erection is attained. In women, vaginal lubrication diminishes because of estrogen depletion, so that artificial lubricants may be necessary during intercourse. However, the capacity for sexual functioning does not disappear. Ongoing sexual behavior will depend on attitudes about sexual activity for this age group, interest, availability of a partner, and health status. Sex becomes a recreative rather than procreative activity. While arousal and orgasm diminish in intensity and frequency, sexual activity can continue to provide a physical and emotional bond that creates and expresses intimacy, affection, and tenderness.[30]

Health problems become an increasing concern. Cardiovascular, pulmonary, and renal problems can be treated medically but may eventually take their toll. Cancer is prevalent in this age group.

COGNITIVE CHANGES. Cognitive changes occur in late adulthood. However, their extent is quite variable. Physical factors such as sensory, neurological, and circulatory changes can interfere with the reception of incoming and outgoing stimuli and increase reaction time.[28] New information may take more time to assimilate, and visual and auditory information may be missed. However, cognitive abilities can be retained into advanced old age. The brain has a reserve capacity that enables older adults to remain relatively unimpaired cognitively because they develop ways to counteract slight memory loss or slowness in learning. The older person is likely to be superior to the younger person in overall factual information and coordination of facts or ideas, all of which enhance or maintain problem-solving skills. Experience, maturity, and judgment may also combine to maintain problem-solving abilities.[29]

Some of what is considered cognitive impairment results from attitudes toward older people. Society expects people to become mentally deteriorated or senile as they age. If this attitude is incorporated by older people, they begin to perceive themselves as cognitively inept, become less willing to use the cognitive skills they do have, and become apprehensive about intellectual activities. Thus cognitive deterioration becomes a self-fulfilling prophecy. In fact, however, older people can maintain cognitive integrity if extra time is allowed for assimilation and mastery, if adequate social stimulation is provided, and if they are valued by themselves and others as a meaningful participants and contributors.

Psychosocial Development in Late Adulthood

Little is known about the older adult psychosocially. There are several theories about certain aspects of psychosocial aging, but inadequate evidence exists to formulate a single theory. According to the *disengagement theory* proposed by Cummings and Henry, aging people and society inevitably withdraw from each other physically, emotionally, and socially. In this process both society and the individual prepare for death.[31] The *activity theory* formulated by Havighurst and others is opposed to the disengagement theory and is currently more popular.[13] According to this theory, the majority of older people maintain a fairly high level of activity and engagement. The degree of engagement or disengagement is influenced more by past lifestyles and social and economic forces than by aging itself. Physical, mental, and social activities are usually necessary for successful aging and should be maintained long as possible.

These theories can be seen as representing opposite ends of a continuum. It is likely that most people fall somewhere between. Although older people reduce activities in some areas, such as work, they may increase activities in other areas, such as hobbies. "Load shedding" occurs as energy decreases. However, selective, meaningful involvement may continue. Neugarten[14] states that level of activity will be influenced by patterns established in younger years. Disengagement may occur involuntarily owing to death of spouse and peers and concomitant lack of social opportunities, lack of finances or transportation, or poor health.

The central psychosocial tasks of late adulthood involve loss and change. Changes in roles, activity, social relationships, finances, and living arrangements frequently occur. Loss is experienced with death of a spouse and friends and decreased independence. The changes noted above can also be perceived as losses if they are extensive or occur in areas of great importance. *Redefining a lifestyle* includes dealing with retirement, death of a spouse, rearrangement of social relationships, loss of independence, and altered living arrangements.

RETIREMENT. Retirement is often a crisis because it threatens identity, integrity, and self-esteem. In a production-oriented society, where (especially for men) one's major social role is occupational, retirement, whether voluntary or forced, may mean loss or reduction of income, influence, responsibility, authority, status, social relationships, creativity, activity, and control over the environment.[10,15,27]

Retirement may be less of a crisis for women who have primarily been homemakers. They have already had to adjust to a form of retirement when child rearing was completed in their late forties or fifties. However, a husband's retirement may result in loss of privacy and increased demands on a woman's personal time. Women who have combined homemaking and a career may also find retirement less of a crisis, since they have undergone many changes in and modifications of roles.

Retirement does not affect everyone in the same way. Several factors contribute to the way it is experienced:

- Degree to which leisure-time activities have been developed and are seen as meaningful and ego-enhancing
- Degree to which attitudes and perceptions of self-worth are determined by one's work
- Degree to which friendships and social involvement have been developed and can be maintained
- Degree to which changes in income will inhibit retirement activity and determine lifestyle
- Degree to which the spouses look forward to increased opportunities for time together and whether these expectations are met

The likelihood that retirement will be experienced as a crisis is increased when a person has been rigidly preoccupied with work, has done no preretirement planning, or has found little order or meaning in life throughout adulthood.[27]

DEATH OF SPOUSE. Women, who outlive men by an average of 8 years, are much more likely to experience loss of a spouse than men. The loss is significant, for it not only involves the death of a lifelong companion but also is an undeniable reminder of one's own mortality. Reaction to the loss of a spouse will depend on the quality of the relationship, how much warning there was of the approaching death, how independent the survivor is, how supportive family and friends are, and what financial burdens exist.

For a woman, the loss of a spouse deprives her not only of a significant other, but also of any identity which she may have achieved through her husband's social and economic position. If a woman has not developed an individual identity, she must now redefine herself socially and economically. For example, a woman who has never learned to balance a checkbook may suddenly have to handle financial matters for herself, or a woman who was married for 40 years may have to enter the dating world in search of companionship.

However, men are more apt to suffer acute loneliness after the death of their wives. The wife is often the husband's only confidant and friend. Men may feel that they must be courageous and unemotional in their bereavement, and they may have nobody with whom to share their grief. Also, some men are less independent. Living alone and taking care of themselves may be difficult: laundry, housecleaning, shopping, and cooking may be unfamiliar tasks. Twice as many widowers remarry as widows—possibly for these reasons, and possibly because women have more opportunities for companionship without remarrying than men do.

ONE'S OWN DEATH. Life, of course, does not continue indefinitely. Some people deal with the prospect of death by denying it; others seem to accept it, saying that they have lived full lives and have no fear of personal extinction. Some cultures—ours included—avoid the subject of death and thus make it difficult for people to verbalize their positive or negative feelings about it. This often leads to suppression of fear, increased anxiety, and maladaptive behavior.[20]

SOCIAL RELATIONSHIPS. Peer groups of old, close friends grow smaller as friends die and move away; and three-fourths of older people live apart from their families. Opportunities for social contacts shrink unless people reach out and form new relationships. It is easy for the elderly to sink into isolation, loneliness, boredom, and despair. At a time when they feel that social connectedness is vanishing and that their worth as social beings is gone, they must repattern their social world so that they do not become isolated. Senior citizens' centers, church groups, "volunteer grandparent" groups, and residential complexes for the elderly are all vehicles for expanding social relationships.

Connectedness with family, particularly children and grandchildren, can be very satisfying if the older adult is not perceived in a negative way by family members, made a scapegoat for family problems, or excluded from an active role in the family.[32] The desire to leave a legacy, to pass something personal along to others in the next generation, can often be accomplished in grandparent-grandchild relationships; grandparents pass on skills, family history, and the wisdom gained through experience to their grandchildren. This enables them to feel a sense of immortality and a link with the future. Such a legacy can also be transmitted through other young people or the community.[5,28]

MAINTAINING INDEPENDENCE. Ongoing health problems and disability may result in dependence on others for care, support, and security. The older adult has fewer support systems. For example, an older adult may live far from family, may be widowed, may be without friends, and may be unaware of community resources. Lack of financial resources also may inhibit the seeking of needed services. Meals-on-Wheels, homemaker services, community health nurses, senior citizen clinics, Dial-a-Ride, and state aid to the elderly are all community services available to help people care for themselves and remain as independent as possible.

ALTERED LIVING ARRANGEMENTS. A need to alter living arrangements can come about because of physical limitations, changes in financial status or family configurations, changed relationships, and deteriorating neighborhood conditions.

Physical limitations can lead to a loss of the ability to live independently. Sometimes only a relatively minor change will solve a problem; for example, a woman who had had a severe heart attack moved from a third-floor walk-up apartment to a lobby-level apartment. But physical disability may also necessitate supervision. The degree of supervision required can vary from a nighttime sitter to a full-time homemaker to a skilled nursing facility. Only 5 percent of the elderly live in institutions; most maintain themselves in community settings.

Changing family configurations most commonly result from loss of a spouse and geographic separation from children. Loss of a spouse through death leaves the survivor alone and faced with a decision to live alone, find a companion, or move in with other family members. In most cases family members are unwilling or unable to have a parent move in. They may feel that this would set the stage for multigenerational conflict between grandparents, parents, and children; or they may not have space for an extra person. Older people themselves may not want to live under someone else's roof, even if invited. They often feel like a "fifth wheel" with no authority, role, or corner to call their own. Older adults must thus come to terms with the decision to remain alone or find a place where they will belong.

Options for altered living arrangements are available to individuals or couples in late adulthood. Many older people leave established neighborhoods and head south to the warmth of Florida, Arizona, and California; others move to senior housing in their own communities. Retirement communities provide transportation, an age-appropriate social network, and sense of community that may be missing for the older adult who remains in a heterogeneous community.

Changes in finances may necessitate a move to more modest surroundings. This may be accompanied by loss of status, prestige, and self-worth, and it may mean separation from any social network that is not accessible with available transportation. Many older adults exist on fixed incomes; when income does not increase with inflation, the older person may become impoverished. This often results in the entrapment of older people in deteriorating neighborhoods, the only ones they can afford. Their living arrangements are substandard; they are often terrorized by neighborhood crime. They huddle in isolation, powerless to help themselves. Community resources can assist such people in locating more adequate, safer housing that is government-subsidized or privately owned.

Despite losses, potential crises, and undercurrents of grief running through their lives, members of this older age group are also concerned with actualizing their remaining possibilities and maintaining integrity and dignity.

Those who do not cope effectively, who do not reach out, become bored and stagnant.[5] Many also become bitter and withdrawn, feeling themselves to be victims of their age. Because processes of decline and growth occur concomitantly but not in equal balance, it is of utmost importance for care givers to examine the symptomatology before making judgments about any client. More than with any other age group, it is necessary to be aware of stereotyped attitudes toward the aging process, the wide variety of individual differences that do exist, and the effectiveness of intervention.

Spiritual Development in Late Adulthood

Spiritual development continues into late adulthood. Although death looms, people still have time to contemplate spiritual issues, especially mortality, immortality, and transcendence.[30]

Religion is a significant factor in happiness, usefulness, and personal adjustment in older people, especially men and those over 70.[33] Research indicates that people who have grown up with a religious affiliation continue it for as long as possible.[34] Very often, activities related to a church or synogogue became the focus of the social world and decrease only when a person becomes ill or transportation is not available. Religious activities within the home may increase as well.

Older people who do not have a religion or an abiding sense of the spiritual may feel purposeless, worthless, unloved, and perhaps abandoned by God, and they may fear death. They may struggle frantically to find some belief that will help them deal with the inevitable end of life. Most people with strong religious beliefs do not fear death; rather, they accept it as an inherent part of life. If they are anxious, it is about the process of dying, not death itself. They fear losing control as death approaches, being unable to obtain help when they need it, and being abandoned.[30]

SUMMARY

Development is a continuous process that represents an evolution toward increasing complexity and diversity; there is no "final stage" of growth or maturity. All aspects of human development are integrated and interrelated. Developmental processes, which are unique for each person, emerge from continuous interaction with the environment. Developmental norms are relative; therefore, development cannot be predicted with absolute accuracy. Norms are more useful as a tool for communication than as generalizations about people.

The life cycle can be viewed in terms of physical, cognitive, psychosocial, and spiritual forces that form a matrix for individual growth and development. The life cycle is divided into nine stages: infancy, early childhood, middle childhood, late childhood, adolescence, young adulthood, adulthood, middle adulthood, and late adulthood. The theories of Freud, Erikson, Sullivan, Mahler, Piaget, Levinson, Lidz, Sheehy, Havighurst, and Neugarten contribute to the understanding of developmental processes. These theorists provide an eclectic base for examining physical, cognitive, psychosocial, and spiritual development throughout each stage of the life cycle.

Nurses need a thorough knowledge base about developmental processes in order to understand the feelings, thoughts, and actions of individuals and families in particular stages of the life cycle as they encounter them in clinical settings. Such a knowledge base is also invaluable for anticipatory guidance and health teaching.

REFERENCES

1. L. Von Bertalanffy, *General Systems Theory*, Braziller, New York, 1968.
2. Martha Rogers, *An Introduction to the Theoretical Basis of Nursing*, Davis, Philadelphia, 1970.
3. Sigmund Freud, *A General Introduction to Psychoanalysis*, Pocket Books, New York, 1972.
4. Harry S. Sullivan, in Helen S. Perry, ed., *Interpersonal Theory of Psychiatry*, Norton, New York, 1953.
5. Erik H. Erikson, *Childhood and Society*, Norton, New York, 1963.
6. M. Mahler, *The Psychological Birth of the Human Infant: Symbiosis and Individuation*, Basic Books, New York, 1975.
7. M. Mahler, "The Rapprochement Subphase of the Separation-Individuation Process," in R. F. Lax, S. Bach, and J. A. Burland, eds., *Rapprochement: The Critical Subphase of Separation-Individuation*, Aronson, New York, 1980.
8. J. Piaget, *The Child's Conception of the World*, Littlefield, Adams, New York, 1963.
9. J. Piaget, "The Stages of the Intellectual Development of the Child," *Bulletin of the Menninger Clinic*, vol. 26, no. 4103, 1962, pp. 120–132.
10. Theodore Lidz, *The Person: His Development throughout the Life Cycle*, Basic Books, New York, 1968.
11. Daniel J. Levinson et al., *The Seasons of a Man's Life*, Ballantine, New York, 1978.

12. Gail Sheehy, *Passages*, Dutton, New York, 1976.
13. R. J. Havighurst and R. Albrecht, *Older People*, Longmans, New York, 1953.
14. Bernice Neugarten et al., *Middle Age and Aging*, University of Chicago Press, Chicago, 1968.
15. K. Freiberg, *Human Development*, Duxbury, North Scituate, Mass., 1979.
16. G. Scipien et al., *Comprehensive Pediatric Nursing*, 3d ed., McGraw-Hill, New York, 1983.
17. K. Berger, *The Developing Person*, Worth, New York, 1980.
18. J. A. Shelly, *The Spiritual Needs of Children*, Inter-Varsity, Downers Grove, Ill., 1982.
19. Robert F. Biehler, *Child Development: An Introduction*, Houghton Mifflin, Hopewell, N. J., 1976.
20. D. Aguilera and J. Messick, *Crisis Intervention: Theory and Methodology*, 4th ed., Mosby, St. Louis, 1982.
21. L. Kohlberg, "The Cognitive-Developmental Approach to Socialization," in D. Goslin, ed., *Handbook of Socialization*, Rand McNally, Chicago, 1969.
22. J. Piaget, *The Moral Judgement of the Child*, Routledge, London, 1932.
23. S. W. Nicholson, "Growth and Development," in Jeanne Howe, ed., *Nursing Care of Adolescents*, McGraw-Hill, New York, 1980.
24. Patricia H. Meyer, "Between Families: The Unattached Young Adult," in B. Carter and M. McGoldrick, eds., *The Family Life Cycle*, Gardner, New York, 1980.
25. M. McGoldrick, "The Joining of Families through Marriage: The New Couple," in B. Carter and M. McGoldrick, eds., *The Family Life Cycle*, Gardner Press, New York, 1980.
26. Paulina McCullough, "Launching Children and Moving On," in B. Carter and M. McGoldrick, eds., *The Family Life Cycle*, Gardner Press, New York, 1980.
27. R. N. Butler and M. I. Lewis, *Aging and Mental Health*, 3d ed., Mosby, St. Louis, 1981.
28. Irene M. Burnside, *Nursing and the Aged*, 2d ed., McGraw-Hill, New York, 1981.
29. Ruth Murray et al., *The Nursing Process in Later Maturity*, Prentice-Hall, Englewood Cliffs, N. J., 1980.
30. R. Ebersole and R. Ness, *Toward Healthy Aging: Human Needs and Nursing Response*, 2d ed., Mosby, St. Louis, 1985.
31. E. Cummings and W. E. Henry, *Growing Old: The Process of Disengagement*, Basic Books, New York, 1961.
32. John J. Herr and John H. Weakland, *Counseling Elders and Their Families*, Springer, New York, 1979.
33. D. Blazer and E. Palmore, "Religion and Aging in a Longitudinal Panel," *Gerontologist*, vol. 16, no. 1, 1976, pp. 82–94.
34. B. A. Devine, "Attitudes of the Elderly Toward Religion," *Journal of Gerontological Nursing*, vol. 6, no. 11, 1980, pp. 679–687.

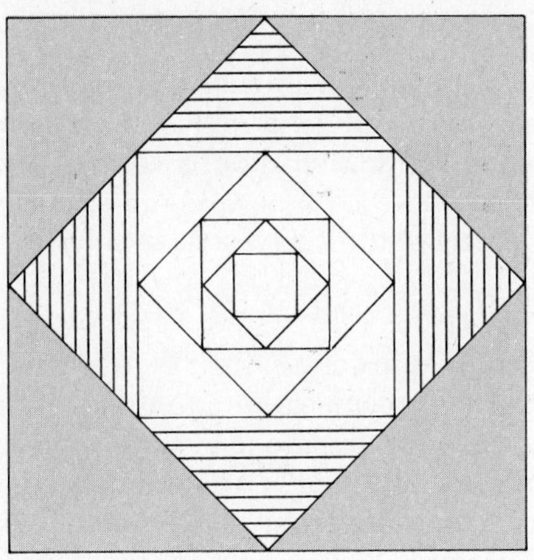

CHAPTER 6
Sociocultural Issues

Mary J. Giuffra

LEARNING OBJECTIVES

After studying this chapter, the student should be able to:

1. Identify the relevance of sociocultural issues in psychiatric–mental health nursing.
2. Define culture.
3. Discuss the characteristics and components of culture.
4. Describe the dominant value orientations of selected American ethnic groups.
5. Define ethnicity.
6. Discuss the effect of positive and negative stereotyping.
7. Compare and contrast a relativistic and ethnocentric cultural perspective.
8. Formulate a definition of *health.*
9. Differentiate between an emic and etic definition of mental health.
10. Discuss the process and consequences of labeling.
11. Describe the nurse's role in the labeling process.
12. Discuss beliefs about health that may be held by the black, Hispanic, and Asian Americans and American Indians.
13. Discuss sociocultural influences on the definition of mental health and illness.
14. Describe sociocultural influences on health care.
15. Identify cultural barriers to the formulation of effective nurse-client relationships.

Nurses assume that they know a great deal about their fellow human beings, particularly their patients or clients. In actuality very little is known. The British psychiatrist, R. D. Laing, proposes that

> I see you and you see me. I experience you and you experience me. I see your behavior. You see my behavior. But I do not [see], and never have [seen], and never will see your experience of me. Just as you cannot "see" my experience of you ... [1]

Laing suggests that all people are invisible to one another. What a humbling thought! This quotation highlights the importance of knowing as much as possible about other people's, other families', and other groups' unique experience of mind, body, and spirit. A logical extension of this thought is that understanding the complexities of clients' unique cultural experiences is important in psychiatric–mental health nursing. The potential for misunderstanding is accentuated when the nurse and the client—whether an individual, a family, or a community—are from different cultural or ethnic groups.[2–6] Misunderstanding, and inability to provide appropriate and effective health care, may arise from differences in beliefs, values, customs, or health practices. Recognition of and sensitivity to these cultural variables is a requirement for the delivery of high-quality health care in culturally diverse situations. The purpose of this chapter is to examine important cultural factors that influence the practice of psychiatric–mental health nursing.

CULTURE

Culture is defined as learned patterns of values, beliefs, attitudes, customs, and behaviors that are shared by a group in a particular social environment. Culture provides a set of rules or prescriptions for daily living and decision making that are valued by a specific group of people. In effect, each of us lives within an invisible sheath we call *culture*. There are many layers to this sheath. Some layers are fashioned by our family of origin and ethnic background. Other layers are formed by our religion, political beliefs, or social class. Climate and geography also affect our sheath of culture. The layers in this sheath touch us, leaving an imprint, lightly or indelibly. Basic characteristics of culture are presented in Table 6-1.

Components of Culture

Components of a culture include subsystems through which beliefs, values, and behaviors are expressed by its members. Communication, religious and political beliefs, values, roles, norms, and ethnicity are an integral part of the expression of culture.

Communication

The goal of a communication system is to transmit the values that help members of an ethnic group or a culture to set priorities and to resolve conflicts. These elements are bound in verbal and nonverbal language and are passed from one generation to the next. For example, Italian culture traditionally gives family needs priority in times of conflict. German culture gives respect for authority high priority. American culture would tend to resolve conflicts on the basis of individual need.

Through communication, children are taught the values and behaviors considered appropriate by the society. Language is culture-bound in that it prescribes what events can be expressed, and what events are negated or denied to the extent that no words exist to describe them or communicate about them.[7] The meaning of *communication* itself varies across cultures. For example, the Japanese client may nod and say *hai* ("yes"); a Hawaiian child may not look you full in the face; a Hispanic client may be late for your appointment. This does not mean that the Japanese person agrees with you, or that the Hawaiian child is evasive, or that the Hispanic person is resisting treatment. Rather, communication patterns, verbal and nonverbal, reflect the cultural prescriptions.[8]

Religious Beliefs

Religious beliefs reflect a culture's assumptions about its members' relationship to a spiritual being. Within most cultures, religious beliefs are structured and systematized. They range from beliefs in magic and superstition to beliefs that are grounded in science and rationality. Each culture has an organizing framework for combining the elements of superstition, religion, and science into a harmonious whole. Certain people in every society are considered religious specialists. They may be priests, rabbis, or shamans. They provide leadership in helping people understand and operationalize the religious beliefs and values of the culture.

Table 6-1 Characteristics That Identify the Nature of Cultures

Characteristic	Description	Example
Culture is learned.	Culture is a learned set of values, beliefs, and behaviors that are shared by a group of people who learn them through formal and informal channels. Culture is not genetically inherited—unlike *race,* which refers to biologically inherited characteristics that are observable in physical traits.	Children learn what, when, where, how, and with whom they will eat.
Culture is transmitted.	Culture is passed from one generation to another by a process called *enculturation.*	Parenting behaviors are transmitted from one generation to the next by informally observing the behaviors of parental role models and the reactions of others to their behavior.
Culture is shared.	Culture is a shared set of assumptions, values, beliefs, attitudes, and behaviors of a group of people. Sharing a common culture allows members of a cultural group to predict one another's actions and to react accordingly.	An assumption of traditional Arab culture is that a woman will not make eye contact with a man other than her husband. All decisions are made by the husband. Since a woman may not be touched by another man, health care may be provided only by another woman.
Individual behavior is not necessarily representative of the culture.	Although the culture defines the dominant patterns of values, beliefs, and behaviors, it does not determine all the behaviors in any group. Variation from the dominant pattern of behavior encountered in one individual is called *idiosyncratic behavior.* The meaning of this behavior within the culture will determine whether it is regarded as normal, eccentric, or deviant. A whole group of people within a society who share values, beliefs, and behaviors that differ from those of the dominant culture is referred to as a *subculture.*	Male and female roles are highly stereotyped in traditional Greek culture. Women are secondary to men. The man is the head of the family. Men work and provide for their families; it is a dishonor if the wife works outside the home. Within this cultural context, a Greek woman who is a proponent of the feminist movement might be viewed as eccentric or deviant, depending on how vocal she is or how much her beliefs disrupt the community.
Culture is integrated.	Universal aspects of culture include religion, politics, economics, art, kinship, diet, health, and patterns of communication. It is difficult, if not impossible, to study only one aspect of a culture because these categories are so interrelated.	When examining the dominant religion of any culture, one must also consider the political, economic, and social forces that have shaped the belief system that has evolved.
Culture contains ideal and real components.	Ideal cultural patterns are called *norms.* They refer to what people ought to do in a particular situation. These norms may be reinforced through legal or social means. Real behavior may diverge from ideal behavior and still be acceptable.	A cultural norm may condemn direct use of alcohol on a daily basis. However, those people who consume alcohol daily, but "hold their liquor well," are looked upon with only minimal disapproval.
Cultures are dynamic entities that are continuously evolving.	Cultural change is an ongoing, but slow process. All aspects of culture do not change simultaneously. Cultural habits and superficial behaviors are easier to alter than are deep-rooted values and beliefs that are acquired early in life.	Changes in economic systems may precede changes in family relationships or political organizations.

Religion validates and reinforces the social order of the culture. A deity is identified as the power behind humanity. This could be an energizing life force, called *mana;* to the Indian it could be the "great spirit"; to central African tribes it could be called *zeza,* or "cherisher." Many gods and spirits are included in the concept of deity.[9] It has been envisioned as being shaped by culture and era. At least one anthropologist believes that people's view of deity is influenced by their view of their parents.

Images of God will change with each generation's experience of parental style. A gentle style of child rearing, for instance, may lead to a view of God as loving, kind, and forgiving.

Religion provides answers to questions such as: "Why am I sick, bereaved, a failure?" Consoling answers may help people toward resignation: "It is God's will." "This is your karma." "This is Allah's will." Some religions see misfortune as punishment by the deity for misdeeds by clients and their families or ancestors. Others see misfortune as a gift from God to those strong enough to accept burdens.

An important aspect of religion relates to the afterlife. What happens after death is conceived of in various ways: nirvana, jodo land, paradise, the isle of the blest, heaven, or hell. But all such concepts involve continued existence of the soul or spirit after death. Belief in an afterlife can solace the bereaved, or it can reinforce guilt and anxiety. It can motivate people to live by the highest values, or it can inhibit personal ambition and social progress.

For generations, religions have used spiritual practices as a form of catharsis. For example, Buddhists, some Christians, and Indians use confession to alleviate guilt and acquire forgiveness. Many clients go to their religious leader before visiting a health professional. No matter what one's personal beliefs about religion are, it is essential to respect, and use, clients' religious beliefs as part of the therapeutic healing process.

Political Beliefs

The legal and the political systems of a culture emphasize its values, in general and at a specific period in history. In a country such as Germany or Japan, the government assumes a great deal of power in organizing people and resources. In others, such as Ireland, political beliefs are strongly influenced by the church. In Italy, for example, church and government are traditionally perceived as allies;[10] and in Greece the church has helped the Greeks to unify politically. In the United States, belief in individual rights is so strong that separation of church and state exists to an extreme. This belief also makes the notion of governmental planning abhorrent to many Americans, who see it in terms of totalitarianism or socialism; the people resist interference with free enterprise or the natural workings of the market.[11] A political leader, especially one who is charismatic, tends to be more influential than his or her political party. The individual, rather than the political party, becomes the focus of interest. It is evident that political beliefs evolve naturally from the basic value system of the culture. Through the political system, the values of the mainstream are supported, and the resulting norms are enforced through the legal system.

Values

Values are individualized rules by which people live. They provide the basis for beliefs, attitudes, and behaviors. Cultural values are those which are acquired unconsciously as one assimilates one's culture during the growing-up years. Because values generally exist on an unconscious level, they are difficult to assess objectively and difficult to alter. Thus, values which reflect one's culture have a pervasive influence. They prescribe the goals that people need to pursue and indicate behaviors that are appropriate in certain situations.

A comparative-values approach examines similar values in different cultures. Kluckhohn and Strodtbeck[12] define value orientations as "complex but definitely patterned principles ... which give order and direction to the ever-flowing stream of human acts and thoughts as these relate to the solution of 'common human problems.'" They propose that, although in all cultures some members will hold value orientations that vary from those of the rest of the group, dominant value orientations can be identified. Kluckhohn and Strodtbeck compare the way in which people of different cultures organize their thinking about time, personal activity, interpersonal relations, and their relation to nature and the supernatural.[12,13]

Temporal orientation divides time into three frames: past, present, and future. All cultures deal with all three, but cultures differ in their emphasis.

Activity orientation perceives the culture as primarily "doing"-oriented (that is, oriented toward achievement) or "being"-oriented. A "doing" orientation implies valuing accomplishments rather than inherent existence. The opposite is true in cultures with a "being" orientation; here a person is valued as a link in the chain between generations.

Relational orientation distinguishes among interpersonal patterns, that is, the ways in which the culture sets goals for its individual members. Relational orientations may be collateral, lineal, or individualistic.

When the *collateral* mode is dominant, the goals and welfare of laterally extended groups such as siblings or peers are of prime importance. In societies such as the Soviet Union and Israel, the goals of the individual are subordinated to those of the group. The group assumes responsibility for all its members.

When the *lineal* mode is dominant, group goals and group welfare are also of paramount importance. However, continuity of the group and orderly succession within the group over time are extremely important. All cultures which value lineality view kinship bonds as the basis for maintaining lineage.

Dominance of the *individualistic* mode suggests the primacy of individual goals over the goals of specific collateral or lineal groups. Each person's responsibility to and place in the total society are defined by autonomous goals. The individual is held responsible for personal behavior and is judged on the basis of personal accomplishments.

People-to-nature orientation has to do with whether people dominate nature, live in harmony with nature, or are subjugated to nature. The view that humans dominate nature suggests that humans can master or control natural events. The view that humans live in harmony with nature suggests that there is integration among people, nature, and the universe. The view that humans are subjugated to nature suggests a philosophy of fatalism: one accepts one's fate as inevitable and believes that nature dominates humans, who are powerless to guide their own destiny. Most cultures combine these three orientations, but one is likely to predominate.

"Innate human nature" orientation distinguishes among three different perspectives on human nature: good, evil, and neutral or mixed (a mixture of good and evil). Human beings can be viewed as having a basic nature that is either changeable or unchangeable. For instance, they can be considered evil and unchangeable, or evil but perfectible, or a mixture of good and evil subject to positive and negative influences. In the United States today, the prevailing view of human nature is a mixture of good and evil (this has replaced the Calvinist view of human nature as basically evil); thus there is a perceived need for control and discipline, but lapses in behavior are felt to be understandable and are not always to be condemned.

The United States, because it contains many diverse ethnic groups, does not exhibit a single dominant value orientation. Although a dominant value system might be identified for middle-class Americans of northern European descent, members of other American culture groups may have considerably different value orientations.[14] Table 6-2 (page 130) illustrates the diversity of traditional tendencies in value orientations among some American ethnic groups.

Roles and Norms

Each culture ascribes certain roles and role expectations based on age, sex, and marital status. *Roles* are patterns of behavior expected of people in certain positions. The concept of a role includes expectations about how one should think, value, act, and so on. A role, whether based on age, sex, or marital status, encompasses the duties of a position. For example, roles can be ascribed to the young, old, male, female, married, and widowed.

Roles are interdependent. A culture defines one person's role in relation to the roles of others. For example, as the role of a woman in a society changes, the role of a man changes simultaneously. Roles are "families of expectancies" about motivations, beliefs, feelings, attitudes, and values. Most people occupy more than one role at a given time. For instance, a competent professional woman may, at the same time, act as a subservient wife. Conversely, a highly demanding successful businessman may also be an obedient son to his father. Different treatment is given to people occupying certain positions, and this is guided by role expectations. There are great differences in role expectations from culture to culture.

Each group has norms which constitute standards for acceptable behavior. *Norms* are rules of conduct specifying what people should or should not do in given circumstances. Underlying shared beliefs about humans, their nature, and their interaction with the environment provide a sense of what is real and right for members of a particular society. For example, while among members of the dominant American culture it is considered polite and indicative of interest to make direct eye contact with a person, among members of Asian cultures it is considered polite *not* to make direct eye contact.

Table 6-2 Tendencies in Value Orientation of Selected American Ethnic Groups

	Orientation				
Ethnic Group	**Temporal**	**Activity**	**Relational**	**People to Nature and the Supernatural**	**Innate Nature of Human Beings**
Northern European Americans	Future over present	Doing	Individualistic	1. Dominant 2. Harmony with nature 3. Subjugated	1. Mixed 2. Evil 3. Good
Black Americans	Present over future	Being	Collateral-lineal	1. Subjugated 2. Dominant 3. Harmony with nature	1. Mixed 2. Evil 3. Good
Mexican Americans	Present	Being	Lineal-collateral	Subjugated	1. Mixed 2. Evil 3. Good
Puerto Ricans	Present over future	Being	Lineal-collateral	Subjugated	1. Mixed 2. Evil 3. Good
American Indians	Present	Being	Collateral-individual	Harmony with nature	1. Good 2. Mixed 3. Evil
Chinese Americans	Past-present	Being	Lineal	Harmony with nature	1. Good 2. Mixed 3. Evil
Japanese Americans	Past-present	Being	Lineal	Harmony with nature	1. Good 2. Mixed 3. Evil

Ethnicity

An *ethnic* group has been defined as people who consider themselves alike by virtue of a common ancestry (real or fictitious), and who are so regarded by others.[15] *Ethnicity* refers to traditions handed down from generation to generation, and to common roots and beliefs that are reinforced by the environment. Ethnicity runs deep; some aspects may even have a genetic basis. It involves conscious and unconscious processes that meet a need for identity and continuity. Ethnicity determines our initial values and beliefs and greatly influences our thinking, emotional responses, and feelings; responses to life events are also colored by ethnicity.

Ethnicity affects people's appearance—skin color and texture, shape of the eyes, form and height of the body, and bone structure. It affects speech patterns and tones, use of language, and vocabulary (words that are included and excluded). Thinking, whether concrete or abstract, and the ways in which people are encouraged to develop are also influenced by ethnicity. Patterns of child rearing, relationships between men and women, careers chosen—all these can be related, in some way, to ethnicity. The god worshipped or negated and the place of worship can be determined ethnically. Books that are read, the way they are written, literary style, the ways they are bound and opened—these too may be guided by ethnicity. Games played and rules used to organize them; holidays and how they are celebrated; homes people live in and the way they are furnished—again, these are things that can be determined by ethnicity. Sexual experiences and reactions to them, and types of marriages or living arrangements can have an ethnic basis. Illnesses and the way people view and cure them and beliefs about death and what lies beyond it are affected by ethnicity. Political and educational systems and people's attitudes toward them can have ethnic underpinnings. Who people are—how they see themselves, their self-esteem, their body image, their leadership styles, and their ways of following leaders—may also be rooted in ethnicity. Foods people eat, use of leisure time, artistic expression—music, art, theater, photography—have been influenced by ethnicity. Since ethnicity is—consciously and unconsciously—so much a part of people's deepest being, it is an essential subject for the psychiatric–mental health nurse to study.

Culture obviously has many components. Nurses need to remember that, although all people are under the influence of their own cultural system, within all groups individuals exhibit various patterns. Thus, although culture can be expressed in communication, religious and political beliefs, values, roles, and norms (among many other things), it is essential not to use culture as a basis for stereotyping people but rather to consider it as a dimension that requires attention when clients and nurses come from different backgrounds.

Stereotyping

Awareness of and sensitivity to cultural differences in clients is essential. However, ethnicity is only one guideline among many for effective delivery of health care. Cultural affiliation can serve as a backdrop or context for approaching clients in a holistic way. But it is important not to overgeneralize or to stereotype people on the basis of culture or ethnicity.

A *stereotype* is a relatively simple picture of a cultural group. Stereotypes are formed from things we *think* are true about other cultures. For example, even today it is not uncommon to hear people say, "Blacks are musical"; "Jews have money"; "The Japanese are good mathematicians"; "The Irish drink too much." These are overgeneralizations—they are founded on incomplete experiences and are not universally valid when individual members of the culture are looked at holistically. For example, European Jews were traditionally moneylenders and bankers because for a long time they were not allowed to own land. The idea that they were, therefore, wealthy was valid in only a few cases; but the stereotype "Jews have money" was perpetuated over the generations and took on negative connotations. Our ideas about members of any ethnic, religious, or racial group can be influenced by stereotypes.

Three types of stereotypes are negative, positive, and traditional. A negative stereotype which is emotionally charged and not easily changed by new information is called *prejudice.* In a classic study, Campbell explored ethnic prejudice.[16] He interviewed 316 white, non-Jewish Americans to obtain information on factors in their private life which were associated with negative attitudes toward Jews. He found that subjects who were dissatisfied with their own economic situation expressed hostile attitudes toward Jews more frequently than those who were satisfied. Only 10 percent of the satisfied subjects expressed hostility in contrast to 38 percent of the dissatisfied subjects. Subjects who were dissatisfied with the current political situation also showed greater hostility. Research like this suggests that prejudice is a way of displacing unacceptable impulses of cruelty, greed, or aggression onto people from another group.

Even positive stereotypes can create problems. For example, studies of the elderly in San Francisco's Chinatown have revealed that a serious erosion of Chinese patterns of kinship and community has occurred in the urban United States.[17,18] These findings are contrary to the stereotyped idea of the Chinese as particularly reverent toward their elders. In this case, as a result of positive stereotyping, actual problems of the elderly may be overlooked.

Another type of stereotyping is indiscriminate characterization of all members of minority populations as traditionalists—that is, the notion that all members of a culture maintain its traditional beliefs, values, and customs. Each ethnic group has members who are more or less like the dominant society or the world at large. *Acculturation* is the degree to which members of a culture other than the dominant culture have internalized the dominant culture's norms and values. It varies greatly, depending on age, sex, education, and generation of immigration, among other factors.

A single comment can bring stereotyping alive. For example, a health care worker said to a female Arab client, "I won't even tell you what your options are until you come back with your husband," not taking time to find out whether or not this woman—who was casually dressed in western fashion—lived on the basis of traditional Arab beliefs or was more Americanized.[19,20] It is wise for nurses to be aware of the fact that their ethnic, racial, and religious stereotypes will be readily communicated to clients. It is not surprising that clients are often hostile toward health care workers and resist intervention—they may bear the scars of stereotyping and discrimination. Nurses should identify and examine their own stereotypes, since cultural and sexual stereotyping makes it difficult to recognize and accept diversity and individuality within a cultural group. Generalization about cultural patterns may be necessary for an overview, but failure to see differences within a culture results in misconceptions and misunderstandings.

The Relative Nature of Culture

Culture is seen from a *relativistic,* or *relative,* perspective when we try to understand others within the context of their background—in health care and in other areas of life. In contrast to this is the *ethnocentric* perspective, from which we judge everyone by the standards of our own culture.

Ethnocentrism characterizes much of our thinking. It is, to put it simply, the idea that the way things are done in one's own culture is the correct way. Ethnocentrism has been described by Simpson and Yanker as belief in the universal validity of one's own ways.[21] As a generalized attitude, it predisposes us to reject values, beliefs, and members of groups other than our own. Adorno defined ethnocentrism as based on

> rigid in-group out-group distinction; it involves stereotyped negative imagery and hostile attitudes regarding out-groups, and a hierarchical, authoritarian view of group direction in which in-groups are rightly dominant, out-groups subordinate.[22]

Dominance is particularly significant in multiethnic health care settings. In American society, health professionals tend to assume a dominant position relative to clients. When the health professional is a member of the mainstream culture, this dominance is accentuated. Jaffe Ruiz studied ethnocentrism among members of a nursing faculty[23] and found that it was correlated with negative attitudes toward culturally different patients. She has suggested that further study is needed to observe whether ethnocentric faculty members adequately convey cultural differences to their students.

In contrast, *cultural relativism* is the idea that judgments are based on experience, and experience is interpreted by each individual in terms of his or her unique cultural experience. As a member of a particular culture, the health professional—say, the nurse—is a biased observer. However, a nurse who takes a relativistic perspective attempts to accept or understand behavior of transcultural clients without making evaluations on the basis of his or her own culture. The relativist strives to understand the client's culture as a whole. A relativistic framework implies cultural acceptance rather than cultural imposition.[24] For example:

> A native of the British West Indies was hospitalized in New York for repair of torn knee ligaments. Following surgery, the man—who had a robust, husky build—appeared downcast and had no appetite. Tray after tray of food was returned untouched. The staff asked him why he wasn't eating. They told him that the hospital had very good food, asked whether he needed help filling out the menu form, and finally told him that if he didn't eat he would have to be fed intravenously. The next day a student nurse who was completing a cultural assessment which contained questions about dietary preferences approached the head nurse and said, "I think I know why Mr. A. is not eating. The foods he described eating at home are not at all like what he can order in the hospital." The head nurse went in to see Mr. A., verified the student's findings, and further discovered that Mr. A. felt intimidated about giving the staff this information and about asking if his wife could bring food from home. Once the staff was able to understand this client within the context of his culture rather than its own, the problem was solved: the staff agreed to let his wife bring him foods that he liked.

DEFINITIONS OF HEALTH

Each culture defines health in its own way; definitions of health are closely linked to cultural beliefs, values, and institutions. Several approaches to a definition of health are current in the literature; these approaches include *holistic, adaptive, wellness,* and *epidemiological*. There is, however, no one definition that completely defines health. Rather, various definitions provide a framework from which providers of health care are able to understand clients' behavior. The following paragraphs summarize definitions of health from these perspectives.

Holistic Definition

A holistic definition of health involves the entire person, not merely the mind or the body. A person is viewed as a unified, integrated biopsychosocial being in constant interaction with his or her environment throughout the life process from conception to death.[25] The definition implies an understanding of the interrelationship of psychological, social, and cultural processes. People are viewed as open systems with a continuous interchange between internal environment and external environment (other people, places, and things).[26]

There are different definitions of the term *holism* itself. But in general, in a holistic approach, the focus is on the client as a whole person. Clients are considered in the context of all their component parts and their interaction with the environment. Arbitrary divisions—such as "physical," "psychological," and "sociocultural" characteristics—run counter to the holistic approach.

The holistic approach implies that functioning or malfunctioning of mind, body, or environment will affect the whole person. A client's own perception of health and illness is considered an essential factor in assessment. Nurses consider multiple aspects of each client when formulating a nursing diagnosis—that is, a perception of health and illness. They consider that illness and health are concepts which vary with cultural norms and mores as well as socioeconomic background.

Adaptive Definition

Dubos defines *health* as a physical and mental state, fairly free of discomfort and pain, which permits us to function as effectively and as long as possible in the environment where chance or choice has placed us. Health, as Dubos sees it, is the adaptive response of the body to environmental stress or disease in order to maintain homeostasis. Homeostasis implies that the body can function well only if it can rapidly make adjustments which keep its internal composition within precisely defined limits. The concepts of homeostasis and adaptation are complementary and apply not only to biological organization but to social groups as well.[27]

Health as a process of adaptation requires a purposefully defined lifestyle. According to this interpretation, as we progress through the life cycle, we adapt to the changing environment and deal with maturation, aging, suffering, and death in an optimum manner.

Wellness Definition

A complete departure from the definition of *health* as merely the absence of disease, disability, or dysfunction can be found in Dunn's concept of high-level wellness.[28] *High-level wellness* is defined as an integrated method of functioning which is oriented toward maximizing one's potential. It requires that one maintain a continuum of balance and purposeful direction within one's environment. It is a state of complete physical, mental, and social well-being, characterized by energy, vitality, and a zest for life, that is an "integrated method of functioning which is oriented toward maximizing the potential."

Data suggest that few people have reached or will reach high-level wellness. However, this theory does clarify the dichotomy between wellness and illness, and it defines health in a positive sense. *Health* can be defined as the ability to cope with the activities of daily living without undue stress. People function at various levels of wellness; wellness is not static, but rather an ongoing process of maximizing one's potential. Illness, then, is defined as absence of the ability to cope with the activities of daily life.[29]

Epidemiological Definition

Epidemiology is a science and a specialized field of public health that concerns itself with the health of whole populations—specifically, with factors related to the distribution and control of disease and promotion of health in identified populations over given time periods. Two terms, *incidence* and *prevalence,* are used in the discussion and definition of health problems. *Incidence* refers to the number of new cases of a disease in a specific population over a specified period of time. *Prevalence* refers to the rate of established or diagnosed cases of the illness in a population at a certain point of time. Prevalence, then, includes the number of newly diagnosed cases of a disease as well as the number of old cases under treatment. Statistics concerning host, agent, and environment are accumulated and used to define the presence or absence of disease and to identify factors relating to the onset and persistence of illness.[30]

In speaking of populations, it is helpful to identify *populations at risk.* These are all the members of a specific population who might, under certain conditions, be vulnerable to a particular disease. Valid and reliable statistics on the incidence and prevalence of a health problem in a population at risk yield valuable information on the need for preventive health services and community programs and are one measure of effectiveness of a health care delivery system.

Although the epidemiological definition of health has value, its exclusive use has several drawbacks. Because health is defined as the absence of disease, little consideration is given to the impact of social, cultural, or personal factors. Likewise, only *reported* diseases are considered; this gives rise to questions about the accuracy of available statistics.

Definitions of Mental Health

There is wide variation in the way mental health and mental illness are defined and identified. From an ethnoscientific approach—that is, when we try to obtain an accurate account of a peoples' view and interpretation of the universe[31]—it seems especially appropriate to distinguish between *emic* and *etic* perspectives. The emic-etic framework, based on the work of Pike, is a way of characterizing how members of a cultural group define *normality* and *abnormality*.[32]

When we take an *emic* perspective, we set out to discover and describe an individual, a family, or a society from within a culture. This is a culture-specific approach which is concerned with how members of a culture order and interpret their world. The emic approach results in a definition of mental illness that is derived from the client's cultural matrix.[31]

In contrast, when we take an *etic* perspective, we focus on cultural universals—dimensions belonging to all cultures. An etic perspective does not involve learning about the cultural viewpoint of those being studied. Using externally derived criteria, the etic researcher examines and compares several cultures.[32,33] Pike calls these criteria "culture-free features of the real world" because they can be applied across cultures. The third edition of *Diagnostic and Statistical Manual of Mental Disorders* (DSM III) uses nomenclature which represents an attempt at a transcultural, etic classification system according to which data from individual clients are analyzed.

Nurses and clients may come to a health care setting with different beliefs about how mental illness is defined, how it is caused, and how it is best treated. The fundamental question that arises is, "Whose definition of mental health or illness is correct?" Because there are cultural variations in defining mental health and mental illness, what is viewed as normal behavior in one culture (or from an emic perspective) might be considered quite abnormal in another (or from an etic perspective). Consider a nurse from the dominant American culture whose Puerto Rican client states that he has been in contact with a dead relative or has been possessed by an evil spirit. From an etic perspective, this client is viewed by the non-Hispanic nurse as having a mental disorder. From an emic perspective, the client may be seen as having had a normal, culturally sanctioned experience of an altered state of consciousness, based on a culturally prescribed belief system that is common in many of the cultures of the world.[24]

THE LABELING PROCESS*

Because different cultures vary greatly in what they consider mentally "normal" and "abnormal," it is incumbent on psychiatric nurses to be aware of factors that combine to create what is called the *labeling process. Labeling* is a term used to refer to assigning a particular impression or diagnostic specification to a client. The labeling of mental illness is influenced by numerous factors. Labels are determined by environmental factors such as culture, economic status, social class, previous exposure to mentally ill persons, and familial attitudes toward mental illness.

Labeling involves another person's response to the behavior in question. How labels are derived determines their validity to a considerable extent. A label implies that others agree with the one doing the labeling. It is the diagnosis and labeling of clients that determine the way in which their illnesses are reported. A diagnostic label is also required in order to receive payment for care.

Frequently, labels determine what care clients receive. For example, because of withdrawn and unsocialized behavior a young adult woman may be labeled *schizophrenic,* then hospitalized, and then placed on psychotropic medication. Another label for the same person may suggest only that she is shy and unsocial and result in no treatment.

* Portions of this section from Deanna R. Pearlmutter and Mary T. Ramshorn, "Socio, Cultural, and Historical Aspects of Mental Health," in the second edition of this book.

In 1973 Rosenhan[34] published a research paper (which caused much discussion in medical circles) about the contextual nature of the labeling process. He examined the reasons for admission of eight sane people who simulated symptoms and were subsequently labeled *mentally ill.* The research gave cause for serious concern about discrepancies in the labeling process.[35]

Uniform Labels (DSM III)

Historically, the labeling process was influenced by both practitioners and clients. The cultural, social, economic, and professional backgrounds of the participants produced labels that were subjective and unscientific. Improvement in labeling began in 1952, when the American Psychiatric Association (APA) published the *Diagnostic and Statistical Manual of Mental Disorders* (DSM I). The second edition, DSM II, published in 1968, based its classification on the *International Classification of Diseases.*[36]

DSM III was approved by the APA in January 1979. It represents a diagnostic classification system that is proposed as clinically useful in a variety of settings, uses reliable diagnostic categories, and is acceptable to clinicians with a variety of professional backgrounds and theoretical orientations. Diagnostic categories are specifically defined, eliminating terminology that has outlived its usefulness but avoiding new terminology and untraditional concepts. Whenever they were available, data from research studies have been used to validate diagnostic categories. DSM III lists clinical features of each disorder. Associated features, age at onset, course of the illness, usual impairment, complications, and predisposing factors are listed when known. Prevalence, sex ratio (relative frequency of a disorder as diagnosed in men and women), and family patterns for each category are included.

A multiaxial system for labeling is recommended; it provides information of value in planning treatment and predicting outcomes. The severity of psychosocial stressors is rated from 1 (none) to 7 (catastrophic). A category for unspecified or unknown stressors is also included. Table 6-3 lists the psychosocial stressors that are considered by practitioners using DSM III to label clients.

Judgments about the highest level of functioning over the past year are included as part of the labeling process. This information provides care

Table 6-3 Psychosocial Stressors

Significant Stressor	Definitions and Examples, DSM III	Significant Stressor	Definitions and Examples, DSM III
Conjugal (marital and nonmarital)	Engagement Marriage Discord Separation Death of spouse	Financial	Inadequate finances Change in financial status
Parenting	Becoming a parent Friction with a child Illness of a child	Legal	Arrest Incarceration Lawsuit or trial
Other interpersonal	Problems with friends, neighbors, associates, nonconjugal family members Discordant relationship with boss Illness of best friend	Developmental	Phases of life cycle, such as transition from puberty to adulthood Menopause
Occupational	Work, school, homemaking, unemployment, retirement School problems	Physical illness or injury	Illness Accident Surgery Abortion
Living circumstances	Change in residence Threat to personal safety Immigration	Other psychosocial stressors	Natural and human disaster Persecution Unwanted pregnancy Out-of-wedlock birth Rape

(Continued.)

Table 6-3 Continued

Significant Stressor	Definitions and Examples, DSM III	Significant Stressor	Definitions and Examples, DSM III
Family factors (children and adolescents)	Cold, distant, or hostile relationship between parents Physical or mental illness in the family Cold, distant, or hostile behavior toward children Parental intrusiveness	Family factors (continued)	Inconsistent parental control Insufficient social and cognitive stimulation Anomalous family situation, such as single parent, foster family, institutional rearing, loss of members of nuclear family

SOURCE: *Diagnostic and Statistical Manual of Mental Disorders*, 3d ed., American Psychiatric Association, Washington, D. C., 1980.

givers with data about prognosis—the probability that clients will be able to return to a previous or adaptive level of functioning. Social relations, occupational functioning, and use of leisure time in the past year are assessed. These are rated on a scale of 1 to 7 from superior (1) to grossly impaired (7). "Unspecified" or "unknown" is scaled as zero (0). Table 6-4 lists and defines these levels of premorbid functioning.

Table 6-4 Adaptive Levels of Functioning before Illness

Level of Social Relationship, Occupational Functioning, and Use of Leisure Time	Definition
Superior	Unusually effective functioning in social relations, occupational functioning, and use of leisure time
Very good	Better-than-average functioning
Good	No more than slight impairment in either social or occupational functioning
Fair	Moderate impairment in either social or occupational functioning, or some impairment in both
Very poor	Marked impairment in both social relations and occupational functioning
Grossly impaired	Gross impairment in all areas of functioning

SOURCE: *Diagnostic and Statistical Manual of Mental Disorders*, 3d ed., American Psychiatric Association, Washington, D.C., 1980.

Consequences of Mislabeling

Because society as a whole remains ignorant about and sometimes biased toward the mentally ill, the consequences of mislabeling are often grave and sometimes even life-threatening.[37] Family members, employers, and others may stereotype a person labeled *mentally ill,* increasing the stress he or she is already undergoing. Labeling may also result in a negation of symptoms ("It's all in his head"), so that the person fails to seek treatment. Moreover, once people are labeled *deviant,* their self-concept may be injured. Some clients will disagree with a diagnosis and be labeled *resistive.* Others may comply, begin to behave as they have been labeled, and thus participate in a self-fulfilling prophesy. Some clients participate in a mislabeling process in order to obtain third-party payment or to avoid employment. Currently, prognoses based on diagnostic labels remain imprecise. Labeling does, however, provide a way for professionals to categorize clients. As the labeling of mental illness becomes more objective and more specific, care given to clients will be more uniform, efficient, and accurate.

Deviance

Deviance is a product of labeling, not an inherent quality. It is a human artifact. The term *deviance* describes behavior that diverges from—is different from—norms established by a group. The concept of deviance is other people's response to behavior and involves a sequence of recognizable roles.

It has been said that deviance is created by society. However, as a rule people within a society do agree about labels. People are labeled *deviant* not simply because they fail to obey established rules, but because their behavior disrupts or threatens the stability of those around them. Society creates deviance because society as a whole makes rules and assigns labels to those who break them. If society did not make rules or socially segregate people who break them, deviance would, of course, not exist. But this does not mean that there is no such thing as deviance or that people who commit crimes are innocent victims of society. Some people choose to engage in criminal behavior which society then labels as *deviant.* The phenomenon of deviance thus requires a look at both the individual and the society. For example, smoking in itself is not deviant. However, certain groups in our society have labeled smoking *deviant* by categorizing it and those who do it as violating group rules.

In any discussion of deviance, several factors should be considered:

1. Classifications of deviant behavior will vary over time. Behavior may be considered chic or avant-garde at one point in time and deviant at another. Some people may react differently to the same behavior at different times. For example, in our society driving while intoxicated has been handled ambivalently. At times it has been regarded as naughty but acceptable behavior with no penalty; at present it is regarded as deviant, and there are severe legal penalties.
2. Cultural background may influence whether a behavior is labeled *deviant* or *normal.* For example, in some cultures hallucinations are considered deviant; in others, people who hallucinate are honored as having special gifts.
3. Social status influences whether a behavior is labeled deviant. For example, upper-class adolescents may be said to be "sowing their wild oats" when they get tickets for speeding, while lower-class adolescents may be labeled *delinquent.*
4. The person or group that feels harmed or threatened by a particular thought, feeling, or action influences whether that behavior is labeled *deviant.* For example, if a hospitalized man from a West Indian culture reports that he has had a hex, or *mojo,* cast upon him by witchcraft, and if he is afraid to eat the food provided by the hospital because it may have been adulterated, this belief may generate anxiety in staff members. The staff may label this behavior as *deviant* or "crazy" and feel threatened because a client is saying "crazy" things.
5. The consequences of behavior also influence labeling. For example, pornography for adults may be considered less deviant than pornography for children.

Deviance is not just behavior that disrupts society. It also serves to preserve stability by clearly defining people who stray from the norm. Deviants are placed outside the bounds of society because they engage in certain socially unacceptable behaviors. When a person is redefined as deviant, that alters status and leads to negative expectations about behavior. The deviant evolves a negative self-image which may influence other people's present and future expectations.

The Nurse's Role in the Labeling Process

The nurse's role in the labeling process should not be underestimated. Nurses, like their clients, are the products of their environment. They, too, have cultural, socioeconomic, and theoretical biases. Nurses may, on their first encounter with the mentally ill, become reactive to their clients, and reactivity may take the form of avoidance, sympathy, or fear and may be the result of previous experience or ignorance. The application of the nursing process to the labeling of the mentally ill will help nurses remain objective in reporting behaviors. Objectivity is achieved and maintained by careful and ongoing self-assessment. Questions that nurses must ask themselves when assessing and labeling clients include the following:

1. How do I define this behavior?
2. Am I being influenced by my cultural, religious, or social environment?
3. Am I attempting to understand the client's behavior from a relativistic or from an ethnocentric perspective?
4. Will this label clearly describe the behavior to others?
5. Is my assessment objective?
6. Am I stereotyping the client?
7. Is my label the result of my need to be in control of this client?
8. Will this particular label be of greater benefit to the client or to myself?
9. Am I being influenced by others (such as family members or team members) I hold in high regard?

10. Can I give objective data to substantiate the label given?
11. Am I expressing a professional assessment or a personal opinion?
12. Does the context in which the behavior has occurred influence the labeling process?
13. Are there underlying political or financial motives for the label given?
14. Is the label valid, or is it given as a way of influencing third-party payers?
15. What will be the results to the client of the label I give to this behavior?
16. Does this client remind me of a family member?
17. Have I ever been injured by a mentally ill person?
18. Am I afraid of injury from this client? What is the source of my fear?
19. Does this client confront some behavioral weakness of mine?

The answers to many of these questions may involve moral and ethical decisions. Nurses often become advocates for clients as a result of this self-assessment process. Others come to the realization that their own personal history may serve as a deterrent to caring for the emotionally ill.

HEALTH BELIEFS OF DIVERSE CULTURES IN THE UNITED STATES

The United States has never really been a "melting pot," where Europeans, Asians, blacks, Hispanics, Indians, Greeks, Celts, and others have become one unified American culture.[38] Instead, ethnically homogeneous communities have often developed in the new world, in which ethnic groups have been able to preserve much of their culture. Among the cultural elements that remain despite varying degrees of acculturation to the dominant American culture are certain beliefs about health and health practices, which may be called *folk beliefs* or *healing practices.* These are culture-specific ways of dealing with physical and emotional problems. An emic perspective is necessary for understanding them. For example, in most western societies disease is viewed as the result of such natural phenomena as microorganisms, chromosomal abnormalities, and chemicals; but many people in third world societies still believe that supernatural forces cause illness, and that cures can be effected by appealing to them through witches or sorcerers or by controlling them with magic.

Being aware of the beliefs and practices of different cultural groups will help nurses to provide more effective health care to specific groups of people. Psychiatric nurses who are culturally aware can use this understanding to facilitate mental health treatment. Some folk beliefs and healing practices of four ethnic groups—black Americans, Hispanic Americans, Asian Americans, and American Indians—will be presented below. These beliefs and practices are given only as examples of concepts and behaviors that *may* be found among *some* members of these groups, so that they can be more readily recognized *if* they are encountered by the nurse. Nurses should remember that not all members of these groups will hold the beliefs discussed here, or follow the practices, and should therefore be careful to avoid preconceived ideas about individual clients.

Black Americans

Black American culture consists of several distinct groups: people descended from antebellum "free persons of color," people descended from slaves emancipated at the time of the Civil War (the largest component of the black population), and black immigrants (and their descendants) from other parts of the western hemisphere (particularly the British West Indies).[39] The three groups differ in history, values, beliefs, lifestyles, and social and economic position.

The folk beliefs and healing practices found among some black people are a combination of African folklore, fundamentalist Christianity, and the Voodoo religion of the West Indies, along with elements of modern medicine.[40] Folk beliefs are more prevalent among blacks whose income is low, who live in the southern United States or in rural areas, or who are recent immigrants; these groups are less likely to have been thoroughly assimilated into the dominant American culture. However, folk beliefs and practices may also be found among other blacks.

Among some low-income black Americans, three major themes seem to underlie folk beliefs. First, the world is perceived as a hostile, dangerous place. Second, a person is vulnerable to attack from external sources. Third, a person is helpless without internal resources to combat such an attack and must depend on outside assistance.[41] Therefore, people—as potential victims—are wise to be suspicious and to mistrust others unlike themselves. The effects of both natural and supernatural forces are to be guarded against because they are potentially dangerous. Supernatural aid may be sought as a protection.

Some African and West Indian blacks in the United States believe in magic and witchcraft. These practices are viewed as a means of nullifying evil spells, harmful magic, disease, or the punishments of an angry God.[42] Black magic, or *obeah*, which originated in the West Indies, is still practiced by some people in the Bahamas and some Bahamians in southern Florida. *Obeah* practitioners utilize plants, ground fibers, ground glass, and herbs to make up folk remedies for various physical, spiritual and emotional ailments. Such mixtures can also be used to put a hex (*mojo*) on another person. A person can be literally frightened to death by a hex. Root doctors, known as *hoodoo* men or women, are believed to be able to neutralize or cause a hex.

Voodoo is a West African word meaning "God" or "spirit." A Voodoo belief is that the spirits of the dead can visit the world of the living to bless or curse people. Haitians combined Voodoo with Catholicism to create a folk system called *Vodun*, which is integral to the religious life of some Haitian peasants. Voodoo priests and priestesses are believed to be able to exorcise evil spirits or injure an enemy by thrusting pins into a wax image. Voodoo and other forms of spiritualism have had an influence on the folk beliefs and healing practices of some black Americans.

Asian Americans

Asian Americans are people whose ethnic heritage is linked to China, Japan, Korea, and southeast Asian islands such as Guam, Samoa, and the Philippines. More recently immigrants from South Vietnam, Cambodia, and Laos have been added to this group.[43] Although there are similarities between these groups, each represents a complex civilization with its own unique values, norms, and traditions. Chinese and Japanese Americans make up the largest Asian population in the United States, and the material in this section has to do primarily with these two cultures. The folk beliefs and practices of all Asian cultures have been influenced by traditional Chinese medicine, which is a well-developed system of medical theory with a strong philosophical foundation.

Chinese medicine evolved from the philosophy that pervades Chinese culture: the belief that each organism in the universe interacts with and is affected by all the others. Human beings are held to derive energy from the *yin* and the *yang*, two opposing forces that must be in perfect harmony for physical, mental, and social harmony to occur.[44] (Figure 6-1 shows the symbol for yin and yang.) The yang is a positive force that produces light, warmth, strength, and fullness. In contrast, the yin is a negative force that produces darkness, cold, and emptiness. Some parts of the body are yin, and others are yang. Excesses or deficiencies in physiological functions are thought to affect the balance of yin and yang, leading to mental illness. Yin and yang are also symbols for hot and cold. Yin is a cold energy force and yang a hot energy force. As one may imagine, hot treatments (such as hot foods and herbs) are used to treat yin illnesses, and cold treatments (cold foods and herbs) to treat yang illnesses. Example of "hot" yang illnesses or conditions are infections, diarrhea, ulcers, and warts. "Cold" yin illnesses include cancer, earaches, headaches, dysmennorhea, and pneumonia.[44]

The holistic health movement has led to a resurgence of interest in Chinese medical practices such as acupuncture, acupressure, massage, and certain principles of nutrition. The goal of all health

Figure 6-1 Yin and yang.

This symbol suggests the opposing but potentially harmonious nature of the yin and the yang.

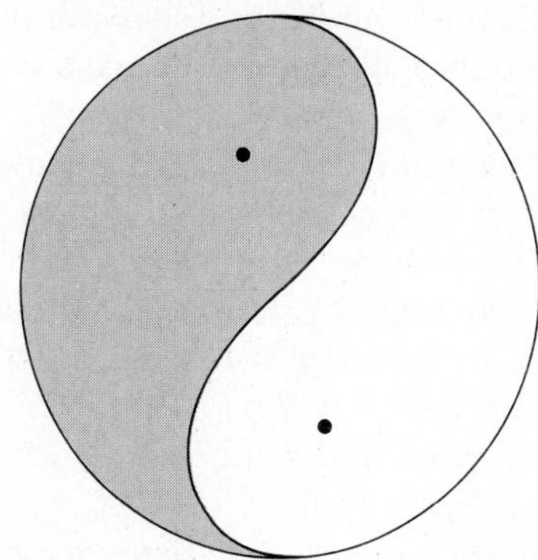

care might be considered the restoration of balance and harmony between yin and yang.

Some Asian Americans go to Asian health practitioners for diagnosis and treatment; some go to herbal pharmacists for prescriptions to treat their symptoms. And clients will also consult western physicians and personally combine herbs, pills, and food as treatment.[45]

Hispanic Americans

Hispanic Americans are people whose origins are in Central and South America, as well as some Caribbean islands. Hispanic Americans speak several dialects of Spanish, depending on the country of origin, and groups also differ in their folk beliefs and practices. However, among some Hispanic people three beliefs about the cause of illness are common: first, that illness is the result of the evil eye, or *mal de ojo;* second, that illness is God's punishment for sin; and third, that "hot-cold" (*caliente-frio*) imbalance of body humors is responsible for disease.[46,47]

The evil eye is thought by some people to be the result of witchcraft—that is, the deliberate casting of a spell. For example, a person may have a spell cast on him or her for openly admiring the beauty of someone else's child. Magical amulets, such as coral, jet, scapulars of the saints, and tiny bags of garlic or salt worn around the neck or wrist are believed to protect one from the evil eye which can cause injury or death.

Some Puerto Ricans, Mexican Americans, and Cubans believe that they can be put in touch with the dead by an *espirista,* or spiritualist. The *espirista* and the Cuban *santero* prescribe folk medicines such as teas, herbs, salves, and lotions, which are sold in a store called a *botanica.* (*Botanicas* also sell articles such as religious scapulars to ward off the evil eye.[48]) A Mexican American family might consult another type of healer, called a *curandero* or *cusandera,* to nullify the "fright sickness" (*susto*) thought to be associated with loss of the soul.[46] Some people believe that health problems caused by natural phenomena such as accidental falls can be treated by *curanderos* but diseases caused by the spirits (*espanto*) can be treated only by witch-doctors (*brujas*). Herbs, prayers, and rituals are viewed as remedies.[49]

Hispanic Americans sometimes espouse a "hot and cold" theory of disease, according to which the four body humors—blood, phlegm, and black and yellow bile—must be balanced in terms of temperature and moisture for a body to be healthy. When the four humors are not balanced, and the body is very hot, cold, dry, or wet (or any combination of these), the body may become diseased.[50] Treatment would consist of the proper hot and cold foods, herbs, or medicines. "Hot" diseases such as liver complaints might be treated by cold foods (such as tropical fruits) and cold herbs (such as sage). Although ideas about hot and cold foods, illnesses, and treatments vary from group to group, clients who seem to hold these kinds of ideas should be questioned about the theory. (The theory of hot and cold is very similar to the Asian philosophy of yin and yang.)

American Indians

Historically, medicine was a rather mysterious concept in American Indian culture, and it was traditionally linked with supernatural, religious experiences.

Some American Indians view disease as a matrix of physical, psychological, social, and environmental forces which are part of the spiritual and religious elements in a person's life. The medicine man, or *shaman,* is, for some, the central healing figure. He conducts tribal healing ceremonies which are a highly ritualized and religious way of coping with illness and death. The shaman may include family members in the healing ritual, because family members are important sources of support during a crisis. Even some families who accept western medical care may feel it important to have the healing ritual carried out at the bedside of a hospitalized person.[51,52] A medicine bundle containing charms to ward off evil; a bag of herbs, roots, or plants to provide the treatment; a drum or rattle; and a special costume for the shaman may all be part of the healing ceremony. The rattle is shaken or the drum is beaten while the shaman chants the remedies revealed by the spirits.

SOCIOCULTURAL INFLUENCES ON DEFINITIONS OF MENTAL HEALTH AND MENTAL ILLNESS

A transcultural perspective on mental health and illness suggests that there is cultural variation in the expression of symptoms of mental illness as well as in how patients are perceived and treated by others.

Evidence of psychiatric disorders has been found in every culture. Common transcultural features that are frequently observed in schizophrenic clients include:

- Auditory hallucinations
- Emotional and social withdrawal
- Delusions
- Flat affect

Common symptoms of psychiatric depression are also evident across cultures; these include loss of interest in social interaction, diurnal mood changes, insomnia, and early-morning awakening. However, other features of depression—such as guilt, suicidal ideation, and somatic complaints like hypochondriasis—are culturally patterned. The content of delusions and hallucinations also varies across cultures.[53,54,55] For example, in a classic study of 30 Irish and 30 Italian clients hospitalized on a psychiatric unit, nearly all the Irish clients exhibited guilt about sex and 75 percent of them had elaborate and fixed delusions. In contrast, the Italian clients did not demonstrate guilt about sex, and less than 30 percent showed evidence of delusions. Instead, the Italian clients had histories of outbursts of violent behavior.[56]

There is also great diversity in the way that clients with the same disorder are perceived and treated by their own cultural group. This is a function of beliefs and values about the disorder. For example, in Greece attitudes toward epilepsy may be linked to the Mediterranean concept of honor and shame. Epilepsy is often perceived as one of the most shameful diseases, and epileptics may be negatively labeled and stigmatized for life.[57] In contrast, among Arabs, many legendary heroes were epileptic. In Arab cultures seizures may be viewed as a sign of leadership, and a person with epilepsy may be highly valued. As a result, epilepsy does not carry the negative connotation that it does for some Greeks.

SOCIOCULTURAL INFLUENCES ON HEALTH CARE

The health care system may not be the first or only choice for help with mental health problems for clients who are not members of the dominant American culture. Nurses must be aware of the fact that for some people in many ethnic groups, the initial route—and the route considered most appropriate—for restoration of mental health may be traditional folk methods.

Some Asian Americans may enter the health care system reluctantly, generally only when all else has failed. Some families will make early, intensive, and prolonged efforts to cope with members who have mental health problems. These efforts might include consulting faith healers about diet and herbal therapies, as well as traditional therapies such as massage and acupressure. A delay in seeking psychiatric help may be explained by several factors:[43,44,58,59]

1. A family's genuine concern for the well-being of a sick member
2. Lack of familiarity with western mental health concepts
3. Internally oriented problem-solving mechanisms
4. Social stigma of "mental problems," which may be seen as shameful by the client and the family.

Folk beliefs and practices, as well as a cultural definition of mental illness, can be a factor in the way members of this cultural group go about seeking help.

Among some blacks, Hispanics, and American Indians, there are strong folk beliefs about the causes of mental problems. Consequently, there may be a tendency to seek help from folk healers rather than from the mental health system. For example, some Hispanics may seek the services of a spiritist or *curandero;* some blacks may use the services of a root healer; and some Indians may seek out a medicine man who will use chants, songs, or sand paintings to effect a cure.[40,60,61] As mentioned earlier, even when some people have entered the health care system as clients, family members may continue to consult with and use folk healers within the community. It sometimes happens that although clients and their families appear to comply with the demands and recommendations of the mental health system, they may actually mistrust it because it seems philosophically opposed to their own world view. For example, an American Indian might hesitate to seek health care because of a fear that the health system disrupts the harmonious relationship between humans and nature. Health professionals may be suspect because they are perceived as misusing power in a way that prevents the restoration of harmony. Mental health practitioners who show an understanding of traditional Indian beliefs about the common order of the universe and people's state of mind and being may be accepted as one component of a holistic therapy.

Familial protocol for responding to an illness can also become a factor in how people seek help for mental health problems. For example, in a field study conducted by Leiniger,[47] it is noted that some Spanish American families first inform the mother of an illness; she then seeks the father's advice, then the maternal grandmother's advice, and then the godparents' advice. Next, lay health workers—the *medicos* or *curanderos*—are approached. As a last resort, professional mental health practitioners are consulted. By the time a nurse sees a client from such a family, he or she may be in crisis.

Even among groups (like the Irish, Italians, and Jews) which are acculturated and whose members routinely use the health care system, some people will consult with respected members of the community, such as priests and rabbis, before seeking assistance from the mental health system.

A primary factor in how health care is sought is the degree to which a person or family is acculturated.[49] The greater the incongruence between the beliefs and values of a person, family, or ethnic group and those of the dominant culture, the greater the reluctance to seek help from professional mental health services. Nurses should not assume that all members of a culture are equally acculturated; they may need to make a conscious effort to link current scientific beliefs with traditional beliefs about health and illness. A sensitive attitude on the part of the nurse—understanding and respecting clients' traditional beliefs—can facilitate clients' ability to move effectively between two cultural health care systems.

CULTURAL BARRIERS TO EFFECTIVE NURSE-CLIENT RELATIONSHIPS

Both psychiatric–mental health nurses and their clients bring to the clinical setting their cultural backgrounds—perceptual matrixes of beliefs, values, attitudes, and expectations regarding patterns of behavior. Their cultural backgrounds may be congruent or incongruent. In a multiethnic country like the United States, nurses will, in all likelihood, work with clients from a number of cultural groups. Because values, beliefs, attitudes, and customs have a major influence on beliefs and practices regarding mental health, nurses need to understand the culture of the client. If the nurse chooses to view the client only from the cultural perspective of the care giver, misunderstandings and frustration on both sides may ensue. Knowledge, acceptance, and incorporation of cultural variables will enable the nurse to understand clients' behavior, formulate a realistic plan of care, and build a mutually respectful relationship.

In all health care settings, the potential for misunderstanding and negative reactions is accentuated when nurses and clients are from different ethnic or cultural groups. As health care providers, nurses are expected to take a leadership role. In a study by Bonaparte,[62] it was found that open-minded nurses, when confronted with clients who held unfamiliar beliefs and followed unfamiliar practices, would seek information about their diet, language, social patterns inside and outside the group, values, and concepts of health and illness. In contrast, closed-minded nurses avoided culturally different clients whose beliefs and practices were incongruent with their own.

Knowledge of health beliefs and practices, and of cultural values, norms, and expectations for behavior, can make the difference between a therapeutic relationship and a stalemate. For example, when the nurse encounters an Asian American client or family, it is essential to know that for Asians mental disorders may bring a sense of shame. Some Asians feel that to reveal such problems to others is to lose face and be disgraced. Sensitivity to the shame and defeat that may be felt by an Asian family entering the mental health system is important. Furthermore, an Asian American family may be accustomed to cultural norms regarding who initiates a conversation, who changes the topic, how direct the conversation is, and how much eye contact there should be. If the family follows traditional custom, it may be appropriate to indicate respect for the father by recognizing him as the family spokesperson. Similarly, direct conversation and eye contact may be inappropriate, and ritualistic small talk might precede intimate questioning. Some Asians have an indirect communication style which can result in a downplaying of symptoms, restrained behavior, and little expression of feeling. Social errors which result in loss of face may lead an Asian family to choose not to return to the treatment setting, rather than express their anger at a health professional who is perceived as "superior" to the family. Consequently, nurses who work with Asian-American families may find that they have to proceed in an indirect rather than a direct manner; directness is seen by some Asians as lack of subtlety, rudeness, and disrespect. This may at times create a feeling of frustration; a nurse may come to realize that an Asian client's smile or "yes" does not necessarily indicate agreement or compliance, but rather is an expression of unwillingness to be disrespectful or impolite. The nurse must beware of labeling such a client as evasive or unwilling to deal with health problems.[43,44]

As was noted in Table 6-2, time, or temporal orientation, differs across cultures. Nurses who are part of the dominant American culture are probably future-oriented and therefore must be aware of cultural differences in the way time is structured. American culture tends to structure time very rigidly. In a clinical setting this means that punctuality is valued and the clock is watched during a therapy session. In contrast, people who are present-oriented may have a more flexible approach to time. For example, Happe and Heller, in studying Mexican Americans, proposed that their orientation to the present time may account for their tendency to be late for appointments.[63] In mental health settings, a present-time orientation may result in a crisis approach rather than a preventive approach. Clients who have immediate needs at home may be late for appointments or miss them altogether; some clients may be reluctant to leave an appointment simply because "the time is up."

Table 6-2 also noted subjugation to nature as a significant cultural variable. In this regard, nurses may encounter Hispanic clients, who, feeling subjugated to nature, have a fatalistic attitude to mental health problems. It should not be surprising to the nurse if they are not optimistic about the benefits of mental health services, if they refuse treatment, or both.

When a client appears to be a member of the dominant American culture, a nurse may be inclined to disregard ethnic background. This, however, can lead to problems in the therapeutic relationship. For example, Irish American clients might grant a great deal of authority to health professionals and try to follow directions exactly. But they may find it difficult to follow directions in a mental health setting where clients are encouraged to express their inner feelings, because this type of expression is not characteristic of their culture. The nurse who does not understand that pride is important for some Irish people and that some are reluctant to reveal emotional issues may not recognize that the client may appear to comply with the nurse's suggestions without genuinely participating in the therapy or believing in its effectiveness. Some Irish people (like people from many other backgrounds) are embarrassed about uncovering and admitting intimate, hostile, and erotic feelings. Therefore, it may be wiser to use a more structured approach that does not include strategies like touching or self-disclosure exercises. The nurse who maintains a friendly, calm distance, who proceeds slowly with intimate questions, who has a sense of humor, who does not swear, and who does not make a display of values different from the client's own is most likely to engage the client and the family in a therapeutic alliance.[64]

In contrast, some Italian families may overwhelm a nurse from a more restrained culture with expressions of emotional intensity; it may even be difficult for the nurse to distinguish between dramatic details and real mental health problems. Some Italians express their feelings in great detail; but their real problems may have a tendency to be expressed as somatic complaints, rather than with words. Some Italian American clients want quick relief for their problems, which may well have reached crisis proportions by the time they enter the mental health system, since they may have already spent much time consulting with family, friends, and priest. Mental health services are perhaps most likely to be sought out when there is a child-oriented problem. With some Italian American clients, the nurse who attempts to uncover difficult issues like a marital problem may encounter resistance because strong efforts are made to maintain the image of a "good" husband-wife relationship. Allowing the family to keep its "secrets" may be important in establishing an effective working relationship.[65]

Obviously, no one can become an expert on all ethnic groups. What nurses should aim for is openness to cultural variability and to the relativistic nature of culture. Nurses will come to understand cultural patterns only by observing differences among people. Understanding diverse cultural groups does not mean squeezing them into stereotypical cate-

Table 6-5 Cultural Assessment

Questions
1. Of what cultural or ethnic group is this client a member?
2. What are the important communication patterns of this culture that might influence the establishment and maintenance of a relationship with this client?
3. What effect would the client's religious and political beliefs have on his or her health beliefs or practices?
4. What is the client's a. Temporal orientation? b. Activity orientation? c. Relational orientation? d. People-to-nature orientation? How does this orientation affect health beliefs and practices?
5. What are the acceptable cultural norms and roles for this client?
6. How does the client's ethnicity affect his or her health beliefs and practices?
7. Has the client been positively or negatively stereotyped by others, such as health care providers? If so, how, and with what consequences?
8. To what extent is the client acculturated? How representative of the culture is the person's behavior?
9. Does the culture define the person's behavior as normal, eccentric, or deviant? If so, with what consequences?
10. How does the client define mental illness?
11. What are the specific folk beliefs and healing practices of the cultural group of which the client is a member?
12. To what degree does the client adhere to such beliefs and practices?
13. Will the folk beliefs and healing practices complement or interfere with the delivery of mental health care? How?
14. What is the cultural influence on the client's health practices?
15. What is the degree of incongruence between the client's cultural health beliefs and values and those of the dominant culture?
16. What are the cultural barriers to establishing a nurse-client relationship?
17. Specific cultural preferences: a. Dietary preferences or needs b. Sleep pattern c. Preferred sex of care provider d. Specific needs regarding modesty e. Specific needs for privacy and space f. Necessary personal effects (religious articles, adjunct healing remedies, charms, amulets, and so on) g. Needs and patterns of nuclear family h. Needs and patterns of extended family i. Specific religious needs

gories, but rather moving beyond rigid boundaries and being aware of general cultural patterns. This will enable psychiatric–mental health nurses to meet and work with their transcultural clients in a more effective way.[66] Table 6-5 presents a cultural assessment that nurses can utilize when working with clients of diverse ethnic groups.

SUMMARY

Psychiatric–mental health nurses need to understand the complexities of each client's unique cultural experience in order to avoid misunderstandings and therapeutic stalls.

An understanding of the nature of culture, as well as its components—communication patterns, religious and political beliefs, values, roles, norms, and ethnicity—provides a foundation for understanding diverse ethnic groups. All people are under the influence of their own cultural system. Within every group, variant patterns are exhibited by individuals. Stereotypes, positive and negative, are incomplete cognitions about cultural groups that perpetuate inaccurate generalizations. Stereotypes may interfere with accurate assessment and effective delivery of health care.

Culture may be seen from a relativistic or an ethnocentric perspective. The nurse who takes a relativistic approach attempts to understand clients' behavior in the context of their cultural experience. The ethnocentric approach sees behavior from the perspective of the health care provider, whose norms are seen as "correct."

Definitions of health are culture-bound and are closely linked to beliefs, values, and institutions. Definitions of health include holistic, adaptive, wellness, and epidemiological perspectives. Definitions of mental health can be derived from an emic or an etic perspective—that is, from a viewpoint inside the culture or from a transcultural viewpoint. Labeling people as mentally *healthy* or *ill* is determined by cultural factors. DSM III attempts to establish etic, objective diagnostic categories for mental disorders. When the labeling process is not objective, people may be mislabeled (for example, as *deviants*); that may have lifelong consequences. Nurses need to be aware of the role they play in the labeling process.

Some ethnic and cultural groups in the United States include members whose beliefs and practices regarding health differ from those of the dominant American culture. Some people in many cultural groups (such as blacks, Hispanics, Asian Americans, and American Indians) adhere to folk beliefs and healing practices instead of, or in conjunction with, mental health care services.

Certain mental health problems and disorders (such as schizophrenia and depression) are common to all cultures. However, there are culture-specific behaviors, and there are also culture-specific ways in which behaviors are perceived and treated. Utilization of mental health services may vary according to the cultural beliefs about mental illness, the health care system, and the protocol for dealing with mental health problems; it may also vary with the degree of acculturation of an individual or family. Barriers to effective nurse-client relationships often exist when there is little congruence between the cultural worlds of nurse and client. As providers of health care, nurses are expected to take a leadership role in forming realistic plans of care and effective relationships. This role can be carried out only if the nurse becomes knowledgeable about and accepts the diverse cultural and ethnic groups that are encountered in a multi-ethnic society like the United States.

REFERENCES

1. R. D. Laing, *The Politics of Experience,* Ballantine, New York, 1967, p. 18.
2. W. S. Tseng and J. McDermott, *Culture, Mind and Therapy: An Introduction to Cultural Psychiatry,* Bruner-Mazel, New York, 1981.
3. M. A. Hautman and J. K. Harrison, "Health Beliefs and Practices in a Middle Income Anglo American Neighborhood," *Advances in Nursing Science,* vol. 4, no. 3, April 1982, pp. 49–64.
4. B. Baumann, "Diversities in Conceptions of Health and Physical Fitness," *Journal of Health and Human Behavior,* vol. 2, Spring 1961, pp. 39–46.
5. M. Bush, J. Ullom, and O. Osborne, "The Meaning of Mental Health: A Report of Two Ethnoscientific Studies," *Nursing Research,* vol. 24, March–April 1975, pp. 130–138.
6. J. A. Smith, "The Idea of Health: A Philosophic Inquiry," *Advances In Nursing Science,* vol. 3, no. 3, April 1981, pp. 43–50.
7. I. Zola, "Pathways to the Doctor—from Person to Person," *Social Service and Medicine,* vol. 7, 1973, pp. 667–684.
8. N. Hutchens, *Recent Italian Immigrants in Brooklyn: Their Social Worlds,* unpublished doctoral dissertation, Rice University, 1977.
9. E. Welts, "Greek Families," in M. McGoldrick et al., eds., *Ethnicity and Family Therapy,* Guilford, New York, 1982, pp. 269–288.
10. H. Winawar-Steiner, "German Families," in M. McGoldrick et al., *Ethnicity and Family Therapy,* Guilford, New York, 1982, pp. 247–268.
11. M. Ferguson, *The Aquarian Conspiracy,* Houghton Mifflin, Boston, 1980.
12. F. Kluckhohn and F. Strodtbeck, *Variations in Value Orientations,* Row, Peterson, New York, 1961, p. 4.
13. M. Giuffra, "Culture, Family Values, and the Individual," *The Family,* vol. 10, no. 2, 1983, pp. 128–138.
14. T. Tripp-Reimer, in J. Bellack and P. Barnford, eds., *Nursing Assessment: A Multidimensional Approach,* Wadsworth, Monterey, Calif., 1984.
15. C. Harris, *The Family,* Praeger, New York, 1969.
16. A. A. Campbell, "Factors Associated with Attitudes toward Jews", in T. M. Newcomb and E. L. Hartley, eds., *Readings in Social Psychology,* Holt, New York, 1947.
17. R. Kalish and S. Yuen, "Americans of East Asian Ancestry: Aging and the Aged," *Gerontologist,* vol. 11 (suppl.), 1971, p. 36.
18. F. Carp and E. Kataoka, "Health Care Problems of the Elderly in San Francisco's Chinatown," *Gerontologist,* vol. 16, 1976, p. 30.
19. Evelyn Shaw, "Female Circumcision," *American Journal of Nursing,* vol. 85, no. 6, June 1985, pp. 684–87.
20. A. I. Meleis and C. W. Silver, "The Arab American and Psychiatric Care," *Perspectives in Psychiatric Care,* vol. 22, no. 2, 1984, pp. 72–76.
21. G. E. Simpson and M. Yinger, Jr., *Racial and Cultural Minorities: An Analysis of Prejudice and Discrimination,* 4th ed., Harper and Row, New York, 1965.
22. T. Adorno et al., *The Authoritarian Personality,* Harper, New York, 1950.

23. M. Jaffe Ruiz, "Open-Closed Mindedness, Intolerance of Ambiguity and Nursing Faculty Attitudes toward Culturally Different Patients," *Nursing Research,* vol. 30, no. 3, May–June 1981, pp. 177–181.
24. T. Tripp-Reimer, "Cultural Diversity in Therapy," in C. Beck et al., eds., *Mental Health–Psychiatric Nursing,* Mosby, St. Louis, 1984, pp. 381–398.
25. Thomas Scheff, ed., *Labeling Madness,* Prentice-Hall, Englewood Cliffs, N.J., 1975.
26. Carolyn Chambers Clark, *Mental Health Aspects of Community Health Nursing,* McGraw-Hill, New York, 1978.
27. Rene Dubos, *Man Adapting,* Yale University Press, New Haven, Conn., 1965.
28. Halbert L. Dunn, *High Level Wellness,* Beatty, Arlington, Va., 1961.
29. Jeanette Lanchaster, *Community Mental Health Nursing,* Mosby, St. Louis, 1980.
30. Morton Beiser, "Psychiatric Epidemiology," in Armand M. Nicholi, ed., *The Harvard Guide to Modern Psychiatry,* Harvard University Press, Cambridge, Mass., 1978, pp. 609–626.
31. L. Moore, P. Van Arsdale, et al., *The Biocultural Basis of Health,* Mosby, St. Louis, 1980, p. 191.
32. K. L. Pike, *Language in Relation to a Unified Theory of the Structure of Human Behavior,* 2d ed., Humanities Press, New York, 1967.
33. M. Segall, *Human Behavior in Cross-Cultural Psychology: Global Perspectives,* Brooks/Cole, Monterey, Calif., 1979.
34. David L. Rosenhan, "On Being Sane in Insane Places," *Science,* vol. 179, no. 4070, 1973, pp. 250–258.
35. David L. Rosenhan, "The Contextual Nature of Psychiatric Diagnosis," *Journal of Abnormal Psychology,* vol. 84, no. 5, 1975, pp. 462–474.
36. American Psychiatric Association, *Diagnostic and Statistical Manual of Mental Disorders,* 3d ed., APA, Washington, D.C., 1980.
37. Robert L. Spitzer and J. L. Fleiss, "A Reanalysis of the Reliability of Psychiatric Diagnosis," *British Journal of Psychiatry,* vol. 125, 1974, pp. 341–347.
38. S. Fava, *Urbanism in World Perspective,* Thomas C. Crowell Co., New York, 1971, pp. 436–440.
39. T. Sowell, *Essays and Data on American Ethnic Groups,* Urban Institute, New York, 1978, pp. 7, 53.
40. M. Tamari, "La Vie, Mon Dieu! A Study of World View and Values in a Rural Haitian Community," *Dissertation Abstracts International,* vol. 45, no. 3, September 1984, pp. 882A–883A.
41. P. M. Hines and N. Boyd-Franklin, "Black Families," in M. McGoldrick et al., eds., *Ethnicity and Family Therapy,* Guilford Press, New York, 1980, pp. 84–107.
42. M. Becker, "The Health Belief Model and Sick Role Behavior," *Health Education Monographs,* vol. 2, Winter 1974, pp. 409–419.
43. S. Shon and D. Ja, "Asian Families" in M. McGoldrick et al., eds., *Ethnicity and Family Therapy,* Guilford, New York, 1980, pp. 208–228.
44. W. Tseng and M. McDermott, *Culture, Mind and Therapy,* Bruner-Mazel, New York, 1981.
45. T. Louie, "Illness Concept and Management Among Chinese-Americans in San Francisco," paper presented June 11, 1974 at the American Nurses Association Biennial Convention, San Francisco, Calif.
46. C. Falicou, "Mexian Families," in M. McGoldrick et al., eds., *Ethnicity and Family Therapy,* Guilford, New York, 1980.
47. M. Leininger, *Nursing and Anthropology: Two Worlds to Blend,* Wiley, New York, 1970, pp. 111–127.
48. R. Ailinger, "A Study of Illness Referral in a Spanish-Speaking Community," *Nursing Research,* vol. 25, no. 1, January–February 1977, pp. 53–56.
49. N. Garcia-Preto, "Puerto Rican Families," in M. McGoldrick et al., eds., *Ethnicity and Family Therapy,* Guilford Press, New York, 1980, pp. 164–186.
50. I. Murillo-Rohde, "Hispanic American Patient Care," in G. Henderson and M. Primeaux, eds., *Transcultural Health Care,* Addison-Wesley, Menlo Park, Calif., pp. 224–238.
51. T. M. Brod, "Alcoholism as a Mental Health Problem of Native Americans: A Review of the Literature," *Archives of General Psychiatry,* vol. 32, 1975, pp. 1385–1391.
52. J. Shore, "American Indian Suicide: Fact and Fantasy," *Psychiatry,* vol. 38, 1975, pp. 87–91.
53. A. Kiev, *Transcultural Psychiatry,* Free Press, New York, 1972.
54. J. Kennedy, "Cultural Psychiatry," in J. Hanigman, ed., *Handbook of Social and Cultural Anthropology,* Rand McNally, Chicago, 1973.
55. B. Good and M. Good, "The Meaning of Symptoms: A Cultural Hermeneutic Model for Clinical Practice," in L. Eisenberg and A. Kleinman, eds., *The Relevance of Social Science for Medicine,* D. Reidel, Voorstraat, The Netherlands, 1980.
56. M. Oppler and J. Singer, "Ethnic Differences in Behavior and Psychopathology: Italian and Irish," *International Journal of Social Psychiatry,* vol. 1, no. 1, 1957, pp. 11–17.
57. R. Blum and E. Blum, *Health and Healing in Rural Greece: A Study of Three Communities,* Stanford University Press, Stanford, Calif., 1965.
58. T. Ling and M. Ling, "Service Delivery Issues in Asian North American Communities," *American Journal of Psychiatry,* vol. 135, no. 4, April 1978, pp. 454–456.
59. F. Cheung, "The Mental Health Status of Asian-Americans," *Clinical Psychologist,* vol. 34, no. 1, Fall 1980, pp. 23–24.
60. R. Boss, "The Validity of Sociocultural Factors in the Assessment and Treatment of Black Americans," in

B. Boss et al., eds., *The Afro American Family: Assessment, Treatment and Research Issues,* Grune and Stratton, New York, 1982, pp. 69–83.
61. D. Trainor, "Shamans and Endorphins," *Psychiatric News,* vol. 2, 1981, pp. 28–29.
62. B. Bonaparte, "Ego Defensiveness, Open-Closed Mindedness, and Nurses' Attitude toward Culturally Different Patients," *Nursing Research,* vol. 28, no. 3, May–June 1979, pp. 166–171.
63. S. Happe and P. Heller, "Alienation Familism and the Utilization of Health Services by Mexican-Americans," *Journal of Health and Social Behavior,* vol. 15, 1974, p. 304.
64. M. McGoldrick, "Irish Families," in McGoldrick et al., eds., *Ethnicity and Family Theory,* Guilford, New York, 1982, pp. 310–336.
65. M. Rotanno and M. McGoldrick, "Italian-Americans," in McGoldrick et al., eds., *Ethnicity and Family Therapy,* Guilford, New York, 1980, pp. 349–363.
66. T. Tripp-Reimer, P. Brink, and J. Saunders, "Cultural Assessment: Content and Process," *Nursing Outlook,* vol. 32, no. 2, 1984, pp. 78–85.

PART THREE
Mental Health Nursing

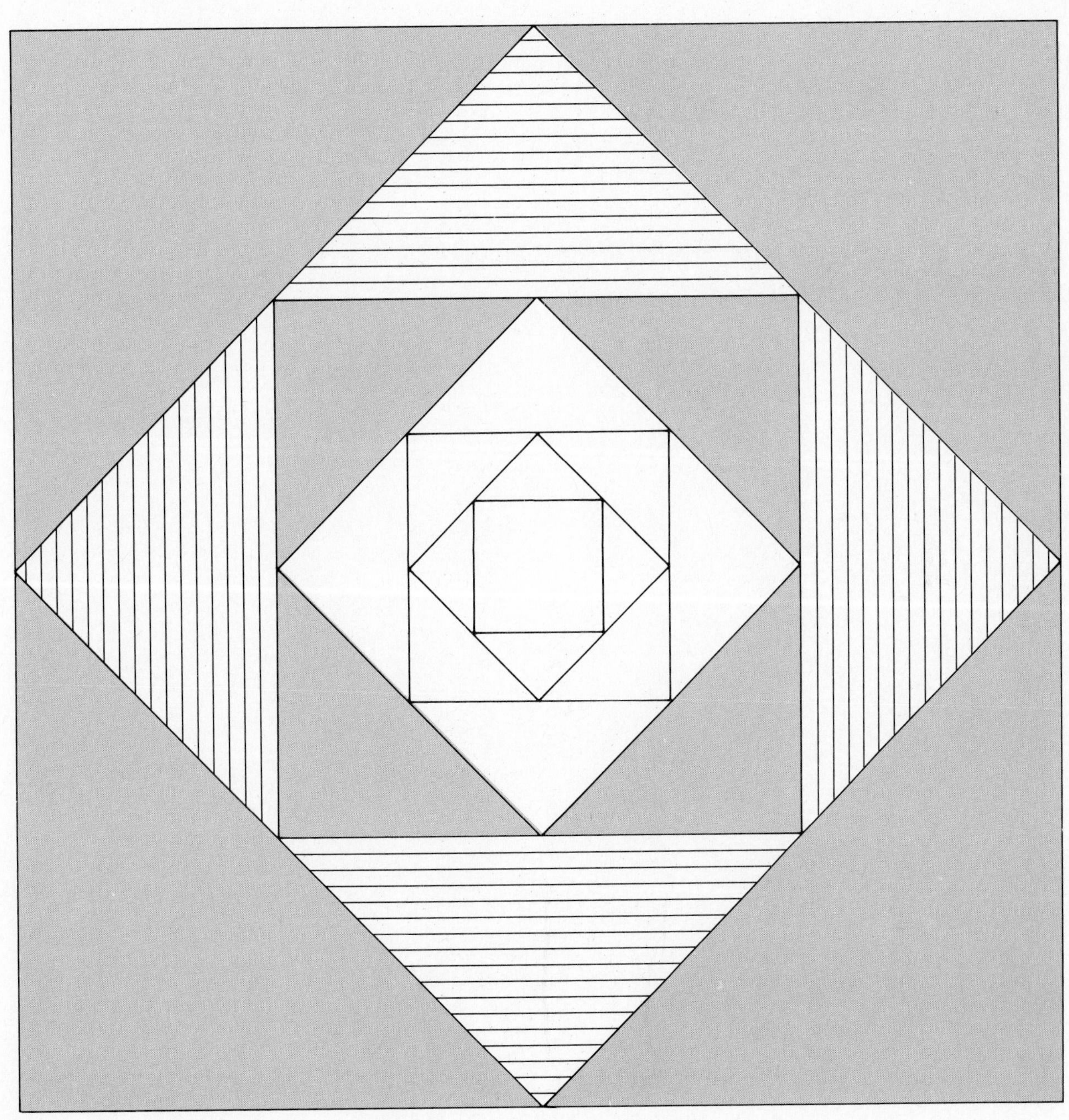

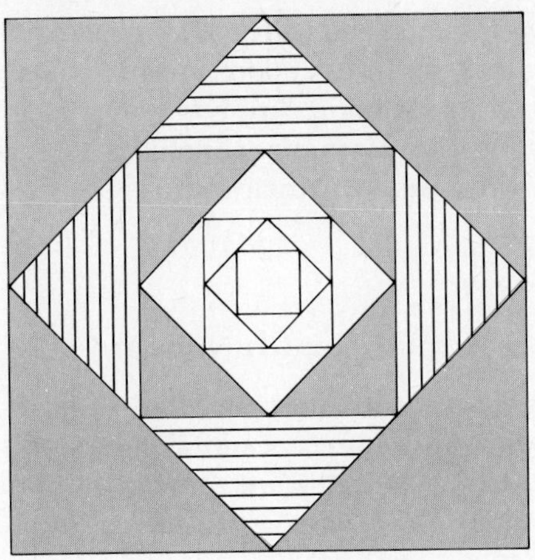

CHAPTER 7
Defining Nursing

Judith Haber
Pamela Price Hoskins
Anita M. Leach
Barbara Flynn Sideleau

LEARNING OBJECTIVES

After studying this chapter, the student should be able to:

1. Formulate a personal definition of *nursing*.
2. Define *psychiatric–mental health nursing*.
3. Analyze the interface between therapeutic use of self and professional self-awareness.
4. Outline the essential elements of the role of nurses in mental health care settings.

The purpose of this chapter is to expand the definition of *nursing* to include the multiple interacting dimensions of holistic psychiatric–mental health nursing. It also provides a conceptual framework for use throughout Part Three. Definitions of *nursing* and *psychiatric–mental health nursing* are included. The requirements for nursing certification are mentioned, and the therapeutic uses of self and self-assessment, which are part of the unique contribution of the nursing profession to the care of clients, are discussed.

THE CONCEPT OF NURSING

Nursing is both a healing art and a precise science. It is a unique and autonomous profession. Nursing practice focuses on the promotion, maintenance, restoration, and rehabilitation of the health of individuals, families, and communities. Nursing interventions are theory-based and promote synchronous patterns of interaction between the client and the environment by using strategies that are supportive-educative, partly compensatory, or wholly compensatory. The goal of such interventions is to facilitate the client's quest for optimal health.

Promotion of health involves nursing activities that facilitate clients' change toward more synchronous patterns of interaction with the environment. *Maintenance of health* involves nursing activities that continue or preserve clients' current health status. *Restoration of health* involves nursing activities that return clients' health status to previous levels. *Rehabilitation of health* involves nursing activities that break clients' dysfunctional patterns and facilitate the establishment of more functional patterns of interaction.[1]

Nurses use the scientific method to systematically assess and diagnose clients' health status, to formulate goals and expected outcomes, to determine interventions, and to evaluate outcomes.

Supportive-educative interventions help clients care for themselves by providing support, guidance, healthy developmental environments, counseling, and teaching. *Partially compensatory interventions* are cooperative, interactive activities shared by nurses and clients. Specific interventions vary with clients' limitations, the knowledge and skill required by the nurse to complete care, and clients' readiness to perform or learn needed activities. *Wholly compensatory interventions* are interventions in which clients have no active role. Nursing care compensates for clients' temporary or permanent inability to care for themselves and supports their role as recipients of care.[1]

Psychiatric–Mental Health Nursing

Psychiatric–mental health nursing is an interpersonal process that promotes, maintains, restores, and rehabilitates mental health. The American Nurses Association (ANA) defines *psychiatric–mental health nursing* as a specialized area of nursing practice that employs theories of human behavior as its science and powerful use of self as its art.[2] Theories of personality, behavioral patterns, and sociocultural and psychological principles are necessary components of the knowledge base of nursing. Communication skills, willingness to correct misunderstandings in relationships, knowledge about legal and ethical dimensions of care, and familiarity with the skills of other mental health disciplines are also necessary for the psychiatric–mental health nurse.

Educational Preparation for Nursing Practice

The nursing profession includes practitioners with different levels of educational preparation and experience. Current educational preparation of registered nurses may include taking courses culminating in a diploma, an associate degree, or a baccalaureate or master's degree in nursing. Practical nurses are prepared for technical roles in nursing. The basic entry-level requirement for professional nurses continues to be controversial, but this has not devalued the consumer's perception of the profession as a whole.

The scope of practice in psychiatric–mental health nursing is defined by the educational preparation of the nurse and, in some states, by the nature of the work setting. As determined by the ANA, the basic certification level in psychiatric–mental health nursing requires a baccalaureate degree in nursing and at least 2 years of supervised practice in a mental health care setting. Basic roles of a psychiatric–mental health nurse include nurturing, coordinating, acting as a socializing agent, counseling, educating, and performing technical tasks.

The clinical specialist's scope of practice includes expertise and competence in individual, group, and family therapy. The psychiatric–mental health clinical specialist is prepared at the master's level and is recognized by others in the nursing profession as an advanced-level practitioner through the certification process. Nurses with doctorates may concentrate on research and thus represent a creative "cutting edge" and provide the leadership needed for the survival of the profession.

Therapeutic Use Of Self

Psychiatric–mental health nursing is a unique, meaningful, healing relationship between nurse and client that involves the therapeutic use of self. Therapeutic relationships necessitate a clear understanding of self, a high level of communication skills, and a commitment to the ethical and legal aspects of nursing.

The concept of *therapeutic use of self* implies that *nurses,* not just procedures or techniques, facilitate the healing process that occurs as clients start to attain self-actualization and become whole. Self-awareness is essential to this process.

Each nurse responds to each client in a unique way. Nurses' emotional and spiritual responses parallel those of clients and significant others, providing many clues to what is necessary to effect healing. Feelings and emotions form a continuum, and nurses, like clients, experience varying degrees of anger, bitterness, faith, fear, frustration, gentleness, guilt, helplessness, joy, love, patience, peace, rage, self-control, and temperance. When a nurse's reaction to a client is spontaneous or not conscious, the resulting communication pattern might be labeled *dysfunctional,* or it might be considered simply a social interaction. On the other hand, if nurses remain aware of the sources of their emotions and feelings, they are better able to interact on a therapeutic level with clients. Aside from providing clues to clients' inner selves, nurses facilitate and hasten clients' healing processes by therapeutically sharing their own positive and hopeful emotional responses. In any case, nurses have a responsibility to care for themselves and to facilitate their evolution toward becoming whole—physically, mentally, and spiritually.

Professional Self-Assessment

Self-responsibility is facilitated by self-awareness. Self-awareness involves ongoing and responsible exploration of physical, mental, and spiritual dimensions of the self and recognition of the freedom to make choices and changes that are congruent with one's self-image. Self-assessment facilitates formulation of a personal philosophy which, for nurses, would include the choice of nursing as their vocation and an integral part of their life purpose. Self-assessment contributes to nurses' quest for wholeness as people and as members of a profession.

Reflection, meditation, and consultation with a supervisor and, in some cases, a spiritual guide are ways in which nurses can grow in self-awareness. The following questions will facilitate the process of becoming self-aware:

Who am I?

What is my purpose in life?

What are my gifts? In what areas is growth needed?

What are my most common interactive patterns with men? With women?

What are my most common interactive patterns with authority figures?

Who are the people I like or dislike?

Are there common behaviors among the people I like and dislike?

How do I express anxiety?

What do I do to relieve anxiety?

Who am I with this client?

What emotions are stirred in me when I interact with this client?

How do I behave with this client?

What consistent patterns of behavior do I exhibit when I am around certain kinds of clients?

With what kinds of clients am I most reactive? Least reactive?

How have I grown in the last week, month, or year?

In what ways have I identified with nursing?

What are the high points of my professional practice? What are the low points?

How do my family's beliefs, values, and attitudes influence the way in which I see this client?

RATIONALE FOR THE ORGANIZATION OF PART THREE

The chapters in Part Three provide the nursing student with a general view of holistic nursing and a specific view of psychiatric–mental health nursing. The historical development of psychiatric–mental health nursing is presented in Chapter 8. Chapter 9 discusses legal issues and ethical processes that become important when a person has made a commitment to the nursing profession and to the care of mentally ill clients. The role of the nurse and the nursing process in mental health settings are discussed in Chapters 10 and 11.

The healing process occurs as people communicate therapeutically with one another and establish therapeutic relationships. Communication theory and the therapeutic nurse-client relationship are presented in Chapters 12 and 13. The theoretical framework for actions and decisions in nursing practice depends upon continuous nursing research. Research in psychiatric–mental health nursing is discussed in Chapter 14.

REFERENCES

1. D. E. Orem, *Nursing: Concepts of Practice,* McGraw-Hill, New York, 1971.
2. American Nurses Association, *Statement on Psychiatric–Mental Health Nursing,* ANA, Kansas City, Mo., 1976.

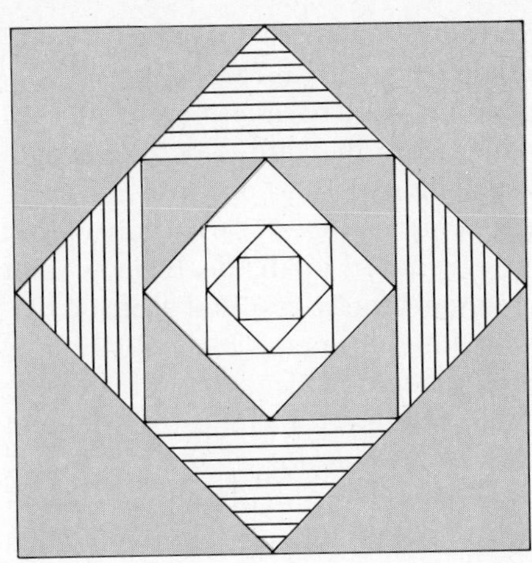

CHAPTER 8
A History of Psychiatric Nursing and Mental Health Care

Doris Troth Sommerfield Lippman

LEARNING OBJECTIVES

After studying this chapter, the student should be able to:

1. Identify major historical trends in the medical care of the mentally ill from before 700 B.C. to the 1970s.
2. Discuss historical trends in the development of psychiatric nursing in the United States in relation to education and the nursing role from 1882 to 1971.
3. Identify significant leaders that have influenced the medical care of the mentally ill.
4. Discuss the influence of nursing leaders in the development of psychiatric nursing in the United States in relation to education and the nursing role.

The purpose of this chapter is to present a brief history of mental health care and of psychiatric–mental health nursing. The chapter traces the evolution of the care of clients once labeled *insane* from the centuries when they were regarded as demons and consequently handed over to an exorcist or even an executioner; through the periods when they were treated like criminals and paupers and were placed in prisons or almshouses; to the present, when the care given is more humane and is provided in hospitals and community health facilities. Psychiatric–mental health nursing has moved from nonexistence, through a time when untrained attendants acted as custodians, to the present, where it exists as a clinical nursing specialty whose members frequently have advanced degrees and function as independent practitioners.

Since a historical orientation is used for this chapter, the mental health events presented date from primitive societies (before about 700 B.C.) to the 1960s. The decades of the 1970s and 1980s are still too recent to be presented historically.

HISTORICAL TRENDS IN THE MEDICAL CARE OF THE MENTALLY ILL

Primitive Societies: Before 700 B.C.

Most primitive cultures thought that the mentally ill were possessed by demons or had violated the moral code. Mentally ill people were starved or beaten in an effort to drive out evil spirits. The mentally ill who were not violent were often allowed to wander about aimlessly, but those exhibiting extremely violent or bizarre behavior were locked away or banished from the community and left to die. Primitive societies based their response to the mentally ill on several different beliefs: a foreign object with magical powers or an evil spirit had entered the body; the soul had fled the body; a taboo had been broken; or a person had sinned.[1]

Classical Civilization: 700 B.C.–A.D. 500

The history of ancient Greek and Roman psychiatry encompasses a period of 12 centuries from the time of Homer onward. Little is known of the practice of clinical psychiatry in antiquity, because the field as an entity scarcely existed and because medical histories were usually transmitted orally, not written.

It is known that the family was the primary caretaker for a member who was mentally ill. People with no family, if they were harmless, were allowed to wander. If they were dangerous or unmanageable, they were jailed, exiled, or put to death.[2]

The Greek Hippocrates (460–377 B.C.), considered to be the father of modern medicine, believed that insanity and mental illness resulted from a disequilibrium of the four "humors": blood, black bile, yellow bile, and phlegm. Phlegm and bile were thought to corrupt the brain, and those maddened by bile were expected to be noisy.[2]

The belief that disequilibrium of humors caused madness was also held by followers of the famous Roman physician Galen (130–200 A.D.); it led to treatments for mental illness that included venesection (bleeding) and purging through the use of drugs that induced vomiting and diarrhea. The humoral theory of disease continued to dictate treatment for both physical and emotional diseases well into the sixteenth and seventeenth centuries.

During the classical period there were some people who denounced bleedings, purgings, starvation, and flogging as treatments for the mentally ill. A Greek physician, Caelius Aurelianus, wanted his patients placed under the best conditions of temperature, light, and quiet. He recommended theatricals, walking, riding, and work during convalescence; and he specifically referred to the behavior of attendants caring for the mentally ill, stating that they should be tactful, avoid antagonism, and use restraint in a limited and cautious way.[3]

The Middle Ages: A.D. 500–1500

With the collapse of the Roman Empire, the Middle Ages began, and in Europe a "cloud of darkness" fell over medicine. The insane were regarded as possessed by evil spirits, or demons. Their treatment consisted of "demonical exorcism" which often took the form of a religious ceremony in which physical punishment and torture were inflicted on "possessed" people in an effort to drive out evil spirits. During the Middle Ages, insane women were often regarded as witches; the punishment for people practicing witchcraft often was to have them burned at the stake.[4]

Although in Europe during the Middle Ages the belief that the insane were possessed by the devil was widespread, in Islamic countries the mentally ill found more understanding and better treatment. In the Islamic east, the torch of medical science lit by Hippocrates was still held aloft; as a result, the darkness of superstition which existed in the European countries was to some extent dispelled. The insane were treated as sick persons and many were cared for in what were probably the first asylums for the insane in the world.[5]

The Modern Era: A.D. 1500–1971

Many American practices in the early colonial days (1500s–1600s) reflected a European influence. Delusions concerning witchcraft existed; but although people were punished for supposed witchcraft, and even put to death, persecutions were not carried out to the same extent as in France and Germany, except perhaps in the New England colonies.

In the American colonies in the latter part of the seventeenth century, witch hunts gave way to incarceration of the mentally ill to protect the public without causing harm to the afflicted. During this period, there were two classes of mentally ill in America: the "propertied" (middle and upper classes) and the poor. The propertied were typically cared for in their own homes, locked away in cellars and strongrooms if they were troublesome, but the poor were the responsibility of the towns in which they lived.[5]

Care of the insane was much more hospital-centered in Europe during the fifteenth and sixteenth centuries. (Life in such an institution is depicted in Figure 8-1.) Colonial America founded its first hospital for the insane in 1752. Located in Philadelphia, it was not founded exclusively for the care of the insane, but it was the first hospital to

Figure 8-1 Bethlem Royal Hospital in London.
(SOURCE: Drawing by William Hogarth, 1697–1764. National Library of Medicine.)

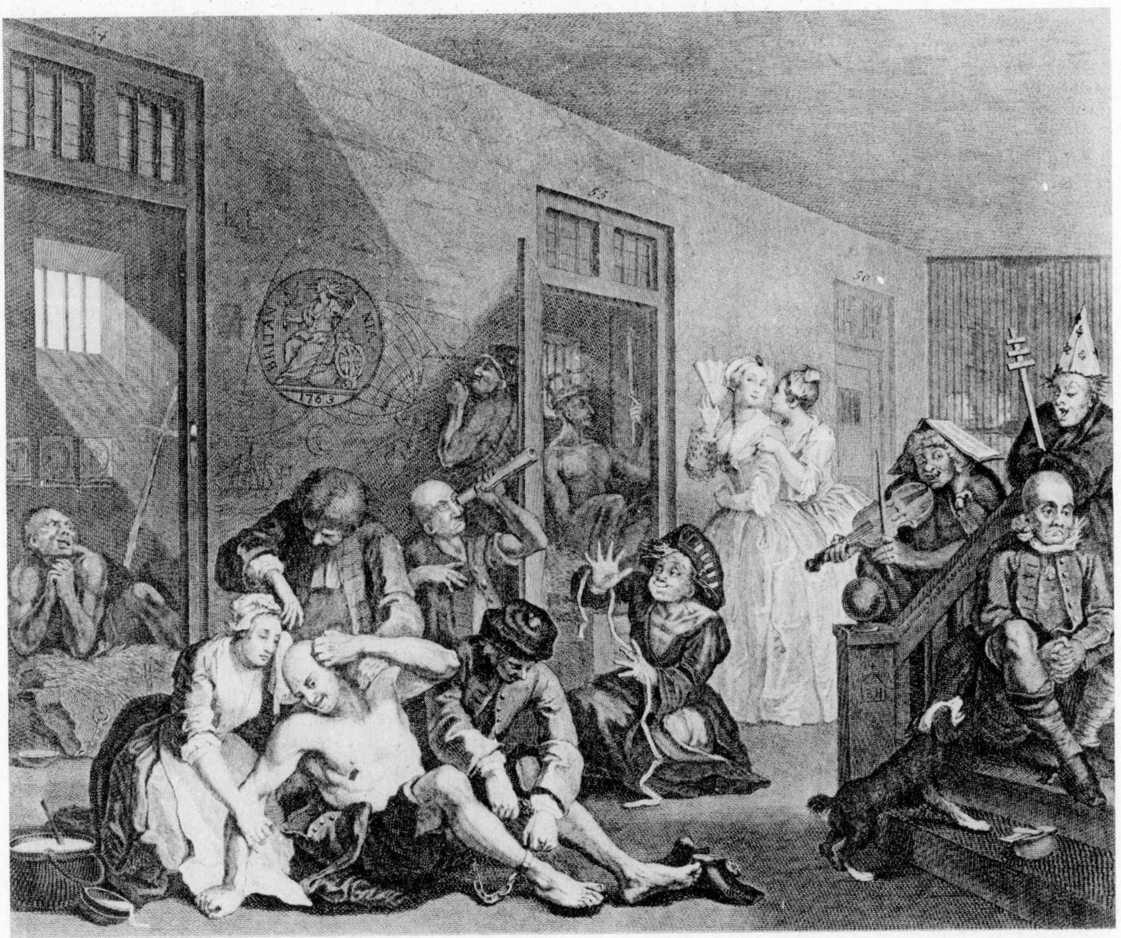

admit the insane. The patients were kept in cells and cared for by a cellkeeper until a wing strictly for the insane was built in 1796.

In 1773, the Eastern Lunatic Hospital, the first public hospital exclusively for the mentally ill, was founded in Virginia. Although early records of treatment methods used do not remain, it is believed that the hospital relied heavily on the use of chains and confinement in cells.[5]

The year 1783 was important in American history not only because it marked the end of the Revolutionary War, but also because it was the year that Benjamin Rush, who would become known as the "father of American psychiatry," joined the staff at the hospital outside Philadelphia. (The tranquilizing chair shown in Figure 8-2 was a common treatment of the time, as were the circulating swing and bed shown in Figure 8-3.) Some of Rush's treatment measures, such as bloodletting and purging, reflected the medical theories of the times; these were still based on ancient Greek and Roman theories which attributed disease to a disequilibrium of humors. However, Rush saw his primary role as a crusader for the humane care of the insane. (Table 8-1 lists suggestions he made for the care of the insane.)

Figure 8-2 Tranquilizing chair.
(SOURCE: National Library of Medicine.)

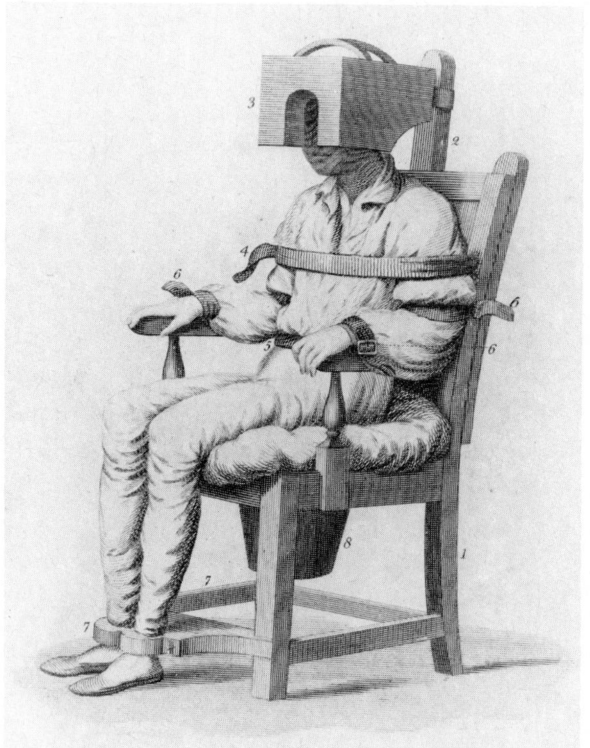

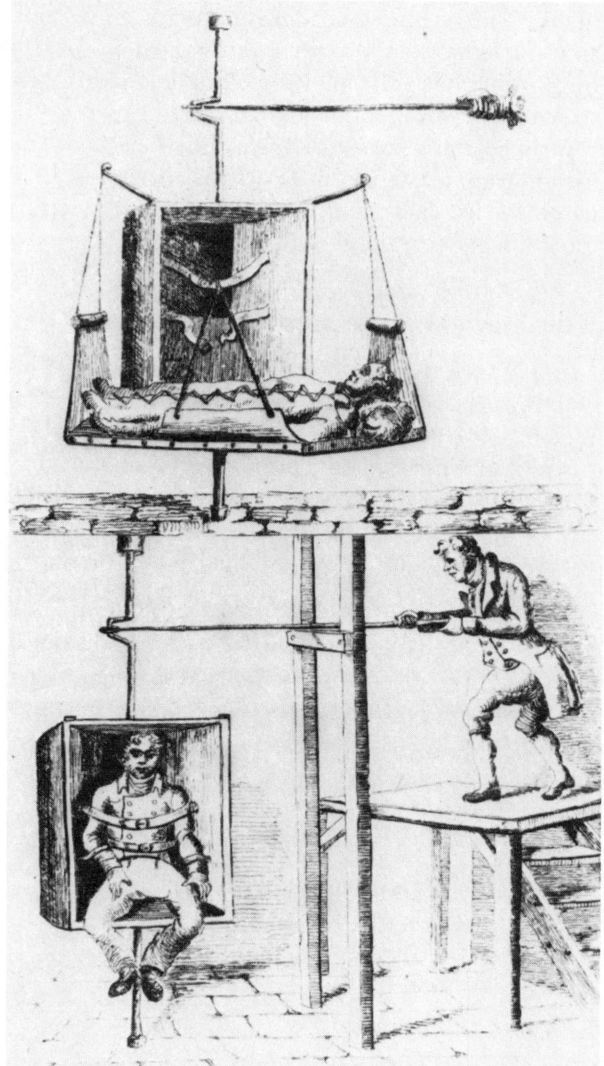

Figure 8-3 Circulating swing and bed.
This device was considered an antimaniacal remedy. It dates from about 1818. (SOURCE: National Library of Medicine.)

The Modern Era: France

One of the first people to take up the cause of the insane in Europe during the modern era was a Frenchman, Philippe Pinel. His interest in the care of the insane began in 1782, when a friend, "who

Table 8-1 Rush: Humane Care of the Insane

Recommendations
Kindness
Heat and proper ventilation
Clean and neat cells
Separate buildings for the insane
Venesection (bleeding)
Purging
Labor, exercise, and amusement
Hiring of intelligent people to care for the insane
Exclusion of visitors who upset patients

Table 8-2 Pinel: "Moral Treatment" of the Insane

Recommendations
Lay aside coercion by chains and blows.
Remove patients to proper retreat in the country.
Adopt a system of humane vigilance.
Attendants should be firm, but kind.
Light food that is easy on the digestion should be served.
Patients should be exercised regularly.
Involve patients in agricultural pursuits.
Introduce patients to entertaining books and conversation.

was tired and overworked, lost his reason and one night rushed off into the woods. The next morning he was found dead—half devoured by wolves who in those days still roamed the forest around Paris."[6] As a result of his friend's death, Pinel began to study, observe, and treat patients in one of the few private institutions for the well-to-do. (A whirling device used to treat the mentally ill at this time is shown in Figure 8-4.)

With the outbreak of the French Revolution in 1789, Pinel, whose humane work with the insane was known to the revolutionaries, was appointed as administrator of Salpêtrière, one of the largest hospitals in Paris; it had a reputation for treating insane patients by shackling them to the floors and walls with irons. The patients were at the mercy of attendants (who were often criminals) armed with whips which they used freely on the inmates.[5] Pinel was extremely distressed by the conditions and treatment. He resolved that the chains must come off and was able to achieve this goal of "unchaining." Pinel also instituted "moral treatment" in the care of the insane; his recommendations for such care are presented in Table 8-2. (A gravure of a painting showing Pinel standing in the courtyard of Salpêtrière surrounded by the patients is shown in Figure 8-5, on page 160.)

Figure 8-4 Whirling device.
The patient seated in the device is wearing a straitjacket. (SOURCE: National Library of Medicine.)

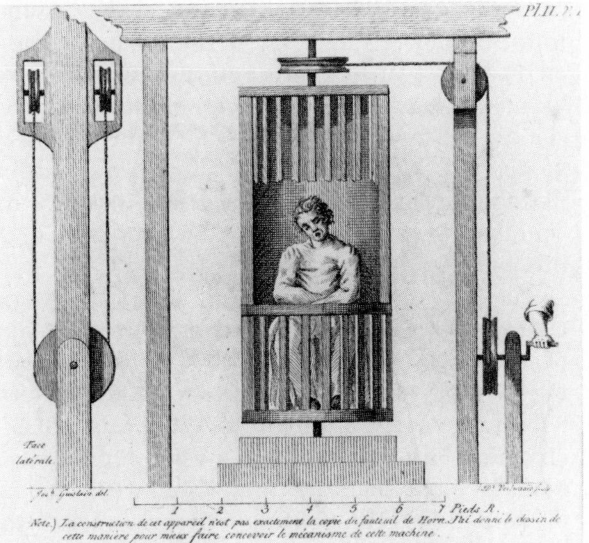

The Modern Era: England

In England, the reformer for the insane was not a physician but a merchant, William Tuke. His work in advocating humane care for the mentally ill was essentially a result of the suspicious circumstances of the death of a woman friend in the York Asylum. In 1796, he opened the York Retreat, which became a model for American institutions such as the Friends' Asylum, the Bloomingdale Asylum, and the McClean Asylum, all founded in the early 1800s. His recommendations for humane care are presented in Table 8-3.

The Modern Era: America

THE 1800s. Pinel's work influenced psychiatric practice primarily in Europe, while Tuke's work played a more influential role in America. Of the eight hospitals that were founded in the United States in the first quarter of the nineteenth century, two were directly inspired by the success of Tuke's York Retreat.

By the end of the first quarter of the nineteenth century, institutions for the insane had been estab-

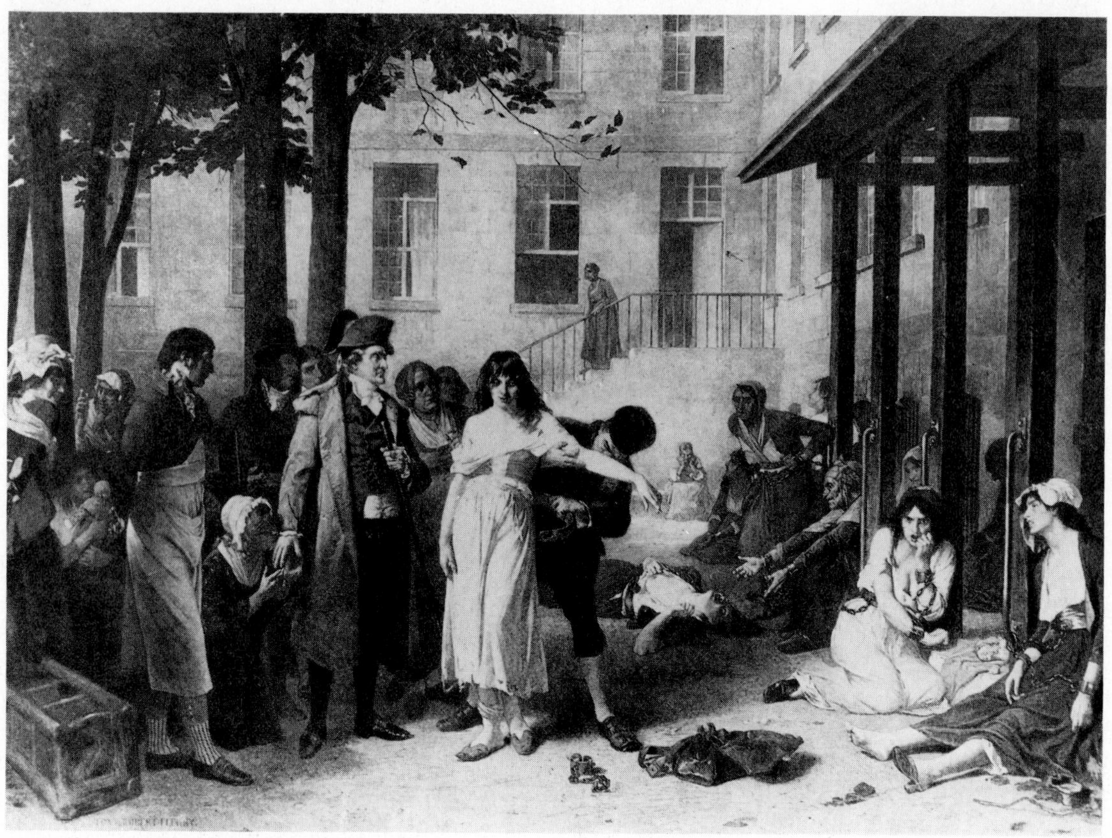

Figure 8-5 Pinel.
Dr. Pinel is shown liberating the mentally ill from their chains at the hospital of Salpêtrière.
(SOURCE: National Library of Medicine.)

Table 8-3 Tuke: Humane Care of the Insane

Recommendations
Use sympathy.
Show kindness.
Encourage gardening for men.
Encourage sewing for women.
Use only leather straps to restrain the violent; no chains are to be used.

lished in eight different states. These institutions represented great strides forward, but they did not house all the mentally ill. Officials responsible for caring for the poor and the insane often placed the "nonpropertied" insane in jails or almshouses at the cost of 50 cents to $1 per week rather than at a private institution, such as the Bloomingdale Asylum, which cost $2 per week.[5]

During the period of the 1830s to 1840s, a "cult of curability" arose. There was a change from the pessimistic attitude, "Once insane, always insane," to an optimistic, "Insanity is the most curable of all diseases." Much of this optimism was, however, based on exaggerated claims; for example, a retired sea captain from the Royal Navy reported cures in 91 percent of the clients he visited in the Hartford Retreat in Connecticut. As a direct result of this "curability craze," there was an increase in the number of mental hospitals being built.

The 1840s also brought other important events. Dorothea Dix, a pioneering crusader in the reform of care of the mentally ill, had her first contact with the mentally ill in 1841 when she agreed to teach Sunday school at a jail in East Cambridge, Massachusetts. She was shocked by the conditions in which the prisoners, many of whom were mentally ill, lived.[7] As a result of this experience, she began a crusade which involved surveying institutions housing the insane in the United States, Canada, and Scotland. Frequently, she found patients "confined in cages, closets, cellars, stalls, and pens, . . . chained, naked, beaten with rods and lashed into obedience."[7] She presented her findings to concerned citizens and legislatures everywhere; as a result, standards of care for the insane were elevated.

In 1844, the Association of Medical Superintendents of American Institutions of the Insane, which would become the American Medico-Psychological Association in 1921 and later the American Psychiatric Association, was founded. Some people think that the history of psychiatry in America parallels the history of this organization.

During the 1840s and early 1850s, with the increased influx of immigrants into America and increased industrialization, the number of poor people who were publicly dependent, including the insane, grew. This became a major social problem in America to which the state legislatures responded by expanding existing asylums and erecting larger ones. Because the patients housed in these institutions were disproportionately drawn from immigrants, many of whom were in advanced stages of mental illness, an attitude of pessimism again began to develop. Chronic mental problems led to overcrowding in institutions; consequently, therapeutic practices were undermined and cure rates dropped. The "curability craze" declined; insanity again became associated with incurability and pauperism.[8]

The period 1850–1870 became a time of reassessment, largely as a result of the work of Dorothea Dix. Alternatives to the care in large public institutions were explored. One imaginative idea, originated by John Gault in 1850 and resurrected after the Civil War, was to replace large institutions with small cottages; but it was largely unsuccessful, and a two-class system of psychiatric care would continue to develop over the next century. The poor insane were housed in large public institutions which offered only custodial care and community protection. The wealthy, nonviolent insane used private facilities which provided care primarily to voluntary mental patients.

THE 1900s. A rise in reform movements—political, social, and economic—occurred with the beginning of the twentieth century. In the field of social welfare, there was a growing conviction that radical measures were required in dealing with the major social ills—poverty, delinquency, and disease. Emphasis was placed on trying to break the vicious circle of poverty-disease-poverty. Therefore, the focus in most areas was on prevention.[5]

The medical discoveries of Pasteur, Koch, and other pioneer "microbe hunters" made it possible to prevent some diseases, such as cholera, bubonic plague, and typhus. The feeling existed that if these diseases were practically abolished, others could be also. In this climate, the American Social Hygiene Committee and the National Committee for Mental Hygiene were organized.

The mental hygiene movement began in 1908 in New Haven, Connecticut, and was founded by Clifford Beers. Beers, as a result of a suicide attempt in 1900, while he was a student at Yale University, spent 3 years in mental hospitals in Connecticut. His experiences as a mental patient made him determined to fight for freedom in the care of the mentally ill. As a first step, he wrote a book titled *A Mind That Found Itself* that described his experiences as a mental patient:

> I was beaten mercilessly, choked, spat upon and reviled by attendants, imprisoned for long periods of time in dark, dank cells and forced to suffer a strait-jacket for as many as twenty-one consecutive nights. . . .[9]

Beers's work mobilized others and was instrumental in founding the Committee for Mental Hygiene.[10] The goals of the committee were many, but its focus was to prevent mental illness and remove the stigma attached to it. The committee renewed the notion of treatability for mental illness and, in particular, the idea of early treatment.

At approximately the same time as the Mental Hygiene Movement began, Freud's ideas began to take hold in America. Up to this time, Kraepelin, the founder of descriptive psychiatry, had been the primary influence on American psychiatry. *Descriptive psychiatry* (as the term implies) focused on describing and classifying the characteristics of mental illness using methods similar to those used to describe and classify a specimen. Freud's approach was different. He hypothesized that important influences or forces at work within and outside the personality produced pathological mental illness. As a result of Freud's work, psychoanalysis gained a strong hold in institutes and medical schools in America. However, because it demanded intense one-to-one contact between a mentally ill person and a physician, it was inefficient as a means of treating large numbers of chronic, institutionalized patients.

It was also during this period that Adolph Meyer, considered the "father of psychobiology," was carrying on his work.[11] *Psychobiology* is the study of a person as a biological unit which reacts uniquely to social and biological influences. Meyer's work is thought of as a link between the early pioneers and present-day practice. From the beginning, Meyer stressed the importance of adequate diet and occupational and recreational therapy. He also championed adequate follow-up and aftercare.[12]

In 1917, the United States entered World War I. At this time, the government called on the National Committee for Mental Hygiene and its director to devise a master plan for treatment of mentally ill soldiers; it included (1) eliminating mentally deficient people from military service, (2) identifying cases of mental disorders in soldiers early on, (3) having psychiatric treatment as close to the fighting front as possible, (4) assigning psychiatrists to base hospitals to treat soldiers experiencing emotional difficulties, and (5) continuing psychiatric care once the soldiers returned home.[10]

The war and the postwar period saw a significant, increased interest in mental hygiene. Care and treatment of the mentally ill were affected not only by the war, but also by the introduction of somatic therapies during the 1930s. These included Metrazol, insulin, and electroshock therapies and were important because they often made patients more receptive to psychotherapy.

Another treatment, the lobotomy (an operation which severs the connection between the thought centers in the frontal lobes of the brain and the emotional center in the thalamus), was also introduced in the 1930s. Because of its irreversibility and (later on) because of the discovery of antianxiety and antipsychotic drug therapies, the lobotomy decreased as a treatment modality.

World War II (1937–1945) acted as a catalyzing agent in the growth and public acceptance of psychiatry in America, for several reasons: a large number of draftees were rejected because of emotional problems; a large number of soldiers were discharged because of severe emotional problems; and there was a high incidence of neuropsychiatric disorders among military personnel.[13]

After the war, in 1946, the National Mental Health Act was passed. This act provided federal funds for research of mental diseases, for expansion and improvement of state mental health facilities, and for training of professional personnel (psychiatrists, psychologists, nurses, and social workers). It provided for the creation of the National Institute of Mental Health. (The act and its impact are discussed in more detail in the next section of this chapter.)

In 1952, the "tranquilizer" (antipsychotic) chlorpromazine was discovered. This drug and its successors had a major effect upon the care of the mentally ill, since many people receiving them became amenable to psychotherapy. The use of other therapies, such as insulin shock, electroshock, and psychosurgery, decreased; and the need for physical restraints also declined considerably. (The effect of these drugs on the role of the nurse is discussed later in this chapter; Chapter 26 deals with current psychotropics and their use.)

The work of Maxwell Jones also took place in the 1950s. His concept of a "therapeutic community" as a means of treating the mentally ill was designed to preserve, or improve, hospitalized clients' sense of self-respect and responsibility for their own behavior.[14] With the advent of the concept of therapeutic community and the emphasis on the psychosocial aspects of mental illness, many hospitals began to change. Nurses and attendants no longer wore uniforms, units functioned as communities with patient-run governments, and decision making became democratic by involving both staff and clients.[14] The extensive use of group therapy, in both inpatient and outpatient settings, had also been stimulated by the success of this treatment with soldiers during World War II.

With the success of psychopharmacological therapy and the therapeutic community movement—as well as new approaches such as halfway houses, family care, and aftercare—enthusiasm for action on mental health care became a national phenomenon in the United States. As a result, the Mental Health Study Act was passed in 1955. This act established the Joint Commission on Mental Illness and Health, whose purpose was to study the existing system of care in terms of both psychiatric personnel and facilities. Its report, *Action for Mental Health,* published in 1961, proposed that a concerted attack be made on mental illness through better redistribution of services, reorientation of psychiatrists to community-based care, greater involvement of laypeople in massive prevention programs, and a progressive shift from institutional to community services with funding shared by federal, state, and local governments.

As a result of the commission's report and efforts of professionals and the public, the community mental health movement was begun. President John F. Kennedy, in his address to the Eighty-Eighth Congress on February 5, 1963, stressed the importance of returning mental illness to the mainstream of American medicine and upgrading mental health services. On October 31, 1963, the Community Mental Health Act was passed. This act mandated that the National Institute of Mental Health be created to establish and fund community mental health centers.

The 1960s were characterized by an optimistic and enlightened view of the problem of mental illness on the part of both professionals and the public: milieu therapy became the focus rather than the context of the psychotherapeutic process; short-term psychotherapy became a distinct form of treatment; family and communication therapies came into their own; and trends toward systems theory and behavior therapy emerged. By the mid-1960s, it seemed that psychiatry was gaining favor in this country.

With the advent of drugs to alleviate the symptoms of mental illness, and with the effects of the Community Mental Health Act, came the deinstitutionalization of large numbers of people. But neither the deinstitutionalized patients nor their communities were ready for this. Many communities did not have enough facilities or enough personnel to deal with the many people seeking care. Also, many people who had been in institutions for most of their lives were not ready to live alone in their communities; they often lacked the ability to carry out even simple activities of daily living. For many chronic patients, the move away from a traditional mental hospital had devastating results, often leaving them stranded and alone. This problem continues to exist.

The decades of the 1960s and 1970s brought many events, such as the Vietnamese war, the outbreak of violence in cities and on college campuses, racial confrontations over school integration and black militancy, the women's movement, concern over survival and the environment, and the rise of the third world.[11] The effect of these events on mental health has yet to be analyzed by historians. These decades are still too close to be viewed from a historical perspective. However, psychiatrists and others in psychiatry and psychiatric nursing (its history will be discussed next) must continue to reassess and to move toward progressive and humane care of the mentally ill.

HISTORICAL TRENDS IN THE DEVELOPMENT OF PSYCHIATRIC NURSING IN THE UNITED STATES: EDUCATION AND ROLE

> It stands to reason that the mentally sick should be at least as well cared for as the physically sick.[15]

Psychiatric Nursing before 1882

Although the concept of nursing has existed for a long time, nursing as an organized profession is relatively new. The specialized practice of psychiatric nursing is even more recent, and it is essentially unique to the United States.

In colonial America until the late 1600s, nursing functions were usually carried out by members of the family, neighbors, servants, or members of religious and charitable organizations. The early hospitals were generally places for the poor. Upper- and middle-class people received care at home.

When hospitals were established, there was a need for people who could attend to the needs of patients. For over 100 years—until the founding of the first training school for nurses in 1872—hospital attendants were usually untrained women, frequently of questionable character and reputation.

The origin of professional nursing and nursing education is generally attributed to the work of Florence Nightingale (1820–1910). She resisted the norms for women of her time and class and pursued a career in nursing. Her work during the Crimean War not only resulted in improved care of the sick and wounded but also led to her founding a school for training nurses at the Saint Thomas Hospital, London, in 1860. It is generally agreed that this date marks the beginning of modern nursing and nursing education.

The American Civil War resulted in the beginning of formalized nursing education here. In 1872, a training school for nurses was established at the New England Hospital for Women and Children. Linda Richards, who would later become a significant figure in psychiatric nursing education, was the first graduate of this school and therefore became recognized as America's "first trained graduate nurse." In 1873, the first three Nightingale-type training schools were established.

By the turn of the century, the number of hospitals in the United States had grown to more than 2500 from 178 in 1873.[16] As the number of hospitals grew, so too did the number of training schools for nurses. In 1880, there were 15 schools with 323 students; in 1900, there were 432 schools with 11,164 students.[16] Although initially hospital administrators thought they had little use for training schools, they soon knew the merit of having a constant supply of nursing students who could provide the hospital with free nursing care.[17]

Psychiatric Nursing: 1882–1914

Education

Although the majority of hospitals during the period from 1882 to 1914 were general hospitals, there were also specialized institutions such as mental hospitals, or asylums. As early as the 1830s, superintendents of asylums were aware of the need to provide instruction for attendants. However, it was not until 1882, 65 years after the McLean Asylum had been established, that Linda Richards and Edward Cowles opened the first training school for "mental nurses" at the McLean Asylum. A year later, in 1883, the first training school for nurses to be founded in a state mental institution was opened in New York at the Buffalo State Hospital. By 1895, there were 38 schools in mental institutions and about 900 graduates.[18]

The opening of schools to train "mental" nurses was significant because generally speaking, until the nineteenth century the insane were simply incarcerated. In the early 1800s, there were no trained nurses and few religious orders, either Catholic or Protestant, available to provide humane care for the mentally ill in the United States. The attendants in asylums, as in the general hospitals, were a haphazard lot; at best they were decent guards or "practical nurses"; at worst, they were crude keepers or "Sairy Gamp" types.

Even though the early schools in mental hospitals were regarded as significant by the medical superintendents who directed them, they were generally held in low esteem; they had lower standards of training than the general hospital schools, had difficulty finding recruits, and often depended on people who were already attendants as a primary source of students.[13] Frequently, their graduates were not recognized or accepted by the public or other nurses, and often they could not gain employment in general hospitals.

Although training programs for nurses in both general and specialty hospitals grew out of the same need, for many years training programs for "mental nursing" developed under the auspices of medicine, not nursing.[19]

Much as the mentally ill were isolated from the physically ill, and psychiatry was isolated from general medicine, "mental" (psychiatric) nursing was isolated from general nursing in both education and service. A review of the curricula in the early training schools associated with nonspecialty hospitals, and a report presented at the 1896 Annual Convention of the American Society of Superintendents of Training Schools of Nursing (ASSTSN) reveals that "mental" nursing was not included in the education of a nursing student.[20]

Early nursing leaders, such as Isabel Hampton Robb, were concerned about the relationship between specialty hospitals and training schools. Although Robb did not support the idea of having training schools in specialty hospitals, she did recognize the need to provide students with an opportunity to receive experience in "mental" nursing, and also to provide students in specialty hospitals with an opportunity to affiliate with general hospital programs. She recommended that cooperative or affiliation programs be developed; but at the time her recommendation went largely unheeded.

The attitude of the nursing profession toward education in "mental" nursing was evident: it was considered unimportant, as can be seen in the criteria for licensure established by the first nursing practice acts. These acts did not require nurses who sat for the licensure exam to have any experience in "mental" nursing.[21]

Schools for "mental" nursing remained isolated in the specialty hospitals. Standards were determined and controlled by psychiatrists—that is, physicians. The nursing profession had rejected "mental" nursing; and the control of this specialty by psychiatrists was reinforced in 1906, when the American Psychiatric Association (APA) established the American Psychiatric Committee on Psychiatric Nursing. This committee was responsible for monitoring and standardizing psychiatric nursing care and education.[22]

There were nursing leaders who fought psychiatrists' control over psychiatric nursing, particularly Euphemia ("Effie") Taylor. In 1913, Taylor became the director of nursing services at the Henry Phipps Clinic, which was considered one of the great centers of psychiatric research and education in the United States and the world.[5] While at this institution, she was influenced by Adolph Meyer and his holistic approach to mental health and illness. Taylor attempted to unite psychiatric nursing with general nursing. She developed a course in psychiatric nursing which was added to the curriculum of the general nursing program at Johns Hopkins. This was the first time a general hospital's nursing program offered such a course under the direction and control of its own faculty.[22]

Role

During the period from 1882 to 1914, the role of trained nurses at mental hospitals in the United States changed very little. The care given by these nurses was mainly custodial, since they had limited training in psychiatry or in the use of psychosocial skills. The nurse focused primarily on meeting the physical needs of patients: ensuring proper nutrition and hygiene, giving medications such as paraldehyde and chloral hydrate, assisting in hydrotherapy, and encouraging patients to participate in ward activities. At this time, psychological care consisted of being kind and tolerant to patients. Laird, matron of the Willard State Hospital, described the duties of the psychiatric nurse in 1900;[23] they are listed in Table 8-4.

Table 8-4 Role of the Psychiatric Nurse in 1900

Duties
1. Humor fancies and delusions.
2. Understand the individual peculiarities.
3. Control excited and abusive patients.
4. Keep the filthy and demented clean.
5. Furnish each patient capable of it with work adapted to his or her comprehension.
6. Prevent the vicious from injuring each other.
7. See that the delicate ones do not overwork.
8. Keep a lookout for sharp implements and knives.
9. Prevent patients from eating grass or pebbles.
10. Enter into various forms of diversion—dancing, ball-playing, assisting at musical instruments, using any talent patients may possess or be able to acquire for the pleasure of those unfortunate people.

SOURCE: S. Louise Laird, "The Work of Nurses in Asylums," *American Journal of Nursing*, vol. 1, 1900, p. 518.

Psychiatric Nursing: 1915–1945

The 30 years from 1915 to 1945 saw many significant events that have had major effects on the world, including two world wars, the great depression, and tremendous advances in medical science.

Education

According to Peplau,

> This era brought an awakening of interest in raising the standards of care in psychiatric work, a growing realization of the role of nurses and the nursing profession in the needed improvements, and gradual inclusion in basic nursing curricula of the dominant psychiatric concepts available at this time.[24]

In 1915, Katherine Tucker confronted nurses with the plight of the insane and their need for nursing care. In an investigation of 41 mental hospitals that had training schools for nurses, Tucker had found that many schools had superintendents who were not nurses. As compared with general hospital training schools, these schools were poorer and had lower standards of education and administration, and their students had longer hours and less adequate living conditions.[25] These findings were corroborated by a study done by the American Nurses Association with financial support from the National Committee for Mental Hygiene.[25]

"Effie" Taylor returned in 1919 from her work during World War I and continued to stress to other nurses the importance of psychiatric nursing in the holistic care of patients.

The great depression, which began with the crash of the stock market in October 1929, affected the entire world, including nurses. Many graduate nurses were unemployed—neither families nor hospitals (which used students as staff) could afford to hire them. Ironically, mental hospitals were in need of nurses, but most nurses were neither trained nor interested in this area.

The impact of the depression also resulted in a decline in the number of nursing schools. As a result of—and in response to—closings of nursing schools, and out of concern for the uniformity of nursing curriculums, nursing educators participated in the development of a third revision of *A Curriculum Guide for Schools of Nursing.* This curriculum guide and others were important for the nursing profession in general, but more specifically for those in psychiatric nursing education because they recommended the inclusion of psychiatric nursing in the general nursing curriculum. *The Standard Curriculum for Schools of Nursing,* published in 1917, specified a 20-hour course in mental and nervous diseases, and the 1927 curriculum guide recommended a 2-month clinical psychiatric nursing experience for each undergraduate. The third edition of *A Curriculum Guide for Schools of Nursing,* published in 1937, strongly recommended the inclusion of psychiatric nursing content in the standard curriculum for any school:

> In addition to the four main branches of nursing (medical, surgical, obstetrical, and children's) it is now considered essential for an adequate preparation that facilities be found for teaching the nursing of psychiatric patients and for experience in nursing and health service in the family.[26]

In addition, for the first time in 1934, the National League for Nursing Education at its thirty-ninth annual convention devoted an entire session to nursing care of patients in state mental hospitals.[27] Important comments made at the convention included the following: there was a dire need for trained nurses in mental hospitals; student nurses needed to continue their affiliation at mental hospitals; postgraduate education in psychiatric nursing was essential.[27] May Kennedy, then Chairman of the Committee on Mental Hygiene and Psychiatric Nursing, noted:

> The well-equipped nurse of today and tomorrow must have knowledge of human nature—the human organism unit has both physical and psychiatric components. . . . Nursing education has been at fault because . . . schools of the past, and many of today, have not given sufficient consideration to the mental and emotional aspects of health and sickness.[28]

From 1940 to 1943, the National League of Nursing Education conducted a series of "roundtables" at its conventions. These meetings provided an opportunity for widespread discussion of various viewpoints regarding psychiatric nursing education. At the 1940 roundtable, Walsh discussed the teaching methods at Bellevue and expressed the opinion that since only one-fifth of nurses choose psychiatric nursing as a specialty, it is crucial that teaching "be directed to the increasing understanding of human behavior which [in turn] can be directed toward all patients. . . ."[29]

With the advent of World War II, several conditions were brought to public awareness: there was an extreme shortage of nursing personnel; there was a large amount of mental illness in the populace, as evidenced by the number of recruits rejected because they were unfit psychologically and by the number of those devastated psychologically by the war; and there was a dearth of trained psychiatric nurses and psychiatrists available to care for the population in need. In response to these acute shortages, the Bolton Act was passed in 1943; it created the United States Cadet Nurse Corps. This led to an increase in the number of available nurses and to an increase in psychiatric affiliations held by nursing students. According to Church, "The Cadet Corps was a major factor in the increased exposure to the development of psychiatric experience as a credible requirement instead of an interesting option for adventurous students."[19] In addition, three university-sponsored programs in psychiatric nursing received financial assistance from funds allocated under the Bolton Act.

Role

During the period from 1915 to 1945, many new developments in the treatment of the mentally ill influenced the role of the psychiatric nurse. The first of these developments was the use of the organism that caused malaria in the treatment of paresis, a psychosis caused by extensive invasion by spirochetes of the brain that once accounted for 10 percent of all admissions to mental hospitals.[11] Because the treatment resulted in high fevers, skilled nursing care was essential. In addition, the somatic therapies introduced in the 1930s required that patients receiving these treatments be given both physical and emotional care.

By the end of this era, Peplau states, "The climate of the nursing profession was more favorable for considering the pressing problems of psychiatric nursing in institutions and agencies of all kinds."[24] However, the predominant attitude held by members of the medical profession toward trained graduate psychiatric nurses seemed ambivalent. They believed that a graduate nurse was the most qualified to direct the care of a hospitalized psychiatric patient, but they generally disliked nurses' independence, initiative, and unwillingness to continue in their previous roles as custodians.[12,24]

Psychiatric Nursing: 1946–1962

This period in the history of psychiatric nursing and nursing education felt the impact of several significant factors: (1) the increase in federal funding for programs that focused on the mentally ill and their care; (2) the discovery of phenothiazines; and (3) the return of control of psychiatric nursing and psychiatric nursing education to the nursing profession.

Education

The era from 1946 to 1962 began with the passage of the Mental Health Act in 1946. It focused on three main areas—research in the field of mental diseases; training of personnel; and assistance to states in developing mental health programs and establishing mental health centers.[30] It also authorized the founding of the National Institute of Mental Health to implement the programs. The institute, aware that there were insufficient qualified personnel, gave priority to training and research. Grants were provided to educational institutions, both public and private, for the expansion of programs and to individuals for advanced study and research.

Collegiate education of psychiatric nurses, supported by training grants, resulted in an increase in (1) nursing faculties trained in psychiatric nursing, (2) nurses trained to do individual and group psychotherapy, and (3) nurses holding graduate degrees in psychiatric nursing.[31] Consequently, the standard of psychiatric nursing care became much higher than it had ever been before. As a result of the influx of funds for education that led to advanced degrees, psychiatric nursing, which in the past had so often been viewed as a stepchild of the nursing profession, grew in stature and strength.

Role

This period brought changes and growth for psychiatric nurses and their roles. With the discovery of chlorpromazine (Thorazine) in 1952, the treatment of psychiatric patients was revolutionized. Many patients who had been chronically psychotic and hospitalized for much of their lives responded to this "tranquilizer," and as a result they became more amenable to treatment.

The advent of "tranquilizers" also affected the role of the nurse. Supervision of sedative baths, cold sheet packs, insulin comas, electroconvulsive therapy (ECT), and restraints was replaced by a focus on administering new medications and, more important, on therapeutic relationships with patients. Nurses began to develop a role in group, occupational, and recreational therapies.

In addition, as the result of the development of psychiatric nursing theories by Mellow, Peplau, and Tudor, psychiatric nurses had a theoretical base for their practice and role. Mellow developed the concept of *nursing therapy* on the basis of her work with schizophrenic patients at Boston State Hospital. Peplau, with the publication in 1952 of her book *Interpersonal Relationships in Nursing,* set forth principles upon which psychiatric nurses could build their skills and base their activities in the nurse-patient relationship. Tudor defined *psychiatric nursing* as a continuous interpersonal process of observation, intervention, and evaluation.[32] In addition, during the 1950s the National League of Nursing was also involved in defining desirable functions and qualifications for psychiatric nurses, by sponsoring regional and national conferences.

The role of the psychiatric nurse was further expanded by Maxwell Jones and his colleagues, who developed the concept of the "therapeutic community." Jones regarded the role of the nurse in this community as very important. He saw it as including setting limits, playing games to help patients learn how to accept others, and transmitting the unit's culture and philosophy to clients.[31]

Another important theorist, Harry Stack Sullivan, who worked extensively with acutely ill schizophrenics, also influenced the role of the psychiatric nurse. His theory focused on the importance of interpersonal relationships and interconnectedness. Nurses in the 1950s adopted Sullivan's theories of interpersonal psychiatry and used them to develop psychotherapeutic nursing approaches.[33]

Federal legislation in the 1950s also affected the development and progress of the role of the psychiatric nurse. In 1955, Congress enacted the Mental Health Survey Act. This act created the Joint Commission on Mental Illness and Health to analyze and evaluate the needs and resources of the mentally ill in the United States, and to make recommendations to Congress for a National Mental Health Program.[14]

In 1961, the report of the Joint Commission of Mental Illness and Health was published. The commission recommended that the treatment of the mentally ill be moved from state hospitals to community health centers.

Psychiatric Nursing: 1963–1971

Education

The Community Mental Health Act of 1963 further encouraged graduate nursing education. The focus of that education shifted as the context of mental health care shifted from large state facilities to community health centers and short-term inpatient facilities. By 1965, 31 colleges and universities in 22 states were conducting advanced programs in psychiatric and mental health nursing leading to master's degrees; 4 also had doctoral programs in psychiatric nursing.[13,34]

Role

The Community Mental Health Act of 1963 had a revolutionary impact not only on the direction of psychiatric nursing but also on the role of the psychiatric nurse. The basic premise of this act was that the mentally ill could and should be treated in their home communities rather than be housed in large state institutions often far from their homes. The act had the effect not only of moving the mentally ill out of institutions but also of moving the psychiatric nurse out of the hospital into the community.

According to Church, the community health movement helped to expand the role of the psychiatric nurse from strictly treating mental illness to promoting mental health.[35] New roles have developed in the community for psychiatric nurses; these include group and individual therapist; consultant in well-child clinics; liaison nurse in pediatric, obstetric, medical, and surgical settings; and private practitioner.[36]

The progress of psychiatric nursing education and the role of the psychiatric nurses during this 25-year period was captured in remarks made by Mary T. Ramshorn at the silver anniversary of the National Mental Health Conference:

> From an era when graduate education was virtually nonexistent, and on-the-job training in state hospitals prepared nurses to practice more custodial than therapeutic nursing, psychiatric nursing has moved into clinical specialization, into community mental health centers, and into graduate programs which offer increasingly sophisticated courses in general systems theory, crisis theory, and community organization. In brief, it would appear from the record that we psychiatric nurses ... have been the long-distance runners of these last twenty-five years.[37]

From a historical perspective it is too soon to evaluate recent events. There have been cutbacks in federal funds for higher education in psychiatric nursing and expanded services for the mentally ill in the community; there is an increasing emphasis on the biological causes of mental illness; interpersonal intervention techniques are being questioned; concern over the effectiveness of deinstitutionalization is developing; the number of professionals other than nurses providing emotional care is increasing. How these factors will affect psychiatric–mental health nursing is not yet known.

There still exist opportunities for the psychiatric nursing profession to continue to move forward and develop. Political, social, economic and scientific forces, however, interact with the nursing profession, including psychiatric–mental health nursing. Progress requires the psychiatric–mental health nursing profession to meet challenges and make them an opportunity for growth.

SUMMARY

The history of care of the mentally ill in the United States involves progression from treatments such as death or abandonment, to treatment such as isolation in prisons or other institutions, to commitments to community care and encouragement of increasing autonomy for patients.

The role of the psychiatric nurse has also advanced from an unacknowledged nursing specialist focusing on custodial care controlled by physicians to an accepted and respected nursing practitioner. Psychiatric nursing education has advanced to the point where graduate education is stressed and independent practice is encouraged.

Although progress has been made on behalf of the mentally ill and many battles have been fought and won, challenges will continue. It seems certain that crucial factors, such as lack of money, lack of adequate facilities, and lack of enlightened public policy, will continue, as in the past, to affect treatment. Ancient prejudices of society may keep the emotionally ill in the chains of misery and neglect.

REFERENCES

1. Nancy L. Hedlund and Finis B. Jeffrey, "Historical Development," in Cornelia Beck, Ruth Rawlins, and Sophronia Williams, eds. *Mental Health Psychiatric Nursing: A Holistic Life Cycle Approach*, Mosby, St. Louis, 1984, pp. 4, 5, 27, 28.
2. John G. Howells, *World History of Psychiatry*, Brunner/Mazel, New York, 1975, pp. vii, 2, 12, 15, 22, 448, 454.
3. David Henderson and R. D. Gillespie, *A Textbook of Psychiatry for Students and Practitioners*, Oxford University Press, London, 1950, pp. 2, 4.
4. Irving J. Sands, *Neuropsychiatry for Nurses*, Saunders, Philadelphia, 1948, p. 275.
5. Alfred Deutsch, *The Mentally Ill in America: A History of Their Care from Colonial Times*, Doubleday, Garden City, N.Y., 1938, pp. 15, 32, 40, 45, 51, 71, 84, 88, 113, 237, 300, 303, 318.
6. Suzanne Loebl, *Exploring the Mind*, Schuman, New York, 1968, p. 162.
7. Josephine Dolan, *History of Nursing*, Saunders, Philadelphia, 1968, p. 207.
8. Joseph P. Morrissey and Howard Goldman, "Cycles of Reform in the Care of the Chronically Mentally Ill," *Hospital and Community Psychiatry*, vol. 35, 1984, pp. 785–793.
9. Clifford Beers, *A Mind That Found Itself: An Autobiography*, Longmans, New York, 1908, pp. 1, 2.
10. Nina Ridenour, *Mental Health in the United States: A Fifty Year History*, Harvard University Press, Cambridge, Mass., 1961, pp. 1091–1093, 1098.
11. Alfred Freedman, Harold Kaplan, and Benjamin Sadock, *Comprehensive Textbook of Psychiatry II*. Williams and Williams, Baltimore, 1975, pp. 70, 71, 72, 629, 1126.
12. J. K. Hall, ed., *One Hundred Years of American Psychiatry*, Columbia University Press, New York, 1944, pp. 21, 131, 284, 285, 293, 500.
13. Esta Carini, Dorothy Douglas, Lois Heck, and Marguerite Pearson, *The Mentally Ill in Connecticut: Changing Patterns of Care and the Evolution of Psychiatric Nursing, 1636–1972*, State of Connecticut Department of Mental Health, 1974, pp. iv, 317, 327, 343.
14. Judith Krauss and Ann Slavinsky, *The Chronically Ill Psychiatric Patient and the Community*, Blackwell, Boston, 1982, pp. 76, 78.
15. Linda Richards, *Reminiscences of America's First Trained Nurse*, Witcomb and Barrows, Boston, 1915, pp. 108–110.
16. Philip Kalisch and Beatrice Kalisch, *The Advance of American Nursing*, Little, Brown, Boston, 1978, pp. 134, 164.
17. JoAnn Ashley, *Hospitals, Paternalism and the Role of the Nurse*, Teachers College Press, New York, 1976, p. 34.
18. Minnie Goodnow, *Outlines of Nursing History*, Saunders, Philadelphia, 1938, pp. 217–222.
19. Olga Church, *The Noble Reform: The Emergence of Psychiatric Nursing in the United States, 1882–1963*, unpublished doctoral dissertation, 1982, pp. 71, 193.
20. Mary Roberts, *American Nursing History and Interpretation*, Macmillan, New York, 1961, p. 263.
21. *Proceedings of the Second Annual Convention of the National League of Nursing Education*, 1896, pp. 10, 17.
22. Olga Church and Kathleen Buckwalter, "Harriet Bailey: A Psychiatric Nurse Pioneer," *Perspectives in Psychiatric Care*, vol. 18, 1980, pp. 62–66, 126.
23. S. Louise Laird, "The Work of Nurses in Asylums," *American Journal of Nursing*, vol. 1, no. 7, April 1900, p. 518.
24. Hildegard Peplau, "Historical Development of Psychiatric Nursing: A Preliminary Statement of Some Facts and Trends," in Shirley Smoyak and Sheila Rouslin, eds., *A Collection of Classics in Psychiatric Nursing Literature*, Slack, Thorofare, N. J., 1982, p. 17.
25. Katherine Tucker, "Nursing Care of the Insane," *American Journal of Nursing*, vol. 16, no. 3, December 1915, p. 198–202.
26. National League of Nursing Education, *Curriculum Guide for Schools of Nursing*, NLNE, New York, 1937, p. 108.
27. "Report of the Committee on Nursing in Mental Hospitals," *National League of Nursing Education Proceedings*, NLNE, New York, 1934, pp. 240–245, 258.
28. May Kennedy, "Psychiatry in Nursing Education," *American Journal of Nursing*, vol. 37, no. 10, October 1937, pp. 1139–1140.
29. "Round Table on Psychiatric Nursing," *National League*

of Nursing Education Proceedings, NLNE, New York, 1940, p. 213.

30. Silvano Arieti, *American Handbook of Psychiatry*, Basic Books, New York, 1959, pp. 12, 19.
31. Marion Kalkman and Anne Davis, *New Dimensions in Mental Health–Psychiatric Nursing*, McGraw-Hill, New York, 1974, pp. 11, 385.
32. Gwen E. Tudor, "A Sociopsychiatric Nursing Approach to Intervention in a Problem of Mutual Withdrawal on a Mental Hospital Ward," *Psychiatry*, vol. 15, 1952, p. 197.
33. Helen Grace and Dorothy Camilleri, *Mental Health Nursing: A Socio-Psychological Approach*, Brown, Dubuque, Iowa, 1951, p. 15.
34. Documents from National League of Nursing, 3 pages (not numbered).
35. Olga Church, "That Noble Reform: A Brief Examination of the Emergence of Psychiatric–Mental Health Nursing," *The History of American Nursing: Conference Proceedings*, Nursing Archives Special Collections, Boston, 1982, p. 72.
36. Catherine Norris, "The Trend Toward Community Health Centers," *Perspectives in Psychiatric Care*, vol. 2, 1983, p. 127.
37. Mary T. Ramshorn, "The Major Thrust in American Psychiatry Past, Present and Future," *Perspectives in Psychiatric Care*, vol. 2, 1983, p. 154.

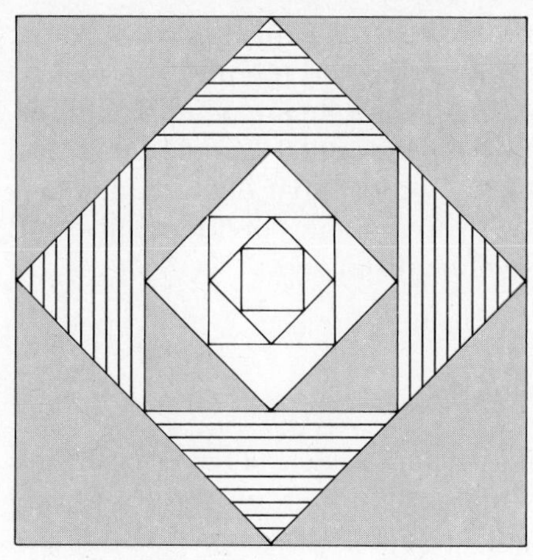

CHAPTER 9
Legal and Ethical Issues

Anita M. Leach

LEARNING OBJECTIVES

After studying this chapter, the student should be able to:

1. Evaluate her or his personal philosophy about the nursing profession.
2. Discuss ethical norms and orientations as they relate to the practice of psychiatric–mental health nursing.
3. Identify ethical dilemmas for nurses and clients.
4. Use an organized process to make ethical decisions.
5. Discuss the meaning of *values* and the values-clarification process.
6. List stages of moral development.
7. Describe various kinds of rights.
8. Identify legal precedents that significantly affect the care of the mentally ill.
9. Discuss the legal and ethical roles of nurses.

Nurses live and work in a world where choices about good and evil or life and death are commonplace. The very nature of nursing creates an atmosphere of tension in which nurses are constantly faced with conflicting values and "terrible" choices. In each interpersonal situation, decisions made by nurses, or decisions they refuse to make, have far-reaching consequences. As nurses assume greater autonomy and responsibility, there is a greater need for moral and legal accountability.

The nursing profession reflects the philosophical positions and values of its members, which include beliefs that people are integrated wholes and that nurses are vital change agents in the lives of clients and as such are involved in the restoration and maintenance of wholeness. Nurses are also whole persons. When engaged in the art of healing, they are called to develop an interdependent and trusting relationship with others and with God or some other power beyond the self, so that they can give compassionate, sensitive, and thorough care to clients and their families.

The study of ethics encourages people to determine what they believe, why they believe it, and how they should act on their beliefs. *Ethics* can be considered as a value system in action. A decision-making process concerning values involves getting to know and to choose what is right or good in each situation. The values of today's society are rapidly changing. Often changes are subtle and people are swept along with the trends without thinking of their apparent logic. Adult values, however, are the result of conscious decisions made after balanced consideration and integration of mental, physical, and spiritual processes.

A person's beliefs or ethics are influenced not only by internal processes but also by the environment. Society influences what is considered "right" in concrete human behavior. This "global rightness" is considered *ethical* because an individual's *choice* of goodness is influenced by the needs and interests that exist in the wider world of other human beings. Ethical values determine how much deviance will be tolerated within a community. Nursing as a profession demands that nurses be accountable for their actions on behalf of clients. Without ethical values, nurses and others cannot arrive at true self-actualization.

The purpose of this chapter is to provide the beginning psychiatric nurse with a framework for ethical decision making. The meanings of *ethics* and *values* are discussed, and the process used by nurses to solve ethical dilemmas is described. Because the law defines societal "good," some legal statutes—particularly those that define a mentally ill client's right to treatment, confidentiality, and competency—will be discussed.

ETHICS

An *ethic* is a standard of valued behavior or beliefs adhered to by individuals or a group. It is concerned with what ought to be rather than what is. *Ethics* is a system of objective norms having to do with the concrete and the present. Ethics deals with questions of human conduct, "right" and "wrong" actions, motives and outcomes of actions, and formulations of principles and standards of conduct for groups of people. Ethics attempts to answer questions about right and wrong, good and bad, and how to achieve the good and avoid the bad. The study of ethics helps to determine what people believe, why they believe it, and how they should act because of their beliefs.[1]

The science of ethics exists only because of human actions or behaviors. The goal of ethics is to ensure that "right" and "good" prevail. Actions are morally appropriate, or "right," when they are in accord with the spiritual nature and the purpose of "being human." For many people, that purpose implies an interrelationship with God or a power beyond the self. Actions are morally inappropriate when they are not in accord with the spiritual self. Morality, then, appeals to the completeness, or wholeness, of human beings in harmony with their environment.[2]

Formation of a system of ethics or morality is a spiritual process in that it transcends the concrete and is impossible without faith and trust in God, a power beyond the self, or other human beings. People who are not professed believers but who are deeply concerned for humanity and human values, by the very nature of their human caring for others, acknowledge an absolute beyond themselves. Attempts to explain the spiritual dimension of people may differ, but a system of beliefs or "oughts" is an inescapable part of the search for wholeness. The study of ethics and ethical discourse becomes possible not because people believe in God, but because holistic human experiences demand recognition of right and wrong.[3]

Nursing, from its very beginnings, was rooted in ethical beliefs. Its normative ethic is selfless concern for others, personal goodness, and rightness of action within society.

Ethical Norms

An *ethical norm* is a standard of behavior which supports nonegotistical conduct—that is, openness to oneself and to one's fellow human beings. For some people, ethical norms grow out of religious writings, such as the decalogue in the Old Testament, the sermon on the mount in the New Testament, the Koran, and other testaments.[2] For others, ethical norms evolve from an understanding that society needs humaneness for survival. Norms evolve from tradition and culture or from the idea that the universe and its creatures are capable of being "cleansed" and improved. Some people believe that such a transformation is possible through a relationship with the creator. Others believe that it is possible through human understanding and insight, human endeavor, planning, reflection, and judgment. Our ability to defend, discuss, expedite, honor, identify, and justify our activities is the result of ethical norms. Without ethical transcendence, chaos, neglect, and evil generally would occur.

Ethical Orientations

An ethical orientation may also be called a *philosophy of life*. A philosophy of life influences what kind of decisions a person makes and how they are made. It is an integral part of human relationships. Ethics or philosophies having to do with health care are referred to as *biomedical ethics*, or *bioethics*. Implementation of bioethics promotes standards of behavior for the delivery of health care by individuals, agencies, institutions, or the system as a whole.

Anyone who thinks seriously about certain important questions can be considered a philosopher; there are people, however, who make philosophy their life work. Much of philosophy—as practiced by these people—involves examination of truths and principles that are important—even essential—to humanity; and many philosophies, such as paternalism, libertarianism, utilitarianism, legalism, egoism, and altruism, are of particular interest to psychiatric nurses. Nurses may also base their actions and their concept of "rightness" on principles of justice as they relate to clients and nurses.[4] Table 9-1 (page 174) defines some philosophical positions and gives an example of each. These positions can serve as a foundation for the development of ethical orientations by nurses.

Ethical orientations are meaningful only if they are *used* and acted upon in the context of situations to which they apply.[5] Nurses can study philosophy, understand various ethical approaches, and say that they hold a certain set of beliefs; but how they act in a given situation depends upon the personal choices they make. Choices are made on a basis of belief in and adherence to principles, on what comes from inside the self, on one's philosophy about life and nursing, and on the environmental context in which they are made.

Personal choice is the exercise of conscience when people do what they do because they feel a moral need to do it. Of course, people may do what they feel is right in order to avoid guilt; then, it is avoidance of guilt that leads to correct actions. In a pragmatic sense, the reasons for actions are not as important as the actions themselves. Ends or outcomes may be similar even if motivating philosophies are in conflict. For example, two nurses may put a client in restraints. One nurse has an altruistic philosophy and believes that the action is a benevolent one motivated by care and concern for the client. No personal guilt is experienced. The second nurse has a paternalistic view and is motivated by a perceived need to protect the client. Again, there is not guilt. These nurses have avoided guilt because of their personal philosophical positions. But the question, "Has good been done?" is not easily answered.

ETHICS AND VALUES IN NURSING

As members of a healing profession, nurses need to answer the questions, "What is the meaning of nursing for me?" and, "What do I value as a person and as a member of the profession?" People's value systems are based on what they *think* is important, what they believe to be true, and what their philosophies or overarching "world views" are. Value systems are expressed through actions or behaviors.

Table 9-1 Ethical Orientations

Ethical Orientation	Philosophical Position	Example and Explanation
Libertarianism (John Stuart Mill)	Belief that people have autonomous power and may make choices without interference from others as long as there is no harm done. People seek solutions that are best for themselves.	Clients may refuse treatment as long as there is no harm done to others. A person may commit suicide if it does not harm others.
Paternalism (Plato)	Belief that some people are subordinate and subject to the regulation of others, much the same way as children are subject to their parents. A person uses coercion to achieve something that is not recognized as "good" by another.	The autonomous rights of a violent client may be overridden and restraints may be used to protect him or her and others from harm.
Utilitarianism (John Stuart Mill)	Belief that a person's actions are "good" or "right" if they promote happiness, and "wrong" if they result in adverse conditions. A person appeals to the "majority rule" and minimizes potentially negative outcomes of her or his actions. The end justifies the means.	The right of a minority, such as the mentally ill, may be overruled for the happiness or good of the whole society. A lesser good or evil may be tolerated if it is done to achieve a greater good and if an evil side effect is not directly intended (principle of double effect). For instance, professionals may violate confidentiality to inform police of the intentions of a psychiatric client to commit suicide.
Formalism-legalism (Kant)	Belief that there are universal principles and basic rules that govern a person's behavior. A person considers the nature of the act itself and applies principles with equality and without regard for changing circumstances.	Clients are treated with love and respect regardless of the nurse's personal dislike for a specific client. Clients are always told the truth about their diagnoses regardless of their ability to accept them.
Egoism (Hobbes)	Belief that one thinks and acts only in self-interest and that the basic drives of human nature are self-preservation and power. A person does solely what is self-gratifying.	Self-preservation dominates a nurse's reactions to a violent client. Clients fail to respect the rules and regulations of the therapeutic environment.
Altruism (Aristotle and Judeo-Christian traditions)	Belief that people should treat one another in a selfless way. A person devotes self to the service of others, sometimes at great personal sacrifice.	Nursing care is characterized by caring and affection for clients. Therapists view their work as a way of creatively transforming clients into whole, responsive, and functioning human beings.

Nurses are not born with a set of values about themselves or about their profession. Rather, they acquire values through personal and spiritual growth. Values emerge from thoughtful consideration of life experiences and from decision making in the face of ethical dilemmas. Figure 9-1 shows a schematic conceptualization of the components of a person's value system and the interaction among them. A person's value system is holistic. External, environmental influences motivate complex internal processes to produce the value itself—a volitional, freely made decision that becomes known externally only when it is expressed in an action.

A value system influences how nurses practice their profession. They may take religious, scientific, or purely humanistic approaches as they practice the art of healing. Regardless of the approach or value system used, nurses must answer the question, "What personal meaning does the healing process have for me?" Nurses are expected to acknowledge their beliefs and practice them on behalf of themselves and their clients.

A value system provides a way to process information, analyze it, and clarify its meaning. It guides the ethical decision-making process and protects the wholeness of the person. When people are not clear about what they value, they communicate their lack of clarity to others—subliminally or directly. For nurses, this results in chaos and harm for themselves and their clients. The ethical person—that is, the person with a carefully thought-out adult value system—respects and protects the needs and rights of others. For example, nurses whose philosophy and value system holds that all

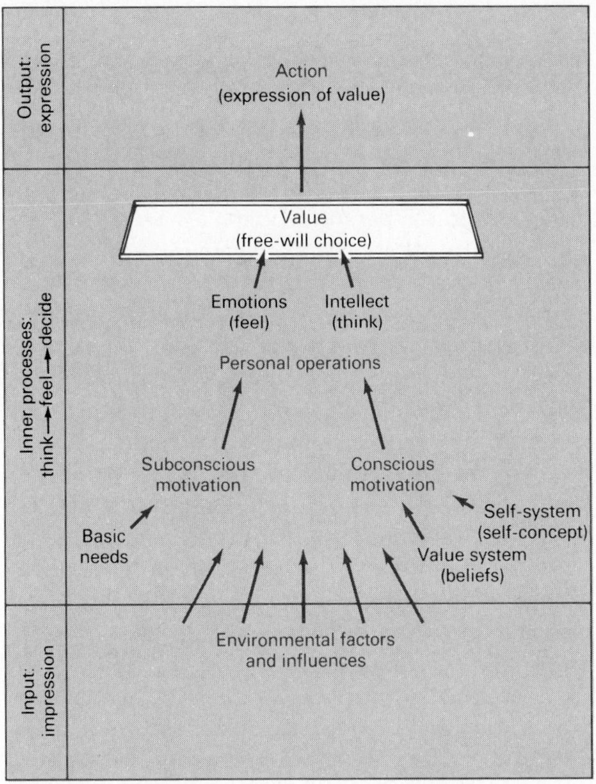

Figure 9-1 Components of a value system.
A person's value system involves many complex processes, including input from the environment, inner processes, and expression through action. The value system may be compared to a sieve through which all decisions and consequent actions are filtered.

life is meaningful will treat clients with great respect. When faced with decisions that involve life itself, such as abortion and euthanasia, they will need to act in congruence with their value system despite economic and societal pressure. To remain true to their value system, they may need to disregard the consequences of their ethical actions. To refuse to work in an abortion clinic or neglect a dying client may cost a nurse his or her job. The act of remaining true to an ethical position—such as respect for human life—by letting it take precedence over job security requires courage. In reality, nurses do not always feel free to act according to their beliefs and may remain in jobs or perform actions which seem to be in conflict with them. This often results in unease or guilt.

The nursing profession has formulated a code of ethics that governs nursing practice.[3] The code, in an abbreviated form, is given in Table 9-2. However, to merely list or memorize a code of behavior does not make it a value system. Thought, discussion, reflection, decision making, action, and sometimes even "trial and error" are needed to clarify adult ethics and values.

Ethical Dilemmas

An *ethical dilemma* is a situation in which there are two or more alternative decisions to choose from, and none is clearly "right."[6] An ethical di-

Table 9-2 Nursing Code of Ethics

Principles
1. The nurse provides services with respect for human dignity and the uniqueness of the client unrestricted by considerations of social or economic status, personal attributes, or the nature of health problems.
2. The nurse safeguards the client's right to privacy by judiciously protecting information of a confidential nature.
3. The nurse acts to safeguard the client and the public when health care and safety are affected by the incompetent, unethical, or illegal practice of any person.
4. The nurse assumes responsibility and accountability for individual nursing judgments and actions.
5. The nurse maintains competence in nursing.
6. The nurse exercises informed judgment and uses individual competence and qualification as criteria in seeking consultation, accepting responsibilities, and delegating nursing activities to others.
7. The nurse participates in activities that contribute to the ongoing development of the profession's body of knowledge.
8. The nurse participates in the profession's efforts to implement and improve standards of nursing.
9. The nurse participates in the profession's efforts to establish and maintain conditions of employment conducive to high-quality nursing care.
10. The nurse participates in the profession's effort to protect the public from misinformation and misrepresentation and to maintain the integrity of nursing.
11. The nurse collaborates with members of the health professions and other citizens in promoting community and national efforts to meet public health needs.

SOURCE: "Nursing Code of Ethics," American Nurses Association, Kansas City, Mo., 1976. Reprinted with permission.

lemma may also be called a *moral conflict.* For nurses, ethical dilemmas may originate from a number of sources and occur on a number of levels. Generally, however, they can be described as involving a choice between two unsatisfactory solutions. For example, a nurse may need to choose between loyalty to peers and what he or she believes to be "right" for a client. Conflicts may occur on an *internal level* for individuals; on a *decision-making* level when nurses interact with physicians, clients, family members, or others; or on a *societal* level when nurses are involved with matters having to do with legislation and social policy. Common ethical dilemmas for nurses include the following:[6]

1. *Conflict between ethical principles.* A nurse may not personally believe in the use of birth control but may work in a clinic where holistic care involves teaching methods of contraception.
2. *Conflict between two possible actions.* A nurse who does not believe professionals should strike may need to decide whether to join colleagues on strike or cross the picket line in order to care for critically ill clients.
3. *Conflict between the need for reflection and the need for action.* A nurse in an emergency may decide to resuscitate a dying client who has had a cardiac arrest although the team has not met to discuss a "no code" policy.
4. *Conflict between two unsatisfactory alternatives.* A nurse may have the choice of using sedatives or arm restraints as an emergency procedure when a client does not respond to verbal calming.
5. *Conflict between role obligations and personal ethical principles.* A director of nursing may value fairness and equality for all persons but be told by an administrator to fire a relative of a person the administrator does not like.

The term *dilemma* implies options about how to act or not act, even though all the options may be in some sense unsatisfactory. When a dilemma exists, people are free to choose a course of action from among several options; the decision that results may be ethical or unethical. The decision-making process involves taking risks and may itself be ethical, but whether the eventual choice is ethical or unethical depends on the decision maker's value system, ethical orientation, and honesty of internal processing.

Ethical Decisions

An *ethical decision* is a freely made personal choice, arising from within, and based on belief in and adherence to principles.[7] Making an ethical decision is a process which is often initiated by an ethical dilemma. Personal choices are influenced by the *agent,* the person who makes a decision and carries it out; the *circumstances,* including intention or motivation; and the *consequences* that result from the decision.[8] Agent, circumstances, and intent determine whether an act is considered ethical or unethical. For example, a nurse who administers a narcotic to relieve a client's pain would almost certainly be seen as acting ethically and morally because the motivation and the consequences of the act are, in the circumstances, good. A street addict who administers drugs to himself or herself with the intention of getting high is likely to be seen as acting unethically or immorally—in these circumstances neither the consequences nor the motivation would be considered good.

In psychiatric nursing, nurses are agents who practice in many environments and under many different circumstances with the intention of healing their clients; the consequences of their actions include change for clients. How easily individual nurses make ethical decisions depends on their value systems, their established values, and their stages of moral and spiritual development.

The Decision-Making Process

Curtin proposed a model for making ethical decisions in nursing.[9] The steps in the process include the following:

- Gather data and information about the situation.
- Study and think about the ethical components of the situation.
- Clarify the rights and responsibilities of the agents involved.
- Define and explore the options available in the situation.
- Apply ethical principles.
- Resolve to act within the context of societal expectations and legal requirements.

This model follows closely a decision-making process proposed by Shelly.[7] She suggests the following steps in the ethical decision-making process. First, in *assessment,* nurses observe, investigate, and interpret the components of an issue and identify their emotional responses and personal biases. Second, *options* available along with alternative choices for action are listed. The issue is thoughtfully considered in the light of each nurse's *ethical orientation,* which may be based on Judeo-Christian tradition, on the teachings of other religions, on the Nursing Code of Ethics, or on the work of philosophers, theologians, and other informed people. An *ethical decision* is then made.

The process of making an ethical decision is not complete until a plan of action has been formulated and communicated to everyone involved. Figure 9-2 illustrates the flow of the ethical decision-making process.

Figure 9-2 Ethical decision-making process. Ethical decision making is holistic and cyclical. Input from the environment motivates people to formulate values. Issues are assessed in light of values. Options for action are listed and considered in light of one's ethical orientation. Decisions are made as values emerge. A value is not incorporated into the self until it is expressed in some form of communication to the environment.

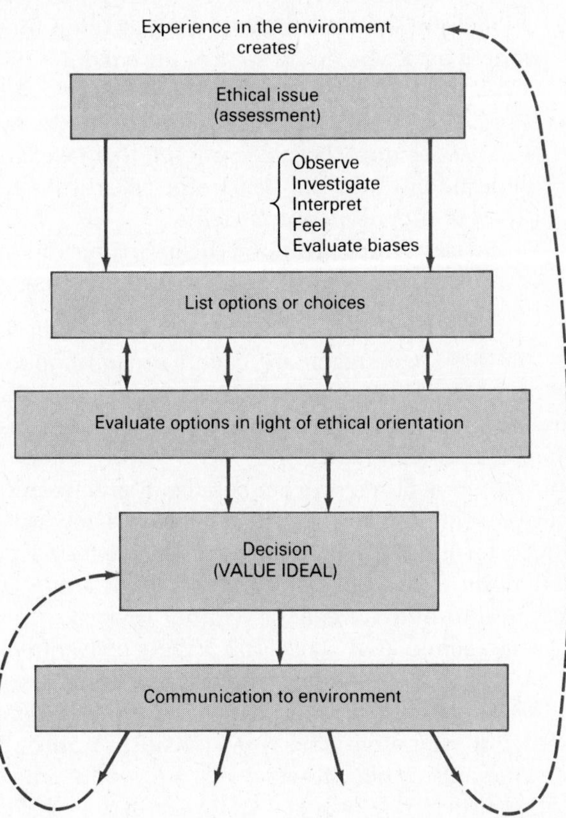

The following vignette shows how the decision-making process operates.

Christine, a nursing student, is assigned to the outpatient obstetrics (OBS) clinic of a Catholic hospital in a large city. Her first client, Jeanne, is a 29-year-old woman who gave birth to her tenth child 6 weeks ago. After examining Jeanne, the doctor informs her that she is in good health and can resume sexual relations with her husband. The woman requests information about an intrauterine device (IUD), saying she cannot afford any more children; she is told that it is against the policy of the hospital to prescribe this form of birth control. The nursing student is upset by her client's plight, knows that information about birth control is part of holistic care, and also knows that such information is available at a competing hospital. She recognizes that an ethical dilemma exists for her.

ASSESSMENT

After Christine observes the woman's plight and receives her request, she checks the hospital's policy and finds that the Catholic church, which supports the hospital, teaches that artificial birth control is a sin. Christine recognizes her anger at the policy and empathy for Jeanne, despite her own personal values, which would not let her practice birth control. But she also believes in loyalty and commitment to the agency in which she is working. She is confused and frustrated. She discusses the issue with her instructor and the pastor of her church.

CONFLICT

Conflicts exist here between two possible actions (to send the client to another agency or do nothing), and between role obligation and personal ethical principles (holistic nursing care and the belief that this form of artificial birth control is wrong).

OPTIONS

Christine can explain to Jeanne that she can do nothing, since hospital policy forbids recommending artificial birth control; Christine can be supportive of Jeanne's plight and refer her to another hospital, or she can become an advocate for change in the hospital policy.

CONSIDERATION

Christine's pastor tells her that her concern for her client constitutes "love of neighbor." He also states, objectively, the position of the hospital and the church—that artificial birth control is wrong. Christine believes that she cannot impose her religious principles on clients.

DECISION

Christine decides that her altruistic value of concern for her client is correct. She recognizes that she risks censure from the hospital and even possible loss of her clinical placement.

ACTION AND COMMUNICATION

Chrsitine refers the client to the local Planned Parenthood clinic. Christine, together with her instructor, begins the process of attempting to modify the hospital's policy so that clients requesting information on artificial birth control will be given data and a referral.

VALUES

Values, which are subjective and personal, are action-oriented, productive, personal beliefs about the truth, beauty, or worth of a thought, object, or behavior. Something may have *intrinsic value,* that is, for its own sake; or it may have *instrumental value,* that is, it may be a means to an end.

Values are ordered hierarchically according to a rational plan known as a *value system.* A value system provides a means for ranking values along a continuum; each ranking reflects the relative importance of a value. In such a system, each value relates to a series of higher values.

Nurses are frequently faced with situations in which one value competes with another. These situations call for them to intelligently appraise the competing values in order to resolve the conflict. Value systems are shaped by education, religion, sex, social system, occupation, culture, and political orientation, among other things. Commitment to a particular hierarchy of values necessitates a corresponding allocation of time, energy, and resources to support it.

Values Clarification

Values clarification is an evolutionary process that facilitates decision making about conflicting values. It is not, therefore, a set of rules. Because values are formed over a period of time,[10] values clarification involves discovering, through feelings and analysis of behavior, what choices to make when alternatives are presented, and identifying whether these choices will be made rationally or on the basis of previous conditioning. The values-clarification process attempts to bring to conscious awareness the values and underlying motivations that guide actions. For nurses, this process sheds light on why their actions have specific outcomes.[11] Values clarification is a dynamic process that fosters understanding of oneself.

Stages of Moral Development

The exploration of one's values is an expression of the search for meaning in life and fulfillment of aesthetic and spiritual needs. People continue to grow as individuals as long as values are maturing and being modified. Like physical, emotional, and spiritual development, moral development is also an important aspect of each person.

Kohlberg[12] defined six stages, or levels, of moral development, or reasons for doing right:

1. Doing right to avoid punishment and discomfort with the superior power of authority figures.
2. Doing right to serve one's own needs and interests.
3. Doing right in order to be a good person in one's own eyes and those of others.
4. Doing right in order to keep an institution functioning as a whole and to avoid breakdown of a system.
5. Doing right from a sense of obligation to the law because of one's social contract to make and abide by laws for the welfare of all and for the protection of all people's rights.
6. Doing right from a rational belief in the validity of universal moral principles and a sense of personal commitment to them.

The first two stages are called *preconventional levels* of moral development. People at these levels are oriented toward obedience to authority because they fear punishment, or they act in the expectation that others will reciprocate equally. Some people's values remain fixed at these levels. They value authority and reciprocity, seldom deviate from legal sanctions, and are restricted in their ability to respond to others freely or without reward.

The second two stages are called *conventional levels* of moral development. People at these levels value conformity and loyalty, and they expend energy to maintain what they consider "appropriate" behavior. They strive for a "good child" image and maintenance of social order for its own sake.

The last two stages are called *postconventional levels.* People at these levels have clearly defined what they value, and they are able to act autonomously and altruistically. They act according to widely accepted moral principles and values: justice, the reciprocity and equality of human rights, and respect for the human dignity of every person.[12]

Moral development, or value formation, is a dynamic, active process that is facilitated by self-assessment, discussion of moral dilemmas, and consequent changes in one's own behavior.[11] The stages of moral development, like other known stages of development, are sequential: people must complete each stage in order to move to the next higher one. One can speculate that ordinary people never reach the last stage of moral development, although great religious figures, such as Jesus Christ, the saints, and Gandhi, are thought to have attained this ideal state. However, most ethical people struggle to reach and maintain a level of moral development that is congruent with their conscience and self-image.

Nurses cannot expect others to have values similar to their own. However, assessing a client's stage of moral development helps to determine what will motivate him or her to change self-destructive behaviors.

Values-Clarification Process

The need to clarify one's values usually originates from one of three situations:

1. Exposing oneself to new information or experiences that are inconsistent with the present value system
2. Being forced to behave in ways that are inconsistent with one's present value system
3. Recognizing, either internally or externally, inconsistencies in one's value system[13]

New information or challenging experiences usually jar existing beliefs and attitudes. People then look at the experiences or the information in the light of *value orientations.* Ideally, feelings and decisions are based on the values from a specific, previously thought-out philosophy. Sometimes, however, people are unclear about what constitutes their value orientation or belief system. Professional nurses encounter many situations which call for analysis, decision making, action, and accountability. If they do not know what they value, or why they value certain concepts, beliefs, attitudes, and behaviors, then they cannot make responsible, ethical decisions. For example:

> Jack, a student nurse, is assigned to a clinic in the ghetto area of a large city and for the first time meets clients who are poor. He is overwhelmed by what he sees and hears. He recognizes an inner need to assess what he believes about the poor and poverty. He has read about poverty and has heard his minister speak about the needs of the poor, but previously he did not need to formulate a value about any of this.

Once the need to formulate a value has been established and a commitment to a value orientation or philosophy has been made, a list of possible alternatives or possible decisions can be drawn up and a choice can be made from among them. Once a value is chosen, it is carefully *considered, prized,* and *cherished.*[10] The key to values clarification is the active choice that is made. A person can think constantly, but until he or she makes a decision, values will not really be formulated. Once a value is chosen, it is reflected in subsequent actions. (Value formation is part of the self-assessment process discussed in Chapters 4 and 7.)

RIGHTS

A *right* is a claim made by an individual or a group to another individual or group; it involves ethical principles or enlightened conscience, but not necessarily the law.[1] Human rights are based on the concept of freedom and self-determination in the context of society. Rights always involve corresponding duties and obligations. Rights have to be consistent with principles of justice; and they are reciprocal in that, for every right of one person, other people have constraints that permit its exercise. Americans generally believe that people have a fundamental right to truth, justice, personal exercise of moral integrity and virtue, propriety in public settings, and the fulfillment of certain basic needs. People retain the freedom to exercise or not exercise rights.

Kinds of Rights

There are several different kinds of rights. When freedom is unrestricted, a right is *absolute.* When freedom is restricted, a *prima facie* right exists.[1] *Legal rights* are those agreed to by society and codified as law. They can be claimed by every citizen. *Moral* or *ethical rights* are based on moral principles; an example would be the right to personal autonomy.[1] Moral and legal rights may be congruent or may conflict with one another.

Legal Rights of the Mentally Ill

Legal rights themselves are of several kinds.[14] Table 9-3 outlines the differences between guaranteed legal rights, nonabsolute legal rights, legal privileges, and legal liberties and gives an example of each.

In 1980, the Mental Health Systems Act (MHSA) adopted into law what had previously been a recommended Bill of Rights for the Mentally Disabled;[15] these were not legislated rights but only recommendations, and it was left up to the states to implement them. Table 9-4 lists the 13 rights, now mandated by MHSA. But even MHSA does not guarantee that clients will know about these rights or know how to exercise them. Nurses have an ethical and legal responsibility not only to inform clients of their legal rights and how they are handled

Table 9-4 Mental Health Systems Act

Recommended Bill of Rights for Clients
1. The right to appropriate treatment in settings and under conditions most supportive of and least restrictive to personal liberty.
2. The right to an individualized, written treatment plan, periodic review of treatment, and revision of plan.
3. The right to ongoing participation in the planning of services, and the right to a reasonable explanation of general mental condition, treatment objective, adverse effects of treatment, reasons for treatment, and available alternatives.
4. The right to refuse treatment except in an emergency or as permitted by law.
5. The right not to participate in experimentation.
6. The right to freedom from restraint or seclusion.
7. The right to a humane treatment environment.
8. The right to confidentiality of records.
9. The right of access to records except data provided by third parties or unless access would be detrimental to health.
10. The right of access to telephone use, mail, and visitors.
11. The right to know these rights.
12. The right to assert grievances when rights are infringed.
13. The right to referral when discharged.

SOURCE: Adapted from *Mental Health Systems Act*, 96th Cong., Pub. L. 96–398, Sec. 9501, 1980.

Table 9-3 Legal Rights

Legal Right	Characteristics	Example
Guaranteed legal right	Grants permission to act Guarantees protection from interference by others Cannot be withdrawn, even with advance notice	A client has the right to refuse medication if there is no threat to self or others.
Nonabsolute legal right	Grants permission to act Guarantees protection for an act Subject to interest-balancing tests; may be withdrawn when it is useful to do so	A client is placed in restraints against his own wishes to protect the interests of the general public.
Legal privilege	Grants permission to act May or may not guarantee protection from interference by others Permission to act; protection may be withdrawn at any time Privilege holder is usually notified in advance	A nurse may lose a nursing license because of unsafe nursing practices, such as working while intoxicated.
Legal liberty	Grants permission to act No guarantee is given against interference by others.	A nurse may teach a client but it is not guaranteed that she will learn what is taught.

SOURCE: Definitions in this table adapted from J. Feinberg, "Rights," in T. L. Beauchamp and L. Walters, eds., *Contemporary Issues in Bioethics*, Dickinson, Belmont, Calif., 1978, pp. 38–43.

in a particular state but also to advocate the implementation of these rights.

Legislation to protect the rights of mentally ill clients has increased dramatically in the last 20 years. Several landmark court cases have given legal status to the ethical rights of clients.[1,3] Table 9-5 lists selected cases, the legal and ethical questions they dealt with, and a brief statement about each decision. Concerns, conflicts, and needs of the mentally ill are coming before the courts more and more; as a consequence, the actions of mental health professionals are being more carefully scrutinized.

The Legal Role of the Nurse

Nurses assume many roles and often play several at one time as they participate in therapeutic activities. They may, for example, be advocates of clients' rights or provide care that helps secure those rights. Nurses are professionals as well as private citizens. Regardless of their role in therapeutic interactions with clients, many legal relationships are involved. It is the individual nurse's responsibility to be familiar with laws and statutes that regulate them both as citizens and as professionals.

Nurses also have rights and responsibilities defined and protected by law. Among the legal rights of nurses are the following:

- To practice their profession
- To compete with others who are equally qualified for employment
- To be compensated for their expertise
- To be advocates for clients
- To be represented in legal and labor matters
- To receive periodic and objective evaluation by peers
- To pursue continuing education
- To participate in the political and legislative decision-making process

Like their clients, nurses have corresponding responsibilities along with these rights. Nurses are accountable for their professional actions and their educational preparation and competence. Providing objective documentation of the care they give and participating in the ongoing development of the nursing profession are among the responsibilities that accompany nurses' right to practice.

Table 9-5 Legal Suits of Significance to Psychiatric Nursing Practice

Ethical or Legal Issue	Legal Case	Decisions
Malpractice	*Pisel v. Stamford Hospital* (1980)	The hospital's policy for monitoring secluded clients did not meet accepted standards of care at the time of the incident. Nurses are bound by current standards of care.
Privileged communication (homicide)	*Tarasoff v. Board of Regents of the University of California* (1976)	A client had told his therapist that he was going to kill Tatiana Tarasoff. The therapist did not warn the victim or her parents. Therapists must warn people of threats that pose a serious danger.
Privileged communication (suicide)	*Bellah v. Greenson* (1978)	The therapist failed to warn the family of his client's potential to commit suicide. There is no responsibility for a professional to notify a family of pending suicide; however, there is a responsibility to notify other professional caregivers of the client.
Right to free speech (right to own thoughts)	*Kaimowitz v. Department of Mental Hygiene* (1973)	Clients have the right to their own thoughts even if they are bizarre or vary from the norm.
Protection against mind-altering effects of medication	*Scott v. Plante* (1976)	Clients are protected against the altering effects of medication.

(Continued.)

Table 9-5 Continued

Ethical or Legal Issue	Legal Case	Decisions
Right to practice religion while institutionalized	*Winters v. Miller* (1971)	A client has the right to refuse medication or treatment on the grounds that it conflicts with religious beliefs.
Protection against cruel and unusual treatment	*Lessard v. Schmidt* (1974)	Institutional conditions such as unsanitary living conditions, inadequate exercise or nutrition, insufficient staffing, and excessive or forced medication are considered cruel and unusual punishment.
Right to due process	*Humphrey v. Cody* (1972)	Clients who are being committed to an institution are entitled to due process of the law.
Right to due process	*O'Connor v. Donaldson* (1975)	Mental illness alone is not enough to justify institutionalization. Donaldson was committed without due process but was not dangerous to himself or others. People not dangerous to themselves or to others and who are capable of surviving safely in freedom by themselves cannot be confined without due process of the law.
Right to treatment and least-restrictive alternative	*Rouse v. Cameron* (1966)	Rouse applied for release from the hospital on grounds that he was receiving no treatment. A client who is institutionalized is entitled to treatment. Criminals have a right to treatment if they are insane or a right to be released if they are no longer insane.
Rights of criminally committed	*Jackson v. Indiana* (1972)	In mandated commitment cases to determine competency, civil commitment procedures are initiated or the client goes free if a significant period of time elapses.
Right to counsel	*Vitek v. Jones* (1980)	Clients have the right to counsel and a hearing when they are changed from confinement in a jail to confinement in a mental hospital.
Informed consent (lack of voluntariness)	*Kaimowitz v. Department of Mental Health* (1973)	An involuntarily committed criminal cannot consent to, or volunteer for, intrusive and irreversable procedures (in this case, psychosurgery).
Right of society to protection	*Mills v. Rogers* (1982)	Emergency treatment can begin without a client's consent. Emergency psychotropic medications can be forced only after other alternative approaches have been attempted.
Right to refuse treatment	*Rennie v. Klein*	An involuntarily committed, competent client has a partial right to refuse treatment. The state may protect other hospitalized clients by forcing medication, but it should provide a review of medication refusal and due process under the law.

SOURCES: Data in this table from J. A. Mappes and J. S. Zembaty, *Biomedical Ethics*, McGraw-Hill, New York, 1981; and B. Bandman and E. L. Bandman, *Bioethics and Human Rights*, Little, Brown, Boston, 1978.

Not all states legally protect nurses' rights, but every state has legislation that defines the scope of nursing practice.[16] The right to practice nursing and intervene therapeutically with clients also carries with it the responsibility to practice competently and in accordance with certain standards of care. Failure to do so may result in harm to clients and may make the nurse vulnerable to malpractice litigation. Claims of negligence are the most common complaints brought against nurses. Nurses are considered negligent if, while they are the legal caretakers, they neglect their responsibilities and the client suffers substantial damages as a result.

Lawsuits against nurses are becoming more common. If nurses follow the ANA Standards of Psychiatric and Mental Health Nursing Practice (see Appendix 1), know their state laws and their corresponding rights and responsibilities, document their care accurately and concisely, and maintain confidentiality as it is defined by legal precedent, they will minimize their risk of being sued for malpractice. If questions or doubts emerge in the course of their practice, nurses should consult with the state nurses' association; if necessary, a state nurses' association will provide a lawyer familiar with the nursing practice act in the state.

Nurses, from a legal point of view, need to be competent and committed to professional standards and the profession. Nurses are legally accountable for their actions. The nursing profession cannot lose sight of the responsibility and accountability inherent in the nurse-client relationship. Professional accountability exists to maintain goals and standards; it is measured by feedback from clients, peer reviews, audits, reevaluation of employment contracts, inspections, and observations of colleagues and superiors. The Nursing Code of Ethics provides further guidelines for accountability.

Nurses are considered competent when they maintain their knowledge base, intervene with clients at a level of practice congruent with their education and skills, and are not impaired by illness, disability, or the use of drugs or other toxic substances.

Commitment to the profession involves mutual support and care for peers, active membership in professional nursing organizations, provision of expert testimony when called upon to do so on behalf of the profession, and political activity on behalf of better health care for clients and for the protection of the rights and responsibilities of the nursing profession.

SUMMARY

The study of ethics encourages people to determine what they believe, why they believe it, and how to act on their beliefs. An ethical orientation is called a *philosophy of life.* Philosophical positions of interest to nurses include paternalism, liberatarianism, utilitarianism, legalism, egoism, altruism, and the principles of justice from which the rights of clients are derived.

People's *value systems* are what they think is important. A value system is formed by what a person believes to be true and the philosophy or "world view" he or she accepts. It provides a way to process information, criticize it, and clarify its meaning. It guides the ethical decision-making process.

An *ethic* is a standard of valued behavior or belief adhered to by individuals or groups. A person's ethical dimension or ethical norms support non-egotistical conduct, that is, openness to oneself and to others. An *ethical dilemma* occurs when an ethical decision involves two or more alternatives, or choices, none of which is entirely satisfactory. An ethical dilemma may also be called a *moral conflict.* Sources of moral conflict for nurses occur when two or more opposing ethical principles, possible actions, or unsatisfactory alternatives are available; when the need for reflection vies with the need for action; and when role obligations interfere with personal ethical principles.

An *ethical decision* is a personal choice, freely made, arising from within the self and based on belief in and adherence to principles. Personal choices are determined by the *agent* (the person who makes a decision and carries it out); the *circumstances* (motivations for the choice); and the *consequences* that may result from a decision. Whether a person can make ethical decisions easily depends on his or her value system, values, and stage of moral and spiritual development.

Values are action-oriented, productive, personal beliefs about the truth, beauty, or worth of a thought, object, or behavior. *Values clarification* is an evolutionary process involving decisions about conflicting values.

Stages of moral development provide a framework for assessing people's motivations. The process of moral development, or value formation, is dynamic and active and is facilitated by self-assessment, discussion of moral dilemmas, and consequent personal change in behavior.

A *right* is a claim made by an individual or group to another individual or group that involves ethical principles or enlighted conscience, but not necessarily laws. Rights may be absolute, prima facie, legal, or moral or ethical. Every right has corresponding duties and obligations. Several landmark legal decisions have given legal status to the ethical rights of clients. The right to practice nursing and intervene therapeutically with clients carries with it the responsibility to practice competently and in accordance with standards of care.

REFERENCES

1. J. A. Mappes and J. S. Zembaty, *Biomedical Ethics*, McGraw-Hill, New York, 1981.
2. J. Fuchs, *Christian Ethics In A Secular Arena*, Georgetown University Press, Washington, D.C., 1984.
3. American Nurses Association, *Code for Nurses*, ANA, Kansas City, Mo., 1976.
4. M. J. Fromer, *Ethical Issues in Health Care*, Mosby, St. Louis, 1981.
5. B. Bandman and E. L. Bandman, *Bioethics and Human Rights*, Little, Brown, Boston, 1978.
6. S. Smith and A. Davis, "Ethical Dilemmas: Conflict Among Rights, Duties, and Obligations," *American Journal of Nursing*, vol. 80, no. 8, August 1980, pp. 1463–1466.
7. J. A. Shelly, *Dilemma: A Nurses' Guide For Making Ethical Decisions*, Inter-Varsity, Downers Grove, Ill., 1980.
8. L. L. Curtin, "Clarity and Freedom: Ethical Issues in Mental Health," *Issues In Mental Health Nursing*, vol. 2, no. 1, 1979, pp. 102–108.
9. L. L. Curtin, "A Proposed Model for Critical Ethical Analysis," *Nursing Forum*, vol. 17, no. 1, 1978, p. 12.
10. S. M. Steele and V. M. Harmon, *Values Clarification in Nursing*, 2d ed., Appleton-Century-Crofts, East Norwalk, Conn., 1983.
11. E. K. Shriver, "Symposium on Bioethical Issues in Nursing," *Nursing Clinics of North America*, vol. 14, no. 1, March 1979, pp. 1–81.
12. L. Kohlberg, "Moral Stages and Moralization," in T. Lickona, ed., *Moral Development and Behavior*, Holt, New York, 1976.
13. S. Sibert, "Ethics In Psychosocial Nursing," *Journal of Psychosocial Nursing and Mental Health Services*, vol. 21, no. 12, December 1983, pp. 29–33.
14. J. Feinberg, "Rights," in T. L. Beauchamp and L. Walters, eds., *Contemporary Issues In Bioethics*, Dickinson, Belmont, Calif., 1978, pp. 38–43.
15. *Mental Health System Act*, 96th Cong., Pub. L. 96-398, sec. 9501, Amendment to Senate Bill 1177, September 23, 1980.
16. S. M. Steele and F. L. Maraviglia, *Creativity in Nursing*, Slack, Thorofare, N.J., 1981.

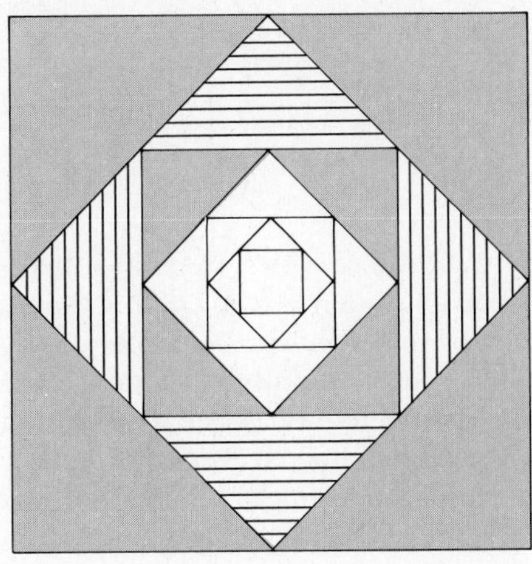

CHAPTER 10
Role of the Nurse

Karen D. Frank

LEARNING OBJECTIVES

After studying this chapter, the student should be able to:

1. Discuss the components of a role.
2. Describe the components of a role.
3. Discuss the concept of *role conflict* as it pertains to psychiatric–mental health nursing.
4. Describe the effect of role blurring in psychiatric–mental health nursing.
5. Define the term *psychiatric–mental health nursing*.
6. Identify subroles in psychiatric–mental health nursing.
7. Describe the role of the generalist psychiatric nurse in an inpatient setting.
8. Describe the role of the generalist psychiatric nurse in an outpatient setting.
9. Compare and contrast the role of the psychiatric nurse in inpatient and outpatient settings.
10. Describe the role of the head nurse and the psychiatric coordinator.
11. Discuss the subroles of the clinical specialist:
    a. Consultant
    b. Provider of liaison services
    c. Systems change agent
    d. Clinical researcher
    e. Independent practitioner
12. Describe the responsibilities of the nurse in relation to:
    a. Accountability
    b. Continuing education
    c. Credentialing
    d. Doctoral education

> Psychiatric–mental health nurses are called upon today to function in many varied ways.... We are administrators, teachers, supervisors, clinical specialists, and although "bedside" hardly seems applicable, we are "client-side practitioners."[1]

Dramatic changes in the nursing profession and in the mental health care delivery system have created a complex, multifaceted role for the psychiatric–mental health nurse. The quotation above—from Suzanne Lego, a pioneer in the expansion of the role of the psychiatric–mental health nurse—makes it clear that today the role of the nurse is indeed multidimensional.

The practice of psychiatric–mental health nursing is based on scientific knowledge which in turn is based on theories of nursing itself, on theories in the behavioral sciences, on concepts of stress as a biopsychosocial phenomenon, and on interpersonal relationships. It is through their various roles that nurses translate this body of knowledge into actions.[2]

Nurses who no longer feel confined to traditional roles have many opportunities to make their roles operational in a variety of settings. Generalist nurses, prepared at the undergraduate level, assume responsibility for providing primary psychiatric nursing care in settings which include short-term psychiatric units in community hospitals, long-term extended-care facilities, public health agencies, and clinics and mental health centers. Nurses with a master's degree or a higher degree function as clinical specialists in a wide variety of settings. Clinical nurse specialists serve as coordinators, supervisors, liaison consultants, private practitioners, researchers, and educators in short- and long-term hospitals, mental health centers, prisons, group homes, private offices, and colleges.[3] Indeed, opportunities for the practice of psychiatric–mental health nursing are nearly limitless. Regardless of the settings in which they work or the level of educational preparation which they have, psychiatric–mental health nurses use their expertise to meet the physical, emotional, social, and spiritual needs of their clients.

The purpose of this chapter is to explore the role of the psychiatric nurse in both inpatient and outpatient settings. The clinical specialist's roles (therapist, systems change agent, consultant, liaison, researcher, educator) will be presented. Responsibility for continuing professional development—including accountability, continuing education, credentialing, and doctoral education—will be explored.

ROLE THEORY

Regardless of the setting in which they find themselves, nurses need an understanding of role theory and the concept of role conflict. Roles frequently reflect goals, values, and sentiments which characterize a situation. Role theory assists in assessing the priorities of an individual, an organization, or an authority structure; determining how decisions are made and labor is divided; and evaluating relationships that have evolved among various components of a system.

A *role* is a culturally defined set of performances (behaviors) and expectations.[4] It provides a strategy for coping with recurrent situations as well as a basis for identifying and placing people in society. When a role is performed, characteristic, patterned behaviors and qualities are exhibited, and expectations are established. A role, then, might be considered a *description*, analogous to (say) a job description. (For example, nurses are often traditionally described as "maternal figures who are warm and friendly.")

Performance of a role is guided by *role expectations*—concepts of what behaviors are appropriate, anticipated and desired by oneself, others, and society.[4,5] Performers adjust their role expectations according to their own perceptions of their actions and their perception of how others are reacting. Nurses today frequently encounter discrepancies between their own role expectations and the expectations of others. For example, a clinical specialist, comfortably functioning in the role of family therapist, will often encounter prospective clients who express surprise that the family therapist can be a nurse. The nurse may have to explain why and how that is possible in order to make the expectations congruent.

Roles exist both in society as a whole and in organizations. Various people may perform a role. In each situation, the nature of a role may vary to some degree depending on the person who performs it, the "audience," and the interaction that evolves between that person and the audience.

Roles, role expectations, and the rights, duties, privileges, and obligations of roles are learned.[5,6] Socialization—planned and unplanned, direct and indirect—begins early and continues throughout life. Observations of and interactions with peers and adults provide children with information about how to behave in various relationships and situations.[4] People learn what is expected of them and what to expect of others. Creating and enacting roles, and attempting to conform to role prescriptions (cultural standards and definitions of roles in social systems such as school and work) also represent learning experiences.

Kinds of Roles

People may take on a variety of roles, and roles may be ascribed, achieved, assumed, or adopted.

An *ascribed role* is one in which a person formally assumes responsibility for carrying out an established set of norms. The director of nursing in a health care setting, for example, has an ascribed role by virtue of the title and job description. The head nurse on a surgical unit has specific role responsibilities.

An *achieved role* is one which is assumed as the result of an accomplishment. The role of nurse is achieved through completing an educational program and meeting state requirements.

An *adopted role* is one assumed for the achievement of a specific goal. For example, a nurse may adopt the role of "stern parent" when setting limits with a rebellious adolescent. How a person behaves in an adopted role may or may not be consistent with his or her ordinary behavior.

An *assumed role* is one taken up or already possessed as an integral part of the personality. The role of nurse is assumed by someone who is employed as a nurse, of course; but it also connotes competence in specific circumstances in a hospital setting (clinically competent nurses often assume the role of distinguished practitioners or awe-inspiring figures in the eyes of students). The nurse-practitioner may assume a leadership role with peers in order to promote improved care for clients.

A role is *internalized* when it becomes part of one's self-concept. Not all roles are internalized. For example, although a nurse can function as a family therapist, someone in this role may think of himself or herself simply as a nurse who conducts family therapy.

Roles may also be formal or informal. A *formal role* is one that is ascribed. For example, a physician-psychiatrist may be the formal leader of a treatment team. The actual leader of the team may, in fact, be a nurse. An *informal role* is one that is achieved: the term *informal leader* refers to the person with greatest influence in a situation. The informal leader may lack ascribed power, but he or she is generally one who has achieved the role.

Performance of a role is affected by the personality of the person assuming it and by the structure of the setting in which it is carried out. For example, an authoritarian person may function in the role of head nurse very differently from someone who is more laissez-faire. And if the structure calls for a dominant person, the authoritarian nurse will have no difficulty assuming the role—but the laissez-faire nurse might have little success with it.

Role Characteristics

Role characteristics are distinguishable, specific, unique behaviors associated with a role.[7] How role characteristics are perceived is influenced by family background, occupation, education, and cultural origin. For example, the role of psychiatric–mental health nurse is perceived in different ways: some people believe that psychiatric nurses are caring and take a holistic approach to their clients; others perceive psychiatric nurses as threats or as uneducated and unskilled.

The characteristics of some roles include gender. For example, the roles of secretary and nurse are generally characterized as female, and the roles of executive and administrator may be characterized as male. Certain other roles have characteristics related to cultural background. Today, it is increasingly felt that gender and culture are not valid sources of role characteristics but are far more likely to be harmful stereotypes. This growing belief is gradually changing the perceived characteristics of many roles that were traditionally stereotyped.

Role Conflict

Role conflict—"friction" between or among two or more roles that a person is expected to perform—can occur under various circumstances.

One source of role conflict is *incongruity*. A role is performed more adequately and comfortably if it is congruent with one's self-concept, values, wishes, and needs. If it is incongruent, the performance will be invalid, unconvincing, inappropriate, and a source of distress; a conflict will exist within the person and between the person and other people or the system. As a result, the role expectations of others, the system, or society as a whole may not be met. For example:

> Ms. A., a nurse, has been hired to work in a day treatment program. She expects to be conducting daily therapy groups—this role represents her self-concept and values. But she finds that she must spend most of her time administering medications; and for her, that role is incongruent. She will experience a role conflict that may cause her to perform poorly, so that she fails to meet the expectations of the system or of other people in it.

Another source of role conflict is *incompatibility*. When a person must perform several roles, the demands of one role may not be compatible with those of another. A person faced with this sort of role conflict may establish a hierarchy, giving one role priority over the others; this is called *role primacy*. Role primacy can be a complicated phenomenon—its consequences may be perceived differently by different people, for one thing—and it may generate even more conflict within the person. Here is an example of incompatibility:

> Ms. B. is a nurse who perceives herself as an advocate for clients but sometimes finds herself in the role of an advocate for the system—the institution. She has a client who, in her judgment, should be referred to Alcoholics Anonymous; as client's advocate she would make the referral. But the system in which she works has a rule that only physicians can make such referrals, and the client's physician will not do so. Ms. B's role as client's advocate is, in this situation, incompatible with her role as system advocate.

Ms. B in this example might resort to role primacy and decide that her role as client's advocate takes precedence over her role as system advocate, or vice versa. But a decision to act on behalf of the client instead of the system obviously has potential consequences, some of them quite serious. A situation such as this can therefore lead to the assumption of a *counterfeit role*—a role that is performed and overtly accepted (in order to avoid a penalty, say) but not really internalized. Incompatibility can also lead to *role strain*—difficulty or stress associated with the demands of a role.

A third source of role conflict is *role distance*—a gap or a contradiction between one's role and one's self-concept. In such a situation, a person may exhibit behaviors that reflect his or her unique personal traits and may resist the prescribed role. For example, a nurse who perceives himself or herself as a "colorful dresser" may come to work each day dressed in a different, eccentric outfit rather than conform to the dress code of the institution or agency. (Role distance might be considered a form of role incongruity, but the two are somewhat different. Role incongruity has to do more with conflicts between perceived roles and actual roles; role distance is a conflict between self-concept and role—it could be thought of as friction between the "private self" and the "public self.")

Role Blurring

Role blurring occurs when expectations and characteristics of roles and associated behaviors are unclear or there is no consensus on them.[4] Role blurring can impair the effectiveness and morale of a system and individuals within it. Perhaps the most common form of role blurring is performance by one person (or group) of a role that others believe belongs to them.

Role blurring is a familiar phenomenon in psychiatric–mental health settings, where therapy is shared by various disciplines. Although each person brings specific expertise to the work with clients, in some treatment facilities there may be little or no way to distinguish the roles of the nurse, the physician, and the social worker. About the most that can be said is that each of them approaches therapy from a different perspective. (For example, in a chemical dependency center, it is difficult to distinguish between what a certified alcoholism counselor—CAC—does and what a psychiatric nurse does when they co-lead clients' confrontation groups.)

Role blurring is often a source of role conflict. Moreover, assumption of roles belonging to others may result in abandonment or rejection of roles and activities that should be performed. This too is common in health care settings. (For example, if a psychiatric unit has a nursing coordinator who effectively monitors its daily functioning, the coordinating psychiatrist may abandon his or her own administrative role.) When personal or interpersonal role conflicts develop among health care professionals as a result of role blurring, collaboration is weakened, and the quality of care diminishes.

Role blurring can lead to *role ambivalence*—that is, conflicting attitudes toward a role. As nurses move out of traditional hospital settings, and as their skills become more comprehensive, they may experience such ambivalence. This is also true of other mental health professionals. There is sometimes considerable uncertainty about who should take what roles and about what consequences are desirable.[8] As was noted above, the nurse's role may appear to be interchangeable with the roles of other mental health professionals. All the following functions, for instance, can be performed by appropriately trained psychiatrists, psychiatric social workers, clinical psychologists, or psychiatric nurses: (1) conducting intake interviews and disposition evaluations, (2) conducting ongoing psychotherapy, (3) conducting group therapy and group discussions, (4) conducting family therapy and family support groups, (5) preparing clients for termination of treatment, and (6) developing aftercare plans with clients. The ability of two or more people to perform similar functions can lead not only to ambivalence but also to professional jealousy, rivalry, competition, and conflict about expectations, status, and performance.[8,9]

From a nursing perspective, role blurring, or role overlap, can be perceived as either a negative or a positive phenomenon. One nurse leader, Dixie Koldjeski, warns that nurses should not be considered interchangeable with other personnel, and that loss of the unique body of nursing practices might ultimately result in a loss of positions for nurses.[10] In contrast, another nurse leader, Claire Fagin, concludes that nursing services are indeed comparable to, if not interchangeable with, services provided by other disciplines and believes that this can have a good effect on the nursing profession:

> Nurses' claims for access to the reimbursement system should be made for those services that are clearly substitutive for services presently reimbursed or where sufficient data exist indicating that [alternative] services to those currently reimbursed will be cost-effective.[11]

Nurses in the private practice of psychotherapy, for example, provide service at least equivalent in quality to that of other mental health professionals such as psychiatrists, clinical psychologists, and psychiatric social workers, and often at a more reasonable fee. Role blurring, therefore, may help nurses get a larger share of reimbursement in this decade of cost-effective health care.

However, if role blurring is considered undesirable, it can be reduced by clearly defining the unique characteristics of the nursing role. Although it is obviously impossible to define nursing so that there is *no* overlap with other disciplines, the conceptual approach of the nurse is distinctive. Members of the nursing profession more than other professions view clients holistically from a biopsychosocial perspective. Thus, a nurse who, for example, administers psychiatric medications to a client is concerned with the physical, emotional, social, and spiritual aspects of the treatment. Observation of *role models*—people who provide an example or a standard for others—can also be useful in defining roles. Nurses who can serve as positive models are those who are familiar with, and expert in, their roles; clinical specialists, head nurses, and senior staff nurses are often role models and sometimes also act as mentors for students or beginning staff nurses. However, a beginning practitioner should not indiscriminately adopt the attitude or point of view of others simply because they have been perceived or labeled *experts*.

ROLES IN PSYCHIATRIC–MENTAL HEALTH NURSING*

Psychiatric nursing is an interpersonal process aimed at promoting and maintaining behavior which contributes to integrated functioning. The American Nurses Association (ANA) has defined *psychiatric–mental health nursing* as a specialized area of nursing practice employing theories of human behavior as its science and powerful use of self as its art.[12] The recommended educational preparation for the role of psychiatric–mental health nurse is a baccalaureate degree in nursing and expertise in psychiatric and mental health nursing. ANA notes that psychiatric–mental health nursing demands knowledge of theories of personality development and behavior patterns, understanding of sociopsychological principles, and ability to communicate

* Portions of this section from Anita M. Leach, "Context of Care," in the second edition of this book.

meaningfully with clients. Nurses also need to know about contributions of other disciplines, dynamics of interpersonal relationships, and theories and methods of treatment of mental illness. Standards for psychiatric–mental health nursing practice are listed in Appendix 1.

In 1976 the ANA issued a statement on psychiatric–mental health nursing practice which delineated two types of practitioners:

1. The *psychiatric–mental health nurse* without a master's degree is recognized through general certification at a basic level of competence.
2. The *psychiatric–mental health nursing clinical specialist* is prepared at the master's level and recognized through special certification at an advanced level of competence.

Professional nurses who practice in psychiatric–mental health settings are identified by the profession as psychiatric–mental health nurses only when they demonstrate its standard of knowledge, expertise, and quality of care.

The nurse's role differs from roles of other mental health professionals because nursing takes a holistic view of its clients. Nurses are educated as generalists, and they see their clients as total beings with interacting physical, emotional, social, and spiritual dimensions. Other mental health professionals, by contrast, perceive clients in a more compartmentalized way; they may focus on only one or two dimensions, such as the emotional and the social. For example:

> When evaluating Mr. Y., a client who reports feeling depressed, the nurse notices that he has dry skin, thinning hair, and a sluggish manner. After considering what these physical observations may indicate, as well as the emotional, social, and spiritual aspects of Mr. Y., the nurse suggests that an endocrine workup may demonstrate a thyroid dysfunction which is manifested as mild depression.

Nurses' broad perspective distinguishes the nursing role in both inpatient and outpatient settings.

Psychiatric–mental health nurses perform a variety of roles. What the specific aspects of each role are depends on the context or environment in which the nurses work; but all their roles have dependent, interdependent, and independent aspects.

Subroles

Only infrequently do nurses function in a single role at a time; they generally have a variety of subroles.[13,14] A *subrole* is a role that follows from or is part of a principal role. Six key subroles can be identified with nursing; each grows out of the multiplicity of clients' needs:

1. Nurturer
2. Coordinator
3. Socializing agent
4. Counselor
5. Educator
6. Technician

The nurse as *nurturer* functions as care giver, protector from injury, source of unconditional acceptance, and growth-promoting agent. For instance, a nurturer may listen attentively to a depressed client and then gently encourage him or her to join other clients in the dining room for lunch.

The nurse as *coordinator* organizes the many activities associated with the care of the client. This involves conceptualizing the plan of care as a whole rather than as unintegrated segments. The nurse consistently assesses clients' progress in the therapeutic process and shares this assessment with team members. A nurse-manager can also help clients coordinate their daily schedules for maximum benefit. (A client who wants to take part in an off-unit outing to the movies, for example, may need help in adjusting his or her schedule to avoid a conflict with a physical therapy session.)

The nurse as a *socializing agent* serves as a "mirror of reality" to prepare clients to leave the more tolerant environment provided by the hospital for the less tolerant environment of society—helping to establish norms for appropriate behavior, teaching them how to relate, and suggesting how unstructured time can be used. (For example, a nurse may remind clients that they are expected to shower and dress appropriately before joining a group for lunch in the dining room.)

The nurse as *counselor* helps clients to examine their patterns of problem solving and develop new ones. Clients who injure themselves superficially when they feel anxious, for instance, are helped to assume responsibility for their own self-control.

The counselor helps clients explore alternative, more constructive behaviors for the relief of anxiety, such as seeking out staff members and staying with the group.

The nurse as *educator* helps clients learn behavior that will promote health. In this role nurses teach clients about structuring daily activities, using medications, and utilizing available community resources.

The nurse as *technician* provides expert nursing requiring specialized skills. For instance, the nurse makes sure that a client doesn't eat or drink before electroconvulsive therapy, carefully monitors the client's vital signs as the effects of anesthesia wear off, and provides reassurance that the memory loss experienced after treatments is usually transient.

These six roles are also characteristic of the nurse's interaction with coworkers. A charge nurse for the day serves as nurturer by carefully listening to a coworker who complains that his or her assignment is unfair. A nurse assumes the role of technician when a coworker asks for help in bringing an out-of-control client to a less stimulating environment such as the unit's quiet room. A nurse serves as educator, or information resource, when a coworker is unsure which of two antidepressants is more cardiotoxic; the nurse and coworker may research the drugs together in a pharmacology text. A charge nurse acts as socializing agent when he or she reminds staff members to discuss personal concerns during meals and breaks only. A nurse serves as counselor when a coworker expresses the desire to be more assertive and self-directed on the job; the nurse and coworker may review together some steps that could be taken in this direction. Finally, a nurse serves as coordinator by making sure that coworkers take scheduled meals and breaks, that they are certified each year to perform cardiopulmonary resuscitation, and that documentation is complete on all clients' charts.

Each subrole is associated with different expectations. Nurses may feel more comfortable or expert in some subroles than in others. For example, one nurse may feel skillful as a technician and educator but less secure as a counselor or nurturer. Although nurses are required to have a basic level of competence for each subrole, they naturally will be more competent in certain roles. It is important for nurses to be aware of their strengths and weaknesses and to take advantage of opportunities for continuing education.

The Generalist Nurse

The Role of Generalist Nurses in an Inpatient Setting

A generalist nurse most often has a staff position in the psychiatric unit of a community hospital, a private psychiatric hospital, or a state psychiatric hospital—settings which offer a restricted environment for clients who have poor reality orientation or impulse control.

The role of the nurse in such settings is to deliver care that promotes functional patterns in clients. Table 10-1 lists common role behaviors of a generalist nurse on the staff of a psychiatric unit.

In inpatient settings where *primary nursing* is the modality of care delivery, one nurse is assigned to coordinate the total nursing care of a client from admission to discharge.[15] This modality of care delivery provides very individualized, comprehensive care with a greater degree of continuity than other modalities can offer. The primary nurse assesses the client's needs, formulates a plan of care to be implemented continuously, and evaluates the results of care. Primary nurses may delegate responsibility for implementation of a care plan in their absence, but they must provide the directions for care through written and oral communication, and they are held accountable for these directions. Primary nurses are also held accountable for all decisions made and actions taken in the nursing care of a client.

Role behaviors of the primary nurse include the six nursing subroles. For example:

> A woman client who has not responded to several trials of antidepressants and regularly scheduled psychotherapy is evaluated by a consultant psychiatrist. Her attending psychiatrist reviews the consultation and recommends electroconvulsive therapy (ECT), but the client is fearful of this type of treatment, and refuses to consent to it. The nurse as counselor explores the client's fears with her. As an educator trying to help the client cope with a difficult decision-making process, the nurse recommends that the client view an educational videocassette which deals with depression and how it is treated. As a socializing agent, the nurse introduces the client to another client who has had ECT, whose depression has lifted, and

Table 10-1 Role Behaviors of the Generalist Nurse: Psychiatric–Mental Health Nurse, Staff Nurse Position

Role Behaviors	Examples
1. Assess new clients upon their admission to unit.	1. Conduct clients' intake interviews. Chart outcomes.
2. Provide for comprehensive, individualized primary care for clients while they are in treatment.	2. Conduct individual nurse-client interactions daily. Chart outcomes. Regularly develop and modify a nursing care plan for each client.
3. Plan, implement, and evaluate clients' group activities.	3. Conduct or colead group therapy, discussion groups, and activity groups. Facilitate clients' leadership of therapeutic community meetings. Chart outcomes.
4. Facilitate satisfactory verbal and written communication among members of different disciplines and among members of the same discipline concerning clients' progress.	4. Share pertinent clinical information in daily team rounds, presentations of clients, clinical conferences, and charts.
5. Implement and coordinate diagnostic and treatment services provided by other disciplines.	5. Administer medications, treatments, or both, when ordered by each client's physician. Prepare clients for physical therapy, laboratory tests, electroconvulsive therapy, or other related services. Report back to other staff members and chart the outcomes of these services.
6. Provide teaching of clients prior to termination of treatments.	6. Teach clients individually or in group settings about medication regimes, available community resources, and follow-up psychotherapy.
7. Monitor and evaluate policies concerning clients which are currently in practice, and propose relevant changes.	7. Participate in nursing department meetings and interdepartmental meetings and committees. Promote ad hoc committees.

who will soon be discharged. As a nurturer, the nurse supports the client's decision-making efforts. Once the client realizes that she, too, may benefit from ECT, no longer fears the treatment, and agrees to have this somatic therapy, the nurse as coordinator schedules the treatment. As a technician, the nurse monitors the client's vital signs, level of consciousness, and responses during and after treatment.

The generalist nurse also tries to help clients perform as much self-care as possible. The nurse may initially have to provide complete daily care for regressed clients, but as the clients become more reality-oriented, they are able to complete certain aspects of daily care with supervision. For example, they may require supervision during a shower, but are able to dress themselves with little or no guidance. They may require structured directions for cleaning their rooms. Eventually, as reality orientation increases and the educational approach of the nurse takes effect, they will be able to complete their daily self-care independently and report this to the nurse, who then assigns them to a discharge group dealing with activities of daily living.

Other role behaviors of the generalist nurse include maintenance of clients' rights, maintenance of a therapeutic milieu, participation in nursing rounds and team meetings, and supervision of other members of the nursing staff. Table 10-2 illustrates each of these.

The role of the generalist will of course vary somewhat from setting to setting. However, the six subroles will be important in any setting. Table 10-3 (page 194) illustrates the role of one generalist staff nurse during a typical week.

The Role of Generalist Nurses in an Outpatient Setting

Psychiatric–mental health nurses prepared at the undergraduate level are employed in a variety of outpatient settings, such as public health agencies, visiting nurse associations, day hospitals, mental health centers, crisis centers, well-child centers, and mobile emergency units. The generalist nurse is qualified to assume a staff or public health role in such settings. Nurses prepared at the master's level or beyond work both in such settings and in private practice; they serve as clinical specialists, primary therapists, consultants, educators, coordinators, and researchers.

A good way to understand the role of a generalist nurse in an outpatient facility is to compare it with that of a clinical specialist working in the same

Table 10-2 Additional Role Behaviors of the Generalist Nurse

Role Behavior	Description	Example
Maintenance of clients' rights.	The nurse is aware of clients' individual rights and is willing to discuss them with clients.	From admission through discharge of clients, a nurse orients them to unit policies and procedures, encourages them to play active roles in planning and evaluating their own treatment, and has them ask questions about anything which is not fully understood. A psychiatric nurse, aware that psychiatric treatment differs from incarceration as a means for treating objectionable behavior, knows that clients must freely consent to admission and treatment before coming to a voluntary psychiatric unit. Once clients are hospitalized, they retain the right to refuse medications, diagnostic tests, and recommended therapies, even if, in the nurse's judgment, these measures will help clients get well.
Maintenance of a therapeutic milieu.	The nurse strives to establish an environment in which clients can learn to identify their positive and negative feelings and express them appropriately; to relate to others in a group and tolerate closeness; and to seek and accept feedback from others in response to their behavior.	On an inpatient unit, one instrument of milieu therapy is the regularly scheduled community meeting. All clients and staff members are encouraged to attend these meetings, which may be scheduled on a daily or weekly basis, depending upon the unit's needs. A psychiatric nurse is responsible for ensuring that the meetings are held as scheduled and that other appointments and activities are discouraged at those times.
Participation in nursing rounds.	During daily nursing rounds, each primary nurse reports all daily data pertinent to his or her clients to members of the nursing staff.	A nurse reports that Mr. Jones, who had been very agitated on admission 2 days ago, had not had any episodes of agitation on any shift yesterday and had been observed sitting quietly but not participating verbally during daytime activities, sitting calmly and talking to other clients at three different times on the evening shift, and sleeping until 5 A.M. Staff members will continue to observe his behavior, gradually involve him in activity groups, and report the observations at team rounds.
Participation in team rounds.	The primary nurse, as a member of the multidisciplinary team, communicates to other team members all nursing data pertinent to his or her clients for the previous 24-hour period. Several times a week each client may be reviewed in-depth by the team. The primary nurse reviews each client's chart and evaluates his or her status from a nursing perspective. The data is communicated to other team members, who share their perceptions based on their involvement with that client. A client may be brought in for a primary nurse to interview in front of the team. Goals and plans for future care are formulated following a review of all data pertinent to that client.	The primary nurse reports that Mrs. Bates, who was hospitalized following a suicide threat, has not verbalized any suicide threats in the past 48 hours. Her affect is more varied and appropriate. No evidence of self-destructive behavior has been observed, but she continues to engage in isolating behavior and sits by herself in a corner. The occupational therapist states that, with encouragement, Mrs. Bates has attended an art class, although she did not participate. The dance therapist has observed Mrs. Bates moving her arms to music while sitting in a chair. The social worker says that Mrs. Bates's family describes her as "a loner." A decision is made to try to set limits on Mrs. Bates's social isolation by firmly involving her in unit activities; however, her involvement will be allowed to increase gradually.

(Continued.)

Table 10-2 Continued

Role Behavior	Description	Example
Supervision and guidance of other nursing personnel.	The professional nurse is responsible for planning, monitoring, and evaluating care for clients given by licensed practical nurses, nursing assistants, new orientees to the unit, and nursing students. The nurse serves as a role model and mentor to other nursing personnel.	A staff nurse who serves as charge nurse for the shift assigns another nurse to a new client who is unknown to the unit. The charge nurse assigns the licensed practical nurse to assist in orienting a second client to the unit who has just been readmitted after being discharged a few months ago. The nursing assistant is assigned to make half-hour rounds, ascertaining where each client is at those times and noting the observations on the rounds' board, and to prepare clients for evening snacks.

Table 10-3 Role of a Generalist Staff Nurse on an Inpatient Psychiatric Unit in a Community Hospital from 7 A.M. to 3 P.M.

Time	Monday	Tuesday	Wednesday	Thursday	Friday
7:00 A.M.–7:30 A.M.	Listen to 24-hour report.	Listen to 24-hour report.	Listen to 24-hour report.	Listen to 24-hour report.	Listen to 24-hour report.
7:30 A.M.–8:30 A.M.	Assist in ECT. Monitor clients in recovery room.	NPI* with primary clients.	Assist in ECT. Monitor clients in recovery room.	NPI with primary clients.	Assist in ECT. Monitor clients in recovery room.
8:30 A.M.–9:30 A.M.	Assist clients with breakfast. Conduct relaxation group.	Prepare, administer, and chart medications for unit.	Assist clients at breakfast. Help orient a new RN.	Prepare, administer, and chart medications for unit.	Assist clients with breakfast. Admit new client.
9:30 A.M.–10:15 A.M.	Daily team rounds and weekend report.	Daily team rounds and presentation of clients.	Daily team rounds and unit administration.	Daily team rounds and presentation of clients.	Daily team rounds and presentation of clients.
10:15 A.M.–10:30 A.M.	Break.	Break.	Break.	Break.	Break.
10:30 A.M.–11:30 A.M.	Therapeutic community meeting.	Exercise group. Small group discussion.	Group therapy. Post-group discussion.	Off-unit outing to bowling alley.	Assist in occupational therapy baking group.
11:30 A.M.–12:00 P.M.	Chart.	Admit new client.	Help orient new RN.		
12:00 P.M.–12:45 P.M.	Lunch break.	Lunch break.	Lunch break.	Lunch break.	Assist clients with lunch.
12:45 P.M.–1:30 P.M.	NPI with primary clients.	Prepare, administer, and chart medications for unit.	NPI with primary clients.	Prepare, administer, and chart medications for unit.	Lunch break.
1:30 P.M.–2:30 P.M.	Take two clients for a walk on grounds.	NPI with primary clients.	Conduct medication teaching group.	Assist with music therapy.	NPI with primary clients.
2:30 P.M.–3:00 P.M.	Chart. Cover nursing station. Give prn medications.	Chart. Cover nursing station. Give prn medications.	Chart. Cover nursing station. Give prn medications.	Admit new client.	Chart.

*NPI: Nurse-patient interaction.

facility (the clinical specialist's role will be taken up in more detail later in this chapter):

> Mrs. C., a clinical specialist, is a member of the interdisciplinary health team of a mental health center. She conducts individual and group therapy with her clients. She is also a consultant for a local well-child center where she assists the staff in designing a preschoolers' parents' education program. Mr. D., a generalist nurse, works in the day treatment program of the center. He is a member of the day treatment program's interdisciplinary team, conducts nursing assessment interviews, participates in the development of treatment plans, conducts groups focused on socialization and activities of daily life, spends one-to-one time with specified clients each day, and acts as a liaison with the halfway house in which many clients live.

Both the generalist nurse and the clinical specialist encounter in outpatient settings clients who have been discharged from inpatient psychiatric facilities and were referred for follow-up care; clients who are initially referred to home health care agencies or outpatient mental health centers; clients who "walk in" to mental health centers or crisis centers with a problem; and clients who telephone a "hot line" for mobile emergency services. Such clients may or may not initially present their problems as psychiatric.

The nursing subroles discussed earlier are relevant in outpatient settings as well as inpatient settings. However, because outpatient settings—and the clients encountered in them—vary so widely, role behaviors will differ considerably from one setting to another. For example, since clients in a day treatment program generally function at a higher level than clients who are hospitalized, the role of nurturer may have a different objective in an outpatient setting—as may the role of educator. Here is an example:

> Richard, a client enrolled in a day treatment program, may require encouragement and approval because he takes two buses each day in order to attend the program. He may also need sophisticated information concerning vocational rehabilitation services available to him upon completion of the day treatment program at the hospital.

It should be noted that an outpatient facility is likely to have a more flexible structure than an inpatient setting; thus, it represents more opportunities for role blurring.

In a community setting, the generalist nurse performs the subroles in a context of promotion, maintenance, restoration, and rehabilitation of health. For example:

> A public health nurse makes a home visit to a client with Alzheimer's disease who needs dressing changes for a diabetic foot ulcer. During the assessment, the nurse notes the following data:
>
> 1. The client has been living with her married daughter for the past 10 years.
> 2. She has had Alzheimer's disease for 4 years.
> 3. The daughter has become increasingly protective as her mother's symptoms—forgetfulness and helplessness—have worsened; the daughter quit her job 1 year ago to care for her mother.
> 4. The daughter describes herself as nervous, exhausted, and short-tempered with her husband and children.
> 5. The daughter's husband says that they have no freedom as a family because the mother requires so much care.
> 6. The family's background is Greek—a culture that places a high value on children caring for the elderly at home.
> 7. The family will not consider referral of the mother to an extended-care facility.
>
> The public health nurse, utilizing psychiatric–mental health principles, realizes that this family, especially the daughter, is at risk of developing physical and emotional problems as a result of the stress of having a family member with Alzheimer's disease living at home. The public health nurse returns to the agency and, after exploring community resources, finds an available adult day care program for the client near her home. The family accepts this respite care, which partially relieves its burden. As a result, through the utilization of community resources the client is able to remain in familiar surroundings a little longer with less stress to the family.
>
> Following this experience, the public health nurse notices an increasing number of referrals from families seeking help with Alzheimer's disease; the nurse decides to initiate a weekly care givers' self-help support group, which is well-attended. The nurse encourages group members to decide how they would like to use the group. After several "ventilation" sessions, the members decide that they want to do something concrete for one another. They contact local nursing homes and find a few which will accept clients for just a weekend or a week at a time for respite care. They also decide to raise funds to make it possible for the existing adult day care program to

accept more clients. The nurse assists the group in obtaining speakers on Alzheimer's disease.

Nurses in the community perform an educational role in various ways—for instance, when they formally or informally provide anticipatory guidance and parenting information to families, and when they serve as members of citizens' action groups whose goal is to improve neighborhood safety and housing conditions for the elderly. They may also participate in early case finding and treatment of high-risk groups when they coordinate identification of, and counseling services for, unwed pregnant teenagers. They perform roles as counselors, educators, and resource people in outpatient crisis units designed to reduce clients' stress and return them to precrisis levels of functioning. Nurses serve as nurturers, socializing agents, technicians, educators, and coordinators for the chronic mentally ill when, during home visits in day-treatment programs or in medication clinics, they help limit the disability associated with mental illness. Table 10-4 provides an illustration of the role behaviors

Table 10-4 Role Behaviors of a Generalist Staff Nurse in a Community Mental Health Center (CMHC) from 8:30 A.M. to 4:30 P.M.

Time	Monday	Tuesday	Wednesday	Thursday	Friday
8:30 A.M.–9:30 A.M.	Attend staff planning and evaluation meeting.	Attend staff planning and evaluation meeting.	Attend staff planning and evaluation meeting.	Attend staff planning and evaluation meeting.	Attend staff planning and evaluation meeting.
9:30 A.M.–10:30 A.M.	Be women's morning group therapy coleader.	Attend therapeutic community meeting.	Conduct intake interview of new client. Write report.	Attend monthly meeting with generalist nurses from CMHC programs.	Conduct Prolixin clinic.
10:30 A.M.–11:00 A.M.	Postgroup rehash.	Post group rehash.	Attend case conference and presentation of client for all team members.		At lunch, speak to school nurses about alcohol and substance abuse.
11:00 A.M.–12:00 P.M.	Meet with nursing students.	Help clients to prepare, run, and clean up after bagel luncheon.		Help clients to prepare, run, and clean up from hot dog luncheon.	
12:00 P.M.–1:00 P.M.	Lunch break.		Lunch break.		
1:00 P.M.–2:00 P.M.	Conduct intake interview with new client. Write report.	Perform individual therapy; two appointments, half an hour each.	Visit CMHC client who has been hospitalized at local inpatient unit.	Perform one-to-one sessions with clients (two appointments, half an hour each).	Conduct intake interview with new client. Write report.
2:00 P.M.–3:00 P.M.	Attend meeting with public health nurses to plan unwed teenage pregnancy program.	Conduct Prolixin clinic.		Attend community mental health center administrative meeting.	
3:00 P.M.–4:00 P.M.			Office hours.	Office hours.	Bring client group to vocational rehabilitation center to spark future interest.
4:00 P.M.–4:30 P.M.	Office hours.	Office hours.		Attend conference with the family of a client suffering from Alzheimer's disease to complete referral to adult day care program.	

of one generalist staff nurse in a typical week in a community mental health center.

Psychiatric nurses who work in community settings must keep in mind that many of their colleagues, such as school nurses, occupational health nurses, public health nurses, pediatric nurses, and nursing midwives, though not psychiatric–mental health practitioners, encounter clients with mental health needs and problems every day. These practitioners need to be aware of, and knowledgeable about, their clients' mental health needs and the mental health resources of the community. Similarly, community psychiatric–mental health nurses need to be aware of other community health nurses. The interaction among all these nurses provides an invaluable referral and resource network that increases the opportunity for collaborative health care. Community mental health nurses must also be aware of, and receptive to, the possibility of collaborative relationships with nurses in inpatient settings. All nurses can perform roles to provide holistic health care for clients, irrespective of the setting.

The Head Nurse and the Psychiatric Nursing Coordinator

To ensure a coordinated, smoothly run unit, the head nurse, a nursing manager, must plan for clients' and staff members' needs on a short- and long-term basis. The nursing coordinator, also a nursing manager, functions as a clinician, educator, and administrator for clients and staff members, and serves as liaison and consultant to other clients and staff members throughout the hospital and in the community.

The head nurse also performs the role of counselor, demonstrating sensitivity to staff problems, conflicts, and ethical dilemmas. Sensitivity on the part of a head nurse encourages staff members to express and solve problems in a group setting or in individual settings. The nursing coordinator often acts as a counselor for the head nurse and as a resource person who supervises staff members' one-to-one nurse-client relationships.

As nursing managers, both the head nurse and the psychiatric nursing coordinator have additional responsibilities. Each employee who reports to the head nurse or nursing coordinator must be continually evaluated. Conferences must be held as needed to point out especially good performances or areas where improvement is needed. (Such conferences should always be documented in writing, in accordance with most hospitals' personnel policies.) In addition, each employee must be evaluated systematically by the nursing manager. The nurse's performance during the past year is reviewed against standards established by the personnel and nursing departments. These conferences help nurses grow and improve, especially if the nursing manager really enjoys the role of mentor.

Both the head nurse and the psychiatric nursing coordinator are usually responsible for hiring and firing nursing personnel working on a psychiatric unit. These functions include facilitating the professional growth of all staff members, developing and implementing orientation procedures for new members, and implementing appropriate disciplinary procedures when performances are not up to standards.

Maintaining cost-effective care within budget constraints is also an important part of the nursing manager's role. Nursing managers need to develop their skills further in this area, especially because nursing care is likely to be covered by prospective payment plans based on diagnosis-related groups (DRGs) in the near future.

In many hospitals, especially those closely linked with a community health center, the psychiatric nursing coordinator has a great deal of responsibility for emergency room clients. The coordinator is often a mental health professional who sees the clients first, conducts the assessment interview, and recommends case disposition (inpatient or outpatient care, transfer, or discharge).

The Clinical Specialist

Roles and Subroles of Clinical Specialists

Psychiatric–mental health nurses who have a master's degree are eligible for certification by the ANA as clinical specialists in child or adult psychiatric–mental health nursing.[16] After certification they are considered expert clinicians who are qualified to perform a variety of leadership roles. In many states they are increasingly eligible for third-party reimbursement from insurance companies for the provision of direct services to clients.

Clinical specialists assume leadership subroles as consultants, liaison nurses, clinical coordinators, primary therapists, educators, and researchers. They perform these subroles in both in- and outpatient settings. A particular job description for a clinical specialist may include several subroles. For example, a clinician working in a community mental health center may have not only the role of primary therapist but also the roles of educator and consultant. Table 10-5 summarizes clinical specialists' subroles, roles, and behaviors and the settings in which the roles are performed. A clinical specialist may have a joint appointment with both a clinical agency and an educational institution—for example, with a college's or a university's school of nursing. Such a clinician spends part of his or her time working in the clinical setting and part in the educational setting. Some joint appointments are designed to promote collaborative research by agencies whose expertise is complementary. For example, several hospital clinical specialists and professors of nursing from an affiliated university might

Table 10-5 Roles of The Clinical Specialist

Subrole	Role Behaviors	Setting	Example
Consultant	Provides consultative, indirect health services to staff nurses in hospitals. Also provides services to community agencies, schools, and organizations.	Hospital-based, community agency; independent consulting firm.	A consultant in a community mental health center is called by a community task force to give advice regarding the development of a domestic violence program.
Liaison nurse	In nonpsychiatric units provides consultative, indirect services to staff nurses and direct care to clients with specific mental health problems. Also serves as an educator regarding mental health issues.	General hospital.	A liaison nurse is called upon to meet with nursing staff members of a medical-surgical unit who are having difficulty managing an aggressive client.
Primary therapist	Provides direct cliental services: individual, group, or family therapy.	Psychiatric unit of a general hospital; psychiatric hospital; state hospital; or community mental health center; solo or group private practice.	As a primary therapist working in a psychiatric hospital, the nurse sees six clients per week for individual therapy sessions and conducts daily group therapy on a predischarge unit.
Researcher	Initiates, facilitates, and participates in the development and implementation of research projects as well as the utilization of research findings in clinical practice.	General hospital; psychiatric hospital; community mental health center; community agency.	A psychiatric nursing coordinator of a 32-bed general hospital's psychiatric unit facilitates the design of a research project initiated by the nursing staff; it investigates how the nurses utilize their time and what their effect is on patient care.
Educator	Develops and conducts educational programs for clients, staff, students, community agencies, and organizations.	General hospital; psychiatric hospital; community mental health center; school; community organizations or corporation.	The clinical specialist as an educator develops and conducts a stress-management program for the local police department, then modifies and conducts it for critical-care nurses at a local general hospital.
Clinical coordinator	Performs as a nursing manager in a psychiatric unit, providing clinical supervision for the nursing staff; acts as primary therapist for specific clients; provides consulting services to other departments, developing the staff's educational programs and promoting research activity.	Psychiatric unit of a general hospital; psychiatric hospital; state hospital.	As a clinical coordinator of a psychiatric unit, the nurse also acts as a consultant to the emergency room staff in the evaluation of potential psychiatric clients.

have joint appointments with the two institutions. Such arrangements are cost-effective and use talent very efficiently.[17]

Irrespective of the setting in which they work or the specific roles that are required of them, clinical specialists always utilize nursing theories and theories from the physical and behavioral sciences as bases for their practice. (Thus, joint appointments are also important because they provide both role and clinical preparation.)

The following sections will explore the role of the clinical specialist as consultant, provider of liaison services, systems change agent, researcher, and independent practitioner.

Consultation

Mental health consultation offered by a psychiatric nurse who is a clinical specialist may be client-centered, group-centered, or program-centered. A referral for consultation is initiated by people in the community who are seeking expert help, such as police officers, school nurses, nursing-home personnel, the clergy, or faculty members.

When clinical specialists provide *client-centered* consultation, they focus on helping find the most effective treatment for clients. For example:

> Miss O., a public health nurse requests consultation for a client who she suspects is hypomanic. The clinical specialist, Miss P., interviews the client, determines that the client is indeed hypomanic, and recommends referral to a lithium clinic. Miss P. also offers behavioral guidelines for evaluating the client after lithium therapy has been instituted.

Here is another example:

> The police request a client-centered consultation for John S., a prisoner in the local jail who they fear may be impulsive and self-destructive. The clinical specialist makes recommendations for minimizing John S.'s risk of self-injury, such as monitoring his belongings, instituting a one-to-one suicide watch, and keeping him out of solitary confinement. The consultant is able to make all these recommendations without meeting John S.

Consultation can also be *group-centered.* A group, such as the staff of a community nursing service or all school nurses within a district, may request consultation with a psychiatric nurse who is a clinical specialist. The consultant can meet directly with such a group to offer expertise on an identified problem (for example, how to help school-age children cope with their feelings when their parents are in the midst of separation or divorce).

Finally, consultation can be *program-centered.* A clinical specialist may be hired to help solve institutionwide problems or provide expertise in developing, refining, or modifying such problems. A consultant may originate new programs or improve existing ones by modifying the structure and function of an organization. For example:

> A teacher in a middle school wants to establish a six-session values-clarification workshop for seventh- and eighth-graders. A clinical specialist, Mr. M., is called in to help develop the program by collaborating with teachers in planning, implementing, and evaluating the lesson plan. Often a consultant leads a pilot project—in this case, Mr. M. leads the first workshop session and thus serves as a role model.

Program-centered consultation may be requested by a general hospital or a community mental health center. For example:

> The head nurse of an oncology unit in a general hospital is planning a program to help children cope with feelings about their parents' serious illnesses. A clinical specialist offers expert advice on how to establish art therapy, play therapy, and self-help (mutual-support) groups for the affected families. Such services will then be offered (for some specified time) by a nurse already on the inpatient staff or by a nurse in the community who has a private consulting practice or works with a consulting firm.[18]

In program-centered consultation, the participants have usually agreed to innovate. However, it is important to note that despite overt agreements, covert resistance to change can develop quickly, since there may be strong differences of opinion regarding the value of a proposed change. Resistance may be especially strong from elected public servants and representatives of vested interests; and communities may be anxious or fearful about changing the status quo. Such resistance can sabotage a consultant's services so that recommended plans are never implemented. Sabotage may take the form of an increase in the bureaucratic workload, or "red tape," or delays in decision making, which lead to a loss of momentum for change.[19] High school faculty members, for example, may fear implementing a suicide education program because they think (however mistakenly) that such a program will encourage suicidal behavior.

Clinical specialists serve most often as consultants within general hospitals where they are on the staff; they are skilled at assessing clients' immediate psychiatric needs, providing direct psychiatric care, and recommending appropriate aftercare or referral. For example:

> A clinical specialist is asked to serve as consultant to emergency room staff members who are not sure how dangerous a client is (to himself or herself or to others), whether voluntary treatment is an option, and what treatment services are available for alcohol and drug abuse. The clinical specialist makes an immediate determination as to whether a psychiatrist needs or does not need to see the client so that an appropriate schedule for administration of psychotropic medication can be initiated.

Liaison Services

Liaison nursing involves provision of direct and indirect care. *Direct care* is defined as provision of services to a client; *indirect care* is defined as helping a nursing staff make its care more therapeutic. Liaison nursing is similar to cliented-centered consulting. Just as a clinical specialist is called for a client whose needs are beyond the scope of, say, a unit staff, a liaison nurse serves as an expert advisor who collaborates with the staff to solve a work-related problem, such as assessment, diagnosis, planning, and intervention with a specific client, family, or group.

The liaison nurse has no administrative authority over the staff which has requested the service and is not usually responsible for implementing a change. Unless the liaison nurse is providing direct service, the user is free to accept or reject any part of the recommendations.

Liaison services exist outside of the regular organization; therefore, they provide freedom for liaison nurses to work with people at any level. The power of liaison nurses rests in their ideas in their acknowledged area of expertise. A liaison nurse whose specialty is psychiatric nursing is skilled in, and knowledgeable about, systems, change, organizations, problem solving, stress, crisis, interpersonal relationships, communication, and sociocultural concepts. As a consultant, such a nurse will identify applicable principles, work collaboratively in a problem-solving partnership with the user, and confirm that the user is ultimately responsible for implementing recommended ideas.[20]

Liaison consultation within a hospital provides help to troubled inpatients.[21] An oncology client, for example, looks forward to a weekly support group led by an oncology clinician and a psychiatric clinical specialist. A couple who are grief-stricken after learning that their baby was stillborn find some comfort in the visit of the liaison nurse and plan to attend the monthly support group for couples coping with this kind of loss. An orthopedic client who is suffering from endogenous depression is relieved to learn that a psychiatrist can prescribe an antidepressant medication. Families of terminally ill clients seek help in working through their feelings of loss, so that they can better help their loved ones.

Clinical specialists involved in liaison work also provide community services. For instance, they may train hospice volunteers to work with a hospital's community nursing service; they may offer parenting classes for the families of pediatric clients; they may plan a conference for laypeople on a mental health problem such as alcoholism and drug abuse.

Referrals for liaison services are generated by networks of professionals who recognize their availability and value. When a liaison nurse is established in a health care agency, much of his or her initial work consists of developing a referral network by educating staff members about the liaison service and its potential value to themselves and their clients. As a network develops, referrals will originate from staff members. For example, a physical therapist may request a visit for a client who has not been motivated to keep up with needed exercises. A physician may request a visit for a client with multiple sclerosis who has suddenly become depressed. A head nurse may request a staff consultation regarding a client who has become increasingly demanding and hostile. The liaison nurse's report is included in nurses' notes, integrated progress notes, or a separate consultant's report. (In some hospitals, it should be mentioned, initiation of a referral must be made in writing.)

Systems Change Agent

A clinical specialist may also plan and implement changes at a systems level; this type of change involves many departments and disciplines. Clinical specialists who hold management positions are likely to serve on a number of policy-making committees among several departments. They must be aware of the psychosocial needs of all clients and employees in the health care setting and propose programs and research projects that will improve their mental health. For example, on an emergency medicine committee, a nurse could promote a change that would streamline the evaluation and treatment of walk-in clients. On a client education committee, a nurse could propose that relaxation techniques be taught to clients on all services. On a health and welfare committee, a nurse could encourage the development of a comprehensive employee assistance program. A nurse who chooses to have high visibility can have a powerful impact on a health care facility.

Following is an illustration of a clinical specialist functioning as change agent at a systems level:

> Ms. R., a clinical specialist, develops a hypothesis that hospitalized people who abuse alcohol, drugs, or both are not being identified and referred for appropriate treatment. She is aware that multiple resources for such referrals are available within the hospital premises but suspects that they are underutilized. She also suspects that some providers of health care are using the resources consistently while others never use them, even though their clients are much the same.
>
> Ms. R. discusses the problem with carefully chosen colleagues in several departments. She finds her hypothesis well received, and so she can begin to set up a support system for a project to examine the problem and deal with it.
>
> She then discusses the project with her manager to determine whether any other departments are working on similar projects. Finding that no action is under way, she proceeds to develop a proposal and a plan for a needs assessment.
>
> The proposal can be simple. A *client in need* is defined as any client who tells a staff member that he or she has a problem with alcohol or drug abuse. A *program* provides that all clients in need receive a brochure listing community services, are shown a videotape from the patient education library, are informed of when Alcoholics Anonymous (AA) and Narcotics Anonymous (NA) hold their meetings on hospital premises, are offered an opportunity to be linked up with an AA sponsor, and are given the names of three psychotherapists who can provide aftercare.
>
> Ms. R. then takes the proposal through appropriate channels, hoping to develop supporters—like-minded practitioners who will volunteer to serve on an ad hoc alcohol and substance abuse committee.
>
> Once the committee is formed, Ms. R. helps move the project along, suggesting goals and deadlines. If necessary, she will recommend expanding the committee membership so that it will be broad enough to implement change effectively. She realizes that all appropriate disciplines—such as medicine, nursing, social work, and psychology—should be represented.
>
> The committee members design a tool for assessing needs and a brochure to give to patients. Once the program is in place, the committee will develop an evaluation mechanism, such as a follow-up questionnaire, to determine whether the program is helpful or not and what future services will be needed.

Clinical Research

Clinical specialists are also leaders who initiate research projects and guide nursing staffs in formulating, planning, and executing research. Both clinical specialists and nursing staffs of clinical units will think of many possible projects; and the clinical specialist can promote an attitude of inquiry and curiosity regarding clients and the context of care.[22]

For example:

> At a weekly staff meeting, one nurse, Barbara J., said to the group, "Have you ever noticed that clients who have met with their aftercare therapist before discharge seem to stay out of the hospital longer than those who don't?" The clinical specialist said, "Why, Barbara, what an interesting observation! Why don't we investigate it more systematically?"
>
> That interchange proved to be the seed of a clinical research project guided by the clinical specialist, in which the entire nursing staff participated. The project was called "An Investigation of the Effect of Predischarge Contact with Aftercare Therapist on Readmission Rates to North 1." Charts of clients who had been discharged from the unit within the previous 18 months were examined and data regarding discharge planning were reviewed. Clients were categorized into three groups: (1) those having no aftercare, (2) those having an aftercare plan but no contact with an aftercare therapist before discharge, and (3) those having an aftercare plan and contact with an aftercare therapist before discharge. Readmissions for clients representing each group were reviewed, as were their demographic characteristics—age, sex, marital status,

socioeconomic level, and employment status. Data on readmission rates and types of aftercare plans were analyzed by the hospital statistician to see if there was a significant difference in readmission rates for the three groups. The results revealed that the readmission rate was significantly lower for the group which had contact with an aftercare therapist before discharge; the readmission rates of the other two groups did not differ significantly.

The staff reported its findings at a meeting with all the unit's personnel. At the meeting, nursing staff members stated that, in light of the nonexperimental, retrospective nature of the study, a cause-and-effect relationship between the variables (types of aftercare and readmission rates) could not be established. Moreover, the figures had not been adjusted for extraneous variables, such as age, employment status, and family support. However, the staff members suggested that the data be used as a foundation for a small, experimental aftercare research project; such a project might provide criteria for an optimal aftercare program.

A clinical specialist can also promote "consumers' skills" with regard to research—that is, the ability to understand and evaluate the findings of completed research studies in terms of strengths, weaknesses, and potential applicability to nursing practice. "Research consumership" is important because research provides the basis for practice. Consumers' skills can be improved in many ways. One possibility is a research journal club where published research reports can be read and evaluated by the staff—with direction and guidance from a clinical specialist if necessary. Clinical research conferences can also be attended to learn about recent findings.[23]

Independent Practice

Clinical specialists in increasing numbers are developing independent practices. Now that a number of states include nurses among the professionals eligible for third-party insurance reimbursement, nurses can practice on equal financial footing with other providers of health care.[24]

A clinical specialist in private practice provides direct services to individual clients, groups of clients, and families. Private practice enables qualified nurses to choose their own treatment modalities and their own settings. This role provides for a maximum of autonomy, independence, decision making, and accountability.[25,26]

To qualify as an independent practitioner, a nurse must have a license as a registered nurse (RN) in the state where the practice will be located, a master's degree in psychiatric–mental health nursing, a strong theoretical foundation, and supervised experience in a variety of clinical settings. The private practitioner demonstrates continuing clinical competence by securing regularly scheduled supervision, peer review, and consultation; continuing his or her education in an advanced degree program or a certificate program; and receiving certification as a clinical specialist by the American Nurses Association.

Legislation regarding nursing practice differs from state to state. Nurses must therefore determine whether their state recognizes an expanded role for the nurse and allows private practice—such a practice goes beyond the traditional, limited role of the nurse.

Each private practitioner, whether he or she works with individuals, families, or groups, should have a sound theoretical framework which guides professional practice. Such a theoretical framework can be psychoanalytic, behavioral, or focused on family systems, or it may be eclectic, combining what seems most useful in each theory. Independent practitioners must guard against becoming isolated from the ideas of others by seeking supervision and collaboration with peers on a regular basis. They can then effectively help clients address problematic issues in their lives, formulate goals with clients for dealing with problems, and intervene to help clients work on options for repatterning specific problems.

RESPONSIBILITIES OF THE NURSE

Accountability

In a time of "quality assurance" and "cost containment," nurses are increasingly accountable for the evaluation of the care they provide for clients. Evaluation involves developing criteria and standards for structures, processes, and outcomes and measurement tools to determine whether standards and criteria have been met.[27]

Diagnostically related groupings (DRGs), now being developed and implemented in conjunction with prospective payment plans, will necessitate careful scrutiny and evaluation of the efficiency of patterns of nursing care. Standards for arriving at formulas for prospective-payment schedules demand that nurses evaluate and document the scope and components of nursing practice in all settings, to ensure accurate estimations of nursing responsibilities. As yet, DRGs do not exist for psychiatry; however, most observers believe that they are coming, and Joel states that they are inevitable in both psychiatry and psychiatric nursing.[28]

Nursing managers should therefore define, qualitatively and quantitatively, the scope of psychiatric–mental health nursing in their settings and establish criteria for its practice. Underreporting any roles or activities (such as assessing and planning) may mean that they will be excluded from cost-estimate equations.

Clinical specialists serving as psychiatric coordinators of inpatient units automatically become members of the departmental audit committees. An audit committee systematically reviews outcomes of nursing practices that have been documented in care plans and notes. This process is integral to a clinical unit's ongoing review of the quality of its nursing care. For example, an audit may focus on whether clients who attended the nurses' weekly medication teaching group have been more compliant about taking their psychotropic medication during hospitalization than those who did not attend. Another audit might review whether nurses' discharge notes consistently specify aftercare plans. Here is another example:

> An audit committee, reviewing a unit's "incident reports," observes that the overwhelming majority of clients' falls within the past 6 months have occurred when they were on psychotropic medication and had a drop in diastolic blood pressure of 20 millimeters or more since admission. The committee formulates a new policy to identify those clients at risk of falling because of orthostatic hypotension which is a result of psychotropic medication. The new policy requires all clients receiving psychotropic medications to have their blood pressure monitored four times daily, sitting and standing, for the first week they receive such medications. Should a client's blood pressure drop 20 millimeters or more, his or her activity will be restricted and supervised.

Monitoring mechanisms are built into the administrative policies and procedures of any health care agency. In hospitals, monitoring procedures are required by accrediting bodies (such as the Joint Commission on Accreditation of Hospitals) or by a state's department of health. For example, the nursing department in every hospital is required to measure "quality assurance" and make recommendations to improve the quality of care; a "quality assurance" committee may therefore be formed to provide peer review of nursing policies and procedures. Such a committee would be broad-based, consisting of nursing managers and staff members from a variety of services. It might review, for instance, how much time elapses before a liaison nurse makes the first visit to a suicidal client on a medical floor, or how long a psychiatric client waits in the emergency room before being escorted to the psychiatric service. On the basis of data collected, treatment protocols and policies would be revised.

Continuing Education

Psychiatric–mental health nurses are responsible for expanding their knowledge to keep up with changes in the field. Nurses, as self-directed professionals, need to seek out academic coursework and continuing education programs which meet their clinical needs.[29]

Nurses should regularly consult a variety of psychiatric and mental health journals (as well as journals from other disciplines) in order to keep abreast of current issues, ideas, controversies, strategies, and research relevant to psychiatric–mental health nursing. The book reviews in these journals are especially useful; they can help nurses make informed decisions about which books to add to their professional libraries.

Membership in professional organizations enables nurses to participate in meetings, special interest groups, and conferences that are professionally relevant. By attending clinical and research conferences, nurses can enhance their professional growth by expanding their scientific knowledge.

Learning experiences with peers—as in journal clubs, clinical case conferences, and support groups—provide valuable feedback which enhances the nurse's self-assessment process.[30]

Another kind of peer review which is characteristic of psychiatric nursing is clinical supervision.[31] A nursing clinician selects another practitioner with equal or superior credentials and experience. The clinician requests that the supervising practitioner be available for a regularly scheduled hour each week. At that time, the clinician discusses ongoing casework and encourages the supervising practitioner to offer feedback. (For example, the supervising practitioner may say, "You really managed to avoid being drawn into that conflict," or, "It seems that your own feelings may have provoked you to make a statement which cut off further discussion.") Such supervision can help nurses increase both their self-knowledge and their expertise; and a clinician may, in turn, provide supervision for another colleague.

Credentialing

Credentialing of psychiatric nurses has developed because their clients—and other professionals—need some way to assess their qualifications.

In most settings today, a master's degree in psychiatric–mental health nursing is required for a nurse to be a clinical specialist. Therefore, a nurse who has completed an approved graduate school program (one which meets the standards of the profession) is considered to have developed a nationally recognized level of expertise and may begin practicing.

In some settings (and particularly when a nurse has established a private practice and seeks third-party payment), a nurse may need to demonstrate, in addition to at least a master's degree, certification as a psychiatric–mental health clinical specialist. To be eligible for this certification, a nursing candidate must pass an examination developed and administered by the American Nurses Association.

Psychiatric nurses with baccalaureate degrees have been permitted to sit for examinations which certify them as generalist psychiatric–mental health nurses. Psychiatric nurses seeking to further their education, develop their skills, and receive additional credentialing can participate in a post-master's certificate program available to nurses and others in the mental health disciplines. For example, nurses enroll in large numbers in family therapy institutes, where they greatly expand their clinical skills in family therapy; they earn a certificate at the conclusion of the coursework.

Doctoral Education

Nurses who choose to pursue a doctorate will acquire several unique skills and increase their theoretical and clinical knowledge. Doctoral education, whether it leads to a Ph.D., an Ed.D., or a D.N.S., is designed to develop nursing scholars in theory, research, and clinical practice. Ph.D. and Ed.D. programs focus primarily on theory and research. Nurses in such programs develop expertise in formulating, testing, and criticizing the theoretical base of nursing science and practice; they also develop sound knowledge of research principles and methods.

Nurses who have either a Ph.D. or an Ed.D. will be likely to assume roles as leaders in academic, research, or clinical settings. For example:

> Dr. E., a nurse with a Ph.D. in theory development and research, teaches nursing theory and research to undergraduate students in a baccalaureate program and serves on a joint nursing research committee sponsored by a college and a local medical center. The committee is currently completing a study of the self-care needs of frail, elderly people who are housebound. Dr. E. is also a family therapist who maintains a part-time private practice. At present, Dr. E. is conducting an independent, basic research project: developing a tool to measure "differentiation of self" (a concept in family theory).

The expertise developed in a doctoral program, added to that gained in a master's program and in postgraduate training (such as family therapy), constitutes a broad knowledge base which will be used in academic, research, and clinical settings.

D.N.S. degree programs are also based on theory and research. However, there is a more pronounced clinical emphasis in such programs. That is, candidates concentrate on *clinical* theory and research, so that they will be able to assume leadership positions in clinical settings. For example:

> Dr. F., a nurse with a D.N.S. degree, is the director of research at a large urban medical center. Dr. F. provides leadership in nursing research, which involves collaborating with the hospital research committee and spearheading research activities within the nursing department. Currently, Dr. F. is coordinating the writing of a grant for a research proposal formulated by a clinical specialist and nurses on the oncology unit. The proposed study will investigate the effect of social support on self-coping in families of terminally ill clients.
>
> Dr. F. works closely with the clinical specialists who, in turn, guide the research efforts of the nursing staff. Dr. F. also supports various research activities undertaken by the nursing staff: specific research

projects, a monthly research journal club, and attendance at research conferences.

Funds for clinical research activities are allocated according to the needs of an entire institution.

Many nurses with doctorates are involved in independent practice, although a doctor's degree is not a prerequisite for such practice. Private practice, whether in an individual or a group setting, affords clinical autonomy to a greater degree than other settings. Clinical expertise already developed in other programs and settings is strengthened either by the clinical focus of a D.N.S. program or by the emphasis on theory and research characteristic of other doctoral programs. Then, clinical practice can become an arena for generating and testing research.

Doctoral education prepares nurses to become leaders and mentors in academic, research, and practice settings. The goal underlying the work of doctorally prepared nurses is to stimulate the development and utilization of nursing theory as a foundation for nursing practice by fostering a spirit of inquiry, critical thinking, and research, all of which will ultimately extend the knowledge base of the nursing profession.

SUMMARY

Dramatic changes in the nursing profession as well as in the mental health care delivery system have combined to create a complex, multifaceted role for the psychiatric–mental health nurse. Nurses assume a variety of roles in many settings.

Role theory provides a base for understanding roles and role expectations. Roles may be ascribed, achieved, assumed, or adopted, and formal or informal. As roles are internalized, they become part of one's self-concept. Role conflict and role blurring are problems that can be resolved through a clarification of role expectations and demands.

Psychiatric–mental health nursing is defined as an interpersonal process aimed at promoting and maintaining behavior which contributes to integrated functioning. It is a specialized area of practice in which there are two types of practitioners, the generalist and the clinical specialist. Subroles of such nurses include (1) nurturer, (2) coordinator, (3) counselor, (4) socializing agent, (5) educator, and (6) technician.

The generalist nurse working in an inpatient setting often has a staff position on a psychiatric unit or in a psychiatric hospital. In addition to this primary role, there are the six key subroles. Generalist nurses in inpatient settings also promote self-care by clients, advocate clients' rights, maintain a therapeutic milieu, participate in nursing rounds and team meetings, and supervise other members of the nursing staff.

The generalist nurse working in an outpatient setting may have a staff position in a community mental health center, a day treatment program, a crisis center, or a public health or visiting nurse association. The six nursing subroles are relevant in these settings; however, specific role behaviors vary because of the nature of the settings. Since these settings are quite flexible, there is considerable opportunity for role blurring.

The head nurse and the psychiatric coordinator are both nurse-managers, but they perform different role activities.

Clinical specialists have subroles as consultants, providers of liaison services, systems change agents, clinical coordinators, primary therapists, educators, and researchers. They fulfill these subroles in a variety of in- and outpatient settings.

Nurses also have responsibilities involving professionalism and personal and professional growth; these may include accountability, continuing education, credentialing, and doctoral education.

REFERENCES

1. Suzanne Lego, ed., *The American Handbook of Psychiatric Nursing,* Lippincott, Philadelphia, 1984, p. xiiii.
2. Beverly Hoeffer and Shirley Murphy, "The Unfinished Task: Development of Nursing Theory for Psychiatric and Mental Health Nursing Practice," *Journal of Psychosocial Nursing and Mental Health Services,* vol. 20, December 1982, pp. 8–14.
3. Sarah Sease, "Grief Associated with a Prison Experience: Counseling the Client," *Journal of Psychosocial Nursing and Mental Health Services,* vol. 20, July 1982, pp. 25–27.
4 D. L. Sills, ed., *International Encyclopedia of The Social Sciences,* vol. 13, Free Press, New York, 1968, pp. 546–556.
5. G. A. Theodorson and A. G. Theodorson, *A Modern Dictionary of Sociology,* Crowell, New York, 1969, pp. 352–357.

6. G. D. Mitchell, ed., *A Dictionary of Sociology,* Aldire, Chicago, 1975, pp. 148–152.
7. B. J. Biddle and E. J. Thomas, eds., *Role Theory: Concepts and Research,* Wiley, New York, 1966.
8. M. Leininger, "Community Mental Health Nursing: Trends, Issues, and Problems," *Perspectives in Psychiatric Care,* vol. 21, no. 4, 1983, pp. 139–146.
9. E. D. Davis and M. Pattison, "The Psychiatric Nurse's Role Identity," *American Journal of Nursing,* vol. 79, no. 2, 1979, pp. 298–299.
10. Dixie Koldjeski, "Mental Health and Psychiatric Nursing and Primary Health Care: Issues and Prospects," *Proceedings of the Fourth National Conference in Graduate Education in Psychiatric and Mental Health Nursing,* American Nurses Association, Kansas City, Mo., 1979. Cited by Deanna Pearlmutter, "Recent Trends and Issues in Psychiatric–Mental Health Nursing," *Hospital and Community Psychiatry,* vol. 36, January 1985, p. 57.
11. Claire Fagin, "Concepts for the Future: Competition and Substitution," *Journal of Psychiatric Nursing and Mental Health Services,* vol. 21, March 1983, pp. 36–40.
12. American Nurses Association, "Statement of Psychiatric Nursing Practice," ANA, Kansas City, Mo., 1976.
13. B. A. Benfer, "Defining the Role and Function of the Psychiatric Nurse as a Member of the Team," *Perspectives in Psychiatric Care,* vol. 78, no. 4, 1980, pp. 166–177.
14. H. Peplau, *Interpersonal Relations in Nursing,* Putnam, New York, 1952.
15. M. Manthey, "Primary Nursing is Alive and Well in the Hospital," *American Journal of Nursing,* vol. 73, no. 1, 1973.
16. S. Kuntz, J. Stehle, and R. Marshall, "The Psychiatric Clinical Specialist: The Progression of a Specialty," *Perspectives in Psychiatric Care,* vol. 28, no. 2, 1980, pp. 51–59.
17. M. Styles, "Reflections on Collaboration and Unification," *Image,* vol. 16, no. 1, 1984, pp. 21–23.
18. C. Chriness, "Creating Consultation Programs in CMHCS," *Community Mental Health Journal,* vol. 13, Summer 1977, p. 133.
19. I. N. Berlin, "Resistance to Mental Health Consultation Directed at Change in Public Institutions," *Community Mental Health Journal,* vol. 15, no. 2, 1979, p. 1119.
20. L. Robinson, *Liaison Nursing: Psychological Approach to Patient Care,* Davis, Philadelphia, 1974.
21. B. Fife, "The Challenge of the Medical Setting for the Clinical Specialist in Psychiatric Nursing," *Journal of Psychiatric Nursing and Mental Health Services,* vol. 21, January 1983, pp. 8–13.
22. D. Schanding, R. L. Garber, and V. Siomopoulos, "A Small Study of How the Staff of an In Patient Psychiatric Unit Spends Its Time," *Perspectives in Psychiatric Care,* vol. 20, no. 2, 1982, pp. 91–93.
23. G. LoBiondo-Wood and J. Haber, *Nursing Research: Critical Appraisal and Utilization,* Mosby, St. Louis, 1986.
24. "New York Law Allows Third Party Reimbursement to All R.N.'s," *American Journal of Nursing,* vol. 85, February 1985, pp. 198–199.
25. R. Willie and K. C. Fredrickson, "Establishing a Group Private Practice in Nursing," *Nursing Outlook,* vol. 29, no. 9, 1981, pp. 522–524.
26. J. C. Geller, "Starting a Private Practice of Psychotherapy," *Perspectives in Psychiatric Care,* vol. 18, no. 3, 1980, pp. 106–111.
27. N. L. Griffith and M. E. Megel, "Quality Assurance: An Educational Approach," *Nursing Outlook,* vol. 29, no. 11, 1981, pp. 670–673.
28. L. A. Joel, "DRGs and RIMs: Implications for Nursing," *Nursing Outlook,* vol. 32, no. 1, 1984, pp. 42–49.
29. M. M. Smith, "Career Development in Nursing: An Individual and Professional Responsibility," *Nursing Outlook,* vol. 30, no. 2, 1982, pp. 128–131.
30. R. Johnson et al., "The Professional Support Group: A Model for Psychiatric Clinical Nurse Specialists," *Journal of Psychiatric Nursing and Mental Health Services,* vol. 20, February 1982, pp. 9–13.
31. D. Perlmutter, "Recent Trends and Issues in Psychiatric–Mental Health Nursing," *Hospital and Community Psychiatry,* vol. 36, January 1985, pp. 56–62.

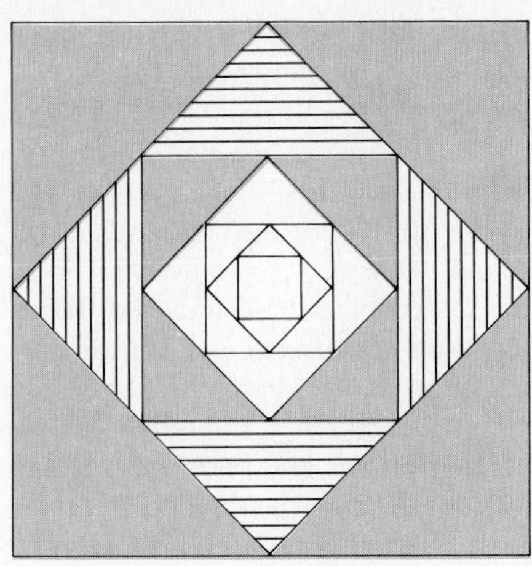

CHAPTER 11
The Nursing Process

Pamela Price Hoskins

LEARNING OBJECTIVES

After studying this chapter, the student should be able to:

1. Describe the purposes and steps of the nursing process.
2. Organize a nursing care plan.
3. Write nursing diagnoses, client outcomes, and nursing interventions that are congruent with assessment data.
4. Identify the appropriateness of selected forms of nursing diagnoses.
5. Relate the use of nursing process to the solution of selected issues.

The *nursing process* is a scientific method used by nurses to systematically assess and diagnose a client's health status, formulate client outcomes, determine interventions, and evaluate the quality and outcomes of care—in conjunction with the client.

All professionals plan the delivery of their services using a goal-directed process. The purpose of this chapter is to provide an understanding of how a plan for nursing care may be formulated. Each step of the nursing process is covered in detail: *assessment, diagnoses, outcome criteria, interventions,* and *evaluation.* Several issues that arise when the nursing process is used within an agency setting will be discussed: (1) Should nurses use the same process, or format, nationwide, or should it be determined by each agency? (2) Should the care plan be focused on the nurse or the client? (3) Should the format be oriented toward problems or toward health status? (4) In what ways can the plan be used to determine quality of care? (5) How can the plan be used to validate payment for services?

PURPOSES OF THE NURSING PROCESS

The nursing process has five main purposes: (1) planning and evaluation; (2) provision of a systematic approach to clients; (3) individualized planning; (4) goal-directedness; and (5) a mechanism for communication. Each purpose is explained below.

Planning and Evaluation

Planning and evaluating the care of clients is the first purpose of the nursing process. The conceptual framework presented in Chapter 1 is relevant to this purpose, since it determines the parameters, or boundaries, of the nursing process itself. In this conceptual framework, the *client* may be a person, a family, or a community; nursing *interventions* are ways of promoting, maintaining, restoring, or rehabilitating health; and *assessment* of the client will involve three dimensions—body, mind, and spirit.

Systematic Approach to Clients

The second purpose of the nursing process is to provide a systematic approach to all clients in all settings. The process—how nurses actually go about nursing—is logical, and in a sense circular. The nurse begins by assessing the client and formulating a diagnosis. Then the nurse collaborates with the client and with other professionals to establish outcome criteria for the client and nursing interventions to be used—that is, to specify what is to be done and what is expected to be achieved. Then, at some specified time (for example, at the time of discharge), both the quality of care the client has received and the outcomes are evaluated. It can be seen that this process begins and ends with a form of evaluation (which might be described as assessment and reassessment or evaluation and reevaluation); that is why it can be considered "circular."

Individualized Planning

The third purpose of the nursing process is to individualize the plan of care for each client, within the systematic approach that has just been described. Each client is a unique configuration: no two clients have exactly the same physical, mental, or spiritual characteristics; no two have exactly the same health status; no two are part of exactly the same environment; and no two will exhibit the same patterns of interaction. Part of the nursing process, therefore, is identifying what is unique about each client and arriving at an appropriate plan for care.

Goal-Directedness

Goal-directedness is the fourth purpose of the nursing process. The client's health is the goal of nursing—everything a nurse does with a client is directed toward promoting, maintaining, restoring, or rehabilitating health. In psychiatric–mental health nursing particularly, it is absolutely necessary that goals represent collaboration between nurse and client. If the client's goals, for example, seem unrealistic to the nurse, or if the nurse's outcome criteria seem irrelevant to the client, then there will be little cooperation between them, and it is unlikely that anyone's goals will be accomplished.

Communication

The fifth purpose of the nursing process is to create a mechanism of communication among nurses working with a client. Today, a model for professional nursing practice is widely recognized; it includes two important ideas (among others): first, that a nurse is responsible and accountable for planning, implementing, overseeing, and evaluating the care of each client; and second, that the client has the right to know who this is. (It has long been assumed that a client will know his or her physician, social worker, occupational therapist, or psychologist; now such identification and accountability have been extended to the nurse.) The nurse who is responsible for a client—the *primary nurse*—uses the nursing process to communicate the plan of care and the outcomes to others, especially when some activities are delegated.

STEPS IN THE NURSING PROCESS

The nursing process (see Figure 11-1) consists of five steps: (1) assessment, (2) nursing diagnosis, (3) client outcomes (or outcome criteria), (4) nursing interventions, and (5) evaluation of outcomes and nursing care. Each step must be congruent with the others, and a change in one will entail changes in the rest.

Figure 11-1 Components of the nursing process. (SOURCE: From Elizabeth Maloney, "The Nursing Process," in the second edition of this book.)

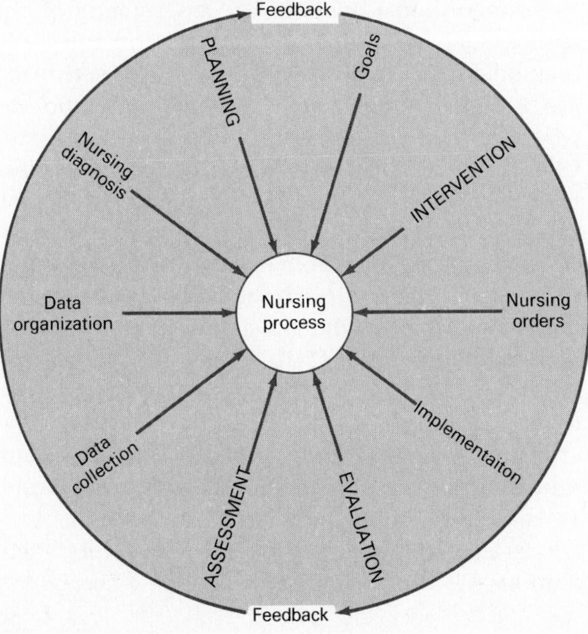

Assessment

Assessment is the systematic collection of health-related data about a client's internal and external environment. When the client is an *individual*, the internal environment is the physical, mental, and spiritual dimensions of the person; the external environment is the family and the community. When the client is a *family*, the internal environment is its structure, functions, and members; the external environment is the community. When the client is a *community*, the internal environment is its structure, functions, and resources, including individuals and families; and the external environment is the larger society and its resources.

Assessment of the Person

Assessment of the individual client—the person—consists of a physical examination, a mental status examination, a spiritual assessment, and a nursing history.

PHYSICAL EXAMINATION. The physical examination is done systematically, though not necessarily from head to toe. Many clients tolerate an examination of the head, including the mouth, eyes, nose, and ears, only after rapport and a sense of comfort have been established with the nurse, possibly because physical closeness is needed to perform such an examination. For instance, extreme closeness is needed to examine the eye; invasion of the body is needed to examine the mouth; and mild physical restraint is needed to examine the ear. Furthermore, the client must "submit" an organ of perception to the nurse, and this requires trust. If the nurse uses the systematic approach to examining, beginning the examination with the client's hands and feet and proceeding to the trunk, and then to the head, that will allow time to establish rapport. Rapport can also be established by conferring with the client or by deciding how to proceed only after completing the mental status examination, spiritual assessment, and nursing history.

MENTAL STATUS EXAMINATION. In a mental status examination the mental functioning of the client is assessed.[1] A mental status examination consists of assessing the client's appearance and behavior, thought content, sensory perceptions, intellect, thought processes, emotions, and insights. Table 11-1 defines each aspect of the mental status examination.

Table 11-1 Mental Status Examination

Aspects of the Examination
1. Attitude, manner, and behavior a. Appearance, dress, facial expression, activity, posture, and demeanor are noted. b. Disturbances include deviations of degree of activity, mannerisms, distortions of motility, and uncooperativeness.
2. Mental content a. This consists of the thoughts, concerns, and trends that are uppermost in the client's mind. b. Disturbances of content include delusions, hallucinations, obsessions, and phobias.
3. Sensorium and intellect a. The degree of the client's awareness and the level of his or her functioning are noted. b. Disturbances of orientation, memory, retention, attention, information, and judgment can be elicited with standardized questions and test materials.
4. Stream of thought a. This includes the quantitative and qualitative aspects of the client's verbal communication. b. Disturbances include over- and underproductivity, disconnectedness, unintelligibility, and incoherence.
5. Emotional tone a. This includes the client's report of subjective feelings (mood or affect) and the examiner's observations of facial expression, posture, and attitude. b. Disturbances include both quantitative deviations (elation, depression, apathy) and incongruence (disagreement among the client's subjective report, behavior, and mental content).
6. Insight This means the degree to which the patient can appreciate the nature of his or her condition and the need for treatment.

SOURCE: Clarence J. Rowe, *An Outline of Psychiatry*, 8th ed., Brown, Dubuque, Iowa, 1984. All rights reserved. Reprinted by permission.

SPIRITUAL ASSESSMENT. A spiritual assessment involves determining a client's sense of meaning and purpose in life, sense of relatedness or belonging, and sense of giving and receiving forgiveness.[2]

A client's sense of *meaning and purpose* in life may, of course, be well-developed and implemented to her or his satisfaction. However, people who are ill usually have problems in this regard. They may never have developed a purpose or meaning for life; or their sense of purpose and meaning may have been lost, forgotten, displaced, or destroyed by tragic experiences.

Relatedness and belonging are patterns established with oneself, with others, and, for many people, with God. These patterns may be firmly grounded, comfortable, and conducive to growth; but they may also be poorly developed and characterized by misconceptions, misperceptions, distrust, lack of commitment, superficiality, distance, and coolness. The nurse needs to know what relationships exist for each client, and what relationships the client wants to establish or strengthen.

Every person has a need to *forgive and to receive forgiveness.* If people are unable to forgive themselves or others, or if they are unable to accept forgiveness, they must continue to live with pain, disillusionment, or a sense of wrongdoing. (As Smedes has expressed it, forgiveness is the only way to heal the hurt that one never deserved.[3]) Forgiveness implies being free of the past, so that energy can be used creatively in the present.

NURSING HISTORY. When preparing a nursing history of a client with mental or emotional difficulties, the nurse focuses on the client's activities of daily living, lifestyle, ability to function, and methods of coping. The purpose of the nursing history is to identify patterns of functioning that are healthy as well as patterns that create problems in the client's everyday life. Table 11-2 gives an analysis of the components of the nursing history and examples of questions.

Assessment of the Family

When a client is a *family member,* his or her assessment must include an assessment of the family. Such an assessment focuses on roles and relationships from both the client's perspective and the family's perspective. Expected roles and the way roles are enacted need to be explored (See Chapter 10, "Role Theory," for a discussion of roles). Family relationships—level of integration, organization of the family, and patterns of interaction—need to be assessed. Table 11-3 outlines assessment of a client's family. It should be noted that the client determines who the family is, since many nontraditional forms of the family exist today.

When the client is a *family,* its structure, functions, and stage in the life-cycle are assessed, as are family members' roles, relationships, and communication in a multigenerational context. (Chapter 19 discusses family patterns and assessment.) A genogram—a diagram of a family over three generations—is very helpful in assessing a family.

Table 11-2 Nursing History and Examples of Assessment Questions

Activities of Daily Living	Lifestyle
Patterns of activity and rest What time do you get up? What time do you go to bed? Do you take naps? What do you do while you are awake? What do you do when you are energetic? What time of the day do you feel most energetic? When do you feel best physically? **Patterns of nutrition and elimination** How often do you eat each day? What times do you eat? What is the size of each meal? How often do you have a bowel movement? What time or times of the day or week do you have bowel movements? **Patterns of roles and role expectations** What relationships are you involved in (with your mother, sister, employee, wife, and so on)? What is entailed in each of these relationships? What feedback do you get from others about your relationship with them? What do you do well in each relationship? What would you like to do better in each relationship? **Patterns of hygiene and appearance** How often do you bathe? Brush teeth? Wash hair? Do laundry? What hygiene products do you use? How do you think you look? Are there areas of personal appearance you would like to change? **Patterns of socialization and isolation** How much time do you spend with other people per day? Per week? How much time do you spend alone? How comfortable are you with members of your family? How comfortable are you with strangers? **Patterns of work and leisure** What do you like to do in your spare time? How often do you engage in these spare-time activities? What kind of work do you do? How long have you been doing this work? How long have you been employed or unemployed? What do you do to keep your job? What do you do to find a job?	**Influence of illness on everyday life** What are your thoughts about your illness? How does it influence your everyday life? Because of your illness, how do you think your life will be 5 years from now? **Health habits, such as exercise, recreation, and nutrition** Do you exercise? How often? What do you do? What kinds of recreation do you enjoy? What kinds of recreation do you participate in? How often? What do you think about the food you eat? Is it healthy? What other activities do you participate in that are good for you? **Illness-producing habits, such as abusing drugs, smoking, drinking, getting involved in violent events** Do you do drugs? Smoke? Drink alcohol? How often? How much? What is your perception of the effect of this habit? Are you involved in fights? Do you start them? What about accidents? How often are you involved in events in which you or someone with you is hurt? **Ability to Function** **Strengths and weaknesses in experience and expression of emotion** What is your favorite emotion? What is the emotion you experience most often? What emotions do you never experience? Why are those emotions absent from your life? What are the good points about your emotional life? What are the bad points about your emotional life? **Initiation of purposeful activity** What activities are the easiest for you to do each day? Why? What are the hardest? What gets in your way? **Will, determination, and perseverance** Would you say you are someone who finishes what he or she starts? Tell me about that. How hard is it for you to make decisions? How hard is it for you to follow through on your decisions?
Lifestyle	**Methods for Coping**
Home situation Where do you live? With whom? What is your home like? Do you have some privacy? When? Under what circumstances? Describe your neighborhood.	Do you prefer to talk or to act? How do you solve your problems or make a decision? Tell me about the last time you were very anxious. How do you handle stressful situations? Do these methods work? How have you tried to solve the problem you have right now?

Table 11-3 Assessment of the Family When the Client Is a Family Member

Continuum of Integration of Client				Patterns of Interaction
Full integration and acceptance	Peripheral membership	Isolation	Scapegoating	Symmetrical equal interactions Complementary, one-up, one-down interactions Combination of symmetrical and complementary interactions
Continuum of Family's Organization				
Flexible organization determined by need	Organization around the sick member	Rigid organization insensitive to family members	Chaotic, random, unreliable organization	

Assessment of the Community

The first step in assessing the client's community is to identify systems relevant to the client—that is, systems with which the client actually interacts and systems with which the client should be interacting. (For instance, if the client was hospitalized for psychiatric problems 6 months ago, it is logical to ask about follow-up plans made upon discharge: "Is the client being seen in an outpatient medication group? If not, why not?") Since the community of which any person or family is a member would have a very large number of possibly relevant systems, the guiding principle to use in assessing is, "What resources does this client need to facilitate achievement of his or her life purpose?" An assessment of a community and its resources for promotion, maintenance, restoration, and rehabilitation of health will include information on the extent to which individuals and families have access to resources. Table 11-4 is an excellent tool for a community assessment. A nurse could use it initially to collect data and then add to it as appropriate.[4]

Table 11-4 Community Assessment Tool: Overview of People, Environment, and Systems

Check (√) Appropriate Column	Strength	Potential Need	Problem	Comments
People				
A. Vital and demographic statistics				
1. Population density				
2. Population composition				
a. Sex ratio				
b. Age distribution				
c. Race distribution				
3. Population characteristics				
a. Mobility				
b. Socioeconomic status				
c. Level of unemployment				
d. Education level				
e. Marriage rate				
f. Divorce rate				
g. Dependency ratio				
h. Fertility rate				
i. Head of household				
4. Mortality characteristics				
a. Crude death rate				
b. Infant mortality rate				
c. Maternal mortality rate				
d. Age-specific death rate				
e. Leading causes of death				
5. Morbidity characteristics				
a. Incidence rate (specific diseases)				
b. Prevalence rate (specific diseases)				
B. History of community (founding, growth)				
C. Ethnic origin				
D. Values, attitudes, and norms				
E. Individual and family living practices				
1. Types of families				
2. Number of children per family				
3. Leisure activities engaged in				
F. Housing (types available by percent, condition, percent rented, percent owned)				

(Continued.)

Table 11-4 Continued

Check (√) Appropriate Column	Strength	Potential Need	Problem	Comments
Environment				
A. Physical				
1. Natural resources				
2. Geography/climate/terrain				
3. Roads/transportation				
4. Boundaries				
5. Housing (types available by percent, condition, percent rented, percent owned)				
6. Other major structures				
B. Biological and chemical				
1. Water supply				
2. Air (color, odor, particulates)				
3. Food supply (sources, preparation)				
4. Pollutants; toxic substances; animal reservoirs or vectors				
5. Flora and fauna				
C. Is this a predominately urban, suburban, or rural community? (How is land used?)				
Systems				
A. Health				
1. Preventive health care practices and facilities (List.)				
2. Treatment health care facilities (i.e., acute care, medical and surgical hospitals) (List.)				
3. Rehabilitation health care facilities (i.e., alcoholism) (List.)				
4. Long-term health care facilities (such as nursing homes) (List.)				
5. Respite care services for special groups (List.)				
6. Hospice care services				
7. Catastrophic health care facilities and services				
8. Special health services for population groups (what and how provided)				
a. Preschool				
b. School-age children				
c. Adults and young adults				
d. Occupational health				
e. Adults and children with handicapping conditions				
9. Voluntary health care resources				
10. Sanitation services				
11. Health work force (population ratios)				
12. Health education activities				
13. Methods of health care financing (approximate percent)				
a. Private pay				
b. Health insurance				
c. HMO				
d. Medicaid, Medicare				
e. Workers' compensation				
14. Prevalent diseases and conditions (List.)				

(Continued.)

Table 11-4 Continued

Check (√) Appropriate Column	Strength	Potential Need	Problem	Comments
15. Linkages with other systems				
16. Health care resources: overall availability				
17. Health care resources: overall utilization				
B. Welfare				
1. Official (public) welfare resources				
a. General (such as Department of Social Services) (List.)				
b. Safety and protection (such as fire department) (List.)				
2. Voluntary welfare resources (List.)				
3. Transportation resources (public and private)				
4. Facilities to meet needs (such as shopping areas, public housing)				
5. Special services for population groups (List.)				
6. Accessibility of resources				
7. Utilization of resources				
C. Education				
1. Public educational facilities (List.)				
2. Private educational facilities (List.)				
3. Libraries (List.)				
4. Educational services for special populations				
a. Pregnant teens				
b. Adults				
c. Developmentally disabled children and adults				
d. Other				
5. Resource accessibility				
6. Resource utilization				
D. Economic				
1. Major industry and business (List.)				
2. Banks, savings and loans associations, credit unions (List.)				
3. Major occupations (List.)				
4. General socioeconomic status of population				
5. Median income				
6. Percent of population below poverty level				
7. Percent of population who are retired				
E. Government and leadership				
1. Elected (official) leadership (List with title.)				
2. Nonofficial leadership (List with title affiliations.)				
3. City offices (location, hours, services)				
4. Accessibility to constituents				
5. Support of community resources				

(Continued.)

Table 11-4 Continued

Check (√) Appropriate Column	Strength	Potential Need	Problem	Comments
F. Recreation 1. Public facilities (List.) 2. Private facilities (List.) 3. Recreational activities frequently utilized (List.) 4. Leisure activities frequently utilized (List.) 5. Coordination with educational recreation facilities and programs 6. Programs for special groups a. Elderly b. People who are handicapped c. Others 7. Accessibility of resources 8. Utilization of resources				
G. Religion 1. Facilities, by denomination (List.) 2. Religious leaders (List.) 3. Community programs and services 4. Accessibility of resources 5. Utilization of resources				
Community dynamics (Describe.) A. Communication (Diagram and describe.) 1. Vertical (community to larger society) 2. Horizontal (community to itself) 3. Specific resources (such as television, radio, newspapers)				
Major sources of community data A. Government (such as local health department, city office) (List.) B. Private (such as chamber of commerce) (List.)				

Questions for the Community Health Nurse

1. In general, are resources readily available and accessible?
2. What does the community see as its major strengths and needs?
3. How self-sufficient is the community in meeting its perceived needs?
4. What does the community health nurse see as the community's major strengths and needs?
5. Health care
   a. How does the community view and utilize the health care system?
   b. What does the community see as its health care needs?
   c. What are the goals and major activities of the health system?
   d. How self-sufficient is the community in meeting its health needs?

Community Health Care: Goals and Activities to Implement Them

Date	Goals	Activities

SOURCE: Susan Clemen-Stone et al., *Comprehensive Family and Community Nursing*, 2d ed., McGraw-Hill, New York, 1987. Used with permission.

When the client is a *community*, its internal environment can be assessed using Table 11-4. Assessment of the external environment of the community takes into account the larger society and its resources. Assessment of how a community interacts with society will focus on congruence or incongruence of value systems, exchanges of people and material resources, and degree of dependence or independence. External resources include physical resources, such as water, sewage disposal, food, and construction materials; mental resources, such as colleges, educational television stations, and other educational institutions; and spiritual resources, such as a sense of belonging, mutual valuing, and cohesiveness with the larger society.

The Process of Assessment*

Assessment is the first step in the nursing process, but it is not completed during the first interview and physical examination. It continues as rapport is established; and it changes as the client changes.

SOURCES OF DATA. The two major types of information, or input, in an assessment are subjective data and objective data.

Subjective data consist of statements made by the client or other informants. The nurse's use of perceptive interviewing skills facilitates clients' articulation of their problems and of contributing factors and possible solutions. When asking clients what they see as their problems, the nurse is offering them an opportunity to answer for themselves, regardless of their condition. Some clients, however, are unable to contribute subjective data—for example, because they are out of touch with reality, deeply depressed, or intoxicated. In this case, to obtain essential data the nurse will move from the primary source of information, the client, to secondary sources, such as the family and the social network. Secondary sources may become primary sources at certain times in the assessment process—for instance, when family perceptions and environmental support systems are assessed.

Objective data are information obtained and verified through observation. They include measurable data, such as laboratory tests and vital signs; nonverbal data conveyed by clients, such as facial expressions, gestures, postures, and movements; and data about the environment—for example, home, employment, and school.

The nurse correlates subjective data and objective data, checking one against the other to identify discrepancies and verify information. Discrepancies between subjective and objective data will lead the nurse to question and investigate the information more completely.

Sources of data other than clients and their families include records of interviews from assessments completed during previous admissions, assessments from other agencies, and assessments completed by school personnel, employers, or community health nurses. Community health nurses can contribute to the data base for clients and families if they act as a liaison between the treatment center and the community.

METHODS OF DATA COLLECTION. Data are collected through (1) interviews, (2) observations, and (3) examinations, whether the client is an individual, a family, or a community.

The *initial interview* is conducted when a client is first encountered in a treatment setting. The intensity of the interview will depend upon whether the client is being admitted for treatment at this setting or referred elsewhere. The purpose of the interview is to establish rapport with the client, the family, or a significant other; provide an opportunity for self-disclosure on the part of the client; and gather data for the nursing care plan. The interviewer utilizes facilitative communication skills and encourages clients to talk openly about themselves. This provides an opportunity for the nurse to learn more about each client as a person. Understanding clients as unique human beings enables the nurse to determine their needs and develop an appropriate plan of care.

The nurse needs to be skilled in interviewing if an accurate view of the client is to be obtained. Interviewing skills are discussed in Chapter 12, which explores facilitative communication techniques; and Chapter 13, which explains the phases of the nurse-client relationship that affect the choice of interviewing techniques. However, a few of these skills should be mentioned here. First, the nurse must help the client to feel safe and comfortable; this is done by listening compassionately and by ensuring privacy. Second, the nurse must allow the

* Parts of this section from Elizabeth Maloney, "The Nursing Process," in the second edition of this book.

client to tell his or her own story; the nurse assists by clarifying and reflecting the story, but the client must be responsible for ordering it, and momentum and initiative are determined by the client. Third, the nurse must trust the client's sense of what to share and what to withhold; pushing and probing create too much pressure on a new, untested relationship with a client.

The following examples illustrate a variety of ways in which the initial interview may take place:

CLIENT A

A 23-year-old woman was admitted to the emergency room with vaginal bleeding. While asking her questions about her physical problems, the nurse observed that the woman was chain-smoking and seemed restless. When asked about how long she had been bleeding, the woman began to cry and told the nurse about her boyfriend, who had been killed in an automobile accident. The nurse questioned the woman further and from this brief initial assessment decided to call the psychiatric liaison nurse for further consultation.

CLIENT B

A 45-year-old man was admitted to the medical service for a gastrointestinal workup because of abdominal pain. During the initial interview, the client said that he did not use drugs or alcohol. However, the primary nurse observed that the client became restless and irritable within 48 hours after admission. The nurse suspected impending alcohol withdrawal syndrome and questioned the man further about his drinking habits. He acknowledged that he did, in fact, drink two to three six-packs of beer a day, but he stated, "That's not booze." The nurse took this assessment information to the medical team and a systematic detoxification program was initiated; alcohol withdrawal syndrome was averted.

CLIENT C

A 55-year-old woman was admitted to the psychiatric unit of a general hospital in a severely depressed state following the death of her mother. After orienting the woman to the unit, the primary nurse interviewed her in order to complete the nursing history. The woman was very withdrawn and quiet, but after gentle, persistent questioning she was able to provide answers to many of the questions. The nurse returned twice the next day to interview the woman and complete the assessment. Each time the woman was more at ease with the nurse and able to supply more data. The nurse then shared this information at a team care conference.

CLIENT D

Billy, a 6-year-old, was noted by his teacher to be wetting and soiling his pants in school. He was a worried-looking child who cried when his work was not praised by the teacher. The teacher communicated this information to the school health nurse, who spent some time talking to Billy about how he felt and how things were going for him at school. The nurse called Billy's mother to determine whether any behavioral changes had occurred at home. The mother stated that Billy had been increasingly withdrawn, and she was frantic about his "accidents" at home. On the basis of an initial assessment of behavior change and regression, the school nurse obtained the mother's consent and initiated a referral to a local child guidance clinic. A total assessment was completed there.

From these examples it is clear that the initial assessment may be either brief or extensive. The assessment may be completed in one interview or in a series of interviews. This will also depend on the ability of the client to communicate and on the availability of other significant people.

Another type of interview is the *informal interview.* Informal interviewing can take place casually at different times during each day, particularly during the course of giving nursing care. It provides opportunities for the client to express thoughts and feelings spontaneously. For example:

As a nurse and client were sitting in a lounge having a cup of coffee, the client (a 14-year-old girl), told the nurse that she didn't take drugs just to feel loose. More important, she explained that when she got into trouble with drugs her parents would stop fighting with each other and begin to work together to solve her problem. She was afraid that if she had no problems, her parents' marriage would break up.

Data gathered informally can be valuable additions to the data base.

Observation is an important way of collecting data. It involves sight, smell, hearing, and touch. When nurses observe, they must recognize the significance of their observations and interpret them using other data.[1] Nonverbal communication can be especially significant. It is important to note whether verbal and nonverbal behavior fit together or whether there are discrepancies. For example:

Maryann W., age 17, was very sad and tearful when talking with a nurse about her parents' impending divorce. Yet when her parents visited Maryann on the unit, she was aggressive and hostile toward them when their divorce was discussed. When the nurse pointed this out, Maryann stated, "Do you think I'd let them know how much I'm hurting? They'd just use it against me." The nurse was able to use those observations and the client's response to help Maryann learn to express her feelings more appropriately without having to present a defensive facade.

A third method of data collection is the *examination.* The physical examination, discussed earlier, includes measuring temperature, pulse, respiration, and blood pressure; listening for chest and heart sounds; and paying particular attention to the client's previous and current health problems and physical complaints. It is necessary for the nurse to establish a relationship with the client before the examination. The examination itself can be a tool for showing concern and enhancing the relationship. The examination, whether done partially or completely by the nurse, will result in findings which are added to the data base; they will complete the assessment of the client.

Nursing Diagnosis

Once data are collected, the nurse synthesizes them to make a *nursing diagnosis*—an abstract statement about the client's health status. The diagnosis is made through a cognitive process carried out by the nurse and validated with the client. A nursing diagnosis is not simply a summary or a restatement of the assessment; rather, the nurse creatively synthesizes nursing theory and the data collected. The diagnosis reflects judgments and decisions about patterns of interaction between client and environment, from which goals and interventions are logically derived. It may make a statement about strengths as well as actual or potential problems. It must present an accurate picture of the assessment data; and the assessment data must support it. If more than one nursing diagnosis is made for a client, the assessment data must support each diagnosis. For example, if a client has two diagnoses—(1) unreasonable fear associated with undeveloped ability to test reality, and (2) poor hygiene related to overwhelming feelings of despair—then an adequate data base must exist to support both diagnosis 1 and diagnosis 2.

The art of diagnosis is the creative engagement of theory and data to gain insight into clients' interactions with the environment. The nurse's background—for instance, philosophy, religion, liberal arts, sociology, psychology, family relations, anatomy, and history—as well as nursing theory contributes to his or her understanding of the client. In fact, the better nurses understand humankind, the more insightful and accurate their nursing diagnoses will be.

Nursing as a profession has not yet adopted a standard format for diagnoses, though many possibilities are being explored. The format used most often in this book was chosen because it is logical, provides direction, and makes the nursing process internally consistent. That is, it links assessment data, dictates logical outcomes and evaluation criteria, and suggests appropriate nursing interventions. A diagnosis in this format consists of three parts: (1) a statement about the client; (2) a statement about the relevant situation, environment, or conditions of the client; (3) a statement about the relationship between the two. Table 11-5 gives several examples of this format.

The statement of relationship (part 3 of the format) may take two forms. The first form, *correlational,* is most common. A correlational statement uses terms such as *associated with* and *correlated with.* It implies no more than a relationship between two things; it does not imply one has caused or been caused by other. (For instance, the diagnosis "inappropriate dependence associated with excessive nurturing by others" does not state that dependence has caused excessive nurturing or that excessive nurturing has caused dependence.) The second form the statement of relationship may take is *causal*; this form is used only when there is a well-established cause-and-effect relationship. The phrase *related to* implies causality in a nursing diagnosis. (For instance, the diagnosis "grieving related to recent death of mother" implies that the grief experienced by the client is *caused by* the death of the client's mother.) Life is complex. Pinpointing one or two causes for a condition is likely to be simplistic; the resulting diagnosis will rarely be an accurate statement of reality.

A second format for nursing diagnosis is sometimes used in this book. It is simply a statement about a client, and it is used when a problem must be recognized and addressed by a nurse, but the situation, environment, or condition is unknown or so universal that it need not be made explicit. (For example, the diagnosis "lethal suicidal idea-

Table 11-5 Examples of Nursing Diagnoses

Statement Concerning Person →	Statement of Relationship →	Statement Concerning Situation, Environment, or Condition
Depressed affect	associated with	sociocultural isolation
Grief reaction	related to	death of mother
Social isolation	correlated with	suspiciousness
Accurate labeling of feelings	related to	adequate intellectual function, appropriate teaching in the family
Statement Concerning Family or group →	**Statement of Relationship →**	**Statement Concerning Situation, Environment, or Condition**
Destructive conflict	associated with	unresolved competition for parents' or leaders' attention
Efficient use of resources	correlated with	maintenance of a common group or family purpose
Developmental crisis	related to	addition of new family member
Statement Concerning Community →	**Statement of Relationship →**	**Statement Concerning Situation, Environment, or Condition**
Lack of community *esprit de corps*	associated with	undefined community boundaries
Vulnerability to financial crisis	correlated with	dependence on a single industry
High rate of drug addiction	related to	disenfranchisement of the youth and minority subcultures

tion" obviously must be addressed by the nurse, but the conditions under which the behavior emerges in this client are not known.)

The examples of nursing diagnoses used thus far have related to individuals, but the same format can be used with families, groups, and communities as well. Examples of nursing diagnoses for families, groups, and communities are found in Table 11-5.

Outcome Criteria

Outcome criteria are statements of measurable goals that are expected to be reached as a result of nursing interventions. These goals are dictated by nursing diagnoses and should be formulated in collaboration with clients or at least with their knowledge.

Evaluation of the client outcomes occurs when nursing service is terminated or at some other time specified as part of the outcome criteria. Outcomes must be client-specific and measurable and must relate to the promotion, maintenance, restoration, and rehabilitation of healthy functioning in the client; otherwise, nurses cannot facilitate them. Table 11-6 gives examples of correct and incorrect outcome statements.

Table 11-6 Evaluation of Statements of Client Outcomes

Statement	Evaluation
Client will complete two job interviews before discharge.	Statement is correct. It is client-oriented and measurable. It specifies what the client must do and gives a time frame.
The nurse will encourage the client to interview for jobs.	Statement is incorrect. It is nurse-oriented and not measurable. No time frame is given.
Relief of depressed affect.	Statement is incorrect. It is unclear whose affect is to be addressed. Statement is not measurable, and no time frame is given.
Client will experience relief from depression in 3 weeks, as evidenced by maintenance of own nutrition and elimination patterns, sleep-wake patterns, activity-rest patterns, and realistic problem-solving patterns. Verbalization of lifting of depression will occur.	Statement is correct. It is client-oriented and measurable. What the client must do is specified. A time frame is given.
Client will participate in group therapy daily until discharge.	Statement is partially correct. It is client-oriented and a time frame is given, but it is not measurable. What level of participation is considered adequate?

Relationship of Client Outcomes to Nursing Diagnoses

Client outcomes, or outcome criteria, relate directly to, and are determined by, the nursing diagnosis. In the format used in the book, it is the first part of the diagnosis—the statement about the client—that is related to the outcome criteria. For example, if the diagnosis is "social isolation correlated with suspiciousness," the client outcome would be "social integration." (However, as Table 11-6 makes clear, although an outcome stated like this is indeed related to part 1 of the diagnosis, it is inadequate as it stands because it is neither client-specific nor measurable. Client A, a successful, 45-year-old professional, would not exhibit social integration in the same ways as client B, a 16-year-old victim of rape. The student may find it instructive to formulate acceptable outcome statements for these two clients.)

Unique Problems Related to Psychiatric Clients

Collaborating with clients to establish outcome criteria may at first seem difficult or impossible in the context of psychiatric–mental health nursing. Often, part of the clients' problems is their inability to commit themselves to goals or work toward goals. They may have perceptual difficulties or dysfunctional patterns of thought that impair their ability to formulate goals; and they may be unskilled in making decisions, setting priorities, or planning in general.

The conceptual framework of nursing can provide the solution to this problem. The client, like any other human being, is seen as a physical, mental, and spiritual being, interacting with the environment (in recognizable patterns) to achieve a life purpose. Therefore, the client—like anyone else—is motivated by something. Psychiatric clients often are less aware of their motivations than people whose patterns are more functional; but nurses can help them discover their motivations—and discovering motives can itself be an outcome to which both nurse and client can make a commitment.

The most useful goals for psychiatric clients are small ones. Let's say a client has been increasingly withdrawn and has not spoken to anyone in 2 weeks. Tolerating the presence of another person sitting nearby for longer periods each day is a small goal, but for the client it is a significant step toward social integration. By setting small goals, celebrating their achievement, and then helping the client move toward the next goal, nurses can help reestablish functional interactions. Moreover, setting and reaching small goals is a way for nurses themselves to experience accomplishment in their daily work.

Interventions

Nursing interventions are activities planned by the nurse—with the client—to achieve the outcomes that have been established. Nurses who are new to the psychiatric setting tend to limit their interventions to talking, but this is an ineffective approach. Nursing interventions must be broad in scope, and—although they must always relate to client outcomes—they can include many kinds of activities: accompanying a client on a bus to town, teaching a client to use a dial or push-button telephone, participating with a client in a game, modeling assertive communication, and praying with a client. Appropriate interventions are based on the client's condition, environment, or situation (as determined by the diagnosis) and are aimed at improving the client's ability to function. Figure 11-2 illustrates the relationship of nursing interventions to nursing diagnoses in the context of the nursing process as a whole.

Evaluation

Evaluation is a judgment concerning the relevance, effectiveness, and efficiency of outcomes achieved as well as of nursing interventions provided. That is, both the nursing process itself and its results are evaluated. Evaluation is relatively easy if goals are measurable and if interventions are specific and documented. Evaluation of outcomes may be used as a new set of assessment data, which in turn can be used to formulate new nursing diagnoses.

It is important to examine the content and the process of the evaluation:

Were outcomes achieved?

If so, were they achieved because of the nursing interventions or for some other reason?

If not, where was the failure? Misdiagnosis? Ineffective interventions?

Did the interventions facilitate the outcome?

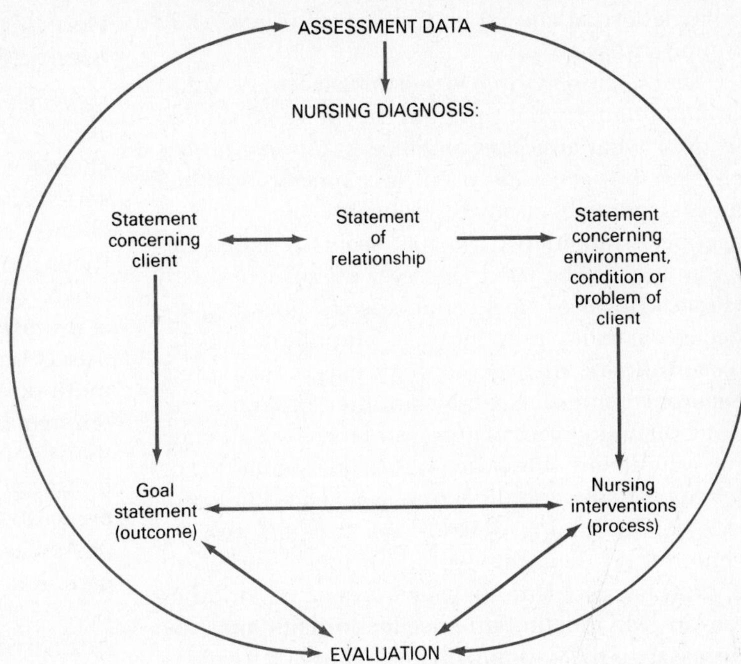

Figure 11-2 The nursing process.

Were there intervening conditions that did not receive adequate attention in the assessment and diagnosis phases?

Was the assessment complete and accurate?

Through evaluation, the nurse is held accountable for the nursing care that was planned and delivered and the outcomes that were achieved. For example:

A nurse, Mark, determined the following outcome with his client, Jerry: "social integration as evidenced by reestablishment of telephone contact with parents, finding a roommate, and eating at least four evening meals per week with another person." Mark planned interventions designed to help Jerry achieve the outcome. At the time of termination of the nurse-client relationship, Jerry and Mark evaluated how well the outcome had been achieved and how well each of the interventions had fostered attainment of the goal.

ISSUES RELATED TO THE NURSING PROCESS

As the nursing process has developed over the past 20 years, and as the profession has come to recognize the importance of writing out a nursing care plan for each client, several issues have emerged. These issues will eventually be resolved by members of the profession, in conjunction with governmental and accrediting bodies and in collaboration with other disciplines; but a few of them are briefly outlined here to stimulate thinking about the nursing process. The issues are:

- Nursingwide format versus institution-specific format
- Nursing-focused format versus client-focused format
- Problem-oriented approach versus strengths-and-challenges approach
- Accountability through auditing
- Payment for outcomes versus payment for interventions

Nursingwide Format versus Institution-Specific Format

The nursing process outlined in this chapter is one of several conceptualizations used to direct nurses' goal-directed activity. All these formats include similar steps, but there are some differences among them. (For instance, some formats have a "problem statement" instead of a nursing diagnosis.) Whether a single format should be used by all nurses is an important issue.

A *nursingwide format* is one that all nurses would use, no matter what program they have graduated from or what area they practice in. An *institution-specific format* is one used by a specific hospital, a nursing home, or any other health care center or agency. A nursingwide format seems sensible, because it could be used wherever nurses work with clients. However, institution-specific formats are becoming more prevalent as computerized data-based nursing management systems are adopted. Different computers and computer programs require different forms of input, and these may dictate the way the nursing process is to be executed. (For instance, many computerized systems do not provide for a nursing diagnosis; a nursing process centered on diagnosis would obviously represent a gigantic problem for such systems.) Another reason why institution-specific formats may be necessary is that—unfortunately—nursing management systems are sometimes designed by people who are not familiar with the way nurses actually plan care. The solution in the future will probably be a nursingwide format with the specific needs of the agency or institution taken into account. Nurses must contribute significant input to the design of systems so that the structure of the systems will adequately reflect the nursing process.

Nursing-Focused Format versus Client-Focused Format

In the past, the nursing process was *nursing-focused*—that is, organized around nurses' work. Today, however, the idea that the process should be *client-focused*—organized around the client—is widely accepted. This has resulted from changes in the health care environment and from consumerism, particularly demands for more individualized care. Client-focused formats specify desired client outcomes; everything nurses do is aimed at achieving these outcomes, and the nursing process as a whole reflects that commitment. For example:

> A client, Marie, is very suspicious. Client-focused nursing would include interventions to make her less so. The nursing staff might, for instance, find that interacting with Marie in a matter-of-fact way is most useful.

Problem-Oriented Approach versus Strengths-and-Challenges Approach

A *problem-oriented approach* to the nursing process (as the term implies) focuses on ameliorating clients' actual or potential problems. A *strengths-and-challenges approach* focuses on maximizing clients' strengths and minimizing the impact of their problems, their weaknesses, and the challenges they are facing. The trend in nursing today is toward a focus on strengths and challenges; and this is logical if the goals of nursing include promotion, maintenance, restoration, and rehabilitation of health. With a problem-oriented approach, there is likely to be insufficient emphasis on promoting and maintaining health. Moreover, focusing on problems can make it difficult to approach clients as whole persons or to formulate plans for care that will affirm and reflect their wholeness.

Accountability through Auditing

An *audit* is a method used to document the extent to which nursing structures and processes have achieved specific outcomes. In general, nursing audits have tended to concentrate on activities and to evaluate them according to predetermined standards. Nurses have been concerned that this approach is superficial, since there is more to nursing than activities. This criticism can be answered by auditing the nursing process as a whole—not only interventions but also planning, implementation, and evaluation. Auditing of the entire nursing process will become more and more feasible as the rationale for specific interventions is validated through research, and as computerization becomes more widespread. For accurate auditing of nursing, not only records but also plans for care during the period each client has received treatment will have to be accessible; computers will simplify the storage and retrieval of nursing care plans.

The Joint Commission on Accreditation of Hospitals (JCAH) evaluates through the use of audits the quality of services provided to hospitalized clients. JCAH revises its standards yearly, and each year they have become more rigorous. This has resulted in higher standards for care of clients; but unfortunately, JCAH, a nonnursing group, is also setting the standards for accountability of nurses. Although JCAH has sought input from nurses for standards related to nursing, nurses do not control their own accountability. This issue will continue to be addressed by state nurses' associations and at the national level by the American Nurses Association.

Another issue related to accountability is interdisciplinary audits versus nursing audits. An *interdisciplinary audit* focuses on all the efforts made to bring about client outcomes; a *nursing audit* focuses solely on nurses' efforts. The advantage of an interdisciplinary audit is its emphasis on outcomes and teamwork. Its disadvantage is that each profession loses some individual accountability. The advantage of a nursing audit is that the effectiveness of nursing care is evaluated in relation to outcomes. Its disadvantage is that specifying the part of the outcome for which nurses are largely responsible is difficult. For instance, suppose that outcome is "social integration, as evidenced by an increase in socially acceptable behaviors, social communication skills, and helpful behaviors." A nursing audit would identify the extent to which the planned interventions were accomplished, but it would be almost impossible to determine exactly what percentage of the outcome was due to those interventions.

Payment for Outcomes versus Payment for Interventions

Payment for nursing services by third parties such as insurance companies has in the past been included with payment for room and board in most states. "Cost containment" is changing this: the cost of nursing services is being separated from the cost of room and board. Since administrators at all levels must document the cost of services, the trend is to document nursing services, listed on a client's bill as a separate item.

Prospective payment for treatment began in hospitals for Medicare and Medicaid clients. It has had an effect on all forms of care provided in communities and hospitals which are paid for by third parties. Psychiatric care is not yet paid for prospectively, but psychiatric professionals and treatment facilities are getting ready for a prospective payment system.

The question for the nursing profession is, "Should charges for nursing services be based on outcomes or on nursing interventions?" As payment mechanisms continue to change, the outcome of services will probably receive increasing attention. Nurses must continue to develop the research base necessary to specify outcomes in relation to interventions. If research ties interventions to outcomes, nurses will have a way to document the cost of outcomes and thus a rational basis for charges.

SUMMARY

The *nursing process* is a method of systematically assessing and diagnosing a client's health status, formulating outcomes, determining interventions to be used with the client, and evaluating quality of care and outcomes of care planned for, and in conjunction with, the client. The purpose of the chapter is to provide an understanding of the nursing process so that a nursing care plan can be formulated.

The nursing process has five purposes:

1. To plan and evaluate care offered to a client
2. To provide a systematic approach to each client
3. To facilitate individualized planning
4. To promote the client's health through goal-directedness
5. To provide a mechanism for communication among nurses working with a client

There are five steps in the nursing process: assessing, diagnosing, determining client outcomes, planning interventions, and evaluating.

Assessment is a systematic collection of health-related data about the client (a person, family, or community) and the environment. Data may be subjective or objective. Data are collected through interviewing, observing, and listening.

A *nursing diagnosis* is a statement reflecting a judgment about the pattern of interaction between the client and the environment, from which goals and interventions are logically derived. The diagnosis consists of three parts: (1) a statement about the client; (2) a statement about the relevant situation, environment, or conditions of the client; and (3) a statement about the relationship between the two.

Outcome criteria are statements of measurable goals that are expected to be reached through nursing interventions. Client outcomes relate directly to, and are determined by, the nursing diagnosis.

Nursing interventions are activities planned by the nurse, with the client's input, that are designed to achieve client outcomes. Interventions must be broad in scope and related to the outcomes to be accomplished; they must include diverse activities (such as accompanying a client on a bus and role-modeling assertive communication).

Evaluation is a judgment about the relevance, effectiveness, and efficiency of the outcomes and the nursing interventions. Evaluation is relatively easy to do if goals are measurable and if interventions are specific and documented.

Several issues have emerged related to the nursing process: nursingwide format versus institution-specific format; nursing-focused format versus client-focused format; problem-oriented approach versus strengths-and-challenges approach; accountability through auditing; and payment for nursing outcomes versus payment for nursing interventions.

REFERENCES

1. Clarence J. Rowe, *An Outline of Psychiatry*, 8th ed., Brown, Dubuque, Iowa, 1984.
2. Sharon Fish and Judith Allen Shelly: *Spiritual Care: The Nurse's Role*, Inter-Varsity, Downers Grove, Ill., 1978.
3. Lewis B. Smedes, *Forgive and Forget*, Harper and Row, New York, 1984.
4. Susan Clemen-Stone, *Comprehensive Family and Community Health Nursing*, 2d ed., McGraw-Hill, New York, 1986.

BIBLIOGRAPHY

Leslie D. Atkinson and Mary E. Murray, *Understanding the Nursing Process*, 2d ed., Macmillan, New York, 1983.

Fay L. Bower, *The Process of Planning Nursing Care: A Theoretical Model*, 3d ed., Mosby, St. Louis, 1982.

B. J. Carmack, "Guidelines for Assessing Mental/Psychosocial Status," *Occupational Health Nursing*, vol. 30, May 1982, pp. 29–34.

Doris Carnevali et al., *Diagnostic Reasoning in Nursing*, Lippincott, Philadelphia, 1984.

Doris Carnevali, *Nursing Care Planning: Diagnosis and Management*, 3d ed., Lippincott, Philadelphia, 1983.

Marilynn Doenges et al., *Nursing Care Plans: Diagnosis in Planning Patient Care*, Davis, Philadelphia, 1984.

Janet W. Griffith and Paula Chuslensen, *Nursing Process: Application of Theories, Frameworks, and Models*, Mosby, St. Louis, 1982.

Bonnie Kawczak Hagerty, *Psychiatric–Mental Health Assessment*, Mosby, St. Louis, 1984.

J. Johnston, "Nursing Mirror Mental Health Forum: The Nursing Process and Psychiatry," *Nursing Mirror*, vol. 158, January 4, 1984, pp. i–ii.

P. Keane, "The Nursing Process in Action - 4. The Nursing Process in a Psychiatric Context," *Nursing Times*, vol. 77, July 8–14, 1981, pp. 1223–1224.

M. J. Kim and Derry A. Mority, eds., *Classification of Nursing Diagnosis: Proceedings of the Third and Fourth National Conference*, McGraw-Hill, New York, 1982.

Josephine Sana and Richard P. Judge, *Physical Assessment Skills for Nursing Practice*, 2d ed., Little, Brown, Boston, 1982.

A. L. Whall, "Nursing Theory and the Assessment of Families," *Journal of Psychiatric Nursing*, vol. 19, January 1981, pp. 30–36.

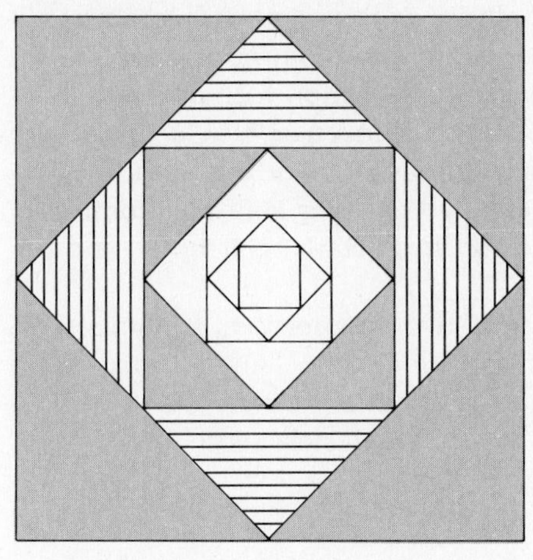

CHAPTER 12 Communication Theories and Application

Judith Haber
Pamela Price Hoskins

LEARNING OBJECTIVES

After studying this chapter, the student should be able to:

1. Define the process and components of communication.
2. Recognize factors that influence communication.
3. Differentiate among levels of communication.
4. Explain the communication theories of Watzlawick, Scheflen, Birdwhistell, Berne, and Ruesch.
5. Define *attending skills.*
6. Describe physical and psychological attending skills.
7. Define *responding skills.*
8. Describe the core dimensions of facilitative communication.
9. Describe responding strategies that facilitate communication.
10. Describe barriers to effective communication.

Communication is ongoing interaction through which people relate to one another. It is a process of discovering and conveying meaning; it is a process of moving toward one's life purpose; it is the way we are known by others and come to know them; and it is one way we learn about ourselves. Human beings are social, and when they interact their communication influences their personal growth and development as well as their relationships with each other.

Everything affects, and is affected by, communication: the environment, other people, and the self. When communication goes awry, people feel devalued and misunderstood; their perceptions are distorted; they cannot understand others; and they may become alienated, bitter, lonely, and frustrated. Through effective communication, people become aware of their problems and learn to solve them.

Understanding the factors that influence communication allows people to communicate more effectively. This understanding is especially important for nurses, because nursing requires excellent communication skills. In order to communicate effectively, nurses must have a knowledge of communication theories, an understanding of environmental and cultural components of communication, an ability to analyze communication, and a sense of purposeful interaction with others. Nurses also help their clients to engage in a process of self-exploration, self-understanding, and change, and that is facilitated by their ability to communicate ideas and feelings clearly, efficiently, and appropriately.

The purpose of this chapter is to facilitate therapeutic communication with clients. It focuses on theories of communication developed by Watzlawick, Scheflen and Birdwhistell, Berne, and Ruesch.

WHAT IS COMMUNICATION?

A Definition of Communication

Communication is a process by which information is transmitted through a common system of symbols, signs, or behavior. This definition deserves close examination.

The first part of the definition expresses the notion that communication is a complex *process*. (See Figure 12-1 for a diagram of the process of

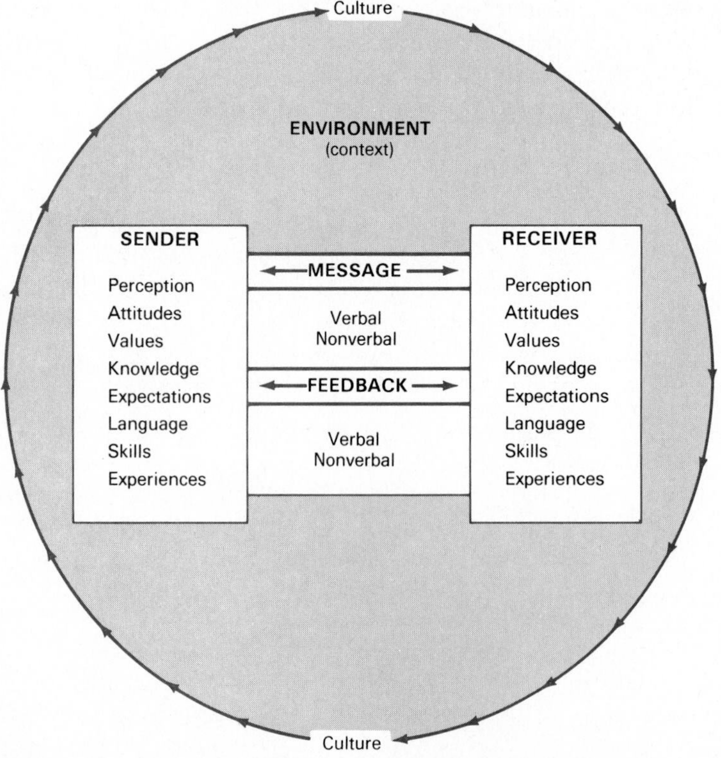

Figure 12-1 The circular process of communication.

communication.) This process is an ongoing experience that has phases; it can be analyzed, but it has no identifiable beginning or end. It is *circular*. (For example, John may think his disagreement with Mary is over, only to discover that she thinks it is just beginning.) The term *process* implies that communication is not a cut-and-dried experience where one says, "You talk first; then it's my turn." Communication is *continuous*, a term which suggests motion and dynamism in situations where people are interacting—sometimes synchronously and sometimes chaotically. It is not a "language process" but a "people process" and a "social process." It is also an *irreversible* process. One cannot take back a message, or "uncommunicate."[1]

The second part of the definition states that *information is transmitted.* The information or message relates not only to facts (such as a client's weight, height, and diagnosis) but also to feelings, perceptions, and thoughts. Facts, however, are more easily communicated than thoughts, perceptions, and feelings. The latter often require complex systems for transmission. Information is transmitted by nonverbal as well as verbal means. A total message or set of information consists of a combination of factors, including body posture, eye contact, nonverbal clues, environment, and spoken words.

The third part of the definition states that a *common system of symbols, signs, or behavior* is required to transmit information. This implies that people *learn* to communicate, and that some people learn one system of communication while others learn another system. There are nonverbal as well as verbal "languages"—none "right" or "better," but each with its own cadence, symbols, and accepted behavior. Nonverbal communication is all behavior that communicates without words. Nonverbal behavior can be as difficult to understand or interpret as a foreign language, and whether or not a "translation" is valid will depend on the context of the message. (For example, shrugging one's shoulders may mean indifference to one sender but indecision to another. A smile may express pleasure or cunning or amusement or many other things, depending on the sender.) Since not everyone speaks the same language—verbally or nonverbally—effective communication requires a clear understanding of what is being communicated, which includes validating messages sent and received.

Verbal Communication

A *symbol* is anything that takes the place of, stands for, or refers to something or someone. It is created by arbitrary agreement or social custom, and it has a universal meaning, but it may be altered by an individual to take on a special meaning.[2] A symbol by itself is meaningless. Meaning is attributed only in context, and only by agreement. Human beings communicate through the use of symbols called *words.* Words have consistent meanings because of tradition and widespread usage.

Verbal communication refers to spoken or written words (words that are "signed" would also be considered verbal communication). In verbal communication, meaning is derived not only from the words themselves but also from the way they are arranged—in sentences, paragraphs, and so on. Some groups of words have specialized meanings or mean more than they actually say; these include figures of speech, proverbs, clichés, mottos, and the like. "The squeaky wheel gets the grease" is an example: it can be interpreted to mean that clients who make the most demands will get the most attention. Sentences and phrases like this have acquired their special meaning over time and can convey a great deal very briefly. Other specialized forms of verbal communication are abbreviations, jokes, and graffiti.

Nonverbal Communication

Messages are also conveyed in many nonverbal ways. In fact, research has indicated that nonverbal messages carry more social and emotional meaning and are more likely to be believed than verbal messages; and nonverbal behavior is used to check the reliability of verbal messages. Nonverbal messages are recognized through observation.[3] Four ways in which they can be expressed are:

1. Kinesics—body movements
2. Paralanguage—voice quality and nonlanguage vocalizations
3. Proxemics—use of personal and social space
4. Appearance—use of clothing and other personal objects to communicate a personal image

Kinesics

Kinesics refers to the study of body movement as a form of nonverbal communication. The face and body are extremely communicative. Even when people are silent, the atmosphere is filled with messages. Facial expressions, posture, gestures, eye movements, and touch provide nonverbal communication.

Facial expressions are perhaps the single most important source of nonverbal messages. For example, a teenager comes home late for dinner, looks at the mother's facial expression, and says, "Mom, let me explain. I can tell you're fuming by the look on your face."

Posture can reveal a great deal about one's self-concept. When a person is stooped, relaxed, awkward, or always erect and at attention, subtle messages are received and responded to by others. The way in which a person walks (gait) relates to posture and also communicates self-concept.

An infinite array of body movements and *gestures* are carriers of emotional messages. Such movements and gestures provide a variety of clues about how people feel about themselves and others. For example, hand gestures can convey indifference, anxiety, relaxation, and impatience. Fidgeting suggests unease, impatience, or a wish to avoid or escape from a situation.

Eye contact can communicate level of interest about or involvement with a current interaction. In western society, direct eye contact usually implies an invitation to relate and communicates positive regard for another person.

Touch conveys a variety of feelings that accentuate the way in which emotions are communicated. Touch communicates a range of feelings from tenderness and warmth to anger and resentment. The use of touch is determined by cultural norms. It is important to understand and be sensitive to cultural as well as personal norms about touch so that personal boundaries are not violated.

Paralanguage

Messages are also conveyed by the way the voice is used. *Paralinguistic behavior,* which includes tone of voice, inflection, spacing of words, emphasis, and pauses, is part of a total message. Paralinguistic behavior also includes nonlanguage vocalizations such as sobbing, laughing, and grunting. For example, people who speak in a loud voice, accent their words, and speak at a rapid rate are often thought to be vivacious. People who speak softly, slowly, and without emphasis might be viewed as wishy-washy. These factors become important qualifiers of verbal messages. Paralinguistic behavior is recognized by listening to nonword vocalizations as well as tone of voice and other factors mentioned above.

Proxemics

Proxemics is the study of spatial relationships during personal interactions. Proxemics is concerned with *territoriality,* that is, the fixed, defined space that is customarily marked off by a person to prevent intrusion by others.[4] It is also concerned with *personal space,* the "portable" territory surrounding the self and acting as an invisible barrier beyond which others are expected not to trespass.[4] When these boundaries are threatened by intrusion, communication alters in direct response. Use of space and territory varies depending on people's cultural background; and it can influence the meaning of a message. Characteristics of territoriality as exemplified by intimate, personal, social, and public space are outlined in Table 12-1 (see also Chapter 3).

Appearance

Appearance refers to the way in which people use clothing and other personal objects to convey an image.[4] Appearance acts as a nonverbal message that can confirm or deny verbal messages. Clothing, hairstyles, makeup, jewelry, beards, and eyeglasses are examples of articles that people put together in unique ways. A change in a person's appearance can be an indication of developing problems. For example:

> Mr. S., a retired man of 70, was always immaculately groomed and wore perfectly coordinated sports outfits. He was clean-shaven and smelled of after-shave lotion and hair tonic. Following the death of his wife, he was frequently observed in the street unshaven, in raggedy, unmatched outfits, with greasy, straggly hair. Shortly thereafter he was hospitalized for severe depression.

FACTORS THAT INFLUENCE COMMUNICATION

Through communication people reveal themselves to one another, sometimes in mutually understood symbols and sometimes in symbols that are misunderstood. Interactions are influenced by cultural

Table 12-1 Characteristics of Territoriality

Space	Distance	Body Contact	Visual Focus	Vocalization	Smell
Intimate	0–18 inches	Inevitable and expected	Sharpened and detailed. Restricted to small area of body.	Low and more frequent	Heightened and distorted
Personal	$1\frac{1}{2}$–4 feet	Close contact possible	Less distorted; clearer. Focus is on full face instead of part of face, or other.	Moderate	Not as perceptible
Social	4–12 feet	Denotes a limit to physical dominance; person is out of reach or touch	Eye contact becomes important. Person can be seen more clearly, inclusively, and in more detail.	Louder	Imperceptible
Public	12–25 feet and beyond	Vacant of personal contact or involvement	Details lost. Individuals not as perceptible; individuality lost.	Louder; pronunciation more careful and exaggerated	Not relevant

SOURCE: Adapted from E. C. Hein, *Communication in Nursing Practice*, 2d ed., Little, Brown, Boston, 1980, p. 151. Used with permission.

background, sex roles, social class, and value system. Relationships between people, the content exchanged, and the environment where an interaction occurs also contribute to the outcome of the communication process.

Culture and Religion

"Culture is communication, and communication is culture."[5] Cultural variables include norms, customs, rituals, myths, religious traditions, and symbolic behavior. Culture prescribes how people come to know their world; preconceptions and generalizations evolve from cultural definitions.

Culture influences all aspects of communication. People are taught by their culture how to communicate through gestures, symbols, rituals, and clothing. Cultural attitudes—including generalizations and stereotypes—influence how people see each other and relate to each other within and across cultural boundaries. Symbols of faiths and ideologies—a cross, a star, a crescent—are given meanings by cultures. Clothing does not differ from culture to culture as much as it once did, but a costume can still indicate a person's nationality, religion, or subculture. Many gestures are established culturally—for example, Japanese people bow when they greet each other, but English people bow to members of the royal family; and a handshake, which expresses a greeting in our culture, can be an invasion of personal space in another cultural context. Understanding how culture affects communication is necessary if communication is to be effective (see Chapter 6).

Sex Roles

Sex roles affect communication in many ways. Two of the most important have to do with reflections of sex roles and sexual stereotypes in the language itself, and with how people's sex actually affects their communicative interactions with others.

The way our language has developed not only reflects but also has contributed to attitudes about gender, as terms such as *manpower, chairman, fireman,* and *bachelor* (on the one hand) and *housewife, weaker sex, apron strings,* and *old maid* (on the other) suggest. Today, as sexual roles and attitudes toward gender are changing, the language is also changing; terms that are not "gender-specific"—*human resources, chairperson, fire fighter, unmarried people*—are an indication that we are moving toward sexual equality.

Gender also influences how people communicate with each other; whether one is interacting with a person of the same sex or of the opposite sex will affect the communication. For example, a man who is generally shy and uncomfortable with other men may compensate by being aggressive and self-assured with women; a woman who is flirtatious or self-conscious with men may be matter-of-fact with women. Obviously, then, the sex of a nurse and a client will have an affect on interactions between them.

Social Class

Social class has a very significant influence on communication. One example of its effect is *semantic reaction:* a spontaneous response to an image which a person forms when confronted with symbols, especially words.[4] Many semantic reactions are linked to social class in ways that can be changed; that is, words which evoke negative reactions can be eliminated in favor of words that evoke positive or neutral reactions. For example, *ghetto* or *slum* can be replaced by *inner city; poverty* can be replaced by *low income; janitor* can be replaced by *sanitary engineer.*

Perceptions

A *perception* is a personal, internal experience of the environment which is processed and received through the senses. It is a way of sensing, interpreting, and comprehending the world. People's individual perceptions of the same situation may differ. (For example, a nurse and a family may have different perceptions of a client's behavior. The family may perceive the client—their adolescent son—as quiet and shy, while the nurse may perceive him as depressed and withdrawn.) An event has different meanings, then, because people's perceptions of it differ.[5]

What a person senses or perceives is not always what actually exists; it may be a misperception. One way in which misperceptions can arise is through the influence of past experiences, which prepare people to see persons, places, and things in certain, and sometimes distorted, ways.

People need to know how their perceptions influence the way they understand their environment and the way they communicate with each other. Particularly, nurses need to understand that the perceptions clients have of them are important in the communication process; and they must also be aware of their own perceptions of clients.

Values

A person's value system influences the way that person communicates. Someone who values politeness will express this in numerous symbolic ways. If a person values education, this will be communicated in numerous ways. Whether health is valued is also communicated. For example, diabetic clients may say with words that they want to control the disease, but consistently abuse their diet. They may be communicating that health lacks value to them.

Relationships

Another factor that influences communication is relationships between people. One aspect of this is known as *level of relatedness.* Husband and wife will relate differently from two persons who are strangers. Clients may communicate with physicians in a way that differs greatly from the way in which they interact with nurses.

A second aspect of relationships is *emotional climate.* Whether the emotional climate is comfortable or tense will affect both *what* is communicated and *how* it is communicated. At a cocktail party a man may interact with his boss in a very different way from at a board meeting, and the same words may convey very different messages. A woman who is having a hard day at work may communicate her needs tensely; on a less stressful day her interactions will be more relaxed.

Content of the Message

The *content* of the message can either charge or defuse the atmosphere of a communication. When a client talks about death or loss, certain feelings are aroused that can affect how the message is sent and received. Taboo subjects will likewise affect interactions, often creating tension and resulting in distorted communication.

Context of the Message

The place where an interaction takes place will influence the communication process. Clients may be unable to discuss their problems while hospitalized but may be willing to confide in a nurse who visits them at home. Saying "I love you" in a crowded elevator will convey a very different message from saying it at a table for two at a quiet night spot. The context or place of the communication is an integral component of the message.

THEORIES OF COMMUNICATION

Theories of communication—such as those of Watzlawick, Scheflen and Birdwhistell, Berne, and Ruesch, discussed in this section—can be useful in understanding communicative interactions. These theories are based on the idea that all behavior communicates and is reciprocal.

Watzlawick's Theory

Communication and Circumstances

Watzlawick, Beavin, and Jackson[1] theorized that the *circumstances* of a communication, particularly the relationship between the people involved, can dictate a certain response. When the circumstances are taken into account, there may be no difference between a normal person's communication and a disturbed person's communication, although the response may be considered "disturbed." For example:

> A client who is undergoing a painful procedure is given no painkillers but is told not to move or make any noise. The client kicks the physician. The response is considered "disturbed"; but since the client was offered no other means of communicating, the behavior makes sense.

Feedback Loop

Another feature of Watzlawick's theory is the *feedback loop.* Relationships are characterized by dynamic communication patterns that remain the same even when the topic changes; and every communication is both a response to a stimulus and a new stimulus designed to elicit a response. This circular pattern, the feedback loop, is shown in Figure 12-2.

Positive feedback is any communication that leads to a change in a relationship; *negative feedback* is any communication that maintains the status quo. The behavior of each person affects and is affected by that of the other; because communication is continuous and circular, any distinction between "beginning" and "end" or "cause" and "effect" is purely arbitrary.

Axioms

Watzlawick and his colleagues proposed five axioms, discussed in the following paragraphs.[1]

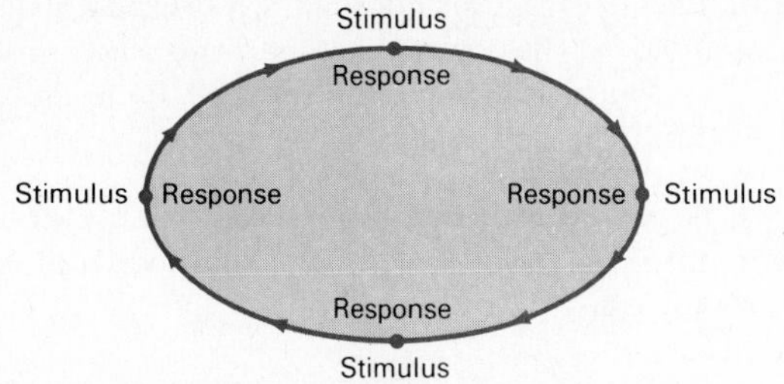

Figure 12-2 Feedback loop.
Every response is at the same time a stimulus evoking another response. (SOURCE: Adapted from P. Watzlawick et al., *The Pragmatics of Human Communication,* Norton, New York, 1967.)

AXIOM 1. *A person cannot* not *communicate.* This axiom has to do with the idea that all behavior is communicative. Since there is no such thing as "nonbehavior," there is no such thing as "noncommunication." Attempts to avoid communication must fail, then: either behavior itself will convey the communication, or the attempt will take the form of somehow trying to avoid behavior—and, that being impossible, a confusing or unorthodox message will be conveyed. Here is a rather simple example:

> A mother does not speak to her daughter for 3 days (during which time the two ordinarily would speak). This is *not* "no communication." It is a message: "I do not want to speak with you."

AXIOM 2. *Any message has two levels, content and relationship.* The *content level* of a message is verbal information; the *relationship level* is information about the relationship between the people involved. There are three kinds of messages at the relationship level: (1) confirming, (2) disconfirming, and (3) rejecting. A *confirming message* is an agreement with another person's message about a relationship; a *rejecting message* is a disagreement with the other person's message about the relationship; a *disconfirming message* tells the other person that he or she does not exist. A message always demands some response to its relationship level; such a response is called *metacommunication*—communication about communication.[6]

When the content level and the relationship level of a message become confused and contaminated; or if they are contradictory, problems arise. For example:

> A mother says, "I love you, son," but backs away from his embrace. The son says, "Mom, you say you love me, but you're backing away from me. What are you telling me?"

The son's response here is an example of metacommunication; he is addressing the relationship level of the message.

AXIOM 3. *"Punctuation" organizes communication patterns and is vital to ongoing relationships.* To an outsider, communications may seem to be uninterrupted, but the participants arbitrarily identify sequences which have beginnings and ends. These arbitrary decisions are called *punctuation.* If two people punctuate a communication differently (identify different sequences), problems will arise in their relationship. For example:

> A husband says, "I drink because my wife nags me." The wife says, "I nag him because he drinks."

AXIOM 4. *There are two kinds of communication, analogic and digital. Analogic communication* is nonverbal; it includes kinesics, paralanguage, proxemics, and appearance (discussed earlier). *Digital communication* is verbal; it is more logical, more abstract, and more complex than analogic communication.

AXIOM 5. *There are two kinds of interactions, symmetrical and complementary. Symmetrical interactions* are characterized by equality and minimal differences between the people involved. When two people escalate their messages to compete with each other in what ought to be a symmetrical interaction, problems will occur. At the relationship level, messages will be rejecting. For example:

> Terry says, "I've had the worst day ever." Teddy responds, "You've had a bad day? Wait till you hear about mine." Relationally, Terry and Teddy will compete with each other until they have a fight about whose day was worse.

Complementary interactions are characterized by a maximum of differences between the people involved; they are sometimes called *one-up, one-down interactions.* When problems occur in complementary interactions, a relationship may become rigid, so that one person is always one up while the other is always one down. In a rigid complementary interaction, a disconfirming message is sent at the relationship level. For example:

> Mary says, "John, I'm going to the store. Do you want anything?" John ignores this message and responds as if Mary has asked his permission: "It's OK with me if you go now, but be back in an hour, honey." John has disconfirmed Mary to maintain a complementary interaction.

It should be noted that a healthy relationship will be characterized by both symmetrical and complementary interactions, used at appropriate times.

These five axioms are believed to apply to all relationships, including the nurse-client relationship, and they can assist the nurse in understanding communication patterns. Symmetrical interactions are appropriate when the nurse is doing an assessment, setting goals with the client, discussing alternative nursing treatments, and solving problems with the client. Complementary interactions are appropriate when the client needs to be protected, when information is being given, and when haste is important for the client's well-being. Some of the most difficult communication problems occur when people disagree about the kind of interaction they want or receive disconfirming or rejecting messages. When such problems arise, the skill of metacommunication becomes important if the nurse is to communicate clearly with the client. Metacommunication is not only clear but also concise and congruent.

The following example illustrates some of the kinds of communication that have just been described:

> A nurse, Rudy Price, approaches a newly admitted client, George Johnson. "Hello, George," says the nurse; "my name is Mr. Price." This is a communication at two levels—relationship and content. It is a complementary interaction, since the names as used by the nurse imply inequality, with the nurse in the one-up position.
>
> The client responds, "I expect to be called Mr. Johnson," conveying a rejecting message at both the content level and the relationship level, and communicating the fact that he expects his interactions with the nurse to be symmetrical.
>
> The nurse now says, "Mr. Johnson. I'll remember that. It sounds as if you're used to making decisions and maintaining control." This is a metacommunication, since the nurse is commenting on the client's

desire or need to maintain an equal relationship; it is also a confirming message for the symmetrical interaction.

Scheflen and Birdwhistell's Theory

Scheflen[7] and Birdwhistell[8] have studied patterns of space and time in communication. Spatial and temporal aspects of communication are nonverbal and often unconscious, but this does not lessen their importance.

Time

Time is a concept, an experience, and a way of perceiving (see Chapter 3). How time is spent is an important issue in people's lives, and thus in their communications as well.

Although people may not often think of it in this way, *silence* is one use of time. For example:

> Meg asks Joe a question. He does not answer. His failure to answer communicates something to Meg—the possible messages include anger, deafness, indifference, and thoughtlessness. (Remember that it is not correct to say that Joe did *not* communicate at all.)
>
> If Meg thinks that Joe's silence is communicating anger, she may repeat her question (a content message) or ask him if he is angry (a relationship message and a metacommunication).

Time may be sensed as motion (passing of time) or duration (length of time). *How long* it takes to visit relatives who live far away and *how often* such visits are made are verbal time-oriented communications about distance. *How long* a relationship has lasted and *when* it might be cut off are time-oriented communications about relatedness.

Communications having to do with time can be of particular importance in nursing. For example, when clients are kept waiting for appointments, a variety of messages may be conveyed. The client may perceive the provider of care to be "too busy." The client may receive the message, "Your time is unimportant and therefore you are unimportant." People who come early may be expressing anxiety, and those who are consistently late may be expressing hostility.

Space

Space may also be used as a form of nonverbal communication. Scheflen and Birdwhistell's thesis is that, as human beings, we learn culture-specific patterns of moving in space that are identifiable and predictable. Scheflen[7] is studying each simple movement of these patterns in an effort to explain the complexity of nonverbal human communication. Space affects interaction; closeness, distance, touch, and confinement indicate some of the spatial dimensions of communication (see Chapter 3).

Behavior in space is often predictable. For instance, in an elevator people all face in the same direction, focus eyes on the floor indicators, maintain equal distance from others, and move to a new spot as more people enter. It is anxiety-provoking to be on an elevator with someone who isn't behaving in this manner, because the person is acting unpredictably.

There are certain prescribed patterns of behavior in the use of space and time that are learned and culture-specific. Conforming to prescribed behaviors communicates a message. Behaving in unprescribed ways communicates a different message. The behavior patterns learned depend on such variables as age, sex, culture, and physical limitations.

Berne's Theory

Another theorist who has contributed to the understanding of communication is Eric Berne.[9] Three aspects of Berne's theory are ego states, transactions, and script theory.

Ego States

Berne believed that all human behavior could be categorized into three states: parent ego state, adult ego state, and child ego state.[10] (These are often confused with Freud's superego, ego, and id. However, Berne's states are all functions of the ego; no aspect of his theory deals with the superego or id.) No ego state is considered more valuable than another at any time. Six-month-old infants can exhibit adult ego-state behaviors; and some of the spontaneity, creativity, and joy of the child ego state will characterize a healthy person throughout life. Healthy people are thought to respond to current situations with ego-state behaviors that promote personal growth, effective relationships, and efficient problem solving. The ego states are shown in Figure 12-3.

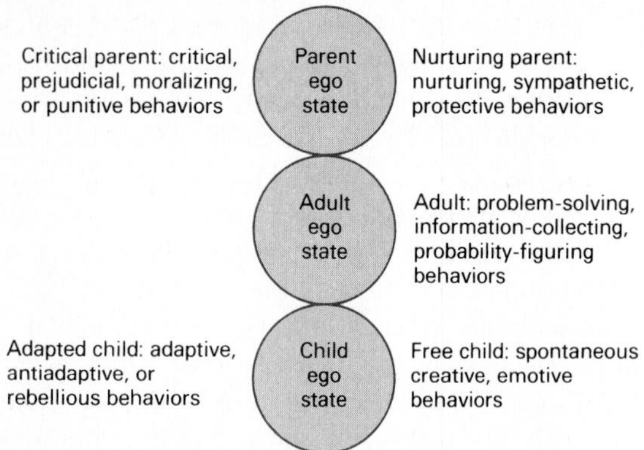

Figure 12-3 Berne's ego states.
(SOURCE: Adapted from E. Berne, *Transactional Analysis in Psychotherapy*, Grove, New York, 1961.

CHILD EGO STATE. The child ego state has two aspects: free child and adapted child. *Free child* behaviors are activities that are spontaneous and creative but also destructive. Any behavior that is free of restraint and socialization is categorized as free child behavior.

Adapted child behaviors are those that are learned. These behaviors are not spontaneous, and they can take the form of either compliance or rebellion. *Compliant* behaviors characterize the socialized person. Some examples are bypassing a mud puddle, saying "please" and "thank you," brushing teeth properly, and washing hands after using the toilet. *Noncompliant* or *rebellious* behaviors include jumping into a mud puddle when told not to, refusing to brush teeth, and assuming a "you can't make me" attitude toward socialization. In order to understand rebellious child behavior, its context must be understood. Laing[6] believed that if the context is understood, no behavior will be seen as rebellious or crazy. Suppose a parent is angry and hateful and often tells the child in subtle and blatant ways to "go play in traffic." Persons receiving this message in their child ego state may comply, a supposedly "good" behavior, and consequently find some way to hurt or kill themselves. On the other hand, they may choose to rebel and refuse to be destructive to themselves. In this case, rebellious child behavior can save a person's life. This example is not as farfetched as one may imagine. Nurses often work with people who are torn between compliance and rebellion and have difficulty expressing free child behaviors.

PARENT EGO STATE. The parent ego state has two functional aspects: critical parent and nurturing parent. The *critical parent* ego state may be perceived as angry, critical, or helpful. Examples of critical parent statements are, "You're no good," "You're a bad person," "You didn't do that right," "You should know better than that," and "Go play in the traffic." Basically, the critical parent is angry and critical. Some helpful critical parent statements are: "Don't touch that!" when someone is about to touch something harmful; "Get in here right now!" when a child is seen being offered candy by a stranger; and "If you play near that cliff once more, I'll blister you!" when a child is showing no concern for safety.

Nurturing parent behaviors show concern and care for the person. "You're special," "Want some hot chocolate?" "Your muffler will make you feel warm," "May I help you?" and "You should take care of yourself," are all examples of nurturing parent statements. Again, although nurturing parent messages sound good to receive, they sometimes are not. For instance, "You don't have to do it if you don't want to," may be constructive for a person afraid of an amusement park ride. It may be destructive when said to someone who has been unable to hold a job.

ADULT EGO STATE. There are no subdivisions in the adult ego state. Adult behaviors consist of thinking, problem solving, decision making, observing, and the like. The adult ego state has been likened to a computer, dealing with information, recognizing but experiencing no feeling. Although the adult ego state is extremely helpful, it is not fun. One would not enjoy being all adult, even if it were possible.

The adult ego state offers alternatives to the perception that one must either adapt or rebel, that one must either be nasty or be smothering. The adult ego state helps the person develop options.

People initiate and respond to communication from one of the three ego states. A person behaves from only one ego state at a time, though one may change ego states in a split second. Ego states are helpful in analyzing intrapersonal, interpersonal, and social communications.

Transactions

There are three kinds of transactions: complementary, crossed, and ulterior.[11] In a *complementary*

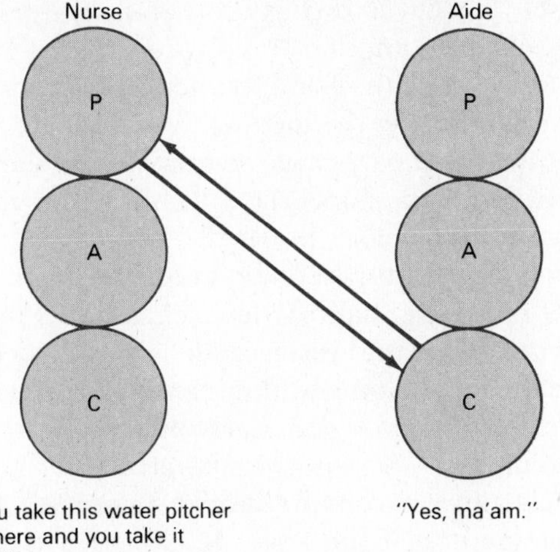

Figure 12-4 Complementary transaction.
A complementary transaction occurs when a person responds from the ego state addressed.

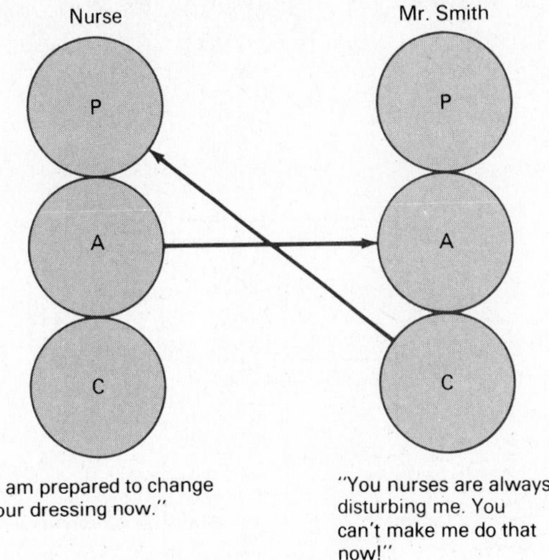

Figure 12-5 Crossed transaction.
A crossed transaction occurs when a person does not respond from the ego state addressed.

transaction, a person responds from the ego state addressed, to the ego state from which the message was received. Figure 12-4 illustrates a complementary transaction:

> The nurse, from a critical parent ego state, says to the nurse's aide (in the adapted child ego state), "You take this ice pitcher in there, and you take it now!" The aide responds from the adapted child to the nurse's critical parent, "Yes, ma'am."

Whenever a person responds from the ego state addressed and communicates to the ego state sending the message, a complementary transaction occurs.

A *crossed transaction* occurs when a person does not respond from the ego state addressed, or when a person does not address the ego state sending the message. For example:

> The nurse, from an adult ego state, says to Mr. Smith, "I am prepared to change your dressing now," expecting to receive a response from Mr. Smith's adult. Mr. Smith, however, responds from the rebellious child state to the nurse's parent state, saying, "You nurses are always disturbing me. You can't make me do that now!"

Here, the transaction has been crossed (see Figure 12-5). A crossed transaction disturbs the flow of conversation because the person receiving the message is stopped short, wondering what happened. This kind of transaction is often the first signal of a fight. On the other hand, crossing a transaction is a good way to stop an undesirable communication sequence. For instance, teenage children tired of being addressed in their child ego state are sometimes successful in being addressed in the adult ego state if they do not respond from the child ego state. Rather, they cross the transaction by responding from their adult and address the adult in the other. For instance:

> When a teacher says, from his or her parent to a student's child, "You just seem unable to get your assignments in on time. I don't know what I'm going to do with you." The student may respond from adapted child, "I'm sorry. I'll try not to do it again." Or the student may cross the transaction and say from the adult ego state, "This is a problem. I'd like to work out a schedule for getting my assignments done on time." The transaction is crossed, and the student may receive an adult response from the teacher.

The third kind of transaction is an *ulterior transaction.* It is more complex because double messages are received and sent. Ulterior transactions tend to occur when role expectations are clear and preclude certain other kinds of behaviors. An example of this kind of communication occurs in the nurse-client relationship. Certain behaviors are expected, while others, such as developing social relationships, are not acceptable. The follow-

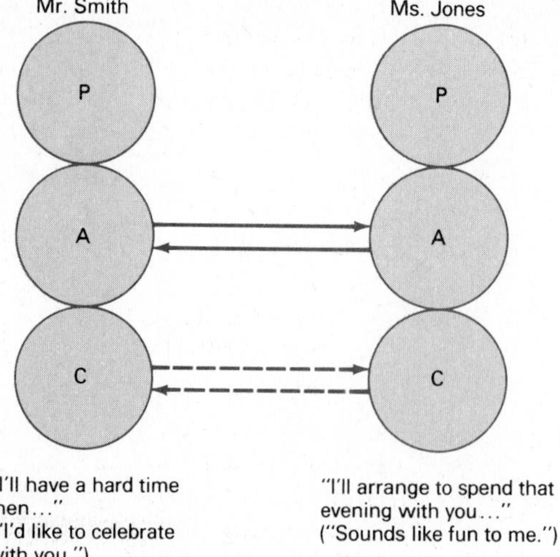

Figure 12-6 Ulterior transaction.
An ulterior transaction occurs when the interaction seems to occur on one level but actually occurs on another.

ing example (see Figure 12-6) will show how an ulterior transaction unfolds in a relationship:

> Mr. Smith, a client being discharged from an alcoholic treatment unit, says to Ms. Jones, a new nursing graduate, "I think I'll do OK except on my birthday. I'll have a hard time then, and some moral support would be a godsend." This message sounds purely informative, originating in Mr. Smith's adult. However, he may also be sending an ulterior child-to-child message, "It's my birthday and I'd like to celebrate with you." Ms. Jones answers, seemingly from her adult ego state, "That will be a difficult day. I'll arrange to spend that evening with you so you won't be tempted to drink." The ulterior message may be a child-to-child response, "Sounds like fun to me."

The difficulty with ulterior transactions is that the ulterior message may be sent unconsciously or may not be recognized as ulterior by the other person. If the nurse in the example above did not recognize the ulterior message and did not send an ulterior response, both persons might have felt misunderstood and alienated. Diagnosis of transactions may be used each time a nurse communicates with a client.

When clients need to express feelings, asking adult questions of the clients' adult ego states will elicit only facts. Clients may *report* feelings but not *express* them. In order to express bottled-up feelings, clients need to know it is acceptable to do so with the helping person. Saying (from the adult ego state), "It's OK to express your feelings," will probably elicit a computer-like response (from the adult state), "Yes, I've been led to understand that." Communicating the message analogically, through the nurturing parent ego state, saying to the client's child ego state, "How did you feel when your dad forgave you before he died?" more clearly communicates nurturance and empathy.

On the other hand, when a client lacks problem-solving ability and resolves life issues by becoming dependent on others, the client's adult ego state needs to be developed. Carrying on a parent-child relationship will not promote growth. Adult-adult transactions have more growth potential. Because dependent persons have developed a pattern of parent-child transactions, they often cross the adult transaction by reverting to the child ego state. The nurse who understands Berne's theory will recognize the need to cross the transaction again and respond in the adult ego state.

Script Theory

Berne believed that clients were capable of deciding what they needed, how their growth should be directed, and how they should live. He developed script theory to explain the control people exercise over their lives. *Script theory* described the process by which a life script is decided on.[11]

At an early age, on the basis of integration of childhood experiences—including fairy tales, comic books, television, and experiences with significant people—children decide what the world is like and choose their places in it. This happens even though the child has undeveloped assessment skills, thinks very concretely, and has inadequate information. People live according to those early decisions, which are like lifelong self-fulfilling prophecies. Scripts can make people feel that they have no choice, even though an early decision is now obsolete and the resulting behavior is troublesome.

Much of the theory of *transactional analysis* uses language that appeals to the child ego state. Since the child has decided the life script, it is the child in the person who must be addressed. The parent and adult ego-state efforts are sabotaged by a neglected, starved child ego state.

The need for *strokes*—gestures of personal recognition—motivates human behavior. Strokes can be *positive* ("I love you"), *negative* ("I wish you had never been born"), or *plastic,* which means that they sound positive but feel negative. One of the first (implicit) questions children ask is, "How do I get strokes around here?" The answer depends on the people in the child's life who give recognition. They may stroke feelings such as happiness, anger, or depression. They may reward behavior such as helplessness, helpfulness, or rebelliousness. The child may decide that exhibiting stroked behavior is the way to get strokes, now and forever. Adults can continue to use those behaviors, fearing that if the strokes stop they will shrivel up and die. One motivation for change is the realization that one is no longer dependent on childhood sources of strokes, that one has many other options as an adult.

Ruesch's Theory

In the process of socialization to the nursing profession, students learn to communicate therapeutically. The ability to develop therapeutic relationships is crucial to the art and science of nursing. It is within a relationship that one learns trust, tries out new behavior, chooses freely, and expresses emotion. A *therapeutic nursing relationship* is a goal-directed process that promotes synchronous patterns of interaction between client and environment (see Chapter 13). Ruesch identified the components of the process as perception, evaluation, and transmission.[12]

Therapeutic Communication

According to Ruesch, *therapeutic communication* is the hallmark of a therapeutic relationship. It is the art and process of reaching a person with messages designed to facilitate health. Therapeutic communication provides healing experiences. Each message is deliberately chosen and considered in relation to a client's need for growth. To communicate therapeutically, nurses assess and diagnose clients' needs. They develop goals in collaboration with each client, choosing communication patterns designed to foster growth and accomplish the goals they formulate. Because each client has unique needs and goals, the nurse communicates therapeutically in a different way with each client.

Characteristics of Therapeutic Communication

There are seven characteristics or messages to be conveyed in the process of therapeutic communication.[12] These messages are rarely communicated verbally but rather are transmitted analogically. Clients receive these messages more clearly when they are communicated in nonverbal form, since nonverbal messages are almost always true. The messages that are transmitted in a therapeutic communication are acceptance, interest, respect, honesty, assistance, permission, and protection.

1. *Acceptance* is a favorable reception of another person. This does not mean approval of the person's behavior; rather, it implies, "You have a right to exist, to live your life, to have somebody care about you." It is only when people feel accepted as persons that any consideration will be given to changing.
2. *Interest* conveys a feeling of genuine curiosity, a desire to know another person. Interest is communicated by asking about those aspects of a person's life that others reject. Nurses demonstrate by their attitude that "everything can be talked about here." This suggests to the client, "I want to know all about you," and communicates a therapeutic message with compassion and skill.
3. *Respect* is the process of showing consideration for another. It is communicated by listening attentively, explaining the intent of the relationship, obtaining informed consent, collaborating on shared goals, calling the client by name, arriving and leaving on time, and keeping one's word. False reassurance is to be avoided; it is a form of disrespect that conveys the message, "Your feelings are unfounded."
4. *Honesty* is sincerity and truthfulness. Honesty without respect, acceptance, and interest is nontherapeutic. There are many responses one may make at any time in a relationship. A nurse communicating therapeutically chooses the message that facilitates the greatest growth in the client. In the context of the relationship, after the client has received the messages of respect, acceptance, and interest, it may be appropriate for the nurse to say, "My mind wanders when you talk about your feelings. How do you feel when you report your feelings?" Clients may be feeling detached from their feelings, and discussing this may open up new avenues for exploration.
5. *Assistance* means being present and helping clients. A therapeutic relationship requires the nurse to commit time and energy and to invest

self in another person. Assistance conveys the idea that the nurse is present and available to the client and has tangible aid to offer. The nurse utilizes theory, research, and selected techniques to communicate in a way that fosters growth.

6. *Permission* in the context of communication is defined as consent or authorization to behave in new ways. Often, clients are afraid to choose freely and to act autonomously. They are bound by their misconceived archaic rules and magical thinking. The person communicating therapeutically conveys the message that it is acceptable to try new ways of behaving.
7. *Protection* is defined as ensuring safety. Permission without protection is nontherapeutic and sometimes dangerous. Clients must feel that the helping person is able to keep bad things from happening. The client must learn to trust the care giver as a child trusts a parent. The nurse assumes the responsibility of working with clients to anticipate trouble spots with the new behavior, thus assuring success of the new behavior. For example, giving permission to a withdrawn person to be assertive, without creating a climate for success, may lead to aggressive, even violent, behavior and subsequent withdrawal from which that individual may never again venture.

Theory forms the basis for communicating therapeutically. Therapeutic communication provides a context within which genuine, goal-directed relationships that facilitate health may be offered.

TYPES OF COMMUNICATION

There are two types of communication: intrapersonal and interpersonal. The two may occur simultaneously. The need for common symbols, shared behaviors, and validating the meaning of messages becomes clear when the two types of communication are considered.

Intrapersonal Communication

Communication at the *intrapersonal* level occurs within oneself and consists of getting in touch with oneself. Planning a sequence of actions toward a goal (for example, when one says to oneself, "First, I will go in and meet the clients, then I'll obtain permission to care for them, then I'll do the nursing assessments . . .") is an example of intrapersonal communication. One also communicates nonverbally at an intrapersonal level. For example:

> June noticed that she had been sitting with her arms and legs crossed, looking over her left shoulder at a person speaking to her. She realized as she received her own nonverbal message that she was annoyed and not interested in listening to the message, though she felt compelled to be polite. What if she had not received the nonverbal message? The message would have remained unconscious, and June would have been unaware of the feelings she was experiencing.

Interpersonal Communication

Interpersonal communication is communication among two or more people. It has both verbal and nonverbal components. Interpersonal communication is simultaneous and complex; it consists of a multitude of factors for each person involved. Verbal and nonverbal messages are being sent simultaneously. Some are received; some are not. Some are understood; some may be misunderstood. Nonverbal messages may be sent unconsciously; verbal messages may be perceived incorrectly. By use of feedback, however, people involved in interpersonal communication remain relevant to one another. There are three kinds of interpersonal communication: social, collegial, and facilitative.

Social Communication

Social communication occurs in everyday settings among people who are friends, acquaintances, and relatives. Topics of social communication include work, politics, social activities, vacations, and family affairs such as child rearing. This type of communication is characterized by lack of a goal, lack of interdependence among participants, and superficiality.

Lack of a goal refers to the fact that social communication does not necessarily have a purpose other than interpersonal contact and enjoyment. *Lack of interdependence* refers to the fact that in this kind of communication people do not expect help or guidance. Varying levels of intimacy and self-disclosure are observed in social communication, but in general, self-disclosure is not encouraged and may even be taboo; therefore, *superficiality* is the norm. People may, of course, have intimate social relationships that move beyond superficial conversation; however, even in such relationships there is no expectation of help.

Collegial Communication

Collegial communication occurs among colleagues. In the context of nursing, these people are helpers whose purpose is to collaborate in the treatment of clients. Although there are both verbal and nonverbal messages in collegial communication, nonverbal messages are validated only when they seem to be breaking down goal-directed verbal messages and thus impairing treatment. Collegial communication in nursing is confidential; that is, discussions about clients and the variables influencing their treatment are not shared with anyone else for any reason unless explicit permission is given.

Facilitative Communication

In the context of nursing, *facilitative communication* takes place between helper and client. The content of facilitative communication is meaningful (not superficial); it moves into the client's areas of concern. As a process, facilitative communication focuses on the client—the person who needs or seeks help. The nurse actively listens to each client and responds in ways that convey acceptance and understanding, thus encouraging clients to talk openly about themselves. Sharing feelings is considered beneficial to clients because it brings their emotions to the surface and leads them to insights about themselves. Moreover, when feelings can be identified in this way, people have more control over them. For example:

> A male client who had had a colostomy was concerned about how others would treat him, and particularly how his wife would respond to him sexually when he returned home. Brooding over this problem magnified his worries and fears. Talking about it with a nurse helped him recognize his own feelings and put them, and his situation, in perspective.

Many people are frightened by intense emotions—their own as well as those of others. They feel that it is better to avoid expressing such feelings, even if not expressing them creates problems. This belief may arise from the fear that others will be intolerant, insensitive, indifferent, or simply reluctant to listen; and that fear is sometimes well founded. If, for example, a client and a nurse have difficulty with the same feeling, each may want to avoid verbalizing it. (For instance, a nurse for whom death is a source of anxiety will have difficulty encouraging a client with a terminal illness to express his or her feelings about it.) On the other hand, a nurse who accepts feelings as natural will be able to encourage clients to share them; and when feelings (such as fears) are expressed to a supportive person who tries to understand the situation, they can be viewed realistically, analyzed, and resolved.

Facilitative communication in nursing has three goals:

1. *Exploration* of one's own feelings, thoughts, behavior, and experiences
2. *Understanding* of the roles played by the client and other significant people that contribute to identified problems
3. *Action* directed at resolving problematic areas of the client's life through the identification and implementation of alternative options[4]

The work of the communication theorists Watzlawick, Beavin and Jackson;[1] Scheflen[7] and Birdwhistell;[8] Berne[9,10] and Ruesch,[12] which was presented in a theoretical context earlier in this chapter, provides a basis for the principles and skills of facilitative communication that will be discussed in the remaining sections.

SKILLS OF FACILITATIVE COMMUNICATION

It is not unusual for a beginning nurse not to know how to respond to a client or what to say next. Relying on social skills (such as those used for developing friendships) has proved to be unsuccessful in establishing a relationship with a client. Therefore, nurses and other health professionals have developed a set of attending and responding strategies, called *facilitative communication skills,* for developing more effective relationships with clients.

Two kinds of skills facilitate effective communication: *attending skills* and *responding skills.* Attending skills involve active listening and observing in order to evaluate verbal and nonverbal communication.[13,14] Responding skills involve verbal strategies that encourage people to communicate.[13,14] The following sections present attending and responding skills that can be used as guidelines for facilitating communication. It is important for the reader to understand that these are *not* intended as a set of rules. Communication and people are too complex for rules to be rigidly applied. Each nurse must modify the skills so that they fit his or her style and adapt them so that they are relevant to each interaction.

Attending Skills

Therapeutic interactions require something that can be called *presence.* Presence involves being with a person both physically and psychologically, and with a certain degree of intensity. *Attending* is using the self so as to communicate to another person that you are paying attention—for example, that you are listening to what is being said. Attending skills involve *physical skills* (making the body attentive) and *psychosocial skills* (making the mind attentive).

Physical Attending Skills

The body plays a large part in interpersonal communication. What is done with the body can emphasize—or, on the other hand, confuse or contradict—a message that is being communicated in words. For example:

> Cindy invites Bill to go sailing, and he turns to her, looks her in the eye, smiles, and says, "Great! When will we go?" What Bill did with his body confirmed his verbal message. However, if Cindy invites Bill to go sailing and he turns away from her, hesitates, hunches his shoulders, looks down, and finally says, "Yes, OK," his body is saying no even though his words are saying yes. In this case Bill's body is conveying the real message, and it's the opposite of the spoken words.

It is impossible *not* to communicate with the body. What is done with the body and how it is done will either facilitate or inhibit the interactive process.

There are six basic physical attending skills:[14]

1. *Facing the other person squarely.* This is the basic posture of involvement. Facing another person squarely says, "I'm available to you; I choose to be with you." Turning the body away from another person while talking lowers the level of involvement with that person.
2. *Adopting an open posture.* Crossed arms and crossed legs can be signs of defensiveness or lessened involvement with others. An open posture, especially open arms, is a sign that the listener is open to the other person and to what he or she has to say. It is also a nondefensive position.
3. *Leaning toward the other person.* This is another sign of presence, availability, and involvement. It indicates that the listener is making a consistent effort to take in what the other person is communicating.
4. *Maintaining direct eye contact.* The listener should spend much of the time looking directly at the other person. Some people object to this idea; they say that this can be frightening or can make the other person uncomfortable. However, there is a difference between staring another person down (which may be an attack) and maintaining the direct eye contact indicative of interested involvement.
5. *Remaining relaxed.* The listener should sit or stand quietly without excessive movement and fidgeting. This does not imply that one should sit rigidly in a fixed position. That would communicate negative tension and discomfort. Instead, a relaxed posture communicates a natural readiness and ease in listening to what is being said. It says, "I feel comfortable with you."
6. *Creating a relaxing environment.* This communicates concern about the physical setting in which communication is taking place. It involves providing for privacy and comfort. Privacy is the degree to which people can interact without interference, distraction, and loss of confidentiality. Privacy is usually ensured by setting apart an area or room for the people who are interacting. Comfort relates to factors such as seating, lighting, noise level, and space. Seating should be comfortable, but not so relaxing that people want to go to sleep. Lighting should be soft, but bright; dim or glaring light is harsh and can be distracting. The noise level should be low so that it is not distracting. Space should meet the territorial needs of the people involved. Placement of people and furniture should reflect boundary needs. For example:

Tom, a nurse, and Mike, a cardiac client, went into the lounge to begin discussing Mike's discharge plans. There were many informal seating arrangements available in which the nurse and the client could have sat next to each other; however, Mike selected a seat at a table with chairs on opposite sides. The second time they met Mike selected the same seat. But the third time they met Mike said, "I'd like to sit over here today." He indicated an area in which two chairs were next to one another. Mike rearranged his chair so that it was touching Tom's and permitted direct eye contact.

It is important to observe how people use interpersonal space. Space can be used to increase or decrease interpersonal distance, and it is often an indicator of intimacy and involvement.

Psychosocial Attending Skills

Active listening is a psychosocial attending skill that involves listening to all the messages the other person is sending. It involves paying attention to two sources of messages: spoken words and nonverbal behavior. This type of listening is an active rather than a passive process; it conveys respect for the other person and thus will facilitate the development of relationships.

THE SPOKEN WORD. The effective listener tries to hear both content and feelings that are being verbally communicated. The listener wants to know about the experiences, behavior, and underlying feelings of the speaker. This material enables the listener to identify patterns and themes that become important keys to understanding the person within his or her own frame of reference. The following psychosocial listening skills relate to the verbal message.[13]

1. *Focusing your complete attention on the speaker.* Do not be preoccupied with yourself. Suspend thinking about your own experiences and problems and suspend personal judgments about the client.
2. *Listening to everything that is being said.* It is important to get a total picture of the person's verbal communication. Selective listening, which is often used to keep the anxiety of the listener in check, is ineffective because it may keep the listener from hearing important information. Examples of selective listening are hearing superficial instead of intimate things, praise instead of criticism, and positive parts of sentences instead of disturbing parts—or vice versa.
3. *Analyzing the verbal message that is being communicated.* A speaker may relate both relevant and irrelevant information. The listener needs to sort it out and come up with the essence of the message so that he or she can begin to make sense of what is being heard.
4. *Identifying themes and patterns in the verbal communication.* After the sorting process has taken place, the listener will realize the there is a structure to what is being expressed. Themes and patterns relate to this structure and convey underlying meanings. Examples of themes and patterns are: feelings of powerlessness at work; excessive reliance on others for positive feelings about self; talking only in a positive way; avoiding talking about personal strengths. Identification of themes and patterns enables the listener to respond with understanding.
5. *Summarizing the content and feelings that have been expressed.* It is important to summarize not only content but also feelings.

NONVERBAL BEHAVIOR. Much of the meaning of a message—65 percent or more—is conveyed by nonverbal behavior,[8] although many nonverbal behaviors are interpreted by verbal symbols. Verbal and nonverbal behaviors complement each other and consequently cannot be examined independently. The four major forms of nonverbal messages—kinesics, paralanguage, proxemics, and appearance—can be seen as ways of:

1. Confirming what is being said
2. Strengthening and emphasizing what is being said
3. Adding emotional color to what is being said
4. Confusing or contradicting what is being said

Verbal and nonverbal behavior, then, fit together and function to confirm, complement, or contradict each other. The listener puts this information into context so that the communication can be understood and responded to appropriately.

Confirming nonverbal behavior. The degree of congruence between verbal and nonverbal behavior often provides clues about the validity of a client's verbal communication.[5] A high degree of congruence between verbal and nonverbal behavior is usually a good indicator that the client means what he or she is saying. For example:

Jane, a depressed client, walked into the nurse's office for her daily session with a disheveled appearance, a slow gait, and stooped posture. She slowly sat down in the chair and hunched over without establishing eye contact with the nurse. In a shaky voice, she haltingly said, "I'm upset about telling my parents that I want to get my own apartment." She sat there trembling and wringing her hands, waiting for the nurse to respond. This client's verbal and nonverbal communications are congruent.

Complementary nonverbal behavior. In some situations not only will a client's verbal and nonverbal communication be congruent, but the nonverbal part of the message will strengthen, complement, or emphasize the verbal part. For example:

John, a client who has identified a problem in being assertive with his family, feels that the family has taken advantage of his unwillingness to say "No" to them. John and the nurse have been working on how he can express himself more forcefully and convincingly. At a family session John's wife says to the nurse, "Oh, John doesn't feel that way about my telling him what to do." John leans forward in his chair, makes direct eye contact with his wife, and points his finger at her. In a loud, firm voice he emphatically states, "I will no longer tolerate your telling anybody how I feel. Those days are *over.* I will be the one to tell you *and* anybody else necessary *exactly* how I feel from now on." He maintains his position and stares at his wife, who sits back with her mouth open.

Often, nonverbal behavior adds emotional color to verbal messages. For example:

Alison has been hospitalized for 4 months following multiple fractures sustained in an automobile accident. When discharge plans are initially discussed, Alison appears reluctant to leave the protective environment of the hospital. She begins to experience various nonspecific physical complaints. After 1 month of working with the psychiatric liaison nurse, however, she is finally ready to go home. She walks up to the nurse's station and, with sparkling eyes, a smile on her face, and a toss of her chin, says to the head nurse in a pleasant tone of voice, "I'm finally ready to fly from your nest, and, as much as I love you all, I won't be sorry to say good-bye!" The nurse smiles, gently touches Alison's arm, and says in a lilting voice, "Alison, I'm just glad that you sound so ready to leave us."

Contradictory nonverbal behavior. When verbal messages do not agree with nonverbal messages, communications become confusing. Often, the sender is not aware that there is a conflict in a message, and the receiver of the contradictory message is uncertain about what the real message is. For example:

A nurse, Ms. M., is working on self-feeding skills with Mr. L., a client who has had a cerebrovascular accident (CVA). Mr. L., attempting to feed himself, spills much of the food on himself and the bed. Ms. M., who wants to convey her acceptance of the situation, says, "Don't be upset. We all have days when it seems as if we're not making much progress." This sounds supportive, but, as she says it, she has a look of disgust on her face, roughly takes the spoon out of Mr. L.'s hand, and begins to feed him, sighing and shaking the crumbs from the soiled linens. Her nonverbal behavior appears to invalidate her supportive verbal statement. The client is likely to become confused and think, "Is it OK to make mistakes? Should I or should I not get upset? Is she saying, 'You're clumsy; you can't even perform a simple task that any bright 2-year-old is capable of doing'?" The nurse has said one thing, but her behavior expresses the exact opposite of her words. The client may very well accept her nonverbal behavior as the truth and begin to see himself as a hopeless case.

A client may also present a nurse with a contradictory message. This is common when clients verbally state what they think others want to hear but simultaneously contradict the verbal message with nonverbal behavior. For example:

A nurse asks Joan N., the wife of an alcoholic, if she would like to attend an AA meeting. Joan, in a low tone of voice, with halting words, and no eye contact, says, "Well, ... sure.... I'm free that night...." Her words are affirmative, indicating that she is available. However, her nonverbal behavior implies her uncertainty and hesitation about going to the AA meeting.

The various functions of nonverbal communication are summarized in Table 12-2.

Responding Skills

Strategies that nurses and other health professionals use when verbally communicating with clients (and colleagues) are refered to as *responding skills.* These skills are used to convey understanding, validate perceptions, and provide feedback, as well

Table 12-2 Functions of Nonverbal Communication

Function of Nonverbal Communication	Verbal Behavior	Nonverbal Behavior
Confirms verbal message	"I'm upset about telling my parents that I want to move out."	Voice is shaky, words are haltingly stated, hands are wrung, no eye contact is established
Strengthens or emphasizes verbal message	"I don't like to be treated that way."	Loud voice, harsh tone, emphatic statement of words, forward leaning, direct eye contact, hands on hips
Adds emotional color to verbal message	"I like you so much."	Words sing, tone is modulated, smiles, direct eye contact is established, arm of other person is touched
Contradicts or confuses verbal message	"Well . . . sure. . . . I think I'm free."	Affirming words, low tone of voice, loss of eye contact, slumped posture, forehead rubbed

as to clarify and maintain a specific focus. Responding skills are a way of creating "verbal presence" and a sense of involvement with a client throughout an interview or relationship. Two components of responding will be discussed here: the "core dimensions" of the nurse-client relationship and responding strategies that facilitate communication.

Core Dimensions of Facilitative Communication

The *core dimensions* of the nurse-client relationship are empathy, respect, genuineness, concreteness, immediacy, and confrontation. They provide a foundation for facilitative communication: each of them describes a way of relating with a client so that effective communication can take place. Relationships with clients are begun, built upon, and maintained through facilitative communication. In Chapter 13, the core dimensions will be explored as aspects of the nurse-client relationship. In this chapter they will be discussed as principles underlying facilitative communication.[13,14]

EMPATHY. *Empathy* is the temporary experiencing of another person's feelings. It involves getting inside another person's world as he or she perceives it.[15] Empathy allows one to understand what someone else has said and then communicate it back to the speaker in one's own words and in terms of expressed and underlying feelings. Responses in facilitative communication should be directed not only at what a person says directly, but also at what the person hints, implies, or communicates nonverbally.[13,16] Empathy is therefore the most important dimension of facilitative communication. Without it there is no basis for meaningful interpersonal exchange and exploration.

Empathy also communicates interest and a sense of caring; it provides an opportunity to accept messages, refute them, or elaborate on them. The door is open for further client-centered communication. Validation of the nurse's perceptions by the client is possible because the client has an avenue for responding, knowing that the nurse cares and will listen. The client feels valued as a person and able to respond; and the nurse will be likely to obtain client-centered data on which to build individualized nursing care.[17]

RESPECT. *Respect* communicates the nurse's availability to work with the client and acceptance of the client's ideas, feelings, experiences, and rights. It conveys belief in clients' ability to solve their own problems—with assistance—and assume responsibility for their own lives. Respect conveys regard for the client as a unique person. Efforts are directed toward supporting and developing individuality and inner resources, not making the client over in the therapist's image. This involves suspending critical judgment about the client and communicating in a nonjudgmental way.[13,14]

GENUINENESS. *Genuineness* is closely related to respect; it is the ability to be real and honest with another person. The expression of genuineness means that the nurse does not take refuge behind a professional mask but instead communicates with the client as an authentic person. This means that:

1. Nurses need to develop their own communication and relationship style.
2. Nurses need to be willing to take risks in *appropriately* disclosing their own reactions and feelings as they occur in an interactional process.

3. Nurses need to develop the ability to be nondefensive. This entails knowing their own strengths and weaknesses. When clients respond negatively to nurses, an attempt is made to examine and understand what the client is thinking and feeling to see if what is being stated has validity. Rather than being self-protective, nurses will utilize self-assessment skills to see if they are, in fact, contributing to a therapeutic stall[13,14] (see Chapter 13).

Genuineness also involves honesty. *Honesty* implies communicating in a consistent, open, and frank way. *Consistency* means that the nurse does not feel and think one thing and say another. *Openness* and *frankness* mean that the nurse uses tact and timing to express thoughts and feelings. Direct feedback is important for clients, but it must be communicated in a way that does not seem like brutal frankness. *Tact* and *timing* involve knowing when to withhold information because the client is not yet ready to hear it—for example, at the beginning of a relationship before trust has been established. Indiscriminate use of honesty will serve only to erect barriers in the development of a working partnership. A client who experiences the nurse's authenticity is encouraged to take further risks with authenticity and genuineness. This will facilitate the therapeutic process of self-exploration and self-understanding, as the client is then more willing to look inside, share discoveries with the nurse, and risk making changes.

CONCRETENESS. *Concreteness* refers to being specific, succinct, and clear when communicating. Concreteness has two aspects. First, it involves eliminating psychiatric jargon from one's vocabulary and using language that clearly expresses what is meant in words the client understands. Second, it involves being specific and to the point. Nurses must be aware of these factors in their own communication as well as in that of their clients. Clients who are permitted to speak in vague, general, unfocused ways will come up with nothing more than vague, general, unfocused statements of problems and solutions. Questions that yield the most concrete information are those that ask "What?" "How?" "When?" and "With what feeling?" rather than "Why?" "Why" questions allude to causes, which are seldom obvious. To ask the client to come up with causes is often to "whistle in the wind." Clients can talk endlessly about causes, but such talk usually does not produce the kind of self-understanding that leads to effective goals and actions.[13,14]

IMMEDIACY. *Immediacy* refers to communication about what is happening here and now in an interpersonal relationship. It is sometimes called *you-me talk* because it has to do with what is happening between client and nurse.

The purpose of immediate responses on the part of the *nurse* is to help clients gain specific and clear understanding of what they are doing and how they are interacting with the nurse. Over time, problematic patterns and themes will emerge from the nurse-client relationship; these can be examined, and modifications of ineffective patterns can be transferred to relationships in the outside world.

The nurse encourages immediate responses on the part of the *client* as well, because they increase clients' awareness of what is being experienced in an interaction and their ability to share this information with the nurse.[13,14]

Because immediacy involves the feelings of the client and the nurse, it is often difficult to put into action. Both client and nurse may be frightened and defensive about what is being communicated, and they may attempt to evade direct responses. This is particularly true when immediacy is attempted before a solid relationship has been established or when the competence of the nurse is shaky and easily threatened—as the exchange with nurse A in the following example shows:

CLIENT: I'm still not convinced of the value of therapy; you sit around and talk a lot, but things don't seem to get much better. It isn't easy to keep talking about yourself.

NURSE A: This whole thing doesn't seem to be going anyplace. I feel frustrated and question your motivation to work at changing right now. (*Nontherapeutic*)

NURSE B: From a number of things you've said so far, I have the feeling that you're not sure whether you can trust me or not. You're still not convinced that I'm on your side. (*Therapeutic*)

If the nurse is skillful, the client first learns to accept direct communication from the helper and then learns how to address the helpful in the same way. If the nurse does not know how to accept immediacy, the client can hardly be expected to learn this skill from the helper.

CONFRONTATION. Constructive confrontation often leads to productive change on the part of clients. *Constructive confrontation* means responsible unmasking of discrepancies, evasions, distortions, games, and smoke screens the client uses to hide from both self-understanding and behavioral change.[13] It calls attention to discrepancies between what the client says (verbal communication) and what the client does (nonverbal communication). It involves challenging clients' undeveloped, underdeveloped, unused, and misused skills and resources. It also helps clients examine the consequences of behavior. Constructive confrontation is *not* attacking or blaming clients "for their own good." Destructive or punitive confrontation may relieve the aggressor of a burden, but it does not help the other person learn to live more effectively.[14]

There are six guidelines to follow when using constructive confrontation:

1. Use personal pronouns such as *I, my,* and *me* when making statements.
2. Describe a person's observable unproductive behavior and its effect on you.
3. Translate your thoughts and feelings into "relationship statements" that express how you think and feel about a person in an interaction.
4. Respond to a person with skills that convey understanding—such as reflecting, restating, and verbalizing the implied.
5. Specifically name feelings to avoid making vague, evasive statements that don't convey clear, precise feedback.
6. Focus the statement on what is said rather than on why it is said.

Confrontation can involve giving and interpreting information. *Informational confrontations* describe observable behaviors of the client. *Interpretive confrontations* describe the nurse's thoughts and feelings about what has been implied by the client. Interpretive confrontation is directed toward underlying patterns and themes in the client's verbal and nonverbal communication from which the nurse makes inferences about the client's behavior. In the examples of constructive confrontation that follow, the client's maneuver is in capital letters, and the nurse's constructive response follows in ordinary type.

DISCREPANCY: I hear you say *yes* with your words, but your body language says *no.*

DISTORTION: My sense of it is that you equate stubbornness with commitment.

GAMES, SMOKE SCREENS: I appreciate your wanting to discuss in private what happened in the group tonight, but I'm a little uncomfortable being singled out like this. I think that all of us should look at the level of trust in the group.

EVASIONS: I have a sense of vagueness when you tell me you're angry with your husband. I don't hear what it is he does that makes you feel unappreciated.

Responding Strategies

Responding strategies are ways of talking with clients that encourage them to communicate. In the nurse-client relationship this becomes an important part of helping clients engage in the process of self-exploration, self-understanding, and change. The reader is reminded that while many of the following strategies are very helpful, there are drawbacks to such techniques if they are overused or used inappropriately. It is important for nurses to identify ways in which these strategies are both assets and liabilities, thereby facilitating more realistic and effective use of them.

BROAD OPENINGS. Lead-in phrases or beginning statements that encourage the client to discuss his or her problem are called *broad openings.* They assist the client in taking the initiative in introducing topics, focusing on feelings, and identifying and thinking through problems. Statements such as, "Is there anything special you would like to talk about today?" and, "What have you been thinking about since our last session?" make it easier for the client to take the lead or determine the focus.[18]

OPEN-ENDED QUESTIONS. Questions that do not influence the direction of a client's responses are called *open-ended.* They are phrased in such a way that a wide variety of answers will be possible. They encourage the client to express, in his or her own way, ideas and feelings on a particular topic. They allow the client freedom to structure the answer in an individual way. (For example, the nurse asks, "How can I help you to be more comfortable at night?")

In contrast, *closed-ended* questions ask for specific data and limit clients' responses. They tend to cut off communication rather than encourage it. Although closed-ended questions are sometimes necessary to elicit clear-cut and precise information (such as name, age, and religion), they have been structured by the nurse and therefore require less thought on the part of the client than open-ended questions do. As a result, the answers will be less revealing than answers to open-ended questions. For example, the question, "With whom do you live?" has only a limited range of possible answers: wife, husband, parents, friends, nobody. A more open-ended way of phrasing the question would be, "Tell me about the people you live with." This would uncover not only who the client lives with but also something about each of them.

CONVEYING INFORMATION. Information is conveyed to a client by making statements that supply data. New input encourages further clarification. Withholding useful information may prevent the client from making informed choices or decisions. When a client is seeking direct information, the nurse should not ask the client what he or she thinks the answer is. If the client knew the answer, the information would not have been requested in most cases. When conveying information, nurses need to avoid giving advice or providing interpretations.

RESTATEMENT. A nurse can convey understanding of what a client has just said by *restating* it. This means that the nurse paraphrases the main content and feeling of the client's message, using new (and probably fewer) words. This indicates that the nurse is listening to the client and is trying to enter and understand the client's frame of reference. Paraphrasing also helps to highlight important parts of the client's message that might otherwise be lost or obscured by details. The following dialogue illustrates restatement.

CLIENT: I don't know what's going on. I study hard, but I just don't get good marks. I think I study as hard as anyone else, but all my efforts seem to go down the tube. I don't know what else to do.

NURSE: It sounds as if you feel frustrated because even when you think you try hard, you fail. Perhaps you also feel a little sorry for yourself.

REFLECTION. Reflection involves two dimensions of communication: content and feeling.[19] *Reflecting the content* of a message means repeating a client's basic statement. This provides the client with an opportunity to hear and think about what he or she has said. The danger inherent in content reflection is that it can become simply hollow repetition, and the nurse can end up sounding like a parrot. If it is misused or overused, it will not be therapeutically effective. Here is an example of content reflection:

CLIENT: I'm so discouraged. I thought I'd be home from the hospital today.

NURSE: You're discouraged today?

Reflection of feelings means verbalizing what is implied or hinted at by a client. In reflecting feelings the nurse seeks to identify the underlying meaning of content. Themes, patterns, and indirect expressions of thoughts and feelings emerge as the nurse considers what the client is really expressing. The nurse goes beyond what the client has explicitly stated and provides additional material for the client to consider. Verbalizing the implied is useful because it provides a more objective picture of the situation and helps the client view problems in greater depth and with more accuracy. It also encourages the client to make additional clarifying comments. Here is an example of reflection of feelings:

CLIENT: I'm so discouraged. I thought I'd be home from the hospital today.

NURSE: It sounds as though you feel discouraged because you're still in the hospital and you expected more of yourself than has happened.

CLIENT: Yes; I thought I would feel fine after surgery. I always expect a lot of myself; my family does, too.

NURSE: The surgery took more out of you than you anticipated.

CLIENT: Yes. In the past, I've always looked forward to going home and picking up my responsibilities, but this time ...

NURSE: It sounds as if this time you're not sure you can do it.

CLIENT: I don't think I can do it. The kids require so much attention—I'm really afraid I'll get sick again.

CONNECTING ISLANDS OF INFORMATION. Nurses attempt to build bridges between, to *connect*, "islands" of feelings, thoughts, experiences, and behavior. This means helping the client connect seemingly isolated phenomena by filling in blanks and establishing relationships.[13] For example:

> A client, Ralph, presents two islands of information: (1) his disagreements with his wife about sex, parenting, and budgeting, and (2) his progressively heavier drinking, which upsets his wife. The missing link might be that the client is using his drinking behavior as a way of punishing his wife. The following response could be directed to Ralph: "I wonder what the relationship is between your drinking and your disagreements with your wife. It sounds as though it might be an effective way of punishing her."

The nurse must strive for accuracy in making such connections and present them collaboratively to the client as theories for consideration, not as statements of fact. It may take considerable discussion between nurse and client for an accurate picture to be established. For example, a nurse and client were working toward identifying factors contributing to the client's social withdrawal, particularly her reluctance to engage in relationships with men. The following interaction took place:

CLIENT: I'm uncomfortable, really anxious, in a social situation. Not so much with adults, people older than myself, but more with my peers.

NURSE: What is it about relating with young men and women (as opposed to older adults) that makes you tense and want to withdraw?

CLIENT: With older people, I feel that I know what to say and how to act. I know the "good little girl" role very well. But with friends . . .

NURSE: Are you saying that a parent-child or adult-child interaction is a known, comfortable situation that you don't feel the same urge to run from?

CLIENT: Yes. It's as if I know they'll take care of me; I may not like it, but it will be basically OK.

NURSE: What do you suppose the connection is between relating with peers, feeling anxious, and needing to withdraw socially?

CLIENT: I have to be adult in that kind of relationship; you know—be responsible for myself. I don't think I can do that. I'm petrified of being an adult with another adult.

This example provides an abbreviated version of the kind of interaction needed to connect islands of information and find a pattern; an actual interaction might take much more time. The nurse and client in the above example might have had to connect many more data before a complete picture was formulated.

STATING OBSERVATIONS. *Stating observations* involves descriptions by the nurse of interpersonal dynamics in the nurse-client relationship. These dynamics explain connections between overt behavior and underlying thoughts and feelings in nurse and client. They enable feelings having to do with transference and countertransference to surface for examination, clarification, and resolution (see Chapter 13). Stating observations is an aspect of immediacy and is most appropriately used when trust has been established in the nurse-client relationship. Following is an example of stating observations:

NURSE: You were telling me about fighting with your mom this weekend, and suddenly you began fidgeting, looked away, and then got up to take a walk. When I called to you, you told me to go to hell.

CLIENT: That's right—shove it.

NURSE: I wonder how you feel when I encourage you to talk about something that makes you uncomfortable.

PROVIDING FEEDBACK. *Feedback* involves giving constructive information to clients about how the nurse perceives and hears them. The nurse describes his or her perceptions about clients' thoughts, feelings, and behaviors in interactions. This offers the clients an opportunity to verify, modify, or correct the nurse's perceptions. It also provides an opportunity for clients to see how others perceive them. Feedback of this kind—a validation system—ensures that the nurse accurately understands the client. It is a method of correcting and clearing up confusing communications quickly. It minimizes the possibility that the nurse will make false assumptions, since misperceptions can be cleared up before they become misunderstandings.

Following is an example of a statement that provides feedback and an opportunity to validate the nurse's perceptions:

CLIENT: My husband doesn't ever find time to spend with me. He's always working or watching television.

NURSE: I hear you saying that he doesn't *want* to spend time with you.

CLIENT: Not exactly. I think he does, but other things come first, and I want to be first in his life.

Feedback also provides clients with an opportunity to examine and integrate their own conflicting or scattered thoughts and feelings.

CLIENT: I don't know what I believe about myself any more. I still hear my dad telling me that I'm destined to be a great achiever. But I also hear him telling me that I'm too weak to stand up under pressure.

NURSE: What I'm hearing you say is that you live with two opposing scripts: a "you will be great" script and a "you will be a failure" script. Those scripts sound contradictory. It's not surprising to me that you feel confused.

CLIENT: That's right. Which script do I believe? Which is the real me? How do I sort that out?

Feedback can also bring to light discrepancies in what both the nurse and client are thinking and open them up for examination, clarification, and exploration of alternatives.

The main guidelines for giving feedback are:[1,4]

1. Feedback should be given in amounts that the client can use. Too many items may overload the client, create confusion, and possibly cause resentment. Feedback given in large amounts is likely to function more as a way for the care giver to express hostility then as a way to help the client.
2. Focus feedback on the behavior rather than on the client. This focuses comments on what the client is actually doing rather than on what one imagines the client is doing.
3. Describe the behavior instead of making judgments about it. Report what is happening instead of making judgments about whether the behavior is right or wrong, good or bad. This leaves the client free to use feedback as he or she sees fit.
4. Focus feedback on conveying information and ideas rather than on giving advice. This helps the client become self-directed in decision making and problem solving. Giving advice denies the client's right and ability to be self-directed.
5. Focus feedback on exploration of alternatives and options, rather than on answers or solutions. Focusing on a variety of alternatives prevents premature acceptance of solutions that may not be self-initiated or appropriate.
6. Give feedback about things that the client has the capacity to change. It would not be helpful to give feedback about physical characteristics or life circumstances which are impossible to change.
7. Feedback should be a prompt response to current and specific behavior, not unfinished business from the past. Feedback that is inappropriate to time and place is often irrelevant and ineffective.

Effective feedback should be nonthreatening so that it does not increase the defensiveness of the client. The more defensive the client is, the less likely he or she is to hear or understand the feedback. When clients receive nonthreatening feedback from people they trust, they are able to fill in gaps in their self-awareness.[20]

STRUCTURING. *Structuring* is a responding strategy that creates order, guidelines, and priorities. The nurse assists the client in identifying problems and establishing their relative importance. This is useful in establishing an order for dealing with them. This kind of structuring is helpful to clients who present a wide array of problems, have no idea of which problems are most important, and don't know where to begin working on them. Structuring can also take the form of establishing contract guidelines for nurse-client interactions, such as time, place, length of treatment, and fee. An example of a structuring statement is:

NURSE: You've described several problems to me. As I hear them, they would be: loneliness, dissatisfaction with your schoolwork, obesity, emotional distance from your father, and an inability to be assertive. Which one would you say is most important, and which would you want to begin work on first?

FOCUSING. *Focusing* involves keeping the flow of communication goal-directed, specific, and concrete. It helps clients to be clear rather than vague, specific rather than general, oriented to reality rather than oriented to fantasy, and purposeful rather than rambling. This facilitates keeping discussions focused on central issues related to important problems. Related techniques, such as encouraging description, placing events in time sequence, and encouraging comparisons, can be used to promote specificity and analysis of problems. An example of focusing would be:

CLIENT: I feel so down today....

NURSE: Describe how you feel right now.

CLIENT: I'm so tired. I feel like lead. I feel sad, too, I could cry at the drop of a hat....

NURSE: How long have you been feeling that way?

CLARIFYING. *Clarifying* is attempting to understand a client's communication when it is vague, confusing, or unclear. Clarification is often necessary because clients' communications are not always direct and straightforward. This is particularly true with clients who are out of touch with reality, intoxicated, or reluctant to share feelings with another person. The nurse should not hesitate to let a client know (tactfully) that something is not understood. A client's communication may be confused, fragmented, disorganized, symbolic, hesitant, or incomplete. If the nurse allows communication to continue in this way without seeking clarification, the client will not know that he or she is not understood. Valuable time will be wasted; opportunities for feedback and correction will be missed, and a serious problem may remain undiscovered. In addition, the client may develop doubts about the nurse's ability to understand. Clients are perceptive; they soon come to recognize nurses who pretend to understand but do not.

Clarifications are often tentative, phrased as general questions or statements: "I'm not sure I'm following what you're saying. Are you saying that ...?" or "Could you go over that again, please?" At other times clarification can take the form of a specific question, asking a client to clarify a particular idea or feeling that is confusing to either the client or the nurse. Consider, for example, an interaction in which a depressed client is attempting to differentiate between what she *wants* to do for herself and what she feels she *should* do for herself.

CLIENT: I just want to break free and do things that I want to do. But I shouldn't want that, because I should be acting like a responsible person.... Oh, it's so confusing....

NURSE: Let's take a moment to clarify what you're feeling. It sounds as though you feel that there is an irresponsible child part of you and a responsible adult or parent part of you, and that you can't fit the two together into a whole person that functions smoothly.

CLIENT: That makes it less confusing. I feel as if I'm going to be either one or the other, either totally irresponsible or entirely responsible. Either extreme is exhausting.

NURSE: Well, what other alternative can you come up with?

SUMMARIZING. Giving feedback to a client about the general substance of an interview or a portion of the interview, as seen by the nurse, is called *summarizing*. This technique unifies a number of pieces of information into main themes of content and feeling. By highlighting the most significant data, the nurse can determine with the client the progress they have made and whether the information obtained is accurate. They can also use these data for making future plans. This cooperative nurse-client interaction gives clients a sense of contributing to the resolution of their problems and thus reaffirms their sense of self-worth. An example of a summary statement is:[19]

CLIENT: (*A middle-aged man fighting alcoholism.*) I know drinking doesn't really help me in the long run. And it sure doesn't help my family. My wife keeps threatening to leave. I know all this. But it's hard to stay away from the booze. Having a drink makes me feel relieved.

NURSE: You're aware of some of the ways that drinking is not very helpful to you (*summarization of content*), yet you feel better, less overwhelmed, after a drink (*summarization of affect*).

SILENCE. Silence is a responding strategy that gives the nurse and the client a way to interact without words. Because it gives clients an opportunity to collect and organize their thoughts, it can increase their awareness of their problems. It can also convey acceptance, concern, support, and the message that talking is not always necessary in a therapeutic relationship. A comfortable silence can let clients see the nurse as a person who is willing to let them give cues as to when the conversation will begin again.

Although silence is an effective communication skill, competence is needed to employ it correctly. Socially, most people do not feel comfortable with silence. If there are lulls in a conversation, people feel that something is wrong. Therefore, it is not unusual for a nurse to feel this way about silence during a nurse-client interaction. Nurses may feel compelled to break silences because they are self-conscious and uncomfortable; and they may need to practice this skill often before they can use it with confidence.[18]

Facilitative communication skills are used throughout the nurse-client relationship—when it is initiated, as it progresses, and when it is terminated. The use of communication skills in this context will be explored in detail in Chapter 13. The skills are also used during the assessment process, when data about client, family, and community are being collected. Facilitative communication in assessment interviews is discussed in Chapter 11. As they work with clients and colleagues, nurses will find that communication theory and communication skills are invaluable in establishing and conducting effective interpersonal relationships.

BARRIERS TO FACILITATIVE COMMUNICATION

In the previous section, skills for facilitative communication were presented. It is important for the nurse to realize that there are also barriers to facilitative communication. Barriers are an inevitable part of the communication process.[4,19] They are protective behaviors that arise when interactions are perceived as threatening and likely to increase self-exposure, insecurity, and helplessness. If barriers are unchecked, they will prevent the nurse and client from continuing the work of the interaction by interfering with each person's ability to attend and respond to the messages the other sends. When barriers to facilitative communication occur, the primary goals for the nurse are to: (1) recognize that a barrier exists, (2) identify the purpose or need served by such a behavior, (3) identify appropriate alternative behavior, and (4) implement the alternative behavior in the interaction so that facilitative communication can be resumed. Table 12-3 summarizes barriers to facilitative communication that are commonly experienced by nurses.[4,19]

Table 12-3 Barriers to Facilitative Communication

Barriers	Dynamics	Nonfacilitative Examples	Facilitative Examples
Giving advice	The nurse offers solutions and advises the client about what course of action to take. This denies the client's ability to formulate solutions to problems and assume responsibility for the direction of his or her life. This devalues the client and keeps the nurse in a position of control.	"Why don't you—" "If I were you—" "It would be best if—" "Let me suggest—"	"I hear what you are saying." "What would you suggest?" "What other alternatives have you come up with?"
Giving reassurance	The nurse offers information to the client that is not based on fact and truth. Reassurance denies the client's right to the feelings being experienced and closes off communication about them. All the client's real feelings remain undiscussed and unexplored. This action shows the client that his or her feelings are not being taken seriously. It is also a protective action on the part of the nurse who is unable to listen to the client's painful feelings.	"Don't worry." "You'll feel better tomorrow. Everybody feels that way." "It's not that bad." "Things always look worse before they get better."	"What worries you about that?" "This is a difficult time for you—" "Tell me what you are thinking." "What's the worst thing about this for you?"

(Continued.)

Table 12-3 Continued

Barriers	Dynamics	Nonfacilitative Examples	Facilitative Examples
Changing the subject	The nurse diverts the focus of the interaction at crucial times to something less threatening. Changing the subject usually occurs when the nurse is unwilling or unable to listen to painful feelings being expressed by the client. This communicates to the client that the nurse cannot stand to hear what the client has to say and is not able to talk about what is important to the client. Communication may remain superficial.	"Let's discuss that later—" "Let's leave that and talk about—" "I forgot that I wanted to ask you about—"	"That sounds important, go on and tell me more." "I know that's painful for you to talk about, but try to tell me how you're feeling." "Let's look at that further."
Being judgmental	The nurse responds to the client with value-laden judgments that come from the nurse's value system. Those are critical evaluative statements that label the client and do not convey acceptance of him or her as a unique person. Being judgmental conveys stereotyped attitudes toward others and lack of acceptance of individual differences. The client is only approved and accepted if he or she conforms to the nurse's values.	"You're wrong." "I should have known; all you men are alike." "You're just another lazy teenager—you have it too good at home." "What right do you have to consider an abortion? You're married."	"Your interpretation is different. I'd like to hear more about how you see the situation." "I've heard other men express that point of view, I'd like to understand where you're coming from when you say that." "How difficult is it for you to be moving toward independence?" "I may not agree with your decision, but I can understand your reasons for arriving at that decision."
Giving directions	The nurse approaches the client with specific directions to be followed and frequently lectures the client about the advisability of following this course of action. This denies the client's ability to think through and arrive at solutions to problems. It reinforces and maintains the dependent-child position of the client. It is a protective maneuver for the nurse who has difficulty sharing control and power.	"That's not the way—" "These are the facts, this is the way it should be done." "You must follow these directions." "Listen to me—"	"Which do you think would be best?" "Let's look at your options." "Can you come up with another way to accomplish this?" "How would you approach this situation?"
Excessive questioning	Excessive questioning on the part of the nurse controls the nature and range of the client's responses. The nurse can be perceived by the client as an interrogator who is demanding information without respect for the client's ability or readiness to respond. Closed-ended questions limit the client's choices of response to "Yes" or "No." Questions that ask, "Why?" tend to make the client feel defensive; often she or he does not know why. Thus a stressful rather than a helpful situation is created. Excessive questioning on the part of the nurse is protective. It initially keeps the nurse's anxiety down, for it fills in gaps in an interaction. However, the client may feel overwhelmed and may ultimately withdraw.	"Why do you feel that way?" "What's the real reason?" "Where have you been?" "Do you feel angry?"	"What was happening when you began to feel that way?" "Tell me more about that—" "I've missed you. You don't have to explain if you don't want to." "Can you describe in words how you're feeling right now?"

(Continued.)

Table 12-3 Continued

Barriers	Dynamics	Nonfacilitative Examples	Facilitative Examples
Using emotionally charged words	The nurse uses emotionally charged words with the client who cannot tolerate or accept such feelings. The client may withdraw physically or emotionally. Clients often have a great deal of shame and embarrassment about their feelings, especially those they perceive as negative, and they have difficulty communicating them to another person. The nurse who uses words like *angry*, *guilty*, and *hostile*, before the client is ready to hear or speak them is misjudging the client's pace and risks losing the client's involvement. When more comfortable with feelings, the client will choose comfortable words to illustrate an experience. The nurse should use low-key words that the client uses and is comfortable with.	"Your mother makes you feel pretty angry." "You feel guilty about what happened." "You describe your wife as acting 'crazy.'"	"How do you feel about what she did?" "I wonder if you feel at all responsible for what happened?" "You describe your wife's behavior as having changed in the past week."
Challenging	The nurse sometimes feels that if the client is challenged to prove unrealistic ideas or perceptions, the client will realize that there is no proof to support such ideas and he or she will be forced to acknowledge what is true. The nurse forgets that unrealistic thoughts, perceptions, and feelings serve a purpose for the client and will not be given up until that purpose can be fulfilled in healthier ways. When challenged, the client feels threatened and tends to cling to and expand such misinterpretations because they provide support for his or her point of view.	"You *can't* be the president of that company!" "You can't really hear the devil saying you're wicked."	"It sounds as though you'd like to be able to think of yourself as an important person." "The voices you say you hear seem to make you feel that you haven't lived up to your beliefs and values."
Making stereotyped comments	Offering trite expressions and meaningless clichés as responses diminishes the value of the nurse-client interaction. Such comments on the part of the nurse imply lack of understanding of this client's uniqueness. Nothing about either the client or the nurse is really communicated by such statements. It is a way of creating or maintaining distance because the nurse is acting in a mechanical way as a substitute for a more personal, considered response. The nurse communicates an unwillingness to delve further into the client's feelings. Behind a nurse's automatic responses may be equally stereotyped attitudes.	"You're looking chipper today, Tom." "Keep your chin up, Mary; it won't be much longer now."	"I've noticed you smiling a few times this morning. Is that an indication of how you're feeling?" "How difficult is it for you to keep your motivation at a high level?"
Self-focusing behavior	Self-focusing behavior is characterized by the nurse's excessive interest in or preoccupation with his or her own thoughts, feelings, or actions. When thoughts or feelings involve total self-absorption, they detract from or interfere with attentiveness toward the client as well as fulfillment of the interview goals. In *cognitive self-focusing*, the nurse devotes less attention to what the client is saying and more attention to wondering if he or she (the nurse) will answer correctly, ask the right follow-up question, or have another question to ask if the first one doesn't work. *Affective self-focusing* occurs when the nurse verbalizes his or her own feelings during an interview and does not focus on those of the client.	(*Thinking to himself* or *herself*) Now what? What do I say, what if he doesn't answer? What did he say he was thinking before? (*Then aloud*) "Oh, excuse me; could you repeat that? I didn't hear what you said."	"If I understand you correctly, Mr. Brown, you said that . . ."

SUMMARY

Communication is interaction—an ongoing process through which people relate to one another. Everything affects communication, and communication affects everything: the environment, other people, and the self. Effective communication skills are essential to professional nursing practice.

Communication is a circular process that transmits information through a common system of symbols, signs, or behavior. Verbal communication, which consists of symbols (words), and nonverbal communication, which consists of kinesics, paralanguage, proxemics, and appearance, are the two forms of communication.

Factors that influence communication and the nature and outcome of an interaction are culture and religion, sex roles, social class, perceptions, values, levels of relatedness, and the context of a message.

Communications theorists include Watzlawick, Scheflen and Birdwhistell, Berne, and Ruesch.

Watzlawick and his colleagues proposed that there is not necessarily any difference between a normal person's and a disturbed person's communications; they focused on the relationships among people, defined communication in terms of feedback loops, and stated five axioms of communication.

Scheflen and Birdwhistell studied patterns of space and time in communication.

Berne categorized human behavior as parent, adult, and child ego states and proposed that people communicate using complementary, crossed, and ulterior transactions. He also described the process by which a "life script" is decided on.

Ruesch identified seven components of therapeutic communication, or messages transmitted in therapeutic communication: acceptance, interest, respect, honesty, assistance, permission, and protection.

There are two types of communication: intrapersonal and interpersonal. Intrapersonal communication occurs within the self and consists of getting in touch with oneself. Interpersonal communication occurs between or among two or more people and has three forms: social, collegial, and facilitative.

Facilitative communication takes place within nurse-client relationships. It focuses on areas of concern for the client and has three goals: self-exploration, self-understanding, and action. Nurses assist clients in self-exploration so that they will gain the self-understanding that will enable them to initiate action—to repattern their problems.

Facilitative communication requires attending skills and responding skills. Physical attending skills are ways of letting someone know that the listener is physically involved. Psychosocial attending skills involve paying attention to both verbal and nonverbal behavior. The context of a message and the feelings expressed in it, as well as the congruence between verbal and nonverbal messages, must be evaluated.

Two aspects of responding skills are the core dimensions of the nurse-client relationship (empathy, respect, genuineness, concreteness, immediacy, and confrontation) and responding strategies. The core dimensions are a foundation for facilitative communication. Responding strategies are ways of talking with clients that encourage them to communicate. In the nurse-client relationship, these strategies are ways of helping clients engage in the process of self-exploration, self-understanding, and change.

Barriers to facilitate communication are protective behaviors that arise when interactions are perceived as threatening and likely to increase self-exposure, insecurity, and helplessness. They can create stalls in nurse-client relationships. Nurses must recognize their existence, identify the purpose they serve, and correct them so that facilitative communication can be resumed.

Facilitative communication skills are invaluable in establishing and conducting effective interpersonal relationships.

REFERENCES

1. Paul Watzlawick, Janet H. Beavin, and Don D. Jackson, *The Pragmatics of Human Communication,* Norton, New York, 1967.
2. Bonnie W. Duldt, Kim Griffin, and Bobby R. Patton, *Interpersonal Communication in Nursing,* Davis, Philadelphia, 1984.
3. Edward T. Hall, *The Silent Language,* Fawcett, Greenwich, Conn., 1959.
4. Eleanor C. Hein, *Communication in Nursing Practice,* 2d ed., Little, Brown, Boston, 1980.

5. Mark King, Larry Novik, and Charles Citrenbaum, *Irresistible Communication: Creative Skills for the Health Professional,* Saunders, Philadelphia, 1982.
6. R. D. Laing, *Self and Others,* Penguin Books, Baltimore, Md., 1975.
7. Albert E. Scheflen and Norman Ashcraft, *Human Territories: How We Behave in Space-Time,* Prentice-Hall, Englewood Cliffs, N.J., 1976.
8. Ray L. Birdwhistell, *Kinesics and Context: Essays on Body Motion Communication,* University of Pennsylvania Press, University Park, 1970.
9. Eric Berne, *Games People Play,* Grove, New York, 1964.
10. Eric Berne, *Transactional Analysis in Psychotherapy,* Grove, New York, 1961.
11. Claude M. Steiner, *Scripts People Live: Transactional Analysis of Life Scripts,* Bantam, New York, 1975.
12. Jurgen Ruesch, *Therapeutic Communication,* Norton, New York, 1968.
13. Gerard Egan, *The Skilled Helper,* Wadsworth, Belmont, Calif., 1975.
14. Gerard Egan, *You and Me,* Brooks/Cole, Monterey, Calif., 1977.
15. Elaine LaMonica, "Construct Validity of an Empathy Instrument," *Research in Nursing and Health,* vol. 4, no. 4, 1981, pp. 389–400.
16. Robert Carkhuff, *The Art of Helping,* Human Resources Development Press, Amherst, Mass., 1973.
17. Elaine LaMonica, "Empathy in Nursing Practice," *Issues in Mental Health Nursing,* vol. 2, no. 1, 1979, pp. 1–14.
18. Carolyn C. Hames and Doyle H. Joseph, *Basic Concepts of Helping,* Appleton-Century-Crofts, East Norwalk, Conn., 1980.
19. W. H. Cormier and L. S. Cormier, *Interviewing Strategies for Helpers,* Brooks/Cole, Monterey, Calif., 1979.
20. Lawrence M. Brammer, *The Helping Relationship,* 2d ed., Prentice-Hall, Englewood Cliffs, N.J., 1979.

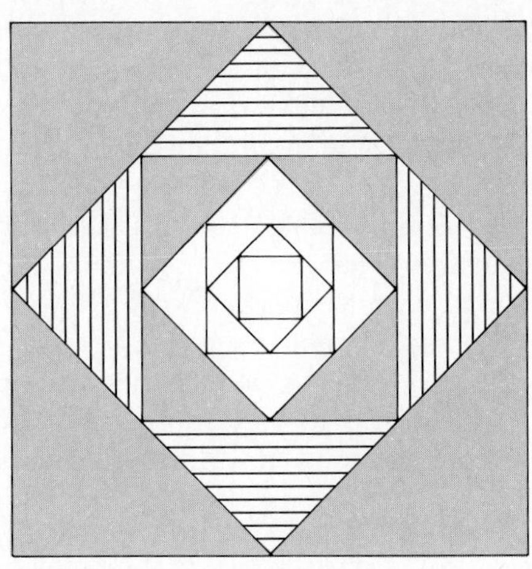

CHAPTER 13
Nurse-Client Relationship

Judith Ackerhalt

LEARNING OBJECTIVES

After studying this chapter, the student should be able to:

1. Describe a personal reason or motive for engaging in a helping relationship.
2. Identify the fears and concerns nurses and clients have at the outset of a therapeutic relationship.
3. Describe the phenomena of transference and countertransference as these occur in helping relationships.
4. Recognize resistance.
5. Differentiate among the stages of a therapeutic relationship.
6. Utilize the core dimensions—empathy, concreteness, confrontation, immediacy, respect, and genuineness—in each stage of a therapeutic relationship.
7. Discuss the ethics of the nurse-client relationship.

Definitions of significant aspects of the nurse-client relationship are often fragmented and unclear. The ability to relate therapeutically is an art but is evolving rapidly into a science. The therapeutic relationship is the cornerstone of client-centered psychiatric–mental health nursing and is characterized by meaningful communication between nurses and their clients, goal-directed nursing interventions, and an atmosphere of collaboration. In no other aspect of psychiatric nursing care is the nurse called upon to be more whole or more in touch with the wholeness of the client.

In a therapeutic relationship, reactions, feelings, sentiments, and dreams are intentionally expressed. Clients as well as nurses bring their uniqueness—their "personhood"—to the therapeutic encounter. The physical, mental, and spiritual dimensions of both are challenged to grow as the process unfolds.

Although every relationship has unique characteristics, all relationships have some common features that can be observed. All clients and nurses have fears and expectations; and if these are not explored, movement through the stages of a relationship can be impeded. Each person brings to a therapeutic encounter a personal history out of which transference and countertransference dynamics grow.

The core dimensions of the nurse-client relationship—empathy, concreteness, confrontation, immediacy, respect, and genuineness—are used in this chapter to provide a foundation upon which nurses and clients can build therapeutic interactions. Nurses interact out of their own unique selves and offer healing to other unique persons. In the process, clients and nurses evolve and grow together. This chapter discusses what psychiatric nurses need to know about therapeutic relationships. The information presented is intended to enhance self-awareness and facilitate meaningful encounters between nurses and their clients.

HISTORICAL PERSPECTIVES

Peplau, in her classic work, *Interpersonal Relations in Nursing*,[1] for the first time presented a theoretical rationale for psychiatric nursing practice, clarified the various roles of the psychiatric nurse, and explained the goals and activities associated with the counseling role. She also discussed the role of the nurse as "participant-observer." She instructed nurses to monitor the behaviors provoked by interactions with clients and to intervene in ways that would encourage growth.

Advances in the conceptualization of psychiatric nursing practice stimulated controversy about the therapeutic use of self. Nurses labored over the question, "Can nurses maintain their nursing identity while assuming a helping role in one-to-one relationships?" Out of this inquiry there gradually evolved a concern about how the nurse performs psychotherapy.[2]

Today, nurses working in a variety of settings are studying concepts, principles, and theories which help to explain human experience. They are looking at, analyzing, and interpreting helping interactions. The goal of their work and research is to make rational modifications of their helping methods and to extend the scope of their technical ability.

In a sense, the same road that psychiatric nursing has taken historically is repeated by each nurse, but in a unique way. Maturing and refining one's professional image requires an intense inner journey. When a nurse engages in the process of self-assessment, examination of professional ideals, values, and responsibilities is essential. Beliefs about the self are subjected to review. Insight and knowledge about *self* in relationship to *others* leads to a deeper understanding of the technical abilities required in the nurse-client relationship.

DEFINITION OF THE NURSE-CLIENT RELATIONSHIP: PROCESS AND OUTCOMES

A *relationship* may be defined as an interpersonal process. The definition and the direction of the nurse-client relationship are derived from actual clinical practices and direct experiences of professional nurses. To understand the true significance of this interpersonal helping process one must recognize the familiar concerns, well-known issues, and real purposes and accomplishments of nurses engaged in one-to-one relationships with clients. Each nurse, as well as each client, has a distinctive, or idiosyncratic, way of experiencing and responding to specific situations in the helping process.

Idiosyncratic experiences, which illuminate the meaning of the nurse-client relationship, involve the following elements:

1. Forces which bring the nurse and the client together, that is, what each initially hopes and expects to gain from the collaborative effort
2. Resultant fears, concerns, and reservations of the nurse and client
3. Resources nurses and clients have for coping with these experiences

Much of what happens when nurses enter a therapeutic relationship with clients is a product of the complex interaction among these personal elements.

The nurse-client relationship can be understood as an organized sequence of activities or events—or as a process—leading toward a planned goal or objective. The terms *goal* and *objective* do not suggest that the future is predetermined; a goal or an objective is, rather, an image of the future which only suggests and legitimizes the events of the helping relationship.

Establishing goals for a relationship requires a nursing diagnosis to be formulated. Goals, or outcomes, are established in conjunction with the client and are set forth in a *contract,* or agreement, during the initial contact between the nurse and client. The contract outlines and clarifies the purpose of the relationship, the role of the nurse, and the responsibilities of the client. The expectations of both nurse and client are explicitly stated. Many clients have misconceptions about the helping relationship; therefore, nurses assume an educative role during the process of making the contract and establishing goals. Concerns of both the client and the nurse need to be identified if the outcome of the relationship is to be therapeutic.

The outcomes established for any therapeutic relationship will be intended to facilitate the client's self-understanding, self-acceptance, and self-respect; to help the client achieve a clear personal identity; to increase the client's ability to form intimate, interdependent relationships; and to enable clients to give and receive love. For each client, unique outcome criteria are established to facilitate improvement in behavior. These goals integrate thoughts, feelings, and behaviors to satisfy individual needs and achieve individual purposes.

THE OUTSET OF THE HELPING RELATIONSHIP: CONCERNS AND EXPECTATIONS

Nurses and clients are subject to many doubts, concerns, and fears when they commit themselves to a relationship. Their action brings them face to face with the necessity of revising their self-image or exposing themselves to real or imagined threats to self-esteem. It is not uncommon for their determination to waver. The nurse-client relationship, like any promising new venture, is not without its risks and impediments. Concerns and expectations of nurses and clients will be explained in this section.

Nurses' Fears and Concerns

Typically, the beginning nurse is fearful and uncertain, although each person responds to the helping relationship in a distinctive way. Novices frequently have difficulty picturing themselves in the role of therapeutic helper. One nursing student, a mature 40-year-old mother of three children, summed up her experience in this way: "I felt like a fish out of water, ... so very awkward. I was certain that the client would see right through me, that he would see how incompetent and ill-qualified I was." During the early stages of the helping relationship, novice helpers are often uncertain as to how to conduct themselves. Lacking a clear definition of their role and a sense of direction, they are likely to perceive themselves as unskillful or, worse, bungling and inept. Beginning helpers may fear that the client will reject them or that they will exploit the client. Nurses may also have fears connected with doubts about their own mental health or with a sense of helplessness; or they may fear that clients will assault them.

Fear of Rejection

A common fear of novice helpers is that the client will detect that they are unaccustomed to the counseling role and will reject their efforts to help. No one likes to be rejected, but the possibility of rejection exists in each new relationship.

Regardless of how nurses really feel about a client who withdraws from a relationship—whether they are secretly relieved or truly disappointed—they ponder the client's motives. Questions such as, "Did I do something wrong?" and "Could I have acted to prevent this from happening?" acknowledge the fact that rejection by a client can be understood only in relation to the helpers' actions. However, although it is true that only in the context of relationship can insight and learning be obtained, nurses and nursing students too often blame themselves alone when a client withdraws. Students often fear that others on the health team will think less of them because they did not maintain contact with their client. Nurses sometimes rationalize a rejection by claiming that a client is unable to accept help or is hopeless; but frequently, nurses whose efforts have been rejected fear that it will happen again and again. For example:

> A nursing student who had succeeded in establishing a firm alliance with a client noted, "During the first 2 weeks of the semester, I lost two clients. They just didn't want to see me anymore. I began to think that I was the only one who couldn't hold onto a client. It seemed as though all the other students were doing OK. Boy, was I jealous. We are really relieved when our clients want to see us again."

Fear of Exploiting the Client

At the outset of a new nurse-client relationship, nurses who regard themselves as novices are likely to discount the skills they have acquired in previous helping relationships. They think less about what they have to offer the new client than about the possibility that they may be exploiting clients. The idea that the nurse-client relationship is a learning experience for the nurse becomes an ethical concern.

When, for example, a client who is mistrustful asks, "Are you using me as a guinea pig?" a novice or student nurse might be at a loss for a response. In such a case, an empathic instructor, a supervisor, or even a group of understanding classmates or peers can often help the nurse to assess the situation more rationally and support whatever interventions occurred. The student is also directed to recognize the value of skills that were learned previously.

This is not to say, however, that the fear of exploiting a client is invariably irrational or groundless. Nurses may sometimes need to be reminded that clients, having made a commitment to the therapeutic relationship, have the right to express their needs and to expect help. Clients also have a responsibility to indicate to the nurse when help is not being given.

Fear of Helplessness

Generally speaking, nurses hope to effect some change in clients' life situations. When clients exhibit extreme forms of maladaptive behavior but appear to be satisfied with the status quo, when their sources of support are minimal, and when the treatment environment is viewed as having many shortcomings, nurses become disheartened. At first glance, it sometimes appears impossible for the nurse to change the client or the client's milieu. When that happens, nurses often feel helpless, powerless, and frustrated.

Setting realistic therapeutic goals will give nurses and their clients a sense of accomplishment. For example, to expect a middle-aged schizophrenic client who has been ill for many years to reverse a pattern of marginal functioning is unrealistic. To help such a client accept and conform to a medication regimen and attend weekly sessions with a therapist is a more realistic goal and less frustrating for both the client and the nurse.

Fear of Physical Assault

Fears of being physically assaulted or verbally abused are common among nurses. A student working with a client who had little control over sexual or aggressive urges described the situation in this way: "I didn't want to do anything to upset my client's balance. It was like walking on eggs. I was terrified of making a mistake." Clients' potential for losing control is only one reason for this kind of fear. Other factors include stereotyped images of the "violent" mentally ill, the fact that some clients are physically intrusive or seek physical contact, and the feelings of alienation and powerlessness which students occasionally experience when, as strangers, they enter a psychiatric unit for the first time.

Fear of Mental Illness

Many clients, though deeply troubled, do not exhibit overt forms of maladaptive behavior. Initially, nurses wonder why these people have been assigned to the client's role. Nurses are likely to compare aspects of their own lives with those of a client who appears "normal." When similarities are noted, nurses may begin to question their own mental health. Questions such as, "Am I mentally ill?" and "How am I different from my client?" are anxiety-provoking and compel nurses to examine the significance of their own experiences as well as those of their clients. Out of this inquiry, new meanings of *mental health* and *mental illness* may emerge, as well as a deeper awareness of the self.

While many nurses have experienced these fears, not all are able to recognize them as a natural result of the therapeutic encounter—a situation which entails taking risks. The nurse-client relationship requires courage, and that comes more easily when fear is accepted as appropriate. The idea that fear is cowardice is mistaken, and an unnecessary burden on nurses. Failure to come to grips with ever-present fear poses one of the most serious barriers to the development of the nurse-client relationship, since clients who elicit fear sense the effect of their behavior. Fears borne in secret are intensified and generalized. Brought out into the open—shared with an instructor, classmate, peer, or supervisor—fears can be named and understood.

Clients' Fears and Concerns

As the helping relationship begins, clients—like nurses—live through moments of fear and uncertainty. Like nurses, clients may not recognize, understand, or own up to their misgivings. Like nurses, they must grapple with a number of threats to their self-image whenever they invest in a relationship which involves receiving help.

Accepting help has a different meaning for each client. For clients with low self-esteem it may imply that they are helpless, that they are not competent to handle their own problems, or that they are inadequate as people. These impressions may then engender fear, anger, resentment, or guilt.[2] Others may expect the helping person to be a "savior" and rescue them from their illness.

A nurse who assumes an encouraging and empathic role can help to alleviate feelings generated by a client's sense of inadequacy. Avoiding any tendency to be overhelpful or attempt to "rescue" clients will help nurses remain therapeutic while reducing clients' resentment and anger.

Clients' fears and concerns may not be clearly stated. But although clients may be overwhelmed, on some level they are likely to be aware of their fears. They may be heard to say, "It's hard to admit to myself that I have problems. It's even more difficult to admit it to others." "It's not easy to trust strangers and be open with them. I hardly trust myself." "My problems are enormous and not easy to solve. How can I share myself with anyone else?" The skillful nurse will listen to these concerns and not move too quickly to reassure clients or to try to change them. Nurses might respond with a general comment such as, "I appreciate how much courage it must have taken for you to be here," thus acknowledging the client's concern and the struggle involved in initiating a therapeutic encounter.

Some clients are overwhelmed by their assumption that there is a stigma involved in seeking help. They may be heard to say, "It's a sign of weakness to have problems. If I share them, I will be thought of as a failure." "It's a threat to my independence to involve someone else in my problems." Clients need at this juncture to know, from a nurse, that to be human is to have difficulties. Generally a statement such as the following can be made: "It is in the midst of our incompleteness and pain that we are most strong. Your presence here in spite of your concerns is evidence of courage."

Another fear which clients sometimes express at the outset of the helping relationship is their fear of what change may entail. They may say: "It is very hard to change. I want to be different, but I'm not sure I want to commit the time or energy necessary to accomplish the change. I might have to view myself differently, or I might have to act differently—and that's frightening." Generally an empathic sharing or reflection such as the following is appropriate: "I understand your fear. It is always painful when we are growing." This comment acknowledges the client's concern and at the same time suggests that the nurse also struggles and therefore knows the pain of becoming whole.

Nurses' Expectations

There are innumerable reasons why people are drawn to the study and practice of nursing. A broad range of interests, values, expectations, and aims motivate nurses to participate in helping relationships. Frequently, however, nurses do not recognize or understand the motivations which have led them into nursing and operate during their relationships with clients. This section will discuss several important motivations which constitute nurses' expectations at the outset of the therapeutic encounter: humanitarian ideals, value clarification, diversion, control, performance evaluation, and self-enhancement.

Humanitarian Ideals

Nurses sometimes perceive helping others as an act of generosity. Those who have succeeded in overcoming internal conflicts or external obstacles may wish to help others find inner peace and satisfaction. Experiences with friends and loved ones who have supplied support and guidance may inspire nurses to share themselves with clients. Feeling fully aware and alive, many nurses would like to introduce their suffering clients to what life has to offer. Studies of the character traits of effective helpers indicate that these people hold strong humanitarian values.[3] Nurses with such values need to be alert to prevent overgiving and "burnout." *Burnout* is a term commonly used to refer to the discouragement nurses experience when performing their role.

Value Clarification

The nurse-client relationship may be viewed as an opportunity to actualize prized beliefs or values. An example of a prized belief is the inner conviction that it is worthwhile to explore and to grasp the deeper meaning of conscious experience. Through participation in the helping relationship, nurses may enable themselves, as well as their clients, to attain greater self-understanding, self-acceptance, and self-actualization.

Maintenance of Self-Esteem

For some people, maintenance or enhancement of self-esteem is a pressing need. Not infrequently, nurses experience increased status when clients perceive them as helpers. Through helping, nurses may hope to gain confidence in their personal well-being. If they are capable of sustaining a client, they may be reassured that they are "OK." By giving help, nurses are able to avoid the anxiety of receiving help.

Diversion

Nurses who are troubled by their own personal problems may wish for a respite. Focusing upon a client's problems, rather than one's own, may provide needed diversion. The helpers are thus able to get their minds off themselves. In fact, some people may seek a career in psychiatric nursing to "avoid" illness and treatment for themselves.

Control

Sometimes people are motivated by the wish to exert power or control over others. Such impulses may be operating when a nurse approaches a helping situation. The nurse may find a client who needs to cling to, or lean upon, someone. The expectation or hope that the role of a nurse or nursing student is more powerful than the role of client may also be present. When nurses accept clients as people like themselves, exerting power or control is discouraged and becomes less of a factor in the helping relationship.

Performance Evaluation

Nurses are often concerned about how their own performance will be evaluated. They feel pressured to demonstrate competence. They want clients to move rapidly toward a designated goal and may be disheartened when this does not occur. When the helping interaction and the client's potential are seen as more significant than the nurse's performance, nurses are under less pressure and can form more useful expectations.

Self-Enhancement

Nurses enter helping relationships with numerous expectations about themselves. They hope to acquire knowledge of the helping process, a repertoire of helping skills, and perhaps an opportunity to try out various kinds of nursing interventions. When nurses recognize that self-enhancement is a motive underlying their participation in the nurse-client relationship, they have a tendency to chastise themselves. They make an "either-or" assumption: one is *either* out for oneself and hence self-seeking *or* acting in the best interest of the other. This assumption is irrational. Most often, self-enhancement is intertwined with its opposite, generosity. To deny either motive is to limit the genuineness of the people involved in a therapeutic relationship.

Clients' Expectations

Clients have both conscious and unconscious expectations at the outset of a helping relationship. When a client is mentally ill, however, therapeutic goals and expectations may not be entirely clear. Nurses need to assess what the client hopes to gain by collaborating in the relationship and clarify what will be most effective in bringing about desired changes. Some clients' expectations represent images of physical well-being and may be limited to medical treatment. Other clients may expect the relationship to result in spiritual growth through ventilation, confession, or counseling. Still others may expect emotional healing and may seek nurturance, control, reality, contact, psychological expertise, psychotherapeutic clarification, or perhaps even social intervention. Some clients relate more to the nurse in his or her capacity as employee and expect only to maintain contact with an agency or have an administrative request granted.

Clients need to clearly identify expectations and make accurate statements regarding their needs. By talking with a nurse about their desires, clients can clarify their desired outcomes. The nurse is thus provided with an opportunity to define how the therapeutic relationship can be most effective. Table 13-1 lists some common expectations held by clients at the outset of a helping relationship.

As the nurse-client relationship evolves, clients' original expectations decline in significance. When clients encounter new aspects of themselves, their values, their desires, and their images of the future

Table 13-1 Expectations of Clients at the Outset of the Helping Relationship

Expectation	Explanation
Medical treatment	Clients are unwilling to share their concerns with anyone but a physician. They may hope that a physician will provide a diagnosis, medication, electroconvulsive therapy, or even surgery. These hopes are reinforced in some agencies where clients' problems are viewed as somatic in origin or where the nurse's role is defined as custodial rather than therapeutic.
Confession	Clients, when they wish to reveal real or imagined transgressions, seek a nurse who will listen in a nonjudgmental way rather than moralize. Clients hope as a result of their revelation or confession to be told that what they have done is not as terrible as they believe it to be. Their motive is to be rid of guilt or shame.
Ventilation	Clients want to unburden themselves to a nurse who will listen. They do not expect the nurse to help them examine or solve the problem.
Advice	Clients hope that the nurse will have the answers to what is troubling them. They want the nurse to come up with solutions to a particular problem or to make a decision for them. By seeking direction, they would like to be told what to do or which way to go.
Clarification	Clients hope to clear up confusing thoughts, to crystallize an idea, or to better understand the meaning of a critical event. Getting things into perspective may be the sole motive for seeking help.
Nurturance	Clients who have sustained the loss of a significant other person upon whom they were dependent for support may feel needy, deprived, or empty and seek out a caring, sympathetic helper. They hope for kindness and support; they need to be "filled up."
Control	Clients are besieged by thoughts of doing violence to themselves or to others. They are seeking protection or someone to set limits and take charge. They are exhausted by the struggle to control powerful aggressive or sexual urges. Disabled by severe anxiety, intense guilt feelings, or paralyzing depressions, these clients frequently claim that they are unable to "pull themselves together," that they are "cracking up," "falling apart," or "going crazy." They foresee and fear a complete loss of self-control and require help in keeping a rein on the direct expression of frightening impulses.
Contact with reality	Clients out of touch with themselves or the world may be motivated by the feeling of unreality or personal estrangement to establish rapport with a nurse. The clients' aim is to make contact with a representative of the real world and to get back in touch with themselves. Such aspirations may be the source of incessant demands made by a person recovering from a myocardial infarction; by a lonely, aging widow; or by a psychiatric client who has spent an afternoon in seclusion.

(Continued.)

Table 13-1 Continued

Expectation	Explanation	Expectation	Explanation
Psychotherapy	Clients who engage in an ongoing relationship with the nurse may hope to discover the relationship between current experiences and past events. Usually, these people believe that by subjecting their experiences to careful scrutiny over a period of time, they will acquire greater self-understanding and self-acceptance. They hope to get more satisfaction out of life.	Referral	Clients hope only to get information about where to go to satisfy various needs. A client may request information about how to make an appointment with another agency and have little or no interest in continuing a relationship once the request is granted and the referral is accomplished.
Psychological expertise	Clients who wish to know why they feel or act as they do may hope that the nurse, whom they see as an expert, will have the answers. When the expected answers are not forthcoming, these persons may claim that the nurse is "holding out" on them. The role of the nurse is to allow clients to grow in insight and recognition of their motivating dynamics. Nurses need to be wary of falling into the "expert trap" and making premature interpretations.	Contact with an agency	Clients may not want anything from any one particular person. Instead, clients who live in a community may want to make contact with an agency or clinic where help has been received in the past. Occasionally, such clients will drop in to visit one of, or all of, the nurses; they are "touching base," not seeking intimate personal relationships. Sometimes, however, such clients are beginning to "decompensate" and will need additional treatment.
Social intervention	Clients underestimate their ability to fend for themselves, and ask the nurse to contact a relative, friend, landlord, or employer. In these instances, the client's expectation is that nurses will actively intervene in a problematic situation on their behalf.	Administrative request	Clients want nurses to exercise authority in helping them to acquire a privilege card, to obtain a weekend pass or a hospital discharge, or to secure legal or financial assistance. Usually, these clients will not acknowledge other concerns until these initial requests are addressed by the nurse.

change. Frequently, as expected outcomes are revised, the one-to-one relationship becomes a way of helping clients strengthen or acquire the qualities essential for self-realization. If a relationship proceeds therapeutically, the client will come to expect outcomes such as independence, spontaneity, trust, self-awareness, honesty, responsibility, and acceptance of reality.

DIMENSIONS OF THE NURSE-CLIENT RELATIONSHIP

Action Dimensions

Two unconscious phenomena, transference and countertransference, occur in all relationships. In psychoanalytic theory *transference* refers to an unconscious phenomenon in which the feelings, attitudes, and wishes originally linked with significant figures in one's early life are projected onto others who have come to represent these people in current life. Generally, transference occurs in the client during the helping relationship. *Countertransference,* on the other hand, is a conscious or unconscious response occurring in the nurse or therapist in response to the client. Wishes and conflicts originating in the helper's own relationships with significant others are transferred onto the client.[4] Transference and countertransference may result in *resistance*—behavior that interferes with the interaction.

Transference

When clients recognize that the nurse is listening and that they are understood better than they understand themselves, they begin to develop transference feelings. These feelings may be positive or negative. The client may begin to project onto the nurse past or present attitudes toward loved ones or persons in authority. Thus, clients may experience nurses as they might have experienced other persons who have played significant roles in their lives. Clients may form an image or a multiplicity of images of the nurse, some of which may be distorted by past events. Accordingly, clients anticipate the roles that both they and the nurse will play in the helping relationship. They unconsciously contemplate the specific techniques that the nurse will employ, and perhaps they think about the duration and outcomes of the interpersonal helping process. Transference on the part of clients interferes with their ability to assess interaction as it exists in the present. They may repeat interaction patterns which were characteristic of earlier relationships.

Transference accounts for both positive and negative expectations which clients have about nurses. Negative or problematic transference evokes the fear that the nurses will treat clients with disrespect or control, punish, stereotype, manipulate, humiliate, or abandon them.

Negative transference is uncomfortable for both client and nurse. It represents a form of resistance to change on the part of the client. The skillful practitioner, however, will use negative transference to intervene with clients. Through exploration of negative feelings the nurse may gain valuable insight and information about the client's past conflicts. By using timely interventions, nurses may help clients gain insight into their behavior. Feelings, thoughts, and behaviors belonging to the current client-nurse relationship are separated from those that represent past experiences. Many researchers and practitioners believe that it is the work accomplished through interpretation of transference reactions which helps reduce clients' anxiety so that positive change can occur.

Countertransference

The term *countertransference* is used to describe all the feelings which nurses experience toward clients.[4] Attraction, warmth, and concern are common positive countertransference reactions; but negative responses to the client—such as discouragement, resentment, boredom, guilt, or anger—are equally typical. Unanticipated changes in the nurse's behavior take place when countertransference is unrecognized or when it evokes anxiety. When this occurs, the overt communication of nurses may be unrelated to their inner feelings. Thus, while nurses may appear to be attending to the client's concerns, their energies are in fact being diverted toward efforts to recapture a feeling of personal security.

Discrepancies between nurses' overt communication and their inner experience result from failure to recognize countertransference. Nurses may respond to clients as parents would to children, conveying a tone of superiority. They may also perceive clients as parental figures from their past and respond in a meek and ineffectual way.

In these instances nurses fail to provide clients with genuine feedback. Some nurses react the way they think they *should*, in a rehersed, "professional" fashion. Recent research suggests that much of what happens in a therapeutic relationship involves the unconscious need of professionals to defend their images at the expense of the client. Clients' rejection of this may be mislabeled as *resistance*[4] (see below). Nurses may suspect that countertransference is occurring if they are ignoring selected data about a client, blaming a client, being smug about their own opinions, or being rigid in the structure of a relationship.[4] In each instance nurses fail to provide clients with any indication of how they themselves feel. This generally has the effect of eliciting defensive responses from clients. Genuine expressions, on the other hand, further the spirit of inquiry. Honest, spontaneous communications, regardless of their emotional content, are usually liberating and contribute to a feeling that one is being oneself.

Transference and countertransference occur not only in nurse-client relationships but also in relationships between nurses. Conflicts and feelings about others in a work environment need to be explored in the light of each nurse's past conflicts, particularly those with parental authority figures and siblings. Self-awareness and admission of the irrational nature of these feelings will help ease work relationships.

Resistance

The existence of transference and countertransference in a therapeutic relationship may result in resistance behavior. *Resistance* is defined as all the phenomena that interfere with and disrupt the smooth interactional flow of feelings, memories, and thoughts.[5] It is a client's or nurse's attempt to remain unaware of anxiety-provoking aspects of the self. People fear being blamed, being shamed, or being found incompetent. Sometimes their feelings of guilt are so painful that they cannot be shared. When such feelings and fears exist, resistance may occur.

Resistance generally results in avoidance behavior by both nurse and client and in the slowing of the work of a therapeutic relationship. Burgess and

Lazare list several "stalls," or blocks, that are encountered by clients and nurses in their work together.[6] These may be viewed as resistance behaviors. Table 13-2 lists stalls and nurse-initiated solutions which will help reestablish movement in the relationship.

Care should be taken by the nurse when labeling a client's behavior as *resistance.* (For example,

Table 13-2 Stalls in the Nurse-Client Relationship

Stall	Solution
Judgmental feelings	Autodiagnosis Acceptance and realization
Ambivalent feelings	Realization of its normality Acceptance and understanding in self and others
Rescue feelings	Avoid secret alliances with client Share responsibilities and goals with others
Pessimistic feelings	Look for client assets, not just problems Set realistic goals Develop optimism about goals of the relationship Give supportive encouragement
Omnipotent feelings	Realize human limitations Realize achievement in a relationship is a partnership Develop humility Develop respect for self and for the client Consult with colleagues and supervisors when necessary
False reassurance	Be supportive rather than reassuring Be honest
Misuse of confrontation	Stay with here-and-now issues Be aware of "timing" when making interpretations
Misjudging independence	Acknowledge the misjudgment Ask what clients *can* do for themselves Reassess client and family capabilities Do not infantilize
Labeling	Acknowledge feelings and reason for label Describe rather than label Remember that diagnostic labeling is only a small part of describing client's behavior
Overidentification	Acknowledge the existence of overidentification Talk over and assist client to look at the problem from all perspectives
Overinvolvement	Recognize that the reason for hospitalization of a client is serious Maintain a therapeutic involvement Do not allow client to deny reality of illness Avoid discussing personal life Avoid social invitations from the client Avoid calling the client at home
Painful feelings	Explore the possible sources of painful feelings (anger, etc.) Avoid isolation and withdrawal when confronted by the client Utilize autodiagnosis Learn to accept and adjust own feelings with other people
Misuse of honesty	Avoid failure to fulfill promise Answer questions directly and honestly; avoid "hedging" Avoid omissions in conversations with the client
Listening pitfalls	Autodiagnosis Avoid excessive verbalization Avoid giving advice and making decisions for the client Avoid faking attention, interrupting, and asking clients to repeat what they have said Maintain eye contact Avoid introducing "intolerable" words Avoid changing the subject; keep the client focused Be alert to repetition Make efforts to clearly understand what is being said

SOURCE: Ann Burgess and Aaron Lazare, *Psychiatric Nursing in the Hospital and the Community,* Prentice-Hall, Englewood Cliffs, N.J., 1973.

clients who are late for appointments may have realistic time constraints to cope with in order to accommodate schedules.) An understanding helper will explore the behavior and attempt to find mutually agreeable solutions to problems. It should also be pointed out that, as noted earlier, unrecognized countertransference may lead therapists to mislabel clients' behavior. A client's rejection of a therapist's defensive behavior is not true resistance.

Nurses help clients to become aware of resistance through awareness of their own avoidance behaviors. This requires honest self-assessment or diagnosis by use of self. Listening, clarifying, and reflecting are ways in which nurses assist clients in understanding and avoiding resistance so that the work of the relationship can continue.[7]

Core Dimensions: Responsive Interpersonal Dimensions

It is impossible to draw a sharp distinction between the anticipated outcomes of the nurse-client relationship and the way in which these goals are accomplished. Investigators have been attempting to identify and operationally define helping behaviors which enable clients to fully experience, explore, and resolve problems and to become self-actualized.

A number of facilitative interpersonal processes have been conceptualized. Each describes a way of "being with" a client so that healing takes place. These core dimensions, or facilitative dimensions, are: (1) empathy, (2) concreteness, (3) respect, (4) genuineness, (5) confrontation, and (6) immediacy.[8] The six core dimensions, each of which can demonstrate the interconnection between helping transactions and specific outcomes, are defined in Table 13-3. They are discussed in depth throughout the remainder of this chapter.

Table 13-3 Core Dimensions

Core Dimension	Definition
Empathy	The temporary experiencing of another individual's feelings; expressions which convey the nurse's accurate recognition of the feelings, motives, and meanings underlying a client's communications.
Concreteness	The clear, direct expression of personally relevant perceptions, values, and feelings as they exist in the present relationship.
Confrontation	Communications which call attention to significant discrepancies in the client's experience; verbal messages which are intended to help a client to recognize information which is not consistent with the self-image.
Immediacy	A dimension of communication which deals with the relationship-building element of the helping process; expressions emphasizing immediacy draw relationships between clients' overt communications and their underlying impressions of what is going on between client and nurse in the here and now.
Respect	Communication of acceptance of the client's ideas, feelings, and experiences; recognition of a client's potential for self-actualization.
Genuineness	Spontaneous expressions conveying an individual's inner experience.

SOURCE: Adapted from R. R. Carkhuff, *Helping and Human Relations*, Holt, New York 1968.

PHASES OF THE NURSE-CLIENT RELATIONSHIP

The helping relationship is a "historical" or temporal process, interweaving expectations and concerns of nurses and clients *over time* with the unfolding core dimensions. While much of the information that follows is intended for nurses involved in ongoing relationships with psychiatric clients, the principles presented may be applied in a variety of settings.

Three distinctive yet interrelated phases of this evolving process can be identified: an initial phase, a middle phase, and a termination phase. Frequently these phases are not distinct but flow into one another. When each phase occurs and how long it lasts can vary widely and depends on the specific context of care. For example, the tasks of all three phases may be accomplished in 3 weeks by clients in a short-term inpatient crisis unit. On the other hand, clients placed in a setting for long-term treatment or for ongoing outpatient therapy may experience the phases much more slowly.

In the discussion of each of the phases, the core dimensions will be utilized as a framework. Each of the core dimensions, or behaviors on the part of the helper, undergoes a transformation as the nurse-client relationship evolves. Definitions and general principles of these dimensions will be explained, and they may be applied in any setting or with any time frame. The tasks to be accomplished in each phase of a relationship will also be discussed.

Initial Phase

Characteristics of the Initial Phase

The initial phase of the nurse-client relationship has been referred to as the *orientation phase,* the *establishing phase,* and the *downward* or *inward phase.* During the initial phase, the crucial tasks to be accomplished are establishment of a working partnership between the nurse and client, identification of the client's chief problem or area of concern, and beginning of self-exploration by the client.

During the first phase, nurse and client, who are strangers to one another, meet. Neither can predict much about the events which are about to take place. The things that will happen throughout the relationship can, at best, only be anticipated.

A number of structural and practical details can facilitate the beginning of a therapeutic relationship. The *initial interview,* the first meeting or conference between client and nurse, is structured so that data can be collected by the nurse and the client can be made to feel at ease. Facilitative communication skills are used to determine the client's needs and goals. Table 13-4 describes the kind of therapeutic environment that will be conducive to progress during the initial interview, with specific ways of creating it.

The initial interview is usually completed within a short time; but whether it is short or long, *rapport* must be established. Nurse and client establish harmonious and sympathetic connectedness that is characterized by a sense of affinity and compatability. Spontaneity, freedom to be oneself, clarity and openness, physical and psychological closeness, and intimacy are the signs of rapport. Both nurses and clients feel peaceful, comfortable, and even joyous when rapport has been established. Rapport is, in a sense, the foundation upon which the remainder of the relationship rests. Some researchers have found that the initial contact seems to determine the success or failure of future therapeutic interventions.

The initial phase of the relationship is also the time when *expected outcomes* are first discussed and the contract for accomplishing them is outlined. The time to be spent with the client is structured and given boundaries. *"Rules" for relating* are formulated. *Trust* is established, and resistance is overcome.

During the initial phase, nurses "connect" with clients and empathize with their problems. Nurses make beginning interpretations; simultaneously, clients attempt their first, experimental changes in behavior.

Identification of Clients' Goals

Identifying clients' goals is an important part of the initial phase; it usually follows the assessment process (which is discussed in detail in Chapter 11). Nurses begin by asking clients to state their wishes and expectations as clearly and directly as possible. Specific and detailed questions are asked as they collect data. More generalized questions convey their willingness to consider clients' individual requests and their intention to deal with problems in ways that will be personally relevant to each client, rather than abstractly or in terms of intellectualizations. Following are examples of questions that facilitate identification of goals:

What specifically is bothering you?

What do you see as the cause of your difficulties?

Why are you looking for help now?

What do you think I can do for you?

What do you think is the best help for your difficulty?

What do you think will happen if you are not helped with your problem?

Nurses must evaluate the feasibility of the clients' requests and share their impressions regarding what might be considered a reasonable outcome of the relationship. Confusion and a sense of lacking direction or purpose result when the nurse fails to clarify and evaluate clients' goals. When nurse and client come to a mutual understanding of the purpose to be served by the relationship, they have established a contract. Much of the confusion and uncertainty which so frequently characterize the experiences of both participants at the outset of their relationship is thereby avoided.

Table 13-4 Therapeutic Environment during Initial Interview

Environmental and Structural Goals	Methods of Achieving Outcomes
Establish a relaxing physical environment	Comfortable seating
	Low noise level
	Soft nonglare lighting
	Private room or area free of interruptions and distractions
	Uncrowded spacing of furniture
Through the use of communication techniques, establish a comfortable atmosphere in which the client feels accepted, respected, and free to share real concerns	Use broad openings such as, "Please tell me what's on your mind," that give the client the initiative in the interview. Use open-ended questions such as, "Can you tell me about your relationship with your parents?" in order to encourage the client to describe and clarify material.
	Encourage the client to tell you more by using statements such as "go on," "um hmm," and "tell me more." Use restatement and reflection with statements such as "She really confuses you," and "You are smiling, but I sense you really hurt inside." Such statements convey understanding of the client's frame of reference.
	Use focusing statements that keep the interview goal-directed and avoid rambling with such statements as, "Can you go back to telling me about how it was for you at school?" Focusing helps clients get in touch with deeper feelings and lets them know that the nurse wants to hear them.
	Use clarifying statements that bring vague material into sharper focus such as, "I'm not clear on how you feel about your job. Could you repeat that and give me an example?" This lets the clients know that you are really interested in understanding them.
	Summarize major bits of content and feelings at the close of an interview. Use concise summarizing statements such as, "From your talk about family, school, and now your new job, you've experienced failure in all of them."
	Use information-giving statements that share factual and objective information during the interview such as telling a client what you know about a particular college in terms of enrollment, types of programs, etc. The client is free to accept or reject this information.
	Use observation skills to correlate verbal and nonverbal communication noticed during the interview.
Structure the outlines of the relationship	Establish the specific time, place, and duration of the interview(s).
	Establish the tentative number of interviews.
	Establish the fee, if any, method of payment, or insurance coverage.
	Clarify the purpose of the sessions and/or the relationship.
	Identify the role and responsibilities of the nurse and the client.
Gather data	Use a nursing assessment guide such as the detailed guide in Chapter 11.
	Use the facilitative communication skills outlined in Chapter 12.
Initiate referral to another agency if the client cannot obtain appropriate services at the current agency or is in need of other coordinating services	Use the community referral index established for the agency.
	Contact other agencies to initiate referral process.

SOURCE: From Judith Haber, "Facilitative Communication," in the second edition of this book.

Structuring

Another significant part of the initial phase is *structuring*—a term used to describe activities that are aimed at establishing a working partnership with a client. From the outset, the nurse must carefully outline the roles and responsibilities of both participants in the helping process. Structuring—which includes indicating the focus, duration, frequency, times, and location of meetings—gives clients an idea of what they can expect. Since it reduces ambiguity, it tends to reduce the anxiety caused by ambiguity. How specific relationships are structured will vary according to the setting. For example, a nurse who is running a self-help group for victims of stroke will establish less rigid time constraints than a nurse who is conducting a psychotherapeutic group.

Core Dimensions in the Initial Phase

The core dimensions listed in Table 13-3 are found in each phase of the helping relationship and can serve throughout it as guidelines for healing and promoting growth. It is important for nurses to understand the core dimensions and their significance at each phase.

People who are unable to solve their problems frequently feel cut off or isolated from their environment—even from potential helpers. It is not hard to understand why these clients often feel as if they are "losing ground." Information which might shed light on their problems is not available to them, because forces within them prevent them from recognizing problematic or inconsistent ideas, feelings, and behaviors. To solve their problems constructively, they must confront elements of their personal experiences that are unacknowledged and threatening. To help clients overcome their feelings of alienation and see themselves more clearly, nurses need to be sensitive to each client's inner world. Use of the core dimensions as facilitative communication processes, as well as the use of attending skills, such as paying close attention to clients' verbal and nonverbal behaviors, facial expressions, tone of voice, and posture, contributes to making this possible.

EMPATHY. Empathy has long been an important concept in nursing. It can be defined as the ability to "get inside another person's skin," and to see the world as someone else sees it. Nurses attempt to enter their clients' worlds not only to understand them but also, in some sense, to share their feelings.

In order to grasp clients' reality, nurses become "participant-observers" in the relationship process. They alternate between subjectively "feeling with" clients and objectively observing behavior. This requires a delicate balance of skills. Nurses' personal memories may facilitate empathic understanding, but recognition of clients' separateness and individuality is essential.

When a nurse formulates a response which is similar in content and "feeling tone" to something a client has expressed, empathy—or *empathic understanding*—is communicated. Clients' responses to such communications enable the nurse to determine their readiness for examining ideas, feelings, or actions. When clients feel understood, they are more willing to risk self-disclosure, thus beginning the task of building trust in another.

Following is an example of an interaction in which a nurse, Ms. R., utilizes empathic understanding.

MR. J.: We have been married only 3 months, and already my wife is beginning to nag me. (*Pause. Client rocks back and forth in his seat.*) She wants too much from me. In some ways she is just like my mother. (*Sounding angry.*)

MS. R.: (*Moving foward to listen more carefully.*) I understand your feelings. Perhaps you would like to say more about your anger.

MR. J.: I guess I really am angry at my wife. She nags me the way my mother did when I was younger.

MS. R.: That must be difficult for you.

MR. J.: Yes, but I love my wife. How can I tell her that her nagging makes me angry?

Several conditions exist when a nurse responds to a client with empathy. Forsyth calls these conditions *consciousness, temporality, relationship, validation, accuracy, intensity, objectivity,* and *freedom from value judgment.*[9] *Consciousness* refers to one's experience of self, another, or the environment. In the example above, Ms. R. was aware or conscious of Mr. J.'s anger. It was acknowledged in the "here and now," with *temporality* (timeliness). *Relationship* implies response, interaction, and reciprocity. In the example, Ms. R., through physical movement toward Mr. J., initiates a response to him. By acknowledging and feeding back to Mr. J. the feelings expressed, Ms. R. is *validating* his experience and feelings about his wife, helping him to own and take responsibility for them. When nurses help clients to separate fact from fantasy, they help them to clarify the meaning of a feeling or experience—that is, to achieve *accuracy. Intensity* is a criterion for empathy; it ranges from high to low, from superficial understanding to life-and-death concern. *Objectivity* is the ability to remain neutral in a relationship. It implies the need to avoid subjective or personalized involvement in the feelings of others. (Avoiding value judgments is an obvious component of objectivity.)[10]

CONCRETENESS. The clear, direct expression of personally relevant perceptions, values, and feelings as they exist in a relationship is referred to by Carkhuff as *concreteness*.[8] In the initial phase of a relationship concreteness is used by nurses when they are attempting to directly influence clients' behaviors. Concreteness is used to help clients focus on specific problems, to sharpen their observation skills, and to help them recall significant details of past or recent experiences, even if these details are painful. Storytelling and recitations of irrelevancies are discouraged.

The following excerpt illustrates the nurse's use of concreteness during the initial stage of helping:

CLIENT: The people here bug me. I'm at a loss about how to deal with them.

NURSE: Name one person here who disturbs you.

CLIENT: Mr. Mills, the attendant, always bothers me.

NURSE: What, specifically, does Mr. Mills do that bothers you?

CLIENT: He always wants me to go to those group therapy sessions. I never know how to respond.

NURSE: Tell me about one time when Mr. Mills asked you to attend a session and you were bothered.

By asking direct, explorative questions, the nurse requires the client to relate detailed and specific information about his discomfort with Mr. Mills.

A client's discovery of solutions to critical life problems is generally preceded by a thorough examination of personally relevant perceptions, ideas, feelings, and behaviors. When the nurse's verbal communications are concrete—that is, precise and relevant—the client's direct expression of significant experiences is facilitated.

CONFRONTATION. *Confrontation* is an interpersonal process used by the nurse to facilitate the modification and extension of the client's self-image.[8] It is a deliberate invitation to clients to examine incongruities in their feelings, beliefs, attitudes, and behavior. Self-image is a broad concept denoting a multiplicity of perceptions which may be consciously experienced or exist on a preconscious or unconscious level: (1) the image of one's value or belief system, (2) one's life goals, (3) the cluster of roles that one enacts, (4) one's sense of worth, and (5) perceptions and feelings about one's body. Information or input which is not harmonious with one's self-image is experienced as threatening and anxiety-provoking.

People tend to avoid anxiety by seeking input which maintains their self-image; therefore, confrontation by the nurse is often perceived initially as painful by the client. People who ignore or suppress potentially threatening information about themselves engage in a form of self-deception which impedes problem solving. Troubled people may wish that someone would help them to perceive reality with greater accuracy, but when a nurse calls attention to significant discrepancies in a client's experience, there is often a defensive response.

The purpose of confrontation is to enable the client to see what is real, that is, to perceive internal and external reality with greater precision and clarity. The initial stage of the nurse-client relationship may be viewed as a preparatory phase with regard to confrontation. The nurse attempts to discriminate between the real person that the client is and the client's idealized self-image. In addition, the nurse attempts to assess clients' readiness to look at the ways in which they have failed to live up to an idealized image of themselves. During this phase of the therapeutic relationship, nurses' success in confronting clients is contingent upon their ability to question or reflect upon clients' behavior without directly pointing out contradictions between their idealized and actual selves.

Several techniques are useful in confrontation. Making personal statements—that is, using the first person (*I, me, my*)—allows nurses to express directly how they think and feel about clients. (Statements such as "*Everyone* says your behavior is destructive" are not personal statements and should be avoided.) Describing behavior, naming feelings, paraphrasing, checking perceptions, and using feedback are other helpful techniques.

IMMEDIACY. Responding to what is happening in a relationship in the "here and now" is called *immediacy*. Present feelings and behaviors are explored and utilized to facilitate the therapeutic process and move toward goals.

Relationships with others, and images of others, are not static. Throughout life, people recast their impressions of others and experience changes in their relations with them. Clients' ever-changing perceptions of significant others shape and reshape their relationships. For example, as an individual's needs evolve, family ties may grow weaker or stronger, and friendships may erode or intensify.[10]

The concept of immediacy is important if nurses' relationships with clients are to be vital and productive; thus nurses frequently find themselves subjecting aspects of these relationships to close and careful scrutiny. While nurses are forming and reacting to their impressions of the relationships, so too are the clients. Throughout the helping process, clients' behaviors are determined, in part, by their varying images of the nurse as well as their personal impressions of the relationship. Clients' perceptions reveal much about their earlier experiences with helpers and persons in authority, their beliefs about the helping process, and their expectations, wishes, and fears.

Most clients, however, do not initially feel free to disclose their impressions or react directly and openly to them. Instead, clients tend to convey their impressions in more indirect ways—for example, through the use of metaphor or behavioral expressions. To establish and maintain a working alliance, nurses need to be sensitive to clients' perceptions of them and become adroit at helping clients express immediate and relevant interpersonal themes.

The following example illustrates the use of immediacy to establish a working alliance between a nursing student and a client.

> The client, a 38-year-old woman named Ellen, rarely uttered a word to Susan, the nurse who had been seeing her twice weekly for 2 months. One day, in a desperate effort to surmount the communication barrier which existed between herself and the client, Susan placed before the silent woman a drawing pad and some crayons. "Draw a picture of whatever is on your mind," the nurse suggested. Much to the nurse's surprise, Ellen picked up a crayon and proceeded to sketch the outline of a house. Notably, the house had no door, the windows were shut, and the shades were drawn. The nurse asked the client to explain the picture. Ellen said that she lived in this house with an imaginary female companion. "The shades," the client explained, "are meant to keep people out."
>
> "Perhaps it is difficult for you to let people know what is going on with you in lots of situations," Susan stated, tentatively.
>
> "Yes; this is true," was the client's response.
>
> "And perhaps you keep me out," the nurse continued. "Even now, you may be telling me with your drawing that it is difficult for you to let me know what you are thinking and feeling."
>
> Looking directly at Susan, Ellen smiled and said, "Yes; it is very hard for me."
>
> "Most of the time," Susan explained, "it is very hard for me to get to know what is on your mind. I want very much to help you, but it is difficult when you don't let me in."

The underlined statements illustrate immediacy. These statements are intended to explain the relationship between the client's behavior—in this instance, remaining silent—and her perceptions of the helper and the helping situation. The client's response suggests that it is hard for her to disclose her inner thoughts and feelings and that *at the moment* she views the nurse as an outsider intruding on her private world. The discussion affords the nurse an opportunity to convey to the client her wish to serve as a helpful ally. It is critical that the nurse explicitly convey support, particularly at the outset of the relationship.

Clients are sometimes prevented from immediately recognizing nurses as sensitive and caring collaborators. They presume that nurses bear malice toward them, that they are going to be judgmental or perhaps overly friendly. Some "blocks" to immediacy and participation with nurses in a therapeutic encounter are discussed in the following paragraphs.

One such block can be created by clients' previous experiences with self-disclosure. Clients must sometimes overcome earlier experiences which have taught them that disclosure of their observations may destroy a relationship or cause resentment. They often fear exposing their secrets. Shame and concern about the social acceptability of certain ideas are powerful deterrents to self-disclosure. A client who feels love or hatred, has sexual or aggressive urges, longs for dependency, or perhaps is suspicious may be therefore loath to share personal impressions with the nurse. Clients may also conceal such thoughts because they view them as signs of weakness.

If clients feel insignificant, that too can represent a block. Sometimes clients' hesitation to reveal their perceptions is rooted in the belief that their impressions, beliefs, or wishes are unimportant. These people often think that they are not really entitled to feel or see things as they do. For example:

> A male client reluctantly told the nurse that he had the impression that the nurse was not really paying attention to what he was saying. After sharing his perception, he immediately added, "But I really shouldn't feel that way!"

Clients may require repeated permission to express their thoughts and feelings. Nurses need to give this permission and, at the same time, focus on clients' resistance or withdrawal.

Clients' perceptions of the nurse and their desire to make the nurse respond in certain ways may also constitute a block to immediacy. Clients' perceptions of the nurse account for many of their actions throughout the helping relationship. Many behaviors are calculated or unknowingly intended to induce a mood in the nurse or to elicit a response which will minimize a perceived threat or gratify a wish. Sometimes a client's actions are motivated by a need for approval or a wish to be liked; and sometimes clients act out of a desire to control certain aspects of a relationship.

Finally, cultural differences can lead to blocks. Clients' cultural backgrounds may sometimes affect the way they behave when they are trying to elicit certain responses from the nurse. Thus, some clients may think that they must display intense emotion if they want helpers to take them seriously; other clients may understate their case, fearing that an emotional display will evoke scorn and rejection.

Blocks like these can impair a relationship and make immediacy impossible. To establish or facilitate immediacy, nurses can ask the following questions:

- How do you think things are going with us?
- Perhaps you are trying to tell me something about yourself in relation to me?
- Are you trying to tell me that you see me as (specify attribute)?
- Are you saying that you feel that I am (*specify attribute*)?
- Sometimes clients see nurses as (*specify attribute*). Could this be the case with you?

Nurses can also make statements aimed at helping clients to examine relationships between overt behavior and inner experiences:

- Perhaps your (*specify client's behavior*) is a way of telling me indirectly that you wish me to (*specify nurse's behavior*).
- Perhaps your behavior is meant to tell me that you see our relationship as (*specify characteristic of relationship*).

Expressions of immediacy are intended to explain connections between clients' behavior and their underlying impressions of the nurse or the helping relationship. By drawing attention to the relationship itself, these expressions sometimes have the effect of intensifying the clients' anxiety and magnifying their distorted perceptions of the nurse. Nevertheless, there are critical times when communications of immediacy are necessary for the development and maintenance of a viable working partnership. Six critical times are listed below.

1. The initial phase of the helping relationship, when nurse and client are strangers to one another
2. Before and after a temporary separation between nurse and client, for example, before and after a vacation taken by either person
3. Before or after the occurrence of an unusual event, such as a change in the fee schedule or location of sessions
4. After the nurse has committed a technical error, such as giving advice prematurely
5. When, for unexplained reasons, the client is unable to share inner experiences with the nurse
6. Before termination of the relationship[11]

RESPECT. People with self-respect view themselves as worthy and capable of solving their problems and acting constructively. When nurses convey their acceptance of clients' ideas, feelings, and experiences and recognize clients' potential for self-actualization, they provide the conditions necessary for development and maintenance of self-respect. Respect demonstrates that the nurse values the integrity of clients and has confidence in their ability to solve their problems.

Respect is expressed in diverse ways as the helping relationship evolves. During the early stages of helping, nurses convey to clients their intentions to hear them out. Nurses' responses lead clients to believe that nurses will listen without judging their clients, depreciating them, telling them how they ought to act, or demanding their compliance with some expectations. Nurses' responses suggest confidence and trust in clients' ability to act on their own behalf and to come to a successful resolution of their difficulties. Within this climate of acceptance and trust, clients will feel free to engage in deeper levels of self-exploration.

GENUINENESS. The ability that nurses and clients have to be real and honest with one another is referred to as *genuineness*. Throughout the interpersonal helping process, the nurse experiences feelings toward the client, the relationship, or both. Genuine expressions which convey the nurse's personal reactions to the client can be used by the nurse to further the client's self-exploration.

To facilitate the expression of genuineness, nurses need to look inward. During the initial stage of the relationship, emphasis is placed on noticing personal reactions to the client, but it is also essential that the nurses intervene with themselves. Self-assessment is discussed in Chapter 4.

Middle Phase

Characteristics of the Middle Phase

The gradual transition to the middle phase of a therapeutic relationship is accompanied by the client's willingness to assume a more active role in self-exploration. Taking into account the client's accomplishments during the initial phase, nurses and clients can pursue activities aimed at enabling clients to cope with, or profit from, exploration of the problematic experiences of day-to-day living. The main tasks to be accomplished during the middle phase are in-depth exploration of significant themes and discovery and testing of solutions which are most appropriate to the client's life situations.

Much of the therapeutic work during the middle phase of a relationship is perceived as boring. Clients will say that "nothing is happening," or nurses will complain that they are tired of dealing with the same issues. Clients need to be encouraged to take risks—since risk is inherent in change—and see the relationship through to a therapeutic end. Maximizing the client's self-awareness becomes the desired outcome.

Core Dimensions in the Middle Phase

During the middle phase of the relationship, the nurse continues to use the core dimensions as guides for intervention.

EMPATHY. The recognition by both client and nurse of the clients' troubled world, acquired during the initial phase of their relationship, provides a foundation for deeper inquiry in the next phase. During the middle phase, nurses' empathic expressions are intended to help clients clarify and extend the meaning of their experiences. When the problem is better understood by nurses than by clients themselves, nurses make tentative statements aimed at calling attention to relevant though previously unexplored thoughts and feelings. Nurses convey feelings which transcend those initially expressed by clients. Thus, they prepare clients for experiencing and fully expressing feelings which were up to this time unacknowledged.

The following conversation is an illustration of empathic understanding during the middle phase of a relationship.

CLIENT: I'm afraid to talk about what is going on between my wife and me.

NURSE: It is difficult for you.

CLIENT: Yes. It's just that sometimes I get so mad that I'm ready to walk out.

NURSE: It really bothers you to get so angry with someone you care for.

CLIENT: I shouldn't be so furious with my wife. I love her and have made a commitment to our relationship.

NURSE: You seem to think that it is not acceptable for a person to have both loving and angry feelings toward another.... You seem to feel you must always express devotion toward your wife.

CLIENT: Yes. Isn't that true?

NURSE: No. Most people experience a whole range of intense feelings toward their marital partners. However, you tend to feel guilty about this.

CLIENT: I think that I may have some unrealistic expectations.

NURSE: Yes. And when you fail to live up to them, you blame and condemn yourself.

CLIENT: Yes. That is exactly what happens to me.

NURSE: Perhaps it is time to stop this self-condemnation and to begin looking at the behavior in the situations that make you angry.

Clients frequently derive benefit from hearing the nurse's impressions of their life situation. However, communications which are intended to convey the nurse's perceptions of the clients' experience need to be differentiated from those which give advice prematurely. Often, an astute nurse will quickly "size up" a client's situation and suggest a course of action. But when advice is not based upon the client's thorough self-understanding, it tends to steer the client away from self-exploration—making the therapeutic encounter more a "directed" process and therefore less helpful. As the nurse and the client acquire deeper comprehension of, and insight into, the client's problem, the real but limited number of available alternatives open to the client becomes apparent, and directionality emerges naturally from the process instead of being imposed on it.

A theoretical understanding of empathy, experience, and supervision helps nurses to gauge the timing of empathic communications.

CONCRETENESS. In problem solving, both nurse and client must speak in concrete terms about the client's future. When plans and expectations are formulated and reviewed in specific terms, rather than in generalities, clients are likely to sense the active role they play in determining their future experiences. On the other hand, when nurses and clients fail to communicate clearly about clients' plans, clients may get the impression that the future is, in fact, governed by fate.

Throughout the nurse-client relationship, misunderstandings on the part of clients frequently stem from nurses' ambiguous responses to clients' inquiries. When clients do not receive concrete answers to their questions, they tend to pursue the inquiry in a more indirect fashion or to "invent" explanations which may or may not be valid. Sometimes, clients will interpret the ambiguity or evasiveness of helpers as an indication that they are withholding a terrible piece of information. In such instances, clients come to anticipate the worst.

Evasive responses by nurses increase clients' anxiety.[12] Table 13-5 lists several evasive strategies used by nurses with examples of each. More appropriate concrete responses are also noted.

CONFRONTATION. Communications conveying high levels of empathic understanding tend to involve confrontations. Clients who seek perfection in themselves and others are frequently resistant to confrontations; they anticipate that confrontations will evoke pain, guilt, or anxiety. Clients' efforts to maintain self-deception are generally proportional to their expectations of discomfort. The following statements, made by nurses, are intended to di-

Table 13-5 Evasion Strategies

Evasion Strategy	Evasive Response	Direct Concrete Response
Nurse confuses who is acting by switching to passive tense.	The idea *was expressed* that ... The question *was posed* ...	*You asked* whether ... *You wonder* if ...
Nurse uses unnecessary qualifiers.	*Apparently,* some confusion exists ... *At this time,* it looks as if ... *From my standpoint* ...	You seem confused. This is how I see it. I think that ...
Nurse broadens the subject.	*Many nurses* claim that ... It has been noted by others that ...	*I* think that ... *I* have noticed that ...
Nurse use analogies or figures of speech.	It is *like a three-ring circus.* We are playing a *cat-and-mouse game.*	It is chaotic. We are being evasive with each other.
Nurse delays answering question.	I first want to discover how an answer will help you.	(Nurse answers question.)
Nurse completely changes subject.	Let's look at something else first.	(Nurse pursues subject at hand.)

minish clients' resistances to confrontations during the middle phase of the helping relationship:

- No one is all good or all bad. People cannot be perfect; neither can the world be a perfect place to live in.
- You are a human being. Human beings are fallible and make mistakes.
- It is not possible to be always good, loving, lovable, or kind. Trying to be this way uses up too much energy and requires that you sacrifice the person you really are.
- Our behavior is often influenced by thoughts and feelings of which we are not aware. Recognizing these inner experiences gives us more control over our lives; we are less the "victims of fate."
- The pain that accompanies self-discovery is temporary. It will not last forever and often is short-lived.
- Feelings are simply feelings, not facts.

The extent of the positive transference in a relationship and the timing and style used by each nurse will determine the extent to which clients hear confrontative interpretations and remain receptive to them.

IMMEDIACY. To make use of immediacy in the middle phase of the nurse-client relationship, nurses take the initiative and originate discussion about the ongoing therapeutic process.

Nurses can start by listening to hidden messages—feelings or thoughts which lurk beneath the surface of clients' manifest concerns. These central ideas underlying clients' overt communication are called *content themes.*

In the following example, a client experiences the pain of separation, and an alert nurse determines the underlying theme and confronts it:

> As the summer months approached, the client, an elderly woman, was becoming increasingly apprehensive about the nurse's impending vacation. Not wishing to appear overly dependent or clinging, the woman made a conscious decision to refrain from discussing her anxiety. When the nurse tried to elicit discussion of the client's reactions to the impending separation, the client initiated a broad and lengthy monologue on stoicism. At no point did she speak plainly of her resolve to remain calm and stoic in the face of sadness and fear. Because the cause of the client's feelings was unconscious, the underlying theme could only be inferred by the nurse. The nurse responded to the experience of the client with immediacy by stating, "I sense that you are upset about my upcoming vacation. Let's talk about your concerns."

Sometimes the way clients convey their concerns indicates how they are perceiving the nurse, the relationship, or both. For example:

> Mr. J., a client who feared being dominated by the nurse, was guarded and defensive when he informed the nurse that he had decided to terminate their relationship.

Clients' interpersonal needs frequently determine their impressions of the helping situation. In this instance, the client's need was to maintain control of himself and the situation.

Another aspect of immediacy is *interaction themes.* Ujhely uses the term *interaction theme*[13] to describe clients' behaviors toward nurses and nurses' responses to these behaviors. Analysis of clinical data and the use of supervision can lead nurses to recognize and label significant interaction themes. Ensuring that these themes are related to present events in a client's life is an important result of the use of immediacy.

For instance, sometimes nurses assume roles which are complementary to those of clients. An example of role complementarity is the situation in which nurses find themselves making numerous decisions for clients who refuse or seem unable to make choices. Assumption of a complementary role may obstruct further development or stall the nurse-client relationship. Identification of such an interaction theme is an initial step in exploring with clients their images of and reactions to the nurse.

RESPECT. The more clients reveal their inner life and personal adventures, the greater is the nurse's opportunity to appreciate each client's unique characteristics. Nonjudgmental recognition of, and positive regard for, the individual ways in which clients perceive and respond to various situations is a form of respect. Such respect is characteristic of the middle phase of the helping relationship.

Messages which convey high levels of respect reduce clients' anxiety and heighten their sense of security. Clients who feel respected are less likely to respond defensively when the nurse directs their attention to ways in which they are not living up to their potential. Many people suppress their need for human contact, smother or conceal vital emotions, kill spontaneity, evade responsible action, and avoid self-sufficiency. By the time the nurse and the client have reached the middle phase of the helping relationship, the nurse sees quite clearly the ways in which clients make choices that tend to stifle their growth. As the middle phase unfolds, the nurse conditionally conveys positive regard, commending clients only when they choose a functional course of action.

As trust and respect between client and nurse deepen, nurses strive to help their clients recognize the incapacitating consequences of restrictive behavior patterns and appreciate the value of self-realization.

GENUINENESS. As the helping relationship evolves, nurses begin to recognize countertransference feelings evoked by clients' verbal and nonverbal behaviors. Nurses can utilize these personal reactions to discover clients' impressions and suppressed feelings about the one-to-one relationship and to facilitate the helping process.

The following excerpt illustrates communication of genuineness during the middle phase of the nurse-client relationship:

CLIENT: It's just no use. Things are never going to change. And all you ever give me is a meaningless bunch of words.

NURSE: You're telling me that you are feeling hopeless. Even though we have shared a great deal, you are not experiencing me as helpful.

CLIENT: No. It's probably my fault that I haven't solved my problem. I should have been more open with you. I always ruin everything.

NURSE: Look, at this very moment I'm feeling frustrated and useless. I have the impression that, in truth, you are angry with me. You want to show me how much you are suffering so that I too will suffer.

CLIENT: I guess I've been afraid that you would punish me in some way if I told you how annoyed I've been with you lately.

In this example the nurse shares feelings of frustration and uselessness and the client is enabled to express anger. In this exchange a "stalled" relationship is "moved" because of genuineness in the communication between nurse and client.

Termination Phase

Characteristics of the Termination Phase

The time just preceding a permanent separation between nurse and client is frequently referred to as the *termination phase* of the helping relationship. Clients' reactions to termination are affected by the meaning they ascribe to it, the duration of the relationship, and the extent to which goals have been achieved.[11] The termination process begins when goals are set in the early stages of a relationship, and is completed when both nurse and client think that their goals have been achieved.

Ideally, the timing of termination is agreed upon by client and nurse. Criteria that can be used to determine when termination is appropriate may include a client's experiencing relief from the problem or problems that initiated the relationship; a nurse's observing increased social functioning and decreased social isolation on the part of the client; a client's establishing a strong sense of self-integration; or a client's achieving certain goals.

In some relationships a stall may have occurred, or resistance, transference, or countertransference may make it impossible to accomplish any meaningful change. Nurses have an ethical obligation to recognize the limits of their helping skills and begin termination of clients with whom they are no longer able to achieve preestablished goals. Sometimes such a course of action "jars" the process and enables meaningful work to continue. In any case, the decision to terminate a therapeutic relationship is a delicate process fraught with anxiety.

As termination approaches, nurse and client are becoming part of each other's past; each is moving into a future in which the other will have no part. The future will bring changes, and both nurse and client will experience *anxiety*—that is, they will respond to the danger or risk that their separation from each other entails. They may also experience *grief*—that is, they may respond to the separation itself. Anticipating the end of the relationship and realizing that it is unlikely to be resumed activates a grieving process. The purpose of the grieving process is separation from the nurse, and the process is complete when the client internalizes the loss of the helping relationship.

The onset of grieving is often marked by the client's preoccupation with the nurse and the experiences shared during their relationship. Grieving clients may begin to experience a variety of somatic symptoms. They may become depressed and preoccupied with guilt. They may wonder whether it was something they did that caused the relationship to end. A stiff manner, designed to hide anger, often develops. For a while, the client may lose the capacity for initiating or keeping up with organized patterns of behavior.

In a study of psychoanalytic treatment of adults who had experienced losses of significant others during childhood, it was noted that the treatment itself, particularly situations occurring during the last phase, activated interrupted "grief work" and helped clients resume the process. Observations of nurse-client relationships correspond with these findings.[3]

Clients' fear of facing grief may impair their ability to find meaning in the relationship as it nears conclusion. To reduce their anxiety, clients may use coping mechanisms such as acting out, dependency, resignation, denial, and reaction formation.

Acting out may occur when clients cannot readily control or contain their anxiety. During the termination phase, some clients leave the hospital on a pass and fail to return. Others sign themselves out of the hospital precipitately, "against medical advice." Some clients abruptly end the relationship by refusing to keep appointments with the nurse. On some occasions, clients who have been hospitalized will "sabotage" discharge plans or behave inappropriately so that they can remain in the hospital. Outpatients may begin to revert to old patterns of behavior as termination approaches. Some clients in clinical settings fail to keep their last appointment in order to avoid formally closing the relationship.

Adult clients who sense their *dependency* upon the nurse in order to feel whole and to feel good about themselves sometimes believe that they have been absorbed by, or have become part of, the nurse. For clients, loss of personal identity is the danger which separation from the nurse entails. Clients who fear that they will not survive without the nurse may use guile or adopt ruses to demonstrate their helplessness. They may regress, reexperiencing former symptoms. It is essential for the nurse to assess the seriousness of a client's decompensation and adjust termination planning accordingly.

Frequently, clients dissociate any thoughts regarding the danger which separation may entail. Instead of concern, these clients report a lack of interest in the nurse and the impending termination. Clients who cope by *resigning themselves* have, in a sense, withdrawn from the situation.

Denial is a defense mechanism in which external reality is rejected and replaced by a wish-fulfilling fantasy. Denial takes various forms, ranging from lasting distortions of clients' perceptions of themselves and their world to limited avoidance of reality during a particularly stressful period. Clients who deny the reality of termination may negate the importance of the nurse, insist on repeating with the nurse a fictional relationship with another who was lost in the past, or refuse to talk about termination. During the termination phase, clients' use of denial may have both negative and positive aims. A negative aim is to increase the perceived distance between themselves and danger. A positive aim is to bring about a necessary change while preserving personal integrity.

Sometimes, clients who are experiencing painful feelings attempt to find fault with the nurse and everything in the setting. Such *reaction formation* may take the form of complaining about food, services, or hospital personnel. Feelings of warmth and attachment are avoided at any cost.

Each of these defenses must be explored using the framework of the core dimensions if the goal of healthy separation is to be accomplished.

Core Dimensions in the Termination Phase

The single most important nursing *intervention* during the termination phase of a helping relationship is alerting the client to the impending separation. The most critical *attitude* of the nurse, which must underlie any intervention taken, is the following: *Leaving is not something the nurse is doing to the client but, rather, something the nurse is doing with the client.* Summarizing situations which occurred throughout the relationship, exchanging memories, and evaluating the relationship are experiences which nurses share with clients to help them to cope with the ending of the helping relationship. It needs to be kept in mind that while the client leaves the nurse, the nurse must also separate from the client.

Nurses' ability and willingness to spontaneously disclose their inner experiences to clients and their capacity for conveying to clients their concern for what is happening between them are particularly critical as the helping relationship draws to a close. Immediacy and genuineness therefore play key roles during the termination phase.

IMMEDIACY. Frequently, clients are aware of the impending termination but will not initiate discussion of the subject. Nurses need to be alert for verbal and nonverbal communications from clients which indicate that they are thinking about termination or that they feel ready to terminate the relationship. Clients may reveal their concerns by alluding to the length of the relationship or by introducing material which relates to separations from significant others.

One interesting reason why clients may be reluctant to introduce the subject of termination is that they sometimes have a false expectation that they should be able to make the transition easily. Although the American value is that people accept and deal with change readily, nurses need to remember that the change represented by termination of the helping relationship can be difficult for clients.

When a client fails to initiate discussion of termination, the nurse can broach the subject by indicating the date of the last meeting, the number of interviews remaining, and the reasons for ending them. Once the subject of termination has been introduced, the nurse may discover how, in fact, the client views the chain of events which has occurred. The client may have trouble recognizing and labeling these events; therefore, it is suggested that the nurse begin to reminisce with the client. With the nurse's encouragement and support, the client can be helped to remember significant events and to clarify the significance of the helping relationship.

GENUINENESS. Sometimes, clients refuse to talk about feelings and thoughts related to termination of the therapeutic relationship. At other times, they release a flood of expressions of despair and accusations of abandonment or rejection. Clients' reactions to termination can wreak havoc with nurses who are out of touch with their own feelings about and responses to the ending of the relationship. During the final phase, therefore, nurses' unrecognized countertransference feelings may preclude genuine communication. Self-awareness is essential at this point, and genuineness becomes particularly significant.

It has been noted that there is a correlation between helpers' attitudes toward their next clinical assignment and their ability to handle termination adequately. Helpers who regard future assignments with displeasure or anxiety have more difficulty handling termination. Supervision can facilitate nurses' examination of their perceptions of the present and the future.

During the final phase of the relationship, nurses tend to look back, and they may recognize factors which have influenced their behavior. For example, nurses frequently recognize therapeutic zeal, a need to cure clients, or a desire to perpetuate clients' dependency. Observations made by a nursing student during the termination phase of a helping relationship illustrate this point:

> If I had done everything right, my client would have gotten better. During the initial and middle phases of the relationship, I made a few mistakes. But there was time left to try to correct these. I could look at my client's suffering and try to alleviate it. Now, if I make a mistake, there is no time left to fix it up. I'm powerless. My client will soon be gone, and he hasn't been cured. I will be able to do nothing more to ease his suffering.

A nurse who has plunged headlong into a relationship hoping to cure a client is in trouble during the termination phase. However, recognition of unrealistic motives and their impact upon the relationship may give the nurse a new sense of clarity and relief. Formulation of realistic goals during the beginning phase of the relationship will facilitate the final stage of therapeutic work.

Discovering that one has acted to perpetuate a client's dependency is, perhaps, a more painful experience for the nurse. Nurses who need to be needed sometimes discourage clients' efforts to move away from the refuge represented by the relationship. It is likely that these helpers never seriously acknowledged their clients' goals or drew attention to goals which were attained. These nurses probably neglected to urge clients to become aware of their growing selves and may have presented themselves as necessary to their clients' adjustment. During the termination phase, nurses who need to be needed sense the loss of a gratifying relationship. Often, these helpers would like to think that clients cannot tolerate living without them. Nurses who have trouble "letting go" may experience guilt over deserting their clients. Consequently, they may discourage clients from venting responses to the impending separation. Genuine expressions of pain, sadness, anxiety, or perhaps anger are thus discouraged. When nurses minimize or avoid dealing with their clients' experiences, the clients' pain and anger are often intensified, thereby increasing the nurses' guilt.

Looking back over a relationship, a nurse may recognize what has been described as an inevitable distortion of the therapeutic process. Throughout the one-to-one relationship, nurse and client may tend to underestimate the client's strengths and overestimate weaknesses. Each may devalue the significance of the relationship and may harbor unrealistic fears regarding the client's ability to cope with loss or to confront the future without the nurse. An initial assessment which includes clients' strengths as well as problems will help to avoid this pitfall.

During the termination phase, progress can be measured in terms of attainment of concrete goals which nurse and client originally planned. Progress can also encompass a deeply felt experience of growth and forward movement which derives from extending and clarifying the meaning of events or situations which occurred throughout the helping relationship. The extent to which nurses help clients find meaning in the therapeutic encounter depends in part upon their own ability to find meaning in it.

ETHICS OF THE NURSE-CLIENT RELATIONSHIP

There is a growing body of evidence to suggest that people designated as helpers may have beneficial or harmful effects on people seeking help. The wish to be facilitative provides a base for nurses' interactions with clients. Ongoing self-assessment is a primary component of ethical relationships with clients. While they do not always attain this end, nurses have an ethical obligation to strive for it by using and applying theory, availing themselves of the supervisory process, avoiding burnout, and protecting the confidentiality of clients.

The Value of Theory

Theory explains relationships between events which occur during helping interactions. Use of theory provides a way of conceptualizing what happens in a relationship and enables nurses to make judgments which guide their practice.[14]

On some occasions, the fears of nurses and clients become painful realities. How do nurses ensure and evaluate their effectiveness as helpers? For the most part, nurses' reactions to clients are spontaneous. Rapidly occurring events render it impossible to think out or thoroughly plan responses. Nurses can never anticipate everything that will happen, nor can they plan all their actions in advance. They must rely on basic concepts of practice which grow out of a sound theoretical framework. With the proliferation of knowledge, it becomes essential that nurses constantly update their theoretical base. One of the primary roles of the clinical supervisor is to assist novices with this updating in order that they may better understand and advance their clinical practice.

The Supervisory Process

Clinical supervision is an interpersonal process aimed at helping nurses to understand and advance their practice through the acquisition of professional knowledge and skill.[15]

The complex psychological interaction between nurses and clients constitutes a major part of the helping process. Empathic understanding, concreteness, confrontation, genuineness, immediacy, and respect are concepts which have been used to describe and explain this psychological interaction. An essential function of the psychiatric nursing supervisor is to enable novice helpers to overcome barriers to the full expression of each of these core dimensions. With the aid of more knowledgeable and experienced helpers, nurses can objectively look at their practice and increase their repertoire of therapeutic skills. In addition, they can hope to attain a higher level of knowledge of self as part of facilitative interpersonal processes.

The extension of one's professional self-image and the understanding and advancement of professional nursing practice are objectives of the supervisory relationship. It is noteworthy that, although the supervisor functions not as a psychotherapist but as a teacher, the most effective supervisors are those who convey high levels of each of the core dimensions.

Awareness of Burnout

One of the hazards experienced by people working in an intense helping relationship is referred to as *burnout,* or disillusionment with oneself and one's clients. Burnout is stress-related and generally manifests itself as one of two extreme interpersonal syndromes: total detachment or overinvolvement with clients.

To avoid burnout, nurses working in intense therapeutic situations need to be in touch with their feelings, trust them, share them, and use them constructively. Use of theory and the supervisory relationship are essential in this process.

When burnout occurs, nurses need to consider a change. Leaving the stresses of psychiatric nursing for a time (or permanently) may be indicative of mature decision making which will ultimately benefit nurses and clients equally.[16]

Confidentiality

In the course of a trusting relationship, clients expose a great deal of personal, painful, and potentially damaging content. Nurses are ethically obligated to keep their interactions with clients confidential. If anything that has been revealed must be shared with teachers, supervisors, or team members who are involved in the treatment of the client, the same obligation for confidentiality is placed on these persons. Explicit permission, in writing, should be obtained from clients before any contact with a family member or another agency is initiated.

When audio- or videotaping of sessions is considered appropriate, permission to monitor interactions in this way must be obtained from the client in writing. When permission is not granted by clients, care must be taken that the therapeutic process is not disrupted. Student nurses may interpret a client's refusal to allow mechanical monitoring as rejection or anger. They may become fearful of disapproval from their supervisor or professor or fail to look at other options available for monitoring their work. Being aware of their own reactions and honestly sharing them with appropriate supervisors, teachers, or team members will help nurses to maintain objectivity and allow relationships with clients to continue unblocked.

SUMMARY

The nurse-client relationship is a reciprocal process that evolves over time toward achievement of planned outcomes. The nurse's goal for every therapeutic relationship is self-actualization of the client and integration of the client's physical, mental, and spiritual dimensions.

Therapeutic relationships always involve subjective experiences of both nurses and their clients. At the outset of the relationship nurses may experience fear of rejection, of exploiting clients, of helplessness, of physical assault, or of becoming or being mentally ill themselves. Clients are concerned about the seriousness of their problems and the threat to their self-image.

Nurses' expectations with regard to the helping relationship include actualizing humanitarian ideals, clarifying values, maintaining self-esteem, finding diversion, and enhancing the self. Clients may expect control, contact with reality, nurturance, granting of administrative requests, institutional contact, and the possibility of ventilation. They may also expect advice, clarification, psychological expertise, psychotherapy, socialization, and referral or medical treatment.

Transference, countertransference, and resistance are characteristics of all nurse-client relationships.

Six core dimensions—empathy, concreteness, respect, genuineness, confrontation, and immediacy—are operationalized by nurses throughout the initial, middle, and termination phases of the nurse-client relationship.

The desire to be facilitative is the basis of nurses' interactions with clients. Although they do not always attain this end, nurses have an ethical obligation to strive for it by using and applying theory, availing themselves of the supervisory process, avoiding burnout, and protecting the confidentiality of clients.

REFERENCES

1. H. Peplau, *Interpersonal Relations in Nursing,* Putnam, New York, 1952.
2. S. Lego, "Psychiatric Nursing: Theory and Practice of the One-to-One Nurse-Client Relationship," presented at a conference on *The State of the Art of Psychiatric Nursing,* April 1974.
3. A. Combs, *Florida Studies in Helping Professionals,* University of Florida Press, Gainesville, 1969.
4. G. Gottsegan and M. Gottsegan, "Countertransference—The Professional Identity Defense," *Psychotherapy: Theory, Research and Practice,* vol. 16, no. 2, 1979, p. 57.
5. J. Clement, "The Helping Relationship: Choices and Dilemmas," *Issues in Mental Health Nursing,* vol. 1, no. 4, 1978, pp. 17–31.
6. A. Burgess and A. Lazare, *Psychiatric Nursing in the Hospital and the Community,* Prentice-Hall, Englewood Cliffs, N.J., 1973.
7. C. Hammond, D. Hepworth, and V. Smith, *Improving Therapeutic Relationships,* Josey-Bass, San Francisco, 1977.
8. R. Carkhuff, *Helping and Human Relations,* vols. 1 and 2, Holt, New York, 1968.
9. G. Forsyth, "Analysis of the Concept of Empathy: Illustration of One Approach," *Advances in Nursing Science,* vol. 2, no. 2, January 1980, pp. 33–42.
10. E. LaMonica, "Empathy in Nursing Practice," *Issues in Mental Health Nursing,* vol. 2, no. 1, 1979, p. 3.
11. B. W. Duldt, K. Griffin, and B. R. Patton, *Interpersonal Communication In Nursing,* Davis, Philadelphia, 1984.
12. A. Pokorney, "When to Talk Fuzzy," *Psychiatric News,* vol. 71, no. 4, 1971, pp. 1–2.
13. G. Ujhely, *Determinants of the Nurse-Client Relationship,* Springer, New York, 1968.
14. I. M. King, *A Theory For Nursing,* Wiley, New York, 1981.
15. R. S. Simmons and J. Rosenthal, "The Women's Movement and the Nurse Practitioner's Sense of Role," *Nursing Outlook,* vol. 29, no. 6, June 1981, pp. 373–375.
16. G. A. Wolf, "Nurse Turnover: Some Causes and Solutions," *Nursing Outlook,* vol. 29, no. 4, April 1981, p. 235.

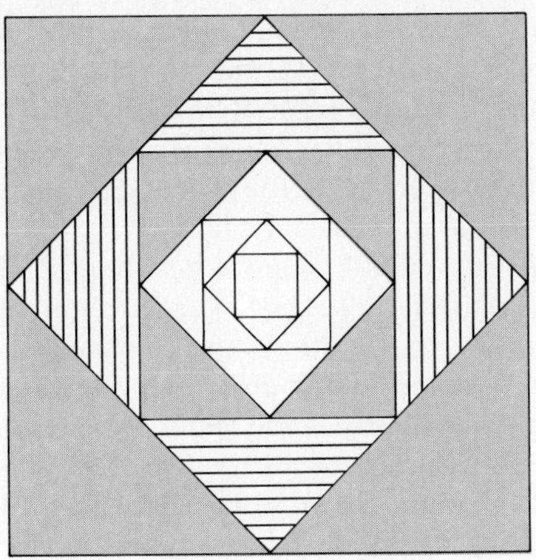

CHAPTER 14
Nursing Research

Judith Belliveau Krauss

LEARNING OBJECTIVES

After studying this chapter, the student should be able to:

1. State the purpose of research in nursing.
2. Define *nursing research.*
3. Differentiate between nursing research and other types of research.
4. Name the steps involved in analyzing clinical nursing problems.
5. Identify at least one major researchable problem in psychiatric–mental health nursing.
6. Differentiate among exploratory designs, hypothesis-testing designs, and measurement designs.
7. Classify areas of nursing practice into their component parts or factors to be studied.
8. List the rights of human subjects participating in research studies.
9. Name at least two major issues which influence the conduct of research in psychiatric–mental health nursing.

Nursing research is the systematic study of the practice of nursing. It uses scientific method to ensure that facts are collected as objectively as possible and that findings and conclusions reflect reality. Its purpose is to describe, and to influence, interactions between nurses and clients; develop appropriate and sensitive methodologies for nursing problems; and develop and test theories which, when implemented, can improve nursing practice.[1–5]

Research is a process—a way of thinking about the problems of nursing practice and assimilating findings through appropriate theories so as to understand how facts are associated and related and predict future events and relationships. Nursing research is a systematic way of examining patterns of interaction among person, family, and community; it involves nursing activities related to promotion, maintenance, restoration, and rehabilitation of health. It focuses on physical, mental, and spiritual dimensions of the person; environmental systems relevant to clients, such as the family; health care delivery systems; interactive patterns of clients and holistic care-giving systems; and the synchronicity or dysynchronicity of such patterns. It contributes to the development of nursing theory and provides a scientific basis for nursing practice.

The purpose of this chapter is to introduce various aspects of nursing research. Some trends in research in psychiatric–mental health nursing—and the need for research in this area—will be discussed. Designs for nursing research will be introduced, and the theory generated by these designs and its applicability to nursing practice will be presented. Problems for nursing research and issues that influence how it is conducted in mental health settings will also be examined. The material covered in the chapter should help readers become knowledgeable consumers of nursing research.

TRENDS IN PSYCHIATRIC–MENTAL HEALTH NURSING

In 1929, Annie Goodrich, the first dean of the Yale School of Nursing, said that the nurse must speak both the language of science and that of the people.[5] In 1982, Paul Starr,[6] a noted sociologist, suggested that the nursing practitioner is an intermediary between science and personal experience. Almost six decades separate Goodrich and Starr, but they would probably have agreed that nursing practitioners must use science to develop technologies that allow them to intervene in the process of illness and to enhance the process of health.

The science of psychiatric–mental health nursing is not very old. In the early 1960s the first substantial psychiatric nursing publications that focused on the *practice* of psychiatric nursing were published. In 1966 the American Nurses Association (ANA) first established the Division of Psychiatric Mental Health Nursing; the division produced a practice statement in 1967 indicating that psychiatric–mental health nurses should perform a wide range of functional roles in the prevention and treatment of mental illness. The statement also indicated that psychiatric–mental health nurses are expected to function in a wide range of settings and use a variety of approaches to care for clients. In the 1970s publications that focused on specific phenomena of psychiatric nursing practice and on problems of care proliferated. By the end of the decade, standards, credentialing, and certification were developed as a means of acknowledging nurses' expertise, distinguishing generalists from specialists, and safeguarding the public.

In the 1980s nurses are likely to witness a reshaping of the practice of psychiatric–mental health nursing. Nursing practice will change because the mental health delivery system as a whole is changing; and the system as a whole is changing because consumers' needs and demands are changing and because the focus is shifting from medical models to psychosocial rehabilitation. It is important to understand changes in the health delivery system because they affect the way psychiatric–mental health nursing care is developed and delivered.

Contextual Approach

Benner[7] argues that a contextual approach must be used in both the practice and the study of nursing. Nurses using such an approach take a holistic view of phenomena and acknowledge that care is dynamic, not static. The basis of psychiatric–mental health nursing is *relationships*. One important premise of psychiatric–mental health nursing *practice* is that the way people talk about their lives is significant, that the language they use and connections they make reveal the world which they see and in which they act, and that the individual must be understood in the larger contexts of family, community, and systems. One important premise of psychiatric–mental health nursing *research* is that phenomena should be studied dynamically, as they occur naturally, and in ways that contribute to the delivery of humane care in a complex environment.

Necessity of Research

The rapid expansion of nurses' roles, coupled with the shift in emphasis of nursing research from educational and administrative studies to clinical studies, suggests that the reasons why nursing research is necessary may be the same as the reasons why nurses themselves are necessary: to improve clients' care and to discover nursing strategies which will assist clients in the attainment and maintenance of health.

Schlotfeldt[8] has suggested that

> systematic inquiry is a responsibility of both practitioners and investigators. Both types of inquirers need the wisdom to select, from among the many hypothetical notions and practical problems that present themselves, those about which inquiry is likely to yield knowledge most important to [humanity]. Both need to understand the nature of objective, systematic inquiry.

Nurses providing care to clients in psychiatric–mental health settings need to use research findings selectively in their practice. They also need to be supportive of nursing research conducted in their workplace.

Nurses and Research

Today, there are several ways in which nurses can be involved in research, directly or indirectly.

First, of course, nurses may actually conduct research. As researchers, they can be seen as falling into two categories, or types. One type creates study designs for scientists working in laboratory settings and tries to fit nursing practice into such designs. Another type is grappling with actual, "live" nursing problems and attempting to create systematic ways of studying them at the same time—or nearly the same time—as they are being experienced; it is this type of researcher who is doing true nursing research.

Second, nurses may work in settings where researchers are conducting investigations. Often, such studies depend on the support of the nurses in the setting—the nurses participate in the research by helping the researchers identify potential subjects and collecting data under the researchers' supervision.

Third, nurses are consumers of nursing research. As consumers, they need to be familiar with all aspects of the research process. Initially, they need to conceive of nursing research as a source of theory on which their practice can be based. Once they understand the research process, they can determine whether the findings of any study can be applied directly to nursing practice or used as a foundation for further study. Nurses also need to know how to evaluate or criticize research—how to assess its weaknesses and strengths and determine whether its weaknesses make it inappropriate or unacceptable for nursing.

Finally, many nurses—particularly those with bachelor's degrees and higher degrees—become involved informally or intuitively in the research process, sometimes without being entirely aware that they are doing so. Their purpose is likely to be practical: to make some process or outcome explicit, to examine some problem that seems "researchable," or to point out some area that seems to need systematic investigation.

WHAT IS NURSING RESEARCH?

Nursing research involves designing studies methodologically, procuring samples appropriately, and measuring clinical phenomena accurately and sensitively. Because each of these aspects presents certain problems, formulating an empirical theory is complex—although not, of course, impossible. The interactions among physical, mental, and spiritual dimensions of the person and among person, family, and environment are complicated in themselves and also give rise to phenomena that are not easily dealt with through controlled research. In a profession such as nursing, which involves *practice*, research is necessarily different from that done in laboratories where variables can be isolated and controlled and measurements can be precise. In nursing research, therefore, researchers must not only study problems but also search continually for appropriate methods of conducting studies.

To understand nursing research, it is helpful to consider it both as a *process* and as *outcomes*. The following sections discuss these two "faces" of research.

Research as Process

The word *research* often conjures up visions of complicated tables and lists of statistics; similarly, a researcher is often pictured as a dusty intellectual tucked away in the library stacks. In other words, research is in a sense equated with *findings*. But nursing research actually means a great deal more than findings; it places researchers in practice settings, and it offers a new way (the best way, some observers would argue) of thinking about and dealing with nursing practice. That is, it is a *process*.

The process of nursing research has several components: identifying and analyzing clinical problems, posing appropriate questions or formulating hypotheses, designing ways to collect data, finding or designing appropriate measurements, collecting data, processing and analyzing data, interpreting findings, comparing findings with results of similar research, and generalizing the findings—that is, applying them to wider situations.

Diers[1] points out that the goal of this process is not simply to find a practical solution to a specific problem but to place a particular clinical problem in a broader framework and relate it to other phenomena of nursing practice. Relating phenomena in this way gives clinicians a broader theoretical understanding of the factors involved and allows them to apply similar solutions or interventions in similar situations.

Generalizing a clinical phenomenon also allows nurses to transfer learning from one situation to another. Diers suggests that when a particular problem can be placed on a more abstract plane, idiosyncrasies are deemphasized and knowledge from a wider context—including literature, previous studies, and relevant theories—becomes available. Thus "client-centeredness" comes to imply a growing base of knowledge about how clients and nurse-client interactions are alike or different; and in any specific circumstances, a well-defined theoretical framework guides nursing practice and enables nurses to make complex clinical judgments that will benefit clients.

Here is an example:*

> Miss A. is a nurse in an outpatient setting for clients with chronic disorders; clinicians in this setting have large caseloads. Over the past year, she has noticed that, apparently, a large number of clients have had to be rehospitalized or have required an increase or a significant change in their medication regimen; and she shares this observation with the nursing supervisor.

In such a situation, a typical response would be to institute certain policy changes: reduce clinicians' caseloads, see all clients more often, change the treatment program, or accept for treatment only clients whose prognosis was good. These immediate solutions are based on untested assumptions about what causes clients to relapse—overworked nurses, insufficient contact with clients, inappropriate interventions, or inappropriate referral of clients. The solutions are only potentially useful; they are random responses to a specific problem, without any systematic examination of the problem within a broader context and without any application of information from other sources.

It therefore seems appropriate to apply the research process; but questions such as these may be raised: "Won't valuable time be wasted using research to find solutions while clients continue to experience difficulties?" "In the long run, will the results really be any different?" To answer these questions, let us return to the example.

> Having noticed that a large number of clients have relapsed, Miss A. feels that there is a discrepancy between the goals of the treatment program and *what has occurred.* The goals of the program are to keep clients out of inpatient settings and to maintain them on low doses of psychotropic medication that will enable them to adjust to community living. But clients are being hospitalized in large numbers and are requiring higher-than-maintenance levels of psychotropic medication, which impair their ability to live in the community.

Up to this point, the clinician, Miss A., has only a hunch or a feeling that something is wrong. How can she be sure? In this situation, it might be a

* This example is taken from the grant "Nursing with Chronically Ill Psychiatric Outpatients," NU 00370-04, USPHS, Slavinsky and Krauss, coinvestigators.

good idea to check records over the last 12 months to validate the impression that large numbers of clients have been rehospitalized or have required major increases in medication. Suppose that such a survey led to the conclusion that 49 percent of all clients in a particular caseload did have a form of relapse in the last year. How does one know that this is a discrepancy that matters? Maybe this situation is peculiar to the caseload or just a chance occurrence. One way to validate the assumption that there is a significant problem is to ask *all* clinicians on the service to systematically check their records over the last year to determine a relapse rate. If all the reported rates are similar, the clinician can determine the average rate for the service over a full year's time. Let us assume that the overall relapse rate turns out to be 48 percent, and return again to the example.

> Since a meaningful average relapse rate (48 percent) has been determined, the problem has moved from the level of a specific caseload to that of the unit as a whole. Now Miss A. turns to the literature, and she discovers that statistics on recidivism (relapse) from local, regional, and national studies suggest that the problem is both widespread and significant. She also learns that relapse in a *chronic* population has been found to be associated with age, sex, living situation, the occurrence of certain kinds of life events, noncompliance with medication, problem-solving ability or social competence, and certain types of symptom exacerbation. But she finds that most of the literature addresses only *untreated* chronic populations—clients who are discharged from inpatient settings with no follow-up or outpatient treatment.
>
> Miss A. and her colleagues now wonder whether the factors identified in the literature as related to relapse would apply to *their* clients, a *treated* chronic population. Further questions then occur: "Which factors, in which combinations, are most likely to predispose clients to relapse?" "Are there adequate tools to gather the necessary information which could be adapted to these clients' capabilities and used by nurses without disrupting their practice?"

A number of other questions might be raised, and statements known as *hypotheses* might be formulated. Hypotheses are predictions that certain events will occur under the right conditions or that certain relationships exist among the phenomena being studied. They attempt to predict certain relationships among facts, on the basis of the researchers' understanding of the literature and previous studies. It is likely that Miss A. and her colleagues will raise so many questions and formulate so many hypotheses that they will have to select those which need to be answered first and for which they have the time, experience, money, and resources to gather, process, and analyze the necessary data.

As this example shows, the research process introduces a way of systematically analyzing clinical problems; it enables the nurse to interact with situations rather than simply react to them. On one level, using research as illustrated in the example is nothing more than good practice. Sound clinical judgments require observations and consistent criteria for describing and interpreting them. Clinicians constantly perform experiments in caring for clients. Although they do not usually regard ordinary care as a type of experiment, every aspect of clinical management can be designed, executed, and appraised with intellectual procedures identical to those used in any experimental situation. The research process illustrated in the example offers one way for nurses not only to observe phenomena but also to process them and to apply criteria in making clinical decisions.

But there is another level beyond that of isolated clinical decisions. The process of research (as was noted earlier) enables nurses to convert their clinical problems into research problems, examining them at a level of abstraction removed from the particular situation and generalizing the learning to similar situations. Table 14 1 (page 286) summarizes the process employed in the example and is designed as a guide for thinking about a clinical problem and converting it into a research problem, research questions, or hypotheses.[1]

It may seem that the quickest and easiest solution for the nurses in the example might have been to institute an immediate change which would seem logically (and intuitively) to address the problem of relapse. For example, Miss A. and her colleagues might have decided that all clients who had relapsed during the previous year would be seen three times per month instead of the usual two, assuming that increased contact would offer the necessary support to decrease clients' anxiety and thus lower their relapse rate. This would be an "experiment" of a sort—trying out an intervention that might or might not produce results. Intuition, or a hunch, or something nebulously referred to as

Table 14-1 Analysis of Clinical Problems

Guidelines
1. Identify and state the discrepancy.
a. Why or how do you know there is a discrepancy? How did you come to feel it as a discrepancy?
b. How do you know it is a difference that *matters*?
c. If the discrepancy were removed, what would the result look like? What are the implications of removing the discrepancy? Of not removing it?
2. Describe the significance of the discrepancy to practice and theory.
a. How big is it? How big a gap is there between what is and what should be, or what is known and what needs to be known?
b. What is this problem an instance of?
3. Analyze the nature of the discrepancy.
a. What are the two conditions?
b. What factors are involved in each?
c. How are the factors related? How do you know?
4. What questions need to be answered to remove the discrepancy?
a. What are the most important questions? Why?
b. How practical will obtaining the answers be? Consider your own resources—energy, time, money, interest, experience.
c. Select the questions to be answered.
5. Specify the type of study that is appropriate.
a. Have you identified factors? Relationships?
b. Do you have hypotheses or predictions or are you looking for them?
c. If you have hypotheses, what form do they take?

SOURCE: Donna Diers, *Research in Nursing Practice*, Lippincott, Philadelphia, 1979.

"previous clinical experience" would guide the clinical judgment and the intervention. But this sort of experimentation—even when it seems to conform to accepted clinical convention or practices, and even when it is carried out by entirely reputable clinicians—may be flagrantly imprecise, vague, and inconsistent. It cannot produce results as vigorous as those arrived at through the research process.

This can be seen by examining just two related aspects of the situation in the example: time and evaluation. Obviously, some time would have to elapse before the clinicians could evaluate the effect of the selected intervention (seeing each client three times a month). In this instance, just about a year would have to pass before the nurses could assess whether or not the intervention had any influence on relapse rates—if they remembered that there was a problem and a solution to be evaluated. However solutions to nursing problems are arrived at, and whatever form they take, time must elapse before evaluation can take place. If the evaluation is not a formal part of the process (as it is in the research process), there is a good chance that it will not take place and nothing at all will be learned from the original situation that could be applied to other situations. The next time a similar problem arises, the nurse will be in the same position, picking a solution and hoping it works. This hit-or-miss process takes time and often leads to inconsistent and ineffective interventions.

The research process clearly takes time as well. It is easy to see from the example that one can generate enough questions about almost any aspect of practice to spend a lifetime searching for answers. Nevertheless, each step of the research process produces usable, transferable knowledge and enables the nurse to establish a network of related theories and data which can explain or predict significant phenomena.

Since all approaches to practice take time, the real question becomes: "Which approach to practice holds the most promise for improving care?" Diers[1] states that in a service profession like nursing, research without practice is sterile and irrelevant, and practice without research is ritualistic and intellectually empty. There can be only one conclusion: good practice is good research, and vice versa. The criteria for each process are the same.

Research as Outcomes

Research can be seen not only as a process but also in terms of its *outcomes*. What outcomes researchers establish will depend to a large extent on how the original problem is analyzed. When problems are analyzed, questions are asked which will ultimately entail different methodological approaches to research.

Since most research problems are discovered by asking questions about practice, it is important to examine the nature of questions which lend themselves to research. Research deals with statements about what is or could be, what relationships exist among facts, and how phenomena can be compared. Research is a way of examining and evaluating work, gathering information, anticipating change, and modifying practice. However, none of these goals will be achieved unless the researcher asks the right questions. Researchers seek answers to questions related to facts—tangible, observable phenomena whose meaning can be validated by others.

Not all questions can be addressed by researchers. Specifically, researchers cannot answer questions about value, that is, questions about what one *should* do or about what is *best* for clients or what may be *better* than something else.[5] Researchers will never tell nurses what they should do; nurses will always have to make important value judgments. Research will only provide nurses with some of the data they need in making decisions. For example, nurses working with chronic psychiatric outpatients often wonder whether medication maintenance, group psychotherapy, individual psychotherapy, social rehabilitation, or some combination of these would be best for their clients. It is not unusual to find psychiatric nurses interested in the question, "What is the *best* treatment for my clients?" No amount of research will provide the answer.

However, a question about value can often be reworded and reformulated into several questions about *fact* which can then be addressed through research. For instance, one could ask, "What are the differential effects of medication maintenance alone versus medication plus biweekly supportive therapy with a nurse-therapist?" Or, "What is the incidence of relapse for chronic psychiatric outpatients treated with medication alone as compared with similar clients treated with medication and weekly individual supportive psychotherapy?" Or, "What factors are related to relapse and symptomatic exacerbation in a treated chronic psychiatric outpatient population?" Answers to these and similar questions of fact would reflect data needed to make policy decisions related to the original question, "What treatment is best for clients?" The answers to the research questions would tell the nurse what effects certain treatment modalities had on certain types of clients. These answers would elucidate the complex set of factors which contribute to remaining asymptomatic or experiencing exacerbation, staying out of the hospital or being rehospitalized, taking or not taking medications, holding a job or losing it, adjusting to community life or withdrawing, and so forth. Obviously, there is no *one* answer, right for all clients and all nurses, to the question, "What is the best treatment for clients?" It is through outcomes of research—the accumulation of answers to questions of fact—that nurses begin to assimilate the data vital to the making of everyday professional value judgments.

RESEARCH DESIGNS

Types of Designs

Various methodological designs can be useful in addressing clinical problems. (Research methodology has been the subject of many texts.[1–4,9,10]) In general, what design is appropriate depends on how much is already known or understood about a problem. When little is known about a problem, or when a researcher wants to take a fresh look at a problem, an *exploratory design* is likely to be used. A *hypothesis-testing design* is—as the term suggests—likely to be used when enough is known about a problem to formulate a hypothesis. Use of a *measurement design* implies the greatest degree of knowledge about a problem, since such a design develops and tests measures employed in gathering data. The following sections discuss each of these designs.

Exploratory Designs

Exploratory designs are most often employed when not much is known about a problem under consideration, or when a researcher is taking a new approach to a long-standing problem. The questions being asked have to do with what facts or factors exist in a situation, how a situation might best be described, or what relationships exist among factors. Thus an exploratory design will be expected to produce descriptions of clinical phenomena, comparisons between situations, discoveries of relationships, development of theory, formulations of hypotheses, and more questions.

An example of an exploratory design is a study conducted by Niemeier,[11] "A Behavioral Analysis of Staff-Patient Interactions in a Psychiatric Setting." The study was concerned with three questions (which have been reworded here):

1. What kind of behaviors do nurses consider desirable or undesirable in clients?
2. How do psychiatric nurses respond to such behaviors?
3. Do psychiatric nurses, psychiatric aides, and other clients respond differently to these behaviors?

To gather data for this study, both rating scales and nonparticipant observation were used. Exploratory designs typically make use of such data-collection techniques to get as broad a view as possible of the phenomena under study; frequently, a situation will be observed in its entirety and field notes will be kept. The way the questions are phrased here is also typical: exploratory designs often ask "what" or "how." The *sample*—that is, the subjects of the study—is typical too: samples in exploratory designs are usually chosen either for convenience or because they represent certain features of the study.

Hypothesis-Testing Designs

Hypothesis-testing designs are used when hypotheses about problems have already been formulated; they are appropriate only when clinical observations, existing literature, and theory all support the logic of a hypothesis. In other words (as was noted earlier), a good deal must be known about a problem before research moves to the hypothesis-testing level. The format of a report of hypothesis-testing research reflects this: first the supporting literature (both empirical and theoretical) is cited; next the hypothesis itself is stated. Clearly, then, the hypothesis must be developed logically from existing knowledge.

A hypothesis being tested is a statement either about *cause and effect* or about *correlations* or *associations* between variables (factors in a situation). Hypotheses about causation are examined through *experimental designs;* hypotheses about correlations are examined through *correlational* or *association-testing* designs.

In an experimental design, researchers must be able to "control" the variables—the factors that are subject to change under different conditions. A factor that is hypothesized to cause (or influence) a change in another is called the *independent variable;* the factor that is hypothesized to be influenced by the independent variable is called the *dependent variable.* When causation is being studied, the independent variable must be applied under rigorously arranged conditions so that what happens to the dependent variable can be observed and recorded. Particularly, all factors other than the independent variable must be kept the same, and time order and "directionality" of changes (that is, whether the independent and dependent variables increase or decrease together or move in opposite directions) must be determined. Cause-and-effect relationships can be found or predicted only through experimental studies.

Correlations, or associations, between variables can be established through correlational or association-testing designs. Such designs can allow researchers to predict or describe relationships, but they cannot determine whether one variable causes another to occur in a certain temporal sequence. They can predict "directionality," however: that is, they can determine whether a positive or negative change in one variable is associated with a positive or negative change in the other.

In general, hypothesis-testing designs require more rigorous sampling methods than those used in exploratory designs—the sample in a hypothesis-testing study must be random or controlled (unlike a sample in an exploratory study, it cannot be chosen for convenience or because it represents some special feature of the problem). A hypothesis-testing design also calls for measuring and monitoring all factors or variables that are known to have an effect on the outcome; and measurements must be rigorous and precise. These criteria are meant to ensure that predicted or observed relationships are caused by, or correlated with, the variables in question and not by other, unaccounted-for phenomena. Following are two examples of hypothesis-testing designs.

Newman and Gaudiano[12] conducted an association-testing, or correlational study, entitled "Depression as an Explanation for Decreased Subjective Time in the Elderly," in which they examined the hypothesis that there is a negative relationship between depression and subjective time (for an explanation of "subjective time," see Chapter 3 of this book): that is, an increase in depression would be correlated with a decrease in subjective time. The researchers measured levels of depression in a sample of women over 65 years old who were participants in a communal meal program; they also measured the subjects' subjective time by asking them to estimate the passage of 40 seconds. They then correlated depression scores with subjective time and found that their results supported the hypothesis. Newman and Gaudiano's study is correlational because the independent variable—depression—could not be controlled: it occurred naturally and randomly in the sample. Therefore, the investigators could not say that depression causes a decrease in subjective time or that a decrease in subjective time causes depression; it can be said only that an increase in depression and a decrease in subjective time are associated.

Godschalx[13] conducted an experimental study entitled "Effect of a Mental Health Education Program upon Police Officers," which examined the hypothesis that police officers' knowledge of and attitudes toward people experiencing emotional difficulties would improve significantly after an 8-hour educational seminar. In this study, the independent variable—the seminar—could be controlled: it was administered to one group (the "experimental group") but not to a second group (the "control group"). Ideally, the researchers should have assigned their subjects (the police officers) randomly to either the experimental group or the control group. Actually, however, they used a "modified random" procedure: the seminar was given to an already-established department, and another existing department served as the control group. (Which department received the seminar was determined by flipping a coin.) Ideally, too, the control group and the experimental group should have been similar; but as it turned out, they were not—the officers in the control group were significantly older and more experienced than those in the experimental group. Both before and after the seminar, the officers in both groups were compared on "attitude measures" and "knowledge measures" to determine the effect of the program. In the experimental group, officers' knowledge about working with people experiencing emotional difficulties increased, but their attitudes were not altered.

Measurement Designs

Exploratory designs are meant, in general, to produce descriptions, hypotheses, and further questions; hypothesis-testing designs are meant to produce explanations, evaluations, statements of causation or association, and—like exploratory designs—more questions or more hypotheses. Measurement designs are somewhat different; they are used to develop and test measures that will be employed in collecting research and clinical data, and they are meant to produce ways of evaluating the reliability, validity, meaningfulness, sensitivity, and precision of measurements.

Reliability of a measure refers to the extent to which it gives the same results each time it is used, and the extent to which two researchers who are using it will get the same results. *Validity* is the extent to which it measures what it claims to measure; *meaningfulness* is the extent to which it fits a situation; *sensitivity* is the extent to which it picks up the full range of events or phenomena along a continuum; and *precision* is the extent to which it distinguishes between events or phenomena.

An example of a measurement design is a series of studies conducted by Dawson, Schirmer, and Beck[14]—entitled "A Patient Self-Disclosure Instrument"—in which they developed and refined an instrument for measuring clients' intimacy values, personal characteristics, and responses to health care, and certain aspects of their lifestyles—factors which, taken together, could be used to define self-disclosure.

To formulate a 50-item instrument, the researchers used existing literature and measures as a starting point. As in most measurement studies, they worked with several samples (groups of subjects) to determine the extent to which their instrument would measure a full range of self-disclosure and variations within the range. They also used statistical techniques to eliminate unreliable or redundant items, to create categories of variables, to measure the extent to which these categories consistently measured the same things as the factors they had identified as significant, and to compare the outcomes found by different raters. They also compared their scale with existing scales that were known to measure the same or similar phenomena; this enabled them to identify other variables that influence self-disclosure.

The final result of this study was a shorter (21-item) rating scale that has demonstrated both reliability and validity and is a useful measure in clinical studies where brevity and accuracy are important considerations. Studies like this can contribute to improving data collection and can lead to useful clinical measures which will enable clinicians to predict certain events as they treat clients.

Designs and Outcomes

Each design, or methodological approach, can lead to a multiplicity of outcomes or results, and each can be utilized to gain a different perspective on parts of the same problem. Some methodological approaches are more rigorous than others and allow knowledge to be transferred from one situation to another with more certainty about its applicability; other approaches produce tentative answers and more questions which must be tested at higher levels before knowledge can be transferred to other situations. But regardless of the design, the outcomes of research enable nurses to test assumptions about practice and about nurse-client interactions. Often, results of research are not in the predicted or expected direction; they frequently challenge long-standing assumptions.

Research in effect transforms nursing from a practice based on assumption and tradition to a profession based on data and theory. One crucial outcome of any research design is to link practice and theory. Theory can be described as a mental invention for the purpose of guiding practice,[15] and the relationship among theory, practice, and research can be seen as circular rather than linear. Practice stimulates theories, which stimulate research; research uses data from practice which test or contribute to theories; theories contribute to different practices and provide a foundation for more advanced research; and practice, once again, validates the results of research and forms the basis for further generation of theory.[1]

Clearly, research designs offer results quite different from, and more far-reaching than, simply practical solutions to individual, isolated problems. Systematic inquiry—research—is essential not only to the survival of the nursing profession but also to the survival and health of the clients nurses serve.

RESEARCH NEEDS

The interaction between psychiatric–mental health nursing and research is so recent that all aspects of practice are still open to study. There are as many questions to ask about practice as there are practitioners to ask them. Keeping that in mind, nurses can use the table of contents of this book to consider potential subjects for research. Nursing theories; person-family-environment interactions in both in- and outpatient settings; and nurse-client interactions related to the promotion, maintenance, restoration, and rehabilitation of health are all subjects that can be characterized in a variety of ways depending on the researcher's interest or on the questions asked; and each individually or in any combination with the others could open avenues for nursing research.

Clients—or "client systems"—might, for example, be examined in terms of (1) demographic characteristics (such as age, sex, race, marital status, and socioeconomic status); (2) diagnoses (such as *organic mental disorder, borderline disorder,* and *substance abuse*); (3) dysynchronous emotional patterns (such as overt anxiety, avoidant anxiety, depression, and elation); (4) dysynchronous patterns of interaction (such as violence and abusiveness); (5) dysynchronous developmental patterns (for instance, in childhood, adolescence, or old age); (6) dysynchronous behavioral patterns (such as suicidal behavior and dysfunctional sexual behavior); (7) dysfunctional patterns of response to illness, disability, death, or dying; (8) becoming a client; (9) self-awareness; and (10) dysynchronous patterns of managing stress.

Family systems might be examined in terms of (1) interactions with clients (or the role of the family as part of the "client system"); (2) theoretical constructs or conceptualizations (such as enmeshment, projection, and multigenerational transmission); (3) dysynchronous patterns of communication or separation, or dysynchronous boundaries; (4) family size; and (5) risk of disruption.

Nurses might be examined in terms of (1) roles; (2) application of the nursing process; (3) relationships with clients (particularly as these are affected by communication, self-awareness, and facilitative processes); (4) legal and ethical issues; and (5) theoretical bases of practice (such as holistic health concepts and theoretical approaches to groups, crises, sexual behavior, and change).

The environment might be examined in terms of (1) contexts of care; (2) dysynchronous patterns of interaction between client and environment; and (3) societal regression.

When any area of nursing practice is being considered as a subject of research, it must be conceptualized in terms of aspects or factors which can be described and compared or contrasted with other factors. That is, the investigator must search out those factors which best characterize the phenomenon or problem under study; this is the point, or level, at which the research process actually begins. For some researchers, this first level will in itself constitute an exploratory study—a study whose goal is to describe a little-known phenomenon in detail. Other researchers will find that the first level has already been dealt with in previous research, that the results have been published, and that these results can become a foundation for research at higher levels with goals such as validating predicted relationships and testing experimental interventions.

To understand research needs better, it will be helpful to consider one example in some detail. The following paragraphs will trace the development of research inquiries which could emerge from aspects of the same clinical problem: relapse in a chronic psychiatric outpatient population. (This is the problem which nurse A. and her colleagues were considering earlier in the chapter.)

Investigators approaching this problem might begin by identifying several relevant or significant aspects: for example, clients, treatment, environments, interventions, nurses, families, and theories. What would they find if they looked at each of these?

- Very little is known about *clients* in this population beyond their diagnosed chronicity and the fact that the population tends to be large.
- *Treatment environments* are likely to vary according to state or local preferences; they may be located in community mental health centers, state institutions, satellite clinics, supportive living-working settings, or general hospital psychiatric clinics, or they may be part of a home-visit service.
- *Interventions* most often employed are medication maintenance, supportive group therapy, social rehabilitation therapy, supportive individual therapy, and various combinations of these.
- *Nurses* have a good deal of contact with the population; and nurses are often the professionals responsible for many aspects of the care of these clients, including supportive individual and group therapy and rehabilitation therapy (when social workers or occupational therapists are not available) and supervision of medication.
- *Families* of these clients often exhibit multiple psychiatric difficulties which may also require therapeutic intervention, and they have problems with integrating the client into the family unit.
- *Theories* which have been used to examine chronicity and relapse include stress theory, life-change theory, social-adjustment theory, and problem-solving theory (among others).

At the outset, then, it is clear that much is still needed in the way of description of phenomena related to chronicity and relapse. An *exploratory study* could be designed which would follow a large number of clients in an outpatient setting who had relapsed during some specified time (say, the previous year) and compare them with the same number of clients who had not relapsed during the same time. Several factors in each client's life might be looked at and described, including certain demographic characteristics (age, sex, race, socioeconomic status, marital status, living situation, diagnosis); the illness in terms of its duration, severity, and symptom patterns; the family setting in terms of size, responsibilities of the client, and its emotional investment in the client; and theoretical phenomena thought to be important, such as problem-solving ability, social competence, and the occurrence of certain life events. Interviews with clients, their families, and their therapists and information from the clients' charts might be sources of data. The data could be compiled so that for each of the factors noted above, similarities and differences between the two groups (relapsed and nonrelapsed clients) could be determined. This would lead to hypotheses about what factors might be related to relapse.

Further descriptive (exploratory) studies could also be conducted. For instance, groups of similar clients in a variety of therapeutic programs could be studied, and symptom exacerbation, life events, relapse, and problem-solving ability might be compared. The outcomes of such a study might include hypotheses about which modalities are related to improved problem-solving ability, lower relapse rates, fewer symptomatic exacerbations, or fewer life events.

Such exploratory studies would provide knowledge which would enable investigators to move on to the next level—testing hypotheses. A *hypothesis-testing study* could be designed to validate the prediction that clients who had low problem-solving ability, experienced many life changes, and had a history of previous relapses would be more likely to relapse than similar clients who had high problem-solving ability, few life changes, and no history of previous relapses. In such a study, the data might be collected through interviews of clients and therapists as well as by reviewing charts, and the prediction—"relapse" or "no relapse"—might be made for the year following data collection. If the predictions proved to be accurate (assuming that they were tested in a variety of settings under similar conditions by several researchers), then another line of study might begin.

One possibility for further research is the "core dimensions" of the nurse-client relationship (see Chapters 12 and 13). These dimensions will remain vague until nurses develop operational definitions and conduct research with groups of clients. However, some significant work has been done on at least one of the core dimensions: empathy. La Monica[16] pursued a line of inquiry concerning empathy in nursing practice which applies to clients with acute or chronic psychiatric illnesses. In reviewing the literature, she identified several conditions, or dimensions, necessary for helpful relationships: empathy, warmth, respect, genuineness, self-disclosure, concreteness, confrontation, and immediacy. Others had demonstrated that empathy is necessary in facilitative interactions; La Monica therefore focused on measuring empathy and on experimental programs designed to increase empathic responses in nurses and nursing students. This work might be used as a basis for studying the effects of empathic interactions on clients with chronic psychiatric illnesses. For example, research might be undertaken to determine whether such clients' responses to empathic interactions are the same as, or different from, those of other clients. Or investigators might examine empathy, intimacy, and distance to see whether these factors interact to elicit predictable patterns of responses in clients with chronic psychiatric illnesses.

It can be seen that even in this one small area of psychiatric–mental health nursing, the possibilities for research are almost infinite. It is obvious, too, that no one study can address all aspects of this, or any, clinical problem. Some researchers will describe a behavior or a phenomenon, others will develop instruments to measure it, and still others will test interventions aimed at altering it. Any of these studies might produce results which would influence the others; and both the measurement studies and the hypothesis-testing studies will have to be repeated several times—in different settings and by different researchers under similar circumstances—before their results can be accepted.

This extended example leads to certain conclusions about nursing research in general. For one thing, it is clear that this kind of effort requires an increase in the number of psychiatric–mental health nurses—not only those engaged directly in research but also those in clinical practice. Second, attempts must be made on local, state, regional, and national levels to identify major problems of nursing care which affect clients' health; and priorities must be established so that nursing research will be conducted in the most crucial areas. Third, systematic research is needed at all levels—exploratory, hypothesis-testing, and measurement—since a holistic approach to care implies that the components of expert practice within the complicated context of clients' lives must be identified. For instance, nurses need to know a great deal more about "recovery trajectories" of clients with chronic mental illnesses, about how these clients are assessed, and about what kinds of interventions—aggressive or protective—are appropriate at certain points during the recovery process. Nurses also need to understand more about early warning signals in psychiatric conditions ("soft signs") that can be used to avert crises and violent episodes when they are working with clients on inpatient units, families of people who have committed suicide, and groups with actively psychotic members. Many other questions could be cited that indicate a need for research: "How do nurses identify the subtle gradations in the behavior of trauma victims that will let them distinguish clients who are coping well from clients who are at risk of moderate or serious psychiatric disturbances?" "What elements of a therapeutic community contribute to improvements in clients' functioning?" "In a general hospital setting, what characteristics of a family suggest that the liaison nurse should actively intervene in the grieving process?" "How do nursing interventions differ—in terms of when they are applied, how they are applied, and how they affect clients?"

A systematic, holistic approach to the study of nursing practice will eventually lead to the identification and description of phenomena that require research at all methodological levels. Psychiatric–mental health nursing is multifaceted and complex, and research into it is equally complex—it may even be so complex that existing methodologies are inadequate. Until nurses uncover and thoroughly understand the phenomena of holistic practice, they will be unable to progress to prescriptive interventions. During the next decades, psychiatric–mental health nursing must devote research to describing and understanding phenomena, setting priorities and research agendas, and establishing programs involving many researchers and national samples. The possibilities for research are endless—and exciting.

RESEARCH IN MENTAL HEALTH SETTINGS: THREE ISSUES

Numerous factors affect the conduct of nursing research in mental health settings—in fact, whole chapters and texts could be (and have been) written about issues which directly influence investigators' ability to carry out research. Three particularly important issues in mental health settings will be examined in this section: (1) access and control, (2) the need for appropriate nursing measures, and (3) the rights of human subjects.

Access and Control

If members of any profession are to conduct research, the problems selected for study must be within the realm of the profession—that is, accessible to it and to some degree under its control. *Access* refers to the training, educational background, and experience (in nursing, this would be clinical experience) which distinguish a profession and enable its members to understand certain phenomena. *Control* refers to the ability of a profession and its members to observe and manipulate certain phenomena which affect practice.

Beginning researchers and professionals are sometimes tempted to try to study someone else's clinical problems.[1] For example, a nurse with no special background in biochemistry or psychopharmacology who attempted to examine biochemical effects of psychopharmacological agents would be choosing a field of study beyond the access and control of nursing. In most states, nurses cannot legally prescribe medications, and nursing education does not provide the necessary theoretical background to conduct such studies. A nurse interested in psychopharmacological intervention might appropriately choose to study the role of the nurse in administering such agents or nurse-client interactions related to their administration. Experimentation with psychosurgical intervention is also beyond the access and control of nursing, but experimentation with the postsurgical management of clients is within the access and control of the profession.

In many psychiatric–mental health settings, the issue of access and control is made explicit by institutional review committees whose purpose is to review research proposals and make decisions as to their appropriateness and usefulness to the setting. Very often such committees make judgments as to whether the researchers possess the capabilities (theoretical and clinical) to conduct the study as well as whether the study fits in with the other research needs of the institution.

Need for Appropriate Nursing Measures

In psychiatric–mental health settings, nurses conducting research most often and most appropriately study aspects of nurse-client interactions. Before assessing, evaluating, or describing such phenomena, they must obtain satisfactory measures and develop impartial, unbiased ways of using them.

There are, of course, many sources of data and many ways to measure them. Nursing, as a profession new to research, has been in the position of simultaneously studying clinical problems and finding ways to measure them; and nurses have had to borrow or adapt measures developed by other professions for different purposes. Borrowed measures, like borrowed methodologies, often shape the problem to the study instead of the study to the problem. For instance, a nurse interested in the effects of a treatment program (conducted by nurses) on the community adjustment of chronic psychiatric outpatients cannot rely on the usual psychiatric outcome measures of symptom exacerbation, days out of the hospital, medication compliance, and so on, to measure the quality of the life a client leads in the community. Psychiatric nurses familiar with community intervention, who understand the problems of everyday living with which clients must cope—and the conditions and standards under which these clients function—need to develop measures sensitive to changes in these areas. Only such measures can identify the effects of *nursing* interventions as opposed to medical interventions.

Measurements are therefore an important issue in psychiatric–mental health nursing research. Measurement studies need to be conducted, and instruments must be developed which will sensitively and accurately measure phenomena which grow out of holistic nursing.

Rights of Participants in Research

Clients have a right to privacy, confidentiality, anonymity, safety, and informed consent. These rights are protected by law and must continue to be safeguarded when clients become subjects of research. In psychiatric–mental health settings (perhaps even more than in other settings), nurses must be particularly careful to ensure not only that clients' rights are protected but that clients understand their rights. Nurses are also obliged to make sure that their clients are capable of making informed choices about participation in research projects.

The issue of privacy in psychiatric settings is a particularly knotty one for researchers. Meltzoff and Kornreich[17] point out that therapeutic relationships are thought to be so individual as to make experiments nonreproducible and so private as to make them inaccessible to outside scrutiny. This, they feel, tends to discourage research and to prevent acceptance of research findings. The therapist-client relationship in psychiatric settings has traditionally been confidential, private, and in some cases anonymous. Many therapists argue that the introduction of anyone or anything (one-way screen, tape recorders, video equipment) into the treatment relationship so drastically alters conditions that progress becomes difficult (if not impossible). Ironically, research studies of this problem are inconclusive; the effects of external recording devices, for instance, are unknown. The findings so far suggest that such devices have some effects, not necessarily detrimental, on the therapeutic process which could influence research results, but not treatment results (see Meltzoff and Kornreich for a thorough review of this literature).

It is possible to conduct research studies and gather data while maintaining confidentiality and anonymity and respecting the privacy of both clients and therapists. Data can be coded so that the people involved cannot be identified; moreover, data can be collected so that there is as little disruption of treatment as possible and so that as much information as possible can be obtained in the time available. Nevertheless, it is clear that nurses and other professionals in mental health settings must allow scrutiny of their most important work if they themselves and others are to benefit from their successes and mistakes and if a body of theory about clinical practice is to be developed.

Informed consent is another issue which requires vigilance in psychiatric–mental health settings. The Department of Health, Education, and Welfare (DHEW) Policy on Protection of Human Subjects, June 16, 1971, defines *informed consent* as "the agreement obtained from a subject, or from a subject's authorized representative, to the subject's participation in an activity."[18]

The basic elements of informed consent are as follows:

1. A fair explanation of the purpose of the study and adequate introduction of the researcher
2. A fair explanation of the procedures to be followed, including an identification of those which are experimental
3. A description of the attendant discomforts and risks
4. A description of the benefits to be expected
5. A disclosure of appropriate alternative procedures that would be advantageous for the subject
6. An offer to answer any inquiries concerning the procedures and purpose
7. An instruction that the subject is free to withdraw consent and to discontinue participation in the project or activity at any time, and instruction that refusal or withdrawal to participate in or to continue with the study will produce no negative consequences at that time or in the future

Most psychiatric and educational institutions now have review committees whose sole purpose is to see that all conditions of informed consent are met and that the research study is within reasonable limits of safety and risk to the human participants.

But a question arises: "Can a committee, however thorough its review may be, monitor by means of written documents a process which must take place between a researcher and a subject?" Ultimately, it would seem that the researcher is responsible for ensuring that the document is dynamically transmitted to any client who must make an informed choice about participating in a project. Nurses who are conducting research must also be skilled clinicians if they are to make judgments about clients' ability to make decisions and understand information being offered. The investigator must offer information in such a way that it can be processed by the client or that the client can seek the assistance of a guardian who could act in the client's best interest in deciding about participation.

A client who has been fully informed and chooses to participate in a research project may be more likely to complete the project. The subject who is not fully informed but agrees to participate out of fear, ignorance, or intimidation may drop out or be unavailable for later interviews. Therefore, informed consent is of benefit not only to the subject but also to the investigator, who can ill afford to lose subjects and valuable data.

It should be clear that the nurse-researcher must be just as strongly motivated toward human welfare as the nurse-clinician. The researcher may more often be concerned with the welfare of groups of people, while the clinician is concerned with the welfare of individuals; but in nursing research, these distinctions become artificial, since the researcher and the clinician are one and the same. Both nursing research and nursing practice must embody sound inquiry, competent interventions, and relevant theory.

SUMMARY

Nursing research is the systematic study of the practice of nursing using scientific methods. Researchers collect and provide facts about nursing phenomena as objectively as possible. The knowledge derived from research provides a theoretical basis for improving practice. Psychiatric–mental health nursing is a comparatively recent development, and research must be based on its contextual approach, its holistic view of phenomena, and its conception of care as dynamic, not static.

Nursing research is needed to improve care and to discover nursing strategies which will help clients attain and maintain health. Nurses need to conduct research, support other investigators, and develop an understanding of the research process so that they can be knowledgeable consumers of research.

The research *process* includes identifying and analyzing clinical problems, formulating questions and hypotheses, designing ways to collect information, designing or discovering appropriate measures, collecting data, processing and analyzing data, interpreting findings, and generalizing results. Research can also be seen as *outcomes*. An outcome depends to a large extent on how the original problem is conceived—that is, on what questions are asked.

Various methodological designs can be useful in addressing clinical problems. There are essentially three major types of methodological designs: exploratory, hypothesis-testing, and measurement. Exploratory designs are used to produce descriptions of clinical phenomena. Hypothesis-testing designs are used to test predictions about cause-and-effect relationships or correlations between variables; outcomes of studies using hypothesis-testing designs are explanations, tested interventions, evaluations, and demonstrations of procedures. Measurement designs are used to develop and test nursing measures that will be useful for gathering data; outcomes of studies using measurement designs are ways of evaluating the reliability, validity, meaningfulness, and sensitivity of measures.

Research transforms nursing from a practice based on assumption and tradition to a profession based on theory. Many aspects of psychiatric–mental health nursing need to be addressed through nursing research; the client, the family, the environment, the nurse, and applications of the nursing process are general areas for study.

Three major issues which directly shape the conduct of nursing research in psychiatric–mental health settings are: (1) access and control, (2) the need for appropriate nursing measures, and (3) the rights of human subjects.

REFERENCES

1. D. Diers, *Research in Nursing Practice,* Lippincott, Philadelphia, 1979.
2. D. Polit and B. Hungler, *Nursing Research: Principles and Methods,* 2d ed., Lippincott, Philadelphia, 1983.

3. C. Waltz and R. B. Bausell, *Nursing Research: Design, Statistics, and Computer Analysis,* Davis, Philadelphia, 1981.
4. H. Wilson, *Research in Nursing,* Addison-Wesley, Menlo Park, Calif., 1985.
5. A. Goodrich, "The Nurse as Interpreter of Life," Reprinted from *Redbook Magazine,* January 1929, in A. Goodrich, *The Social and Ethical Significance of Nursing,* Yale University School of Nursing, New Haven, Conn., 1973.
6. P. Starr, *The Social Transformation of American Medicine,* Basic Books, New York, 1982.
7. P. Benner, *From Novice to Expert,* Addison-Wesley, Menlo Park, Calif., 1984.
8. R. Schlotfeldt, "Cooperative Nursing Investigations: A Role for Everyone," *Nursing Research,* vol. 23, November–December 1974, pp. 452–456.
9. M. Leininger, ed., *Qualitative Research Methods in Nursing,* Grune and Stratton, Orlando, Fla., 1985.
10. C. Sellitz, L. Wrightsman, and S. Cook, *Research Methods in Social Relations,* 3d ed., Holt, New York, 1976.
11. D. Niemeier, "A Behavioral Analysis of Staff-Patient Interactions in a Psychiatric Setting," *Western Journal of Nursing Research,* vol. 5, no. 4, 1983, pp. 270–281.
12. M. Newman and J. Gaudiano, "Depression as an Explanation for Decreased Subjective Time in the Elderly," *Nursing Research,* vol. 33, no. 3, 1984, pp. 137–139.
13. S. Godschalx, "Effect of a Mental Health Educational Program upon Police Officers," *Research in Nursing and Health,* vol. 7, 1984, pp. 111–117.
14. C. Dawson, M. Schirmer, and L. Beck, "A Patient Self-Disclosure Instrument," *Research in Nursing and Health,* vol. 7, 1984, pp. 135–147.
15. J. Dickoff and P. James, "A Theory of Theories: A Position Paper," *Nursing Research,* vol. 17, 1968, pp. 197–203.
16. E. La Monica, "Empathy in Nursing Practice," *Issues in Mental Health Nursing,* vol. 2, no. 1, 1979, pp. 2–13.
17. J. Meltzoff and M. Kornreich, *Research in Psychotherapy,* Atherton, New York, 1970.
18. Yale School of Nursing Guidelines for Master's Thesis, Institutional Guide to DHEW policy on Protection of Human Rights, June 16, 1971.

PART FOUR
Mental Health Environment

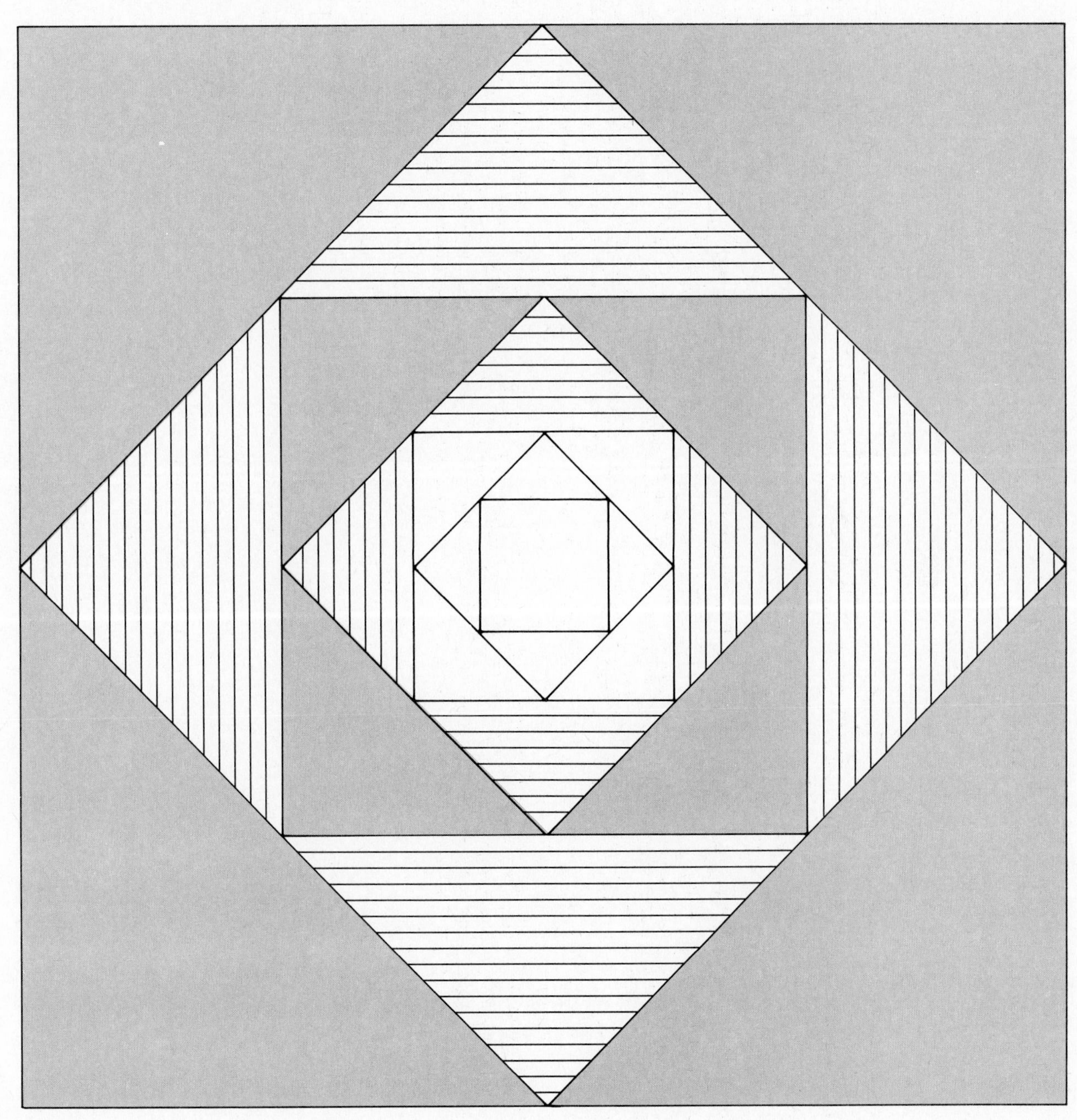

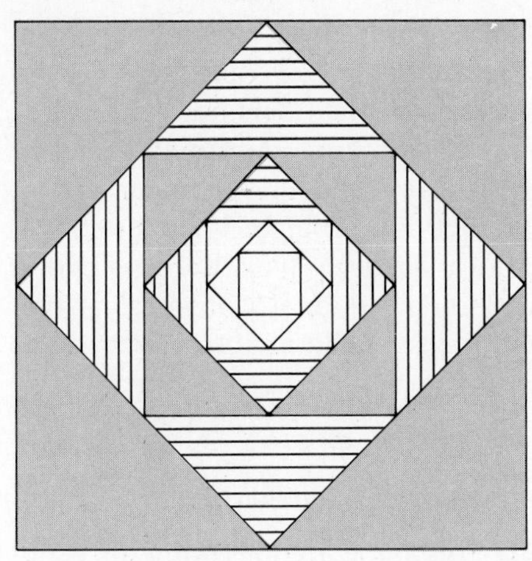

CHAPTER 15
Defining the Environment

Judith Haber
Pamela Price Hoskins
Anita M. Leach
Barbara Flynn Sideleau

LEARNING OBJECTIVES

After studying this chapter, the student should be able to:

1. Elaborate on the definition of *environment*.
2. Analyze the concept of person-environment interactions.
3. Relate the definition of environment to the concept of health.

The purpose of this chapter is to expand the definition of *environment* and provide a conceptual framework for Part Four. Persons, places, and objects will be considered as components of the environment. Simultaneous interactions of people with their environment and the impact of environment on health will be discussed.

THE CONCEPT OF ENVIRONMENT

Environment is a broader concept than just places in which treatment occurs or places where clients live. It is defined as all relevant systems and processes external to clients but interacting with them. It is the patterned wholeness of all that is external to the client. The broadest definition would be the universe and would include all objects, places, and persons as subsystems; but that is hardly practical. When environment is defined as *relevant systems and processes,* it becomes a most useful concept for psychiatric–mental health nursing. The environment in this context includes systems that affect clients and are simultaneously affected by them. It can be thought of as *systems, processes, human interactions,* and a *factor affecting health.*

Systems

In the context of psychiatric–mental health nursing, *systems* are organized structures that influence and are influenced by clients. Which systems are relevant for each client can be determined in collaboration with the client. For example:

> For Mary B., a 45-year-old recently widowed woman with three adolescent children, relevant systems include her family, her church, the nurse, the schools her children attend, her neighborhood, and any support groups she enrolls in to assist her through the mourning process, such as a bereavement group and Parents Without Partners.

Processes

Processes are organized, purposeful patterns or operations. They include the dynamics and interactions of individuals, families, groups, and communities. Processes of particular significance in psychiatric–mental health nursing include satisfaction of needs, self-actualization, and growth and development. For each client, relevant processes emerge from significant interactions. People and their environments continuously exchange matter and energy. When this exchange is goal-directed and patterned in an orderly way, the interaction process is considered functional. Conversely, when an exchange is aimless, chaotic, dissonant, or dysynchronous, it is considered dysfunctional.

Person-Environment Interaction

The interaction of people with environments is not static but continuous and dynamic. It is characterized by patterning and repatterning of both clients and their relevant environments. Any change in a part of a system or process will affect the whole. Everyday experiences make it obvious that people simultaneously affect and are affected by other people, places, and objects in their environment, even if they are not always aware of this.

Human Ecology: The Environment and Health

The study of person-environment interactions is known as *human ecology.* In the health care system, health may be seen as a balance between people and the environment. Proper nutrition, preventive health services, and control over pollution and hazards are believed to have a positive effect on people, who in turn will have a positive effect on the environment. When patterns of simultaneous interaction are disrupted or become dysynchronous, problems arise. From an ecological viewpoint, mental health is a synchronous interaction between people and the environment; psychopathology is a dysynchronous interaction—as when resources are insufficient or when individuals' needs or behaviors demand more than the environment can provide. The idea that environment influences behavior, attitudes, and moods has a long history and is now being supported by research. Human behavior can to some extent be described as a function of the environment, and prolonged exposure to a specific environment can result in human qualities that correspond to those of the environment.

RATIONALE FOR THE ORGANIZATION OF PART FOUR

Part Four, consisting of 11 chapters, presents a variety of environments with which clients interact.

The process by which clients become part of a treatment environment is described in Chapter 16. The inpatient environment is described in Chapter 17; Chapter 18 presents an overview of various outpatient environments.

For many clients, the family is the major component of the environment. Theories about family structure and function and the application of family theory to nursing are discussed in Chapter 19.

Groups and organizational systems are an integral part of the therapeutic environment. Chapters 20 and 21 discuss the dynamics of groups and organizations and how these can be used by nurses in the care of their clients.

Chapter 22 discusses clients who require only a brief encounter with the mental health care environment in the form of crisis intervention.

Sexual partners and other aspects of sexual life constitute a significant part of a client's environment. Chapter 23 discusses psychosexual development, sexual lifestyles, and sexual theory.

When clients seek help from the health care system, various therapies are prescribed for them. Although these are aimed at producing inward changes, they are usually external in nature and thus become part of the clients' environment. Therapies that prescribe change through behavioral repatterning and education are described in Chapter 24. Chapter 25 discusses therapies that represent alternatives to the more traditional individual, group, and family therapies. These approaches can be utilized alone or as adjunct treatments and may influence clients' environments or the clients themselves. Psychopharmacologic agents and electroconvulsive therapy (ECT) result in dramatic changes in clients and repatterning of their behavior. Chapter 26 discusses the nursing care of clients being treated with psychopharmacologic agents or electroconvulsive therapy.

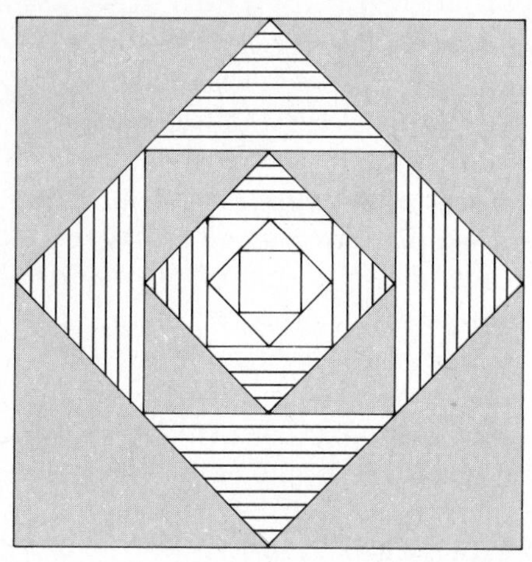

CHAPTER 16
Becoming a Client

Luc Reginald Pelletier

LEARNING OBJECTIVES

After studying this chapter, the student should be able to:

1. List five reasons for seeking help from the mental health care delivery system.
2. Describe a situation in which a client would approach the mental health care delivery system for prevention.
3. Discuss how ability to pay is related to access to psychiatric services.
4. Compare voluntary and involuntary hospitalization with regard to precipitating events and clients' rights.
5. Discuss the nursing diagnosis *powerlessness* as it relates to hospitalization; list four nursing interventions and two outcome criteria for clients.
6. Discuss the process of discharge or termination from an inpatient psychiatric setting.

Few people pass through life without experiencing a personal conflict or crisis—a situation in which life purposes and physical, mental, and spiritual patterns of interaction with the environment have become dysynchronous. This dysynchrony may be evident primarily within the person or may extend to the environment, where interactions with family and community can be sources of dysynchrony. Many people who find themselves in dysynchronous patterns may need professional psychiatric–mental health nursing services.

Identification of a mental health problem is the first step in seeking assistance from a practitioner. Kadushin[1] lists three other, related stages: discussion of the problem with friends and relatives, choice of type of professional healer, and selection of a particular practitioner.

To see oneself in need of assistance from someone else is to feel vulnerable and dependent. This is very painful for some people, especially those who value and thrive on independence. But it should be recognized that independence includes the ability to identify one's needs and seek out appropriate resources to help in fulfilling them. A person who is experiencing a spiritual or theological conflict may seek out a minister or priest; a person in conflict with the law may consult a lawyer. It seems only natural, then, that in a personal crisis one would seek assistance from a mental health practitioner. Why are people so reluctant to approach the mental health system? Social influences from the past give us many reasons.

Although mental illness is not stigmatized now to the extent that it was a century ago, earlier images are difficult to change. The prevalent image of psychiatric institutions was formed from books and films that gave striking, and terrifying, pictures of the pain and chaos experienced there. Most of us are familiar with scenes in which therapeutic procedures are performed in dimly lit, dirty hallways, accompanied by shrieks. Women in white, starched uniforms restrain clients with the assistance of tall, bulky male aides. Their faces are expressionless as clients kick, bite, and spit at them. Bearded psychiatrists sit behind large wooden desks; their speech is slow and purposeful; they puff on cigars or pipes. There is seemingly no personal interaction between client and clinical staff. These depictions could keep anyone from the psychiatric–mental health setting. Only recently have there been any portrayals that could be called hopeful or that reflect the more humane, caring approach which characterizes psychiatric settings today.

The purpose of this chapter is to describe the process of becoming a client and the feelings associated with such an experience. Factors such as ability to pay and components of the mental health delivery continuum are discussed.

WHY DO PEOPLE SEEK HELP FROM THE MENTAL HEALTH CARE DELIVERY SYSTEM?

People seek treatment from the mental health care delivery system for many reasons; the most common is an identified need for help with a problem. Others include a need for environmental change or for protection, a need for relief of psychiatric symptoms, and a need for nurturance. Some people seek treatment because they have been ordered to do so by a court; and some admissions, although not court-ordered, are mandated by laws (for example, some people who are intoxicated are brought directly to a community mental health center by the police, and people in prison may be judged dangerous to themselves or others and transferred to a psychiatric facility). The short vignettes that follow illustrate why people seek assistance.

NEED FOR ENVIRONMENTAL CHANGE

Myra, a 58-year-old woman, has been a "street person" on and off for twenty years. She presently lives with two other women in a suburb of Los Angeles, where she leads a sedentary existence. She has been hospitalized numerous times in the past 30 years. Myra is supposed to visit a local clinic two times a month for maintenance treatment with fluphenazine decanoate (Prolixin Decanoate). Recently, however, she has not visited the clinic for her medications, because her feet are so swollen that she is immobilized. Myra has become violent toward her friends, and since the clinic is closed evenings, she is brought to the emergency department (ED) of a medical center. When asked by the admitting nurse why she came to the ED today, Myra states: "They kicked me out of my apartment."

Myra is suffering from an exacerbation of her psychiatric symptoms. Her transient existence has been supported by two other women who live with her and who are now assisting her in seeking psychiatric help. Recent stressors—being evicted from an apartment and a deteriorating physical condition—have prevented her from receiving her usual maintenance doses of antipsychotic medication. Myra will need to be assessed to determine her mental state and physical condition. Hospitalization will provide pharmacological intervention, protection, refuge, and rest until her acute psychiatric and medical conditions are relieved.

LEGAL SYSTEM

Bob, a 22-year-old assistant electrician, has recently been arrested and charged with indecent exposure. He appeared before a judge who ordered him to seek psychiatric help or be jailed for 30 days. Bob does not think he can afford to be out of work for 30 days, since his wife of 4 months has recently given birth. Bob enters treatment via a mental health outpatient clinic, stating: "I have a problem, and I don't know what to do about it."

Legislation over the past 10 years has given courts responsibility in assessing defendents' need for psychological services. Since mental health treatment is an effective means of altering deviant behavior, judges tend to opt for treatment instead of incarceration when such a course is feasible. In essence, the legal problem is seen as an illness and therefore as treatable. Psychiatric treatment becomes a means of protecting the public by keeping the offender from doing more harm.

RELIEF FROM SYMPTOMS

Mark, a 16-year-old son of a divorced couple, has recently exhibited a marked change in behavior. He is not eating, sleeps poorly, and has no interest in joining his friends in their usual activities. Mark is found crying for long periods of time during the day. His mother is horrified and discouraged after finding Mark in his room alone with his father's loaded gun.

Mark is experiencing suicidal ideation and intent as part of a clinical picture of depression. He does not presently have the internal control necessary to protect himself from harm. People like Mark are hospitalized when they feel "out of control" and when family members do not have the resources to ensure their safety.

NURTURANCE

Eric, a 19-year-old, approaches a community mental health center with a major complaint of anxiety related to a recent homosexual experience. A male friend accompanies him and speaks of his concern over Eric's state of intense anxiety. Eric is seen by the evaluating nurse, who refers his case to a clinical nurse specialist in the outpatient department of the center.

Eric is experiencing a developmental crisis which can be treated on an outpatient basis. His problem is a common one that will first require exploration of his perceptions and establishment of a trusting and nurturing relationship with a therapist.

Lazare[2] studied clients' requests in an outpatient setting. He found that the two most common requests had to do with clarification and psychodynamic insight. Table 16-1 illustrates 14 categories of requests, with definitions and sample items from the patient request form used in the study. When a patient is admitted, the nurse's familiarity with these request categories can be of value in several ways. Familiarity with the categories allows the nurse to anticipate common requests and respond appropriately to clients who seek reassurance and understanding.

WHEN DO PEOPLE SEEK HELP?

Some clients seek mental health services when they expect events in their lives to be stressful, or because they want information on resources in the community. These people can attend seminars, workshops, self-help groups, or classes in specific areas of interest. Examples of classes offered by university continuing education programs include "Menopause and the Potential of Midlife," "Taking Charge of Feelings," "Accentuating Personal Strengths," and "Fathers and Daughters."[3]

However, it is usually arriving at a "point of pain" that motivates people to seek help from a mental health professional. A good example would be a person in crisis who perceives the stressors as intolerable and finds no relief in sight. Crises can be maturational (developmental) or situational. Although *developmental crises* are normal and common, people experience higher levels of stress and anxiety at these times.[4] People may become overwhelmed during such a crisis if they do not receive support and nurturance. It is understandable that people may seek assistance from the mental health professional during certain developmental periods.

Table 16-1 Categorization of Clients' Requests with the Two Highest-Ranking Items from Each Category in an 84-Item Patient Request Form

Request Category and Definition	Item
Clarification: Clients want assistance in putting thoughts, feelings, and behaviors in perspective. Problem is usually acute in nature.	I came to the clinic so that I can figure out what to do. I want to clear things up to make the best decision for myself.
Ventilation: Clients want to get things off their chest and believe this will relieve their burdens. This does not involve confession; clients do not feel guilty or seek forgiveness.	I need to get something off my chest. I want to get some painful feelings out of my system.
Psychodynamic insight: Clients believe their problems are psychological in nature, are repetitive, and stem from early childhood. They want to be active in discovering the meaning of the problems.	I realize that my problem is me, not someone else; and I want help to know why I get the way I do. I believe that my present troubles are only a symptom of what is wrong; I want to learn the deeper causes so that I can change.
Contact with reality: Clients believe that they are losing hold of reality. They want to talk to someone who will reassure them that they are thinking clearly and not "losing their mind."	I want to feel I am thinking straight. I want to talk to someone so that I won't feel I am losing my mind.
Advice: Clients have formed an opinion but want guidance about a personal or social matter. They may want to share the decision.	I would like your guidance about what I should do about a problem. I think I know what to do about my situation, but I would like to get some professional advice.
Succorance: Clients feel empty, alone, and not cared for. They want warmth and caring from the mental health professional.	I want to feel that someone cares about me. I want to talk to a person who is warm and giving.
Control: Clients feel overwhelmed and out of control. They may fear that they will hurt themselves or others. In seeking help, the client is saying: "Please take over. I can no longer manage."	I want someone to help me regain control over myself. I want you to stop my feelings before they overpower me.
Confession: Clients feel guilty about what they have said, thought, or done and hope that by talking to the therapist they will feel better.	I feel guilty about hurting someone (or people) and want to talk about it. If I can feel less guilty, I will be helped.
Psychological expertise: Clients believe that the source of their problems is psychological rather than physical or situational. They are asking the professional to explain why they think, feel, or act the way they do. The clients expect to play a passive role in the interaction.	I would like an expert to tell me why I feel the way I do. If someone could explain to me what causes my emotional problems, I would be helped.
Community triage: Clients request information about community resources.	I would like you to direct me to the agency in my community which can help me with my problems. I would like someone to tell me where in my community to get help.
Medical: Clients see their problems as physical in nature. They often refer to their problem as a "nervous condition." They expect medical intervention such as pills, electroconvulsive therapy, hospitalization, or medical advice. They assume a passive role in their treatment.	I want treatment of my nervous condition. I want someone to examine me to figure out the cause of my nervous condition.
Social intervention: Clients see the problem as residing in people or situations around them. They ask the clinician to intervene on their behalf by bringing social influence to bear.	My problem is other people (family, friends, coworkers, etc.). I want you to do something about them. I want you to speak to the person or people who are giving me trouble.
Administrative request: Clients seek administrative or legal assistance to help them with their current problems. The specific request may be to provide a disability evaluation, a draft deferment, a medical excuse to leave work, etc.	I need the clinic's legal power to take care of a difficult situation for me. I need the clinic's authority to deal with a certain agency I am having trouble with.
Nothing: Clients may want help but are not prepared to state a specific problem.	I do not need psychiatric help. I do not know why I'm here.

SOURCE: Adapted from A. Lazare and S. Eisenthal, "A Negotiated Approach to the Clinical Encounter," in A. Lazare, ed., *Outpatient Psychiatry: Diagnosis and Treatment,* Williams and Wilkins, Baltimore, 1979, pp. 142–144.

Situational crises are defined as events that are unanticipated and traumatic. The usual social supports (such as families and friends) are not able to relieve discomfort, pain, and anxiety. The client becomes aware of this and seeks help, or is prodded by family members or significant others. Situational crises may be treated in a short period of time using crisis intervention techniques; but developmental crises may take longer to treat, especially if developmental tasks of earlier stages have not yet been accomplished.

Clients may seek help when psychic pain is so great that it has affected many areas of their life. Anxious or depressive symptomatology may be so great that activities of daily living cannot be performed. Clients at this juncture seek help because their lives are disintegrating and no other options are available. One client described this experience as follows:

> Initially, I thought I could do it myself. I started jogging and tried to eat more natural foods. But the feelings persisted and got even worse. I had never felt this down in all my life. I would cry for no reason, and people said that I was irritable all the time. Finally, I couldn't take care of myself; getting out of bed in the morning was impossible. My husband brought me to a friend's psychiatrist.

Recent federal and state legislation requires some clients to seek psychiatric–mental health services as part of their sentencing. These clients have been convicted of child molestation, rape, and various other violent acts. Detention centers also employ psychiatrists as part of their rehabilitation programs.

HOW DO PEOPLE SEEK HELP?

Patterns of Referral and Their Relationship to Social Class

There are various patterns of referral to the mental health care delivery system. Traditionally, socioeconomic status has been a major factor in determining access to and quality of mental health services. The poor have access only to whatever the public sector will provide; availability of care is often inadequate, and quality of care is variable. Middle-class people have difficulty in choosing services because of limitations in private insurance coverage. The rich, of course, have the most access to psychiatric care and the widest range of choices.

Ability to pay for services determines the type of care and setting. Psychiatric–mental health treatment can be paid for by various means, including payment by the clients themselves, private insurance, and Medicare. Although private insurance covers some expenses, the amount reimbursed usually does not match actual expenditures by the client. Some states have mandated mental health insurance which puts mental health coverage at parity with medical coverage. (Studies now show that mental health treatment may affect the use of medical services covered by insurance providers.[5] In states that have mandated mental health coverage, use of medical services has decreased.) In addition to these methods of payment, some large university hospitals have teaching funds for clients who cannot pay for hospitalization. These originate from federal funding from the National Institute of Mental Health.

Various people may become definers of mental illness. An individual client may identify a problem, for instance, and go on to seek help from a private practitioner, an emergency department, an outpatient clinic, or some other agency. Socioeconomic status can affect who defines a problem and who is first approached as a client seeks help. Definers of mental illness other than the clients themselves include physicians and other health care professionals (such as nurse practitioners and social workers); members of the client's social network, including families and friends; social agencies such as schools and home health care agencies; and legal agencies such as the police, probation officers, lawyers, and courts.

Care Providers and Their Relationship to Social Class

Private Practice

As has been mentioned, ability to pay is a crucial factor in choosing a mental health practitioner or setting. The client who can afford a relatively expensive fee will seek mental health services from a private practitioner. Professionals in private practice include psychiatrists, clinical nurse specialists, social workers, and psychologists. Although their fees may range from $35 to $120 per session, some private therapists provide a sliding scale in charging for services rendered. Frequency of sessions depends primarily on the diagnosis and the severity of the illness. The diagnostic categories of the *Diagnostic and Statistical Manual of Mental Disorders* (DSM III)[6] are used by all practitioners to assign a diagnosis, since this is a requirement in most states for third-party reimbursement.

With regard to which practitioner is best suited to treat which illness, the little clinical research that has been done is inconclusive. However, a nursing research study has found that nurse psychotherapists most commonly treat women with diagnoses of anxiety neuroses and depression.[7] Generally, clients who require psychopharmacologic intervention seek treatment from a psychiatrist. However, there are many nonmedical practitioners who treat clients in collaboration with psychiatrists. For example, it is common for nurse psychotherapists to seek collaboration with psychiatrists in instituting a medication regime. If medication is indicated, the relationship between psychiatrist and nurse continues to be collaborative, and there is shared responsibility for the client's care.[8]

Community Mental Health Agency or Clinic

Some clients seek services in community mental health agencies or clinics. These agencies provide various services such as individual psychotherapy, group psychotherapy, family therapy, socialization and occupational groups, and medication clinics. Fees are calculated on a basis of ability to pay (a sliding scale). Services are provided by a variety of mental health practitioners including psychiatrists, psychiatric nurses (generalists and specialists), psychiatric social workers, and mental health workers.

Typically, clients with certain acute illnesses (such as acute anxiety, some forms of depression, and posttraumatic syndromes) are treated in an outpatient setting, or by a private practitioner connected with the agency or clinic. Clients with chronic, uncomplicated illnesses are also treated in outpatient settings, in groups and medication clinics. Both kinds of clients are referred to inpatient settings if their symptoms warrant closer observation by professional staff.

A recent trend in community services is the provision of psychiatric–mental health services in the client's home. Psychiatric home care was developed to fill a gap in services between hospitalization and outpatient treatment. Visiting nurses' associations and home health care agencies are now available for psychosocial interventions. These programs are covered by Medicare, some private insurance companies, and prepaid health plans. (Medicare and third-party payers define psychiatric-mental health nursing services and qualifications to practice broadly enough to include nurses at the associate, baccalaureate, and master's level.) Since clients almost always have medical problems along with psychiatric ones, home-care nurses may be expected to provide medical and community care in addition to psychiatric–mental health care.

Indications for referral by a physician to a psychiatric home-care program include the following:

- Recurrence of past psychiatric symptomatology or sudden change in a client's mental status
- Need to monitor the effects of medication and compliance with medication
- Need to assess the client's social milieu and family structure to determine if these factors inhibit the client's participation in treatment[9]

The provision of psychiatric home care has broadened and diversified mental health services (see Figure 16-1).

Specialty Programs

Over the years, various specialty programs have been developed to meet the needs of particular

Figure 16-1 Mental health treatment model.

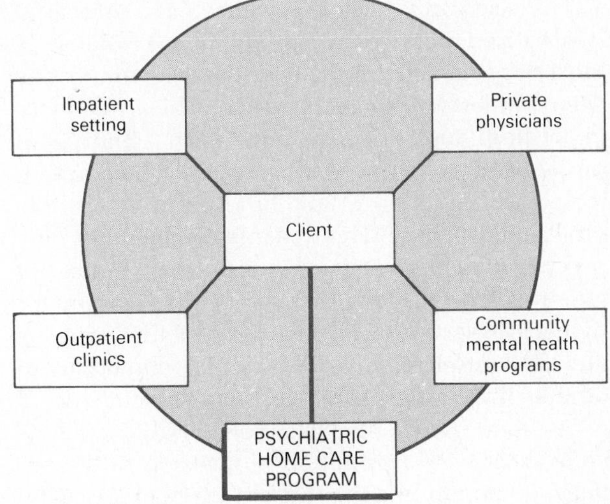

groups of clients. Clients with problems associated with alcohol or drug abuse who want help will usually enter a detoxification program lasting anywhere from 5 to 28 days. While their physiological needs are monitored, these clients' emotional needs are addressed in group and individual counseling. Alcoholics Anonymous is a support and rehabilitation group known nationwide for its effectiveness in treating alcoholism. Clients with drug problems can be treated in much the same way, and usually in the same residential settings, as alcoholic clients. Outpatient follow-up includes Narcotics Anonymous and methadone clinics. Other specialized support groups in the community include postcancer groups, bereavement groups (for example, Parents of Murdered Children), and eating-disorder groups. Growing national concern about kidnapped children in the last 10 years has given rise to many support groups for parents of missing children.

Hospitals

Traditionally, most clients have been treated in hospital settings, and admission has, for the most part, depended upon ability to pay. These settings include psychiatric units within general hospitals, private psychiatric hospitals, and state and federal psychiatric hospitals. Hospitalization provides security and protection that might not be possible with a private practitioner or in an outpatient program. Clients are usually admitted to a hospital when it is feared that they may harm themselves or others. (For clients who are acutely suicidal, the nurse makes safety a focus of the initial interventions.)

The decision to seek hospitalization comes after it is realized that personal resources are exhausted. Most hospitalizations occur voluntarily; that is, the client requests or consents to mental health services in writing. Such consent implies that the client understands what services are available and can leave the institution at any time. Involuntary hospitalization occurs when clients are deemed by a psychiatrist (some states require the testimony of two psychiatrists) to be incapable of caring for themselves (gravely disabled), are suicidal (dangerous to themselves), or are homicidal (dangerous to others). Involuntary admissions are subject to legal review, and the clients have certain rights (such as court hearings). Involuntary admission is, essentially, detention in a psychiatric setting against the client's will. Clients are detained for an initial period and reevaluated. If the circumstances that led to admission have not improved, the client is kept for a longer period of time, usually 14 days.

All clients, whether voluntary or involuntary, have rights that protect their worth and dignity[10] and are informed of these rights as part of the admission procedure. If a right is suspended for clinical purposes, the client must be informed of this, and a progress note must be entered in the medical record by the treating physician. For example, use of the telephone may be restricted if the client's symptoms include making threatening calls to public figures or ordering expensive merchandise which he or she cannot afford.

HOW IT FEELS TO BECOME A CLIENT: PERSONAL, FAMILY, AND COMMUNITY PERSPECTIVES

The Client's Perspective

Clients experience many feelings as they consider seeking treatment from the mental health care delivery system. Initially, doubt may predominate, as clients ask themselves and others, "Can they help me?" Clients fear the unknown. "What will it take to feel better?" "If medications are used, will there be side effects?" "Who will treat me?" "Are they qualified?" "Will I lose control?" "Will I be rejected?" "Will family secrets be revealed?" One concern expressed by all clients is, "How long will it take for me to feel better?" Many clients are confused and bewildered. On the other hand, clients who have just left an abusive environment may feel calmer and safer. Clients need to be oriented to the setting they enter, and they also need to express their feelings. Expectations and requests require exploration by the nurse, and outcome criteria must be established early in the treatment process. Clients must explore their feelings about the stigma of being labeled a *client* or *patient*. Although some socioeconomic classes have begun to accept mental illness in much the same way as they do physical illnesses, there continue to be socioeconomic and cultural factors that cause mental illness to be considered "bad" and not openly discussable. The clients, having struggled with identifying a problem, must also prepare for questions asked by relatives, friends, their bosses or coworkers, or peers at school.

The Family's Perspective

Along with the client, the family must struggle with the stigma associated with mental illness as they consider what will happen if others find out about the client's plight. "What should we tell people?" is a common question asked of care givers. This question is usually accompanied by feelings of dread, shame, guilt, and embarrassment. Although the client is the focus of treatment, it is essential at times (especially in the hospital setting) to include family members in assessment, treatment, and planning for discharge. In this light, the family as a unit becomes the "client," and many of the feelings the client initially experiences may be felt by the family as a whole.

The Community's Perspective

Since there is an uneasy feeling about mental illness in general, it is understandable that people in the community (in the school or workplace, for instance) might feel awkward when they visit clients in the hospital or see them after discharge. "What can I say?" and "What shouldn't I say?" are common questions. With these questions come a protective stance; coworkers, for example, do not want to offend or harm the client. People also have fantasies about what behaviors clients may have exhibited during hospitalization. Did they "go crazy"? Did they require "lots of drugs"? Were they ever put in a "padded cell"? People are often more cautious around clients than they should be. A supportive, nonjudgmental stance is best. Silence can be as destructive as "saying the wrong thing." General questions, such as, "What was it like for you?" are open-ended enough to allow clients to share factual as well as affective responses to their hospitalization. The client senses the uneasiness and withdrawal of friends and coworkers. It is important for the nurse to anticipate these responses and suggest ways of dealing with them before the client leaves the hospital or clinic setting. Clients, once returned to the community, usually want to be treated with the same respect and dignity they received before treatment.

THE TRIAGE PROCESS

The triage process occurs when clients first enter the mental health care delivery system and a decision is made about what setting will best meet their needs. As was mentioned earlier, admissions to various mental health settings are affected by factors such as severity of illness, ability of a setting (resources) to treat certain illnesses, voluntary or involuntary status, and ability of client to pay for services. The process of determining clients' needs and placing them in the most appropriate setting is called *triage*. Descriptions of various settings follow.

Inpatient Setting

Although inpatient settings may have various designs and differ from other medical settings, certain general features characterize effective programs.[11]

1. Staffs which can tolerate *less* order and organization on the unit
2. Nursing staffs with as little shift rotation as possible
3. Lower percentage of socially passive clients
4. Higher percentage of clients off the unit
5. Higher percentage of clients who do not require antipsychotic drugs at discharge
6. Clients on low dosages of minor tranquilizers.

The following treatment modalities are common in most inpatient programs:

Individual psychotherapy

Group psychotherapy

Family therapy and multiple-family therapy

Occupational therapy

Rehabilitation (physical therapy, speech therapy)

Recreation, movement, art therapies

Various other supportive therapies

The client may be seen in the emergency department (ED) or assessment unit before admission to the actual inpatient unit. Once accepted for admission, the client signs consents and financial agreements with the institution. The ED staff then hands over further admission functions to the psychiatric unit staff.

The admission process includes identifying clients' problems and exploring their fears, concerns, and expectations. Factors such as locked doors and community living arrangements may affect clients' initial experiences. It is common for clients to complain of feeling closed in during their first few days in the hospital. The nursing staff provides most of the orientation, shows clients the physical layout of the unit, and introduces personnel. It is useful for clients to be told what will be happening in the first 24 hours on the unit. Most clients are too anxious to retain long descriptions of treatment and other matters on the first day. The nurse should assess what clients can understand, given their emotional state at the time of admission. Further, on the basis of information gained while taking a client's history, the nurse anticipates the clients' perceptions of and responses to admission.

A feeling of powerlessness may be a part of the clients' experience as they enter the hospital setting.[12] Powerlessness can be manifested in behaviors such as apathy, anger, and depression. Interventions for clients diagnosed as feeling powerless in the hospital setting are outlined in Table 16-2.

The nurse orients the client to the primary nursing role within the context of interdisciplinary planning of treatment. On admission, the nurse also establishes what outside sources can be called upon if further information is required or if the client needs support from a family member or friend. Nurses must encourage clients to ask questions as they arise and establish an environment conducive to a trusting relationship.

Outpatient Setting

Clients entering the mental health system through an outpatient setting may very well experience feelings similar to those of hospitalized clients. Like inpatients, they may fear the unknown and be anxious about what the treatment process will be like and how long it will take. The sense of confinement, however, may be missing. The client in the outpatient clinic need not be concerned about locked doors or problems of living in a community. On the other hand, outpatients are not provided with the protection, nurturing, or therapeutic environment that inpatients have. Therefore, resources that will help outpatients successfully negotiate their environment outside the hospital must be explored. The nurse must deal with special problems in this area, such as, "Will the client be able to reach someone if he or she has a problem at night?"

DISCHARGE PLANNING

Just as the professional staff is concerned with what events brought the client to seek help, it is also concerned with where clients will go once they have been treated. Discharge planning or disposition should be considered when the client first enters the mental health care system. Initially, clients may not be able to discuss leaving, or the future in general, because they are preoccupied with their symptoms. Common statements at this point are, "I can't begin to think about plans for the future when my life is in the process of falling apart," and "I'll never be well enough to go home." In responding to these comments, the nurse needs the ability to convince clients that symptomatology is temporary. As discharge approaches, anxiety and fear may reappear; the client wonders, "What will I do without the people here?"

Often, discharge plans include posthospitalization treatment. Referrals are made to private practitioners, individual or group psychotherapy in clinics, or home health care. A major goal of hospitalization is that clients learn new coping and problem-solving skills. The client has had a chance to practice these newly learned skills in the therapeutic community. Although psychiatric symptomatology usually subsides over the course of treatment, it is not uncommon to see a recurrence of symptoms at discharge. Discharge is often a reactivation of a loss or rejection that the client has already experienced (such as maternal separation or death of a loved one). It is the role of the nurse to assist the client in reminiscing about and analyzing the hospitalization and reviewing such matters as initial hesitancy in seeking treatment, the process of identifying specific problems to work on during the hospitalization, and the increased insight gained by learning new coping strategies.

When the client is referred to another agency, the nurse must supply information relevant to the client's past and present physical and emotional state. A review of the nursing care plan and its effectiveness is an excellent means of providing data to the next care giver. If possible, to ease the transition, the nurse might arrange a meeting with the client and the new therapist or group leader before actual discharge. In the event of referral to Alcoholics Anonymous, for example, the nurse might accompany the client to the first meeting. Groups have been developed on some inpatient units to ease the transition from hospital to community. Clients are referred to the group by the treatment team 2 weeks before discharge and come back to the hospital for three visits after actual discharge.

Table 16-2 Powerlessness Related to Hospitalization*

Assessment

Subjective data

The person reports:
- Feelings of lack of control

Objective data
- Anger
- Sadness
- Apathy
- Hostility
- Lack of participation in regimen

Outcome criteria

The person will experience a decreased sense of powerlessness, as evidenced by:
- Identification of factors that can be controlled by him or her
- Making decisions regarding his or her care, treatment, and future when possible

Interventions

A. Assess for causative and contributing factors
- Lack of knowledge
- Previous inadequate coping patterns (e.g., depression)
- Unsatisfactory health care provider's routines
- Locus of control (internal or external)

B. Eliminate or reduce contributing factors if possible

1. Lack of knowledge
   - Increase effective communication between person and health care provider
   - Explain all procedures, rules, and options to person
   - Allow time to answer questions; ask person to write questions down so as not to forget them
   - Provide children with
     a. Opportunities to make decisions (e.g., setting time for bath, holding still for injection)
     b. Specific play therapy before and after a traumatic situation
   - Provide a specific time (10–15 minutes) each shift that person knows can be used to ask questions or discuss subjects as desired
   - Keep person informed about condition, treatments, and results
   - While being realistic, point out positive changes in person's condition, such as serum enzymes decreasing after myocardial infarction or surgical incision healing well
   - Be an active listener by allowing person to verbalize concerns and feelings: assess for areas of concern
   - Provide consistent staffing
   - Single out one nurse to be responsible for 24-hour plan of care, and provide opportunities for person and family to identify with this nurse
2. Unsatisfactory health care provider's routines
   a. Provide opportunities for individual to control decisions
   - Allow person to manipulate surroundings, such as deciding what is to be kept where (shoes under bed, picture on window)
   - Keep needed items within reach (call bell, urinal, tissues)
   - Do not offer options if none exist (e.g., a deep IM Z-tract injection must be rotated)
   - Discuss daily plan of activities and allow person to make as many decisions as possible about it
   - Increase decision-making opportunities as person progresses
   - Respect and follow individual's decision if you have given options
   - Record person's specific choices on care plan to ensure that others on staff acknowledge preferences ("Dislikes orange juice," "Takes showers," "Plan dressing change at 7:30 prior to shower")
   - Keep promises
   - Provide opportunity for person and family to express feelings
   - Provide opportunities for person and family to participate in care
   - Be alert for signs of paternalism/maternalism in health care providers (e.g., making decisions for patients)
   - Plan a care conference to allow staff to discuss methods of individualizing care; encourage each nurse to share at least one action that he or she discovered a particular individual liked
3. Locus of control
   a. Assess the person's usual response to problems
   - Internal control (seeks to change own behaviors or environment to control problems)
   - External control (expects others or other factors—fate, luck—to control problems)

   b. Provide person with internal locus of control the needed information to alter behavior or environment
   - Explain the problem as explicitly as the individual requests
   - Explain the relationship of prescribed behavior and outcome (e.g., need to restrict salt, physiological effects of exercise, effects of bed rest on impaired cardiac function)

   c. Monitor a person with external locus of control to encourage participation
   - Have the person keep a record for you (e.g., food intake for 1 week; weight loss chart; exercise program—type and frequency; medications taken)
   - Use telephone contact to monitor if feasible
   - Provide explicit written directions to follow (e.g., meal plans; exercise regimen—type, frequency, duration; speech practice lessons—for aphasia)

C. Initiate health teaching and referrals as indicated (social worker, psychiatric nurse/physician, visiting nurse)

*This specific diagnosis should be restricted to use for individuals exhibiting objective data, not all hospitalized persons.

SOURCE: L. Carpenito, *Nursing Diagnosis: Application to Clinical Practice*, Lippincott, Philadelphia, 1983, pp. 335–336.

Types of Discharges

Generally, there are three types of discharges: absolute, conditional, and judicial. An *absolute discharge* means that the client formally cuts ties with the hospital or other mental health setting. Such a discharge can occur when a client has made enough improvement in mental state and interpersonal functioning to have derived what is known as *maximum hospital benefit* (MHB). However, when a client leaves the hospital *against medical advice* (AMA), the discharge is also considered absolute. An absolute discharge can also result from utilization review processes: Medicare and third-party payers may limit the number of treatment days for any psychiatric diagnosis.

A *conditional discharge* means that the client must meet certain obligations before formal termination of ties to the treatment setting. Monthly home leaves from a state hospital and weekend visits to an acute care setting are examples of conditional discharges. The goal of this type of discharge is gradual, purposeful transition and reintegration into the community.

Judicial discharges are court-ordered discharges. A psychiatrist's decision to hospitalize a client is subject to judicial review if the client appeals the decision. (Clients, may, if they wish, come to court with members of their families or the professional staff.) If the court decides that there are no legal or clinical grounds for detaining the client, then the client is released into self-custody or the custody of family or friends.

Planning

Family, friends, and others can often provide important information about clients. If the client agrees, the nurse and treatment team should try to establish a good working relationship with these support systems. Where there is no family, perhaps a significant other can be included in the treatment process. The family usually has information about the client's idiosyncracies and can in many instances inform the clinician as to whether a certain approach is likely to be more effective than another. As mentioned earlier, the family must be involved in discharge planning, since it may be a significant support system for the client after discharge.

Families may covertly or overtly sabotage treatment plans when they do not agree with the treatment team's recommendations. Early discharges or AMA discharges are often a sign of clients' or families' disagreement or displeasure with treatment or discharge plans, or of collusion to resist treatment. Resistence to treatment may develop when therapeutic approaches alter family dynamics and disturb family equilibrium. (For example, if family stability depends on one member's being the "identified patient," a therapeutic approach that changed this role would be resisted.)

Treatment Team

In most inpatient psychiatric units, treatment is planned by an interdisciplinary team. The team is usually headed by a psychiatrist. Other mental health practitioners provide valuable information which is used to develop a comprehensive treatment plan. The team includes the nurse, psychologist, social worker, occupational therapist, recreation or movement therapist, nutritionist, and pharmacist.

Clients may at first be bewildered by the number of care givers. It is, therefore, essential for all those involved in providing care and discharge planning to introduce themselves at the outset and explain their role in the treatment. (For example: "Mr. Jones, I am your primary nurse. My name is———. I will be responsible for planning your nursing care during your hospitalization.") Usually, clients want to know who their assigned nurses are for each shift. An effective nursing plan maintains consistency for clients. Placing an information board in a conspicuous place on the unit allows clients to find out for themselves who their care givers are; it might list the names of the primary nurse, the associate nurse, the physician, and other care givers for each client.

Members of the treatment team use their various areas of expertise to develop a realistic, comprehensive discharge plan. The social worker investigates community resources and visits board and care homes (halfway houses) with the client. The team carefully reviews the successes and failures of past discharge plans and placements and uses this information to offer alternatives to the client.

Availability of Resources

Treatment teams are having increasing difficulty placing clients in settings that meet their needs for housing, employment, and leisure-time activities. One reason for this is the fact that federal funds for community mental health services have not been sufficient to develop comprehensive programs for clients after hospitalization. Group homes, halfway houses, and transitional living centers have been established; but these are crowded (applicants must often be placed on a waiting list), and access to them is often contingent on ability to pay. The team must try to find aftercare services which the client can afford. State disability funds may be available for clients who have few resources.

When placement in another setting is necessary after discharge, the supportive role of the nurse will include explaining alternatives to the client. The nurse is also the one who supplies information to the agency receiving the client. This information, usually in the form of a nursing care plan, must specify nursing diagnoses, treatment received during the course of hospitalization, and the client's response to interventions. A description of the client's strengths and weaknesses, interpersonal style, and participation in group settings will help the receiving agency to become familiar with the client.

SUMMARY

Many people at some time in their lives will require help from a psychiatric–mental health professional. This usually happens when supports such as families and friends are not enough to relieve psychic pain. Although some clients seek out psychiatric and community resources for preventive purposes, most turn to these sources when psychiatric symptoms (such as anxiety and depression) are impairing their functioning at home, at school, or at work. In general, people enter the mental health care system because they need environmental change, relief from symptoms, or nurturance, or because they have been ordered to do so by a court.

There are various patterns of entry into the mental health care delivery system, and access to services depends upon many factors, including socioeconomic status of the client, severity of psychiatric symptoms, and resources available in the delivery system. On admission, a triage process is begun to determine which services are most appropriate for the client. Since clients and their families experience anxiety as they enter the system, the nurse's role includes identifying affective responses and intervening as necessary.

Discharge planning is a focus of the treatment team from the time of admission. Families and significant others should be involved in the planning of both treatment and discharge, and care givers must work with both the client and the family if positive outcomes are to be realized.

REFERENCES

1. C. Kadushin, *Why People Go to Psychiatrists*, Atherton, New York, 1969, p. 12.
2. A. Lazare and S. Eisenthal, "A Negotiated Approach to the Clinical Encounter," in A. Lazare, ed., *Outpatient Psychiatry: Diagnosis and Treatment*, Williams and Wilkins, Baltimore, 1979, pp. 142–144.
3. UCLA Extension Catalog (USPS 646–760), Vol. XVIII, 2/13/85, P.O. Box 24901, Los Angeles, Calif., 90024.
4. L. Hoff, *People in Crisis: Understanding and Helping*, 2d ed., Addison-Wesley, Menlo Park, Calif., 1984, p. 342.
5. E. Mumford et al., "A New Look at Evidence about Reduced Cost of Medical Utilization Following Mental Health Treatment," *The American Journal of Psychiatry*, vol. 141, October 1984, pp. 1145–1158.
6. American Psychiatric Association, *Diagnostic and Statistical Manual of Mental Disorders*, 3d ed., APA, Washington, D.C., 1980.
7. L. Pelletier, "Nurse-Psychotherapists: Whom Do They Treat?," *Hospital and Community Psychiatry*, vol. 35, November 1984, pp. 1149–1150.
8. American Psychiatric Association, "Guidelines for Psychiatrists in Consultative, Supervisory and Collaborative Relationships with Non-Medical Therapists," *The American Journal of Psychiatry*, vol. 137, November 1980, pp. 1489–1491.
9. Personal communication with Colleen J. Hewes, R.N., C., M.S.N., and Richard VanGorder, R.N., C., M.S.N.
10. California Administrative Code, Title 22, Section 71507 and Title 9, Section 860–868.
11. J. Collins et al., "Treatment Characteristics of Effective Psychiatric Programs," *Hospital and Community Psychiatry*, vol. 35, June 1984, pp. 601–605.
12. L. Carpenito, *Nursing Diagnosis: Application to Clinical Practice*, Lippincott, Philadelphia, 1983, pp. 335–336.

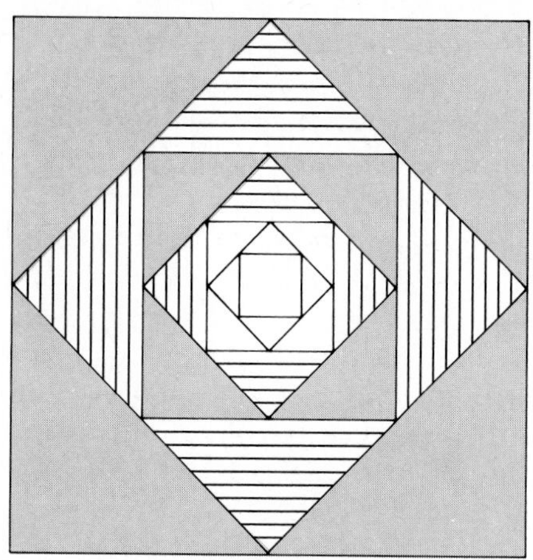

CHAPTER 17
Inpatient Contexts of Care

Anita M. Leach

LEARNING OBJECTIVES

After studying this chapter, the student should be able to:

1. List the purposes of hospitalization of mentally ill clients.
2. Describe the people in inpatient psychiatric hospital environments.
3. Identify the members of the mental health treatment team, their educational preparation, and their usual roles.
4. Define *environment* as it relates to clients' behavior.
5. Describe a therapeutic environment.
6. Discuss concerns the nurse has about clients' safety and comfort in inpatient settings.
7. Describe the psychiatric nursing role in an inpatient setting.

The majority of psychiatric nurses in the United States are employed caring for mentally ill clients in formal inpatient settings. Such settings are usually units in general hospitals or specialty hospitals organized to deliver around-the-clock mental health services to a specified group of clients.

In an average lifetime of 65 years, one out of every four Americans will need some form of mental health intervention, and one out of every four of these will require hospitalization. The current trend is toward shorter hospital stays and more outpatient treatment. However, although the number of institutionalized clients has been drastically reduced since the passage of the Community Mental Health Act and the introduction of psychopharmacologic therapy, 25 percent of all hospital beds in this country remain occupied by mentally ill clients. Inpatient treatment of behavioral symptoms may take place in public mental hospitals, state institutions, or psychiatric units of general hospitals. More affluent clients can afford treatment in private institutions for the mentally ill, or in *sanitariums.* Ten of every 10,000 Americans will at some point in their lives receive care in a federal or state mental institution. Currently, about 50 percent of hospital admissions for mental illness are initiated by clients themselves.[1]

The clinical placement of student nurses during their study of psychiatric nursing is frequently in inpatient settings. The purpose of this chapter is to communicate information about the experience that a hospital environment provides for clients. The environment, or ecological system, of both client and nurse is discussed, since the environment frequently determines the roles nurses assume and the quality of care clients receive. The role of the nurse as creator of a therapeutic milieu is emphasized.

PURPOSES OF HOSPITALIZATION

Clients are admitted to hospitals in various ways and for various reasons. Clients may initiate their own hospitalization, actively oppose it, or be ambivalent about it. In all cases, admission to and discharge from mental health inpatient treatment settings is regulated by state law.

Several reasons are cited for admitting clients for inpatient treatment. While the exact route of entry or reentry into the system will vary for each client (since every person is unique), there are some general purposes for hospitalization.

First, admission may be necessary for the *security* of clients, their families, and the community. This is the most common reason for involuntary admissions. Clients who are dangerous to themselves or others need the security and structure of a hospital; thus people who are actively suicidal and people whose behavior is violent are generally admitted for reasons of safety.

Second, clients may be admitted for *observation* when they have committed crimes and their competence and emotional status need to be determined by experts.

Third, clients may be admitted so that a *differential diagnosis* can be made. For example, the behavioral manifestations of temporal-lobe epilepsy and agitated psychotic depression are very similar. Observation and intensive studies are needed to make a correct diagnosis and determine appropriate treatment.

Fourth, clients may be admitted for *initiation of psychopharmacologic treatment* and titrating of appropriate medication. This is particularly true for the elderly and for clients who are beginning an antidepressant agent or lithium therapy.

Fifth, clients may be hospitalized in *response to a crisis,* such as might occur after the death of a spouse.

Sixth, some clients seek a structured setting for purposes of *healing,* and clients who have spent many years in hospitals may continue to seek out the familiarity of the institutional setting for *solace* and *care.*

Regardless of the purpose served by a structured inpatient environment, the goal of nursing treatment is always promotion, maintenance, restoration, and rehabilitation of clients' physical, mental, and spiritual health. The fundamental purpose of hospitalization is to heal broken bodies, minds, and spirits.

PERSONS IN THE INPATIENT ENVIRONMENT

A therapeutic environment is not just a place or a system; it is a setting created in part by the people, or subsystems, who inhabit it. Clients, their families, nurses, and other members of the health team are the subsystems that interact to form the whole which is called a *therapeutic environment.*

The Client

Clients, once admitted to a hospital, represent individual systems as well as a collective group or subsystem within the hierarchical system of the hospital. Their mental, physical, and spiritual comfort, both as individuals and as a group, is a direct result of the socialization process that begins when they first seek help or are urged or compelled by others to receive it.

Generally, what clients need—particularly in the initial stages of hospitalization—is a secure, structured environment with direct care and management by professionals 24 hours a day. Clients who need the security of a hospital are for the most part acutely ill or in immediate need of services that cannot be provided on an outpatient basis. Today, clients admitted for inpatient care are sicker than those admitted in the past, and their stay in the hospital tends to be shorter.

The mix of clients, with their different ages, personalities, and diagnoses, affects the environment and each client's comfort within it. Adolescents, for example, may be uncomfortable in a setting where there are few people of their own age; and manipulative clients frequently generate anger in those around them. Moreover, clients sometimes form cliques, creating friction with others in the setting. When potential clients are being evaluated, the existing "client mix" is frequently a criterion for admission to a particular setting.

The Family and Significant Others

"Significant others," especially family members, are part of a client's past, present, and future environment. These people expect the client's behavior to be repatterned and changed, but they are not always aware that they too will be affected. Not only spouses, parents, and children but also friends and employers will be affected by whatever change occurs in the client and need to be included in a comprehensive treatment plan.

Family members of clients also contribute to the environment of a particular setting. Some families are supportive of clients; others remain aloof or absent themselves from the treatment process. Some family members support each other; others are indifferent or openly hostile. Inpatient settings frequently have, as a part of treatment, structured multifamily group meetings in which families of hospitalized clients share concerns, frustrations, and creative approaches to helping the clients.

Two additional points are of particular importance with regard to clients' families. First, people on the mental health team respond to clients in much the same way as clients' significant others. For example, if a nurse becomes angry with a client because of his or her manipulative behavior, it is very likely that the behavior also angers a spouse or some other family member. If a client elicits an overresponsible or nurturing response from the nurse, the family is probably responding in a similar way. Second, discharged clients who have supportive families and social networks remain out of the hospital for longer periods of time.

The Mental Health Team

In inpatient settings, nurses are the people who are most crucial in creating a therapeutic atmosphere, and the 24-hour-a-day presence of nurses is the major factor in managing and changing clients' behavior. However, most clients in conventional institutions are treated by a team or group of professionals.

The psychiatric mental health team consists of psychiatrists, nurses, nursing assistants or technicians, social workers, clinical psychologists, and cooperating adjunct therapists. *Adjunct therapists* are people who utilize the arts and other specialized approaches to therapy. Among the specialists who may be on the team are art therapists, occupational therapists, psychodrama therapists, and recreational therapists. Specialists have also been trained to use pets, poetry, and books as adjuncts to therapy. Vocational and educational therapists may be part of a team. Chaplains attend to the spiritual needs of clients. Dietitians contribute to the treatment of food-related illnesses and provide nutritionally sound menus. Table 17-1 lists the people who make up a mental health treatment team, their functions, and their educational backgrounds.

The role of the nurse as a team member has evolved slowly. Nurses' early roles were limited to providing custodial care, monitoring somatic ther-

Table 17-1 Members of the Mental Health Team

Team Member	Educational Preparation	Function on the Team
Psychiatrist	M.D. with residency in psychiatry	Physician who specializes in the treatment of mental diseases. Considered the leader of the team. Has both administrative and care-planning responsibilities; diagnostic and medical functions are the psychiatrist's main tasks.
Clinical psychologist	Ph.D. in clinical psychology	Specializes in the study of mental processes and treatment of mental disorders. Utilizes diagnostic testing to assist the team in differentiating the causative factors in client's behavior. Treats clients, using both individual and group methods.
Psychiatric social worker	Master's degree in social work (M.S.W.)	Evaluates families; studies the environment and social causes of the client's illness. Practices family therapy as a natural outcome of assessment. Works in the intake office and admits new clients.
Psychiatric nurse	R.N. (diploma), A.A., B.S.; advanced preparation at the master's level for independent practice	Environmental management and 24-hour-a-day care. Carries out individual, family, and group psychotherapy; coordinates team activities. Supervises technicians or psychiatric assistants. Primary, secondary, and tertiary role activities in the community.
Psychiatric assistant or technician	High school education, special on-job training in setting of employment	Works under the direct supervision of a professional nurse. Assists nurses in providing for the basic needs of clients. Carries out nursing functions, including maintenance of a therapeutic environment. Supervises leisure-time activity. Assists with individual and group psychotherapy.
Occupational therapist	Advanced degree in occupational therapy	Assesses client's skills for rehabilitative planning. Encourages clients to perform useful tasks. Responsible for socialization therapy and vocational retraining.
Art therapist	Advanced degree and specialized training in art therapy	Utilizes procedures that make use of spontaneous creative work of the client. Works with groups, encouraging members to make and analyze drawings, which are often expressions of their underlying problems. Adjunct to a mental health team in diagnosis and treatment of children.
Recreational therapist	Advanced degree and specialized training in recreational therapy	Provides leisure-time activities for clients. Teaches hospitalized clients useful pastimes which can be utilized when they return to the community. Participates in pet therapy, psychodrama, poetry, and music therapy.
Dietitian	Advanced degree and specialized training in dietetics	Provides attractive, nourishing meals for clients. Involved in direct treatment of such food-related illnesses as anorexia nervosa, bulimia, pica, rumination, and eating-control disorders.
Auxiliary personnel (housekeepers, volunteers, clerks, secretaries, etc.)	Various backgrounds and on-job training	Assist clients in participating in activities of daily living and other practical jobs. When properly educated, invaluable in helping the client to enter into and participate in the therapeutic program.
Chaplain	Seminary pastoral counselor or rabbinical education	Attends to the spiritual needs of clients and their families. Pastoral counseling and marital counseling when chaplain has advanced education.

apies, and functioning as unit managers and role models. But the team concept and the nurse's role have changed rapidly since the team itself was first recognized as an important therapeutic approach in 1949 by the National Institute of Mental Health,[2] and since the number of advanced psychiatric nurse-clinicians has increased.

The team concept is now widely accepted. Professional competition and rivalry, struggles for turf, and the traditional role of the physician as leader have been supplanted by more democratic and more practical processes. The team concept promotes cooperation among colleagues rather than individual professional autonomy.

A clinical team, as it functions today, provides a forum where psychiatrists, social workers, psychologists, nurses, and others can democratically share their professional expertise and develop comprehensive therapeutic plans for clients. The optimally functioning team has several characteristics:

1. Leadership is clear and democratic.
2. All members have an equal opportunity to share what they have learned about clients.
3. The goal—developing a comprehensive treatment plan for clients—is clear.
4. All team members are recognized as professionals who can make unique contributions.
5. Roles of team members are clearly defined for each setting.
6. Mutual respect and understanding characterize communications among members.

THERAPEUTIC ENVIRONMENTS

Environment is defined as relevant systems external to and in interaction with a client. It is the patterned wholeness of all that is external to the person. The environment includes relevant people, places or spaces external to the person, and objects within those spaces. A *therapeutic environment* is based on the concept that everything external to clients, or everything that happens to them in their environment, is potentially therapeutic or antitherapeutic.

Psychiatric clients who are severely ill generally require treatment in protected environments. Conventional or formal settings for such care include large institutions (such as state and federal hospitals), inpatient units in general hospitals, day hospitals, and night hospitals. A *day hospital* is a structured, protected environment that provides treatment during the day; clients, who are generally chronically ill or in transition back to the community, return to their homes or some other shelter for the night. A *night hospital* provides supervision and treatment at the end of the day for clients who spend daytimes at a job, with their families, or at a rehabilitation center in the community.

Physical Environment

Physical features of a therapeutic environment are designed to facilitate healing and provide safety and security. Maintaining both safety and the overall physical space as such in an inpatient setting is generally the responsibility of nurses. Table 17-2 describes how basic needs can be met in ways that promote a secure atmosphere conducive to healing.

There are several significant features necessary in the physical environment. In considering these, it is important to bear in mind that safety and security are crucial, not only from the point of view of the professional staff but also for the clients. Some clients see the hospital—with its therapeutic, safe atmosphere—as a refuge; in fact, this attitude contributes to increased recidivism and frequent readmissions. Other clients seek a secure setting because they are afraid that they will lose control of themselves. For example, a psychotic client may feel unsafe on an "open" unit of a general hospital and request transfer, or behave in such a way as to require transfer, to a more secure, locked setting.

Sensory stimulation is one important aspect of the physical environment. Objects in the environment are sources of sensations and thus of input to the brain. Either sensory overload or sensory deprivation can distort this input; moreover, colors, lighting, and sounds affect the behavior of clients. Nurses are therefore mindful of sensory stimuli. For example, nurses manage disturbed clients by moving them to a *"quiet room"* where sensory stimuli are reduced. The lighting in a quiet room should be subdued; the room is likely to be decorated in colors (pale blues, pale greens, and shades of purple) which have a soothing effect; and noises and distractions are reduced to a minimum. Visitors are limited; and staff members working in the area should curtail their conversations with clients and maintain a silent protectiveness. When sensory input is reduced in these ways, clients are more likely to regain self-control. *Sound* in general is another kind of sensory stimulation that requires attention. Both clients and staff on a unit are often noisy. Nurses should be aware that a quiet, calm, and orderly manner will modify clients' behavior and add to their comfort. Loud noises, therefore, should be avoided whenever possible. A third type of sensory stimulation is *odors:* nurses should be alert to odors in a unit and take steps to eliminate offensive ones.

Dangerous objects, and potentially dangerous objects, are another aspect of the physical environ-

Table 17-2 Atmosphere Needed to Meet Basic Needs

Needs	Atmosphere to Be Created	Needs	Atmosphere to Be Created
Physiological Food, oxygen, water, sleep, sex	**Dining room** Cheerfully decorated, arranged for maximum socialization, noise factor at minimum, background music **Bedroom** Cheerfully decorated, subdued lighting and colors, reading light, desk, quiet, arranged for maximum privacy, planned for individualization and safety **Outdoor space** Planned so client can enjoy fresh air, can walk or sit **Snack kitchen** Snacks and coffee available, arranged for informal socialization **Bathroom** Provide privacy while maintaining safety needs	**Love and belonging** Affection, identification, companionship	**Common room** Homelike, comfortably furnished Furniture groupings conducive to socialization—tables for game playing, etc. Bright, cheerful color scheme
		Esteem and recognition	**Interviewing rooms** Conducive to establishing a caring, therapeutic relationship, quiet, conducive to uninterrupted time with clients **Group rooms** Chairs in round circle, no table in center, quiet, conducive to uninterrupted time with clients and their families
Safety Security, stability, order, physical safety	**Seclusion or quiet room** Place for restricting clients, controlled space confinement, subdued lighting, subdued color, safe room free from objects that can do physical harm **Locked space** To protect clients from themselves and others **Boundaries** Knowledge of limits of a client's personal space **Bulletin boards** For posting schedules, notices, and client assignments. (Use tape, not sharp tacks or pins)	**Self-actualization** Self-fullfilment, achieving one's potential, realizing one's capabilities	**Occupational therapy room** Background music, woodworking and crafts equipment, freedom to explore interests, supervised and secure **Art therapy room** Background music, supervision, ample supplies of oil paints, watercolors, tempera paints, clay, finger paints, and other materials **Music and entertainment center** Equipped with records for all types of listening, television set **Library** Quiet, comfortable chairs, reading lights, variety of books, newspapers, magazines
		Aesthetic Order, harmony, beauty, spiritual goals	Quiet, nondenominational, meditative atmosphere, place to be alone

ment which requires monitoring. Within the limits of safety and practicality, hospitalized clients are encouraged to decorate their living space with personal objects. However, some objects which are commonplace elsewhere must be used with care in psychiatric settings in order to protect clients from their own or others' rage or suicidal impulses. Clients who are suicidal or out of control, for example, can hurt themselves or others with objects that are usually employed safely or even considered harmless. Sharp objects, such as nail files, razors and mirrors, need to be limited in psychiatric treatment settings. Furniture purchased for these settings should be sturdy and have blunt edges. Lighting should be recessed when possible, and light bulbs and tubes should be made of unbreakable material. Scissors, sewing and crocheting needles, and other sharp craft tools should be used only with supervision. In a "quiet room," all potentially harmful objects should be removed, and furniture should have no sharp edges.

Time—although it is not always thought of in this way—is another aspect of the physical environment. Therapeutic environments have structured schedules. Time is provided for therapy, for activities on and off the unit, for meals, and for activities of daily living. Free time and quiet time are also incorporated, generally on a basis of individual clients' needs. Evening and weekend schedules are less busy than weekdays and are frequently the sole responsibility of the recreation and nursing staff. Flexible scheduling permits each client to collaborate with the staff to make choices that reflect individual needs and are conducive to recovery. Table 17-3 is a sample of a typical schedule for clients in inpatient settings.

Emotional and Spiritual Environment

A therapeutic environment is one in which healing of mind, body, and spirit can occur. As has been noted, it has certain physical characteristics; but it

Table 17-3 Clients' Schedule

Time	Monday	Tuesday	Wednesday	Thursday	Friday	Saturday	Sunday
8:00	Rising	Rising	Rising	Rising	Rising	Rising	Rising
8:30	Breakfast	Breakfast	Breakfast	Breakfast	Breakfast	Breakfast	Breakfast
9:00	Quiet time Staff meeting	Quiet time	Quiet time	Quiet time	Quiet time	Free time	Church service
10:00	Bowling or art therapy	Art therapy or newspaper group	Library or bowling	Woodworking or bingo	Community meeting		
	Individual sessions →						
11:00	Group therapy (Group B)	Group therapy (Group A)	Group therapy (Group B)	Group therapy (Group A)	Discharge planning meeting (staff and assigned clients)	Activity planning meeting of weekend staff and clients	Activity planning meeting
12:30	Lunch →						
1:30	Vocational Rehabilitation →						
	Woodworking or bingo	Shopping	Movie	Dance therapy	Patient government	Unit activity →	
2:30	Outdoor activity	Shopping	Movie	Dance therapy	Cooking group	Unit activity	Unit activity
4:00	On-unit college courses Typing class	Medication group Individual sessions	Outdoor activity	On-unit college courses Typing class	Free time (house-keeping chores)	Special entertainment when scheduled	Newspaper sharing group
5:30	Supper →						
6:30	Television →						
7:30	Television night Family therapy sesions	Outdoor activity Family therapy sessions	Family night	Movie	Family discharge planning meeting, selected clients and their families	Television or movie	Social hour with family
8:30	New admissions; orientation	Family therapy sessions	Multifamily groups	Movie	Free time	Television or movie	Unit meeting Weekend rehash
9:30	Bedtime				Unit refreshments	Television or movie	Bedtime
10:30 11:30	Lights out →				Bedtime and lights out	Bedtime and lights out	Lights out

NOTE: Individual and family therapy sessions are scheduled by the primary therapist.

is also, and to a much greater extent, an atmosphere, an intangible sense of a "good" place, that evolves out of the interaction of many subsystems. *Milieu therapy* is the process of utilizing aspects of a treatment setting which are known to have a positive influence on the behavior of clients.[3] The environment is structured to provide human relationships that satisfy emotional needs, reduce psychological conflicts and deprivation, and strengthen impaired ego functions. The concept is based on the assumption that the social milieu itself can be the instrument of treatment.

A therapeutic atmosphere is achieved by scientific manipulation of the environment to limit or expand the behavior of clients. It is an environment in which all that occurs is used therapeutically to intervene with clients. The goal of creating a therapeutic milieu is to prepare clients to live productive and successful lives in the community when they are discharged. This purpose is best served by establishing close relationships between the therapeutic community and the outside community. Use of community facilities such as recreation centers, libraries, general hospitals, and churches prevents the treatment facility from becoming isolated. An active volunteer group can be an invaluable resource in bridging the gap between treatment center and community.[2]

It is not unusual for an environment with a therapeutic atmosphere to be seen as a utopia by clients. The hospital is experienced as benevolent, secure, and relatively free of stress. It is a place where clients are the focus of concern and attention and where companionship abounds. It is an environment that is predictable and consistent and provides a balance of work and play. Clients do not feel "different" but are with others like themselves. For some clients, it is the healthiest place they have ever lived. Clients may therefore want to remain indefinitely and may sabotage treatment plans or be generally uncooperative in order to avoid recovery and discharge to an often uncertain and disorganized world. The staff needs to assess clients' dependency on the therapeutic environment and work to prevent unhealthy attachment.

Characteristics of a Therapeutic Environment

A therapeutic environment differs from ordinary treatment settings in the way an institution's total resources are *purposefully* pooled to provide and improve care. The creation of a therapeutic milieu begins when clients are admitted. It is characterized by an orientation program which facilitates clients' entry into the system, democratic processes, participatory governance, opportunities for problem solving, participation by clients in treatment, and therapeutic discharge planning.

Orientation Program

Orientation of clients and their families to the therapeutic milieu is of prime importance in providing a healthy, safe environment. A well-planned orientation program is also one factor in preventing dependency on the institution. A therapeutic orientation program gives clients and their families initial personal contacts with the nursing staff and other team members. Each client requires unique interventions at this point, including information about the setting and the processes involved in becoming a client in the specific system. Discharge planning is initiated, and clients are given detailed information about negotiating within the system and becoming responsible, committed members of it.

Details of an orientation plan depend on the specific environment, but in general any such plan has certain necessary features. These include the following:

- Providing information on various scheduled events
- Introducing the people within the setting
- Defining the roles and responsibilities of significant people
- Explaining where various events take place
- Establishing the expected length of stay in the setting
- Describing the expectations the institution has for the client and the family
- Initiating the discharge planning process
- Explaining what support resources are available to the client and the family

Providing information to clients and their families helps keep already increased anxiety at a minimum.

Democratic Processes

A therapeutic environment is different from a more traditional, asylumlike hospital, but it is not a democracy run by elected officials. Democratic processes do exist, and clients have some part in decision making and formulation of policy. However, authority and responsibility for the care of clients remain with the staff. No amount of persuasion, group decision making, consensus, joint consultation, or freedom of expression can obscure this fact or excuse nurses from exercising their authority appropriately.

In therapeutic environments, then, the staff does not relinquish responsibility but learns to share it with clients. Including clients in democratic processes is considered a part of treatment. Clients participate and collaborate with the staff in practically all information-sharing processes of the unit. Their opinions are sought about matters such as other clients' readiness for passes and discharges. But the fact that staff and clients have equal rights as human beings in such a community in no way implies that their function, role, or status is equal. Roles, relationships, and expectations are frequently examined and discussed to help clarify role perceptions and to determine what behavior is appropriate in the setting.

A therapeutic environment emphasizes socialization, group interaction, and communication as opportunities for learning. All aspects of the clients' lives are seen as presenting opportunities for growth toward wellness. The emotional climate should be one of warmth, friendliness, acceptance, and optimism. In a setting that is functioning well, group members, as individuals, consider themselves active participants in productive group endeavors. Nurses play a major role in providing and maintaining a safe, conflict-free environment through role modeling and group leadership.

Participatory Governance

An important feature of a traditional therapeutic community is the *community meeting,* also called a *unit meeting* or *large-group meeting.* In a therapeutic environment, community meetings are held regularly and provide opportunities for clients to participate in the management of the environment. They are attended by all staff members and clients who work or live on a unit.

Community meetings have several functions. They provide a setting in which the group deals with social and behavioral problems using techniques such as "exposure," "shaming," and "reality confrontation." Examination of roles, discussion of administrative matters, planning of activities, and review of housekeeping functions are other components. In a broad sense, the meetings are used to inculcate values, norms, and attitudes deemed therapeutic by the leaders of the group. An element which is not part of the community meeting itself but is characteristically associated with it is the staff's "rehash." Staff members meet to discuss and clarify the "social barometer," plan therapeutic strategies, and interpret covert and overt content and processes of the meeting.

For members of all the mental health disciplines, working in a consistently therapeutic atmosphere requires reexamination of the traditional roles for which they have been trained; their formal education may not have prepared them for the role blurring that is common in such a milieu. The therapeutic environment and especially the community meeting lend themselves to a continuing process of in-service training.

Opportunitites for Problem Solving

A therapeutic environment is one in which it is safe for clients to test newly learned behaviors and creative ways of dealing with troublesome relationships or situations. In such a setting, staff members and clients feel free, as individuals, to confront ineffective and inappropriate behavior, and clients are able to plan and execute new ways of relating. For example:

> Mary, a 23-year-old client, learned in group sessions that she tended to monopolize conversations, causing those around her to "tune out." She planned with her therapist to try to listen more, both in the group and at mealtimes, and let others have a chance to speak. Mary asked the group for help with this, and after a time she was given positive feedback about the changes she was attempting. The other clients also encouraged her by good-naturedly reminding her of her behavior whenever she began to monopolize discussions. Later, she was able to work at balancing "overtalking" and "undertalking."

A therapeutic environment also gives clients opportunities to reach out to others. For example:

> A client named Sam has an elderly roommate, Ed, who is regressed and verbally noncommunicative. Sam, without being asked, begins helping Ed get dressed each day. This is a sign of progress for Sam, who generally remains isolated. As time goes on, Sam begins to tell Ed about a bench he is making in the activity room. Sam is both surprised and rewarded when one day Ed thanks him. Before long, Ed is telling

others on the unit how much Sam's care has meant to him. Helping Ed has facilitated a breakthrough for Sam and marks the beginning of an ability to take more risks in other relationships.

Clients' Participation in Treatment

One of the basic rights of clients is to participate—or, if they choose, to refuse to participate—in their own treatment. A structured environment may provide rules and regulations that facilitate healing, a skilled and committed professional team, and an ideal therapeutic atmosphere, but if a client is actively or passively uncooperative in the treatment process, little or no change will occur.

Once a client's symptoms have subsided, and even while they persist, the client and his or her family can begin to participate in formulating an individualized treatment plan. The goal from the outset is discharge to the community. As clients recover, they should take on more responsibility for themselves; ideally, they spend less time under direct supervision and more time engaged in autonomous activities. The more regressed a client is, the more structure is needed. For the staff, facilitating clients' responsibility and autonomy is a gradual, stepwise process; and for the clients themselves, becoming responsible and autonomous is a process with stages much like the stages of human development. Some clients make rapid progress through a planned schedule; others need more time for the healing process. Some clients never regress; others do, and must begin the process again.

Participation by clients in treatment can be achieved in various ways. For example, in some settings small groups are formed to encourage participation. The clients are assigned to these groups according to their level of functioning, which is defined in terms of a hierarchy of needs. The most regressed clients are placed in groups where physical needs and safety are the focus of care; more intact clients are placed in groups where the focus is on social and aesthetic needs and the need for self-actualization.[3]

A second way to promote participation in treatment is through the use of rewards. In some settings, a "token economy" is used to motivate clients to participate; in others, intangible rewards are given when clients participate actively in their treatment and gain control of their behavior. For example, a client with a disorderly room may be told that the reward for keeping the room neat will be a pass to go to town for an afternoon. Ideally, socially acceptable behavior—in this case, keeping one's room orderly—will be internalized by the client and will continue even after tokens or rewards are no longer offered.

A third way to encourage participation is through the use of "client government." Some therapeutic environments have structured client governments which facilitate clients' participation in managing the milieu and help them develop responsibility. Officers are elected by the group, and meetings are held regularly, generally once a week. The agenda usually includes such issues as assigning housekeeping chores on the unit; planning activities for large groups, special events, and "surprises"; and welcoming new clients and saying good-bye to clients who are about to be discharged. The officers learn to enact new roles and to accept responsibilities and follow through with them. For all clients, involvement in "client government" facilitates participation and helps to bridge the gap between hospital and community.

Therapeutic Discharge Planning

Clients in a therapeutic environment participate in the formulation of a comprehensive discharge plan, and planning for discharge begins when the client is admitted. In some institutions, health professionals, particularly nurses, are assigned the role of "discharge planners." When this role is not well established, discharge planning and follow-up care become the responsibility of the client's primary care giver or primary therapist, or some other person on the mental health care team. Generally, the person who is responsible for discharge planning coordinates the efforts of all members of the mental health care team.

The ideal discharge plan takes into account all the basic needs of clients and creates a supportive social network that will enable clients to meet these needs. Discharge planning involves work with the client, the family, the staff members who are currently involved with the client, and each of the agencies that will be involved with the client in the future. Cucuzzo used a mnemonic device, METHOD, which can ensure that clients are properly prepared for discharge.[4] The name, an acronym, stands for the elements needed for discharge planning: *m*ed-

Table 17-4 METHOD Discharge Plan for Psychiatric Clients

Discharge Need	Goals for Psychiatric Clients
Medication	Clients and their families will know the name, purpose, and side effects of their medication.
	Clients and their families will know doses, how often to take their medication, what precautions to take, the side effects, and what problems to report and to whom they should be reported.
Environment	Clients will have adequate shelter and economic support.
	Support services will be made available to clients and their families.
	Families will be prepared for the clients' return to their homes.
	Clients and their families will know what services are available in the community for leisure activities, preventive health, continuing education, etc.
Treatment	Clients and their families will participate in individual, family, or group therapy.
	Clients and their families will demonstrate that they understand the need for follow-up therapy.
Health teaching	Clients and their families will know which support services to use to meet basic needs.
Health teaching (continued)	Clients will be able to describe the behavioral signs and symptoms of their disease that require medical treatment.
	Clients and their families will understand psychiatric illness and how it affects self and others.
	Clients and their families will be able to describe elements of preventive mental health.
Outpatient referral	Clients and their families will know when appointments for therapy are scheduled.
	All necessary referral procedures will be completed.
	Follow-up therapy will be appropriate to the client's needs and be financially affordable.
Diet	Clients and their families will be able to describe the components of a healthy, balanced diet.
	Clients and their families will be able to describe dietary restrictions.
	Written copies of restricted foods, beverages, and medications will be made available to clients.
	When appropriate, typical prescribed menus will be given to the client.

SOURCE: Adapted from A. Cucuzzo, "METHOD Discharge Planning," *Supervisor Nurse,* vol. 7, no. 1, 1976, pp. 43–45.

ication, *e*nvironment, *t*reatment, *h*ealth teaching, *o*utpatient referral, and *d*iet. Table 17-4 adapts this system for use with psychiatric clients. The more carefully chronically ill clients are prepared for discharge, the less frequently they will need hospitalization again.

It should be noted that during the discharge planning process, changes in behavior may occur which indicate that clients are anxious about returning to the community, or that they do not feel ready to return to situations they left when they were admitted. Some clients will also feign physical symptoms as a way of remaining in the hospital, a place they perceive as free from the worries and troubles they will face when they are discharged. A thorough discharge plan will allow time for evaluating and working through such anxiety, and both staff members and clients should have ample opportunity to rethink plans that clients are unwilling or unready to accept.

ROLE OF THE NURSE

Nurses are regarded as "guardians of the milieu." They are pivotal in the creation and maintenance of the therapeutic environment. Their responsibility is for 24-hour maintenance of the environment and awareness of the processes occurring in it.

Nurses assume many direct and indirect roles in inpatient settings. *Roles* are goal-directed, culturally influenced patterns of behavior. *Direct roles* involve nurses in promoting, maintaining, restoring, and rehabilitating clients' physical, mental, and spiritual health. *Indirect roles*—roles that are not directly related to care of clients—involve nurses in the administration and management of therapeutic settings.

Roles and the Therapeutic Environment

Roles in nursing are defined and modified as a consequence of interaction of nurses with their environment. The roles they assume will be influenced by personal, family, and cultural history; by previous experience; and by their level of education.

The interplay of a setting and the roles enacted within it create the atmosphere of an environment. For example, a nurse who assumes the role of an "energizer" may be a factor in transforming a less-than-ideal setting into a therapeutic milieu; and a physically abusive client who takes the role of an "aggressor" may create an atmosphere of fear in an inpatient setting that is not secure enough to handle violent behavior. "Energizer," "aggressor," and other roles of nurses and clients observed in therapeutic settings are listed in Table 17-5 and categorized as conducive to growth, as tending to vitalize groups, or as tending to inhibit growth.[5]

In the interplay of setting and roles, physical space is an important factor, because roles are influenced by space. For example, when nurses are performing functional, or indirect, roles, the physical environment provides legitimate distance and space in the form of a nurses' station. But when nurses are performing direct roles—interacting with clients—they are physically closer, and this closeness facilitates the therapeutic relationship.

Table 17-5 Roles Observed in a Therapeutic Milieu

Role	Behavior	Role	Behavior
Growth-producing roles		**Vitalizing roles**	
Initiator	Offers new ideas and suggests solutions.	Gatekeeper	Encourages and facilitates participation of others.
Information seeker	Seeks clarification of suggestions.	Standard setter	Expresses standards for the group.
Opinion seeker	Seeks clarification of values about an issue.	Follower	Goes along passively as a friendly audience.
Information giver	Offers facts or generalizations which are authoritative	**Growth-inhibiting roles**	
Opinion giver	States beliefs or opinions relevant to the issues.	Aggressor	Deflates status of others; may express disapproval of values, acts, or feelings of others; jokes aggressively.
Elaborater	Gives examples; develops meanings and explanations.	Blocker	Is negativistic and resistive in an unreasonable and stubborn manner.
Coordinator	Clarifies relationships among ideas, suggestions, and activities of individuals.	Recognition seeker	Tries to call attention to self. Boasts about personal achievements.
Orienter	Defines the goals of a setting and orients others to them.	Self-confessor	Uses the milieu to express personal feelings and insights.
Evaluator	Relates the standards of the milieu to a problem.	"Playboy"	Displays lack of involvement and cynical nonchalance.
Energizer	Motivates others to action and decision making.	Dominator	Asserts authority; manipulates the group or individuals.
Procedural technician	Performs routine tasks.	Help-seeker	Tries to get sympathy from others; expresses insecurity, confusion, or depreciation of self beyond reason.
Recorder	Writes down topics, decisions, and actions resulting from discussion.	Special-interest pleader	Speaks for the underdog while masking feelings of bias and prejudice; actions are contrary to verbalizations.
Vitalizing roles			
Encourager	Praises, agrees with, and accepts others' ideas.		
Harmonizer	Mediates quarrels and relieves tension.		
Compromiser	Operates from within to resolve conflicts.		

SOURCE: K. B. Benne and P. Sheats, "Functional Roles of Group Members," *Journal of Social Issues*, vol. 4, no. 2, Spring 1948, pp. 42–49.

Another factor in the way setting and roles combine to create an atmosphere is a phenomenon known as *parallel processes.* When nurses assume growth-producing and vitalizing roles, the atmosphere or "tone" of a setting will generally be calm, peaceful, and therapeutic, and clients will sense that the environment is one where healing can occur. On the other hand, when nurses are authoritarian, block clients' initiative, or behave aggressively, clients also display these tendencies, and unrest, upset, and insecurity become evident.

The atmosphere created on a unit is not tangible and cannot be measured. Rather, it is sensed intuitively. It is not unusual to hear experienced nurses remark, "Something's up!" This is a response to the *mood* of a system, and investigation will usually uncover a reason for it. Because nurses are responsible for the environment 24 hours a day, they are obliged to follow up such hunches. In addition to constant responsibility for nursing tasks, nurses need a collegial relationship with other members of the mental health team, autonomy, and the authority to make decisions. Decision making by nurses should imply freedom to follow professional standards within a particular context or structure, to participate in making policy about salaries and staffing, and to establish appropriate nursing procedures.

Role Activities

Nurses employed in inpatient settings are involved in activities that promote, maintain, restore, and rehabilitate clients' health. These activities include intake screening, evaluating clients, making home visits, supervising the administration of medication, preventing suicide, making somatic interventions, intervening in crises, conducting therapy (individual, group, and family), and maintaining the therapeutic milieu.[6] Activities designed for rehabilitation of clients in an inpatient setting include making referrals for vocational and career counseling, arranging and organizing aftercare, and facilitating clients' transition back to the community.

SUMMARY

A large number of clients receiving psychiatric treatment are hospitalized. Clients may be hospitalized for reasons of security (because they need to be in a safe, controlled setting, or because they are perceived as dangerous to themselves or others); for differential diagnostic workups; to regulate medication; to determine competency; or to carry out mandated observation. Clients may also be hospitalized because they are chronically dependent on an institution.

Clients may be admitted voluntarily, or "informally." "Formal" admission, or commitment, is an admission that is facilitated by someone other than the client.

Environment is defined as relevant systems and processes external to and in interaction with a client. A client's environment in the hospital includes his or her "significant others" (especially family members), other clients, and professionals who contribute to the maintenance of the therapeutic milieu, places or spaces within the setting, and the objects within these spaces. A *therapeutic environment* is one in which healing of mind, body, and spirit can occur. *Milieu therapy* is the process of utilizing aspects of a treatment setting which are known to have a positive influence on the behavior of clients.

A therapeutic environment is characterized by a well-planned orientation program for clients and their families; democratic processes; participatory governance; opportunities for problem solving; participation by clients in treatment; and a therapeutic discharge process. Nurses are considered "guardians of the milieu"; they are pivotal persons in the creation and maintenance of a therapeutic environment.

REFERENCES

1. H. Templin, "The System and the Patient," *American Journal of Nursing,* vol. 82, no. 1, January 1982, p. 108.
2. F. Luthans, *Organizational Behavior,* McGraw-Hill, New York, 1977.
3. K. Skinner, "The Therapeutic Milieu: Making It Work," *Journal of Psychiatric Nursing and Mental Health Services,* vol. 17, no. 8, August 1979, p. 38.
4. R. Cucuzzo, "METHOD Discharge Planning," *Supervisor Nurse,* vol. 7, no. 1, 1976, pp. 43–45.
5. K. B. Benne and P. Sheats, "Functional Roles of Group Members," *Journal of Social Issues,* vol. 4., no. 2., Spring 1948, pp. 42–49.
6. American Nurses Association, "Statement on Psychiatric Nursing Practice," ANA, Kansas City, Mo., 1976.

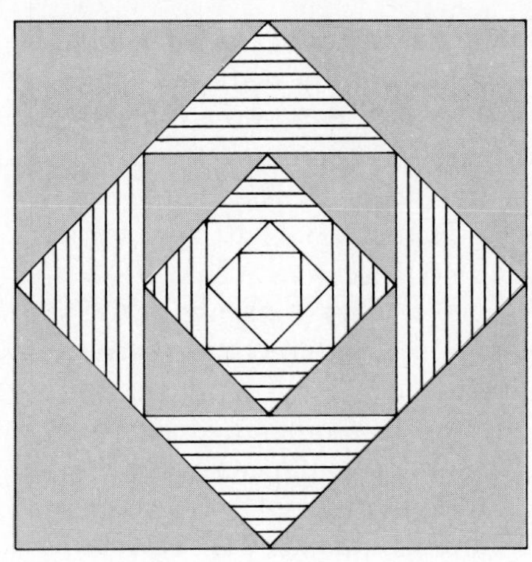

CHAPTER 18 Outpatient Contexts of Care

Pamela Price Hoskins

LEARNING OBJECTIVES

After studying this chapter, the student should be able to:

1. Define *community, community mental health,* and *community mental health status.*
2. Describe the purposes of community mental health services.
3. Compare and contrast *clients* and *providers of services.*
4. Differentiate between mental health resources and community services.
5. Classify community services as direct, semidirect, and indirect.
6. List the principles of community mental health.
7. Apply the characteristics of a therapeutic milieu to the community.
8. Analyze two approaches of nursing in the maintenance of a therapeutic community milieu.
9. Give examples of the three roles of the nurse in community mental health.
10. Discuss the issues involved in the development of the nursing role in community mental health.
11. Discuss the limitations of the community as a treatment setting for both clients and nurses.

An *outpatient context of care* consists of all relevant systems and processes external to the hospital and in interaction with the client, including the client's community. *Community* is defined as an identifiable group of people living in the same locality and under similar conditions, or as a group having common interests, or both. The community is often the context, environment, or situation in which treatment for mental health problems occurs.

This chapter provides an understanding of the community as a setting for treatment and describes principles of community mental health. The purposes of community mental health services are presented, and resources available in the community are explored. The concept of a *therapeutic milieu* in the community, nurses' roles in community services, and issues in community mental health are also examined.

COMMUNITY MENTAL HEALTH: CONCEPTS AND DEFINITIONS

Although the community mental health movement is now about 25 years old, there are still different ideas about what *community mental health* means and what the focus of the movement should be. Therefore, it will be helpful to begin this chapter by defining three basic terms: *community, community mental health,* and *community mental health status.*

Community

A *community* may be thought of physically, mentally, and spiritually. *Physically,* the term *community* may imply a geographic location with fixed boundaries, and its weather and terrain, buildings, and public services—such as the police, the fire department, and stores (groceries, service stations, etc.)

Mentally, the term *community* may refer to people living under similar conditions, obeying the same laws, and sharing similar norms and a similar atmosphere. Someone who wanted to describe the mental aspects of a community might say, "Toytown has a small-town atmosphere; everybody knows everybody's business, and people try to help each other. You can be your own person in Toytown, but not to the point that the rest of us are hurt. When Jack Jones had trouble with drinking, we all tried to help him. And when he ran over the stop sign at Baker and Eleventh Streets, we made him go to the hospital for help."

Spiritually, the term *community* may refer to groups who share common interests and purposes. A "spiritual community" cannot be described in physical terms. The orthodox Jewish community, for example, is worldwide and has a common heritage and purpose and common goals; a member of this community may have more in common with Jews in another country than with his or her gentile neighbors.

For the purposes of this book, a *community* has physical, mental, and spiritual dimensions; it is defined as an identifiable group of people living in the same locality under similar conditions, and sharing common interests, purposes, and goals.

Community Mental Health

Community mental health is commonly defined in two different ways. First, it may be considered as the mental health of an individual within a community; the focus of this definition is on the individual as a client, and the community as a setting. Second, it may be considered as the mental health of the community itself; this definition focuses on the community as both client and setting.

As used in this book, the term *community mental health* has both of these meanings. It refers to synchronous interactions between and among individuals in the community and within the community as a whole, reflected primarily in mental indicators such as acceptable norms, an open atmosphere, socialization that fosters pursuit of life purposes, healthy relationships with others, and freedom to pursue a spiritual life, such as a personal relationship with God. Community mental health is influenced by and reflects the mental health of persons within it.

Parts of this chapter were originally developed by Anita M. Leach, "Context of Care," in the second edition of this book.

Community Mental Health Status

A community is a living, ever-changing system. *Community mental health status* is also always changing; it is dynamic, and it is influenced by circumstances, available resources, and patterns of interaction within it and between it and the larger environment.

For example:

> James, Oklahoma, may be considered as having a high degree of community mental health. It has a low crime rate, enough businesses and industries to provide community resources and jobs for most of the townspeople (the unemployment rate is only 3.4 percent); a community identity to which all the citizens can relate; and a wide range of civic and social activities in which everyone can participate. Its businesses and community services have cooperative relationships and work well together. There is appropriate, friendly competition which has helped provide the creativity and energy needed for community growth.
>
> However, when a disastrous fire swept through the business section, community mental health was dealt a severe blow. The community suffered financially; more than half of the business owners couldn't afford to rebuild, because their insurance was inadequate. The unemployment rate during the time of rebuilding jumped to 29.6 percent. Everyone seemed preoccupied with the devastation caused by the fire, and the community's faith in itself was shaken. Families began to move to larger cities in nearby states, where the job market was better. People who remained in James grieved over the loss of their community and their neighbors. Some of them began to think that there was no reason to stay in James and rebuild. Competition for business and dollars became fierce, and friends began to turn against each other. The community mental health status became unhealthy.

Who is responsible for the mental health status of a community? Providers of health care and their clients share this responsibility. Moreover, all levels of organization share responsibility: individuals, families and groups in the community, and the community itself must join together to address and be accountable for community mental health. There are several reasons why this is so:

- Community mental health is influenced by, and reflects, the mental health of the people within it.
- The family is the basic unit of society and has the greatest influence on a person's mental health.
- Some mental health needs are met more effectively and more efficiently when individuals, families, and groups join together to provide services at the community level.

Because the people, families, and groups within communities, and the communities themselves, are complex, a wide variety of services are offered. A client can choose and coordinate services with the assistance of a mental health worker.

The following example can be considered in terms of community, community mental health, and community mental health status:

> Mary Smith moved to Watchnee, Oregon, to marry a man she had recently met. Although she knew no one in Watchnee, she was looking forward to her new life and the prospect of new friends, a new job, and marriage. Within a week of relocation, however, her fiancé broke off the engagement and refused to see her again. Mary was left with no support system, an abrupt termination of her plans, and many questions about her own worth and the meaning of her life. The arrangements she had made were temporary, pending the marriage. She now had to make many decisions, consider financial problems, and find a new sense of meaning and purpose. Mary went to a crisis intervention center, and a community mental health nurse helped her establish priorities, provided some support, and suggested community resources with which Mary was unfamiliar. Mary joined a group of single and newly divorced people in a new church; through this group, she found a job; she rented an apartment close to her work (through an apartment locator); she leased a used car; and she joined a ski club and a bridge club to build social contacts.

In this example, a person facing a crisis is able to resolve it by putting together for herself, from a wide variety of community resources, a coherent support network. In the process, she contributes to the mental health of the community—not only because she has used its resources effectively but also because she has improved her own mental health.

The example can also be considered in terms of how community mental health services—that is, outpatient services—differ from services in inpatient settings (see Table 18-1).

Table 18-1 Mental Health Services: Differences between Inpatient and Outpatient Settings

	Inpatient Settings	Outpatient Settings
Determination of services	Agency and its personnel select relevant services.	Client identifies and chooses services.
Services provided	A few well-developed services are available to clients on an inpatient basis when appropriate.	Client chooses services from an indefinite number of available services; some services may not be available in the community.
Locus of control	Agency provides safety and control and chooses healing experiences for the client.	Client provides for his or her own safety and control; client chooses healing experiences on the basis of need, availability, and acceptability.

THE COMMUNITY AND ITS SERVICES

Purposes of Community Mental Health Services

The purposes of community mental health services may be categorized as promotion, maintenance, restoration, and rehabilitation of mental health. Actions designed for these purposes range from wholly compensatory to supportive or educative. These are somewhat arbitrary distinctions because the same service may promote the health of one person and serve to restore the health of another. Nevertheless, the distinctions are helpful in understanding community mental health services.

Promotion of Mental Health

A service that *promotes* mental health facilitates positive relationships and life experiences. It need not be directly tied into a network of mental health services.

An example of such a service is a group formed by Planned Parenthood for mothers and their preteen daughters to discuss the challenges of womanhood; anticipating the challenges of physical, mental, and spiritual growth into womanhood is an aspect of promotion of health—as is the recognition that young women need their mothers' guidance and that adolescence places strains on the relationship between mother and daughter.

Maintenance of Mental Health

A service that *maintains* mental health is usually used briefly, is goal-directed, and in general is meant to help people remain mentally healthy when they are faced with difficult circumstances. Maintenance of mental health is assisted by early identification of problems.

The example described earlier illustrates maintenance: Mary maintained the level of mental health she had before the crisis. An example of a service designed for maintenance is a group of supportive parents whose infants died of sudden infant death syndrome (SIDS); such a group helps maintain families' mental health in the face of SIDS. Nurses are often responsible for conducting support and crisis groups of this nature.

Restoration of Mental Health

A service that *restores* mental health is usually meant for short-term use and is designed to help people through the painful process of discovering life's meaning and purpose and developing responsible interdependence with others. Programs for restoration of mental health are those traditionally categorized as "mental health services"; such services are usually funded through insurance, taxes, and grants and are staffed by mental health professionals.

An example of a restorative service is the psychiatric unit of a general hospital. Another example would be a halfway house for abstaining alcoholics which helps them learn to handle family stresses without resorting to drinking.

Rehabilitation of Mental Health

A service that *rehabilitates* mental health is designed primarily for chronically ill clients. It is meant for long-term use, and the care it provides is intensive enough that clients can live in the community without having to meet unrealistic demands for performance. Rehabilitation services are comprehensive and include housing, medication, training in social skills and job skills, and ongoing therapy. Nurses work closely with clients in community rehabilitation programs.

Following is an example of a nurse's work in rehabilitation services:

> June works with a visiting nurse service in Calgary, Minnesota. Her caseload includes 80 chronically mentally ill clients for whom she provides case management. June spends two mornings a week at a day care center where 40 of the 80 clients are enrolled. She has an opportunity to check on these 40, and to assess how well they are functioning socially, how effective their medication is, and whether their personal hygiene is adequate. She also works with the staff to provide opportunities for growth for these clients; and she runs two support groups for the clients' families. She identifies clients who need individualized assistance and follows up with home visits.
>
> June is also the nursing member of a health team assigned to cover 10 "room and board" homes in Calgary; 20 of June's clients live in these homes. A visit every other week to each of these homes gives June an opportunity to visit her clients and provide input to the staffs.
>
> June also works with 8 clients who live in a nursing home in downtown Calgary. She consults with the staff members at the nursing home to help them improve the health of all the clients, including those with whom she works.
>
> In addition, June makes home visits and work visits for clients who are well integrated into the community but who still need some follow-up.

A community mental health center is a good example of a facility that offers comprehensive outpatient services designed to rehabilitate mental health. (Such a health center would also offer services to promote, maintain, and restore health.)

Persons in the Community

As far as community mental health services are concerned, the world is divided into two groups of people: clients and providers. These two groups are discussed below.

Clients

Virtually every person in a community is a consumer of mental health services in the sense that everyone seeks access to services necessary for promoting, maintaining, restoring, or rehabilitating his or her own mental health. Approximately 7 million people are actually clients of a community mental health system at any given time.[1]

DEFINITION OF CLIENTS. The term *client* can be defined in various ways; and a client may be an individual, a family, a group, or an entire community. When an individual client is considered not in isolation but rather in conjunction with his or her family and relevant elements of the environment, responses of the mental health system are more likely to be holistic and to address future needs as well as immediate interventions.

The following example illustrates this broader definition:

> Mr. K. is a 47-year-old married father of two with a diagnosis of manic-depressive illness. He has been on lithium for several years. He was admitted for medication adjustment because of diarrhea, an elevated lithium level, and uncontrollable tremors. Mr. K. is employed in a highly stressful public relations job.

To consider Mr. K. a client in the narrow sense would be to imply that once his medication has been adjusted, the goal of treatment is accomplished. To define Mr. K. as a client in a broader, "community" sense implies intervention that includes (1) a family assessment and possible referral for family therapy; (2) an assessment of the appropriateness of continuing a stressful job, with possible referral for vocational rehabilitation; and (3) health teaching that stresses adequate diet, exercise, and the necessity of frequent medical checkups. A broad "community definition" of clients places them within a holistic context, making more comprehensive care possible.

CLIENTS IN THE COMMUNITY. When clients are discharged from a hospital, some return to a supportive network; others are faced with the loneliness of single-room-occupancy (SRO) residences. Some return to parents after years of married life in another household; some live with friends and acquaintances or in halfway houses. Clients who have never been hospitalized but are in need of mental health services may live in nursing homes, adult homes, hospices, or other home-care facilities.

Providers of Services

Clients receiving health care within the context of home and community will, as their needs are addressed, interact with numerous health care professionals.

The *community health nurse* performs numerous functions: case finding, continuing assessment of clients' mental health, counseling, and providing skilled care and specialized treatment (such as medication and health teaching). Frequently, it is the community health nurse who refers clients for institutional services when there is a change in their health status or when there is a previously undiagnosed mental health problem.

Physicians, vocational rehabilitation specialists, pharmacists, physical therapists, teachers, family therapists, social workers, government officials, recreation therapists, chaplains, and other health care professionals are available to support mentally ill clients at home.

Neighbors, employers, family members, and *friends* are also resources for clients in the community.

Providers of services offered through the community mental health system have varying levels of preparation. "Grass roots" workers may have little academic preparation, but they do have significant life experiences, common sense, and an understanding of community norms. Some personnel may have a liberal arts education and receive on-the-job training for certain functions. The mental health system has a large number of jobs for people with little or no formal preparation for mental health work; they are supervised by a nurse or another professional. Nurses working in community mental health are expected to have a bachelor's degree in nursing; clinical nursing specialists have earned a master's degree in psychiatric–community mental health nursing (see Chapter 10). Some positions require an earned doctorate in a field leading to practice in mental health. Since mental health services receive little financial support, matching academic achievement and experience with jobs and pay scales is very important.

Supportive Resources in the Community

The environment of a nonhospitalized client is the community. This section examines *supportive resources* in the community that have an impact on mental health. Two kinds of community resources—*mental health resources* and *community services*—will be explored.

Mental Health Resources

Mental health resources in the community consist of a network of mental health centers, practitioners, living arrangements, and support groups, offered to clients on an outpatient basis.

COMMUNITY MENTAL HEALTH CENTERS. A community's single most comprehensive mental health service is the community mental health center (CMHC). The Community Mental Health Centers Act of 1963 provided federal funding to move mental health treatment from institutions to communities. Community mental health centers were funded to provide at least five essential services for their catchment areas: (1) 24-hour emergency care, (2) inpatient care, (3) day or night hospitalization, (4) aftercare, and (5) consultation and education designed to prevent mental disorders. Emphasis was placed on comprehensive care, continuity of care, innovative treatment approaches, and the use of teams of professional and paraprofessional mental health workers. The act was amended in 1975 to require the provision of additional services by centers receiving federal funding: (6) comprehensive services for children and the elderly; (7) screening services for community agencies, (8) more systematic follow-up services, (9) transitional services for clients discharged into the community, and (10) treatment and rehabilitation for people suffering from drug and alcohol addiction.

Communities were supposed to take over funding once the importance of the centers to the communities was established. This has not happened; funding of the centers has varied since they were first established, and that has affected the types and quality of services offered. However, CMHCs continue to be the most affordable source of mental health treatment in the community.

MENTAL HEALTH PRACTITIONERS. Mental health practitioners include private practitioners and professionals who develop mental health services in conjunction with other community agencies. Private practitioners usually provide a small number of services, including individual psychotherapy, family therapy, and group therapy. These practitioners have advanced educational preparation and maintain certification standards to ensure the quality of the services they offer.

Professionals may create agencies in conjunction with other agencies, with community institutions (such as churches and schools), or with both. For instance, a school with a high incidence of adolescent suicide may decide to offer a suicide prevention program in conjunction with, but not under the aegis of, the school; mental health professionals may develop the program and its services and offer the program to the entire community. Cooperative efforts by community institutions and private practitioners are needed to provide innovative services.

LIVING ARRANGEMENTS. Clients with mental disorders may not be able to live either independently or with their families, for various reasons. Therefore, living arrangements, either transitional or permanent, must be available.

Transitional living arrangements include halfway houses and foster care. *Halfway houses* are homes in which psychiatric clients are placed temporarily to gain experience in cooperative living. Clients in a halfway house may have been discharged from a hospital or may come from problematic family or independent living situations. *Foster care* is also meant to enhance skills of cooperative living, but clients are placed in families. People who provide foster care are paid for each client they take, and they are expected to attend training classes. A foster home may become a permanent living arrangement.

Permanent arrangements include group homes, nursing homes, room-and-board facilities, and single-room-occupancy dwellings (SROs). These are used when clients recognize that independent living is unrealistic for or unacceptable to them. *Group homes* provide permanent living arrangements in which residents share responsibilities associated with home life, such as cooking, cleaning, building maintenance, and care of grounds. A group home may be supervised full time or part time, depending on the residents' needs and availability of funding for supervision. *Nursing homes* provide permanent living arrangements in which residents have no responsibility for tasks associated with home life; some residents, however, may have an opportunity to participate in such tasks as part of their treatment program. In nursing homes, paraprofessional staff members are supervised by registered nurses, and physicians make visits to the home when they are needed by the residents. A nursing home may be "transinstitutional," the first step out of a hospital on the way to a transitional living experience; in such a situation, a nursing home is considered a temporary placement. *Room-and-board facilities* (as the term implies) provide room and board, and some states require some supervision of their clients—who have no responsibilities to the facility beyond courteous behavior. *Single-room-occupancy dwellings* provide rooms and bathroom facilities. The clients are usually expected to vacate their rooms during the day.

SUPPORT GROUPS. Support groups are self-help groups designed for individuals, families, or communities (see Chapter 20 for further discussion of groups). Some groups are formed to help people become stronger and, in turn, help others. (Alcoholics Anonymous is an example.) Some are formed to help people maintain their mental health while coping with difficult circumstances; an example would be a group of families with members who are receiving prolonged dialysis. Other groups are formed to help restore mental health—groups of bereaved parents, for example. Still others are formed to help rehabilitate mental health; advocacy groups whose members are former mental patients are one example. There are also groups whose goals have to do with changing the community; one example is a group consisting of professionals and physically handicapped people whose goal is to create a "barrier-free" society. Mothers Against Drunk Drivers (MADD) and the National Association for the Advancement of Colored People (NAACP) are other self-help groups that promote individual, family, and community mental health. Some self-help groups—such as Children of Aging Parents (COAP) and groups for relatives of people with Alzheimer's disease—are run by professionals.

Community Services

Community services are supportive resources which promote, maintain, and restore individual, family, and community well-being, and thereby make a contribution to health and mental health.

Archer and Fleshman[2] categorized community services in terms of community nursing practice, as *direct*, *semidirect*, and *indirect*. *Direct services* are those in which there is a personal relationship between the nurse and the client. (The client may be an individual, a family, or a community.) A public health nurse who visits a client and the client's family at home once a month, for example, is providing a direct service.

Semidirect services facilitate the activities of people who are providing direct services. Archer and Fleshman note that nurses who are involved in providing semidirect services "must themselves be expert care givers, since much of their job is to assist [providers of direct care] with challenging clients and to serve as role models."[2] Following is an example of a nurse who is providing semidirect services:

> Mrs. L., who has a Bachelor of Science in Nursing (B.S.N.) degree, supervises two home health aides who provide housekeeping services and prepare meals for 20 clients each week. The aides describe changes in these clients' behavior or home situations that may alert Mrs. L. about impending problems. Mrs. L. also directs the aides in observation and intervention and helps them improve their therapeutic skills.

Indirect services, according to Archer and Fleshman, involve administration, research, public relations, procurement and allocation of resources, and formulation and implementation of policy.[2]

Leach has applied these three categories of nursing practice to the services themselves. *Direct services* refers to "hands-on," physical services and to nonphysical services such as counseling and crisis intervention. Health teaching is also considered a direct service if it is necessary for clients' survival or optimal health. *Semidirect services* prepare or equip clients to receive direct services. Providing transportation to a clinic for treatment is an example of a semidirect service; people who organize or supervise direct care are also providing semidirect services. *Indirect services,* as in Archer and Fleshman's analysis, are essentially administrative or concerned with research.

There are many community services available for people with problems having to do with mental health; however, not all such services exist in every community. Table 18-2 lists some services that are widely available and can be used to build a social network for clients. It should be noted that specific criteria must sometimes be met before a client may use a service (WIC is an example of a service for which criteria must be met).

Table 18-2 Examples of Community Services

Client	Services
Individual	Rape crisis center
	Churches and synagogues
	Job training agencies
	Art shows
	Libraries
	Recreation clubs (such as chess clubs and automobile clubs)
	Adult education programs
	Literacy programs
	Employment agencies
	Meditation groups
	Renewal centers
	Meals on Wheels
	Colleges and universities
	Mental health agencies
Family	Women, Infants, and Children (WIC) Nutritional Services
	Community "welcome wagon"
	Sex counseling agencies
	Family planning agencies
	Recreation centers
	Children's groups (such as Camp Fire Girls)
	Church groups
	Day care centers for children, the disabled, and the elderly
	Family recreation centers and groups
	Shelters for victims of domestic violence
Community	Fresh Air Fund
	Environmental groups
	Education groups (such as American Lung Association and March of Dimes)
	Utility companies
	Community emergency shelters
	Government agencies
	Police department
	Fire department
	Fair housing bureau or agency
	Prisons
	Performing arts centers
	Public forests and parks

To understand the strengths a community has and the challenges it faces, as well as its mental health resources and the services it provides, the nurse should perform a thorough community assessment. A format for such an assessment is given in Chapter 11.

COMMUNITY MENTAL HEALTH NURSING

Principles of Community Mental Health

A *principle* may be defined as a basic truth, law, or assumption. Four principles concerning community mental health provide the rationale for community mental health nursing.

Principle 1

Community mental health is influenced by and reflects the mental health of the individuals and families within the community. People, families, and the community as a whole are part of community mental health. Every subsystem, or part of the system, influences the system, and the system influences all its subsystems; a change in any part changes the whole, and a change in the whole changes all the parts. For instance:

> As individuals incorporate "affirmation" into their behavior toward others, families are influenced positively; affirming, positive families and individuals make the community as a whole "feel" more affirming; and this "feeling" encourages community norms of involvement and commitment, providing opportunities for individuals and families to become more involved in community life.

Principle 2

Persons, families, and the community must be treated holistically. Holistic treatment has two aspects.

First, physical, mental, and spiritual aspects of individuals, families, and the community must be considered. Neglect of any aspect of any system reduces understanding of the whole and may make intervention tangential, irrelevant, and ineffective. For example:

> A public health nurse visited Mr. M. in his home once a month for 6 months. During each visit, the nurse discussed with Mr. M. his activities of daily living, his coping mechanisms, and his handling of stresses. During this period, Mr. M. complained of tiredness, palpitations, tremors, and lack of coordination. The nurse interpreted these symptoms as manifestations of anxiety. Later, however, during a hospitalization, Mr. M. was diagnosed as having tardive dyskinesia, a condition that could have been prevented if his symptoms had been identified early enough. If the nurse had performed a physical examination as well as focusing on the mental and spiritual aspects of Mr. M.'s life, tardive dyskinesia might have been averted.

Second, although the parts are necessary, they must be synthesized into a whole. Dehumanization results when a person, family, or community is treated serially, or by parts. For instance:

> A nurse working in a birthing center may be tempted to treat a woman in labor physically, then mentally, and then (if necessary) spiritually. Once the mother is taken care of, the nurse focuses on the father and possibly the siblings and grandparents; if there is time, the nurse finally focuses on the impact of this birth on the community.

Such an approach is fragmented, time-consuming, dehumanizing, and ineffective. A holistic approach implies that in this situation, the nurse is to treat the birth of a baby into a family, with birth considered as a physical, mental, and spiritual process; and that the community is seen as the essential context of the family. More specifically, not only is a baby born physically into a family; new roles, structures, and responsibilities are created. (For example, an only child may become a sibling or an elder brother or sister, and an older child may become the eldest son or daughter for the first time.) Rearrangement of the family may depend on community resources such as La Leche League, baby-sitting services, a church's "mother's day out," and a community library program on the "fulfilling role of grandparenting."

Principle 3

Promotion, maintenance, restoration, and rehabilitation of community mental health require the mobilization of all community resources. This principle focuses attention on the resources within the community: its people, its heritage, its natural resources (such as water and land), and its unique character. The idea is that health is achieved when a community uses on its own behalf, or mobilizes, all that it has. This does not suggest that a community should not use external resources; temporary use of external resources may be necessary, but permanent dependence on them works against a high level of community mental health. Responsible interdependence among communities is necessary for community mental health, and working out such interdependence is part of the development of the mental health of a community.

Principle 4

Nursing promotes, maintains, restores, and rehabilitates community mental health by providing direct, semidirect, and indirect services as well as by working with and through the health care system. The needs of the community that influence mental health are sufficiently complex to require a comprehensive health plan. The United States has yet to develop such a plan, but each mental health discipline attempts both to offer relevant, effective services and to coordinate with other disciplines to form a comprehensive network of services. Nursing offers necessary, relevant, effective mental health services and also works closely with other disciplines on behalf of the community's mental health. Nursing services are planned, implemented, and evaluated using the nursing process.

Therapeutic Milieu in the Community

What Is a Therapeutic Milieu?

Because a community is a system—a changing whole with a life of its own—it has a spiritual aspect. This spiritual aspect is called the *community milieu.* A community milieu may be conducive to health, or *therapeutic;* or it may be conducive to illness, or *nontherapeutic.*

A therapeutic community milieu is in many ways comparable to a therapeutic inpatient milieu (described in Chapter 17). The characteristics of a therapeutic community milieu are:

- Democratic processes
- Protection of human rights
- Orientation to significant aspects of the community
- Consistent, fair rules
- Opportunities for people to participate in governance

Here is an example of such a milieu:

> Christo, Montana, has a therapeutic milieu. Most aspects of the city government are concerned with service; employees act as if the satisfaction of the citizens of Christo is their most important product. Christo has reduced bureaucratic red tape considerably and has a citizens' committee dedicated to finding ways to streamline its services even more. But established procedures apply to everybody in town; exceptions must be requested in writing. Translators are available to people for whom English is a second language. Each subculture in Christo has formed a group to welcome newcomers and smooth their transition into the community by clarifying which older ways can be retained and which ones should be changed in order to get along in a new environment. (For instance, even though Christo offers a good deal of bilingual help, it is an English-speaking town, and everybody is expected to learn English as soon as possible.) There are many community hearings; elected officials have an open-door policy; and the voter turnout rate is 78 percent. (The citizens of Christo want to register every eligible citizen and eventually to have a turnout rate of 100 percent.) Each citizen's right to choose his or her own level of civic participation is respected.

The Nurse and the Therapeutic Milieu

In a hospital, nurses are responsible for maintaining a therapeutic milieu; in a community, however, the nurse shares that responsibility with many other people. But sharing responsibility does not reduce the nurse's obligation to monitor the milieu, to work diligently to make it therapeutic, and to use it to improve community mental health. The nurse meets this obligation in two ways: as a provider of care in the community, and as a policymaker.

NURSES AS PROVIDERS OF CARE. As a provider of care, the nurse is responsible for upholding clients' rights to participate in programs offered; identifying rules and structures that denigrate clients or deny their rights; participating in establishment of goals and agreeing to costs of treatment; participating in the development and evaluation of services; providing adequate orientation for participants in programs; and formulating fair, consistent rules with fair, consistent rewards and punishments. The nurse also keeps an eye on the process of programs and services to see if they are accomplishing their stated purposes. (For instance, a goal of a program may be "to socialize clients to community expectations"; but the nurse may find that clients are becoming passive and compliant—an outcome which is not socialization but is sometimes confused with it.)

NURSES AS POLICYMAKERS. As a policymaker, the nurse is expected to participate as a citizen and a provider of health care on committees and in groups that influence the community milieu. Therefore, one nurse may seek an appointment to the United Way Funding Determination Committee, whose purpose is to allocate funds among the many agencies supported by United Way. Another nurse may seek election to a school board; and a district nurses' association may participate in planning a community health fair or a voter-registration drive. There are many ways to participate in the life of a community to improve its milieu and its health status.

Roles of the Nurse in Community Mental Health

The roles of the nurse in community mental health are varied and depend on the needs of the community and the organization of agencies providing nursing services to it. However, all services provided by nurses may be categorized into three basic types of roles: direct care, epidemiology, and referral.

Direct Care

Direct care provided by nurses—the first of the three basic roles—was defined earlier in this chapter; it is face-to-face service for individuals, families, or the community itself. Direct care implies accountability for the services provided. These services may take the form of individual counseling, medication and support groups, network therapy, and advocacy in a variety of settings.

Case management may be considered another aspect of direct care. "*Case management* is a method of assigning responsibility for systems coordination to one person, who works with a given client in accessing necessary services."[3] A case manager performs six functions:

1. Identification of and outreach to clients
2. Individual assessment
3. Planning of services
4. Linkage with requisite services
5. Monitoring of delivery of service
6. Client advocacy

Epidemiology

Epidemiology is a science and a specialization within the field of public health; it is concerned with the health of whole populations—specifically, with the spread and control of disease and with populations at risk of certain diseases. (*Populations at risk* are groups of people especially vulnerable to a disease under particular conditions.) Incidence, or prevalence, of a disease within a population may be used to describe the disease as "present" or "absent" and to identify factors related to its onset and persistence; therefore, data on incidence are also a concern of epidemiology.

The epidemiological role of the nurse (the second of the three basic roles in community nursing) encompasses *gathering statistics, case finding, identifying populations at risk,* and *providing primary, secondary, and tertiary preventive services* for such populations.

Gathering statistics entails keeping accurate records on the clients served, completing surveys, and occasionally participating in data collection for epidemiological studies.

Case finding entails participating in screening of populations, in community activities designed for people at risk (such as a community education program on abuse of the elderly), and in other activities that will help identify individuals and families who have begun to develop disorders.

Identifying populations at risk entails recognizing, from available data, a problem that was not previously noted or a population that was not previously considered vulnerable to a disorder. (For instance, until recently women were thought to have little risk of heart disease. When statistics on heart disease among women began to change subtly, a discerning person suggested that statistics on women who held positions as executives be examined separately. Factoring out that specific population from all women validated the idea that women executives are a population at risk of heart disease.)

Providing primary, secondary, and tertiary preventive services entails focusing resources and efforts on the prevention of disorders. *Primary prevention* consists of efforts to keep a disorder from occurring at all. Health education is the most effective method of primary prevention. *Secondary prevention* consists of attempts to interrupt the development of a disorder that is still in its early stages. Crisis intervention is an effective method of secondary prevention. *Tertiary prevention* consists of efforts to limit the disabling effects of a fully developed disorder. Rehabilitation services have been effective for tertiary prevention.

Referral

Referral—connecting clients with community resources needed to promote, maintain, restore, and rehabilitate health—is the third basic role of nurses in community mental health. The referral process can be seen as having nine steps; these are outlined below.

STEP 1. The referral process begins with the identification of a specific need which the nurse is unable to address adequately.

STEP 2. The nurse validates the existence of the need with the client and asks the client to determine a priority for meeting that need. For instance:

> A nurse, Ms. N., who has a B.S.N. degree, identifies a need for sex counseling for a client, Ms. O., but recognizes that sex counseling is beyond the scope of her role as nurse. Ms. N. shares her recognition of this need with Ms. O., who agrees that she is sexually dysfunctional and that the problem is creating a severe strain in her marriage. Ms. O. asks Ms. N. to identify some services available to address the problem.

STEP 3. The third step in the referral process is matching the client's need with the appropriate community service. If need and service are ill-matched, the client will not be helped and will feel frustrated and hopeless, and the community service will be wasted. (For the O. family, for example, sex education will not meet the need; agencies that provide sex counseling are therefore the only agencies considered by Ms. N.)

STEP 4. The fourth step is to determine whether a client is eligible for the community service that seems most appropriate. Every agency has some criteria, and it is useless for a nurse to refer clients to services for which they are ineligible.

STEP 5. The fifth step is for the nurse to make contact with the agency to be sure that it provides the needed service and to confirm that the client is eligible. This step is particularly important if the nurse is unfamiliar with the agency. Moreover, the nurse's knowledge of resources and providers of health care in the community expands greatly when this step has been accomplished for several clients. While discussing the possibility of making a referral, the nurse also ascertains whether or not there are other resources available to deal with the problem and obtains specific information about fees, hours, kinds of therapy offered, and protocols or forms for referrals. At this point, the client's identity is not revealed to the agency.

STEP 6. The nurse now shares all the information gathered with the client and identifies up to three resources that will effectively meet the client's need. The nurse encourages the client to consider the information and make an informed decision. (In the case of Ms. O., her husband may need to be involved in the decision.)

STEP 7. Once the client has made a decision, the nurse and the client decide which of them will approach the agency. If the agency requires paperwork or disclosure of information by the nurse, the nurse asks the client's permission to comply with this requirement and then gives the client a copy of the information provided. When possible, however, the client should be the one who discloses information, although the nurse may accompany the client to the agency or be available for moral support.

STEP 8. If the client is able to contact the agency independently, the nurse should stay out of the situation entirely, ascertaining only that the client's problem is being addressed.

STEP 9. The final step is following up with the client to find out how the referral is working. If the client is dissatisfied, the nurse asks the client's permission to contact the agency or to arrange a three-way meeting to address the problem and achieve a more workable solution. (Agencies are usually willing and sometimes eager to receive feedback about their services.) It may turn out, however, that a referral to some other service is needed; if so, assessment, contact, and follow-up should ensure a better outcome. The more nurses learn about community resources, the more effective their referrals will be.

Issues in Community Mental Health Nursing

There are two major issues in community mental health nursing: the development of the nursing role, and the limitations of the community as a setting for treatment.

Development of the Nursing Role

Two influences on the development of the nursing role in community mental health are entry into practice and clarification of the role itself.

ENTRY INTO PRACTICE. The comprehensive educational preparation for psychiatric–community mental health nursing is offered in Bachelor of Science in Nursing (B.S.N.) programs. Only a nurse with a B.S.N. degree is really prepared to deal with the complexity of communities either as settings for treatment or as clients. However, until the nursing profession has implemented minimum educational requirements for entry into practice, nurses without a B.S.N. may continue to be hired for community mental health positions. Thus the full range of nursing services may not be available to the community, because not all nurses are prepared to provide them.

CLARIFICATION OF THE NURSING ROLE. The second influence on the development of the nursing role in community mental health is the need to clarify the nature of that role. The field of psychiatric–community mental health calls for components of two roles: psychiatric nursing and public health nursing. Thus the role of the psychiatric–community mental health nurse is extremely complex. The nurse must maintain a balance between a focus on mental health (the psychiatric nursing role) and a focus on community health (the public health nursing role).

Psychiatric–community mental health nurses must truly be generalists. They must be able to work with the chronically and the acutely ill, the young and the elderly, individuals and the family—promoting, maintaining, restoring, and rehabilitating health. The breadth of the role of the psychiatric–mental health nurse in the community is so great that the nurse may have difficulty establishing clear goals and priorities.

In addition, what services are considered appropriate for the psychiatric–mental health nurse to carry out may vary from community to community. For example, in a poor rural community, where nurses are the only providers of health care, the nurse may deliver a baby, knowing that providing this service, without the proper credentials, would lead to a reprimand in a community with obstetric practitioners. Such differences in what is expected of a nurse can lead to confusion. The nurse may have difficulty identifying precisely what the job consists of, and may feel a lack of clear role identity.

Moreover, in actual practice there is often little or no distinction between mental health nursing and community health nursing. For instance, performing a physical assessment may seem to be part of the role of community health nurse, but the mental health nurse must be able to perform physical assessments. Helping dying clients and their families come to terms with grief and loss may seem to be part of the role of mental health nurse, but the community health nurse must be able to intervene with clients in this way. Community mental health nurses therefore need to be able to tolerate a sense of ambiguity; and, since others may sometimes see them as "all things to all people," they need to respond to numerous—sometimes even inappropriate—demands.

Finally, because the nursing role is so extensive, maintaining a sufficient knowledge base, though necessary, represents a considerable challenge.

It should be said, however, that despite the difficulties of the role, community mental health nursing is an exciting and rewarding field for people who can organize themselves and their work, bring order out of chaos, set priorities when there are no external controls, and feel a sense of accomplishment in the face of all that remains to be done.

Limitations of the Community as a Treatment Setting

The second issue in community mental health nursing is the limitations of the community as a setting for treatment. These limitations affect both clients and the nursing role.

LIMITATIONS FOR CLIENTS. The community is the least restrictive setting for treatment and the most appropriate setting for the majority of psychiatric clients. However, a community may not have the programs needed by a client. Also, providers of care in the community sometimes lose contact with clients and therefore cannot give follow-up treatment. Clients who are chronically mentally ill and are treated as outpatients have difficulty "bonding" with providers of care and services, and they simply may not continue to return for treatment. A third problem is that payment mechanisms for community services are poorly developed, and some clients cannot afford treatment in the community.

LIMITATIONS FOR THE NURSING ROLE. The community setting can limit the nursing role in three ways: (1) there may be inhibitions, or restrictions, on the delivery of nursing services; (2) there is considerable role blurring in community settings; and (3) there is too little funding for community mental health in general and community mental health nursing in particular.

Restrictions on nursing services are created by some community agencies, which may be structured in ways that inhibit the delivery of the broad range of services nurses can offer. For instance, although nurses can give injections, agency regulations may prohibit a nurse from giving an injection of vitamin B_{12} to a client in the course of a home visit.

Role blurring—an overlap of nursing with other disciplines—can also represent a limitation for the nursing role. (See Chapter 10 for a discussion of role blurring.) When functions overlap, or are seen as overlapping, nurses may be expected to provide certain services that other disciplines offer. For example, a public health nurse who works with chronically mentally ill clients and sees them in their homes might be expected to assess their financial resources and to initiate and follow up on applications for Medicare, Medicaid, and unemployment or disability insurance. Social workers perform these same functions for their clients; therefore, it becomes difficult to distinguish clearly between social work and community mental health nursing on the basis of services provided.

Insufficient financial resources reflect the fact that there is insufficient appreciation on the part of policymakers of the importance of community mental health, and especially of the need for promoting and maintaining mental health. Nurses, of course, are aware that these goals are crucial; but the people who formulate policy, allocate resources, and determine what services will be funded have not yet developed the same understanding.

The issues facing community mental health nursing—how the nursing role will develop and in what ways the community is limited as a setting for treatment—represent both a challenge and an opportunity. The limits of the community need to be addressed and resolved, and the nursing role needs to be developed so that the contributions of nursing to community mental health will be maximized.

SUMMARY

The purpose of this chapter has been to develop an understanding of the community as a treatment setting and the principles of community mental health. A *community* has physical, mental, and spiritual dimensions and can be defined as an identifiable group of people living in the same locality under similar conditions and sharing common interests, purposes, and goals. *Community mental health* is commonly defined in two different ways: first, as the mental health of individuals in the community (a definition which focuses on the individual as a client and the community as a setting); second, as the mental health of the community itself (a definition which focuses on the community as both client and setting). *Community mental health status* is dynamic, ever-changing, and influenced by circumstances, available resources, and patterns of interaction within the community as well as between the community and the larger environment.

Individuals, families, groups, and the community itself must be jointly accountable for community mental health. Because of the complexities of individuals, families, and groups within a community, and the complexity of the community itself, a wide variety of mental health services are offered. The purposes of these services may be categorized as promotion, maintenance, restoration, and rehabilitation of mental health. Services that promote mental health facilitate positive relationships and life experiences. Services that maintain mental health are usually meant to be used briefly by any client, are goal-directed, and help the client to maintain mental health in the face of difficult circumstances. Services that restore mental health help clients to discover life's meaning and purpose for themselves and to develop responsible interdependence with others. Services that rehabilitate mental health are long-term and comprehensive in nature and maintain clients in the community setting.

From the standpoint of health services, the world is divided into clients and providers. A *client* may be a person, a family, a group, or a whole community. *Providers* are persons prepared through education, experience, or both to offer mental health services.

Community health services are categorized as mental health resources and community services. *Mental health resources* are a network of community mental centers, private practitioners, programs, living arrangements, and support groups. *Community services* are services which promote, maintain, and restore individual, family, and community well-being, thereby making a contribution to health in general and mental health in particular.

Community mental health nursing is one discipline offering mental health services; these services may be described as *direct, semidirect,* and *indirect.*

Four *principles*—basic truths, laws, or assumptions—are the basis of community mental health nursing.

The spiritual life of a community is called the *community milieu.* Nurses share with people in other disciplines the responsibility for maintaining a therapeutic community milieu. Nurses fulfill this responsibility in two ways: as providers of care and as participants in policymaking.

The roles of the nurse in community mental health include direct care, epidemiology, and referral.

Two issues facing community mental health nursing are (1) development of the nursing role and (2) limitations of the community as a treatment setting. Development of the nursing role is affected by criteria for entry into practice and by the need for clarification of the role. As a treatment setting, the community can be limited in terms of both the nursing role and the services available to clients.

REFERENCES

1. Howard H. Goldman, "Epidemiology," in John A. Talbott, ed., *The Chronic Mental Patient: Five Years Later,* Grune and Stratton, New York, 1984, p. 17.
2. Sarah Ellen Archer and Ruth P. Fleshman, *Community Health Nursing,* 3d ed., Wadsworth Health Sciences, Monterey, Calif., 1985, pp. 98–99.
3. Irene Shiffren Levine and Mary Heming, *Human Resource Development: Issues in Case Management,* National Institute of Mental Health, Washington, D. C., February 1984, p. *i.*

BIBLIOGRAPHY

Susan Clemen et al., *Comprehensive Family and Community Health Nursing,* McGraw-Hill, New York, 1981.

Elaine Anne Pasquali et al., *Mental Health Nursing: A Holistic Approach,* 2d ed., Mosby, St. Louis, 1985.

Judith Allen Shelly et al., *Spiritual Dimensions of Mental Health,* Intervarsity, Downers Grove, Ill., 1983.

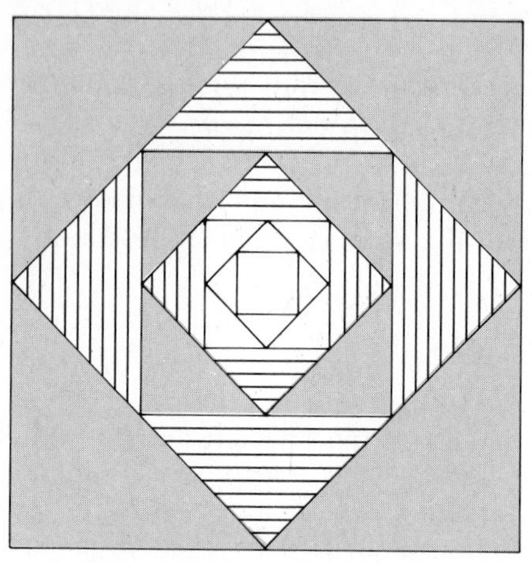

CHAPTER 19
Family Theory and Application

Judith Haber
Anita M. Leach

LEARNING OBJECTIVES

After studying this chapter, the student should be able to:

1. Discuss assumptions and myths about the family.
2. Define *family*.
3. Describe family structures.
4. Describe the functioning of healthy families.
5. Analyze the stages of development in families.
6. Identify the concepts and principles of Bowen's systems theory.
7. Describe the processes involved in structural family therapy.
8. Discuss the elements of strategic family therapy.
9. Construct a genogram.
10. Apply the nursing process to families across the life span.

Every client—like every nurse—is a member of a specific group of people called a *family*. Nursing considers the family the primary focus of health care. Individuals are best understood within the context of the family—which transmits biological and genetic traits; contributes to the emotional, social, and spiritual strength or vulnerability of its members; and therefore has a significant influence on a person's ability to achieve and maintain optimum wellness. To assess an individual without a family context, then, is to consider only a fraction of the person.

Nurses consider the family holistically, as a system. This approach has two implications. First, when a family is seen holistically, it can be said to have three dimensions analogous to those of the person: a "family mind," a "family body," and a "family spirit." Second, as a system the family consists of parts—its members—and any alteration in one part of a system results in a corresponding alteration in the whole. Thus when a family member—one of the parts of the system—is physically, mentally, or spiritually dysfunctional, the family system as a whole is affected: family functioning is disrupted, and the family's energy becomes focused on the dysfunctional member.

Nursing as a profession interacts with families on three levels: (1) Nurses, of course, are themselves members of families; they have family histories and family experiences that can influence them in functional or dysfunctional ways. Nurses need to be aware of how their unique experiences as family members affect their personal and professional relationships. (2) Generalist nurses study their own families and family theory and have knowledge of community agencies available to help families. Thus they are prepared to see clients in a family context, to recognize functional and dysfunctional behavior patterns, and to refer families to appropriate community resources. (3) Nurses with specialized advanced educational preparation—that is, nurses at or beyond the master's level—may function as qualified family therapists or consultants.

This chapter discusses the family as an environment—perhaps the most significant environment—of people in general, but of nurses and their mentally ill clients in particular. Its purpose is to provide a holistic approach to assessing clients within the context of the family. Nurses examine both the effects clients' dysynchronous patterns of interaction have on the family system, and the influence family dynamics have on the development of alterations in clients' behavioral patterns.

THE FAMILY

Assumptions and Myths about the Family

Mistaken assumptions in both popular and scholarly writings contribute to the difficulty of understanding the biopsychosocial unit labeled *family*. Although anthropologists and social scientists, as well as nurses, have attempted to universalize the family by formulating a single definition, most have concluded that no single definition will hold across all times and places; all-embracing definitions are, therefore, not particularly useful. The invasion of the home by television and other media and the rising number of single-parent families have further complicated the process of finding a simple definition. Images of family life today are more complex and varied than they were in the past, and people make many erroneous assumptions about what constitutes family life. Such assumptions, or myths, must be changed before growth can occur.

To assume that a "normal" family consists of heterosexual parents and their children is to contribute to the myth that the *nuclear family* is universal. Erroneous ideas about what is "normal" or "natural" have subtly influenced people to think of deviations as "sick" or "perverse." For example, a nurse who believes that a family consists of a husband, a wife, and their minor children, living in the same household, might be inclined to view an unwed mother, or a single adoptive parent, or an extended-family household—or any other variation—as "abnormal."

Another assumption about the family is that it is a place where individuals harmoniously fulfill their own needs and those of society. One has only to reflect seriously on one's own family to realize that *family harmony* is a myth. Love and joy are of course found in family life; but the myth of family harmony omits the conflicts and struggles that are also found there. In the family, the full range of human emotions are expressed. In such a highly charged atmosphere, conflict is inevitable. Conflict is also inevitable because (as professionals who work with families recognize) each family unit is in reality at least two families: a couple who come together to form a new family, for example, are joining two families of origin and creating a third; a single parent represents a family of origin plus a new family; an extended-family household represents several families of origin. Even so-called "normal" families, then (however *normal* is defined), are environments where meaningful interaction can be difficult. The idea of "family harmony" is therefore unrealistic; a more accurate idea is that families form a continuum of harmony and discord. At one end of the continuum are families in which harmony prevails because factors such as open communication maintain conflict at a reasonable level. At the other extreme are families in which conflict is out of control—families where, for instance, incest and even murder occur.

Another myth is *parental determinism:* the idea that parents are the sole influence on their children. In an age of high technology and extensive communications, parents are no longer the only influence on the socialization of their children and may not even be the most important influence; nor are children (if they ever were) simply passive receptors of their parents' instruction and modeling.[1] Children are exposed to a wide range of outside influences. They learn from the world around them. Schools, religious organizations, and neighborhood environments are strong factors in children's development; even more notable is the powerful influence of the media. Children today are both passive and active recipients of strong stimuli from television, radio, video, and computer technology. At very early ages children have experiences with the media, and some of these are experiences their parents have never had.

The frequently heard laments about the *breakdown of the family* are evidence of another myth. It is widely assumed that in some earlier era the family was more stable than it is today and provided its members with a healthier environment. Recent historical studies cast doubt on this idea; they have found that premarital sexuality, illegitimacy, incest, generational conflict, and infanticide have existed for a long time. What has changed is the amount of attention given to these problems, perhaps especially by health care systems and by the media. A more accurate concept is that new family structures have evolved, and that these issues are best studied as part of the increasing complexity of family life.

Still another myth is that a shift from "community concern" to increased "materialism" has contributed to the *isolation of individuals and families* and has fostered preoccupation with the self rather than concern for the community. There is some truth in this; but, paradoxically, as family isolation has increased, an expressed need for intimacy among individuals has also increased. As a family improves its economic base and lifestyle, it may be able to "buy" privacy but at the same time may set itself apart from earlier support systems of neighborhood and community. A family member may be able to "buy" a relationship with a therapist but may be unable to form meaningful relationships within the family or community.

Definition of "Family"

A *family* (for the purposes of this discussion) is a small social system, made up of people held together by strong reciprocal affections and loyalties and (in some senses of the term) living in a permanent household that persists over some time. Members enter the family through birth, adoption, marriage, or legal cohabitation and leave through death, divorce, or establishment of new homes.

There are many ways in which nurses can approach the study of the family. This book looks at the family as a system or whole which is made up of interacting parts or subsystems and is greater than the sum of its parts. The family in turn is seen within a larger context: the societal system. An eclectic, developmental approach is taken because it allows nurses to consider a family over time; that is, the individual client is viewed at a point in his or her development, but within the context of a family that has a continuous history and a long-standing, unique set of behaviors, attitudes, and values.

Families may be viewed in terms of their structure and functioning. The *structure* of a family is its "membership configuration"—that is, family organization and the pattern of relationships among family members. Family *functioning* is the processes by which a family operates; and analysis of *developmental processes* is essential to an understanding of family functioning.

Family Structure

Definitions of *family* based on systems or developmental approaches view the family broadly, sometimes in terms of family structures. A family structure usually consists of subsystems that are linked by "overlapping" members—individuals who belong to one or more of these subsystems.

Family structure may be considered in terms of *household structure.* In this sense it is (as was noted above) the "membership configuration" of a family, or (to put it another way) the family's organizational dimension. The nuclear family—a man and a woman who are legally married, living with their minor children—was once considered the "normal" household structure and the basic unit of society. Today, however, the concept of household structure has been expanded to include single-parent households, extended sibling groupings, homosexual cohabitation, extended-family households, communes, and other arrangements. Table 19-1 lists household structures and defines them in terms of membership and legal boundaries.

Family structure may also be considered in terms of *kin networks* or *extended families.* A kin network or extended family generally includes members of a family, in different kinds of relationship to each other, living independently in different household configurations but in close geographical proximity, and characterized by a system of exchange of goods and services.[2] Although adult members may have authority within each of their own households, the elder family members are consulted for advice, support, and authority in family affairs. For example:

> Sam and Mary are grandparents who live on the first floor of a house which they have owned since they were married and where all their children were raised. A daughter, Anne, who is divorced, lives with her teenage children in an apartment on another floor in the same house. Another daughter, Judy, lives with her husband and children on the next street. A son, John, lives in the next town with his family. When a second son, Peter, is widowed, Sam and Mary suggest that Anne care for Peter's children.

A third way family structure can be considered is in terms of *family of origin*—that is, the family in which a person grew up. In the example above, Anne, Judy, John, and Peter's family of origin would have consisted of the four of them and their parents, Mary and Sam.

Internal structures of the family, as described by Minuchin and others, are discussed later in the chapter.

Table 19-1 Household Structures

Type of Family	Household Composition and Legal Status
Nuclear family	Legally married. Husband and wife and their children living in the same household.
Dyadic nuclear family	Legally married. Couple with no children living in their own household who voluntarily choose not to have children.
Reconstituted nuclear family (also known as *blended family* or *stepfamily*)	Legally married husband and wife, each previously married, living with children from one or both previous marriages as well as any offspring of the present marriage.
Single adult	Person living alone, or with someone outside the family of origin who may or may not wish to marry.
Single-parent family (custodial)	Legally single. One parent, widowed, divorced, abandoned, or separated, living with legally-controlled dependent children, or one parent, never married, living with biological or adopted children.
Single-parent (noncustodial)	One parent living alone or with new partner, but without daily contact with offspring.
Three-generation family	Three generations of a family—usually grandparents, parents, and children—living in the same household and sharing goods and services.
Aging family	Legally married. Elderly retired couple whose children have been "launched" into career, marriage, or college.
Institutional family	Children cared for by professionals in orphanages or other institutional housing.
Commune family	Household that includes more than one monogamous couple with children, sharing services, talents, and economic resources. Socialization of children is a group activity.
Group marriage commune	Household of adults and children who are their offspring. Boundaries between couples are fluid. Children are socialized by all the adults.
Cohabitation dyad or family	Unmarried couple who may or may not have biological or adoptive children. Considered a legal union after 9 years of cohabitation.
Homosexual family	Homosexual couple living together with or without biological or adopted children.

Family Functioning

Families may be studied not only in terms of their structure but also in terms of their functions or, more specifically, in terms of how functional they are. Here, *functional* is a term that implies a judgment: it describes the utility of the structural or behavioral patterns a family uses to achieve its objectives. *Functions*, on the other hand, is a more neutral term, referring to objectives that are universal or at least widespread among families.

What functions must a family provide? The basic needs of a family—the things it must have in order to survive—are obvious: they include clothing, food, and shelter sufficient for safety and growth. When these basic needs are not met, the family unit is not only physically deprived but also under a severe emotional strain. A more complex function of the family is to foster emotional and spiritual development and the socialization of the young. At very early ages, children learn the overt and covert behavioral patterns of their parents or other older people in the home. They also evolve personal identity, sexual identity, and some sense of social responsibility, even if older people at home do not seem to be taking specific actions to direct or shape these processes. Young girls often pretend to be grown-up women, and they may dress in their mothers' clothing and imitate their mothers without any prompting by adults; boys, too, spontaneously copy the behavior of their male role models. Cultural norms and religious processes are learned similarly but may be intentionally taught or overtly modeled by adults.

What makes a family functional? That is, what enables it to meet the physical, spiritual, intellectual, and social needs of its members? Many researchers have studied the behaviors that families evolve; they have found that functional, healthy families are generally made up of members whose patterns of behavior are nurturing and caring and are characterized by love and loyalty, and that relational bonds are intense and continue over the life of the family. The healthy family thus creates an environment in which its physical, spiritual, affectional, and social functions can be carried out.

Barnhill[3] has attempted to synthesize various descriptions of the healthy family and has identified eight interrelated functional dimensions: (1) individuation, (2) mutuality, (3) flexibility, (4) stability, (5) clear perceptions of members, (6) clear role definitions, (7) role reciprocity, and (8) clear generational boundaries. Dysfunctional families, in contrast, are enmeshed, isolated, rigid, and disorganized and have unclear or distorted perceptions of their members; in dysfunctional families, roles are unclear, role conflicts increase, and generational boundaries become diffuse or are nonexistent.

Beavers[4] used nine variables to describe optimal family functioning: (1) a systems orientation, (2) clear boundaries, (3) contextual clarity in communications, (4) a clearly defined hierarchy of power and equality, (5) processes for achieving intimacy, (6) encouragement of autonomy, (7) joyful and comfortable styles of relating, (8) high-level negotiation skills, and (9) significant "transcendent values." The following paragraphs describe Beavers's variables.

To say that a family has a *systems orientation* implies that each individual is interdependent with other family members in forming a whole, and that causes and effects are interchangeable.[5] Family members recognize their relationship with one another and realize that what they do or say affects everyone in the system. (For example, if one family member becomes jealous, he or she recognizes that others will respond with feelings of rejection and anger, in turn causing someone else to react with hostility, and so forth. The idea may be compared to the ripples and waves that appear when a single pebble is dropped into a pool of water.) A systems orientation also recognizes the limitations of human nature. No one is viewed as absolutely helpless or absolutely powerful in a relationship. Rather, self-esteem comes from achieving relative competence in the family system by using one's unique talents and gifts.

The functional family has *clear boundaries*, both around the family unit as a whole and around its individual members. A boundary is a real or imagined barrier or limit that encircles a family unit or member. Boundaries that are healthy allow for a balanced flow of energy and interaction between the family unit and the environment and among family members themselves. Internal boundaries around members of highly functional families give them freedom to agree or to disagree with one another. The arts of negotiation and compromise develop when boundaries are clear. Generational demarcations exist between parents and children, facilitating mutual respect and intimacy. Enriching interactions between the internal life of a family and the world beyond it are evident in functional families.

Functional families are also characterized by *contextual clarity;* that is, they are perceived by society as unified, optimistic, and clear about their identity. Their members share certain "themes," and these themes and the families' social roles, though flexible, are also clear. The families are seen as "together"—not as deviant or dysfunctional—and they see themselves the same way.

A clear *hierarchy of power* exists in the functional family.[6] Leadership is in the hands of parents or other responsible parental figures. Stress, which can cause increased levels of anxiety in the family, is resolved because loving rather than coercive relationships exist among members. Each member maintains control over his or her inner self and consequently has little need to control others or look to others for self-fulfillment.

Intimacy is another characteristic of the functional family. Role complementarity and role differentiation are marks of growth in intimacy and thus of optimal family functioning.

The functional family encourages and fosters *autonomy* in its members. Autonomy is essential to the development of a satisfactory ego identity. The ability of children to break away and separate from their family of origin is a direct outgrowth of autonomy. The functional family is strong enough to tolerate imperfection and uncertainty. Consequently it is able to develop a climate in which mutual trust flourishes, and this facilitates autonomy.

Members of functional families *relate to each other comfortably and joyfully.* Personal boundaries are respected, but members' needs for sexual expression, intimacy, and assertiveness are recognized and affirmed. "Feeling tones" are intense, warm, and optimistic, and these feeling tones are revealed in overt behavior, tone of voice, verbal content of messages, and overall patterns of communication. There is a high level of empathy.

Functional families also have a highly developed *ability to negotiate.* Members can resolve differences, accept directions, and work together to reach goals. When a conflict arises, healthy families confront the issue directly and use well-established interactive patterns of caring and genuineness to compromise or reach a consensus.

Finally, the functional family is able to *transcend* its own experience and knowledge to envision its possibilities. Change is not threatening; new input is welcomed, examined, and evaluated. Functional families are characterized by openness and by a spiritual ability to tolerate the stress and pain of growth, development, aging, and death.

Family Developmental Processes

Analysis of family processes is basic to an understanding of family functioning. *Family processes* are not physical processes; rather, they are intangible methods used by individual family members to determine how family structure evolves, how decisions are made in the family, and how the family maintains itself as a unit.[7] Family health is a function of family processes rather than of tangible outcomes. How well stresses and crises are resolved, how family members deal with conflict, and how families achieve goals—all these depend on whether the negotiation of family processes is successful or dysfunctional.

Families, like individuals, move through stages of emotional growth and development. In a person, emotional growth is a subjective internal experience; the stages of family development, by contrast, are marked by the accomplishment of specific tasks or by specific events that can be observed objectively by family members and others. *Family development* is defined as the process of progressive structural differentiation and transformation over a family's history. Family development involves active acquisition and selective discarding of roles as family members seek to fulfill the changing functional requisites for survival, and as the family adapts as a holistic system to recurring life stresses.[8,9]

Family development can be analyzed in different ways; Duvall[9] proposed a framework based on family developmental tasks, and Carter and McGoldrick[8] focused on transitional points and changes in family status. These two analyses are discussed below.

A *family developmental task*—the concept underlying Duvall's framework—is a responsibility, having to do with growth, that arises at a specific stage in the life of a family. Theoretically, successful accomplishment of tasks at one stage leads to satisfaction and success with tasks that arise at later stages; failure to accomplish tasks leads to unhappiness in the family, disapproval by society, and difficulty at later stages of family development.[9] For example, if a newly married couple—at the "establishment stage" of the family—fail to make a commitment to their own identifiable system and instead remain too close to their families of origin, they have failed to complete a task of the establishment stage. They will, predictably, have difficulty in subsequent stages when children become part of the system. Because the family is a complex system, it must accomplish developmental tasks in ways that satisfy requirements for biological growth, cultural imperatives, and individual members' personal aspirations and values. Table 19-2 outlines stages, developmental processes, and tasks over the family life span.

Carter and McGoldrick approach family development by using "key transition points" and "second-order changes in family status" as criteria—requirements for proceeding developmentally.[8] They emphasize emotional processes or movement toward goals within families rather than accomplishment of specific tasks. According to Carter and

Table 19-2 Stages of Family Development

Stage	Definition	Emotional Processes and Tasks
Establishment	Joining of two extended family systems through marriage. Begins with the official engagement or plan to marry and continues until first pregnancy.	Formation of marital system. Commitment to new identifiable system. Establishment of a workable philosophy of life as a couple. Realignment of relationships with extended families to include spouse. Realignment of relationships with friends, associates, and community agencies. Negotiation of issues such as eating and sleeping patterns, living space, finances, sexual contact, and use of time. Decision making about parenthood.
Postestablishment or expectant family	Family preparing for the birth of a child. Begins with first pregnancy and continues to the birth of the first child.	Acknowledging that a child is expected. Acquiring knowledge about and planning for pregnancy, childbirth, and parenthood. Adjusting sexual relationships to the patterns of pregnancy.
Childbearing family: Family with infants	Family with infants. Begins with the birth of the first child and continues until that child is 3 or 4 years old.	Adjustment to the stresses and responsibilities of parenthood. Emotional integration of the child into the family unit. Adjustment of parents and grandparents to new roles. Reestablishment of a workable marital relationship that incorporates the new child. Planning for additional children.
Childbearing family: Family with toddlers	Family with preschool children. Begins when eldest child is age 3 and continues until that child starts school.	Incorporation of additional children into family. Socialization of children. Sharing responsibilities for ongoing marital relationship and nurturing of children. Adjustment by parents and child to breaking away and separation.

(Continued.)

Table 19-2 Continued

Stage	Definition	Emotional Processes and Tasks
Childbearing family: Family with schoolchildren	Family with school-age children. Begins when eldest child starts elementary school and ends when that child reaches adolescence.	Acceptance of outside influences. Development of peer relationships by children. Adjustment by parents to child's activities at school and in the community. Integration and adjustment to children's peer groups and other community influences. Continued renegotiation of the marital relationship. Adjustment to expanding extended family.
Childbearing family: Family with adolescents	Family with teenage children. Begins when the eldest child reaches age 13 and continues until the adolescent leaves home or becomes "emancipated."	Adaptation to rapid physical, emotional, spiritual, and sociocultural changes occuring in the family. Adjustment by parents to children's increasing autonomy. Recognition and acceptance of the conflict between physical dependence of adolescent children and their increasing emotional independence. Collaboration between parents and consistency with regard to setting limits for children. Beginning reallocation of responsibilities among older children. Renegotiation of marital goals. Widening career choices and options. Increasing responsibility for elderly family members (grandparents). Beginning preparation for retirement.
Launching	Family with children in the process of "breaking away." Begins with the departure of the first child from the household and continues until all the children have left or are physically, emotionally, spiritually and financially independent.	Adjustment to increased financial burdens (college, etc.). Reallocation of responsibilities among adult members of household. Adjustment by parents to taking care of their aging and increasingly dependent parents. Maintaining extensive communication with systems outside the family (schools, colleges, peer groups, jobs, recreational facilities, etc.). Negotiation of shift from "parent-child" to "parent-separated adult" roles. Renegotiation of marital relationship. Preparation by parents and adult children for the "empty nest."
Middle adult family	Couple in middle adulthood. Begins with the "launching" of the last child and continues through the retirement of one adult.	Negotiation of concrete plans for retirement. Incorporation of the needs of elderly parents. Realignment of communication patterns with children to include their in-laws. Adjustment to grandparents' role. Adjustment to increased leisure time as a couple. Renegotiation of marital roles. Beginning adjustment to decreased physical energy.

(Continued.)

Table 19-2 Continued

Stage	Definition	Emotional Processes and Tasks
Aged adult family	Family with a member over the age of 65. Begins with retirement and ends with the deaths of both spouses.	Adjustment to retirement. Preparation for the death of oneself and one's spouse. Maintaining relationships with adult children, grandchildren, and great-grandchildren. Adjustment to narrowing range of relationships. Realignment of physical and mental resources and energies. Enjoyment of marital companionship.

SOURCE: Adapted from E. Duvall, *Marriage and Family Development*, 5th ed., Lippincott, Philadelphia, 1977.

McGoldrick's schema, the following emotional processes are to be completed:

- Accepting separation of parents and children
- Becoming committed to newly formed family systems
- Accepting new members into the family system
- Increasing the flexibility of family boundaries to include children's independence
- Accepting many exits from and entries into the family system
- Accepting changes and shifts in roles from generation to generation

Stages of development, on this analysis, are generally determined by the age of the eldest child in a family; but stages may overlap or be repeated as successive children are integrated into the family system, and at any point a family may be considered a "multistage family" (a family whose eldest child was an adolescent with siblings in elementary school and parents expecting another child would be an example of a multistage family) or may be at one specific stage. Sudden transitions between stages are held to be stressful: for instance, if all the children in a family were adolescents for several years and the family suddenly shifted to the child-bearing stage or "launched" all the children within a short time, increased stress would be very likely.

The concept of family development, and a developmental framework, can be useful to nurses and others who work with or study families. However, it is evident from a review of recent literature that much of the published information about predictable developmental stages and the family life span is applicable only to middle-class American families and families that closely resemble them.[1] There are at least two ways in which a developmental framework is limited: first, as has already been noted, the "nuclear family" as traditionally defined is by no means universal; second, there are cultural differences between American society and many other societies. Therefore, developmental concepts should be applied cautiously—never rigidly—to strata of American society other than the middle class and to families in markedly different cultures, particularly those in less developed societies.

With these qualifications, though, the developmental approach is valid and practical for nurses. First, it can serve as a *guide for assessment and for setting goals.* Second, it allows nurses to *focus on a family throughout its history,* seeing each member's interactions with other members and observing how individuals and the family unit itself interact and influence each other at different stages. Third, it enables practitioners to *recognize* a family's experiences at a given stage and to *identify* and highlight critical periods of family growth and development.[8] (For example, a family which is just starting the establishment stage is likely to experience more stress than a family which is well established; and a family with adolescent children may be experiencing more crises than a family in the middle years.) Fourth, developmental parameters may be used to *predict* what a family will experience at any period in its life span. This is of major interest to nurses: predictive ability allows them to teach coping strategies and focus on prevention. Finally, the developmental approach reveals both *universal characteristics* of families and *differences* among families, and the ways in which families and society influence one another.

MODELS FOR FAMILY THERAPY

Family therapy is practiced today in a wide variety of clinical settings. Nurses working in both psychiatric settings and other settings will be exposed to it in an ongoing or episodic way. For the practitioner without a graduate degree, understanding the theoretical models of family therapy will be valuable in several ways. First, certain principles of these models will be applicable in work with clients who have been hospitalized for psychiatric or medical reasons; these principles can help the nurse to understand the client within a family context and to promote effective modes of coping with stress and illness for individuals and families. Second, knowledge of the models will increase the nurse's ability to observe clients and families accurately, to identify problems within the family system, to select effective nursing interventions, and to evaluate the effectiveness of interventions designed to promote growth and change. Third, familiarity with the models will increase the nurse's awareness of when, why, and where to initiate referrals for family therapy.

Three theoretical models for family therapy—*family systems therapy, structural family therapy,* and *strategic family therapy*—will be presented in this chapter. Each model represents a major approach to family therapy, and each is based on a theoretical framework developed from clinical research with families; but the three models are distinct from each other. Which model will be selected for use by a nurse-clinician will depend on the practitioner's theoretical orientation.

Family Systems Therapy

Concepts of Family Systems Theory

Family systems theory is one of the major schools of thought underlying the development of family therapy. The family systems approach was developed in the early 1950s by Bowen and takes a biological, evolutionary perspective. Two fundamental premises of this approach are that a family is a fluid, ever-changing system and that a change in one part of the system is followed by a compensatory change in other parts of the system.[10,11] From a systems perspective, the family is seen as a web of parts, or subsystems, which can be understood only as a whole; that is, it is more than and different from the sum of its parts.[10,12]

Family systems theorists explain emotional dysfunction, or the appearance of symptoms in a family member, as a reflection of an acute or chronic disturbance in the balance of forces in the family relationship process. Symptoms in any family member, whether physical (such as asthma, alcoholism, and diabetes), emotional (such as depression and marital discord), or social (such as homicide and delinquency), are viewed as manifestations of dysfunction in the family relationship process.

Bowen proposes that emotional dysfunction can be described as a continuum ranging from "severely dysfunctional" to "highly functional." The difference between dysfunction and function is, then, quantitative rather than qualitative. Therefore, *degree* of impairment is what counts. For example, in terms of dysfunction, the difference between a schizophrenic adolescent and a delinquent adolescent would be one of degree rather than kind.

Bowen views the family as a multigenerational system characterized by patterns of emotional interaction. There are eight interlocking concepts that describe family systems functioning in terms of emotional patterns and interaction: (1) differentiation of self, (2) triangles, (3) the "nuclear family emotional system," (4) the multigenerational transmission process, (5) the family projection process, (6) sibling position, (7) emotional cutoff, and (8) societal regression. All these concepts apply to all families to some degree. To understand a family within this theoretical framework, the nurse must understand each of the concepts and their interrelationship within the individual and within the family.

DIFFERENTIATION OF SELF. According to family systems theory, the individual and the family are intimately connected. Individual family members may seem unique, but they have more similarities than differences. The process underlying this similarity of family members is Bowen's "cornerstone" concept: differentiation of self.

Differentiation of self (like emotional dysfunction) can be described as a continuum. In this case, the continuum ranges from low levels of differentiation ("fusion") to high levels ("clearly defined sense of self"). Bowen conceptualizes it as a scale from 0 to 100. People at the low end of the scale demonstrate the lowest level of functioning; people at the high end exhibit the highest level. Most people fall somewhere in the middle.

What Bowen means by *differentiation* is the degree of separation or fusion between the intellectual and emotional systems. Members of families with low levels of differentiation are unable to distinguish between the intellectual ("thinking") system and the emotional ("feeling") system. It is as if thinking and feeling are so fused or blended that it is impossible to separate thoughts from feelings—especially when anxiety is high. Members of poorly differentiated families commonly say, "I feel" or "We feel," rather than, "I think" or "I believe." Such families direct their efforts toward promoting "togetherness" and agreement; they avoid statements of opinions or beliefs that would establish one family member as different or separate from the rest of the family. In contrast, members of families with high levels of differentiation demonstrate separation between thinking and feeling; that is, they are able to think flexibly and thoroughly and to formulate opinions, values, and beliefs that allow them to guide their lives without being overwhelmed by their emotions. Members of highly differentiated families have a stronger, more solid sense of self that allows for and encourages individual differences.

A person's level of differentiation evolves out of the family relationship system. A family's level of differentiation evolves over several generations as the family creates an environment that either facilitates or inhibits movement in the direction of higher differentiation.

Fusion, or "undifferentiation," is present in all families to some degree, but in some families it is particularly evident. It is most commonly observed as a remarkable emotional "oneness" or "togetherness" that Bowen has referred to as the *undifferentiated ego mass.* Such families live in a world which is dominated by feelings and in which everybody accepts the family "party line." Family members tend to think, feel, act, and live alike. Their emotional closeness or fusion may be so intense that they believe they can read each other's thoughts.[11,13,14,15] Families with a low level of differentiation strive to avoid anxiety and therefore establish relationships that "feel good." These relationships are characterized not only by overcloseness (which would, of course, be expected) but also by a somewhat paradoxical pattern of cyclical closeness and distance: closeness increases until it becomes overwhelming or smothering and is then followed by distancing behavior that attempts to reestablish a sense of self. Such relationships may be functional when the family system is undergoing only minimal stress; but they represent a delicate balance which is easily upset by more significant stresses, such as the birth of a child or the death or illness of a significant other. Members of families characterized by considerable evidence of undifferentiation are prone to physical, emotional, and social problems, particularly when they are under stress.

In other families, evidence of undifferentiation is almost imperceptible. Such families experience feelings of anxiety but are not dominated by them. For members of these families, family relationships are an important part of life but do not become the focus of existence. Family members rely less on each other for self-definition and emotional sustenance; as a result, relationships have a "you-me" quality rather than a "we" quality. People can function autonomously and responsibly together or alone. During periods of stress, the more differentiated person or family is not as vulnerable to dysfunction. Although symptoms of dysfunction may appear, differentiated families tend to recover from stress and anxiety more quickly than undifferentiated families.

The level of differentiation is the background against which a family and its members live. It is quite stable and varies only slightly as it is passed from generation to generation.

TRIANGLES. The concept of "triangles" (the second of Bowen's eight concepts) is important for understanding family interactional patterns and processes. An emotional triangle is a way of describing relational patterns among persons, objects, or issues. Bowen[16] has called the triangle the "basic building block of an emotional system."

A *triangle* is an emotional configuration consisting of three members. The members of a triangle may be three people; or two people and an issue (such as money or infidelity), a group (such as a religious affiliation or Alcoholics Anonymous), or an object (such as a house or a car). What defines a triangle is that a person, issue, group, or object at one "point" has emotional significance for the people at the other points. Triangles can develop between generations or within generations.

Triangles can be thought of as patterns which—when they are not rigid—involve "movement." To visualize this, it is useful to think of a rubber band stretched around three pins; if the pins are moved so that their configuration changes, the rubber band will change shape. "Movement" in an emotional triangle is related to level of differentiation and level of anxiety in a family.[17] Ideally, in a triangle the three points are equidistant, but the people involved are able to move "toward" or "away" from another point at any time. When differentiation decreases and anxiety increases, however, a triangle tends to become both more rigid and more serious.

How and why is a triangle formed? One very common reason for the formation of a triangle is to restore balance or stability in a system that has been threatened by stress. For instance, consider a two-person system that is stable only as long as things are calm. If anxiety increases, a third person, a group, an issue, or an object may be "pushed in" emotionally to create a triangle and thus reestablish stability. The problem with this pattern is that it sometimes allows people to achieve a degree of calm and comfort without having dealt with the underlying problem. For example:

> Lillian's husband Charles had a coronary bypass 8 years ago. He has had no further symptoms of angina since then and has been able to lead a very active life. Yesterday, however, he casually told Lillian that he had some chest pain while playing tennis, but that it was nothing; he then telephoned a friend to make another tennis date. Lillian is very anxious about the possibility of losing her husband; today she calls her oldest daughter to express her fears about Charles's symptoms—but she swears her daughter to secrecy.

Lillian has created a "detour triangle" (illustrated in Figure 19-1) by pulling in her daughter, who forms the third point. This new configuration prevents the dyad—Charles and Lillian—from dealing directly with the situation (Charles's symptoms and Lillian's upset); moreover, the daughter is now caught between her parents. These three people may be able to create an "ideal" equilateral triangle; but it is likely that Charles will move to a position distant from his wife and daughter.

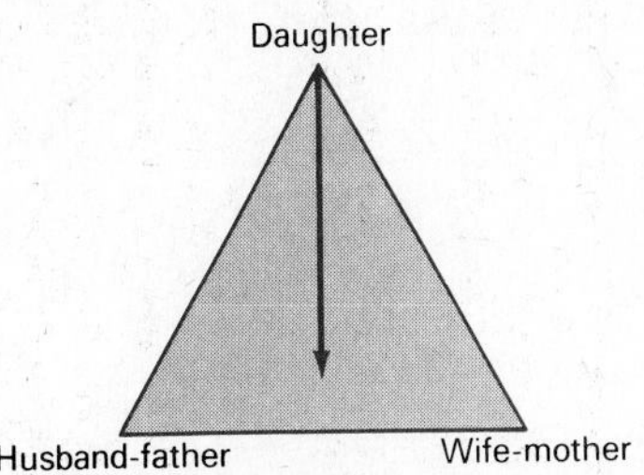

Figure 19-1 Detour triangle.
Lillian (wife-mother) avoids dealing directly with the anxiety and threat posed by the reoccurance of Charles's (husband-father's) cardiac symptoms by "triangling in" their daughter, to whom she expresses her feelings rather than to Charles.

What kinds of triangles can form? Triangles have different configurations and different components, depending on family interaction processes, levels of anxiety, and levels of differentiation. Here is an example of a "husband-wife-issue" triangle:

> Mike has just been promoted to a management position which will require considerable travel. His wife Barbara, although she is proud of him, feels increasingly lonely and empty without him; she has always looked to him for emotional oneness and completeness. When he is home, she pursues him for attention, affection, and recognition. Mike, who is undergoing stress, feels frazzled and tells her, "Leave me alone. Can't you see I'm beat?" Eventually, she stops pursuing him and deals with her anxiety by immersing herself in the children, who initially respond positively to her interest and attention. After a few weeks, Mike begins to notice that Barbara appears withdrawn and busy with the kids even when he is home. They begin to argue: "How come you and the kids are never home when I get back from a trip?" "Why should we be? You care more about your promotion than you do about your wife and children!" "You want a lot of luxuries and then blame me for having to work hard and long hours!"

The triangle that Barbara and Mike have formed is illustrated in Figure 19-2. This is a very common configuration; it allows them to focus on an issue—Mike's work, which is the third point of the triangle—rather than on their emotional life as a couple. Their feelings become oriented toward the issue, which in this case is a false issue; it is not so much

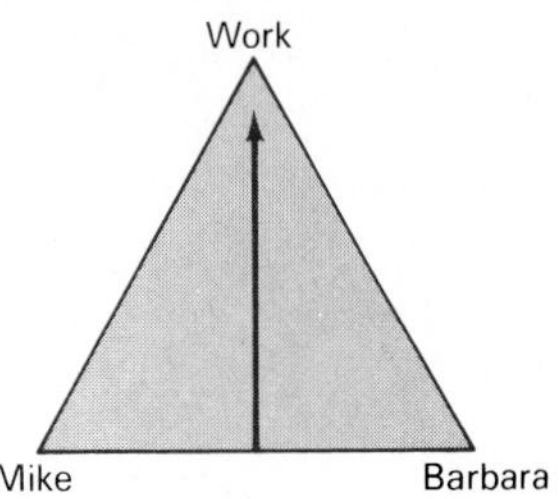

Figure 19-2 Issue triangle.
Barbara (wife) and Mike (husband), focus on Mike's overwork as an issue between them rather than on sensitive emotional issues (such as feeling unloved, not respected, or unappreciated).

Mike's work as Mike and Barbara's relationship which is the problem. Because they focus on the false issue, these two people have shifted their attention away from themselves and their own part in their problems, and thus they avoid any change in themselves.

Another triangular pattern—perhaps the most common pattern—is "mother-father-child." When such a triangle forms, there is usually an unresolved conflict between husband and wife, who avoid their discord or distance by focusing on their "problem" child. Here is an example (illustrated in Figure 19-3):

> Edna and Cary avoid marital conflict by focusing on their 10-year-old son Alan, who is having problems in school. Mother and son avoid dealing with their overcloseness by making the father a common enemy. Father and son are distant, then—but Cary and Alan avoid dealing with their distance (and at the same time perpetuate it) by using Edna as a go-between.

How do triangles function? Triangles are "reciprocal"—that is, when two people "triangle in" a third person, an issue, a group, or an object, they

Figure 19-3 Mother-father-child triangle.
The husband and wife avoid their marital discord by focusing their attention and concern on a child and his or her physical, emotional, or social problems.

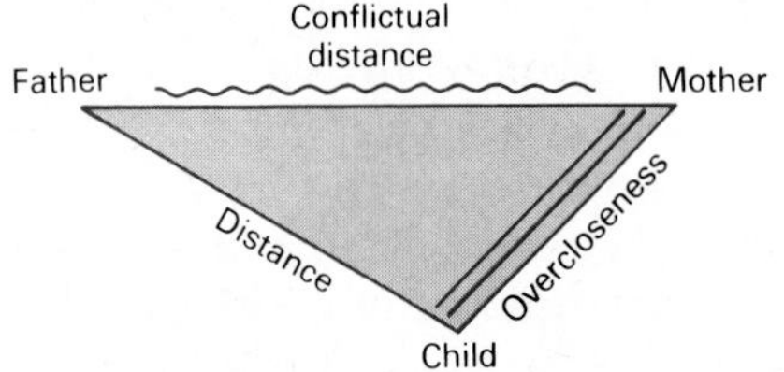

are equally responsible for the situation. When the third "point" of the triangle is a person, that person too may share equally in the responsibility. The example above—the triangle formed by Cary, Edna, and Alan—shows clearly how each member can participate in creating and maintaining the pattern. However, not all triangles reveal this so unambiguously. For example, if a husband distances himself from problematic issues in his marriage by "triangling in" an extramarital affair, it may be difficult for his wife to see that she too is a participant in the triangle. She may find it hard to relinquish a self-righteous position as the "betrayed woman" and thus may be unable to see that, say, overinvolvement with her children is serving to distance her from the marital relationship. Many activities, issues, groups, or objects can serve the function of distancing people in a triangular relationship, including work, hobbies, alcoholism, depression, sex, physical illnesses, and symptoms of psychosis.

Are triangles inevitable? It is impossible to stay out of triangles; they are simply a fact of life in family relationships. They form and reform around different issues and events as families deal with stress, anxiety, and tension. A person's position in a triangle can change, depending on the issue involved; for example:

> Lou and his wife May are in conflict and distant over the issue of Lou's gambling; but they are united and close over the issue of their daughter's drug problem.

Although triangles are unavoidable, some are more problematic than others. The most problematic are those in which the points are no longer equidistant, and this configuration becomes rigid over time; such triangles are likely to involve deep friendships or family relationships. Here is an example (illustrated in Figure 19-4):

> Larry and his daughter Ann have become overclose; at the same time, Larry and his son Roy are distant. Ann and her brother are also at a "conflictual distance."

How does differentiation affect triangles? A family's level of differentiation will significantly influence the degree to which anxiety becomes an unbalancing force, the degree to which patterns of interaction become fixed, and the degree to which rigid triangles must be formed to maintain the status quo. In less differentiated families, members are so fused—and react emotionally to each other

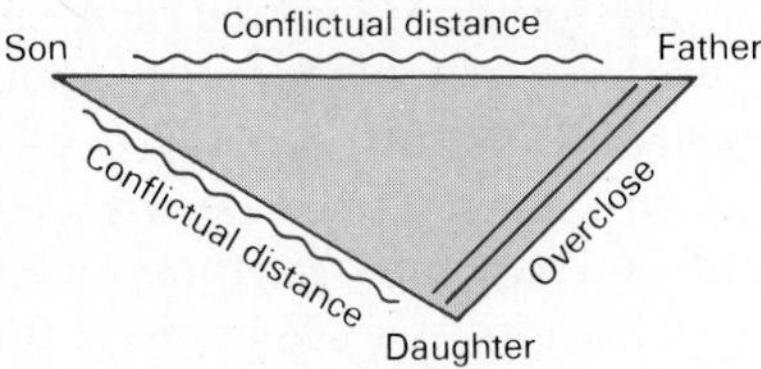

Figure 19-4 Conflictual triangle.
A father initiates and maintains a conflict of unknown origin with his adult son, which results in a distant relationship. The daughter, who is overclose with the father, maintains a similar position with her brother. They have not spoken in 10 years.

to such an extent—that their relationships tend to look like the triangle in Figure 19-5. This triangle is so rigid that there is little opportunity for movement either within it or outside it. A configuration like this perpetuates and increases emotional intensity within the family and decreases the possibility of meaningful relationships outside the family. Thus a rigid triangle can represent a fused, undifferentiated system of relationships, similar to what might be observed in a schizophrenic family.

"NUCLEAR FAMILY EMOTIONAL SYSTEM." The third of Bowen's descriptive concepts is what he calls the *nuclear family emotional system*—the patterns of emotional functioning in a nuclear family.[16] The term *nuclear family* traditionally refers to a husband, a wife, and their minor children. The basic patterns of behavior that are observed in a nuclear family often repeat patterns that occurred in the spouses' families of origin. The lower the level of differentiation in a family, and the higher the level of anxiety, the greater the likelihood that patterns of emotional interaction will pass from generation to generation, although family members are unaware of them.[18]

The formation of a nuclear family's emotional system begins with a marriage. Dating, courtship, and marriage involve an intense attraction between

Figure 19-5 Rigid triangle.
This illustrates a fused, undifferentiated relationship system similar to what would be observed in a schizophrenic family.

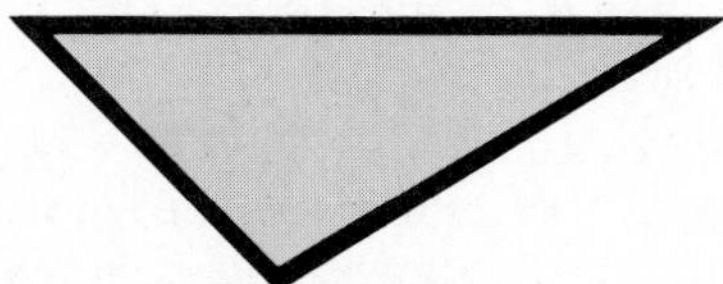

two people which is related to the forces of the emotional rather than the intellectual system; and people with equivalent levels of differentiation tend to marry each other. These two facts imply that the lower the level of differentiation of the partners, the greater the potential for problems in the marriage. If, as Bowen[16] proposes, people with higher levels of differentiation have fewer problems in life, then it is logical to assume that a marriage between two people with a low level of differentiation would be vulnerable to problems.

People with higher levels of differentiation tend to use both the intellectual system and the emotional system in making decisions about marriage. Such people, having a solid sense of self, are better able to make choices about lifestyles and goals in life on the basis of principles, ideas, and values. They are also more accurate in their evaluations of themselves and others, even when they are in love. As a result, they are aware of an intense emotional attraction and, despite this intensity, they are able to examine the relationship in terms of its potential as a marital partnership and to evaluate the congruence of principles, values, and goals.

In contrast, people with lower levels of differentiation make decisions about marriage largely through the emotional system. For such people, courtship is often not only intensely emotional but also chaotic. Undifferentiated couples use each other to meet needs related to dependency and self-esteem. They perceive that they will complete each other; it is through the other that each will feel fulfilled and whole. Impulsive decisions, made on the basis of what "feels good" at the moment, are common. There is often an element of blackmail ("If you really loved me ... ") or rebellion ("I don't care what you think; I love him ...") in the choice of a partner. When a marriage is launched in this way, it is likely to founder: it does not represent a decision based on carefully considered options.

When two people have married, and thus are no longer able to terminate their relationship easily, "fusional forces" begin to operate. Fusion—the emotional merging of two people into a "common self"—is illustrated in Figure 19-6. As would be expected, the degree of fusion is inversely related to the level of differentiation. That is, the more solid two people's individual sense of self is before they are married, the less likely they are to fuse into a common self after marriage.

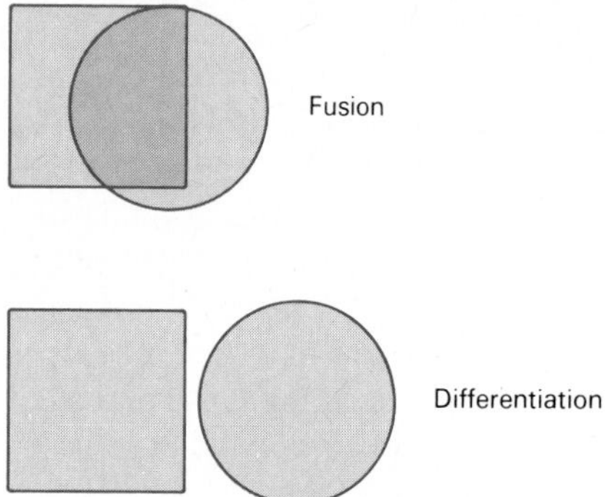

Figure 19-6 Fusion and differentiation.
Fusion is emotional merging of two people into a common self. Differentiation is the maintenance of intact boundaries which enable people to freely move toward or away from each other.

Married people who fuse or blend into each other focus their energy on their relationship to the extent that they have little energy left for developing as separate individuals. Such couples may say things like, "I never have time to see my friends anymore," and, "I've changed so much since my marriage that I'm just not interested in a lot of things anymore"—statements that reflect their shift of energy. "Togetherness," harmony, and agreement become more and more important; this development is reflected in the formation of "we" positions. For example:

> A newly married woman, who used to spend most of her leisure time playing tennis, refused an invitation to a tennis party, saying, "Thank you, but we don't think I ought to spend time playing tennis anymore. John likes it better when I'm with him."

Who will dominate the common self, or merged self, becomes an issue. A merged self implies a degree of "togetherness" that eventually becomes suffocating and fraught with tension as each spouse monitors the emotions of the other. The obvious solution is distance; but distance only creates other problems. For one thing, it channels energy away from the relationship to the point where communication is inadequate and emotional issues are avoided. Couples who have reached this point complain that they aren't as close as they used to be and that they never seem to have time for each other. The relationship becomes increasingly troubled because it is difficult for the partners to find a satisfactory balance between closeness and distance. A less obvious response for fused couples is for one spouse to pursue closeness and the other distance; but in such cases, both spouses have difficulty arriving at a functional level of closeness.

Symptoms of marital fusion can be observed in patterns of relationships in the nuclear family. Three symptoms are marital conflict, dysfunction of a spouse, and projection of anxiety onto the children—with subsequent impairment of one or more children. These three symptoms are described in Table 19-3.

MULTIGENERATIONAL TRANSMISSION PROCESS. The multigenerational transmission process (Bowen's fourth descriptive concept) is the process by which patterns of interaction are passed along from generation to generation.[16] Each generation is linked to past and future generations through family relationships. Bowen holds that family characteristics such as norms, values, behaviors, problems, issues, and patterns of relationships are transmitted from one generation to another. By using the concept of multigenerational transmission, it is possible to trace patterns through several generations of a family, regardless of the behavioral manifestations that are evident in family members. (A three-generation genogram presents information about generational patterns in a way that is graphic and easily understood. It also serves as a guide for following issues, events, and actions of a family over three generations. A complete discussion of the genogram is given in the section "Assessment of the Family" later in this chapter.)

A family's "relationship system" is the expression of its emotional system. Depending on its level of differentiation, the family develops emotional patterns which can be traced over generations. For example, one generation may develop a pattern of one type of emotional expressiveness—say, aggression. In the next generation, the pattern may be passivity. Although these two patterns—aggression and passivity—may appear different, they reflect the same underlying "emotional style," an inability to express anger in constructive ways. The less differentiated a family is, the more likely it becomes that emotional patterns will lead to serious impairment of one or more family members in the course of several generations.

FAMILY PROJECTION PROCESS. The family projection process (the fifth of Bowen's descriptive concepts) is a process through which parental undifferentia-

Table 19-3 Symptoms of Fusion in the Nuclear Family Emotional System

Symptom	Characteristics	Example
Marital conflict	Occurs when neither spouse will assume the adaptive position and allow the other to dominate the fused common self. The cycle of conflict evolves through periods of closeness and conflict, which provide the necessary emotional distance. All marriages contain an element of conflict. However, in high-conflict marriages the predictable pattern is one of frequency and intensity. Conflictual marriages are sometimes stabilized by "triangling in" a third person, group, issue, or thing.	Marie and Frank fight about how he feels smothered by her wanting all of him for herself. They distance themselves from each other for 3 to 5 days and then gradually move back toward each other, to a close position, until he once again feels smothered by her emotional demands. The cycle begins again with another fight. Kelly has designed her life around being emotionally and physically available to John and their 2-year-old son, Jamie. As a musician, John works unusual hours. When John is not working, Kelly is very happy being with him and Jamie; she plans her schedule so that they can spend as much time together as possible. However, when John is working, Kelly becomes lonely, anxious, and upset; Jamie has nightmares and wets the bed. When John comes home, Kelly invariably starts a fight in which the issue of "being available as a parent," is "triangled in."
Dysfunction of a spouse	Occurs when one spouse assumes the adaptive position and allows the other spouse to assume the dominant position in the common self. The dominant spouse is allowed to make all the decisions for both partners. The couple appear never to disagree, because the adaptive spouse agrees with what the dominant spouse thinks, feels, or does. The dominant spouse appears much more functional, because he or she has gained the appearance of strong selfhood at the expense of the spouse who has let some of his or hers go, functioning less and less effectively. In reality, the partners' basic level of differentiation is similar, even if their level of functioning is not. The "dominant spouse–adaptive spouse" relationship usually continues unless the adaptive spouse stages a revolution and, saying, "I've had enough of this," refuses to participate any longer. It is not uncommon for the dominant spouse to slip into the adaptive position as the formerly adaptive spouse regains a more solid sense of self.	When Carol and Bill got married, they both had successful careers and had successfully lived on their own before marriage. Both had friends and a number of leisure interests. Since their marriage, Carol has become preoccupied with being a perfect wife. She supports the advancement of Bill's career at the expense of her own. She travels with him on business trips and entertains his clients. She has less and less interest in her own career, friendships, etc. Bill has gradually begun to make all the decisions for both of them. As this pattern has developed, Carol has become increasingly depressed. Bill covers up for the fact that she spends most of her time doing nothing by hiring a housekeeper and taking on more responsibility himself. Carol's depression becomes more and more severe. One day, she attempts suicide, leaving a note that says, "I am an empty shell."

(Continued.)

Table 19-3 Continued

Symptom	Characteristics	Example
Projection of anxiety onto children	Occurs when symptoms develop in one or more children as the couple project their marital anxiety to the children through a "mother-father-child" triangle, where it is safer for the symptom to reside. The greater the anxiety projected, the greater the impairment of the child. The lower the level of differentiation, the greater the likelihood that fusional forces will be operating as a rigid "mother-father-child" triangle. Better-differentiated parents are able to contain their anxiety; they do not have to pass it on to their children to obtain relief. Factors influencing which child will become a scapegoat (the "problem" child) are: (1) parents' anxiety during conception, pregnancy, and delivery, which affect how the child is perceived; (2) intense positive or negative feelings toward the child by virtue of sex, sibling position, physical appearance, or state of health; (3) "nodal events," such as death, sickness, and divorce, which occurred around the time of the child's birth and which may confer a special status on the child.	Following the stormy exposure of her father's extramarital affair, Gail's behavior has begun to change, even though her parents have resumed their distant but polite relationship. She is quiet and withdrawn, and sleeps during the afternoon after school. A notice is sent home from school stating that Gail, formerly an excellent student, is failing four subjects. Her mother tries to find out what is wrong, but Gail is uncommunicative. One day, while cleaning Gail's room, her mother finds large quantities of pot and pills, but she accepts Gail's explanation—that they belong to a friend. Three weeks later, Gail is arrested for possession of cocaine. The family is referred for family therapy by the court as part of Gail's treatment program. At the third therapy session, the therapist asks Gail what purpose is served by failing at school and taking drugs. She tearfully responds, "The only time my parents talk to each other warmly is when I'm in trouble. I've wondered how bad I'd have to get for them to really make up and not just act as if things are OK."

tion impairs one or more children and operates within the father-mother-child triangle. It results in emotional impairment of a child; or it can superimpose itself on some defect or chronic illness or disability in the child. The projection process exists in all gradations of intensity and is present to some degree in all families. (This process is also noted in the sections "Nuclear Family Emotional System" and "Triangles.")

SIBLING POSITION. Bowen has incorporated Toman's[19] work on sibling position into his family systems theory as a sixth descriptive concept. *Sibling position* refers to the place and role one assumes or learns in a family. A person tends to assume this role outside the family as well. Sibling position is established by birth order and sex. On the basis of his research, Toman formulated a personality profile for each sibling position. (For example, an oldest sister of brothers or sisters tends to be a responsible, caretaking person, who is most likely to marry a younger brother who is used to being cared for and likes the caretaking behavior of an oldest child.) Toman's work makes it possible to predict, fairly accurately, marital discord or harmony on issues of rank and sex. Recognizing such patterns and their potential for conflict can help couples live with their similarities or differences in sibling position. Considering the sibling position of family members helps nurses to obtain a more complete picture of the entire family system.

EMOTIONAL CUTOFF. Emotional cutoff (the seventh concept in Bowen's theory) is the process of becoming physically or emotionally separated or isolated from one's family of origin, or denying its importance.[16] It is a dysfunctional response to fusional forces within a family.

All people have some unresolved emotional attachment to their parents. The way in which people separate from their family of origin to begin a new life as a new generation is related to their level of differentiation. Physical distance is not always an accurate reflection of differentiation: people who are geographically removed from their family may be as emotionally fused as people who never leave home at all (in fact, people who must remove themselves physically in order to have a sense of separateness are probably considerably fused). Moreover, family members can live in the same area—even in the same town or on the same street—and still be emotionally cut off from each other; they may see each other rarely (or never), or relate to each other only superficially.

Some people need emotional closeness but are unable to deal with it functionally. People who cut themselves off from their family of origin deny their actual fusion by acting as if they were uninvolved with the family and independent of it; in reality, they are not autonomous, even if they have moved thousands of miles away.

There are degrees or gradations of emotional cutoff. The more each member maintains some kind of meaningful emotional connection with the family, the more orderly and functional life and family processes will be over the generations. The more intense an emotional cutoff is, the more intense fusion is—and the more vulnerable a family becomes to experiencing cutoffs again in future generations.

SOCIETAL REGRESSION. The eighth descriptive concept in Bowen's theory is *societal regression*—the idea that emotional problems in families are similar to emotional problems in society. Regression in a family occurs when the family is subjected to chronic, sustained anxiety. At such times, families tend to lose the ability to guide their lives according to the principles of the intellectual system and resort instead to the emotions. Bowen[20,21] postulates that the same process may take place in society. For example, periods of social unrest due to economic, political, or racial upheaval create a high degree of anxiety; at such times decisions and behavior are often dominated by the emotional system. An example of regression in society might be a demonstration which escalates into a riot; something that was originally based on ideology has become an emotionally driven situation. Another example of regression might be an adolescent who abuses drugs or alcohol as a response to tension and anxiety within the family—again, this is emotionally driven behavior, and the family's anxiety may reflect environmental anxiety.

Family regression and societal regression, then, not only are similar but also may influence each other. That is, a family's level of anxiety may be a function of the level of anxiety in the environment—in society—and families' anxiety (and other conditions in families) will have an impact on society. Severe conditions in families can send a shock wave through society; severe conditions in the society can send a shock wave through families.

A family's health is a function of the degree to which the family system and the family members are differentiated from societal and generational problems and tensions. A functional family is characterized by a sense of "system integrity": there is enough positive feedback to make the family identifiable as such and enough negative feedback to give the individual members a sense of separate identity and to give the family a sense that it changes over time. Actions by the family, directed toward society (and, similarly, actions by society, directed toward the family) need to be evaluated in the context of a communication process and accurately interpreted. Only when these conditions are fulfilled can families balance emotional and intellectual systems in a societal context.

Therapy Using Family Systems Theory

The goal of family therapy based on family systems theory is to work with a family system to achieve a more functional level of differentiation in family members. In each family member as well as the family as a whole, both the forces of fusion and the forces of differentiation are instinctive; a continuous effort is needed to balance these forces. When anxiety is present, achieving a balance becomes more difficult. The family therapist tries to help families remain connected without submerging individuals in a "family we-ness," and to help individuals draw boundaries and hold functional positions so that they will not be weighed down by the system.[16]

Families seek help when they are confronted with issues that inhibit the effective functioning of the family system. These issues may have to do with maturational crises (such as the birth of a child, the death of a significant other, and the "empty nest" syndrome), situational crises (such as unemployment, relocation, divorce, and serious illness), or other stressful events (such as marital conflict, younger children's problems in school, and setting limits for adolescents). Family therapy should be considered the treatment of choice for dysfunctional families characterized by marital conflict, dysfunction of a spouse, or projection of anxiety onto a child or children.

A family therapist may meet with only one member of a family, some members, or all members; but in any case he or she will conceptualize the presenting problem from a family systems perspective—that is, the therapist will consider the totality of interacting forces within the family that have contributed to the emergence of the identified problem.

A three- or four-generation genogram will allow the therapist to trace family processes over several generations; for a description of genograms, see "Assessment of the Family" later in this chapter. In assessing the family, the therapist will identify nodal events, relevant patterns of behavior, patterns of relationships, "toxic" family issues, and the family's "operating principles," styles of coping, and level of differentiation. This information enables the therapist to identify the "triangles" that are operating within the system and contributing to dysfunction in family members. When the family assessment has been completed, the therapist can formulate a plan for intervention.[22,23]

Following the assessment, the therapist reframes the presenting problem as a family problem. For example:

> The K. family presents its problem as an acting-out adolescent daughter. The therapist reframes this as a family problem in which Mr. and Mrs. K, the parents, have relinquished their authority and control because one of them acts as the "nice guy" and the other as the "heavy"; and in which the daughter is trying, dysfunctionally, to separate from the nuclear family.

Here, the therapist has reframed the problem so that it can be expressed as a situation in which the entire family is having trouble coping with the issue of separation. This strategy establishes the family (rather than any individual) as the client.

The therapist also explains how triangles operate to perpetuate dysfunctional patterns of relationships. Demonstrating how *all* members of a three-person triangle contribute to it is central to this intervention. For example:

> Alison M., when she feels neglected by her husband, Nick (who works long hours), goes to her mother (Irene P.) to complain. Irene lectures Nick about his responsibilities as a husband. Nick, who feels unappreciated, works even longer hours and moves further and further away from his wife—which leaves Alison and Irene in an overclose position. Alison, Nick, and Irene never discuss these problematic issues, and so the issues remain unresolved.

The therapist would encourage "detriangulation" by promoting a one-to-one relationship in each dyad involved. The husband and wife would be encouraged to talk to each other directly about their feelings instead of "triangling in" the wife's mother or the husband's work as a distancing maneuver. The daughter and mother would learn to talk to each other about themselves rather than about the husband. The husband and mother-in-law would establish communication about issues in their own relationship rather than issues in the marital relationship. All this would promote more flexible, more appropriate "relationship boundaries."

Movement toward a higher level of differentiation of self is crucial in any intervention plan.[23] The therapist works back and forth between the generations, "coaching" family members about how to move back into family relationships in a less emotionally reactive way. For example:

> Marlene and Steve are contemplating a divorce. Steve has been an inattentive, achievement-oriented husband; moreover, he was not Marlene's first choice as a spouse. She married a safe, secure man rather than the love of her life, who was a risk. She is currently having an affair with a second "love of her life" and is planning to leave Steve to live with him. The nurse urges her to explore her extended family history before making a decision on the basis of emotionality rather than rationality. The nurse "coaches" her to talk with her mother, her grandmother, and her sister—each of whom (she learns) married a "safe" man and later regretted the choice. Marlene has to ask herself if, in opting to leave her "safe" husband for her "romantic" lover, she is making a decision on her own behalf or for the collective "we" of all the women in her extended family who made a safe, but regretted, choice. After many months of active work on many family relationships, Marlene is finally able to arrive at a differentiated

"I" position: "I may not be madly in love with my husband, but my priorities are such that the best decision for me is to remain married to Steve and try to make my marriage better." A parallel process is carried out with Steve and his family to explore and resolve his emotional distancing as well as his frantic drive for success, which has precluded important personal relationships.

Family systems therapy extends over a prolonged period of time. The therapist works with a consistent or shifting family membership, depending on what needs to be accomplished and by whom. The ultimate goal is the development of personal relationships within the family in which there will be less reactivity and a more solid sense of self, reflected in a better balance between the intellectual and emotional systems. These qualities enable people to move together and apart flexibly and functionally and to guide their lives effectively, particularly when anxiety is high.

Structural Family Therapy

Concepts of Structural Family Theory

The theoretical foundation of structural family therapy is the premise that individuals as well as families are embedded in social contexts within which they act and react.[24] A basic assumption of this theory is that behavior is a consequence of the organization and structure of the family and of patterns of interaction between and among family members. The organization and structure of the family "screen" and qualify family members' experiences.[24] According to this theoretical framework, the family does not totally determine an individual's inner processes. Rather, the individual influences his or her context, and the context influences the individual in recurring sequences of interaction. Therefore, changing a family's organization and structure contributes to changes in the inner processes and behavior of members of that family system. When a therapist works with a family, he or she becomes part of the context. Minuchin and others associated with the Philadelphia Child Guidance Clinic are most closely identified with this theoretical approach.[24]

Family structure influences the level of function or dysfunction exhibited by a family. From a structural perspective, function and dysfunction are determined by the "fit"—or "goodness of fit," as it is often described—between a system's structural organization and the requirements of particular circumstances. *Structural organization of families* refers to relationship patterns common to all families, modified by the idiosyncrasies of each family, with its traditions and its cultural and socioeconomic situation, and by each family's adaptations to meet its functional requirements. *Functions* have to do with all areas of human social activity. *Circumstances* refers to the context—that is, the time, place, and social parameters within which families or family members operationalize the structure in carrying out a function.

Dysfunctional structures are not symptom-specific, since it is the "fit" of a family and its subsystems to the requirements of functions in particular circumstances that determines whether a problem will or will not arise. For example, suppose that a young girl has school phobia. To say that she is not going to school because she is "locked into a stable coalition" against her father does not in itself explain the problem. One would also need to understand the structural pattern of these relationships and the functional purposes it serves for the family and the social context. The nature and purposes of a structure "maintain" a dysfunction.

Components of Structural Family Therapy

Three components are central to the structural model:

1. Families as social systems in transformation
2. Families as social units passing through predictable series of developmental stages that require adaptive restructuring
3. Major elements of family structure: power, sets of relationships, boundaries

Each of these components contributes to understanding and predicting family phenomena from a structural perspective.

THE FAMILY AS A SOCIAL SYSTEM IN TRANSFORMATION. The family is a social system that is always undergoing transformations; that is, the family constantly changes in ways that parallel societal changes. The family system must maintain its integrity and continuity so that family members can grow and change; at the same time, it must adapt to both internal and external stressors. Family functions, then, serve two different needs: (1) psychological protection and support of family members; (2) accommodation of the family to a culture and transmission of a culture to family members.[24]

The ideas of ongoing transition and an ever-present need for family members to accommodate to change are integral to the structural model. Behavior that might be labeled *pathological* by a traditional therapist would be seen by a structural therapist as a manifestation of normal anxiety that characterizes transitional stages and accommodation to new circumstances.[24]

FAMILY DEVELOPMENTAL STAGES. The family goes through predictable stages of development over time, and each stage requires adaptive restructuring. At every stage, there are developmental tasks that must be accomplished before the family can move on to the next stage. This notion is analagous to the stages of the family life cycle described by Duvall and Carter and McGoldrick[8,9] (discussed earlier; see Table 19-2). A functional family adapts to new developmental tasks and restructures itself in order to continue functioning. Families which are unable to transform themselves over time and instead continue to adhere inappropriately to previous structural schemas are those in which stress builds up and symptoms develop.

MAJOR ELEMENTS OF FAMILY STRUCTURE. The major elements of family structure are power, sets of relationships, and boundaries. A structure can become dysfunctional in any one of these areas.[25]

Power. Every family has a structure of power. As in any organization, there is a hierarchy of power—that is, an arrangement of different levels of power and authority—and this hierarchy is necessary for effective functioning. Power can be described or defined as the *relative* influence of each family member on the outcome of an activity;[26] structurally, it is comparative, not absolute. (For example, a mother's influence on her adolescent children's behavior may be effective at home, but minimal in terms of their social behavior outside the home.) Power is generated by the way which family members combine, both actively and passively, to determine the outcome of a transaction. (For example, a mother's authority is, in part, a function of the cooperation of her husband and the acquiescence of her children.)

Power is an "action dimension"; it defines family members in terms of boundaries (inside or outside the system) and alignment (for or against an issue). For example, when power is considered in terms of boundaries and alignments, the parents in a family are viewed as the disciplinarians; the mother may be the rule maker, and the father may play a supportive role. *Alignment* would indicate on which disciplinary issues they agree or disagree with one another and with their children. *Power* would indicate which of the parents would prevail if they disagreed, and whether they could impose their discipline on the children even when they did agree.

Sets of family relationships. Sets of family relationships are formed by subsystems. Subsystems are formed within a system; they consist of individuals or dyads and can be formed according to generation, sex, interest, or function.[24] Each family member belongs to various subsystems with different levels of power. Each subsystem has functions to fulfill and interpersonal developmental tasks to accomplish.

Individuals who are carrying out particular subsystem functions define their own and each other's roles with respect to the operations of a function. Parents, for example, have roles in relation to their children which they choose for themselves and which society will define; these roles will determine what tasks parents themselves do for their children, what tasks they share with others, and what tasks they hand over completely to others. Table 19-4 summarizes the functions and tasks of specific family subsystems.

Boundaries. The concept of boundaries is basic to an understanding of subsystem functions. The boundaries of a subsystem define the participants in subsystem functions and determine how they accomplish tasks.[24]

In order for families to function effectively, boundaries must be clear and firmly established. They must be defined precisely enough to prevent intrusion by other subsystems, but not so rigidly as to preclude emotional connectedness among family members. (For example, the parent subsystem must establish clear boundaries in terms of parenting functions that are not intruded upon by the grandparent subsystem, which may think it knows better how to discipline children.)

Families with boundary problems are described as either enmeshed or disengaged. In an *enmeshed* family, boundaries are diffuse, permeable, and fluid. Development of autonomy and competence is in-

Table 19-4 Tasks and Functions of Family Subsystems

Subsystem	Tasks and Functions
Spouse subsystem	The spouses must develop patterns in which each spouse supports the other's functioning in many areas. They develop patterns of complementarity that allow each spouse to "give in" without feeling that he or she has "given up." Both spouses accommodate to each other and yield part of their separateness to gain in "belonging." This manifests itself in functional interdependence which fosters learning, creativity, and growth. A spouse subsystem with a firm boundary that protects it from intrusion by other subsystems becomes a haven or refuge from the demands of life.
Parental subsystem	The parental subsystem must accommodate the addition of children and must learn the task of nurturing and socializing a child without losing the mutual support that should characterize the spouse subsystem. It must adapt to new factors impinging on the tasks of socialization such as the emerging needs of growing children for autonomy. The parental subsystem must exercise flexible, rational authority and establish rules that change as children reach different developmental stages. Ultimately, it must nurture, guide, and control the children in a process that encourages the development of autonomy.
Sibling subsystem	The sibling subsystem is the arena in which children learn how to be functional people. They experiment with peer relationships and in this context learn from each other the fundamentals of peer interaction—that is, how to support, isolate, "scapegoat," cooperate, negotiate, and compete. The sibling subsystem is one arena for learning about power, alliances, and boundaries. Children use what they have learned in the sibling subsystem (as well as other subsystems to which they belong) when they relate to subsystems outside the family.

hibited by the diffuseness of the boundaries. Perceptions of self and others are poorly differentiated.[27] A child in such a family may be so sensitized to conflict in the marital subsystem that he or she develops a school phobia. A highly enmeshed subsystem of mother and children can exclude the father, who becomes extremely disengaged; the resulting undermining of the children's independence might lead to the development of symptoms. In the subsystem, the behavior of one member immediately affects others, and stress experienced by an individual reverberates strongly across boundaries and is echoed in other subsystems.

In a *disengaged* family, boundaries are inappropriately rigid. Such a family will exhibit poor and minimal communication between subsystems. Supportive or protective contact is also minimal. Members of disengaged subsystems may appear to function autonomously; however, they have an exaggerated sense of independence, and they lack feelings of loyalty and belonging and the capacity for interdependence.

Therapy Using Structural Family Theory

The goal of structural family therapy is to solve problems by changing the underlying structure of the family system. A structural family therapist views a problem to be dealt with as sustained by the current structure of the family, the environmental context, or both. Therefore, whatever the history of the problem, the dynamics that maintain it are currently active in the structure of the system, manifesting themselves in the transactional patterns of the family.[28]

The therapist initiates the therapeutic process by *joining* the family—that is, temporarily becoming part of the family system by adapting his or her behavior to its rules and styles. In joining the family and accommodating to its organization and style, the therapist experiences the family's transactional patterns and can evaluate their intensity. For example, the therapist should be able to feel a family member's pain at being excluded or made a scapegoat, as well as pleasure at being loved, depended on, or otherwise "confirmed" within the family system. Table 19-5 summarizes methods of joining families.

As the therapist joins the family, *assessment* begins. The assessment process consists of identifying the problem, determining its location in the

Table 19-5 Methods of "Joining" Families

Methods	Description	Example
Mirroring or mimicking	The therapist matches the family's mood, pace, communication patterns, or kinesthetic cues.	The nurse adapts a family's slow tempo of communication by accommodating to its pattern of long pauses and slow responses.
Respecting values and hierarchies	The therapist confirms and supports the family's values and structural hierarchies.	The nurse acknowledges the parents' executive position in a family by directing the first questions to them or temporarily accepting their labeling of the "identified patient."
Highlighting elements of cultural or developmental similarity	The therapist confirms that therapist and family members are human beings who have common experiences. This helps the family to develop a sense of kinship with the therapist.	Following the Smiths' description of their problematic adolescent, the therapist states, "I have two adolescent children, myself."
Observing a family's strengths	The therapist searches for any evidence (even the minutest) of characteristics or behaviors in family members that can be identified, confirmed, or supported as actual or potential strengths, thereby bolstering a member's position in the family.	The nurse might comment on a perceptive remark made by a child in the family, praise the way a family member coped with a situation, or compliment a family member on a new outfit or hairdo.
Supporting the structure of family subsystems	The therapist encourages appropriate boundary functions by supporting specific subsystems within the family.	The nurse encourages the spouses to support each other in dealing with the adolescent subsystem or supports an adolescent subgroup in a large sibling subsystem by recommending that younger children not attend certain sessions.
Tracking	The therapist follows the content of the family's communication and behavior by asking for elaboration of details and examples pertaining to specific content under discussion in order to be able to explore the family's structure.	The nurse "tracks" a comment on the part of a father that the house in which the family lives is too small by asking him in what way is it too small. He responds by saying he has no place to call his own. This comment is "tracked" to the point of finding out that there is an enmeshed mother-child subsystem which has excluded the father, who feels disengaged from the family.

"family-environment matrix," and identifying the structures that sustain the problem.

The knowledge needed to formulate a *diagnosis* and begin restructuring dysfunctional transactions is available quickly. Structural family therapy does not explore or interpret the past. It is active and present-oriented. Diagnosis in structural family therapy is based on the therapist's joining the family and observing and experiencing its interactional patterns as well as his or her impact on it. An "interactional diagnosis" is not static; it changes as the family accommodates to or resists a therapist's interventions, and it will depend on which family subsystem is actively involved in the therapeutic process at any time. To this extent, assessment, diagnosis, and intervention are inseparable.

Intervention begins as the therapist joins the family, while maintaining a leadership position. The goal of restructuring interventions is to transform the dysfunctional transactional patterns that maintain symptomatic behavior in one or more family members. However, the therapist strives for more than relief of symptoms. Equally important is changing the organization of the family so that a symptom is not passed on from one family member to another. Areas of family organization that do not maintain symptoms are not dealt with in the therapeutic process. The primary focus of treatment is the nuclear family, unless there is a specific indication that extended-family subsystems should be included.

Seven categories of restructuring interventions have been identified by Minuchin:[24]

1. Enacting family transactional patterns
2. Marking boundaries
3. Escalating stress
4. Assigning tasks
5. Using symptoms
6. Manipulating mood
7. Supporting, educating, and guiding

Table 19-6 summarizes the restructuring interventions and provides an example of each. Such inter-

Table 19-6 Restructuring Interventions

Intervention	Description	Example
Enacting transactional patterns	Family members are encouraged to discuss an issue among themselves rather than describe it to the therapist. Thus the therapist is able to disengage from the interaction, observe the family, and thereby understand the structure that underlies the interaction.	An adolescent boy begins to tell the therapist that his mother treats him like a baby. The therapist tells the boy, "Talk with your mother about that."
Marking individual and subsystem boundaries	In enmeshed families, boundaries are strengthened to facilitate the individuation of family members; in disengaged families, the rigidity of boundaries is decreased.	The nurse instructs family members that they are to speak to each other, not about each other; that no one speaks for another; that no one may interrupt; and that no one acts as another's "memory bank."
	Individual boundaries are delineated by imposing simple rules as overall guidelines governing the family unit. Subsystem boundaries are encouraged by the therapist's inclusion or exclusion of various subsystems attending a session as well as by the assignment of subsystem tasks.	The nurse asks the children to leave (or not attend) a session that will focus on effective parenting patterns. The nurse assigns the husband and wife the task of going out one night of the week without their children. This is designed to strengthen the boundaries of the spouse subsystem.
Escalating stress	Stress is escalated in order to force family members to develop alternative, more functional ways of dealing with it. Dysfunctional transactional patterns of handling stress have developed around the symptomatic member. Maneuvers that produce stress include: blocking usual transactional patterns; emphasizing differences the family is glossing over; making covert conflict overt and temporarily joining in alliance or coalition with a family member or subsystem.	In the D. family, the mother translates the children's communications to their father and his to them. The nurse intervenes, saying, "Excuse me, Ruth," and, "Go ahead" to the father, who had been interrupted by his wife when starting to talk to his son. In the R. family, there is a need for all family members to agree about everything. The nurse, attempting to highlight differences, asks each family member for his or her opinion. The J. family has developed a "method" for defusing conflict rapidly: their child, Luke, throws up whenever his parents enter into conflict. The therapist intervenes by blocking the child's interference in the parental conflict, thus allowing it to escalate. In the P. family, the nurse allies with the wife in her attacks on her husband in order to escalate the conflict to the point where he cannot diffuse it by making their son a scapegoat. The husband is forced to address the conflict between himself and his wife.

(Continued.)

Table 19-6 Continued

Intervention	Description	Example
Assigning tasks	Tasks are assigned to establish an alternative structure for transactions. The goal is to alter a specific dysfunctional pattern. It is important to give each involved member a portion of the task to complete. This decreases the likelihood that one member will sabotage the new behavior of another if each is focused on himself or herself. It is also easier for each person to relinquish a dysfunctional behavior if there is a new one available to replace it.	In a family in which the wife always disciplines the children, excluding the father, the discipline functions are reassigned to the father. The wife is instructed to handle only emergencies, informing her husband of any infractions he does not observe himself. The wife is instructed not to interfere with her husband's disciplinary tactics, even if she disapproves. She is to observe the effect of the discipline on the children's behavior. This intervention equalizes the authority in the parental subsystem.
Using symptoms	Existing symptoms may be used to restructure dysfunctional transactions by focusing on them, by exaggerating them to increase their intensity and thereby mobilize family resources, or by redefining them. By proceeding in one of the above directions, the symptom's effect is changed.	Minuchin describes a family in which the daughter is a fire setter. The "symptom focus" remains on the daughter, but the mother is instructed to spend time daily teaching her daughter how to light matches safely. This promotes a closer mother-daughter relationship (which was previously obstructed). The mother is indirectly forced to interact with the daughter in a competent, educative manner.
Manipulating family mood	The therapist uses an exaggerated imitation of the family's affect to trigger "counteraffect" in the family, thereby stimulating a wider range of affective expression. The therapist may also act as a role model for more appropriate affect in the family. This promotes more appropriate emotional responsiveness on the part of family members.	In a family with an overcontrolling father who yells to force his adolescent children into obedience, the therapist becomes even more aggressive toward the children, forcing the father to soften his mode of contact and give them more autonomy. In a family that is very anxious and controlled, the therapist may want to model a calm, relaxed, accepting mood.
Supporting, educating, and guiding	This type of restructuring operation may consist of modeling, assigning tasks, or sharing concrete information. It serves a healing, nurturing, and support function in families. Members who grew up with transactional defects may have to be taught them now.	In an enmeshed family, the nurse may have to teach the parents how to respond differentially to their children. A therapist may have to teach a child the "tricks of the trade" in getting along at school.

ventions confront and challenge a family in an attempt to force a therapeutic change.

Structural family therapy is used to assist families in changing the organization of the whole family and allowing individual members to have new experiences within it. Restructuring of family transactional patterns occurs in a defined way; it either promotes existing functional subsystems or helps dysfunctional subsystems to reorganize so that new subsystems that will be more functional and growth-promoting can be formed.

Strategic Family Therapy

Concepts of Strategic Family Theory

Strategic family therapy, also referred to as *problem-solving therapy* or *brief therapy,* has its origins in communication theory. The pioneering work of Bateson, Weakland, Haley, and Jackson focused on the nature of observable, face-to-face verbal and nonverbal communication among members of a family and its significance in shaping actual behavior.[29,30] The early communications theorists proposed that all behavior—verbal as well as nonverbal—is communication; and that, since there is no such thing as "nonbehavior," it is impossible *not* to communicate.[31] (See Chapter 12.) They also proposed that most communication does not consist of simple declarative messages. Instead, there are several levels of meaning between sender and receiver. The verbal and nonverbal levels of messages modify and qualify each other. The significance of a message is a function of how it is "confirmed," "contradicted," or "positioned" by preceding or subsequent messages, of the setting in which it is conveyed, and of the relationship between the sender and the receiver. All these factors make up a context that needs to be considered when a message is being interpreted.[30] Communication theorists have also proposed that communication is an ongoing process; it has no beginning and no end but rather is a highly patterned, circular process of repetitive interactions by people in "relationship contexts."

Communication theory suggests that the potential for pathology is high when a family system consisting of two or more people is dysfunctional in its communication. Several forms of pathological communication have been identified by researchers studying the communication patterns of schizophrenic families; these are summarized in Table 19-7.

On the basis of early communication theories of behavior, the goals established for family therapy were to correct pathological modes of communication and to facilitate functional patterns of communication between family members. Functional communication would be characterized by clear, direct messages and by the requesting and receiving of feedback. Behavioral change would occur, and dysfunctions within the family system would be resolved, as a result of direct, clear, unambiguous communication.[31] Communications theorists extended their theoretical formulations, which were based on research with schizophrenic families, to families with other clinical problems; they found that the communications model was also useful in understanding families with psychosomatic, marital, and child-focused problems. This theory, grounded in "here and now" observation of communication patterns in families, was a bridge to the formulation of strategic family therapy.

Weakland, Fisch, and Watzlawick, of the original communications theory group, established the Brief Therapy Center at the Mental Research Institute

Table 19-7 Pathological Communication Patterns

Form	Description	Example
Disqualification	This includes contradictions, inconsistencies, changes of subject, misunderstandings, "tangentializations," incomplete sentences, obscure speech mannerisms, and literal interpretation of metaphor.	A son says to his mother, "I want to go to Johnny's after school today." The mother responds by saying, "What did you say you wanted for dinner?"
Disconfirmation	This involves ignoring or invalidating essential elements of a significant other's perception of himself or herself, of a situation which he or she has experienced, by saying, "You don't really feel the way you say you feel, need what you say you need, or experience what you say you experience."	Susan tells her mother, "I want to go on a vacation with my friends instead of with the family this summer." Her mother responds, "You're just saying that. You can't really want to do that. You'd have much more fun with us."
Incongruent messages (double-bind)	This consists of delivering two conflicting messages simultaneously. The receiver is in a "double bind," of not knowing which message he or she should respond to. It is usually the case that the receiver is in a "no win" situation; if the receiver responds to either message, he or she is "mad" or "bad."	A father offers his son a job immediately following graduation from college. As the son accepts the job offer, the father says angrily, "What's the matter? Don't you have enough ambition to look for a job on your own?"

SOURCE: From P. Watzlawick, J. Beavin, and D. Jackson, *Pragmatics of Human Communications,* Norton, New York, 1967.

(MRI) in Palo Alto, California. They believed that therapy could be short-term and still be effective. Therefore, they looked constantly not only for strategies to effect change but also for strategies to shorten treatment. They focused on the function rather than the meaning of behavior—on "what" rather than "why." At the same time, the work of Haley on the east coast established the validity of a problem-focused approach to family therapy. The work of Milton Erickson[32] on "paradoxical instruction" became an integral component of structural family therapy. Palazzoli-Selvini[33,34] and her associates in Milan, Italy, have refined the use of paradox as an essential tool of strategic therapy. The focus of strategic family therapy today is on understanding how symptoms arise and how they are resolved, particularly with the use of "paradoxical intention."[35]

Therapy Using Strategic Family Theory

The primary goal of strategic family therapy is to remove presenting symptoms through directives or tasks in conjunction with the use of paradox. A *paradox* is defined as an intervention which "prescribes the symptom" or uses reversal and carries the message, "Do more of it" or "Do not change." A *symptom* is regarded as a communicative act, with characteristics of a message, which serves as a contract between two or more people and has a function within an interpersonal network. A symptom usually appears when a person is locked into a pattern of communication with the rest of the family or significant others and cannot envision a nonsymptomatic way of changing the pattern. The symptom serves a function in the family; it maintains the status quo. As a result, the individual cannot change unless the family system changes.

It is not necessary for a family to have "insight" about a problem in order to change. Strategic therapists are not concerned with the history of problems or the motivation behind them. Little distinction is made between acute and chronic problems. The presenting problem and the family behaviors that maintain it are of primary importance.[36]

Communication theorists borrowed from cybernetics in identifying a "positive feedback loop" in human interaction (see Chapter 12). This is a vicious circle that develops when family members or "identified patients" make misguided efforts to improve or stop problematic behavior. For example, a family with a depressed father may try frantically to cheer him up. In such a case, the family may be unable to see, and the father may be unable to say, that what their help amounts to is a demand that the father have certain feelings (joy, optimism) and not others (sadness, pessimism). As a result, what for the father may have been only temporary sadness now becomes laden with feelings of failure, despair, and guilt; the family's attempt to alleviate the problem has only exacerbated it. Resolution of this situation would require changing behaviors that maintain the problem; such change would take the form of interrupting the positive feedback loop.[36,37]

Because strategic therapy is short-term and problem-focused, assessment, diagnosis, and intervention are integrated or "telescoped." Entry into the system begins either with an "identified patient" or with some other member of the family, depending on who is most concerned about or uncomfortable with the problem and thus most willing to change. Effective intervention (breaking the positive feedback loop) can be made through any person in the system.

Strategic therapists often work with a consultation team; members of this team either view the sessions from behind a one-way mirror or are present in the therapy room. In either case, they interrupt at significant moments to consult with the therapist or communicate as a "Greek chorus" with the therapist and the family, to facilitate change.[38]

Since the goal of strategic therapy is to change a dysfunctional sequence of behaviors, the therapist and the consulting team begin by observing interactional sequences of problematic behavior. For example, if the members of a family say, "We are too emotional; we fight all the time," the therapist will first elicit a detailed description of what "being too emotional" means to them and will try to concretely identify all the elements preceding and following the problem (who does what and when) and to identify potential behaviors to be changed. The therapist also wants to find out what solutions the family members have already tried. This provides a clue about what remedies to avoid and also reveals "problem-maintaining" behavior. The family would be asked to identify a minimal goal for treatment—that is, what smallest identifiable change would be evidence of progress or success. "Global" goals, such as, "We'd fight less," "We'd be less emotional," and "We'd be happier," are too vague. Action-oriented behavioral goals that delineate observable behavioral changes are required.

The therapist reframes the problem in language that is congruent with the family's world view—that is, places the problem in another "frame" that fits the "facts" of the situation equally well, thereby changing its meaning.[36] For example:

> A family consisting of a mother, a father, and an acting-out teenage daughter, Jane, identify the problem as the child's delinquent behavior and the conflict that ensues about it. The parents are "verbally killing" each other because of disagreements about how to deal with Jane's behavior. The therapist reframes this as a disagreement between two people who care for each other and their child.

The heart of intervention in strategic family therapy is directives in the form of paradoxical injunctions. (As was noted above, the use of paradox is closely associated with Haley and Erickson, among others; however, Selvini-Palazzoli and her associates in Milan have gained increasing recognition for their refinement of the use of paradox in strategic family therapy.) *Paradoxical* interventions are those which appear absurd because they are apparently contradictory; a family may be required to do what in fact it has been doing, and sometimes to do more of it, rather than changing (which is what everyone else is demanding).[39] This is based on the premise that families will instinctively resist change, as well as a therapist's efforts to initiate change, in order to preserve the status quo. If the therapist "prescribes the symptom"—that is, the status quo—families will resist that directive (and the therapist who has given it) and begin to change. The family will move toward the goal by proving that the therapist is wrong. Paradoxical directives can be given to one, several, or all family members. For example:

> A boy who had stomachaches when his parents left him alone was instructed to try to get sick at a particular time, while the parents were instructed to go outside the house together for at least 10 minutes at the same time.

If a client improves too rapidly, or if the therapist has reason to expect that symptoms will recur, a relapse may be prescribed.

In the strategic therapy model, the therapist is an active, purposeful change agent who formulates a strategy, sometimes in collaboration with a consultation group, that will effect change in the family system. The therapeutic process ends when the problematic symptom is alleviated; this may occur after 3 to 20 sessions.

Strategic therapy is often described as "insincere," "gimmicky," and "manipulative." Strategic therapists acknowledge that these descriptions have some validity. However, research on communication has made it clear that it is impossible *not* to communicate, and a logical extension of this idea is the idea that it is impossible *not* to influence others. Acting on this premise, strategic therapists influence a person or family to change "spontaneously" by arranging a situation in which the people involved will initiate the change in behavior, and thus accomplish the goals of therapy.[40]

NURSING PROCESS

Regardless of the theoretical model that is utilized to conceptualize—that is, think about and understand—a family's functional and dysfunctional behavior patterns, the nursing process provides a framework for organizing assessment data about families, diagnosing family problems, formulating treatment goals and interventions, and evaluating outcomes.

Assessment of the Family

Several assessment models may be utilized by nurses who need information about clients and their families. A comprehensive model involves holistic evaluation of the structural, functional, and developmental aspects of the family. The family is viewed as a system characterized by phenomena that can be described in terms of triangles, projection, closeness, and cutoff. Information about structural elements will include household composition, boundaries, subsystems, culture, and family of origin. Information about the developmental stage of a family will include marriages, ages of children and grandchildren, functional and dysynchronous patterns of behavior, attachments, cutoffs, processes of socialization evident in the family, and if and how developmental tasks are being completed.

Information about functioning will include allocation of work, daily routines, roles, and communication patterns. Information about the larger external structure, or social environment, will include the culture, religion, social class, and potential social mobility of a family. Information about the immediate environment will include the family's dwelling, neighborhood, and access to community services. An assessment will also note how the nuclear family interacts with its extended family network.

A *genogram* provides the nurse with a helpful way to outline a family's internal structure; an *ecomap* depicts a family's outside contacts. *Family processes* also need to be assessed.

Tools of Assessment

GENOGRAM. A genogram is a diagrammatic historical "map" of a family over three generations.[41] Figure 19-7 is a genogram of a three-generation family, the S.'s.

DESCRIPTION OF A THREE-GENERATION FAMILY: THE S. FAMILY

Bob S., a 48-year-old, married, middle-class Jewish male, is admitted to a coronary-care unit (CCU) in acute cardiac distress. His wife, Joan, a 47-year-old housewife, is recovering from a mastectomy following a diagnosis of breast cancer. Their children, Eric and Peter, ages 18 and 20, are (respectively) in the freshman and junior year of college.

There is a family history of coronary artery disease among male members of Bob's family. His father, grandfather, natural uncles, and only brother all died of heart disease before age 50. Bob is the only surviving male in his family other than his sons. Joan has a family history of death from cancer. Her mother and maternal aunts died of breast cancer. Joan's mastectomy was done 6 weeks before her husband's heart attack.

Joan is an only child. She and Bob are the last surviving members of their families of origin. Three months ago, Joan and Bob's youngest son Eric left home to begin college; he is unhappy at school.

During the interview when Bob is admitted to the CCU, Joan describes herself as a high-strung worrier

Figure 19-7 Three-generation genogram.
This genogram is based on assessment data from the S. family.

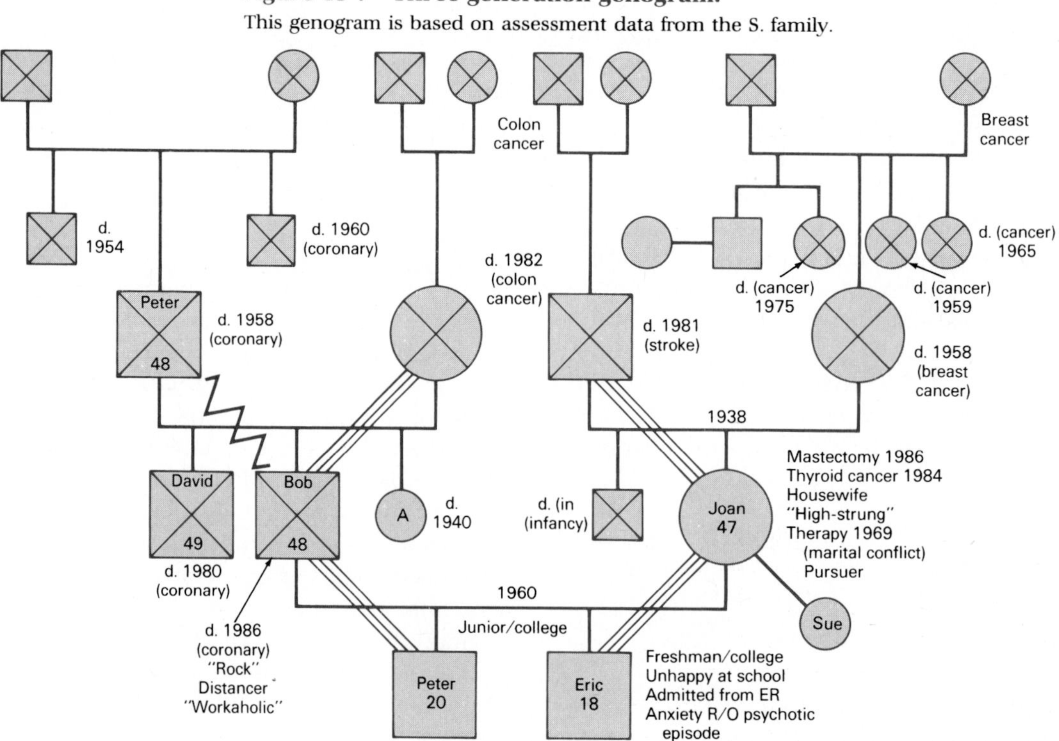

who leans on her husband for everything; she describes Bob as her "rock." Financially they are comfortable. He is self-insured. She has worked part-time in his business, and she is active in their local temple and as a volunteer in the town literacy program. As a couple they have an extensive social network. Bob is a division chairperson for United Way. They have a family membership in the local Jewish center, where they have both participated regularly in the exercise programs.

Three days after his admission to the CCU, Bob has a fatal myocardial infarction while Joan is alone in the CCU waiting room. She faints when she is told of Bob's death. When she is revived, she wails, "How could he do this to me? I'm all alone." She sits in the corner of the waiting room, weeping, as she waits for her sons to arrive. But at one point, she storms into the CCU and screams at the nurses, "You did this to him. He shouldn't have died. He's too young. I'm too young to be alone. I'm the one who was supposed to die. My sons need a father. What will they do?" One nurse matter-of-factly escorts her back to the waiting room and sits with her comfortingly until the sons arrive. They literally carry her to the car.

Joan's eldest son Peter and friends of the family make the funeral arrangements. Her friend Sue and Peter's fiancée Debbie organize the house for the mourning (*shiva*) period, and friends are organized to provide food and companionship. In fact, Sue sleeps with Joan for the entire week. Joan is basically immobilized by her grief and unable to participate in much of the mourning ritual. She is sedated with Valium, which controls her hysterical crying.

Eric, who has a history of anxiety attacks, hovers at his mother's side. Two nights after the funeral, he wakes up diaphoretic with palpitations and chest pain. He feels, he says, as if his body is about to explode. Peter, his brother, immediately calls an ambulance, and Eric is taken to the emergency room, at the same hospital where his father died. A physical examination reveals a normal electrocardiogram and no organic basis for his symptoms. However, he tells the nurse that, like his mother, he does not want to go on living without his father—that he wishes his body would disintegrate. The nurse observes his agitation and preoccupation and suggests admission to the psychiatric unit for further observation.

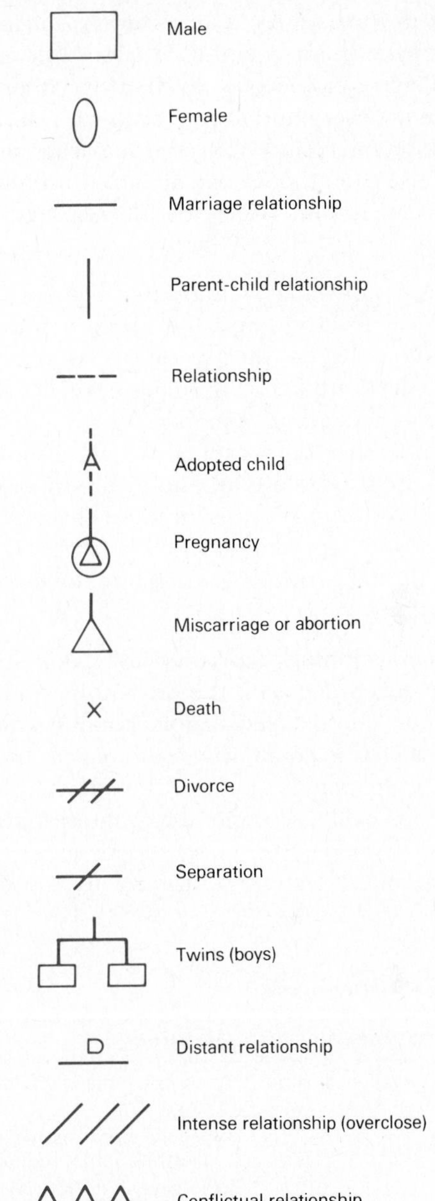

Figure 19-8 Genogram symbols.
(SOURCE: From E. Pendagast and C. Sherman, "A Guide to the Genogram," *The Family*, vol. 5, no. 1, 1976, pp. 101–112.)

Preparation of a genogram begins during the initial interview with a client. The genogram utilizes universally recognized symbols to note facts about a family; some of these are shown in Figure 19-8. The symbols are a kind of shorthand, understood by professionals who use this form for taking histories.

It is ideal to have all family members present for the initial interview; however, nurses most frequently obtain necessary information from individual clients themselves or from one other family member. (In the case of the S. family, for instance, most of the information about Eric was obtained from Peter, who accompanied his brother to the emergency room and stayed with him during the admission interview.) When the goal is to work with the family, even though not all family members are present for the interview, the following guidelines are helpful:

1. Leave empty chairs for absent members. (A chair was left for Joan, and the nurse made several references to her during the interview.)
2. Make it clear that no information will be withheld from absent family members.
3. When appropriate, explain which absent members are expected to attend future meetings.
4. Ask those who are present to invite and encourage absent family members to attend. (The nurse asked Peter to bring his mother to the next family meeting.)

At the beginning of an interview, the first task of the nurse is to focus on the presenting problem of the client. The detailed history obtained needs to be connected in some way to the reason the client is seeking help: for instance, "The information I am asking for will help me understand how your problem developed," and, "My experience has taught me that many factors contribute to a problem." Statements like these begin the process of creating a "systems attitude" toward the problem. The focus of attention is shifted from the "identified patient" to the family system as a whole, and thus the preparation of the genogram helps to reduce anxiety in the family. For example, in the case of the S. family the nurse might say to Eric, "Tell me about your father's family. It will help me to understand what you are feeling if I know more about them." The nurse might also ask Peter to talk about their mother. The focus is shifted from Eric's symptoms to the whole family.

To prepare the genogram, nurses ask a series of questions. As the genogram takes shape, facts such as names, nicknames, sexes, ages, sibling positions, and nodal events fill in the framework—the structure of the family. Level of functioning and emotional processes in the family are recorded as they are disclosed by family members. Table 19-8 includes the facts needed for the genogram, together with questions that facilitate gathering information and uncovering underlying family processes.

The initial process of data collection generally takes two or three meetings—or more, if a family is (like the S. family) experiencing a crisis. The genogram, however, is in a sense a "living map" and is never complete. New information is uncovered as data collection continues and the family

Table 19-8 Genograms

Information	Questions
Names, nicknames, family titles	What does that name signify to you? What does that name signify to other family members? Who gave you that title? What privileges or difficulties do you experience because you have that name, nickname, title, or label?
Ages	What else was happening when . . .?
Dates of nodal events (deaths, births, marriages, separations, divorces, moves, promotions, jobs)	How did you and your family respond to the event? Do you notice any coincidences? Do you see any relationship between your birth and grandmother's death?
Physical location of family members	How close or distant are you to ______? How close is "too close"? How and when do you contact ______? What were the reasons for the move? Where are members of the extended family located? Have any family members moved closer? When? What were the circumstances of that move?
Frequency of contact between members of the extended family and the quality of emotional contact	Do you receive surprise visits? How long do family members stay? Do the rules of visits vary for various family members?

(Continued.)

Table 19-8 Continued

Information	Questions	Information	Questions
Frequency of contact between members of the extended family and the quality of emotional contact	How do you communicate with each family member? Do you write, telephone, use audio cassettes, visit? Is reciprocity required? Suggested? Unimportant? Is there a clearinghouse for family information? Where is it? Who contacts whom? Is family business handled only at special events or holidays? How do people keep others informed about personal and life changes?	Characteristics of relationships (pursuit and distance)	Who is the pursuer? Who chased whom? Who ran away? Are you the pursuer or the distancer? How does that vary? When do you pursue or distance from others? How does that vary? Is there a difference for men or women? Is there a difference with age? Are pursuers and distancers in the family like anyone you know outside the family? Which issues do you pursue on? Which do you distance on? Are there family members with whom you have a "hearsay" relationship? (You hear about them but have no direct contact). Are there family members you have never met? What part do you play in the "family drama"? Which role do you pursue or distance from?
Closeness and distance on each generational level	In what ways are you close or distant? To which person in your own generation are you closest to or most distant from? In your grandmother's generation? Do you feel a difference in closeness to your children? Who is overly close? What are similarities in relationships? Differences? What is your style of closeness or distance? When you move toward distant family members, what happens? To you? To others? Which people in your family make your insides twitch? Which relationships are safe?	Emotional cutoffs	Who is cut off? When did that happen? What was the event? Does anyone talk to the cut-off family member? Who? When? What else was going on in the family at the time of the cutoff? What is still going on that allows the cutoff to continue? What would happen if the cutoff was healed?
Sibling position (the oldest is placed on the left in a genogram)	Who is oldest? Who is the "boss"? Who is the "baby"? Which family member is overly responsible? What are the patterns of behavior in the oldest of each generation? The youngest?		

SOURCE: Adapted from Eileen Pendagast and Charles Sherman, "A Guide to the Genogram," *The Family*, vol. 5, no. 1, 1976, pp. 101–112.

evolves, expands, or contracts over time. A useful way to include new information is to add it, with date, in a contrasting color.

ECOMAP. An ecomap is an overview of a nuclear family system within the context of the larger world—neighborhood and community.[42] It shows the relationship of family members to society and systems outside the structural boundaries of the nuclear household.

Figure 19-9 shows an ecomap of the S. family. The large circle at the center represents the nuclear

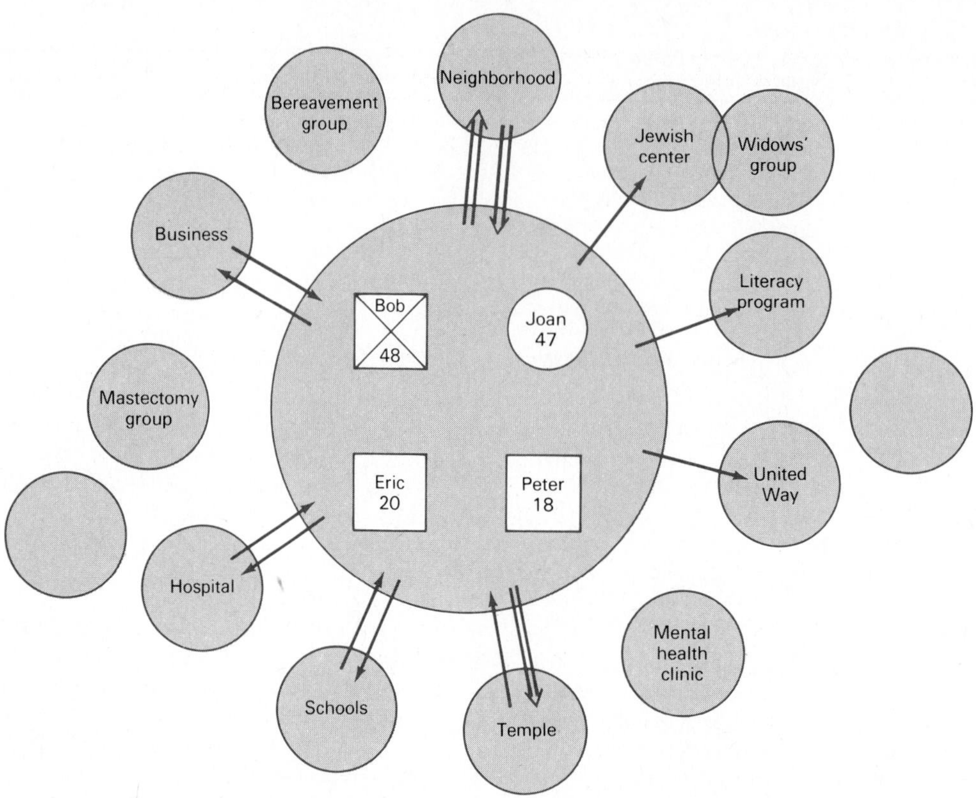

Figure 19-9 Ecomap.
This ecomap is based on assessment data from the S. family.

family. The smaller outer circles represent significant people, agencies, or institutions that make up the family's larger environment, or "context." In this case the "context" includes a neighborhood support group, a hospital, and a Jewish center. Lines are drawn between the circle at the center and the outer circles to indicate both the strength and the direction of connections.

Ecomaps are particularly helpful for nurses working with families that have multiple problems; they also serve as a guide to networking and consolidating services for families and can alert the nurse to social isolation or cutoffs. Potential networks can be sketched in one color and changed to another when contact has been made.

PROCESS ASSESSMENT. Although the genogram and the ecomap are useful in gathering and consolidating facts about families, it is also important for nurses to assess family processes. Levels of family functioning and stages of development are not always immediately clear. As time passes, however, clues are given, and these can provide the nurse with the needed data base. To obtain information, questions are organized to assess the congnitive, emotional, and spiritual "climate" of a family. Decision making, problem solving, and formation of goals are *cognitive* processes of families. Levels of differentiation of family members, degrees of interaction, triangles, and internal conflicts give clues to the *emotional* climate. The *spiritual* dimension of a family is assessed by asking about values and beliefs, ability to dream, productivity, plans for the future, and religious practices. Assessment questions include those listed in Table 19-9.

Analysis of Assessment Data

Assessment data—whether in the form of a genogram, an ecomap, information about family processes, or all three of these—need to be assessed

Table 19-9 Family Assessment

Questions	Questions
Physical functioning	**Emotional functioning**
How clear are family boundaries?	Is there mental illness in the family?
What is the cross-generational evidence of physical illness in the extended family?	What triangles have formed in the family?
What impact has physical illness had on the family system?	Are triangles rigid or fluid?
What is the family's lifestyle?	Are there indications of fusion (If so, identify them.)
Are family members isolated from the community?	What overt behaviors are observed?
Do cultural norms influence the family?	What behaviors do family members describe?
Is there evidence of physical illness in the family?	What emotional issues are revealed by the genogram?
What role does physical illness play for family members?	How are these issues played out in the family?
How are family members' concerns about health expressed?	To what degree do family members interact with harmony or conflict?
	What issues keep the family divided?
	Are there emotional cutoffs in the family?
Cognitive functioning	What are the cross-generational patterns of interaction?
How are decisions made?	Which members of the family are close?
Who has power in the family?	Which members are emotionally distant?
What are characteristics of the family decision-making process?	Are there coalitions within the family? (If so, who is involved in them?)
Are decisions clearly communicated?	Do communication patterns affect family functioning?
Are any family members eliminated from the decision-making process?	**Spiritual functioning**
How does the family handle financial problems?	What is the predominant "mood" of the family?
What intellectual resources do family members have?	How content do family members say they are?
What are the educational levels of family members?	What are the family's beliefs about life? About death?
Are these different from those of previous generations?	What values are evident in the family?
What is the developmental stage of the family?	What do family members believe in?
Are family roles enacted adequately?	What dreams and plans do family members have?
Is the developmental stage appropriate to the age of family members?	Do family members profess a particular religion? If so, what place does religion have in the family?
Are family rules clearly defined?	Do family members regularly attend a church, synagogue, etc.?
Who mediates interactions in the family?	What are the cross-generational spiritual patterns?

so that a nursing diagnosis and outcome criteria can be arrived at.

For example, the data about the S. family, described in the preceding sections, reveal several important patterns:

1. For three generations, all males on Bob's side of the family have died of coronary artery disease before age 50.
2. Joan's grandmother, mother, and maternal aunts all died of breast cancer at a relatively young age. Joan had a mastectomy, following a diagnosis of breast cancer, 6 weeks before Bob's death. (She also had thyroid cancer 2 years earlier).
3. There have been three significant deaths in the family (Bob's mother, Bob's brother, and Joan's father) in the past 5 years.
4. Peter and Eric are the only surviving males on either the paternal or the maternal side of the family.
5. Joan is a dependent, "nervous" person.
6. Eric, the youngest child, has just left home for college and has been unhappy at school.
7. Eric has had periodic anxiety attacks since he entered adolescence.
8. The family has no living blood relatives. The remarried husband of Joan's late aunt lives 500 miles away, and Joan maintains little contact with him.
9. The family has a very strong and extensive network of friends.

Following is an analysis of the assessment data for the S. family:

> A midlife family, with a family history of fatal coronary disease among males and breast cancer among females, has just experienced the unanticipated loss of an important family member—the husband and father. This loss has generated high levels of anxiety in the family. The mother is just recovering from another potentially fatal illness, one that has prematurely ended the lives of all her female relatives. This suggests the presence of a potential triangle including a "toxic" family issue: death.
>
> Joan, a dependent, tense woman, now has to cope with the loss of her husband (whom she described as her "rock"), her own health problems, the lack of an extended family, and the "empty nest" stage of the life cycle. Her sons have to deal with anxiety surrounding the loss of their father, the potential loss of their mother, and their paternal hereditary endowment, as well as the developmental tasks associated with leaving home and consolidating their identity as young adults.
>
> The family's anxiety appears to be expressed through Eric, the "anxious" child in the family, who has become increasingly dysfunctional since his father's death. It is probable that Eric has been involved in a mother-father-child triangle and that family anxiety has been projected onto him.

Table 19-10 The S. Family

Nursing Diagnoses
Actual problems
1. Grief reaction associated with the unanticipated death of the husband-father.
2. Severe anxiety of a child related to the projection of family anxiety.
3. Dependency related to history of role of emotionally underfunctioning spouse.
4. Lack of coping resources associated with incomplete recovery from mastectomy.
5. Absence of extended family support related to lack of living extended family.
Potential problems
1. Dysfunctional mourning related to feelings of abandonment.
2. Fear of living alone related to dependency needs.
3. Coping with "empty nest" syndrome associated with recent departure of youngest child and death of husband.
4. Fear of returning to school associated with history of unhappiness at school and overcloseness of mother and son.
5. Anxiety related to fears about recurrence of breast malignancy.
6. Difficulty in managing financial resources related to lack of experience and knowledge.
Strengths
1. Presence of a strong friendship network.
2. Strong nuclear-family relationships.
3. Spiritual connectedness with a local temple.
4. Involvement in community activities.
5. Successul launching into young adulthood of the older son.
6. Presence of financial resources.
7. Joan's work experience in Bob's business.

Diagnosis

Nursing diagnoses for families should include actual and potential family problems as well as strengths. Using data about the S. family, for example, a nurse would be able to formulate several diagnoses, which appear in Table 19-10.

Outcome Criteria

In working with families, short-term, intermediate, and long-term outcomes can be set. Usually, the nurse will initially encounter families when they are in crisis. The anxiety level of family members is high, forces of undifferentiation are ascendant, and thus dysfunctional thoughts, feelings, or behaviors are likely to be present in one or more family members. Family functioning may be disrupted or disorganized. In many cases, the family has tried using coping mechanisms, but without success. Consequently, the overall short-term outcome for such families would include evidence of ability to function on a daily basis. Intermediate outcomes are directed toward behaviors associated with initiation of the change process. Long-term outcomes are directed toward change in dysfunctional patterns of family interaction. Such patterns, created over time, may involve multiple physical, emotional, spiritual, and social factors and therefore will take longer to resolve.

For example, appropriate *short-term* outcomes for the S. family might include these:

- Family members verbally express feelings related to the death of the husband and father.
- Eric verbally expresses his suicidal thoughts.
- Eric uses physical activity to reduce anxiety.
- Joan uses the rabbi and her friends as a support system.

- Joan participates in household tasks such as cooking and marketing.

Appropriate *intermediate* outcomes for the S. family might include these:

- Eric utilizes relaxation exercises to reduce anxiety.
- Joan joins a bereavement group and a mastectomy group.
- Peter does not assume an overly responsible "parental" role.
- Eric makes plans to transfer to another college next semester.
- Joan consults with a financial planner.
- Joan returns to work.

Appropriate *long-term* outcomes for the S. family include these:

- The family confronts the "toxic" issue of death.
- Joan explores her dependency needs and her fear of independence.
- Joan verbally expresses her rage about abandonment.
- Joan and Eric verbally explore their overclose relationship.
- Peter reevaluates his relationship with his fiancée.
- Eric reduces his anxiety to a mild to moderate level through a relaxation and medication regimen.
- Eric returns to college.

A nurse who is involved with a family in an acute-care setting may not participate in the formulation or realization of all such outcomes. (Nurses' educational preparation, role, and exposure to families do not always make such involvement appropriate.) However, nurses who are knowledgeable about family theory and its application have a framework for understanding families, visualizing, their problems, and participating in the formulation of realistic outcomes.

Intervention

Nurses are often the first people who interact with families—during home visits, clinic appointments, or hospitalization. Nurses who are sensitive to family issues are in a position to intervene with families in a variety of ways. Generalist nurses commonly identify family problems during the assessment process. The type of intervention that is appropriate will vary, depending on their educational preparation and clinical expertise. For example, a staff nurse who identifies the presence of marital conflict in a mother-father-child triangle or alcoholism in a family member would intervene by referring the family to an appropriate community resource. On the other hand, a clinical specialist with postgraduate training in family therapy might become the therapist who works directly with the family on an ongoing basis. Nurses have many opportunities to intervene with families in primary (promotion and maintenance), secondary (restoration), and tertiary (rehabilitation) health care settings.

Promotion and Maintenance of Health

Primary prevention consists of intervening with healthy families to promote and maintain the health of the family system.

Nurses who work with childbearing families in prenatal or obstetrical settings can utilize a family framework. For example, the birth of a first child is an important nodal event. A dyad (the spouses) becomes a triad, moving from an adult relationship to one that must incorporate the child. As with any addition to or subtraction from a family, this event has implications for family health. Nurses can explore with the expectant couple the "meaning" of this baby, their plans for its care, and how it will change the relationship with each other and their extended family. Families benefit from education about developmental processes and about the fact that a baby will change their life. Predicting some of the common experiences and feelings that new parents encounter helps to normalize their experience as it occurs (see Chapter 47).

Restoration of Health

Secondary prevention consists of early case finding, prevention of serious family dysfunction, and restoration of functional health patterns. Nurses working in obstetrical, pediatric, medical, surgical, and psychiatric settings can utilize family theory when intervening with clients.

For example, secondary prevention strategies could be used with the S. family after the death of the husband and father, Bob, and Eric's acute anxiety attack. The family—Joan in particular—could be referred to a bereavement group to prevent serious dysfunction associated with dysfunctional grieving. Joan could also be referred to a mastectomy group. The family could be referred for family therapy to explore "toxic" family issues—death, dependency, and overcloseness between Joan and Eric—in order to prevent the family's anxiety and fusional forces from escalating dysfunction.

Pediatric nurses may intervene with families of sick children. A family with a sick child is vulnerable to fusional forces. For example, if a child has a health problem like asthma, the family will often respond in terms of guilt and blame. Parents may blame their own genetic history, their actions during pregnancy, their lack of skill as parents, or the health professionals who are caring for their child. Through health teaching and counseling, and by clarifying the meaning of a diagnosis, nurses can help such a family understand the true nature of the illness and take steps to stop projecting anxiety, or to reduce the intensity of projection. Parents also need information to help them deal with their own needs as a couple and with the needs of their other children. (Couples with a sick child may tend to forget their own needs and to ignore other children.) Furthermore, because the mother tends to become the caretaker of the ill child, the father may feel distant and uninvolved while the mother feels trapped and overburdened. The nurse should try to include the father in educational sessions and discussions as well as in the care of the child.

Rehabilitation of Health

Tertiary prevention consists of minimizing the sequelae of chronic physical and mental health problems. Nurses who work in tertiary psychiatric health care facilities will have opportunities to intervene with families in both inpatient and outpatient settings. For example, nurses working with clients who have chronic mental illness (CMI) and their families will have opportunities to help families cope with having such a client living at home—especially by guiding them in the development of a schedule for daily living that meets the needs of all family members. Referral to support groups, day treatment programs, and family therapy may also be appropriate components of a comprehensive treatment plan that is sensitive to family issues and needs (see Chapter 53).

Regardless of the setting, the nurse's ability to provide comprehensive care is enhanced by an understanding of family theory. Families concerned with promotion of health as well as families in which there is an acute or chronic health problem can all be assisted by nurses who are knowledgeable about family theory.

Therapeutic Use of Self

Perhaps the most important factor in working with families is the nurse's ability to maintain a differentiated self. Nurses, like other people, come from families and are therefore vulnerable to "triangling," anxiety, and other feelings evoked by particular families. In order to remain therapeutic, nurses must be able to maintain their self-boundaries. They must be sensitive to the way a family's characteristics, issues, and patterns of interaction can trigger their own anxieties. But identifying a "trigger" is an emotional response to a family that can represent a stall in the nurse-family relationship. Nurses need to pause and engage in a self-assessment process which enables them to understand how their own family history interacts with the family in treatment to create triggers, raise anxiety, blur boundaries, and bring about a potential or actual impasse. The goal is for the nurse to identify problematic issues and differentiate between those that belong to the nurse and those that belong to the family. It is only then that the nurse will be able to resume a therapeutic role.

Evaluation

Evaluation of interventions with families involves the outcomes that were established with each family and the degree to which they have been accomplished. Evaluation may be needed at periodic intervals because some of the outcomes are short-term or intermediate.

For example, a short-term outcome for the S. family is the verbal expression of feelings related to the death of Bob. To the extent that the family does this, the outcome is achieved; other evidence might be Joan's joining of a bereavement group, an intermediate outcome. (Such a group would provide a different arena for her "grief work.") A long-term outcome, confrontation of a "toxic" family issue—death—would be accomplished if there is a decrease in anxiety; but this goal may take a long time to accomplish, since the issue is complex.

SUMMARY

In nursing, the family is the primary focus of health care. A *family* is a small social system made up of individuals held together by strong reciprocal affection and loyalty; the term often refers to a permanent household that persists for some time. Members enter a family through birth, adoption, marriage, or legal cohabitation and usually leave through divorce or death; adult children may leave a household to establish their own homes. The structure of a family, its "membership configuration," may be considered an "organizational dimension."

Functional, healthy families are generally characterized by life-giving, nurturing patterns of behavior and by love, caring, and loyalty. A healthy family provides an environment in which physical, spiritual, affectional, and social functions are carried out. Functional dimensions of healthy families include individuation, mutuality, flexibility, stability, clear perceptions of members, clear role definitions, role reciprocity, and clear generational boundaries. Beavers used eight variables to describe "optimal" family functioning: a systems orientation, clear boundaries, contextual clarity, a clearly defined hierarchy of power and equality, processes for achieving intimacy, encouragement of autonomy, joyful and comfortable styles of relating, high-level negotiation skills, and significant "transcendent values."

Family development is defined as the process of progressive structural differentiation and transformation over a family's history and active acquisition and selective discarding of roles as family members seek to fulfill the changing functional requisites for survival, and as the family adapts as a holistic system to recurring life stresses. A family *developmental task* is a responsibility, having to do with growth, that arises at a specific stage in the life of a family.

Family systems theory, developed by Bowen, is the basis of *family systems therapy.* Bowen views the family as a multigenerational system characterized by patterns of emotional interaction. The interlocking concepts that describe family functioning in terms of emotional patterns and interaction are differentiation of self, triangles, the nuclear family's emotional system, the multigenerational transmission process, the family projection process, sibling position, emotional cutoff, and societal regression.

Minuchin, who pioneered the structural approach to intervention with families, believed that behavior is a consequence of the organization and structure of the family and of patterns of interaction among family members. In *structural family therapy,* the therapist "joins" a family by mirroring or mimicking, showing respect for family values and hierarchies, highlighting elements of cultural and developmental similarity, observing the family's strengths, supporting the structure of family subsystems, and "tracking" processes. Restructuring is accomplished by enacting transactional patterns, marking boundaries, escalating stress, assigning tasks, using symptoms, manipulating mood, and supporting, educating, and guiding.

Strategic family therapy, also referred to as *problem-solving therapy* or *brief therapy,* has its origins in communication theory. Behavior—both verbal and nonverbal—is communication. Weakland, Fisch, Watzlawick, Beavin, and Jackson are proponents of communication strategies; and Palazzoli-Selvini refined the use of paradoxical injunction as a technique of strategic therapy. The strategic therapist is an active, purposeful change agent who works with a family using strategies based on "double-bind" messages, the "Greek chorus," and "feedback loops."

When the nursing process is applied to families, genograms, ecomaps, and family processes are important parts of assessment. Genograms and ecomaps are pictorial representations of families and their place in the community. The assessment of processes involves physical, emotional, cognitive, and spiritual elements in the family system. Nursing diagnosis consists of identifying actual and potential strengths and problems of a family system. Outcome criteria include short-term, intermediate, and long-term goals which are periodically reevaluated as the family evolves and changes. Intervention with families takes place in a variety of inpatient and outpatient settings. Intervention by a generalist nurse consists of assessment and diagnoses of family problems and referral to appropriate community resources. Intervention by a clinical specialist with advanced educational preparation may include conducting family therapy. Nurses may provide families with primary, secondary, or tertiary health care. Nurses who work with families must engage in a self-assessment process that enables them to maintain the clear sense of self that is required when working therapeutically with families. Evaluation relates to the outcomes established with the family and the degree to which these outcomes have been accomplished.

REFERENCES

1. V. Trifte and B. Meyerhoff, eds., *Changing Images of the Family,* Yale University Press, New Haven, 1979.
2. J. R. Miller and E. H. Janosik, *Family Focused Care,* McGraw-Hill, New York, 1979.
3. L. Barnhill and D. Longo, "Fixation and Regression in the Family Life Cycle," *Family Process,* vol. 17, no. 4, December 1978.
4. R. W. Beavers, *Psychotherapy and Growth: A Family Systems Perspective,* Brunner/Mazel, New York, 1977.
5. M. Bowen, *Family Therapy in Clinical Practice,* Aronson, New York, 1978.
6. J. M. Lewis, R. W. Beavers, J. T. Gossett, and V. Austin-Philips, *No Single Thread: Psychological Health in Family Systems,* St. Louis, Mosby, 1981.
7. F. Walsh, ed., *Normal Family Processes,* Guilford, New York, 1982.
8. E. A. Carter and M. McGoldrick, *The Family Life Cycle: A Framework for Family Therapy,* Garner, New York, 1980.
9. E. Duvall, *Marriage and Family Development,* 5th ed., Philadelphia, Lippincott, 1977.
10. M. Bowen, "The Use of Family Therapy in Clinical Practice," in M. Bowen, ed., *Family Therapy in Clinical Practice,* Aronson, New York, 1978.
11. M. Bowen, "On the Differentiation of Self," in M. Bowen, ed., *Family Therapy in Clinical Practice,* Aronson, New York, 1978.
12. L. Von Bertalanffy, *General Systems Theory,* Braziller, New York, 1968.
13. M. Bowen, "Intrafamilial Dynamics in Emotional Illness," in M. Bowen, ed. *Family Therapy in Clinical Practice,* Aronson, New York, 1978.
14. M. Bowen, "Family Psychotherapy with Schizophrenia in Hospital and Private Practice," in M. Bowen, ed., *Family Therapy in Clinical Practice,* Aronson, New York, 1978.
15. T. Fogarty, "Fusion," *The Family,* vol. 4, no. 2, 1977, pp. 49–58.
16. M. Bowen, "Theory in the Practice of Psychotherapy," in P. Guerin, ed., *Family Therapy: Theory and Practice,* Gardner, New York, 1976, pp. 42–90.
17. T. Fogarty, "Triangles," *The Family,* vol. 2, no. 4, 1975, pp. 41–49.
18. S. Miller and P. Winstead-Fry, *Family Systems Theory in Nursing Practice,* Reston, Reston, Va., 1982.
19. W. Toman, *Family Constellation,* 3d ed., Springer, New York, 1976.
20. M. Bowen, "Society, Crisis and Systems Theory," in M. Bowen, ed., *Family Therapy in Clinical Practice,* Aronson, New York, 1978, pp. 413–450.
21. M. Bowen, "Societal Regression as Viewed through Family Systems Theory," in M. Bowen, ed., *Family Therapy in Clinical Practice,* Aronson, New York, 1978, pp. 269–282.
22. M. Kerr, "Family Systems Theory and Therapy" in A. Gurman and D. Kriskein, eds., *Handbook of Family Therapy,* Brunner/Mazel, New York, 1981, pp. 226–264.
23. Anonymous, "Toward the Differentiation of Self in One's Own Family of Origin," in M. Bowen, ed., *Family Therapy in Clinical Practice,* Aronson, New York, 1978. pp. 529–547.
24 S. Minuchin, *Families and Family Therapy,* Harvard University Press, Cambridge, Mass., 1974.
25. J. Steidl and J. Wexler, "What's a Clinician to Do with So Many Approaches to Family Therapy?" *The Family,* vol. 4, no. 2, 1977, pp. 59–64.
26. H. J. Aponte, "Underorganization in the Poor Family," in P. Guerin, ed., *Family Therapy: Theory and Practice,* Gardner, New York, 1976.
27. S. Minuchin et al., "A Conceptual Model of Psychosomatic Illness in Children," *Archives of General Psychiatry,* vol. 32, no. 8, 1975, pp. 1031–1050.
28. H. J. Aponte and J. M. Van Deusen, "Structural Family Therapy," in A. Gurman and D. Kniskern, eds., *Handbook of Family Therapy,* Brunner/Mazel, New York, 1981, pp. 310–360.
29. G. Bateson et al., "Toward a Theory of Schizophrenia," *Behavioral Science,* vol. 1, no. 1, 1956, pp. 251-275.
30. J. Weakland, "Communication Theory and Change," in P. Guerin, ed., *Family Therapy: Theory and Practice,* Gardner, New York, 1976.
31. P. Watzlawick, J. Beavin, and D. Jackson, *Pragmatics of Human Communications,* Norton, New York, 1967.
32. M. Erickson, "The Identification of a Secure Reality," *Family Process,* vol. 1, no. 2, 1962, pp. 294–303.
33. M. Palazzoli-Selvini, L. Boscolo, G. Cecchin, and G. Prata, *Paradox and Counterparadox: A New Model in the Therapy of the Family in Schizophrenic Transaction,* Aronson, New York, 1975.
34. M. Palazzoli-Selvini, *Self-Starvation: From Individual to Family Therapy in the Treatment of Anorexia Nervosa,* Aronson, New York, 1978.
35. P. Watzlawick, "Some Basic Issues in Interaction Research," in J. Framo, ed., *Family Interaction,* Springer, New York, 1972.

36. M. D. Stanton, "Strategic Approaches to Family Therapy," in A. Gurman and D. Kriskein, eds., *Handbook of Family Therapy,* Brunner/Mazel, New York, 1981.
37. P. Watzlawick, J. Weakland, and R. Fisch, *Change: Principles of Problem Formation and Problem Resolution,* Norton, New York, 1974.
38. P. Papp, "The Greek Chorus and Other Techniques of Paradoxical Therapy," *Family Process,* vol. 19, 1980, pp. 45–97.
39. R. Hare-Mustin, "Paradoxical Tasks in Family Therapy: Who Can Resist?" *Psychotherapy: Theory, Research and Practice,* vol. 13, no. 1, 1976, pp. 128–130.
40. J. Haley, *Problem-Solving Therapy,* Jossey-Bass, San Francisco, 1976.
41. E. Pendagast and C. Sherman, "A Guide to the Genogram," *The Family,* vol. 5, no. 1, 1976, pp. 101–112.
42. M. Stanhope and J. Lancaster, *Community Health Nursing: Process and Practice of Promoting Health,* Mosby, St. Louis, 1984.

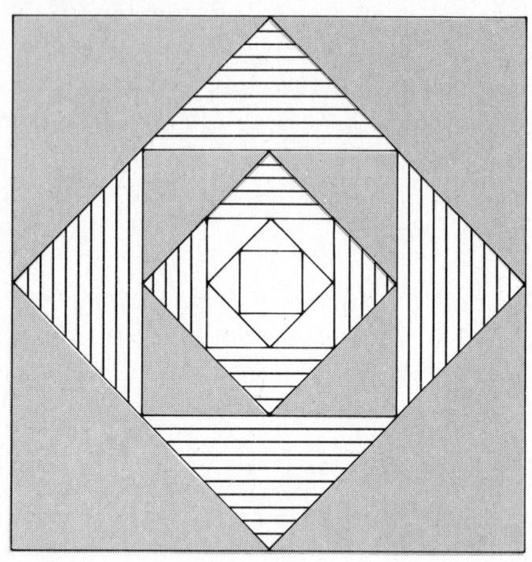

CHAPTER 20
Therapeutic Groups

Suzanne Lego

LEARNING OBJECTIVES

After studying this chapter, the student should be able to:

1. Discuss the principles of group psychotherapy.
2. List the types of group psychotherapy.
3. Describe the role of the leader in group psychotherapy.
4. Identify leadership styles in groups.
5. Describe common problems of beginning group leaders.
6. List the phases in group development.
7. Understand the interrelationship between group content and group process.
8. Recognize the signs of group cohesiveness.
9. Understand the concepts of transference, countertransference, resistance, acting out, subgrouping, and insight.
10. Know the criteria for termination of group therapy.
11. Discuss the goals and types of support groups.
12. Describe the differences between support groups and psychotherapy groups.

Group psychotherapy is the therapeutic process of treating clients in groups. Nurses help clients by observing and commenting on the dynamics created by the relationships and reactions of group members. Group psychotherapy is effective in a variety of settings and with nearly all psychiatric disorders. Group psychotherapy has evolved through many phases. Today, there are as many different schools of group psychotherapy as there are schools of personality development. They range from conservative, long-term group psychoanalysis at one end of the spectrum to short-term crisis groups at the other.

Support groups are composed of relatively healthy people who meet regularly to discuss specific problems that are common to all of them.

The purpose of this chapter is to compare and contrast the therapeutic potential of psychotherapy and support groups.

GROUP PSYCHOTHERAPY

Types of Group Psychotherapy

The various types of group psychotherapy can be categorized under four general headings: (1) activity therapy, (2) educative therapy, (3) repressive-inspirational therapy, and (4) reconstructive therapy.

Activity Therapy

Activity therapy is generally employed with children ages 7 to 14. The focus is on the acting out of impulses, conflicts, and deviant behavior in a group setting. A group of 9-year-olds organized around a theme such as "fun" or "self" is an example of an activity group. The therapist uses the activity to teach appropriate group behavior.

Educative Therapy

In educative, or lecture-discussion, therapy the leader presents content in the form of a lecture or written material which is then discussed by the clients. Examples are ADL (activities of daily living) groups, medication education groups, and women's awareness groups. Fairly large numbers of clients can be reached at one time by use of this method. Individual needs, however, cannot usually be met.

Repressive-Inspirational Therapy

Repressive-inspirational therapy uses clients' present ego strengths and further reinforces them through inspiration in order to help clients repress problems more successfully than they have done previously. This type of therapy, which requires a minimum of specialized training on the part of the leader, is widely practiced by laypersons and paraprofessionals. The disadvantages are that (1) no effort is made to explore a client's specific dynamics; (2) relatively good ego strength is required on the part of clients; and (3) neurotic defenses are reinforced, making the clients more vulnerable, in some respects, to future life crises.

This is probably the most common type of group psychotherapy practiced both in inpatient facilities and in the community. Weekend marathons, joy groups, and encounter groups fall into this category. These groups tend to offer members a "high" but do not have a lasting effect because of their failure to deal with individual personality characteristics. Repressive-inspirational therapy is *not* indicated for clients with weak ego structure, for example, schizophrenic or borderline clients.

Reconstructive Therapy

In reconstructive therapy, intervention is based on exploration and analysis of both individual intrapsychic structures and the group process. The advantage of this type of therapy is that individual and group characteristics are explored in depth with a view toward permanent change in the individual. Each member's behavior within the group is constantly examined, keeping in mind the idea that the group is a microcosm of the larger world. By bringing to light the members' secret wishes and conflicts, and the motivations of their behavior in the group, the therapist can help them understand more about their total mode of being in the world.

The Group

Selection of Group Members

There are many opinions about whom to select for a psychotherapy group. In general, members of an adult group are 21 years old and older. In intensive psychotherapy, a *heterogeneous* group is an advantage. That is, gender, age, and personality dynamics should vary as much as possible. The advantage of this is that members will interact on a deep emotional level if there are multiple stimuli. In a *homogeneous* group, where all the clients are, for example, alcoholic, homosexual, or obsessive people, there is a tendency for the members either to discuss common problems or to support one another's defensive systems. Many psychotherapists believe that certain types of clients, such as schizophrenics, cannot be treated in groups of this kind. This is certainly not the case; many schizophrenics respond positively to group treatment, though it may take a long time to notice a response. It is generally agreed, however, that certain types of clients should not be included. These are brain-damaged or severely retarded clients and those who are destructively paranoid or psychopathic.

All prospective members should be seen by a therapist at least once before being admitted to a group. The more times they are seen individually before entering a group, the better. In general, clients who are in group therapy should be in individual therapy as well. Clients who have not had previous psychotherapy tend to hold back the group or become so threatened by the group sessions that they leave shortly after beginning. Therefore, it is best to see future members individually for some time before they enter the group and to continue to see them individually while they are in the group. This will cut down a great deal on attrition.

When entry into a group is discussed between client and therapist, as little as possible should be revealed about the specific composition of the group. This is to allow for spontaneous and often irrational responses to occur and be explored. If the member knows who will be present, the reaction upon meeting the other members will be controlled. For example:

> Mary might exclaim, upon entering a group, "I had no idea men would be here!" This might lead to exploration of her feelings about men.

The same is true about bringing new members into an ongoing group. The group should not be prepared, as this prevents spontaneous reactions.

The new member should not be told how to behave in the group, as this again will undermine spontaneity. Therefore, the leader should not say, for example, "You will be expected to tell the group about your difficulties." Instead, the leader might say, if asked what group therapy is about, "It's a chance to relate and react to people, and to explore your behavior with them." This answer is vague enough to allow spontaneous responses.

Creation of the Group

There are a number of factors to consider in creating a group. First, the number of members should be not more than 10 to begin with. Research has shown 7 to be an ideal number, and there should never be fewer than 5 people. Since attrition occurs frequently, 10 is a good beginning number. If 4 or fewer members appear for a session and the group is not well-established, the session should be canceled. There is too much pressure on the members to talk when so few attend.

As for the physical setting, no table should be used, for a table sets up a physical barrier. When no such barrier exists, members feel more exposed, are more anxious, and are more likely to act irrationally. Furthermore, a table blocks some nonverbal communication, which is useful to note and explore at times.

The leader should change seats at each meeting so that members are forced to take different seats. This helps prevent any client from finding a comfortable niche where he or she can "blend into the furniture." Each session should last 1½ hours if the group meets weekly, because it takes about 45 minutes for members to loosen up. Sessions should always begin and end on time. Members pace themselves, and this pacing is in itself interesting to note and explore. It is sometimes tempting to run overtime when something valuable is happening, but the leader should avoid the temptation. If a client is very upset at the end of a session, an individual session can be arranged with the client.

Outpatient groups and groups in long-term institutions should meet once or twice weekly. Groups held on short-term inpatient units should meet daily for 1 hour. The same person should lead the group each day because productivity is reduced when a different leader appears for each session or when outsiders are permitted to sit in on the group. If, as in teaching centers, students must observe the group, they should do so through a one-way mirror or on closed-circuit television with the group's knowledge. The presence of a mirror or camera is less inhibiting than that of a person.

In reconstructive group psychotherapy, open-ended groups are preferable to closed-ended ones. An *open-ended group* is structured so that the membership changes every so often, as one member leaves and another joins. This creates anxiety and evokes irrational responses that often lead to important exploration. For example, the introduction of a new member often stimulates a client to recall the birth of a new sibling.

Group Leaders

ROLE OF THE LEADER. The American Nurses' Association (ANA) sets standards by which to judge the qualifications of a leader of a reconstructive psychotherapy group. The ANA suggests that the role of group psychotherapist be limited to nurses with master's degrees in psychiatric nursing. Additional criteria include formal study of group theory, supervised experience as a leader of a psychotherapy group, and personal experience with groups over an extended period of time.

The leader's behavior has a profound effect on the members of the group and on their productivity. The most effective leader is one who does not lead in a heavy-handed way but rather stimulates the group to develop its own direction. The following poem states this well:

A leader is best
When people barely know that he exists.
Not so good when people obey and acclaim him,
Worse when they despise him.
"Fail to honor people,
they fail to honor you;"
But of a good leader, who talks little,
When his work is done, his aim fulfilled,
They will all say, "We did this ourselves."

Lao Tzu, "Leadership"

Joseph Geller,[1] a group psychoanalyst, has devised a chart which shows the effect of three different kinds of leaders—the *boss*, the *guide*, and the *stimulator*—on the interaction and productivity of groups (see Table 20-1). It is important to note that the leader who acts as a boss severely inhibits the natural process of the group, while the leader who is a stimulator helps the group to develop beyond the leader's individual capacities. Group leaders do not always predict the capacity of a group accurately. This is particularly true of psychotherapists who are leading groups of schizophrenic clients; the leader tends to do far more "for" clients than is actually necessary.

There are certain expectations which the leader has of the group members. Table 20-2 lists these expectations, possible behaviors of clients, and appropriate interventions by the leader.

When a new group is being formed, the leader should keep in mind that the first session sets the stage for all that is to follow. It is extremely impor-

Table 20-1 Relationship between Leadership of Group and Group's Development

Type of Leader	Group Interaction Phenomenon	Productivity of the Group
Boss: Plans, controls, directs, and decides autocratically	Group submits, conforms when told what to do, has little influence on things except in a passive way.	Support of leader's irrational needs
Guide: Plans, controls, and steers, usually subtly and indirectly	Group can register differences, initiate complaints, and make requests. Group participates in thinking and forming opinions; makes minor decisions. Group has some active influence but little responsibility.	Limited to leader's capacity
Stimulator: Educates, facilitates productivity and communication, balances group forces, and shares leadership	Group generates ideas, sets limits, and establishes methods. Group stimulates productivity and development of members. Group has primary responsibilities, uses self-evaluation, has healthy group spirit, is creative and productive.	Can be expected to go beyond leader's capacity to members' maximum potential

SOURCE: Joseph J. Geller, "Group Psychotherapy in the Treatment of the Schizophrenic Syndromes," *Psychiatric Quarterly*, vol. 63, 1963, pp. 1–13.

Table 20-2 Leader's Expectations about Clients, Possible Behaviors by Clients, and Appropriate Interventions by Leader

Expectation	Possible Behavior by Clients	Appropriate Intervention by Leader
Members will attend every session or tell leader beforehand if they must miss one. (Expectation voiced by leader.)	Leave messages with other clients, secretary, or answering service.	Tells members they must speak to leader directly. Explores need to avoid leader in this case.
	Miss sessions without notice.	Asks members about absence. Explores meaning if appropriate.
	Call to cancel with vague excuses. ("I'm not feeling up to it.")	Strongly encourages members to come anyway, pointing out that not feeling well may be related to feelings about the group.
Members will be as open as possible. (Not voiced by leader.)	Commit conscious deception. Members feel one way (for example, angry) but act another (for example, sweet).	Points out inconsistency: "You look angry, but you're acting sweet."
	Commit unconscious deception. Members seem to feel one way but do not seem aware of it and act another way.	Points out inconsistency or questions in a gentle way: "Are you sure you're not angry?"
No physical violence will occur. (Not voiced by leader.)	Members threaten violence.	States that physical violence is not allowed, but encourages verbal exploration of reason for violent feelings.
Members will not discuss group matters outside the group with those who are concerned in these matters. (Not voiced by leader.)	Members break group confidentiality.	Explores this in the group.
Members will not meet outside the group, or if they do, they will discuss their meetings in the group. (Not voiced by leader.)	Two members form a sexual relationship.	Explores in the group the meaning of the relationship with regard to the group itself, the leader, and past relationships with significant others.
	Two members of the group appear to be attracted to one another.	Explores the relationship in the group, as above, in order to "nip it in the bud" and deal with the motivation rather than have it acted out.

tant that the leader be as accepting and nondirective as possible. If the leader can manage to sit back and let the group start itself, members will realize from the outset that the group is their responsibility. On the other hand, if the leader adopts an "I am the expert" attitude, the group members will sit back and wait for the therapy to be "done to" them. This is antithetical to the principles of group psychotherapy. A rule of thumb for group leaders is that they should never do for the group what the group can do for itself.

The leader's most important task is to watch the evolving group process and to stimulate the members to act within the context of this evolution. This often involves making overt that which is covert. The leader must be constantly alert to the covert or latent process and stimulate its emergence in relation to members' intrapsychic lives. Table 20-3 outlines growth-inhibiting behaviors to be avoided and some growth-promoting alternatives which may be used by leaders.

In addition to the therapist leader, there are emergent leaders in groups. These are group members to whom the others turn for guidance. Homans has referred to the emergent leader as the person who best embodies the group norms.[2] It is the emergent leader who has observed the needs and wishes of other members and is able to help the group move in the direction of these wishes. Norms occur in two different areas of group life; therefore, two different emergent leaders often appear in a group. The first is the task leader, who helps the group to accomplish its tasks. If the group is a psychotherapy group, the task leader may seem to

Table 20-3 Growth-Inhibiting and Growth-Promoting Behaviors of Leaders

Growth-Inhibiting Behavior	Growth-Promoting Behavior
Starting sessions by introducing members or explaining the purpose of group therapy	Waiting for members to begin on their own Avoiding lengthy explanations of anything
Bringing food or drink for group members	Exploring dependency needs in the context of the group and the members' lives outside the group
Calling on specific members to talk	Allowing silences to continue until a group member breaks them, or commenting on the silence after a few minutes Allowing other members to deal with consistently silent members
"Going around" the group, requiring that each member talk in turn	Allowing members to talk at random as they please
Pushing for closure on a topic or summing up sessions at the end	Realizing that there is no "final solution" Allowing issues to be discussed, explored, examined by anyone in the group, with interest and respect shown to all Allowing sessions to end "up in the air," with some members feeling anxious

be a kind of "cotherapist" or assistant therapist. The second emergent leader is the social leader. This group member is usually the most popular because of his or her ability to relieve tension.

PROBLEMS OF BEGINNING GROUP LEADERS. Beginning group leaders should be aware of the fact that they will experience a level of anxiety based on their need to maintain a good self-image and to maintain control of the group. Table 20-4 lists some of the common irrational and unproductive needs of beginning group psychotherapists. Fears are expressed by inexperienced leaders in a variety of ways. This can be problematic for both clients and leaders. Supervision is essential in helping new leaders understand what is occurring within themselves and how it affects the group process.

Table 20-4 Common Irrational and Unproductive Needs of Beginning Group Psychotherapists

Need to Maintain a Good Self-Image
Need to be liked
Need to avoid exposing self as "human"
Need to impress group with knowledge and authority
Need to Maintain Control of the Group
Need to prevent group disintegration
Need to prevent regressive behavior
Need to prevent resistance
Need to prevent expression of hostility
Need to prevent acting out
Need to avoid taboo topics
Need to prevent intensive, multiple transference reactions
Need to prevent the examination of individuals' or subgroups' problems
Need to restrict process that does not "go through" the therapist

Purpose of the Group

The group's purpose is examination and exploration of the behavior of the group members, as it occurs, with a view toward permanent change of dysynchronous behavior. One of the ways in which clients are helped to behave in their most basic "real" or "irrational" way is for the group leader to create a situation that provokes some slight anxiety. If clients are allowed to remain comfortable and relaxed in a group, their defenses will continue to operate in an optimal way and they will not change. If they are anxious, however, their defenses will be so sharply exaggerated that group members will notice them and begin to explore them. The technique of creating anxiety may be thought of as "stirring up the dust to see how it settles."

The group leader is constantly alert to group process and offers comments from time to time. For example:

> One member of a group, Claudia, mentioned that she had extensive group experience and was interested in seeing how the leader would operate. The leader asked her later, "Am I doing all right so far?" This comment by the leader had the effect of stimulating the group to notice the process, but it was not a heavy-handed and pedantic remark like, "I notice that you want to compete with me." This comment would evoke a fierce denial, while the first one would tend to bring a laugh and then a quiet consideration of what had just happened.

Phases of Group Development

Group development can be divided into four phases. These are *uncertainty, overaggressiveness, regression,* and *adaptation.* While new groups move through these stages sequentially, there is overlapping of behaviors from one phase into another. New members coming into an ongoing group will also move through these stages.

UNCERTAINTY PHASE. The uncertainty phase lasts up to approximately 20 sessions. It is the time in the life of the group when many demands are made on the leader. Table 20-5 outlines the dynamics often present in the uncertainty phase. In this phase, members often feel that comment or interpretation by the leader means that they should not continue to do what the leader has observed. Therefore, the leader must often remind the group that only an observation and not a criticism has been made.

OVERAGGRESSIVENESS PHASE. When a group or a new member in a group has overcome the feeling

Table 20-5 Uncertainty Phase

Behavior by Clients	Example	Intervention by Leader
Initial anxiety	Pacing the floor. Leaving and returning. Hallucinations and delusions. Excessive intellectualization. Organization of a "group plan."	Comment about the anxiety. Question what members fear happening in the group.
Demands on leader to explain purpose or provide structure	"Do we begin now?" "What is supposed to happen here?" "How does this work?"	Communicate to members that it is their group. ("Let's see how things go.")
Competition	Comparison among members of past group experience, past number of years of psychotherapy, knowledge of the leader, etc.	Point out that competition is taking place, being careful to communicate that it is not wrong and should not necessarily stop just because it is noted.
Excessive politeness	Members feel anxious and angry about the lack of structure from the leader, but they are afraid to show this. Instead, they react with inappropriate kindness. To a monopolizer: "You certainly are talkative today."	Note the covert feeling and ask if it is present. ("Are you a little irritated by all that talking?") Encourage openness rather than politeness.
Silence	All members sit for 5 minutes staring at the floor or occasionally glancing at each other.	Comment on the silence. ("I guess everyone is afraid to start.") Comment on some nonverbal behavior. ("Mary, I notice you're staring at John. Do you wish he'd speak?")
Questions about the leader's personal life, qualifications, and competence	Member asks, "Are you a parent?" Member asks, "Are you an M.D.?"	"No. Are you afraid I won't know how to care for you because I'm not?" "No, I'm a psychiatric nurse. Are you afraid I won't know enough to do things right?"
Avoidance of involvement in the group	Schizophrenic member talks to voices instead of other group members. Members intellectualize about their problems. Members adopt roles which were used in their families to reduce anxiety but which are not appropriate in the current group (for example, the buffoon, the boss, the incompetent person, the ingenue).	Comment that these are methods to avoid reacting emotionally to the current group. Explore why this is feared and avoided.
Strong, irrational reactions to the leader	The leader is seen as a "savior" with all the answers. The leader is seen as using power to manipulate or humiliate members and as having a secret reason for every comment or move.	Explore why a "savior" is necessary. Explore the meaning of these ideas in the context of the members' lives.

Table 20-6 Overaggressiveness Phase

Behavior by Clients	Example	Intervention by Leader
Criticism of one another	One member who is very lonely but leads the life of the happy, sophisticated "swinger" is critical of another member whose isolation and loneliness are all too stark and evident.	Ask whether the "swinger" is reminded of himself or herself by the isolated member. Explore their similarities and the resultant anxiety.
	One member becomes enraged when another acts stubborn and impenetrable.	Ask whether there was someone else in the member's life that he or she could not "get through" to.
Anger at one another for using their own defenses in clumsy ways	One obsessive member begins sentences with, "Please don't think I'm trying to be controlling, but . . . ." Another obsessive says, "Don't warn us so obviously. It only calls our attention to the fact that you are trying to control us!"	Point out that people feel their own defenses should be used only in their own unique ways and are spoiled or "exposed" if used "incorrectly."
Ganging up	One member who is secretly anxious about almost everything arrives late to group each week, giving various weak excuses. He refuses to acknowledge that he might have wanted to miss part of a session or that he may have wanted to stir everyone up. All members begin to criticize him.	Examine and explore both sides of the process, why the member is so provocative as well as why members cannot resist being provoked.
Hostility toward the leader	Clients distort the leader's behavior. ("You do nothing to help us.")	Accept their hostility in a nondefensive way. Avoid a win-lose approach. Weaknesses and eccentricities may be acknowledged freely. It is often a great relief to members to see that the leader is human and does not mind if this shows.
	Clients point out real eccentricities of the leader. ("You are too compulsive!")	

of uncertainty and grasped how the group will operate, there follows a phase of overaggressiveness. This occurs as a defense against what is to follow, that is, regression and adaptation. In this phase of group development, hostility is often displayed toward other members and toward the leader. Frequently the hostility which members display toward one another is actually meant for the leader. In addition, attractions are beginning to take place between members, and this is frightening to them. Such an attraction may be the seed of an intimate relationship, which is anathema to most clients who are beginning group therapy. Table 20-6 lists the dynamics experienced in the group during the overaggressiveness phase.

REGRESSION PHASE. The third phase of group development, regression, comes about when clients are no longer afraid to regress. The earlier defenses are put aside, and the members experience pure anxiety, anger at more primitive sources, dependency, fear, longing, envy, jealousy, and other forms of pain. There is no longer a felt need to pretend to be in control. Regression does not arise from a desire to manipulate others but occurs spontaneously. At first, other members may feel anxious and may even begin to cry themselves or want to leave or stop the member who is regressing. It is important at this time for the leader to move in and question the regressed member about what is being experienced, what led to this feeling, and so on. Actually, this is an extremely important period in psychotherapy, for it is in these regressed states that heretofore repressed or dissociated material can come into awareness. For example:

> A client, Helen, who had never felt love or acceptance from her parents but rather had felt like the "ugly duckling" in the family, perceived her brothers and sisters as more attractive and successful. During a session, she began to feel that all the other members were more "loved" by the therapist and that she was "rejected." She began to cry and to express the pain she was experiencing. Other members of the group offered their support. She was surprised, having believed previously that to lose control would lead to disaster.

This is not an uncommon reaction when such a process occurs. The other group members commonly begin to like the regressed member better after such an episode has occurred. They begin to feel they share a common bond of humanness.

During the regression phase the leader often takes on a new image and is seen as an expert resource person, not as an "idol" or "enemy" as before. Just as the other members' humanness has begun to be tolerated, so is the leader's.

ADAPTATION PHASE. In the fourth stage of group development, adaptation, members accept one another in spite of their weaknesses and faults. While their behavior to one another is fairly nonthreatening, it is nonetheless explored in depth and in a relatively nondefensive way. This does not mean that members in this phase never respond to one another irrationally; if this were to happen, the therapeutic effectiveness of the group would be sharply decreased. Therefore, the leader must continue in this phase to "stir up the dust" and poke away at unresolved conflicts and wishes.

The relative stability and comfort of this phase can be a disadvantage. This is one reason why open-ended groups are preferable to those in which all members start together and remain together. In open-ended groups, where the membership varies every so often as one member leaves and another member joins, there are more new stimuli to react to, there is more exposure of more aspects of the personality, and hence there is more exploration. For example:

> A very narcissistic client will evoke rage and indignation at first. Then, eventually, the other group members will react with acceptance and tolerance. This toleration may decrease the amount of "work" done in relation to the client's narcissism. However, a new client in the group will be astonished by the first member's narcissism and by the group's tolerance of it. This client will shake things up a bit and lead the group members to further exploration of both their own and the narcissist's experiences.

Central Concepts of Group Psychotherapy

A number of concepts combine to form the essence of intensive group psychotherapy. They are *content and process, cohesiveness, transference, countertransference, resistance, acting out, subgrouping, insight,* and *termination.* Each of these will be considered separately.

Content and Process

In group psychotherapy one of the most important concepts is that of the relationship between group content and group process. Group *content* refers to that which is *said* in a group, while group *process* refers to that which is *done* in a group or that which is implied through actions. These actions include nonverbal behavior, the tone of voice of members, the order in which topics occur, who speaks to whom, and other kinds of group actions. Thus, group interaction continues on two levels, that which is said and that which is done. Even when there is no content (no one is speaking), there is always process. This is because one cannot *not* communicate. Even when group members are not speaking out loud to one another, they are communicating.

Content and process, the two levels of interaction, are constantly interweaving and giving the group its fabric. In early group meetings, when a group is forming, the members often feel uncertain and anxious about their places in the scheme of things. While this is what is *happening* in the group, what is *said* might be something about the confused state of the world today. Moreover, in early sessions, members experience feelings about the leader but either are unable to voice these or actually are unaware of them. Instead, they might discuss other "authority figures" at great length, for example, the President of the United States.

Here is an example of the interweaving of content and process:

> In one group session, Milly, a member, was accused of constantly defending her friend Ann. Upon hearing this accusation, Milly replied, "Ann needs no defending!" The members broke into spontaneous laughter, since Milly was denying in content what she was doing in process. Later in the same session, she was accused of acting too sweet and "Pollyanna-ish" at times when she "should" have been angry. She replied to this, "Thank you; that is very helpful to me!" Again, the content and process were the same.

The group leader must be alert constantly to the relationship between content and process, because it is content that gives constant clues to what is actually happening in the group.

Cohesiveness

Another group phenomenon is *cohesiveness.* Festinger has defined cohesiveness as "the resultant of all forces acting on members to remain in the group."[3] These forces may come from a variety of sources, the first of which is the group itself. As a group develops, a kind of "belongingness" arises which leads members to want to be together. When they learn that one member wants to leave the group, they will invariably urge this member to stay. When members tell the leader that they wish to leave, the leader should encourage them to discuss the matter in the group. This is done not only to increase the pressure on the member to stay but also to promote exploration of the reasons why the member wants to leave.

A second source of pressure on members to stay is their tie to the leader. For this reason, it is a good idea for group psychotherapists to see group members individually as well as in group sessions. Then their tie to the leader helps members to remain in the group and also to be more open and comfortable in group sessions.

A third source of pressure to remain in the group may come from outside the group. The members may feel, as they compare groups, that they would rather belong to this group than any other. Or significant others may be encouraging each member to remain in the group, as they realize that the group is helping the client.

There are a number of stages of group development which must occur before true cohesiveness appears. The group members must be free to expose positive as well as negative feelings toward each other. Simmel has written that a group attains unity not through harmony alone but rather through a combination of conflict and harmony.[4] Members must experience both love and hate toward one another and toward the leader before true cohesiveness arises. Table 20-7 lists the signs which indicate that a group is becoming cohesive.

The more cohesive a group is, the more likely its members will be to express hostility in a direct manner.[5] It is important to keep this fact in mind, as group leaders who fear hostility themselves will often subtly prevent such direct expressions of feeling and instead promote a kind of pseudo cohesiveness based on mutual "love."

Cohesiveness cannot be produced artificially, nor can its appearance be hastened. Group members must come to know and appreciate each other for their own uniqueness and in spite of their faults. This is part of the natural evolution of the group.[6]

Table 20-7 Group Cohesiveness

Sign of Cohesiveness	Example
Meetings outside the group	Members have coffee together after meetings.
Resentment of new members	Old members act closer than usual and discuss, without explanations, matters which are unknown to new members or that are sexually or highly emotionally charged.
Rescuing the leader when he or she is under attack	When one member is critical of the leader for giving "bad advice," other members point out that it was not advice but rather exploration.
Control of monopolizers	When one member monopolizes, the others point this out and do not permit it to continue.
Looking down on those outside the group	Members state how lucky they are to be in this particular group.
Acceptance of other members even though they are disliked	One member is domineering. The others work around her bossiness and, without strong hostility, cheerfully tease her about it.

Ways to promote cohesiveness are listed in Table 20-8 (page 392).

Transference

Transference occurs when the client transfers onto the therapist or other group members feelings, wishes, conflicts, and so forth which were originally felt in relation to the parents or significant others. Usually this is an unconscious process at first. The client begins to experience feelings about the therapist and other group members which are distortions of reality. When this happens, other clients will notice and talk about it. The client who is doing the transferring or distorting will, at first, defend this perception of reality; but when confronted by a group of surprised faces, he or she will frequently begin to question it. It is then that the client may recall earlier treatment by a parent or significant other which was similar to that which is being experienced in the present. Often other clients will remember something helpful about the client who is experiencing the transference. Through this process, the client is enabled to see the distortion and to begin to experience reality.

Table 20-8 Promoting Cohesiveness

Way to Promote Cohesiveness	Example
Make group personally rewarding.	Clarify observations about group or individual behavior which help members understand themselves better.
	Point out to members that they seem healthier or different.
Promote usefulness of other members whether they are liked or not.	Point out that an unpopular member is only a symbol of a significant other or oneself and therefore useful in helping work out one's own conflicts.
	Point out the "good" qualities of an unpopular member.
Make activities attractive.	Subtly rewarding clients for helping others recognize distortions or clarifying issues by saying something like, "Mary has a good point."

SOURCE: Jerome Frank, "Some Determinants, Manifestations and Effects of Cohesion in Therapy Groups," *International Journal of Group Psychotherapy*, vol. 7, 1957, pp. 53–62.

Here is an example of transference:

A client, Kristy, who had been a "parent" to her parents operated as a chronic helper in the group. She was attentive to other members, offering suggestions and helping others explore their problems. When the focus was on her, she was quick to point out the needs of her close friends and relatives but was not aware of her own needs until the issue was raised by others.

Countertransference

Countertransference occurs when the therapist transfers onto the client feelings, wishes, conflicts, and so forth which originated with the therapist's own parents or significant others. In other words, the therapist begins to experience feelings about the client which are distortions of reality. This usually begins when the therapist notes a feeling of anxiety or anger in regard to a particular client. For example, there may be a feeling that the client is a "jerk" or, the converse, that the client is "special." In either case, the therapist is experiencing some kind of distortion which can be either helpful or destructive to the client.

Here is an example of countertransference:

A beginning graduate nursing student started to work with a group of chronic schizophrenics. One young man in the group, Herb, had a history of violence and frequently acted out on the unit; he even had sustained a broken arm a few weeks after the group began. The nurse, Adele, came from a chaotic family where anger was not discussed but was acted out by a disturbed brother. Adele found herself dreading the group meetings and fearing Herb.

Countertransference can be helpful to the client if the therapist is aware of it and uses it to better understand the client and to help the client explore his or her own personal problems. Countertransference becomes destructive only if (1) the therapist is not aware of his or her powerful reaction to the client and reacts automatically or (2) the therapist is aware of the countertransference but cannot stop reacting. In the latter case, the situation should be discussed carefully with a supervisor or another knowledgeable, disengaged person. Countertransference is most frequently present in the beginning therapist but generally decreases in amount and intensity as the therapist matures. Its existence, however, is one good reason why group psychotherapists should receive personal psychoanalysis as well as supervision over time.

Resistance

Resistance occurs when powerful unconscious forces prevent the client from giving up distortions and from experiencing reality. Clients may feel unable to understand what others are saying about them and may instead feel "blank" or even angry. More subtle forms of resistance are operating when the client is habitually late or absent or feels reluctant to come to sessions. This resistance usually increases when the client is under pressure to experience reality; this pressure can come from others, from the self, or from both. For example, as a client begins to improve and feel more open to life, there is a kind of internal pressure to experience more and more of life. As others observe this about the client, they move more toward relating to him or her in a realistic way.

Here is an example of resistance:

Eleanor, a tough, flippant young woman, kept people at a distance with wit and sarcasm. She began after some time to miss sessions of her group and to hate coming when she did appear. This coincided with the group's first glimpses of her toughness as a mask, a time when they began reacting to her in an unintimidated manner. Unconsciously fearing this closer, more intimate way of relating, she did not want to continue.

It is not uncommon for clients to resist just when they are growing closer to others or are improving in other ways. At these times, the therapist must help clients to notice what is frightening them so that the resistance can be overcome and they can progress to more rewarding levels of experience.

Acting Out

Acting out occurs when the client relives or reproduces—through actions rather than words—feelings, wishes, or conflicts which are operating unconsciously. Instead of talking about buried conflicts, feelings, and wishes, the client dramatizes them in a disguised form. For example:

One client secretly wished for a close, special relationship with the therapist. Instead of talking about this, the client entered into a sexual relationship with the member of the group who was most like the therapist.

In cases of acting out, the therapist must try to understand the symbolic meaning of the behavior and explore it in depth with the clients involved. The symbolism may be very evident if a client is schizophrenic. For example:

Tom, a client, vomited during a session of the group. The therapist asked, "What is it here you can't stomach?"

The purpose of analyzing the acting out is to help the person experience directly the wishes and conflicts that are disguised. If they are simply acted out and not interpreted, they can never come into conscious awareness and will prevent the client from growing.

Subgrouping

It is not uncommon for small groups or even pairs of group members to find more satisfaction in the interaction among themselves than they find with the group as a whole. This is known as *subgrouping*, or formation of cliques. Members of subgroups tend to think of themselves as better than members of other subgroups and often compete with other subgroups or with the leader. Subgrouping can be constructive when members of a pair are able to see, through exploration, how their attraction to one another constitutes a reenactment of unconscious wishes.

Here is an example of subgrouping:

Two group members, Joy and Betty, paired up and began defending each other constantly and acting as allies in all situations. Joy's behavior in the group was that of a "tough person"; she often made caustic, stinging remarks to others. Most members feared her and kept their distance. Betty, however, endlessly pointed out to others that there was a heart of gold under Joy's tough exterior and that her toughness was merely a defense. She used as an illustration the fact that Joy was consistently kind to her.

Through exploration and analysis, it became evident that Joy represented, to Betty, Betty's own mother, who had been very cruel and frightening to her as a child. Betty had attempted to comfort herself throughout her childhood by telling herself that under the cruelty was a "heart of gold." She had also acted this out outside the group by choosing men she called "diamonds in the rough" whom she tried to rehabilitate. Joy's relationship with Betty was also useful to Joy, as it allowed her to explore her tender side, which she felt obliged to hide from most people.

While this is an example of a positive use of subgrouping, it would be destructive to group growth if it were to go unexplored, for this "mutual admiration society" excluded others and put Joy and Betty out of the other members' reach.

Insight

Insight occurs when the client is able to see the connection between unconscious feelings, wishes, and conflicts and conscious behavior. In order to make this connection, the client must first fully experience these feelings, wishes, and conflicts in conscious awareness. This then produces *emotional* insight, which is distinctly different from *intellectual* insight. In the latter case, the client "knows" intellectually why certain behaviors occur but is powerless to stop them. When true emotional insight occurs, the problem behavior vanishes.

Here is an example of insight:

Pat, a client, may know intellectually that she is resisting group interaction because of her fear of closeness. One evening she attends the group and feels a kind of shakiness and fear accompanied by a desire to be close to the others. This marks the beginning of emotional insight.

Intellectual insight almost always precedes emotional insight. Clients often say, "Now I *know* why I do this, but I can't stop, so what good does it do?" Of course there is no simple answer, but the therapist can encourage clients by saying, "The rest will come" or "It does take time."

Another example of emotional insight follows:

A client, Rosa, became depressed following her graduation from a Ph.D. program. This milestone came after years of arduous work, and she could not understand why the symptoms of depression persisted. One night in group she became aware of a terrible longing to be a child again and realized that she was experiencing the graduation as an end to childhood. After this, the symptoms subsided.

Termination

Therapists vary in their opinions about when termination of intensive group therapy should properly occur. It is generally agreed that both the client and the therapist should feel ready at the time of termination. Freud once stated that termination occurred when one was "able to love and work." In general, it is hoped that the client will be able to relate to others in a basically nondefensive way and that there will be other signs of healthy self-esteem. At termination, the client should feel satisfied with life on the whole and be able to recognize the unsatisfying parts that cannot be changed. The client should find contentment in self-directed pleasures as well as happiness in relationships with others. All these criteria can be observed in the group. Other members can be helpful to clients who wish to terminate by pointing out resolved as well as unresolved areas.

SUPPORT GROUPS

A *support group* is a group of relatively healthy people who meet regularly to discuss specific problems that are common to all of them. The main differences between support groups and psychotherapy groups are that members of support groups are *not* psychiatric clients and that, by and large, they have strong, intact ego function. These clients meet together because of some disruption in their individual lives.

The goals of support groups are:

- To promote well-being through shared support
- To increase self-esteem through satisfying interpersonal relations
- To provide education about problems discussed

Table 20-9 Support Groups

Examples
Clients undergoing or recovering from:
Bereavement
Chronic pain
Divorce
Heart attack
Hemodialysis
Terminal illness
Health workers in:
CCUs and ICUs
Colleges
Oncology units
Psychiatric units
Others:
Families of clients with mental or physical illness
Women's consciousness groups

Types of Support Groups

Support groups fall into three categories. Members may be (1) clients who share a common problem, (2) nurses who work together and share group problems, or (3) special groups. See Table 20-9 for examples of support groups.

Differences between Support Groups and Psychotherapy Groups

The conduct of support groups differs from that of psychotherapy groups with psychiatric clients. Because the members of a support group are less anxious, the content is likely to be less "symptomatic." The focus is usually on the problem or issue which brings the members together. Table 20-10 gives a brief overview of the differences between psychotherapy groups and support groups.

SUMMARY

Group psychotherapy is a method of intervening with psychiatric clients in groups. It provides participants with opportunities to relate and react to people while exploring their behavior with one another. The purpose of group psychotherapy is

Table 20-10 Differences between Psychotherapy Groups and Support Groups

Concept	Psychotherapy Group	Support Group
Membership	Psychiatric clients.	Individuals who share a common problem or who work together in a stressful situation.
Duration of group	Is usually open-ended; sometimes closed to 10, 20, or 30 sessions.	May be open-ended or closed.
Use of content and process	Both are used to help clients explore interpersonal and intrapsychic problems.	Emphasis is on content. Process may be used occasionally.
Cohesiveness	Takes longer to develop, as clients often fear closeness and commitment.	Develops quickly, as members come to group with common problems.
Transference and countertransference	Are discussed or used in understanding clients.	Occur but usually are not discussed.
Resistance	Occurs when a client is on the brink of insight or change. Is discussed to help clients understand why they fear changing.	Is an ongoing, subtle, unconscious process, as members begin to change. Is usually not discussed in depth.
Acting out	Occurs frequently and is discussed to promote self-understanding.	Rarely occurs, as members are able to discuss thoughts and feelings relatively openly.
Insight	Occurs over time and is the major goal of group.	May already be present or may occur in some members as group progresses.
Termination	Occurs when symptoms are no longer present.	Occurs when problems have been resolved to clients' satisfaction.

to examine and explore behavior of group members as it occurs with a view toward permanent change.

There are four types of group psychotherapy: activity therapy, educative therapy, repressive-inspirational therapy, and reconstructive therapy.

Selection of members of a group requires awareness of the advantages and disadvantages of homogeneous and heterogeneous groups, as well as awareness of which clients are unsuitable for group treatment.

The leader's behavior has a profound effect on the group. There are three types of leaders: boss, guide, and stimulator. The type of leader will influence the level of productivity and the type of interaction in the group.

The irrational and unproductive needs of beginning group psychotherapists include their need to maintain a good self-image and to maintain control of the group through preventing regressive behavior, resistance, expression of hostility, acting out, and introduction of taboo topics.

Group development can be divided into four sequential phases: uncertainty, overaggressiveness, regression, and adaptation. Central concepts of psychotherapy groups include content and process, cohesiveness, transference, countertransference, resistance, acting out, subgrouping, insight, and termination.

Support groups are groups of relatively healthy people who meet regularly to discuss specific problems common to all of them. These groups offer support, increased self-esteem, and education.

REFERENCES

1. Joseph J. Geller, "Group Psychotherapy in the Treatment of the Schizophrenic Syndromes," *Psychiatric Quarterly*, vol. 63, 1963, pp. 1-13; and unpublished material.
2. George Homans, *The Human Group*, Harcourt, Brace, and World, New York, 1950.
3. Dorwin Cartwright, "The Nature of Group Cohesiveness," in D. Cartwright and A. Zander, eds., *Group Dynamics*, Harper and Row, New York, 1960.
4. Georg Simmel, *Conflict and the Web of Group Affiliations*, Free Press, New York, 1960.
5. Albert Pepitone and George Reichling, "Group Cohesiveness and the Expression of Hostility," *Human Relations*, vol. 8, 1955, pp. 327–337.
6. Jerome Frank, "Some Determinants, Manifestations and Effects of Cohesion in Therapy Groups," *International Journal of Group Psychotherapy*, vol. 7, 1957, pp. 53–62.

BIBLIOGRAPHY

Eleanor Rodio Furlong, "Women's Awareness Groups for Chronic Psychiatric Clients," in Suzanne Lego, ed., *The American Handbook of Psychiatric Nursing,* Lippincott, Philadelphia, 1984.

Suzanne Lego, "Group Therapy," in Suzanne Lego, ed., *The American Handbook of Psychiatric Nursing,* Lippincott, Philadelphia, 1984.

Suzanne Lego, "Psychoanalytically Oriented Individual and Group Therapy with Adults," in D. Critchley and J. Maurin, eds., *the Clinical Specialist in Psychiatric Mental Health Nursing: Theory, Research, and Practice,* Wiley, New York, 1985.

Nada Light, "Group Therapy with Children," in Suzanne Lego, ed., *The American Handbook of Psychiatric Nursing,* Lippincott, Philadelphia, 1984.

Rachel Parios, "Activities of Daily Living Groups," in Suzanne Lego, ed., *The American Handbook of Psychiatric Nursing,* Lippincott, Philadelphia, 1984.

Nancy Sargent, "Teaching Self-Medication," in Suzanne Lego, ed., *The American Handbook of Psychiatric Nursing,* Lippincott, Philadelphia, 1984.

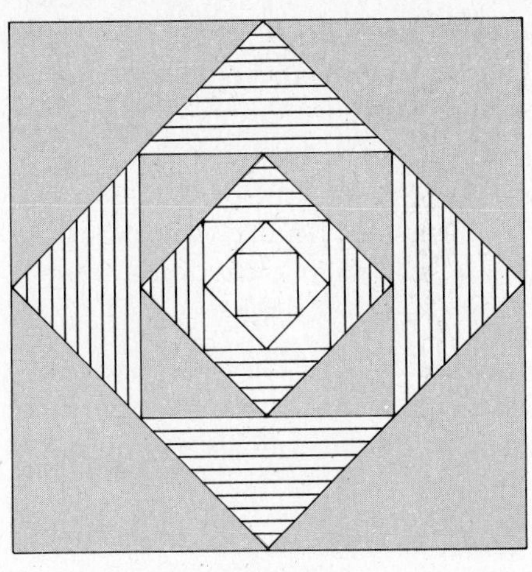

CHAPTER 21
Group and Organizational Theory

Marie Cella Smith

LEARNING OBJECTIVES

After studying this chapter, the student should be able to:

1. Relate the conceptual framework to group and organizational theories.
2. Relate members' behaviors to effective functioning of work groups.
3. Relate leaders' behaviors to effective functioning of work groups.
4. Use Bion's theory of groups to analyze the functioning of work groups.
5. Describe growth-producing, group-vitalizing, and growth-inhibiting roles of group members.
6. Determine the influence of cohesion, groupthink, lack of cohesion, and competition on group functioning.
7. Discuss the classical and modern approaches to organizational structure and functions.
8. Discuss the types and uses of power in organizations.
9. Discuss the relationship of members' needs and various leadership styles.
10. Apply the parallel process in nursing practice.
11. Analyze the approaches to the management of conflict in organizations.
12. Apply the three strategies of planned change to nursing practice.
13. Assess a work group or organization.

Nurses, like other people, are members, and sometimes leaders, of various groups. They were born into families, are members of communities, have attended school as members of classes, and have chosen to join a professional group. Nurses may practice their profession in any of several contexts, including bureaucratic organizations, home-based community agencies, and private practice.

Nurses are simultaneously members and leaders of a number of groups. They are members of a professional nursing group, members or leaders of an interdisciplinary team, members of a management or staff nursing group, collaborative participants in peer groups, and leaders of groups of clients. In each of these groups they function within the philosophy of the group or a larger organization as they deliver or direct care.

The structure of the setting where care takes place is an important factor influencing the nurse's role and function. The administrative structure of organizations, particularly nursing administration, directly influences nursing practice. Organizational philosophy and the quality of relationships between nurses and the administration affect the way in which staff groups and treatment teams function. Team functioning in turn directly affects the quality of care given to clients and their families.

The purpose of this chapter is to develop an understanding of how to work effectively in work groups and organizations. Theories of work groups and organizations will be presented; and dynamics of work groups and organizations will be explored.

CONCEPTUAL FRAMEWORK

Members of a work group or an organization are individuals, with their own life histories, physical and intellectual strengths and limitations, spiritual desires and understanding, and purposes in life. An individual's pursuit of life purposes usually motivates employment in an organization; in the course of a job interview, both the applicant and the potential employer will try to learn whether the applicant's goals and the organization's goals are congruent. However, it is when an individual becomes a member of a work group that the person's pursuit of goals becomes most important. A work group must operate day by day to achieve the organization's goals; and it has its own "life," its own rules, and its own power to reward and punish its members.

The individual, the work group, and the organization all have phases of growth and development, structure, functions, purposes, and meaning. To work effectively within organizations, nurses need to recognize:

- The person's existence, goals, and methods
- The work group's existence, goals, and methods
- The organization's existence, goals, and methods

WORK GROUPS

Definitions

A *group* is defined as more than two persons, interacting with one another in such a way that each person influences and is influenced by the others. A *group goal* is an end state desired by a majority of the members of the group. A group may have a single goal or multiple goals. A *group task* is something that must be done in order for the group to achieve its goal or goals.[1] The *basic drives* in any group are the members' need to belong to the group, their need to achieve in the group, and their need to be recognized by other group members. When drives are frustrated, *group apathy* occurs; it is defined as lack of enthusiasm and inability to mobilize.

Nurses as a group are individuals who interact with one another, influencing care given to clients and being influenced by those around them. As a group, nurses aim to provide optimal care for their clients. This goal is achieved by the performance of a large variety of tasks. Some nurses perform hands-on tasks; others direct or manage clients' care. They collaborate and cooperate in family, client, and work groups.

Kinds of Groups

Groups have been categorized in a variety of ways: as formal or informal groups, for instance. Groups may also be defined in terms of processes, including tasks, assumptions, and dynamics. This section will examine formal and informal groups.

Formal Groups

Formal groups are groups formed for specific purposes to which members are committed; members are selected and agree to be members; leadership is formal and positional; and the boundaries of the groups are clear and known by the leaders and members. Work groups and therapeutic groups (discussed in Chapter 20) are examples of formal groups; organizations are also considered formal groups.

Informal Groups

Informal groups form among people who work together; they satisfy members' needs. The relationships that develop between members provide a sense of affiliation, identification, emotional support, assistance, and protection; these are, basically, the purposes of the informal group. The boundaries of an informal group are unclear; membership is difficult to define exactly. Leadership shifts, depending on the needs of individuals and the group. An informal group provides a certain amount of comfort for its members; but it can also create discomfort when conflicts arise. The degree of comfort and discomfort experienced by members has a direct effect upon the group's performance of tasks.[2]

Informal groups often develop within work groups (and within organizations). For example, a group of nurses from various units may try to eat together in the cafeteria. The dynamics of informal groups influence both work groups and organizations.

Social groups are informal groups which form so that their members may experience companionship and satisfying relationships with friends. They focus on enjoyment and a mutual meeting of needs. "Leaders" are generally called *hosts* or *hostesses.* They select or invite guests on the basis of considerations of friendship or social obligation. A country club and a hiking club are examples of social groups. The existence of social groups within a work group or organization makes it very difficult to focus on tasks and goals.

Work-Group Theory

Small-Group Theories

Small groups, whether formal or informal, have certain characteristics in common. Several theoretical approaches have been developed to describe and explain behavior in small groups.[1,2,3] Some approaches are outlined in Table 21-1.

Table 21-1 Small-Group Theories

Theory	Theoretical Orientation
Field theory	Behavior in a group is seen as the result of a field of interdependent forces.
Interaction theory	Group is viewed as a system of interacting individuals. Group behavior is understood by grasping the relationship among the individuals in terms of activity, interaction, and sentiment.
Systems theory	Group is a system of interacting individuals who exhibit interlocking elements such as positions and roles. Emphasis is placed upon group input and output.
Sociometric theory	Emphasis is placed on the interpersonal choices of individuals.
Psychoanalytic theory	Analysis of the group is concerned with the motivational and defensive processes of individuals as they relate to group life.
General psychology theory	Behavior in the group is analyzed utilizing the individual processes of learning, motivation, and perception. It views individual behavior within the context of a group.
Empirical-statistical theory	The basic aspects of group behavior are viewed from a statistical analysis of data about individuals.
Formal models theory	Formal models of group behavior are constructed using mathematical procedures. Natural situations are compared with the model.
Reinforcement theory	Interpersonal behavior in the group is explained in terms of the outcomes for group members.
Transactional theory	Group members are viewed as making contributions that are valued by group members; the group process is seen as having the potential for healing.

SOURCES: Eric Berne, *The Structure and Dynamics of Organizations and Groups,* Grove, New York, 1966; Dorwin Cartwright and Alvin Zander, eds., *Group Dynamics: Research and Theory,* 3d ed., Harper and Row, New York, 1968; Marvin Shaw, *Group Dynamics: The Psychology of Small-Group Behavior,* 3d ed., McGraw-Hill, New York, 1980.

Bion's Theory of Groups

Bion[4] has described two basic processes that occur in groups: the *work-task process* and the *basic-*

assumption process. These processes do not define or distinguish different kinds of groups; rather, they operate in any group. (Other theorists have described the same phenomena as *content* and *process.*) Work-task dynamics in a group are goal-directed and reflect a rational, scientific approach. Basic-assumption dynamics of a group include unconscious fantasies of the leader and group members having to do with dependency; fight-flight behavior; and pairing. In addition to the "basic assumptions," work groups are also characterized by certain *operational assumptions.*

WORK-TASK PROCESS. Task and work processes accomplish specific goals agreed to by the membership of a group; they constitute one aspect of group functioning. Methods for achieving a task are clearly specified. Work is reality-oriented and goal-directed. In some groups, the work or task is the reason why the group is formed; in such a situation, assigned leaders identify the task, clarify communication, and enable the group to work. A work group knows its purpose and can define its task; a rational, scientific approach is valued; and members learn through experience.[4]

BASIC-ASSUMPTION PROCESS. The second aspect of group functioning is the basic-assumption process. A basic assumption is one which seems to be held by a majority of the group and which, when identified, makes otherwise illogical, contradictory behaviors seem coherent and orderly. Bion described three kinds of basic assumptions: dependency, fight-flight, and pairing.[5] These basic assumptions are usually outside the conscious awareness of individuals in a group.[4]

The basic assumption of *dependency* has to do with obtaining security, support, and direction from outside the group—most often from the leader. Members may act as if they knew nothing and as if the leader were omnipotent. A group of chronically ill, dependent clients led by a giving, overresponsible nurse is an example of the influence of a dependent assumption. When group members present themselves as weak, inadequate, and dependent, they want the leader to take care of them and relieve their feelings of insecurity. They are disappointed and hostile when these expectations are not met and usually abandon the leader and search for an alternative. More ambitious group members may assume the leadership role and experience the same fate as the original leader. Conflict may exist between childlike dependency and the needs of the group members as adults, between a desire to persist in a dependent state and a desire to accept consequences maturely. Resentment at being in a dependent state may develop. When members of a dependent group feel deserted by the leader, they forget internal conflicts, close ranks, develop group cohesiveness, and experience a temporary sense of comfort and security.[4]

The *fight-flight* assumption enables a group to preserve itself by fighting or by running away from someone or something. Action is essential and takes one of these two forms. Individuals are abandoned for the sake of group survival, and the leader is viewed as one who can mobilize the group for attack or lead it in flight.[4] Flight and fight both offer an immediate opportunity to express emotion.[4] Groups whose members avoid tasks by coming late, being absent, or engaging in a multitude of other activities are probably experiencing fight-flight dynamics.

The third basic assumption in a group is *pairing,* or the forming of a couple. When a couple forms, the group acts as if its function is to find strength from within itself. No leader is necessary, but the group expects a new leader, new thoughts, or a kind of new life or utopia to emerge. An air of expectation prevails.[4] Focus is on the future, and phrases like, "Things will be better when . . . ," are heard frequently. The group enjoys a sense of optimism and hope, and members' feelings are consistently agreeable.

The basic-assumption process is almost always present in groups. In a work group, the group's behavior is understandable when one also considers the emotional aspects of the group. The group may act as if it is paralyzed and helpless to do anything toward a goal unless outside resources are made available. At one point, the group may act as if it is fighting, trying to kill, strangle, or destroy a task or problem; the group may also run away from a task, expending multiple resources but moving no closer to accomplishment. At another point, the group may be excited, energized, acting as if the group has the answer and can creatively achieve the work set before it.

Individuals play a part in this balance between group work and the group's basic assumptions. Bion called the individual's contribution *valency* and defined it as the individual's characteristics that determine participation in the emotional life of the group.[4] For example:

> Nancy was involved in a grievance committee formed on her unit to address the expectation that staff members routinely work double shifts. The other members' ideas depended on the administration to solve the problem (dependency). Nancy was extremely uncomfortable with this dependency and created group conflict by opposing the other members' suggestions. Her valency influenced her behavior in the group, and she tried to force the group from a basic assumption of dependency to one of fight or pairing.

OPERATIONAL ASSUMPTIONS. In addition to basic assumptions, work groups are characterized by several operational assumptions:

- Thought must be translated into action.
- Environmental change is believed to be sufficient without any corresponding change in individuals.
- The leader of the group is not the only one with the skills needed to accomplish a task.
- Members of the work group cooperate as separate and discrete individuals to accomplish the group task.
- Membership in a work group implies a choice to see that the task is accomplished.[4]

These assumptions emphasize rationality, problem solving, and accomplishment.

Work-Group Dynamics

Since work groups have the same dynamics as small groups in general, work-group dynamics can be understood in terms of small-group theory. The development of effective groups is facilitated by the recognition of boundaries; by the structural dynamics of rank and status, norms and goals, and roles; and by the functional dynamics of cohesiveness and competition.

Boundaries

An effective group is one in which its members have a common purpose and recognize internal and external boundaries. *Internal boundaries* are those that exist around individual members in the group, while *external boundaries* are those which separate the group's position and function in relation to other groups.[2] Effective groups have sensitive leaders who recognize and elicit creative group participation. They are able to absorb new members and lose old members while maintaining group identity. Individual members are valued for their unique contributions and are encouraged to express needs and thoughts.

Rank and Status

There are a number of concepts which have to do with a member's position in the group. One of these is *rank,* the position of a member relative to the evaluation of other members of the group. If all members were asked to rank one another according to some dimension such as "the person I like best," a rank order of popularity among members would result. While this is seldom done explicitly, members are indeed ranked by others implicitly. The rank order of a member has an influence on group behavior. Members who rank high on participation tend to have a higher group rank and more influence on group behavior.

Another phenomenon having to do with a person's position in a group is *status,* the prestige attributed to particular positions in a group. Homans describes status as a collection of rights and duties.[6] Status, in part, may come from the world outside the group and be brought into the group by the member. For example:

> John, a new member of a research committee group, brought to a meeting a research design completed outside the group. He was creating a position of status for himself inside the group that was comparable to one he believed he occupied outside it.

If members of the group are impressed by a person's qualities, that person is granted status in the group. As an example, in a group of nurses, experienced nurses come into the group with status. Status is also attributed to members as a result of behavior within the group. A person who exhibits the ability to relieve tension is given the right and duty to do so as well as the status of social leader. Status also may be assigned to an individual by the group; for example, a work group may not begin until its selected "status person" arrives.

Norms and Goals

Norms are rules of conduct or standards which specify appropriate behavior in a particular group. A norm is an idea in the minds of group members which may be in the form of a statement specifying what the members are expected to do under given circumstances. *Goals* are explicitly stated outcomes which the group expects to achieve. Group norms are frequently confused with group goals, and sometimes they are in conflict. For example:

> A work group may set a goal that all nursing care plans be completed within a week. Everyone may agree verbally to this goal. However, the norm may be to make sure nobody is left behind, so members may make sure no one works too quickly or makes anybody else's work look bad. When the time for completing the task arrives, not all the care plans are finished, and excuses are made. The norm in this group has hindered the goal.

Norms in a group change subtly as the group evolves. All members are involved in this process of development and change. Neither the leader nor any one member can set the norm for the group.

Roles

A group *role* may be thought of as the function or part a person assumes as a member of a group. A role involves a set of responsibilities assigned to a specific position or job. Role has been called the dynamic aspect of status. When a group member performs a role, he or she is putting into effect the rights and duties granted by the other group members. In a work group, the role acted out by a member may or may not be useful for the task. For example, the status of a member may be that of "group incompetent." The rights and duties that go along with this status may include the need for constant clarification, the need for repetition of the agenda, and the need for ongoing reassurance, especially from the leader. It is important to explore such behavior with the member who acts out roles that are not helpful to the group.

Roles may facilitate, inhibit, vitalize, and produce growth in groups. Benne and Sheats list a number of roles that are assumed in work groups.[7] Table 21-2 identifies several roles and the behavior that is characteristic of each (this table is also given in Chapter 17; it is reproduced here for the reader's convenience).

Cohesiveness

Group cohesiveness is defined as the degree of a group's internal strength; it is the result of the forces that motivate group members to remain in or to leave the group. Cohesive groups are characterized by "we-ness" and esprit de corps. The success of a group depends on its internal strength; internal strength is determined by the degree of each individual's desire to be in and remain in the group, the degree of support the group provides its members, and the degree to which stable values and standards of behavior develop.

FACTORS INFLUENCING COHESIVENESS. Group cohesiveness is a complex phenomenon that is determined by many factors. It varies with the group process and the characteristics of group members. The following variables are known to influence group cohesiveness:

- Attractiveness, to those wishing to join, of the members and goals of the group
- Members' needs for affiliation
- Success or failure of the group in achieving its goals
- Clarity of goals
- Outcome of conflicts
- Nature and timing of feedback to members
- Communication among members
- Readiness of members to be influenced by others in the group[6]

CONSEQUENCES OF GROUP COHESIVENESS. Cohesive groups have high levels of productivity and may produce outcomes in keeping with the organization's expectations. Cohesive groups perform above and beyond expectations. Unfortunately, cohesive groups also may develop group norms which undermine expectations.

Cohesiveness is related to both the quality and the quantity of group interaction. Less cohesive groups have diminished communications, and their interactions are more negatively oriented. Members of highly cohesive groups generally communicate more readily, and the content of their interactions is oriented toward positive ends. For example, nurses who are united around a specific issue will communicate more positively than those who are divided or in conflict about the issue.

Groups characterized by friendliness, cooperation, and attractiveness of members exert strong social influence on members to behave in accordance with group expectations. When a person is attracted to a group, he or she is motivated to behave in accordance with the wishes of other

Table 21-2 Group Roles

Role	Behavior	Role	Behavior
Growth-producing roles		**Vitalizing roles**	
Initiator	Offers new ideas and suggests solutions.	Gatekeeper	Encourages and facilitates participation of others.
Information seeker	Seeks clarification of suggestions.	Standard setter	Expresses standards for the group.
Opinion seeker	Seeks clarification of values about an issue.	Follower	Goes along passively as a friendly audience.
Information giver	Offers facts or generalizations which are authoritative		
Opinion giver	States beliefs or opinions relevant to the issues.	**Growth-inhibiting roles**	
Elaborater	Gives examples; develops meanings and explanations.	Aggressor	Deflates status of others; may express disapproval of values, acts, or feelings of others; jokes aggressively.
Coordinator	Clarifies relationships among ideas, suggestions, and activities of individuals.	Blocker	Is negativistic and resistive in an unreasonable and stubborn manner.
Orienter	Defines the goals of a setting and orients others to them.	Recognition seeker	Tries to call attention to self. Boasts about personal achievements.
Evaluator	Relates the standards of the milieu to a problem.	Self-confessor	Uses the milieu to express personal feelings and insights.
Energizer	Motivates others to action and decision making.	"Playboy"	Displays lack of involvement and cynical nonchalance.
Procedural technician	Performs routine tasks.	Dominator	Asserts authority; manipulates the group or individuals.
Recorder	Writes down topics, decisions, and actions resulting from discussion.	Help-seeker	Tries to get sympathy from others; expresses insecurity, confusion, or depreciation of self beyond reason.
Vitalizing roles			
Encourager	Praises, agrees with, and accepts others' ideas.		
Harmonizer	Mediates quarrels and relieves tension.	Special-interest pleader	Speaks for the underdog while masking feelings of bias and prejudice; actions are contrary to verbalizations.
Compromiser	Operates from within to resolve conflicts.		

SOURCE: Kenneth B. Benne and P. Sheats, "Functional Roles of Group Members," *Journal of Social Issues*, vol. 4, no. 2, Spring 1948, pp. 42–49.

group members and to conform to group norms and standards.

When new graduates select a work setting, social influence is frequently an important factor. The person will attempt to "fit in" by conforming to established norms and standards. For example, new nurses who feel accepted by and a part of the group they have joined will work hard to produce the group goal of high-quality client care. The opposite is also true; in less cohesive groups, productivity is lessened. Members of highly cohesive groups are generally more satisfied with achievements than those who participate in less cohesive groups. This can account for the variability in job satisfaction that exists between staff groups on different units of the same hospital.

CHARACTERISTICS OF COHESIVE GROUPS. Several variables can be observed and evaluated to determine the level of cohesiveness in a group. Positive responses to the following questions would indicate a high level of cohesiveness in a group. The characteristics of cohesive groups are set in *italics*.

- Do group *members like each other?*
- Are members *friendly* and *willing to interact?*
- Do members appear *supportive* of one another?
- Do members provide *feedback* and *praise for accomplishments?*
- Is *participation* in group activities evident?
- Is there *commitment to group goals* by the members?
- Is the *leadership democratic?*

- Is there evidence of *high group productivity?*
- Do members show *cooperation* and *interdependence* when a task needs to be accomplished?
- Are *norms adhered to* and protected?
- Do members of the group experience *increased self-esteem* as a result of their membership?
- Are members *satisfied with the work* of the group?
- Are individuals *satisfied with other members* of the group?
- Are members of the group *influenced by one another?*
- Are *tasks accepted readily?*
- Are *roles accepted readily?*
- Do members *trust* each other?
- Is there evidence of *loyalty* to the group?
- Is there a *low turnover* of members in the group?
- Are *group goals consistent with those of individual members?*
- Do members *attend the group regularly?*
- Are members *prompt?*
- Is *risk taking evident* in the group?

GROUPTHINK: OVERCOHESION. Janis coined the word *groupthink* to describe the mode of thinking engaged in by persons who are members of a highly cohesive in-group in which uniformity and agreement are given such priority that critical thinking is impossible or unacceptable.[8] Groups experiencing groupthink develop group norms around the maintenance of unity and loyalty regardless of cost to individual members or consequences to the group as a whole. Janis describes eight symptoms of groupthink. These are listed with their characteristic behaviors in Table 21-3.

Table 21-3 Symptoms of Groupthink

Symptom	Behavior
Invulnerability	Group members believe there are no dangers. They are overoptimistic and take extraordinary risks.
Rationale	Members collectively construct rationalizations in order to discount warnings and negative feedback.
Morality	Ethical and moral consequences of decision making are ignored by group members.
Stereotypes	Competitive group leadership is viewed as the enemy. Members believe that negotiation is impossible because leaders of "enemy" groups are weak or ineffective.
Pressure	There is pressure on individuals to conform and remain in the group.
Self-censorship	There is no deviation from what is perceived as a group consensus. Doubt and misgivings are minimized and unexpressed.
Unanimity	Members of the group speak in favor of the majority position, creating an illusion of unanimity. The minority position on an issue is never heard.
Mind guards	Individual members of the group appoint themselves to protect the leader and other members from adverse information that may undermine the confidence the group shares in its effectiveness and morality.

SOURCE: Irving Janis, "Groupthink," *Psychology Today,* November 1971, pp. 71–89.

When groupthink exists, there is too much cohesiveness. Members are looked at and perceive themselves as an in-group. Members may be headed toward disastrous decision making but are unable to challenge each other because of the strong norm for loyalty and unity. Decisions made on the basis of groupthink are less reliable than decisions made in a consensual way and should therefore be viewed with caution.

Nurses may avoid groupthink by encouraging critical thinking, open inquiry, and impartial probing of the issues presented to them. Avoiding an in-group and "unity at all costs" attitude encourages positive cohesiveness and prevents the negative outcomes that result from groupthink. The ability to challenge the majority position or the views of "core" members and introduce alternative plans will lead to more objective decision making.[8]

Competition

Competition is rivalry among individuals in a group. Just as cohesion can have positive and negative effects on the achievement of group goals, competition can foster maximum effort or become a destructive force in the work group; that is, it may have positive or negative consequences. For example, competition to improve the quality of services and to have such improvement acknowledged can have extremely beneficial results for group members and the whole organization; acknowledgment for a job well done has far-reaching positive effects upon the morale of work groups. On the other hand, the destructive aspects of competition show themselves when conflict is perpetuated and energy is diverted from achievement of goals. Conflict frequently occurs over who has control in a situation. For example, one nursing shift may compete with another over who controls or has the final say about the care of clients. Such competition is destructive to group membership as well as to group productivity.

Destructive competition is characterized by intimidating communication, use of force and cleverness, and suspicious and hostile attitudes. Competition that is positive is characterized by increased productivity, compromise, and positive and goal-directed attitudes.

ORGANIZATIONS

Organizational Theory

Organizational theory attempts to describe and analyze the structure and function of organizations. This section will examine classical and modern organizational theory.

Classical Organizational Theory

Classical organizational theory describes the organizational structure that was the focus of Weber's work, the bureaucracy. A *bureaucracy* is a systematized and centralized organizational structure.

Weber's bureaucratic model is characterized by specialization and division of labor, a hierarchical arrangement of positions, a system of abstract rules, and a management style characterized by impersonal relationships.[5] Other concepts, including flat, decentralized structures and the staff concept of organization, have been developed to extend and modify Weber's principles of organizational theory.

ORGANIZATIONAL STRUCTURE. An *organizational structure* is a systematic and goal-directed arrangement of the work of an organization. An organizational chart, or *organigram*, is a visual representation of the organizational structure. It shows the positions in an organization as they relate to one another. Figure 21-1 shows a nursing department's organizational chart.

Figure 21-1 Organizational chart for a nursing department.
(SOURCE: Linda Bernhard and Michelle Walsh, *Leadership: The Key to Professionalization of Nursing*, McGraw-Hill, New York, 1981. Used with permission.)

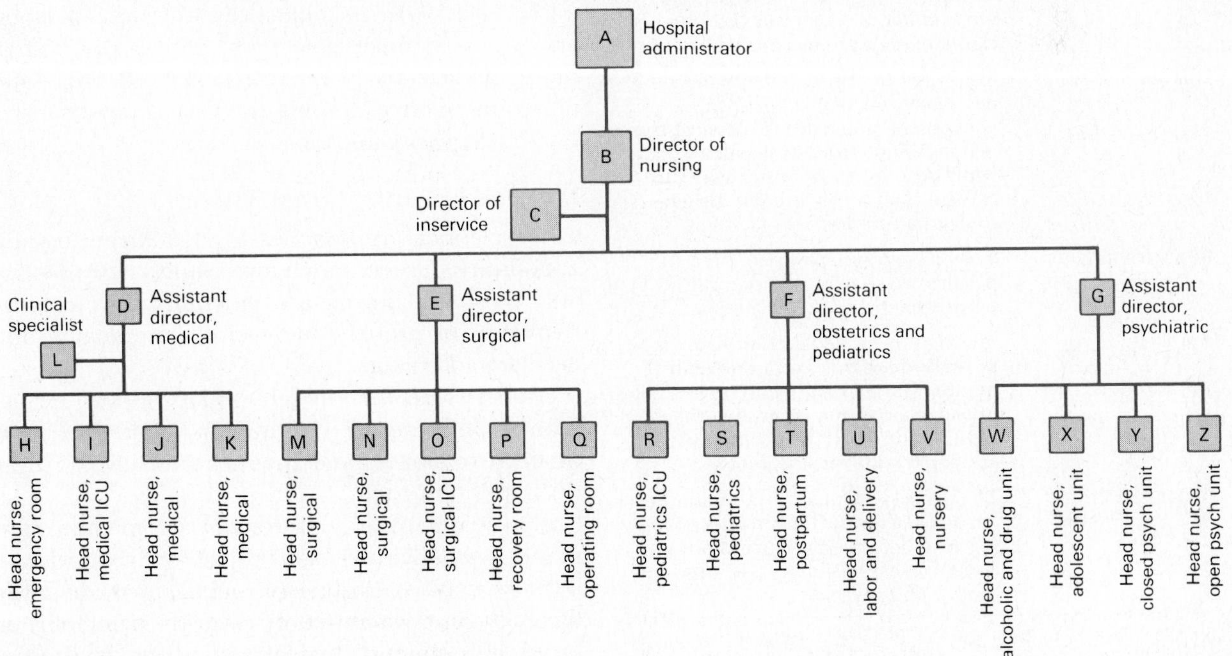

BASIC CONCEPTS OF CLASSICAL ORGANIZATIONS. Institutions organized under classical theory, or bureaucracies, emphasize rigid, centralized control of workers in order to promote high productivity, efficiency, and effectiveness in accomplishing goals.[9] The concepts that underlie classical organizational structure are defined and explained in Table 21-4.

Table 21-4 Concepts Underlying Classical Organizational Theory

Concept	Definition
Scalar chain	Vertical growth of an organization. It consists of a number of levels or steps in the structure known as the *hierarchy*. Tasks are graded according to the degree of authority and responsibility of the individuals at each step.
Functional process	Horizontal growth of an organization. It is a division into different kinds of tasks at the same level in the organization.
Line	The hierarchy of personnel that extends from the chief executive officer (CEO) at the top to the workers at the bottom. Line workers are responsible for performing or supervising the direct primary functions of the organization.
Staff	Persons who function to support those in the line organization. Staff workers support and facilitate the work of line workers but have no rights of decision or command.
Span of control	The number of persons a manager can effectively supervise. A short span is characteristic of classical theory and leads to what is called a *tall*, centralized organizational structure. A wide span leads to a *flat*, decentralized structure.
Responsibility	The obligation individuals have to perform an assigned or delegated task to the best of their ability.
Authority	The right of designated individuals to make decisions and issue commands. *Power* is the moral and physical force that maintains the right to authority. Authority must be *delegated* with responsibility.
Accountability	The process of answering to another for one's actions. It involves reporting whether one has carried out an assigned responsibility, and used authority appropriately.

SOURCE: Linda Anne Bernhard and Michelle Walsh, *Leadership: The Key to the Professionalization of Nursing*, McGraw-Hill, New York, 1981.

CHARACTERISTICS OF A BUREAUCRACY. Classical theory includes the concepts of specialization and the division of labor. All workers become specialists at their own jobs. They do their jobs, and no one knows as much about their jobs as they do. The division of labor defines each worker's area of specialization and responsibility. For instance, one nurse may be assigned responsibility for respirators, and when he or she is off duty, others feel that they lack expertise and may be somewhat concerned about doing this job.

Positions are arranged in a vertical hierarchy in which each lower office is under the control and supervision of a higher one.[5]

There are formal, well-understood rules and regulations. Formal rules ensure uniformity and coordination of efforts in organizations, because rules continue, whereas personnel changes over time.

Managers in a bureaucratic system avoid emotional attachment to subordinates and clients in order to facilitate rational decision making. Their relationships are characteristically impersonal. For example, a head nurse might be friendly with the staff members on a unit but would not socialize with them.

The large size of organizations is the single most important condition in the development of a bureaucracy. Breaking a large system into smaller parts, each with its objectives (division of labor) and ways to meet objectives, makes the system more manageable.[10] Table 21-5 lists, defines, and illustrates with examples the characteristics of a bureaucratic organization.

Modern Organizational Theory

While classical approaches to structuring organizations are still very much in evidence, new theories and structural forms are emerging to meet the demands of growth, increasing complexity, and accelerated change.

Modern *theories* match organizational design with environmental conditions. Table 21-6 lists modern organizational theories and gives a brief description of each.

Newer organizational *designs* are meeting dramatically changing needs. Project, matrix, and free-form structures (discussed below) provide more flexibility but violate such classical principles as unity of command, specialization, and division of labor.

Table 21-5 Characteristics of a Bureaucratic Organization

Characteristic	Definition	Example
A clear chain of command	All individuals from the bottom to the top of the organization know the supervisor to whom they are accountable.	The staff nurse reports to the head nurse.
Unity of command	Each person in the chain of command is accountable to one and only one person.	The staff goes to the head nurse before the supervisor is called.
Clarity of delegation	The superior assigns specific tasks to particular subordinates.	The supervisor asks the head nurse to interview applicants for the head nurse's unit.
Completeness of delegation	For every organizational activity, someone must be responsible.	Every daily operation of the client care unit is assigned to someone.
Sufficiency of delegation	Those delegated responsibility also have authority to implement it.	The head nurse is responsible for client care and has the authority to order supplies from another department.
Nondelegatable responsibilities	Authority can be delegated but responsibility cannot be delegated.	The supervisor assigns certain activities to the head nurse, who in turn assigns these to a staff nurse. The supervisor holds the head nurse accountable and responsible for their completion.
Specialization	Proficiency is shown in a specific skill or task as opposed to a broad range of responsibilities.	The psychiatric–mental health clinical nurse specialist identifies determinants of a client's behavior but does not oversee a unit's picnic in the park.

SOURCE: Ross A. Webber, *Management Pragmatics*, Irwin, Homewood, Ill., 1979.

Table 21-6 Modern Organizational Theories

Theory	Description	Theory	Description
Balance theory	A behavioral theory that stresses organizational equilibrium or balance. There is a balance between the inducements to join the organization and the contributions each participant makes to it.	Group theory	This theory posits that there are group-to-group relationships in an organization. Individuals serve as links for the organizational units above and below their own units. Every individual is a member of two groups. Communications, supervision, influence, and goal attainment are focused upward. Lateral links are needed for communication, influence, motivation, and coordination.
Fusion theory	There is a give-and-take arrangement between the individual and the organization. Role expectations change relative to the demands of the organization and the role perceptions of individual participants. There are "bonds of organization" that include functional specifications, the status system, communication system, system of rewards and penalties, and the organizational mission.	Systems theory	This approach stresses the interrelatedness and interdependency of the elements of an organization. An "open system" consists of inputs, a transformation process, and outputs. The simple open-system concept has universal applicability. Subsystems are organized in such a way that they lead to optimal attainment of goals or output.
Role theory	A role is a set of expectations one has of a position. Each individual in the organization has certain expectations of himself or herself and of others. When there is the role of "benevolent supervisor," there is the corresponding role expectation of "grateful subordinate." The "paternalistic employer" supervises individuals who are expected to play the role of "childlike employees."	Contingency theory	There is focus on environmental variables. The type of technology used and other organizational factors affect the structure of an organization.

SOURCE: Fred Luthans, *Organizational Behavior*, 4th ed., McGraw-Hill, New York, 1985.

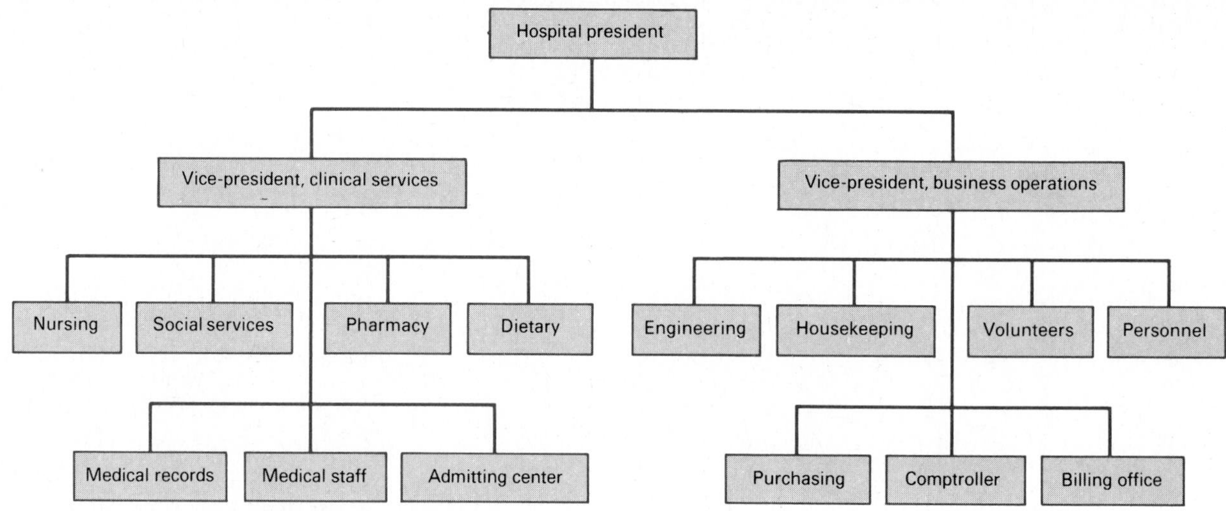

Figure 21-2 Aggregate project organization.
(SOURCE: Fred Luthans, *Organizational Behavior*, McGraw-Hill, New York, 1977.)

PROJECT STRUCTURE. A *project structure* is one in which management decides to focus a great amount of talent and resources for a given period of time on a specific project or goal. A project (1) is definable in terms of specific outcomes, (2) represents a unique effort, (3) calls for a complex interdependence of tasks, and (4) is extremely important to the organization as a whole.[11] There are four types of project structures: individual, staff, intermix, and aggregate.

The *individual* project structure consists of only the project manager. Managers have no personnel reporting to them and no responsibility for activities outside the scope of the individual project. A clinical nurse specialist conducting a study in a hospital setting may be considered an individual project manager. The *staff* project structure provides staff to back up project activities. For example, a nurse may be assigned the task of organizing a picnic for clients; he or she is told to enlist staff members to complete the project. In an *intermix* project structure, staff members report to the project manager and to selected department heads, who also report to the project manager. A nursing coordinator assigned to open a new unit who will be reported to directly by the nursing staff and the managers of the housekeeping, recreational therapy, and dietary departments is a participant in an intermix project structure. In an *aggregate project structure* all necessary personnel report to the project manager, giving the manager full authority over the entire project. Directors of nursing who have all subordinates reporting to them are aggregate project managers. Figure 21-2 illustrates an aggregate project organizational structure.

MATRIX STRUCTURE. A *matrix structure* incorporates project organization and bureaucratic organization in an eclectic manner. It adds a lateral dimension to the traditional vertical organization. Matrix organizational structures are said to provide a better balance of time, cost, and performance because of a built-in system of checks and balances and the continuous negotiations carried on between the project itself and the vertical organization.

Matrix organizations depart from the traditional organizational principles of hierarchy and unity of command. While elements of a vertical chain of command exist, emphasis is on horizontal work flow. Business is conducted as required by the legitimate needs of the task; project managers cross functional and organizational lines to accomplish a common objective. A matrix structure exists in hospitals, although it is frequently not formalized. Head nurses are able to call on department man-

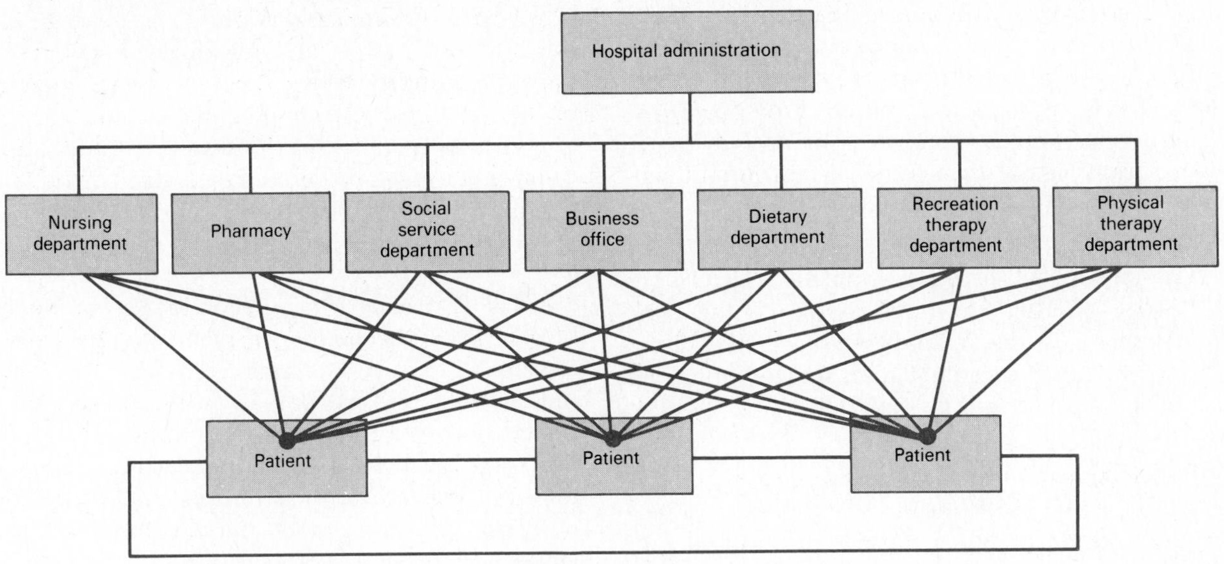

Figure 21-3 Matrix organizational structure.
(SOURCE: Linda Bernhard and Michelle Walsh, *Leadership: The Key to Professionalization of Nursing*, McGraw-Hill, New York, 1981. Used with permission.)

agers other than those in nursing in order to obtain necessary and life-saving services for clients (the project). Figure 21-3 illustrates a matrix organizational structure.

FREE-FORM STRUCTURE. *Free-form structures* are sometimes called *naturalistic,* or *organic, structures.* The free-form structure is based on the premise that the purpose of an organization is to facilitate change. This implies a high degree of adaptability and flexibility. Rigid roles are nonexistent, and internal structures are not allowed to solidify. Participation, self-control, individual initiative, independent judgment, open communication, and sensitivity are encouraged and facilitated.[12]

There are two major characteristics of free-form organizations:

1. They make extensive use of computerized information systems, especially for the purpose of evaluating the performance of organizational units.
2. They are populated by young, dynamic managers who are willing to take calculated risks.

A food cooperative formed by neighbors may be an example of a free-form organization. A group private practice set up by nurses who allow the organization to remain flexible would be another example.

Organizational Dynamics

Organizational dynamics are influenced by power, conflict, and change. Each is defined and explored below.

Power

Power is defined as any force that results in behavioral change. It is the ability of one person to influence another. The manner in which people are influenced is determined by the influencer's personal qualities, growth and development, and self-esteem, and by the interpersonal cooperation that encourages others to be influenced. The person who possesses power has the ability to manipulate and change another person's behavior or to change circumstances which, in turn, alter another's previous position or behavior.

Power is an interaction. If there is no one to influence, then there is no power. A person can be influenced if personal needs are met. The receiver of influence accepts that influence or power because it meets one or more needs. Power is dynamic; it has multiple causes and effects; it is multidimensional; and it is difficult to quantify.

TYPES OF POWER. There are several recognized types of power.[3,13] They are interrelated, and the same person may use different types of power at different times and under different circumstances. The types of power are outlined in Table 21-7.

AUTHORITY. *Authority* makes power legitimate. It is defined as the legitimate right of a person to take action. Administrative or formal authority is generally given to a position, and the person occupying the position is expected to execute that authority judiciously. For example, the director of nursing has legitimate authority and, consequently, the right and responsibility to carry out the goals of the nursing department.

Informal or functional authority is based on the personal qualities of an individual who is designated an authority because others perceive that he or she has expertise or potential power. For example, a person with experience in psychiatric nursing may be considered an authority in the care of emotionally disturbed clients and have informal authority.

LEADERSHIP. *Leadership* is defined as a set of actions or processes that influence members of a group toward setting and attaining goals. It is multidimensional and encompasses the wise use of power, managerial functions, and human-relations processes. Leadership in an organization is a relationship which is contingent upon the interaction of leaders' attitudes, tasks, and environmental variables.[9]

Leadership is not granted solely by a hierarchical structure. Rather, leadership is contingent upon three factors:

- The followers' acceptance of the leader; without followers, there can be no leader.

Table 21-7 Types of Power

Type	Explanation	Example
Representative	Based on delegation of power to a leader by a group with an agreement to follow as long as the leader consults the followers and leads in the direction they want to go	Team members determine a nursing care plan for a client, and the team leader presents the plan at a meeting of the entire staff.
Expert	Based on the perception of followers that the leader is an expert and has expertise which is useful	The clinical nurse specialist is asked to interview a client and contribute to a nursing care plan.
Referent	Based on the desire of the follower to identify with a charismatic leader. The leader is usually followed with blind faith	The staff nurse selects a graduate program because she likes the personal and professional qualities of the program chairperson.
Legitimate	Based on the follower's assessment that the leader has a right to lead and the follower has an obligation to follow; refers to positions which are endowed with formal authority	The staff nurse follows direction from the head nurse because the head nurse has the right and responsibility to give direction.
Reward	Based on perceptions that the leader has the power to reward followers in a satisfying manner	The nurse believes that if performance is exemplary, a raise in status and salary will come from the head nurse.
Coercive	Based on the belief that the influencer has the power to punish and that punishment will be unpleasant and frustrate a need	The nurse believes that the head nurse will fire her if she makes another medication error.

SOURCE: John R.P. French, Jr., and Bertram Raven, "The Bases of Social Power," in Dorwin Cartwright and Alvin Zander, eds., *Group Dynamics: Research and Theory*, 3d ed., Harper and Row, New York, 1968.

- Clearly defined goals with specific procedures to meet them.
- The formal authority of a position in a hierarchy; with authority comes the ability to reward or punish group members.

Research has determined the effects of leadership on organizational performance. A process of joint determination rather than an autocratic one leads to improved creativity and maximum commitment to the work. Participative leadership moves beyond the leader's power and encourages the followers' power to emerge. The expertise of the members is combined with that of the leader so that decisions are jointly reached and implemented. Lego has pointed out that group leaders who are facilitators produce results which go beyond the capacity of any individual in a group (see Chapter 20). The facilitation of maximum participation by members increases the members' attachment to the work group and fosters cohesion among members.

Informal leadership. In addition to the appointment of a formal leader who is responsible for the work of a group, informal leaders emerge from within the membership. The emergence of informal leaders occurs as a result of the interaction of the members and not by any formal selection or voting procedure. The personal and professional qualities of the informal leaders are the main determinants of their group roles.

Benne and Sheats have identified two types of informal leaders in groups. The *task group leader* facilitates communication concerning the task and goals of the group. This informal leader speaks for the members and represents the wishes or norms of the group. The *social leader* balances the forces of conflict and relieves tension. The sharing of leadership with the formal leader helps build cohesion and enhances the productivity of the group.[7]

Theories of leadership. There are several theories of leadership; some theories seem more valid than other, less sophisticated ones. Some of the better-known theories are found in Table 21-8 (page 412), with characteristics of each.

Leaders have a variety of styles of leadership from which to choose. When selecting a leadership style, the leader should consider his or her own characteristics and the characteristics of the group and the environment. The characteristics of followers in relation to leadership styles are outlined in Table 21-9.

Delegation of leadership. Delegation is the process of assigning part or all of one's responsibilities to another person; it is necessary because no one leader can do all the work assigned. When a task or activity is delegated, the accountability for action remains with the leader. Leaders who are unable to delegate are generally overworked and quickly become tired and ineffective. Delegation is also important for group members; group members who are not delegated enough responsibility become bored, lazy and unproductive.

Parallel process. When the behavior of clients mirrors the staff's behavior, or when the staff's behavior reflects clients' activity, *parallel process* is taking place.

In all settings, and especially in psychiatric nursing, when parallel process is operative, the members of the care-giving group respond to clients in a manner similar to the way that leaders respond to the care givers; care givers model the behavior of their supervisors. For example, when the leaders are autocratic, the followers will be dependent, subservient, and hostile. When autocratic supervision of the staff exists, the staff members exhibit a marked degree of control over clients' behavior, and clients, too, are dependent, subservient, and hostile. In contrast, when participative leadership is utilized, the followers are interdependent and productive. With participative leadership, the staff members are less controlling of clients, and the clients participate more and are less dependent and hostile.

When clients influence the staff, there is an upward parallel process. For example, clients who are excessively controlled and are lowest in the hierarchy will influence the staff members with their anger, hostility, and passivity, causing the staff members to exert more control. In addition, the staff members will continue the upward process to the supervisor, who will respond more autocratically.

Parallel process that facilitates a healthy work environment is built around the core dimensions of a helping relationship outlined in Chapter 12 and Chapter 13. Examples of healthy parallel process using these core dimensions are given in Table 21-10 (see page 413).

Table 21-8 Leadership Theories in Relation to Conceptual Framework

Theory	Characteristics
Focus on individual leader	
"Great man" theory	Some persons are born to lead, others to be led.
Traitist theory	The characteristics needed by a successful leader are determined by studying the personality traits of established leaders.
Managerial theory	The leader influences group behavior by planning, organizing, directing, and controlling it.
Focus on group and environment	
Situational theory	The leader is in a position to institute change when a situation demands or is ready for change.
McGregor's theory X and theory Y	The leader utilizes basic assumptions about motivation. Theory X states that individuals dislike and avoid work. Theory Y states that individuals are self-directed and will engage in goal-directed behavior by choice. These are not opposites but separate philosophies.
Focus on interaction of leader, group, and environment	
Interactional theory	Leadership is determined by the interaction of the situation and the personality of the leader.
Styles-of-leadership theory	Forces within the leader, the group members, and the situation determine the amount of control a leader utilizes. Styles of leadership include (1) an autocratic, paternalistic style; (2) a collaborative, democratic, collegial style; and (3) a permissive, liberal, laissez-faire style.
Focus on interaction of leader, group, and environment	
Zaleznik's executive functions theory	Executive functions are homeostatic, mediative, and proactive. Homeostatic functions are those that maintain the status quo. Mediative functions include conscious efforts to alter behavior and attitudes in response to environmental forces. Proactive functions induce change by employing resources creatively.
Management by objectives (MBO) theory	This is a process by which leader and subordinate jointly identify goals and designate areas of responsibility. The key elements are setting goals, planning actions, assessing one's performance, and periodically reviewing progress.
Path-goal theory	Looks at the effect a leader's behavior has on a group. The conditions under which a leader's behavior affects members' satisfaction are specified.
Fiedler's contingency model	Measures leadership effectiveness by looking at group productivity.
Theory Z	Views employees as valued, trusted, integral parts of the organization, and relies on egalitarianism, trust, and commitment more than power to encourage employees to pursue organizational goals.

Table 21-9 Characteristics of Followers in Relation to Leadership Styles

Needs of Followers	How Followers Are Influenced	Necessary Leadership Style	Leader's Power Base
Achievement, competence	Self- and group-determined	Participative	Representative
Power, autonomy, esteem, prestige	Rational agreement and faith	Persuasive	Expert
Social contact, affiliation	Tradition and blind faith	Authoritarian	Referent Legitimate Reward
Safety and security and physiological needs	Fear and hope	Autocratic	Reward Coercive

SOURCE: Ross A. Webber, *Management Pragmatics*, Irwin, Homewood, Ill., 1979.

Table 21-10 Examples of Parallel Process Using Core Dimensions of a Helping Relationship

Core Dimension	Supervisor to Nurse	Nurse to Client
Empathy	"You feel at a disadvantage when I don't tell you what I expect?"	"You feel angry when your wife ignores your requests to talk?"
Concreteness	"Specifically, what days of the week do you wish to work?"	"What in particular does your son do that disturbs you?"
Confrontation	"I understand that you would like more say in how we do our jobs, yet yesterday I noticed that you were not present at the staff meeting."	"While you say you don't like your treatment plan, you agreed to it yesterday when we met."
Immediacy	"Are you telling me that you see me as inconsiderate when I make additional assignments without discussing them with you?"	"Perhaps your use of contraband is your way of telling me you would like me to spend more time with you."
Respect	"I'm interested in knowing your thoughts on the new performance-appraisal form."	"I'm interested in knowing your thoughts about being placed on constant observation."
Genuineness	"Right now, I'm too tired to focus on your request."	"Sometimes I feel frustrated when I have to repeat what I say to you."

Conflict*

Conflict is defined as the clash that occurs when one person actively strives for his or her own preferred outcomes; conflict can also be a clash within one person. Conflict results when two or more sides attempt to gratify their incongruent needs.

Conflict may mean different things to different people. It may involve a minor difference, such as people deciding who should have a weekend off, or a major confrontation, such as a group of nurses deciding to go on strike.

All conflicts serve a purpose. Often, conflict is perceived as a negative occurrence reflecting dysfunction and lack of control. However, conflict has positive functions that promote growth and progress. Conflict performs the following positive and useful functions:[14]

1. Prevents stagnation
2. Promotes growth and change
3. Stimulates interest and curiosity
4. Is the medium through which problems can be explored, analyzed, and solved
5. Is the basis for personal change
6. Is part of the process of testing and assessing the self and increasing self-awareness
7. Demarcates the self and helps define boundaries and establish distinct identities
8. Balances power
9. Clarifies objectives
10. Facilitates the development of norms

SOURCES OF CONFLICT. In organizations, three sources of conflict directly influence functioning and attainment of organizational goals. Conflicts develop around goals, around roles, and around relationships.

Goal conflict. Conflict about goals frequently occurs within individuals and in organizations. Three types of goal conflict are generally identified; approach-approach conflict, approach-avoidance conflict, and avoidance-avoidance conflict.[11]

Approach-approach conflicts can be mildly distressing for individuals. Festinger's theory of cognitive dissonance offers one way of explaining how an approach-approach conflict is operationalized. The theory states that persons experiencing dissonance about two or more desirable goals will be highly motivated to reduce or eliminate the conflict.[15] For instance, suppose that a successful nurse

* Portions of this section from Roberta Mattheis, "Holistic Health Concepts," in the second edition of this book.

feels forced to choose between taking a more challenging, time-consuming position and remaining in the current position and beginning a family; in order to reduce cognitive dissonance, the nurse will find good reasons to choose one alternative and will identify all the negative factors related to the alternative not chosen.

Approach-avoidance conflict occurs when a single goal contains both positive and negative characteristics. Prolonged internal conflict may cause indecision and physical and emotional dysfunction among decision makers.

Avoidance-avoidance conflict, on the other hand, does not have an impact on an organization's behavior. Faced with two negative goals, people generally resolve the conflict by leaving the situation. An exception may be people who hate their jobs but avoid leaving them because jobs are scarce at the moment.

Ensuring compatibility between personal and organizational goals is one way of avoiding goal conflict.

Role conflict. Role conflict occurs when personal characteristics and desires are incompatible with the demands of a role or position. Role conflict is a clash between opposing forces and may be conscious or unconscious, intrapersonal or interpersonal. For example, a person whose highest value is personal freedom may have difficulty deciding when to use restraints to control patients' behavior. Role behaviors are the links that hold an organization together. When role conflict becomes overwhelming, individuals experience frustration, low job satisfaction, reduced productivity, and reduced commitment to the group. This leads to decreased effectiveness in organizational functioning. Webber identified several conditions that lead to role conflict.[10] These conditions and the circumstances characteristic of each are listed in Table 21-11.

The reduction or resolution of role conflict occurs when something happens to make the demands of the role more compatible with the person's characteristics and desires—for example, when the role is expanded as a person grows in the position:

> Miriam, a clinical specialist given the job of assessing and improving health care in the hospital, begins with consultations on a specific unit. Soon, she begins to experience role conflict because she wants to have a greater impact on the organization as a whole. Eventually her assignment is expanded to include other units and the establishment of a program for continuing education.

Because competing goals are evident in role conflict, stress and frustration result. There are several ways to respond to the stress and frustration of role conflict; these responses, along with an explanation and example of each response are given in Table 21-12.

Table 21-11 Conditions That Lead to Role Conflict

Name of Condition	Circumstances	Example
Misassignment	Occurs when role demands are outside the capacity of the individual	An associate nurse is placed in a leadership position.
Demand overload	Occurs when a position's responsibilities are too great for one person	The clinical supervisor is responsible for all operations, policies, hiring, on-the-spot supervision, and in-service educational programs.
Conflicting demands	Occurs when there are different expectations, which are contradictory and inconsistent, of the same role	Head nurses are viewed by administration as members of management while the staff members with whom they work during shortages perceive them as peers.
Ambiguous demands	Occurs when an individual does not know what is expected of him or her	The supervisor accepts a position in administration without a job description and is told to spend a major portion of time on one function. The associate director later asks for an annual review for several functions.

SOURCE: Ross A. Webber, *Management Pragmatics*, Irwin, Homewood, Ill., 1979.

Table 21-12 Responses to Role Conflict

Response	Explanation	Example
Passive stance	Most debilitating response. The person accepts excessive demands and endeavors to overcome them by working harder. Hazard to physical and mental health.	The head nurse attempts to meet all of the staff's demands in addition to complying with requests from the administration and the staff psychiatrists.
Resignation	Withdrawal from the situation. Occurs physically or psychologically. Complete escape from role demands is impossible short of insanity or death.	The head nurse who initially took a passive stance throws her hands up and resigns without attempting to find alternative ways of dealing with excessive demands.
Attempt to modify demands	Most constructive approach. Confrontation and bargaining are used to request simplification and clarification of demands.	The head nurse agrees to consider individual scheduling requests only after the entire staff works out on paper a suggested time schedule for unit staffing.
Change of desires	A mature decision that leads to clarification of values and life purpose.	A head nurse gives up having all nursing care plans done one way in exchange for a staff-developed method of documenting nursing care.
Selective withdrawal	Usually manifests as somatization. Illness diverts attention from the excessive demands and the persons imposing them.	Many sick calls are received from the nursing staff members who work on a busy admitting unit, where they are in general overworked.
Response to power	Represents meeting the demands of the people who are in a position to give one the most grief or pleasure. Difficulty occurs because more than one person makes demands at the same time.	The head nurse accepts understaffing in spite of the fact that the staff is overloaded with assignments; this pleases the supervisor but does not meet the needs of the nursing staff.
Compartmentalization of demands	The development of arbitrary schedules to suit strictly personal needs.	The staff nurse insists on a 10:15 A.M. coffee break regardless of assignment, refusing to take it at 9 or 11 A.M.
Frustration and dissatisfaction	Occurs when employee's job expectations do not match reality.	The recent graduate with a baccalaureate expects to be a team leader upon employment. Assignment as a staff nurse results in feelings of frustration and dissatisfaction.

SOURCE: Ross A. Webber, *Management Pragmatics,* Irwin, Homewood, Ill., 1979.

Interpersonal conflict. Conflict exists among individuals in an organization. Interpersonal conflicts may be veridical, contingent, displaced, misattributed, latent, and false.

A *veridical conflict* is one that exists objectively and is perceived accurately by both participants. It is difficult to resolve amicably unless there is sufficient cooperation between the participants for them to act collaboratively.

A *contingent conflict* is dependent upon circumstances that could be easily and quickly rearranged, thus resolving the conflict. The participants, however, do not recognize this fact and fail to perceive alternatives. The conflict is a product of circumstances which are not necessarily as fixed as the participants believe.[14]

A *displaced conflict* is a dispute that occurs over the wrong issue. The participants initiate and dispute an issue which is symbolic of an underlying and more basic or fundamental issue. The participants avoid confronting the basic issue by using the indirect and tangential issue as a safer way to express their dissatisfactions and strong feelings related to the basic issue. The basic conflict cannot be resolved, because it never becomes the focus of discussions or negotiations. The presenting manifest issue may be resolved, but since it is a pseudo issue and the basic issue remains intact, other manifest issues arise and the conflict continues.[14]

A *misattributed conflict* is a dispute between the wrong participants; as a consequence, this conflict is usually over the wrong issue. In this situation the people who should be in conflict are removed consciously or unconsciously from the dispute by their own and their stand-ins' actions. Such a conflict can never be resolved successfully, because the wrong people are negotiating the wrong issue.[14]

A *latent conflict* is a dispute that should be occurring but is not. Either or both of the participants may not be consciously experiencing the conflict as such. There is no awareness, because the circumstances of the conflict have been repressed, displaced, or misattributed; or the conflict does not yet exist psychologically, because it has not yet been perceived. As long as such a conflict remains latent, efforts cannot be made that would resolve it.[14]

A *false conflict* occurs as a result of misperception or misunderstanding. There is no objective basis for the conflict. Communication directed toward resolving the apparent conflict may or may not produce a resolution, depending upon whether the misperceptions and misconceptions are revised to reflect reality.[14]

TYPES OF CONFLICT. Whatever their source, conflicts fall into certain categories, or types, several of which take the form of pairs of opposites: (1) realistic and unrealistic conflicts; (2) institutionalized and noninstitutionalized conflicts; (3) primary (or face-to-face) conflicts and secondary (or mediated) conflicts; (4) conflicts over rights and conflicts over interests; and (5) ideological conflicts.

Realistic conflicts are characterized by opposed means and ends which arise from incompatible objectives, values, and interests. Wants and needs seem to be or to become incompatible because of other influential factors such as the availability of resources. *Unrealistic conflicts* arise from the need to release tension which has arisen from deflected hostility, from tradition, and from ignorance or error. Dispute often continues long after the precipitating issue has been resolved. This continuation of the conflict is a product of imbalances and ambiguities that are not readily available or accessible for revision.

Institutionalized conflicts are characterized by explicit rules, predictable behavior, and continuity. Collective bargaining and the judicial system exemplify institutionalized management of conflicts. In contrast, *noninstitutionalized conflicts* are disorganized, unauthorized, and only partially supported by the participants. There are no preestablished ground rules, and the behaviors of the participants are unpredictable.

Primary (face-to-face) conflicts are personal disputes between individuals and groups that involve direct interpersonal confrontation and interaction. *Secondary (mediated) conflicts* are impersonal objective conflicts which are carried out through the use of chosen representatives.

Conflicts over rights are concerned with the application of previously agreed upon standards or values to situations for which they are appropriate. When concerns are focused on altering or removing these standards or initiating new standards, *conflicts over interests* develop.

Ideological conflicts arise when conceptions of what is desirable and the associated prescriptive norms and beliefs that do or should govern behavior are in disagreement. Belief systems, rational and irrational, support each opposing position. The ideology is personalized and incorporated into the participant's identity. This lack of objectivity and heightened subjectivity intensify and sometimes escalate the conflict. Characteristically there is a lack of inhibitions that is reflected in personal attacks made by the opposing parties. Resolution of such conflicts is particularly difficult because the issues are enmeshed in emotionally charged systems of values and beliefs.

RESOLUTION OF CONFLICT. Many factors influence the resolution of a conflict. Forces that influence the resolution process arise from both the participants and the context in which the conflict occurs. Issue-oriented conflicts are resolved when the issue is settled in the eyes of the participants. Change need not occur in the structures of either of the conflicting systems or in the supersystems of which they are a part. Structure-oriented conflicts, however, are not resolvable unless the structure of either or both of the parties or the supersystem is changed. For example, a conflict concerning how nursing care should be delivered to meet the goal of individualized planning must be resolved at the structural level; the issue of team nursing versus primary care will have to be settled.

If competition occurs, each participant in a conflict may define the opponent as an "enemy." Such a perception redefines the conflict as a "fight" and sets up an attitude of "us against them." Threats to autonomy or even existence may be perceived. Such threats elicit behaviors aimed at "killing off" the enemy. An open destructive fight or a flight from the situation occurs. The participants believe that the resolution of the conflict is a win-or-lose process, even when one participant flees. The conflict may appear to be resolved if one side wins and the other loses or flees. However, the resolution is only temporary. The loser "lives to fight again another day." Each battle becomes a segment of an ongoing cycle. A win-lose approach to conflict resolution militates against finding a solution that is satisfactory to both parties.

Deutsch identifies two approaches to resolution of conflict: destructive resolution results from competition; productive resolution results from cooperation.[14]

Competition: Destructive resolution. Destructive resolution is characterized by a tendency on the part of the participants to expand and escalate the dispute. The conflict becomes independent of its initiating cause and is thus likely to persist long after the original issue has become irrelevant or been forgotten.

Competitive processes operate in the following ways:[14]

- Increase the value and number of principles and precedents that the participants see as at stake
- Increase the costs participants are willing to bear
- Increase the intensity of negative attitudes toward the opponent
- Increase the use of power tactics: threat, coercion, and deception
- Cause a shift away from persuasive and conciliatory strategies
- Maximize differences
- Negate goodwill on the opponent's part

Three interrelated and interacting processes operate in the development and continuation of destructive resolution of conflict:[14]

1. Competitive processes are involved in the attempt to win the conflict.
2. Processes of misperception and biased perception operate.
3. Processes of commitment to winning arise out of pressures for cognitive and social consistency.

These processes interact and reinforce a cycle of actions and reactions that intensifies the conflict. Through the interaction of these processes, communication between opponents becomes impoverished and unreliable. Consequently, misperception and misunderstanding become more prevalent and aggravate the situation. Competitive processes also support the view that the resolution of the conflict can only be imposed by one of the participants through the use of superior force or power, deception, or cleverness.

Suspicious and hostile attitudes develop and increase when competitive processes influence the conflict. Sensitivity to differences increases, and awareness of similarities and common interests and concerns decreases. A conflict may be minor in nature and easily resolvable initially; however, if communication is impaired or minimal, competitive processes may develop quickly, and the distorted views that come from inadequate communication feed the growth of these processes. In the heat of an escalating conflict, the contest may become blurred and eventually obscured. When this happens, contextual influences that would facilitate resolution become ineffective.[14]

Participants become highly motivated to legitimize their positions and in doing so categorize the opponent's position as illegitimate and therefore not worthy of further discussion. This leads to further distortions and increasing pressure for self-consistency and social conformity.

Stress is inherent in conflict and increases when competitive processes develop. This increase in stress further impairs perceptual and cognitive processes needed for resolution that would be satisfactory to both sides. High levels of stress decrease the range of perceived alternatives and lead to a black-or-white, polarized view of alternative solutions that reflects a win-lose mentality. This polarized perception of events tends to lead to stereotyped responses. Time perspective also narrows, producing a fixed focus on the immediate moment rather than a consideration of long-term consequences. People experiencing high levels of stress in conflict situations become susceptible to intense, unrealistic feelings of fear or hope, and are thus more defensive. Gullibility to rumors and increased sensitivity to perceived gains and losses heighten this emotionality. Anxiety and fear increase the need for structure and support. Increased levels of stress decrease the use of intellectual resources for problem solving. Impulsiveness dictated by emotionality occurs.

People tend to act according to their beliefs. When what one believes does not match the way one acts, *cognitive dissonance* occurs. To resolve this dissonance, people tend to make their beliefs and attitudes agree with their actions. This comes about because of the pressure for self-consistency. Actions "should" reflect beliefs and attitudes. Therefore, there is a need to justify one's actions to oneself and others. A person initially may support a particular position in relation to a conflict. Later, the person may disagree with this position; however, the commitment has been made. If the conflict escalates and expands, the need to defend one's position becomes greater, as does the need to save face.

Cooperation: Productive resolution. Cooperative processes facilitate productive resolution of conflict. These processes are characterized by:

- Open and honest communication and exchange of information
- Recognition of the legitimacy of the other's interests
- Recognition of the necessity to search for a solution responsive to each party's needs
- Increased sensitivity to similarities and common interests
- Tendency to minimize the importance of differences
- Tendency to limit rather than expand the scope of conflicting interests
- Tendency to minimize the need for defensiveness
- Tendency to be issue-oriented rather than person-oriented
- Tendency to promote mutual power
- Efforts to promote convergence of beliefs and values
- Commitment to finding a mutually agreeable solution

Open and honest communication facilitates an exchange of information, prevents misunderstanding and mistrust, and allows for the correction of misperceptions. Such communication also facilitates recognition of the manifest and latent issues and confrontation of the false issues. Consequently, definitions of problems are more likely to be accurate.

When participants recognize the legitimacy of each other's position, there is also a tendency to see that any solution must address the significant needs of both participants. The win-lose solution is therefore viewed as neither satisfactory nor useful. Collaboration is seen as more desirable, and the necessity of limiting the scope of the conflict and remaining issue-oriented is understood. A collaborative interpersonal climate also reduces the need for defensiveness and power struggles and allows for joint, creative problem solving.

An important factor that contributes to reducing the size of the conflict is the participants' abilities to remain issue-oriented. Sticking to the issue and the here and now helps to avoid focusing on personalities. The ability to stick to the issue and negotiate the resolution of differences is influenced by the rigidity with which the participants view the issue, the centrality of the issue, the size of the conflict, the degree of consensus on the importance of different subissues, and the consciousness of the issues.

Problems in perceiving satisfactory alternatives may be related to adherence to a strict definition of the issue. Perceptions that are fixed and narrow may preclude a satisfactory resolution. If the participants are able to reconceptualize the issue in various ways, however, a variety of other alternatives may become available. The context in which the conflict occurs influences the "rigidity" of issues. Environmental resources enhance the ability to implement cooperative processes. Thus, the participants may need to seek out and bring these resources into the process of identifying alternative solutions.

The centrality of an issue is determined by its infringement on both parties' physical well-being, self-esteem, socioeconomic position, or defenses against anxiety. Redefinition of the issue, which requires flexibility, effective communication, and recognition of the legitimacy of the other's position, helps to prevent the participants from becoming locked in a life-or-death struggle.

Larger conflicts tend to be more destructive than smaller ones; however, large conflicts are often an amalgamation of several smaller conflicts. When cooperative processes are operating, an apparently large conflict is broken down into several smaller, more manageable conflicts. Reducing the size, interdependence, and number of conflicts is likely to diminish the importance of the interaction and the outcomes. The smaller and more well-defined the conflict, the greater the possibility that shared interests, concerns, beliefs, and values will be identified. The recognition and acknowledgment of commonalities further supports collaboration and productive resolution.

Isolating subissues and working sequentially on several smaller conflicts may facilitate consensus and allow each participant to meet vital needs. Rather than one major win-lose outcome, multiple shared successes occur and power is shared.

Awareness and recognition of the basic issues in a conflict are vital aspects of cooperative processes inasmuch as they prevent displaced, latent, or repressed conflict. Exchange of perceptions, thoughts, and feelings increases the potential for awareness, recognition, and cooperation. People can seek solutions only when they are aware that a problem exists and recognize the fundamental issue which should be the focus of the dispute.[16]

Table 21-13 outlines the steps of the compromise method of resolution and gives illustrations.

Change

Change is a continuously occurring phenomenon that results in an alteration of the objects of change. It is an emotionally charged word that often connotes a threat to security. Some changes occur imperceptibly, such as the constant replacement of cells in the human body. Some changes occur rhythmically, such as the cycles of day and night and the seasons. Changes may be planned, as the result of conscious decision making, or they may just happen, as is in the case with fate or accidents.

"Planned change is a conscious, deliberate, and collaborative effort to improve systems ... through

Table 21-13 The Compromise Method of Resolving Conflicts

Step	Illustration
1. Identify the problem. a. Verbalize the other's side of the conflict. b. Use active listening.	1. Practical nurses ask the administration for a higher salary. a. The administration believes a raise would be overcompensation for the job. b. Practical nurses believe they perform the same functions as professional nurses and do not get adequate recognition; the administration believes that these nurses are functioning out of their job descriptions.
c. Be sure that both sides accept the definition of the problem.	c. Both sides see the problem as recognition of the contribution of practical nurses as evidenced by the job description, the reality of their functioning on specific occasions, and their salaries.
2. Generate alternative solutions. Competition for solutions indicates that the problem needs redefining.	2. Alternatives are: a. Change the job description to include functions previously given to professional nurses and increase the salary. b. Keep the job description as it is with no increase in salary. c. Add one section to the job description for experienced practical nurses which would allow for limited additional responsibility, and introduce a special pay scale for those practical nurses who function in the absence of a professional nurse and have more responsibility.
3. Evaluate the alternative solutions.	3. Alternative *a* is unacceptable to the administration. Alternative *b* is unacceptable to the practical nurses. Alternative *c* is feasible to both groups.
4. Make decisions by consensus only.	4. All members agree verbally to accept alternative *c*.
5. Implement the solution.	5. The administration will see that supervisors record the names, days, and hours that practical nurses work without a professional nurse and submit the information to the payroll office.
6. Evaluate the implementation.	6. A target date is set to check back with both groups.

SOURCE: Thomas Gordon, *Leader Effectiveness Training*, Bantam, New York, 1980.

the use of knowledge."[17] When change is planned, the agents and targets of change coexist in a collaborative relationship for the express purpose or goal of improving or altering a system. Change in any part of the system results in change of the whole.

The term *target of change* refers to that which must change in order to produce change in policy, procedure, or place. Targets include people's knowledge, attitudes, and behavior. Knowledge is changed by learning. Change in attitude occurs as a result of new knowledge or a conscious effort to alter attitudes through clarification of values or therapy. Behavioral change may result from new knowledge, from a change in attitude, or from altered expectations, or as part of the process of growth and development.[18]

The person responsible for initiating change is called a *change agent.* The agent is an objective person who monitors the change process. He or she may be a recognized expert or consultant from outside a group or organization (*external* change agent) or a person from within the group or organization that will be affected by the change (*internal* change agent).

STAGES OF CHANGE. Certain conditions must exist in a group or organization before permanent change can occur. The change must be compatible with the needs of the group. Effective change is also known to be positively related to the degree of participation of group members in a decision to change. Change occurs in three stages.

Stage 1: Dissatisfaction, or unfreezing. During this stage doubt is cast on old behaviors, and members feel a need for change. When a situation is painful or when members are in a crisis, change occurs most readily. If members are not dissatisfied with current conditions, the change agent creates dissatisfaction through consciousness-raising. Support for old behavior and attitudes is removed, and a new structure that supports the change is proposed.

Stage 2: Conversion, or moving. Actual change is implemented and new methods of operation or new behaviors are tried during the conversion stage. Well-defined strategies are used. Over time the group or organization practices the changes and experiences the benefits of the new attitudes, knowledge, or behavior. The agent of change serves as a role model; members change through identification and emulation of the role model's behavior. Group members learn expected behaviors through planned learning experiences. The structural changes that support the other changes are implemented.

Stage 3: Stabilization, or refreezing. The moving stage ends when change has occurred and is internalized and practiced by group members. Support and ongoing feedback continue to reinforce changed behavior during the refreezing stage to prevent the natural tendency to revert to old behaviors.[19]

RESISTANCE TO CHANGE. *Resistance* is any force that interferes with the process of change. Resistance to change may occur at any stage in the process, may take many forms, and may be active, passive, or apathetic. Active resistance is overt opposition to change; while passive resistance is covert and hidden undermining of the change process. When apathy exists, there is a lack of enthusiasm and a failure to mobilize and implement the change. Generally, apathy occurs when the change is perceived by the target of change as unimportant.

Resistance to change may be viewed as reactions intended to protect individuals from perceived threats to the satisfaction of their needs. Any change may be feared and resisted if it threatens the fundamental needs of security, social relationships, self-esteem, and status. Resistance to change is not necessarily negative. Resistance facilitates sound thinking and planning, creative approaches, and participation in planning by those who will be affected. Resistance that is managed creatively may result in a win-win resolution.

STRATEGIES FOR CHANGE. There are three strategies for planned change: empirical-rational, normative-reeducative, and power-coercive.[17]

The *empirical-rational strategy* is aimed at the mental aspect of the person; it is based on the belief that people are rational, follow patterns of self-interest, and will change if they are shown that they will benefit from the change. For example, nurses are offered increased salary and a more rewarding job if they pursue more nursing education.

The *normative-reeducative strategy* operates when there is direct intervention by an agent of change in the values or spiritual aspect of the person. The change occurs because of a new attitude or a change in belief. For example, a therapist may explore current destructive patterns of behavior with a client. The client and therapist participate actively in the process of exploring the unconscious motivations for the destructive behavior. For example:

> Fred, the client, discovers that he believes he is all bad and there is nothing good in him. This discovery allows for exploration and change of belief about himself, which allows for new, constructive behaviors. Ruby, the therapist, supports the client through the uncomfortable process of gaining insight and begins educating Fred about new ways of behaving.

The *power-coercive strategy* uses power to force compliance with change. The power-coercive strategy is considered a physical maneuver because it entails force against one's will. The strategy "feels" physical even when no direct physical threat is made. For example:

> A supervisor "pulls" staff members from the intensive-care unit to the psychiatric unit to cover an emergency, and threatens immediate dismissal if they refuse to go.

The strategy used is often influenced by the target of change. Frequently, not one but a combination of techniques is utilized when change is planned. Regardless of the strategy taken, the agent of change will find several basic principles helpful in overcoming resistance to change:*

- Make only necessary and advantageous changes. Excessive change produces insecurity.
- Move slowly. Accelerated or rapid change frequently fails. Change is difficult and frequently takes a great deal of time.
- Prepare for the change. What is not fully understood is feared.
- Communicate clearly the needs and reasons for the change as well as what is expected of the target of change. Unclear communications result in sabotage of the change.
- Explain the benefits of the change. When change is perceived as benefiting only the agent of change, it is resisted.
- Understand the change fully before explaining it to others. Inability to answer questions about the change will lead to resistance. Establish an ongoing dialogue with targets of change. One-way communication increases resistance.
- Evaluate and solicit ongoing feedback about the effectiveness of the change. Unresolved complaints or grievances result in anger and hostility.
- Establish a reward system. Lack of recognition for good performance leads to resistance and decreased feelings of satisfaction.
- Whenever possible, encourage participation in the change decision. Pseudo participation, however, results in feelings of abandonment and mistrust.

* From Anita M. Leach, "The Supervising Nurse as Change Agent," in the second edition of this book.

NURSES AS CHANGE AGENTS. Nurses assume the role of change agents in a variety of ways and in numerous settings. They are advocates of change within their practice settings, and they interact with clients and families as facilitators of behavioral change. Nurses assume leadership roles in organizations where they initiate change that improves care. Through self-assessment, they change themselves and ultimately the environment. Nurses with advanced education serve as organizational consultants, applying and imparting to others their understanding of the nature of change and diagnosing and resolving resistance to change.

EVALUATION OF ORGANIZATIONS AND GROUPS

Multiple forces modify and shape systems. Physical environment, territoriality, personal space, cultural background, color, noise, lighting, and spatial arrangements are some of the factors that influence group and organizational functioning. Leadership, decision-making processes and methods, levels of trust, degrees of cohesion, and power are among the less tangible forces that operate in all groups and organizations.

For any group or organization to be effective, it must accomplish its goals, maintain its own cohesion, and develop and modify its structure in ways that improve productivity. Table 21-14 outlines an evaluation of a group or organization, giving the factors that should be evaluated, specific questions for the evaluation process, and expected outcomes when the group or organization is functioning effectively.

Table 21-14 Evaluation of a Group or Organization

Factor	Questions	Expected Outcomes in an Effective Group
Atmosphere	What is the atmosphere? Are there signs of boredom or tension?	The employees are comfortable and relaxed. Members are interested and involved. The atmosphere is conducive to productivity. Space and lighting are adequate. There is privacy, and noise is minimal.
Setting goals	Do the employees understand the purpose of the group? What are the group's stated goals? Are the goals acceptable to the members?	Group goals are clearly understood. Modification of goals occurs with participation by employees.
Leadership	Who are the appointed leaders? Does any one person dominate in the group?	Leadership is assumed by different members at different times. The appointed leader is aware of group happenings and group process.
Membership	What is the level of participation of each member? (Under this factor in an evaluation, one would also include the characteristics of group members—age, sex, occupation, etc.)	Employees participate in a manner appropriate to the circumstances. Each member has several group roles that are also shared with others.
Roles	What kinds of roles are assumed by the group members?	Growth-producing and group-vitalizing roles are in predominance.
Communication	How does communication take place? Are there listeners? Is the verbal communication compatible with nonverbal expressions?	Communication is open and two-way. Ideas and feelings are expressed freely. There is congruence between verbal and nonverbal communication.
Decision making	Who makes decisions? Are employees involved in the decision-making process? How does the group arrive at a consensus?	Most decision making is by consensus. The decision-making process is clear to the membership. There is a plan for implementing group decisions.
Conflict	Is there tolerance for conflict? What issues cause conflict in the group? Is conflict avoided, denied, or suppressed?	There is evidence that disagreement and controversy are viewed positively. Basic unresolved disagreements are accepted and tolerated. Conflict is used as opportunity for personal and organizational growth.
Problem solving	Who solves the problems? What kinds of problems occur? Is there constructive criticism? Are genuine efforts made to solve problems?	Group membership has evolved a clear methodology for problem solving. Constructive criticism is frequent, frank, relatively comfortable, and oriented toward problem solving. Problems relate to group tasks.
Cohesion	Are the positive elements of cohesion present? Is there evidence of trust, liking, and support among the members? Are there any of the symptoms of groupthink? (See Table 21-3.)	There are high levels of membership inclusion, trust, and liking. There is mutual support for all members. Creativity and a wide range of thinking styles are supported.
Power	Who holds the power in the group? What types of power are exercised? (See Table 21-7.)	Influence and power evolve from the members' participation in goal-directed activity. Power is shared by the membership.
Self-evaluation	Is there an evaluation process? Do individuals evaluate their behavior? Who evaluates the group and the individuals in the group? Are changes made as a result of the evaluation process?	There is ongoing evaluation of the group's ability to function. Members openly examine their behavior in the group. All members participate in the evaluations of the group. Decisions are made to improve the functioning of the group.

SUMMARY

The purpose of this chapter was to develop an understanding of how to work effectively in work groups and organizations. The person, work group, and organization and the interaction among them must be recognized to increase effectiveness.

A *group* is defined as more than two persons interacting with one another in such a way that each person influences and is influenced by the others. Groups are established to accomplish specific goals and tasks. The basic drives in any group are the members' need to belong to the group, their need to achieve in the group, and their need to be recognized by other group members.

Groups may be categorized as formal and informal. *Formal groups* are formed for a specific purpose to which members are committed, and include work groups and organizations. *Informal groups* are formed among people who work together, and they satisfy needs for their members.

Bion described two processes that are relevant to work groups: the *work-task process* and the *basic-assumption process.* The work-task process accomplishes specific goals agreed to by the membership. The basic-assumption process involves the unspoken, often unconscious assumptions held by a majority of the group that profoundly influence the group's behavior. The three basic assumptions are dependency, fight-flight, and pairing.[4] Individual characteristics, called *valency,* also influence the interplay between the work-task process and the basic-assumption process.

Work groups have the same dynamics as small groups. Dynamics that influence groups are: boundaries, rank and status, norms and goals, roles, cohesiveness, and competition.

A classical organization, or *bureaucracy,* is a systematized, centralized organizational structure characterized by specialization and division of labor. While classical approaches to structuring organizations are still very much in evidence, new theories and structural forms are emerging to meet the modern demands of growth, increasing complexity, and accelerated change. Project, matrix, and free-form structures provide more flexibility but violate such classical principles as unity of command, specialization, and division of labor.

Power, conflict, and change are the dynamics that operate in organizations.

There are several types of *power,* and they all may be used at different times by the same person. Authority makes power legitimate. Formal and informal leaders influence members of groups; there are a number of theories of leadership and styles of leadership.

Conflict results when two or more sides attempt to gratify incongruent needs. All conflicts serve a purpose. Conflict can be negative or positive. Conflicts in organizations develop around goals, roles, and personal relationships. There are several types of conflicts. Resolution of conflict can be productive or destructive. Destructive resolution results from competition; productive resolution, from cooperation.

The process of *change* goes on all the time. Change may be planned or unplanned. When it is planned, the agents and targets of change coexist in a collaborative relationship for the express purpose or goal of improving or altering a system. Change occurs in three stages: dissatisfaction, conversion, and stabilization. Resistance to change often occurs, but agents of change can use different strategies for planned change. Nurses often act as change agents.

Multiple forces modify and shape organizations and work groups. For any group or organization to be effective, it must clarify its goals, maintain its own cohesion, and develop and modify its structure in ways that improve productivity.

REFERENCES

1. Marvin Shaw, *Group Dynamics: The Psychology of Small-Group Behavior,* 3d ed., McGraw-Hill, New York, 1980.
2. Eric Berne, *The Structure and Dynamics of Organizations and Groups,* Grove, New York, 1966.
3. Dorwin Cartwright and Alvin Zander, eds., *Group Dynamics: Research and Theory,* 3d. ed., Harper and Row, New York, 1968.
4. Wilfred Bion, *Experiences in Groups,* Basic Books, New York, 1959.
5. Max Weber, *The Theory of Social and Economic Organization,* Talcott Parsons, trans. and ed., Free Press, New York, 1947.
6. George C. Homans, *The Human Group,* Harcourt, Brace, Jovanovich, New York, 1950.
7. Kenneth B. Benne and P. Sheats, "Functional Roles of Group Members," *Journal of Social Issues,* vol. 4, no. 2, Spring 1948, pp. 42–49.

8. Irving Janis, "Groupthink," *Psychology Today,* November 1971, pp. 71–89.
9. Linda Anne Bernhard and Michelle Walsh, *Leadership: The Key to the Professionalization of Nursing,* McGraw-Hill, New York, 1981.
10. Ross A. Webber, *Management Pragmatics,* Irwin, Homewood, Ill., 1979.
11. Fred Luthans, *Organizational Behavior,* 4th ed., McGraw-Hill, New York, 1985.
12. Dalton McFarland, *Management and Society: An Institutional Framework,* Prentice-Hall, Englewood Cliffs, N.J., 1982.
13. Mary A. Trainor, "A Helping Model for Clinical Supervision," *Supervisor Nurse,* vol. 9, no. 1, January 1978, pp. 30–42.
14. M. Deutsch, *The Resolution of Conflict,* Yale University Press, New Haven, Conn., 1973.
15. Leon Festinger, *A Theory of Cognitive Dissonance,* Stanford University Press, Stanford, Calif., 1957.
16. Thomas Gordon, *Leader Effectiveness Training,* Bantam, New York, 1980.
17. Warren G. Bennis, et al.: *The Planning of Change,* Holt, New York, 1969.
18. L. B. Welsh, "Planned Change in Nursing: The Theory," *Nursing Clinics of North America,* vol. 14, 1979, pp. 307–321.
19. Kurt Lewin, *Field Theory in Social Science,* University of Chicago Press, Chicago, 1951.

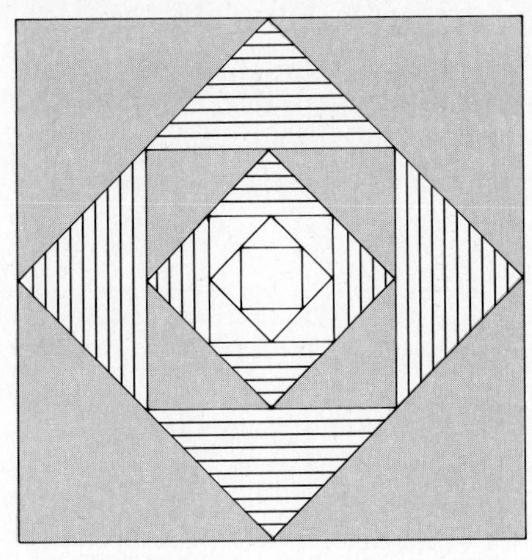

CHAPTER 22
Crisis Theory and Application

Judith Haber

LEARNING OBJECTIVES

After studying this chapter, the student should be able to:

1. Define *crisis.*
2. Discuss the historical development of crisis theory and intervention.
3. Discuss the elements of a crisis.
4. Define three types of crises:
   a. Maturational
   b. Situational
   c. Social
5. Discuss examples of maturational, situational, and social crises.
6. Discuss the crisis intervention process.
7. Discuss the roles nurses play in crisis intervention.
8. Identify methods of crisis intervention.
9. Formulate a plan of intervention for a client in crisis based on a crisis intervention model.

Human beings must solve problems continually in order to maintain an equilibrium or balance between stress and the mechanisms available for coping with it. If there is an imbalance between a problem as perceived by the person experiencing it and the person's available repertoire of coping skills, a crisis may be precipitated. All human beings face such crises from time to time in their lives.

A *crisis* is an internal disturbance that results from a stressful event or a perceived threat to self-integrity.[1] It occurs when a conflict, problem, or situation of basic importance is perceived as threatening and not readily solvable by means of methods that have been successful in the past.[2] As a result, anxiety and tension increase, effective cognitive functioning decreases, and behavior becomes disorganized. The person becomes even less able to find a solution to the problem and feels incompetent to deal with it effectively. Tension continues to rise, and discomfort is experienced, along with such feelings as anxiety, depression, fear, guilt, shame, and helplessness.[1] As anxiety continues to increase, coping skills become less available and less effective. The precipitated crisis, then, is a result not of the event itself but of the person's inability to cope with it.

The essence of a crisis is that a person feels that life has stopped in midstream. The order, purpose, and meaning of life are lost, and efforts to restore them have been futile. The person's usual coping styles have been ineffective. This is extremely anxiety-provoking, particularly to people who have felt comfortable with the meaning and purpose of life and at least somewhat in charge of its direction. The imbalances represented by a crisis, and by the person's inability to restore order, meaning, and purpose, are manifested biopsychosocially. People facing crises need time to regroup and assistance in redefining the order, purpose, and meaning of life and in reinvesting themselves in the effective pursuit of their goals.[3]

Crisis theory provides health professionals and people in crisis with a framework for assessing and alleviating stressful situations in which customary ways of solving problems or making decisions are not adequate. *Crisis intervention* is a form of brief, community-based therapy that takes a problem-solving approach to deal with the immediate situation in a growth-promoting way.

The purpose of this chapter is to help the nurse work effectively with clients experiencing maturational, situational, and social crises. The chapter will discuss the historical development of crisis theory, a paradigm for viewing the development of a crisis, types of crises, and the role of the nurse in crisis intervention.

CRISIS THEORY

Historical Background

The concept of crises and early formulations of crisis theory originated in the field of preventive psychiatry in the early 1940s. *Preventive psychiatry* is concerned with the maintenance of mental health and the prevention of mental illness. Specialists in this field used psychoanalytic theory as a base for a theoretical framework that explored brief intervention for persons having stressful life experiences. People experiencing particular stressful life events were noted to exhibit a characteristic sequence of reactions and outcomes. Intervention strategies for particular stressful life experiences were developed to minimize negative outcomes and maximize resolution of the problem in a growth-promoting way.

Foremost among those involved in preventive psychiatry was Eric Lindeman.[4] Lindeman studied the bereavement seen in the surviving relatives and friends of the hundreds of people who died in the disastrous Coconut Grove nightclub fire in Boston in 1943. He hypothesized that numerous threatening situations might arise in a person's life and that the person either adapts to the situations or fails to adapt and has impaired functioning. His observations provided a theoretical framework for understanding the behavior of people facing crises and their aftermath. He formulated a model for intervention during bereavement that could be applied to other potentially stressful events that people experience throughout the life cycle, such as marriage and the birth of a child. Lindeman visualized crisis intervention as taking place within the community, and set up a communitywide crisis program in Massachusetts called the Wellsley Project.

During this same period, military psychiatrists were observing and treating war-related emotional problems. They found that soldiers who received immediate emotional first aid for stress-related experiences at the front lines were able to return to duty and did not require further treatment in inpatient settings. Later studies and observation during the Korean war substantiated these findings and added to a knowledge base about stress-related human behavior and the benefits of immediate, brief intervention in preventing entrenched patterns of dysfunctional behavior.

Later, in the early 1960s, Gerald Caplan[2] defined crisis theory and described crisis intervention. He utilized principles of preventive psychiatry—primary, secondary, and tertiary prevention—as a basis for his work.

He viewed *primary prevention* as a vehicle for promoting mental health and reducing mental illness. Crisis intervention as a form of primary prevention utilizes social and interpersonal actions. Social action involves working with social and political groups to obtain needed community reforms that would help people cope with crises such as inadequate housing, education, and health care services. Interpersonal action involves helping people deal with a specific stress such as death, illness, or job loss.

Caplan saw *secondary prevention* as a means of reducing the number of existing cases of mental illness through early diagnosis and treatment. Secondary prevention includes screening programs, prompt referral, improvement in the use of diagnostic tools, and prompt treatment. The majority of mental health problems in this area are short-term and acute. Mental health services must be available to provide short-term therapy that would produce a change in communitywide incidence rates. Secondary prevention includes primary prevention in that it aims at successful resolution of crises, restoration of mental health, and reduction in the number of existing cases of mental illness.

Tertiary prevention was seen as a vehicle for reducing the rate of chronic disability resulting from mental illness. Tertiary prevention includes rehabilitation programs designed to restore the person to a maximum level of well-being. Tertiary prevention includes both primary and secondary prevention insofar as it aims at prevention and reduction of chronic disability and its inherent crises through maximum rehabilitation.

A report by the Joint Commission on Mental Illness and Health in 1961 supported a need for crisis intervention services.[5] The report noted a lack of adequate short-term community facilities to treat significant numbers of community residents in need of mental health services. The report stated that when people were in crisis, almost 50 percent sought out helpers who were not mental health professionals, such as a member of the clergy or a family doctor. If people in crisis did seek professional help, they were usually placed on a long waiting list, rather than receiving immediate attention. When they did receive help, it was often given too late or offered in the form of extended psychotherapy, which is often not helpful to people in crisis. Paraprofessionals with minimal training and interested laypeople in the community had been ignored as additional effective resources for helping people in crisis.

Soon after the publication of this report, considerable federal funds were made available for community-based mental health programs. The availability of federal funding for short-term treatment programs, designed to serve large numbers of people within a community, resulted in the establishment of in- and outpatient crisis services throughout the country. The large proportion of funds available for short-term treatment has helped support and shape this concept of treatment.

Immediate, short-term intervention with individuals, families, and groups has been shown to be effective in reaching and helping larger numbers of people in distress and cutting down on the harmful effects of long-term hospitalization. Crisis services have become an integral part of the mental health services offered by communities; they have become more firmly established and organized; and they continue to provide funds for mental health care.

The major problem currently associated with crisis theory is that the theory, although widely used in clinical settings, has never been validated empirically by research findings.[6,7] Several authors state that the fact that the concept of crisis lacks clarity and has not been operationalized impedes the conduct of meaningful research. Brownell[6] states that descriptive and exploratory research studies must be conducted to provide a scientific knowledge base for crisis theory and its application. Consequently, today, the major task in nursing and other health-related professions is the empirical validation of crisis theory. This will generate a more discriminating perspective about an area of knowledge that is currently only assumed to be valid by those who utilize this framework in their clinical practice.

Recently, the clinical focus has been on developing strategies for intervening with the sequela of social crises, the posttraumatic stress disorder. Some veterans of the Vietnamese war are still experiencing stress. Acts of terrorism which include highjacking, bombings, and kidnappings have necessitated the development of strategies to deal with those affected by such events.

Development of a Crisis

Crises are usually precipitated by periods of *loss, transition*, and *challenge*.[8] Losses may include death of a spouse, divorce, or loss of a job. Transitions may include moving to another community, graduation from school and entry into the world of work, marriage, and birth of a child. Challenges may include job promotions or career changes. Often there is a combination of precipitants in operation at the same time. For example, the loss of divorce is often accompanied by a transition to being single as well as the challenge of returning to work and achieving financial independence. Rapaport states that in each of these situations emotional strain is generated and stress is experienced. When such situations arise, a series of behaviors are activated which lead either to mastery of the situation or to the emergence of a crisis.[9] Aguilera states that when solutions are not forthcoming, such events become crises for those who by personality, previous experience, or other factors in the current situation are particularly vulnerable to the stress and whose coping resources are taxed beyond their customary capacity.[1]

Phases of a Crisis

Crises do not occur instantaneously. There are identifiable phases of development, psychosocial in character, which lead to an active crisis state. Caplan[2] describes a four-phase sequence in the development of a crisis as follows.

PHASE 1. *The perceived threat or event produces an increase in anxiety.* Attempts are made to cope with and to resolve the crisis through usual problem-solving methods. If efforts at this stage are ineffective, the person moves on to the second phase.

PHASE 2. *Increased anxiety and disorganization occur as a result of the failure of coping mechanisms in phase 1.* As they become increasingly disorganized, people may feel frantic; their thoughts race, they can't think clearly, they can't figure out what to do, they may feel as if they are falling apart. They may now engage in random, hit-or-miss efforts to cope and reduce feelings of discomfort. These efforts may result in further failure. If they do, the person moves on to the third phase. It is at this point that people are most likely to seek professional assistance.

PHASE 3. *The person mobilizes internal and external resources and tries out new problem-solving methods or redefines the threat so that old ones can work.* Resolution can occur in this phase if new or old problem-solving methods are put into action and are effective. Resolution of the crisis can lead to an increase or decrease in the person's level of functioning that was evident in the precrisis period. If resolution on some level does not occur, the person moves on to the fourth phase.

PHASE 4. *When efforts to resolve the crisis in preceding phases fail and the problem continues, anxiety may escalate to severe or panic levels.* Extensive cognitive, emotional, and behavioral disorganization may occur.

Crises are temporary and are generally resolved positively or negatively with a 6-week period.[10] Crises have an inherent growth-producing potential. People who master crises independently or with professional assistance can develop a new, broader repertoire of problem-solving skills that helps them deal effectively with life situations.

A Crisis Theory Paradigm

Aguilera and Messick[1] have developed a crisis theory paradigm that provides a framework for examining the presence or absence of balancing factors in a crisis. The *balancing factors* include the person's perception of the event, situational supports, and coping mechanisms. Effective resolution of the crisis is more likely to occur if:

1. *The perception of the precipitating event is realistic rather than distorted.* If the event is perceived realistically, there will be recognition of the relationship between the event and feelings of stress. Problem solving can then be appropriately directed toward reduction of tension and resolution of the stressful situation. If the perception of the event is distorted, there may be no recognition of the relationship between the event and feelings of stress. Attempts to solve the problem will be ineffective, and tension will not be reduced.
2. *Situational supports are available to the person; people in the environment can be depended on to help solve the problem.* When situational supports are not available, the person may feel alone, vulnerable, and without an anchor.
3. *Coping mechanisms that alleviate anxiety are available.* Over a lifetime, all people develop coping mechanisms—which can be cognitive, emotional, or spiritual. Available coping mechanisms are what a person usually does when he or she has a problem. They have been found effective in maintaining emotional stability and have become a part of the person's lifestyle in dealing with the stresses of daily life. When a new stress-producing situation arises and learned coping mechanisms are not effective, anxiety is experienced. The person engages in efforts to "do something" to relieve the discomfort of anxiety.

The balancing factors described above are presented in Figure 22-1 in the paradigm developed by Aguilera and Messick.

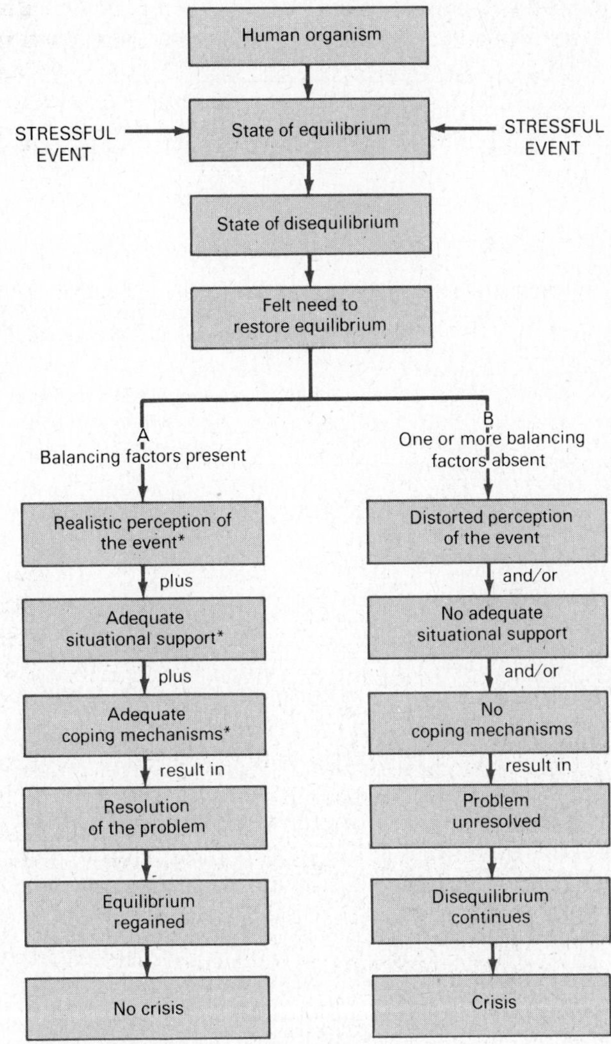

Figure 22-1 Crisis theory paradigm.
Effect of balancing factors in a stressful event.
(SOURCE: Adapted from D. Aguilera and J. Messick, *Crisis Intervention: Theory and Methodology*, 4th ed., Mosby, St. Louis, 1982.)

Types of Crises

Three types of crises can be identified: anticipated maturational crises of the life cycle, unanticipated situational crises, and unanticipated social crises. Table 22-1 (page 430) defines and gives examples of each type. It is not uncommon for a person to experience more than one type of crisis at the same time. A person experiencing an anticipated maturational crisis can simultaneously have a situational or social crisis which compounds the stress experienced during the maturational crisis. For example, a young woman who is having difficulty adjusting to the role changes involved in first-time motherhood might, at the same time, experience the suicide of her own mother.

Maturational Crises

Maturational crises, sometimes called *developmental crises,* are predictable life events which normally occur in the lives of most people. A person's life is continually changing because of the ongoing process of maturation. Aguilera states that potential crisis areas are the periods of physical, social, and psychological changes which are ex-

Table 22-1 Type of Crises

Type	Definition	Example
Maturational (anticipated, normative)	Crises that occur in response to stresses inherent in predictable life transitions and events	Infancy, early childhood, school age, adolescence, young adulthood, adulthood, middle adulthood, late adulthood Marriage, parenthood, job changes, retirement, last child leaving home, menopause
Situational (unanticipated)	Crises that occur when unanticipated events threaten a person's biological, social, or psychological integrity	Death of significant person, physical or mental illness, job loss, divorce, birth of a premature or disabled child
Social (unanticipated)	Crises that occur with uncommon, unanticipated events that involve multiple losses or extensive environmental changes	Flood, fire, war, earthquake, civil riot, volcanic eruption, nuclear contamination, violent crime

perienced during the normal growth process.[1] These changes occur as aspects of the biological and social role transitions that occur during infancy, childhood, adolescence, young adulthood, middle adulthood, and late adulthood. Table 22-2 highlights the maturational crises inherent in each stage of the life cycle. These crises are discussed in depth in Chapter 5.

The onset of a maturational crisis is gradual and occurs over time as the person moves through a period of change. Such transitional periods are characterized by internal disequilibrium and disorganized behavior. The person may experience mood swings and variations of normal behavior in terms of roles and relationships. The nature and extent of the maturational crisis are influenced by four factors:

1. *The success with which previous life transitions have been mastered.* If previous stages of maturational change have been mastered successfully, the residue of unresolved developmental issues is minimized and the person is able to move on to the next transition with a firmer foundation for future growth. People who have unresolved maturational issues from the past often experience greater stress in current life transitions that involve old "unfinished business" than people who are not burdened or vulnerable in this way. Unresolved maturational issues include dependency and authority conflicts, value conflicts, sexual-identity confusion, and lack of capacity for emotional intimacy.[11,12] Examples of these unresolved maturational issues are outlined in Table 22-3 (page 432).
2. *Adequate role models.* These provide the person with examples of how to act in the new role. Teachers, parents, mentors, and peers are examples of people who can act as role models.
3. *Interpersonal resources.* These offer the person a cast of characters with whom to try out new behavior and skills in the attempt to achieve role changes.
4. *The degree to which others accept or resist the new role.* This influences the ease with which role changes are made. The greater the resistance of others, the more difficulty the person experiences in making the change.

Resolution of maturational crises occurs gradually, with and without professional assistance. For those who experience life transitions with normative amounts of stress, resolution may occur without professional assistance as the person experiments with new feelings, roles, and behaviors until a "comfortable fit" is achieved. For those who experience life transitions with intense stress, who have unresolved issues from the past, who do not have adequate role models or interpersonal resources, and who meet resistance to changing roles, crisis resolution may require professional assistance to help them develop ways to cope with and resolve problematic situations.

People who experience average or intense stress have the potential to use maturational crises for personal growth and emerge from them with a new

Table 22-2 Maturational Crises throughout the Life Cycle

Maturational Stage	Crisis Stressors
Infancy	Separation at birth Separation from symbiotic relationship
Early childhood	Giving up certain pleasures Conforming to social demands Separation and autonomy Gender and sexual identity
School age	Separation from the nurturing person Interaction with new authority figures Formation of peer relationships Group cooperation
Adolescence	Change in body image Consolidation of psychosexual identity Heterosexual relationships Educational demands Parent-child separation Independence from parental supports
Young adulthood	Preparation for work and career Commitment to intimate relationships or parenthood Psychosexual maturity
Adulthood	Pursuit of career goals Marital or other intimate relationships Sexual relationships Childbearing and child rearing Independence and interdependence
Middle adulthood	Launching of children or empty-nest syndrome Work stressors (promotion, end of the line, loss of job, retirement) Illness or death of a parent Physical changes Changes in marital status
Late adulthood	Unproductive, less valued role of the retiree Declining physical health Adaptation to chronic health problems Loss of spouse and peers Economic problems Loss of independence

level of maturity. Negative resolution of a maturational transition period may result in a developmental stall. The term *developmental stall* refers to unmet needs, unresolved issues, or unmastered tasks of a particular developmental stage that keep the person focused on the issues, needs, and tasks of that stage. This inhibits developmental movement to other stages and may be reflected in the emergence of dysfunctional behavior patterns. The stall may interfere with the person's self-concept, relationships with others, and control of the environment.

Transitional periods during adolescence, marriage, parenthood, midlife, and retirement are common times for maturational crises to occur. A crisis related to parenthood is presented in the following example:

Anne and Michael J. were referred to the crisis intervention unit of the local mental health center by a nurse-midwife 6 weeks after the birth of their first child, a son, Michael Jr., because of Anne's feelings of depression. Her symptoms included difficulty falling asleep, loss of appetite, unexplainable crying spells, and thoughts of harming the baby. Anne, a small, 22-year-old woman, looked much younger than her age. Michael, age 27, looked mature and appeared calm. Michael was a sales representative for a large computer corporation. After graduating from college, Anne had worked for the same company as a computer programmer, but she left her job when the baby was born.

Michael was the oldest of four children and had helped with the care of the younger children because his mother had always worked. Anne was a sheltered only child who had little experience with children because she had no siblings and her parents had never allowed her to baby-sit. They both came from the same town, had no family nearby, and had no friends with children.

The pregnancy was unplanned. Anne and Michael had planned to wait 4 years before starting a family so that their careers would be well established. Instead, the pregnancy occurred 6 months after the marriage. Anne was initially shocked and then excited about the pregnancy. Toward the end of her pregnancy, she began to feel lonely and worried about being able to take care of the baby, since she had never been around babies before.

After the baby was born, Michael's mother came to help Anne take care of the baby. When Michael's mother left, Anne felt that she basically knew how to take care of the baby, but became upset if he didn't

Table 22-3 Unresolved Maturational Issues

Unresolved Maturational Issue	Example
Dependency conflict	Rob, a 28-year-old college graduate with a master's degree in special education, had taught for 1 year and then had been involved in several other career endeavors which all resulted in personal dissatisfaction, financial problems, and the consequent need to move back to his parents' house. He was experiencing intense stress around a decision to move to another part of the country in order to take advantage of another business opportunity.
Value conflict	Jody, a 21-year-old college senior, went to the college counseling center because of pervasive and intense anxiety and tension. She discussed difficulties relative to her values, particularly moral and religious values. She described her parents as quite religious and morally proper; as people who dominate without being dominating personalities. Jody had developed an idealized image of herself that reflected parental expectations and values to an excessive degree. She was currently struggling with decisions around moving in with her boyfriend and whether to take a year off before applying to graduate school. She felt that her parents would disapprove if she did either one, and she was unable to identify her own value position.
Sexual-identity confusion	Bruce, age 32, was seen at the crisis clinic because he felt severely depressed following the breakup of a 3-month relationship with a woman. Bruce's father died when Bruce was 5 years old. He was raised by his mother and widowed grandmother. As a youngster he was not encouraged to participate in "boyish" activities. As a teenager he had had several homosexual advances made toward him. From that time on, he had worried about his sexuality. He had dated women, but never had a long-lasting relationship. The breakup of this first long-term relationship brought his long-standing worry and confusion about his sexuality to the surface. He was struggling with the concern that perhaps he was homosexual and hadn't realized it and that perhaps this was why he hadn't been able to have successful relationships with women.
Lack of capacity for emotional intimacy	Peter was a 40-year-old successful lawyer who came to the crisis clinic 1 week after he had separated from his wife of 3 years. Peter's wife had asked him to leave, saying, "You don't care about anybody but yourself—you're incapable of loving anyone." Peter stated that he was very involved with himself and his work; he had never found it easy to move toward people even as a child. He stated that his parents were divorced when he was 8 years old; he described his parents as cold and distant. He was now anxious because of the long string of casual relationships before his marriage, which he always ended when they got too heavy, and now the breakup of the marriage. The attendant relief of having his freedom back seemed to point toward his inability to participate in an ongoing intimate relationship. He was relieved to be unencumbered by the emotional demands of his wife, but was intensely worried that he had inherited a tragic flaw.

stop crying when she took care of him. When Michael was home, he helped take care of the baby, and the baby rarely cried after Michael took care of him. Michael's apparent competence and ease made Anne feel even more inadequate and concerned about her ability to be a mother.

The crisis was precipitated on a day when Anne could not get the baby to stop crying. She walked up and down the apartment, holding him, but could not quiet him. Michael entered the apartment at 6 P.M., walked into the living room, and saw Anne shaking the baby and crying while saying, "Shut up, just shut up; all you ever do is cry; I'll shut you up." Michael took the baby from her arms. Anne sat down with her head in her lap, continued crying, and said, "I didn't mean it; he just wouldn't stop crying, no matter what I did." Michael put the baby in his crib; sat with Anne for a while, reassuring her; and then called their nurse-midwife, who referred them to the crisis center.

ASSESSMENT

A young woman who had unresolved dependency needs of her own was now in the unplanned position of being a parent. Her perception of herself as a mother was unrealistic; she had no nearby situational supports; and coping methods that had previously worked were inadequate.

A crisis in relation to retirement is presented in the following example:

Jack W., age 68, came to the crisis clinic complaining of a "nervous stomach," insomnia, and fatigue. His symptoms had begun 1 month before, after he was forced into retirement by business reverses that resulted in the unexpected sale of a previously successful business. All of Jack's friends and acquaintances still worked, as did his wife. His lifetime involvement with work had left little time for or interest in the development of recreational pastimes. He now found himself sitting at home each day by himself with little to do besides read the newspaper and watch television. Although he did little each day, he felt exhausted and nervous. He felt directionless, useless, and lonely. He consulted his family doctor for his "nervous stomach," and she referred him to the crisis clinic.

ASSESSMENT

An older man who was having difficulty dealing with an abrupt transition into retirement. His self-worth was tied to his involvement with work, and he was unprepared with alternative interests to provide meaning in his life. He had no situational supports or role models to ease the transition. His former coping methods were ineffective in this situation.

Situational Crises

Situational crises occur when unanticipated events threaten a person's biological, social, or psychological integrity.[13] There is an accompanying degree of disequilibrium. The person's coping mechanisms become ineffective, or chosen solutions prove to be impractical. The stressful event involves a fundamental loss or deprivation which threatens the person's self-concept. A situational crisis is precipitated by the loss of a systematized support that had enhanced the person's feelings of security and control and was essential to maintaining the integrity of the self-concept. Examples of situational crises include loss of a loved one, loss or change of a job, change in financial status, geographic move, school failure, divorce, unwanted pregnancy, birth of a premature or disabled child, and physical or mental illness. Each of these crises has the potential to create stress, initiate grieving, threaten feelings of self-worth, create conflict and role change among family members, and precipitate loss of emotional support systems.

Caplan states that the unpredictable nature of these events introduces an element of *hazard* that does not exist in the anticipated maturational crises. The element of unpreparedness increases the potential for disruption of lifestyle. The degree of disruption will influence a person's control and ability to cope in such a situation.[2,14] One's perception of situational events influences the point at which a hazardous situation becomes a crisis. Additionally, situational crises can either disrupt many related areas in a person's lifestyle or promote growth and change. Crises create ripple effects, like stones tossed into a pond. The total configuration of disruptions becomes the concern of crisis intervention, as in the example below of a family financial crisis.

John F., age 45, was offered a vice presidency in a California engineering firm that had just secured a large government contract. The offer was too good to refuse. His family, consisting of his wife and three children, ages 12, 15, and 17, reluctantly moved from their lifelong Connecticut home to Los Angeles. After 6 months of work, the contract fell through. John's firm went bankrupt, and he was out of a job. At the same time, John's wife was depressed and lonely, 3000 miles from family and friends. Now she was faced with financial insecurity as well. The children were having difficulty adjusting to a different academic program and making new friends. The financial crisis led John to begin drinking heavily; he was embarrassed to call his old firm in Connecticut, had few business contacts in the area, and was not making any new job connections. The family's savings were being depleted rapidly.

ASSESSMENT

The job change and geographic move initiated a sequence of events that involved all family members. The hazardous situation became a family crisis when John lost his job. Financial stress and loss of self-worth, followed by heavy drinking, school problems, and loss of extended family connections, combined to create a network of situational crises that would have to be confronted before resolution could take place.

Another example illustrates the stresses associated with an unwanted pregnancy.

Patty A., age 19, came alone to the general hospital emergency room on a Saturday night. She paced the waiting room in an agitated manner, crying and muttering to herself. When interviewed by the triage nurse, she complained of abdominal pain and two missed menstrual periods. As she spoke, she began to sob, saying that she was afraid that she was pregnant. She was afraid to tell her parents because they'd throw her out. She was afraid to tell her boyfriend because he would insist that they get married and she didn't want to marry for that reason. She attended a local community college and didn't know what she would do with a baby if she had one. She didn't want to quit school and didn't know if she wanted an abortion. She finished by stating, "My head is in a whirl. I never had so much to decide, and I have no one to talk to who could help me."

ASSESSMENT

An unmarried young woman, with no situational supports, attempting to make major decisions about commitments, roles, and lifestyles with no previous coping experience in this or a related area.

Social Crises

Social crises are accidental, uncommon, and unanticipated crises that involve multiple losses or extensive environmental change.[15] Examples of social crises are natural disasters such as fires, floods, volcanic eruptions, and earthquakes; national disasters such as wars, riots, racial persecution, and nuclear contamination; and violent crimes such as rape and murder. Social crises do not commonly occur in the everyday lives of people. When they do occur, the stress level is so high that the coping resources of each person are maximally challenged.

Tyhurst[16] in his study of individual responses to community disasters found that victims experience three overlapping phases (see Table 22-4):

1. Period of impact
2. Period of recoil
3. Posttraumatic period

During social crises mental health workers must reach out to the community and intervene with a large number of people. An example of the effect of a social crisis on a community follows:

In a small city of 75,000, it had been raining heavily for 3 days. Power failures were widespread, and telephone lines were down in several parts of town. Many rivers and streams had overflowed, flooding many main streets. People were wondering how the dam at the edge of the city would hold in this downpour. They reassured each other by saying, "The old dam has been there for a hundred years; it has withstood worse than this." Many people left their homes to move to higher ground. Others, however, stayed, clinging to the belief that, "It couldn't happen to us." They sat by their radios and waited and listened in the darkness.

Early on the fourth morning, people were awakened by a deafening roar. A huge torrent of water was pouring downhill, overturning everything in its path. People raced to second floors, attics, and roofs. It was too late to get away. They watched neighboring houses break loose from their foundations. They heard the screaming voices of friends and neighbors, adults and children alike, who clung to anything that would keep them afloat in the churning water.

Table 22-4 Phases of a Disaster

Phase	Definition	Characteristics
Impact	The period in which people are hit with the reality of what has happened. This phase lasts from a few minutes to 1 or 2 hours.	Calm, effective action; shock and confusion; hysteria, confusion, or paralyzing fear
Recoil	The period in which there is at least a temporary suspension of the initial stresses of the disaster. Lives are no longer in danger, although many stresses remain, including gradual awareness of the full impact of the disaster.	Looking for connection with support systems such as surviving friends or relatives; desire to be taken care of; desire to share the horror of the experience; weeping
Posttrauma	The period in which survivors become fully aware of what occurred during the impact phase—loss of families, homes, belongings, security. Resolution of loss and reconstruction of lifestyle will occur to lesser and greater degrees. This phase can last for the rest of a person's life.	Guilt, nightmares, anger, frustration, anxiety reactions, reactive depressions, psychotic episodes

The massive flood caused by the dam break destroyed houses, stores, and schools; everything in its path was ruined. Hundreds of people were trapped and drowned in their houses or trying to escape, especially those living in the lower parts of town. Survivors, many of whom had failed to save their loved ones, slowly made their way to higher ground, where they found makeshift emergency shelters. Many appeared numb, in shock; many couldn't describe in a coherent way what had happened. They either sat rigidly still, paced agitatedly, or busily involved themselves in rescue work. Some wept hysterically about lost family members, homes, and business; others were unnaturally calm and contained; still others alternated between the two affective states. Many people had sustained physical shock and needed minor or extensive medical treatment. Rescue assistance arrived by helicopter, because the city was cut off from other transportation routes. The critically injured were evacuated to regional medical centers; those less seriously injured remained in emergency shelters. The unhappy task of cleaning up the city began: finding and burying the dead, cleaning debris, fixing the dam, and rebuilding the city.

ASSESSMENT

Unanticipated natural disaster which destroyed a city and resulted in the death of hundreds. Following the impact phase, emergency interventions were instituted to deal with shock and acute disorganization. In the posttrauma phase, survivors will have to be observed for later sequelae such as persistent intense fear; phobias about weather; apathy, depression, despair; preoccupation with thoughts of dead relatives; guilt about survival; vivid memories and dreams; constricted living patterns; diffuse rage reactions. Such behaviors would be the evidence of ineffective mourning, anxiety, and intense feelings of helplessness and lack of control.

CRISIS INTERVENTION

Role of the Nurse in Crisis Intervention

As a community-based form of short-term therapy, crisis intervention takes place in structured and unstructured settings. It extends the availability of mental health services to larger numbers of people within a community and minimizes the detrimental effects of long-term hospitalization.[2]

Nurses practice in a variety of settings in which crisis intervention is the therapy of choice. Nurses who work on general hospital units deal with crises resulting from the stresses of hospitalization, illness, and death on a daily basis. Nurses who work in obstetric, pediatric, adolescent, or geriatric settings deal with families undergoing maturational crises. Emergency rooms are deluged 24 hours a day with clients in crisis. Community health nurses observe and identify families in crisis in the home setting. More frequently now, nurses are being placed in the role of primary therapist and are, therefore, becoming more involved in the direct process of crisis intervention. Nurses work in collaboration with interdisciplinary crisis teams. The members of a crisis team are representatives of many professional disciplines, including nursing, medicine, psychology, social work, and theology.[17] Others, who work in the community—such as police officers, fire fighters, teachers, bartenders, and rescue workers—are often present when a crisis occurs and can be valuable resources to the crisis team for crisis intervention.

Nursing Process: Phases of Crisis Intervention

According to crisis theorists, during the 4- to 6-week crisis period, a person is psychologically less defended and is consequently more amenable to change.[2,11] The distress experienced during this period and the wish to alleviate it serve as motivating factors that make the person more willing to look at the problem differently and find other ways of dealing with it. The person is ready to engage in an active problem-solving partnership.[18] The goal of crisis intervention is to reestablish a level of functioning equal to or better than the precrisis level. Implicit in this goal is restoration of order, purpose, and meaning in a person's life.

Morely, Messick, and Aguilera[19] have identified four phases of crisis intervention: assessment, planning, intervention, and evaluation. These phases closely parallel the steps of the nursing process.

Assessment

Assessment is the first step of crisis intervention. It involves collection of data about the nature of the crisis and its effect on the client and significant others.[8,18] The assessment phase is also used to establish rapport and a collaborative relationship with the client that is conducive to mutual problem-solving efforts. The nurse should assess three specific areas related to the balancing factors that are important in the development and resolution of a crisis. These three areas are:

1. The precipitating event and the client's *perception of the problem*
2. The client's strengths and *coping skills*
3. The nature and strength of the client's *situational supports*

The assessment should focus on the immediate problem and not delve into a myriad of other problems that may exist.

PERCEPTION OF THE PROBLEM. The nurse's task is to obtain data from the client that clarify the precipitating event, the point at which the symptoms appeared, factors influencing the precipitation of the crisis, and the meaning of the problem to the client.

Questions relating to the precipitating event and symptom formation that are asked of the client include the following:

Why did you come for help today?

What happened in your life that is different?

When did it happen?

Can you describe how you feel now?

When did you begin to feel that way?

Is there a connection between how you're feeling and the events you're describing to me?

The precipitating event has usually occurred within 10 to 14 days before the person seeks help. It is not unusual for something to have happened the day or the night before, such as threat of divorce, discovery of a child's drug abuse, loss of job, or an unwanted pregnancy. Symptoms usually appear after the stressful event. As the client connects life events with symptom formation, understanding of the precipitating event can occur.

Questions relating to the meaning of the problem to the client and factors influencing the occurrence of the problem are also asked of the client:

How does this problem affect your life right now?

How do you see this problem affecting your future?

What effect is this problem having on others around you?

What other factors could be influencing the way you are seeing this problem?

The nurse assesses how realistically or unrealistically the client perceives the problem and the factors that influence those perceptions. Current issues of concern are often linked to past issues of concern. Current issues reawaken old unresolved issues that become influential factors in the precipitation of a crisis. For example:

Louise G. came to the crisis center "feeling thrown out of whack" because of an impending divorce. She stated that it was unlike her to be so upset. The nurse, on questioning her about recent related events, found that Louise's mother had died of cancer 3 years ago. Louise felt that she had never really grieved for her mother, to whom she felt very close, because that kind of emotional display was unacceptable in her family of origin. Thus, the unresolved loss of her mother was influencing the meaning of loss in her current impending divorce.

Since most crises involve actual or potential losses, the issue of loss is commonly expressed. The nurse, therefore, looks for issues from the past that connect with and influence current events.[11,12]

COPING SKILLS. *Strengths* and *coping skills* refer to the ways in which a person acts to solve problems.[1] It is equally important to determine how the client acts when a problem is encountered that he or she cannot solve. Since coping skills are very individual, the client must be asked:

Has anything like this ever happened to you before?

How have you handled other crises in your life?

How do you usually decrease tension and anxiety?

Have you tried the same method this time?

If not, why not, if it usually works?

If it was tried and didn't work, what kept it from working?

What else do you think might work?

As stated above, coping skills are very individual. People use coping skills such as sports, playing a musical instrument, crying, talking to a friend, or going off by themselves to think through a problem.

SITUATIONAL SUPPORTS. *Situational supports* are important people in the client's relationship system that are available resources for helping the client. Assessment of support systems will reveal the presence or absence of important people, networks, or institutions in the client's life.[1] Data are collected about current and potential sources of support. The client is asked:

With whom do you live?

Is there someone with whom you are particularly close?

Do you have friends? Do you have a best friend?

Who is available to help you?

Who understands you?

Whom do you trust?

Are you involved in community activities?

Assessing the support system may help the nurse determine who should come to the crisis therapy sessions. Presence and availability of family members may indicate a need for their involvement. Absence of family or friends may indicate the need for a crisis therapy group so that the support from other group members can be elicited. Once the assessment process is completed, the planning phase can begin.

Planning

Planning is the second step of the crisis intervention process. During this phase, the data from the client, family, school, or other professional agency are organized and analyzed, and specific interventions are proposed.[8] Preliminary hypotheses are advanced about dynamic issues that underlie the problem as information about the precipitating event is contrasted with past experiences. Alternative solutions to the problem are explored, and methods for accomplishing them are outlined. The nurse decides on the situational and environmental supports that can be used and the coping skills that need to be developed or strengthened.

Intervention

Intervention is the third step of the crisis intervention process. It involves implementation of the plan.[1] Intervention is characterized by goal-directedness. It focuses on the problem at hand and usually consists of six to eight structured interviews. At other times, crisis work is completed in 48 to 72 hours and the client is referred to another agency for ongoing therapy. The nurse conveys an attitude of authority, responsibility, and concern, keeping the client focused on issues relating to the problem that is causing the current disequilibrium.

Several steps are followed in resolving the problem. First, the nurse labels his or her perception of the problem and checks it out with the client's perception of the problem, and then both nurse and client explore their perceptions of it. Connections are made between the meaning of the event and the resulting crisis. Clarification is used to clear up any misconceptions on the part of the nurse or the client. Second, the multiple feelings accompanying the crisis are observed and acknowledged. This helps the person to sort out feelings and thoughts, to express them, and to have them validated as normal and acceptable. Third, the nurse and client explore alternative problem-solving behaviors and coping skills such as reaching out to others and verbalizing feelings and expectations. Fourth, the nurse and client test or rehearse new approaches to problem solving in order to arrive at a comfortable fit. This will reinforce new behaviors and coping skills, give the client positive feedback, and enhance the client's self-esteem. Throughout the process, the therapist acts as a role model for open, direct communication; innovative thinking; flexibility; and self-awareness.[18]

Throughout the intervention process the nurse utilizes a variety of related strategies to facilitate effective resolution of the crisis. Two common strategies that are used with the problem-solving approach are environmental manipulation and anticipatory guidance.

Environmental manipulation is a strategy which directly changes the client's physical or interpersonal situation in order to provide situational supports or alleviate stress.[11] For example, a client whose husband has died and now lives alone may have a son, daughter, or grandchild move in for a week. A client who has no social network may be involved in a crisis group for situational support. An older couple living in a deteriorating neighborhood in which they have been mugged may be moved to a housing project for the elderly.

Anticipatory guidance is a strategy for responding to crises involving normative life events such as bereavement, divorce, marriage, birth of a child, and retirement.[11] Anticipatory guidance means helping a person in crisis to anticipate certain internal or external events and to prepare for these events in an adaptive way. The nurse can outline for the person the expected normative thoughts, feelings, and behaviors that might predictably occur to most people in the same situation. The client has the benefit of being able to anticipate and have time to prepare for the impact of change by planning and mobilizing effective coping strategies in advance. The client also has an idea of what it is "normal" to experience in what may be an unusual situation; anxiety is reduced because the number of unknowns is decreased. This process facilitates movement through periods of transition. It applies a specific method that has been effective with large numbers of clients whose similar crises follow the same predictable pattern. Several generic patterns for crises of anticipated life transition have been identified, for example, the stages of dying and the process of adjustment to divorce.

Evaluation

Evaluation is the fourth step of the crisis intervention process. Through evaluation nurses determine the effectiveness of the planned intervention. The goals should be compared with the behavioral outcomes. If the intervention has been successful, the client will experience a decrease in distress and will return to a precrisis level of functioning. The client will be able to identify the events and feelings that caused the disruption, evaluate changes in lifestyle, and implement these changes to the satisfaction of client and nurse. Evaluation provides an opportunity to consolidate learning that has occurred to date, identify emerging unmet needs, and test the client's capacity to initiate activity to meet these needs. Not all learning may take place within the 6 to 8 weeks of the crisis therapy; true integration may occur only after the actual sessions are completed. Then, although the contract time is over, the nurse should remain available for future consultation. Clients with additional areas of concern are often referred to other agencies for long-term counseling once the current crisis has been resolved.[1,18]

Following are two case studies which illustrate the phases of crisis intervention. The first case study describes intervention in a maturational crisis—the crisis of late adulthood.

Robert W. called the crisis unit of the mental health clinic after finding the number in the telephone book. He asked whether the unit could help him and his wife. At the first interview, Robert and Ethel, both in their seventies, related their problem.

ASSESSMENT

They live in a small apartment in a five-story walk-up building in what has become a transitional neighborhood. The incidence of crime in the neighborhood has reached epidemic proportions, and they are afraid to go out alone. Most of their old friends have either died or, if financially able, moved away. Robert was a tailor for many years until failing eyesight forced him to retire. He and his wife now support themselves on a small pension and Social Security. Their two married children have moved to the suburbs, have their own problems making ends meet, and visit only occasionally. Ethel has a heart condition; she is increasingly unable to climb the stairs or clean their apartment. Robert helps her, but his near blindness makes it increasingly difficult for him to go out and do the necessary errands. They are feeling trapped by their aging bodies, lack of money, and inadequate living quarters.

Just when they were feeling very blue, they got a telephone call from their daughter-in-law telling them that their son had been laid off from his job. Ethel said, "Oh, my God. What is happening? We can't help ourselves, much less our children." She sat crying for days, refusing to get out of bed.

At the interview, the nurse recognized that the W.'s were experiencing feelings of inadequacy, powerlessness, helplessness, and hopelessness. The crisis-precipitating event for the W.'s was their children's disaster, which accentuated their own helplessness and generated guilt because they were unable to help themselves, much less their children. They felt that their situation could not be altered in any positive way and were unable to identify any situational supports.

PLAN

A plan was formulated to help the W.'s develop a more objective view of their parental role and identify their strengths and liabilities. Environmental manipulation would be used to arrange for more satisfactory living arrangements, needed medical services, and use of social and community support systems.

INTERVENTION

Intervention was directed toward helping the W.'s to express their feelings, examine their expectations of themselves, look at the problem realistically, and arrive at alternative solutions. First, it was necessary to help the W.'s examine their feelings of responsibility for their children. Once they acknowledged that their middle-aged children's financial status was not their responsibility, they were able to begin focusing on their own needs and problems. They identified their liabilities—blindness, heart condition, financial strain, etc.—that were interfering with their ability to cope. Their strengths were their solid marital relationship, their willingness to socialize, and their independence. They explored requirements for suitable living quarters such as safe neighborhood, no stairs, accessible shopping, and a senior citizens' center.

EVALUATION

By the third week, Robert and Ethel, with the assistance of the nurse, had located a housing project for the elderly with a senior citizens' center attached to it in a safer part of the city and were placed on the waiting list. Medical services were also found, and Robert was scheduled for a cataract operation to correct his eyesight. Ethel was being evaluated for a medical regimen to monitor her heart condition. The W.'s felt more hopeful about their future but were apprehensive about making a move to a new neighborhood and about Robert's impending surgery. The children were contacted, and their son agreed to stay with his mother during his father's hospitalization. He said that he had not realized how difficult life had become for his parents. The W.'s were assured that they could return to the crisis clinic if help was needed in the future.

The second case study illustrates intervention in a situational crisis, divorce:

Marie S., age 34, arrived at the mental health clinic crying and saying that she felt she was losing control of her life. During the first session, she gave the following information.

ASSESSMENT

She and her husband, Don S., age 36, were planning to divorce following her recent discovery that he had been having numerous extramarital affairs. Don had not denied the involvements but had simply said, "So what? All I get from you is nagging. I have to have fun somewhere." A fight ensured, and Marie told him to get out.

In the month after Don left, their two children, ages 6 and 9, had nightmares and problems at school. The younger child did not want to let Marie out of her sight. Marie was having money problems and should have been out looking for a job, but she found herself crying when she looked at the job ads. In addition, she said that she sill loved Don. She felt that they had gradually grown apart. They seemed to be moving in two different worlds, hers at home and his at work. She felt increasingly unable to play a role in his more dynamic life. Don's acknowledged infidelity, which Marie had suspected for a while, was the crisis-precipitating event.

Marie was experiencing feelings of depression, worthlessness, and guilt, believing that she had been a "bad" wife and now was also incompetent as a mother because her children were having problems. Although her family lived in another state, Marie had several situational supports, including a number of neighbors and friends who had reached out to her. But she had reacted to her problem by giving up and becoming immobilized.

PLAN

A plan was formulated using anticipatory guidance to identify and explore the normative grief process experienced by adults and children in loss situations such as divorce. Marie needed to reevaluate realistically her role in the marital conflict. Situational supports were to be used as social resources and more effective coping mechanisms such as part-time work would be explored.

INTERVENTION

Intervention was directed toward helping Marie express her feelings and look at the problem in a more realistic way. It was necessary to diagram the relationship to see the points at which it had gone awry and to define how each partner had contributed to the discord. The nurse was able to provide anticipatory guidance, describing the concept of loss and grief involved with divorce and outlining the predictable responses. Marie could expect to experience. Once Marie realized that her feelings were normal and that she was not going crazy, she was able to acknowledge that she was not completely at fault and was able to begin identifying her strengths. For example, she had been a good mother and homemaker, her children had friends and did well in school, she had been an effective worker in community activities, and she had a number of good friends. She also had a professional skill, teaching. As she began to see her strengths more objectively, she began to feel less depressed. She was able to talk with the children more and help them explore their feelings about the separation.

EVALUATION

By the fifth week Marie had applied for work as a substitute teacher and had been called for a job. Don had called her, and they were considering a reconciliation. Marie and the nurse explored alternative behaviors in the relationship. Plans were made for couples' therapy at the center. At termination, Marie was teaching part time, had joined an evening book-discussion club, had had her hair restyled, and had found that the children's symptoms had decreased. Marie and the therapist reviewed the adjustments she had made, the insight she had gained, and her needs regarding future plans. She felt more confident that even if the divorce went through, she would be able to cope more effectively with her life.

Other Methods of Crisis Intervention

Crisis intervention utilizes a variety of strategies in formulating a comprehensive but short-term treatment plan. The methods of crisis intervention presented below represent initial, additional, or alternative intervention strategies.

Telephone Crisis Counseling

Crisis intervention centers rely heavily on telephone counseling to initiate contact with clients in crisis. Telephone counseling on a hot line is successful because it offers clients in crisis immediate contact with a helping person. A client may call the hot line experiencing severe anxiety and disorganized thinking. The person may feel overwhelmed—unable to cope or identify any situational supports. The telephone counselor will endeavor to maintain contact with the caller, utilizing facilitative communication skills to decrease anxiety and elicit information from the person about the problem. Sometimes, the telephone counselor is powerless. The client may refuse to give his or her name and address, may give false information, or may hang up suddenly. At other times, after obtaining essential information, the counselor will assess the situation as highly dangerous and dispatch expert crisis workers to the caller's home.

The telephone counselor is often instrumental in initiating involvement in treatment. The counselor identifies the appropriate community resources and refers the client to the agency that can meet his or her needs without delay.

Telephone counseling may be set up in a crisis center. Telephone counselors are often community volunteers who have received extensive in-service training in interviewing, crisis theory, and intervention.

Emergency Room Crisis Counseling

The nurse working in the emergency room continually encounters people in crisis. Daily, the nurse observes attempted suicides, rape and assault victims, accident victims and their families, people with sudden-onset illness such as a heart attack, and people with chronic anxiety who present with a myriad of physical symptoms. All these people are candidates for crisis intervention. The role of the nurse in the emergency room is to assess and define the problem. The nurse can then implement brief intervention measures such as approaches designed to reduce anxiety (see Chapter 29). If the nurse is not in a position to work with the client on an ongoing basis, a referral for crisis therapy in another setting can be made.

Home Visits

Home visits are usually made by the community health nurse. The community health nurse observes and assesses clients in their own environment. Potential high-risk families can be observed, identified, and referred (see Chapter 48). Families with new babies, sick members, a recent death or divorce, or a history of difficulty in coping are among those potentially in need of crisis intervention. The nurse often has an ongoing relationship with the family and can intervene effectively in a crisis using interventions described earlier in the chapter. Home visits are also made by crisis teams from crisis centers to obtain additional information about the client's home situation or to reach a client with whom contact is unobtainable in any other way. Frequently telephone contact with a highly suicidal caller who is unwilling to come to the crisis center will result in an immediate home visit by the crisis team.[20]

Family Crisis Therapy

Family crisis therapy utilizes a temporary, brief-therapy model that is problem-focused. It does not delve into general family issues and problems. Rather, it focuses on a specific problem that a family is currently encountering.

Family crisis therapy involves the entire family unit. The family is viewed as a system, with family members involved in an interactive process. A crisis affecting any family member affects all members, producing shifts in the family balance. Thus, the crisis is defined as a family problem regardless of whom the family identifies as having the problem.[21,22] For example:

> If a young child is afraid to go to school and wants to stay home with the mother, it is assumed that the mother participates in the process because of her loneliness and need for this child to remain overly close. The father may participate by traveling extensively for business and being home only on weekends. The child, lonely for the father and sensitive to the mother's upset about these frequent absences, moves closer to the mother in order to have emotional needs met and to calm the mother's upset feelings. Intervention is directed at giving the family tasks that will restructure the dysfunctional interaction and role patterns. The father would be instructed to take charge of getting the child ready to go to school and to spend more "relationship time" with the child. The mother would be instructed to do some other task not involving the child while this was taking place. The family members are taught other ways of meeting each other's needs, so that they can take responsibility for change.

Crisis Groups

Crisis groups are short-term groups that also utilize the problem-solving method of crisis intervention.[23] People are referred to crisis groups after severe and panic-level anxiety has been reduced with other crisis intervention methods.

Leaders and members of crisis groups have several tasks:

1. The nurse acts as a leader and role model for effective problem solving.
2. Group members assist each other in problem resolution. They encourage exploration of feelings and solutions to problems.
3. The group provides an arena for experimentation with new behaviors. Group members reinforce the client's new problem-solving behaviors.
4. The group acts as a support system for the client. This aspect of the group is particularly useful for clients without a peer or family network.
5. The group can be used to give feedback to members about their behavior. This is important because often there will be striking parallels between the way the client acts in the group and his or her problematic behavior patterns in everyday life.

Here is an example of the fifth task:

> After two group sessions, it became obvious that Mitch K. would challenge and argue any point made by a group member. The major reason for Mitch's crisis was that at age 50 he was extremely lonely and had no lasting relationships. The members commented on his behavior in the group and questioned him about a relationship between his argumentativeness and his inability to sustain relationships.

SUMMARY

A *crisis* is an internal disturbance that results from a stressful event or a perceived threat to self-integrity. Crisis theory provides a framework for viewing those stressful life situations or events for which a person's customary methods of solving problems and making decisions are not adequate. Whether or not a hazardous event is defined as a crisis depends on the person's perception of the problem, situational supports, and coping skills, because it is the person's inability to cope with an event that precipitates a crisis, not the event itself.

Crises involve losses, transitions, and challenges. *Maturational crises* are the anticipated transition points of the life cycle, such as adolescence, marriage, parenthood, and retirement. *Situational crises* are unanticipated events such as death, illness, and divorce. *Social crises* are uncommon, unanticipated events such as floods, fires, and nuclear contamination that lead to extensive loss and environmental change.

Crises are dealt with by crisis intervention. *Crisis intervention* is a community-based form of brief therapy that addresses resolution of a current stressful life event in ways aimed at helping the person develop a new, broader array of coping skills. This short-term, problem-solving approach uses a four-step process: assessment, planning, intervention, and evaluation. Nurses intervene with clients in a variety of inpatient and outpatient health care settings in collaboration with a crisis intervention team. Specific methods of crisis intervention include telephone counseling, emergency room crisis counseling, home visits, family crisis therapy, and crisis groups.

REFERENCES

1. Donna C. Aguilera and Janice M. Messick, *Crisis Intervention: Theory and Methodology*, 4th ed., Mosby, St. Louis, 1982.
2. Gerald Caplan, *Principles of Preventive Psychiatry*, Basic Books, New York, 1964.
3. J. A. Shelly, S. D. John, et al. *Spiritual Dimensions of Mental Health*, Intervarsity Press, Downers Grove, Ill., 1983.
4. Eric Lindeman, "Symptomatology and Management of Acute Grief," *American Journal of Psychiatry*, vol. 101, 1944, p. 141.
5. Joint Commission on Mental Illness and Health, *Action for Mental Health*, Basic Books, New York, 1961.
6. M. J. Brownell, "The Concept of Crisis: Its Utility for Nursing," *Advances in Nursing Science*, vol. 6, no. 4, 1984, pp. 10–21.
7. E. M. Geissler, "Crisis: What It Is and Is Not," *Advances in Nursing Science*, vol. 6, no. 4, 1984, pp. 1–9.
8. Deanna Goldstein, "Crisis Intervention: A Brief Therapy Model," *Nursing Clinics of North America*, vol. 13, no. 4, 1978, pp. 657–663.
9. Lydia Rapaport, "The State of Crisis: Some Theoretical Considerations," in Howard J. Parad, ed., *Crisis Intervention: Selected Readings*, Family Service Association of America, New York, 1965.
10. Howard J. Parad and Gerald Caplan, "A Framework for Studying Families in Crisis," in Howard J. Parad, ed., *Crisis Intervention: Selected Readings*, Family Service Association of American, New York, 1965.
11. Bruce A. Baldwin, "A Paradigm for the Classification of Emotional Crises: Implications for Crisis Intervention," *American Journal of Orthopsychiatry*, vol. 48, no. 3, 1978, pp. 538–551.
12. L. R. Barnhill and D. Longo, "Fixation and Regression in the Family Life Cycle," *Family Process*, vol. 17, 1978, pp. 469–478.
13. L. A. Hoff, *People in Crisis: Understanding and Helping*, 2d ed., Addison-Wesley, Menlo Park, Calif., 1984.
14. S. Panzarine, "Coping: Conceptual and Methodological Issues," *Advances in Nursing Science*, vol. 7, no. 4, 1985, pp. 49–57.
15. B. C. Chamberlin, "The Psychological Aftermath of Disaster," *Journal of Clinical Psychology*, vol. 41, no. 7, 1980, pp. 238–243.
16. J. S. Tyhurst, "Individual Reactions to Community Disaster," *American Journal of Psychiatry*, vol. 107, 1951, pp. 764–769.
17. J. Lieb et al., *The Crisis Team*, Harper and Row, New York, 1973.
18. Lorna M. Barrel, "Crisis Intervention: Partnership in Problem-Solving," *Nursing Clinics of North America*, vol. 9, no. 1, 1974, pp. 5–17.
19. Wilbur E. Morely, Janice M. Messick, and Donna C. Aguilera, "Crisis: Paradigms or Intervention," *Journal of Psychiatric Nursing*, November-December 1967, pp. 531–544.
20. Christine Hatch and Lydia Schut, "Description of a Crisis-Oriented Psychiatric Home Visiting Service," *Journal of Psychiatric Nursing and Mental Health Services*, vol. 18, no. 4, 1980, pp. 31–34.
21. Diane Cronin-Stubbs, "Family Crisis Intervention: A Study," *Journal of Psychiatric Nursing and Mental Health Services*, January 1978, pp. 36–44.
22. E. A. Carter and M. McGoldrick, *The Family Life Cycle*, Gardner, New York, 1980.
23. Anita Finkelman, "The Nurse-Therapist: Outpatient Crisis Intervention with the Chronic Psychiatric Patient," *Journal of Psychiatric Nursing and Mental Health Services*, vol. 15, no. 8, 1977, pp. 27–32.

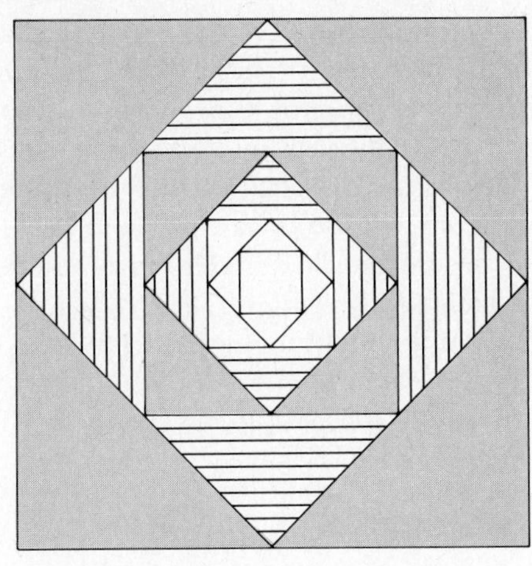

CHAPTER 23
Sexuality Theory and Application

Fern H. Mims

LEARNING OBJECTIVES

After studying this chapter, the student should be able to:

1. Discuss the evolution of values regarding sexuality.
2. Define *sexuality*.
3. Identify expectations for growth and disturbances of growth in each of the stages of psychosexual development.
4. Discuss theories of the development of gender role and identity.
5. Discuss the meanings of intimacy.
6. Discuss the relationship between sexuality, intimacy, and love.
7. Identify motivations for sexual expression.
8. Describe the advantages and disadvantages of various methods of sexual stimulation.
9. Identify various coital positions.
10. Discuss sex-role behavior in today's society.
11. Describe the influences of lifestyle on sexuality.
12. Identify values with regard to sexuality.
13. List techniques for enhancing therapeutic communication about sexuality.
14. Apply the nursing process to sexual health.

Sexuality is an integral part of the self. It involves the mind, body, and spirit, and in that sense it permeates every aspect of life.

Laws governing sexual conduct in this country were derived from and still reflect Judeo-Christian doctrines, and they indirectly affect the sexual standards people set for themselves. In the past two decades there have been changes in the ways people seek sexual fulfillment and increasing acceptance of individual variations. In the 1960s a revived women's movement was in the forefront of a widespread attack on traditional sexual attitudes and values. Since that time, women's rights, homosexuality, abortion, and rape have become highly publicized and controversial issues; divorce rates have increased dramatically; and sexual therapy has become a legitimate form of treatment for sexual dysfunction.

The interplay between men and women and their surroundings is not stagnant; it is an ever-growing and evolving process. People's sexual identities, the sum of their feelings about sexuality, and their role relationships are part of this process.

The purpose of this chapter is to highlight for students the theoretical aspects of sexuality and to familiarize them with the physical, mental, and spiritual dimensions of sex-role behavior.

WHAT IS SEXUALITY?

A person's *sexuality* is the culmination and coming together within the individual of physical, mental, and spiritual influences that result in sex-role behavior, or sexual expression of self.

Sexual expression may have a self-focus, may be motivated by love, or may emphasize the sensuous aspects of sex. People with a *self-focus* believe that sexual fulfillment is a basic need that is highly individualistic despite existing legal, moral, and cultural norms.[1] People who focus on *love* tend to advocate a liberation of sex, but only in the context of a deep emotional bond between two people; the sexual component of love is the desire for shared orgasmic release. People who focus on the *sensual aspects* of sex believe that restricting sex to those in love is repressive.

The author gratefully acknowledges the contributions of Anita M. Leach to this chapter.

Perhaps many people believe and practice a combination of the three orientations. Some people whose sexual needs are met in a love relationship will find both the relationship and sexual activity rewarding. If there is no love relationship, then the sensual aspect of sex will be rewarding whether it involves the self or another person. Moreover, there are those who claim that sexual freedom has decreased people's enjoyment of sex and has increased anxiety. Perhaps all these points of view serve a purpose in helping people develop a set of useful sexual values.

COMPONENTS OF SEXUALITY

Sexuality is an expression of the whole self. The physical, mental, and spiritual dimensions of a person interact in the development of sexuality, and it is important to keep that in mind; however, for the sake of clarity, the three dimensions will be discussed separately here.

The *physical* dimension of sexuality includes the anatomy and physiology of the reproductive system with its hormonal cycles. The stages of psychosexual development and gender role and identity constitute the *mental,* or *cognitive,* dimension of sexuality. Values regarding sex, love, and intimacy make up the *spiritual* dimension.

Physical Aspects of Sexuality

The terms *physical sexuality* and *biological sexuality* refer to the chromosomes, hormones, and primary and secondary sex characteristics of males and females. Mood and environment influence the expression of sexuality, but researchers are finding increasing evidence that physical functioning plays the major role.

The external male genitalia include the penis, scrotum, gonads (testes), epididymis, and parts of the vas deferens. The internal male genitalia consist of other parts of the vas deferens, the seminal vesicles, the ejaculatory ducts, the prostate gland, and Cowper's gland. The external female genitalia include the mons veneris, labia minora, labia majora, clitoris, and vaginal orifice. The internal female genitalia consist of gonads (ovaries), fallopian tubes, uterus, and vagina.

Many hormones are involved in the sexual maturation process. They are produced in sex glands, or gonads (ovaries or testes), and are controlled by the secretions of the pituitary, or master, gland. Hormones influence the development of secondary sex characteristics during puberty and also control the reproductive functions of sperm and ovum formation and the menstrual cycle. A list of the sex hormones and their functions follows:

Follicle-stimulating hormone (FSH). Stimulates ovaries to manufacture female sex hormones.

Luteinizing hormone (LH). Stimulates the production of estrogen and progesterone in the female.

Interstitial cell–stimulating hormone (ICSH). Stimulates manufacture of testosterone in the male.

Progesterone. The female hormone influential in maintaining pregnancy and the menstrual cycle.

Estrogen. The female hormone that stimulates development of secondary sex characteristics during puberty, influences menstruation, and stimulates growth of the glandular surface of the endometrium.

Testosterone. The male hormone responsible for the development of secondary sex characteristics during puberty.

Students are encouraged to consult one of the many fine anatomy and physiology texts for a more complete discussion of the physical aspects of sexuality.

Mental Aspects of Sexuality

The mental aspects of sexuality discussed here include the stages of psychosexual development, and gender role and identity. While these two areas have much in common, they have been separated here to facilitate students' understanding.

Stages of Psychosexual Development

Psychosexual development is the psychic maturation and physical development of sexuality from birth through adulthood. Although social, cultural, and ethnic differences affect sexual development, there are commonalities shared by the majority of people. However, it is wise to avoid arbitrary assignment of labels based on age alone. Sexual behavior throughout the life cycle is a unique experience for each person.

Normal and *average sexual behavior* is described as what is most typical for the majority at a given point in time.[2] A summary of expectations for normal psychosexual development and possible disturbances is given in Table 23-1.

Table 23-1 Stages of Psychosexual Development

Stage of Development	Expectation for Sexual Growth	Disturbance in Sexual Growth
Embryonic period	Fertilization determines chromosomal sex: Female: XX Male: XY	Chromosomal error causing: Turner's syndrome: XO Kleinfelter's syndrome: XXY Other anomalies
Fetal hormonal period	In XY, testes form at 6–7 weeks gestation and produce androgen In XX, ovaries form at 12 weeks gestation and produce no androgen	Androgen insensitivity syndrome (testicular feminizing syndrome) causes XY genotype to develop female external genitalia Adrenogenital syndrome causes XX genotype to develop male external genitalia Ambiguous genitalia caused by hormone excesses or enzyme deficiencies
Birth	Gender assignment	Error in assignment due to ambiguous genitalia

(Continued.)

Table 23-1 Continued

Stage of Development	Expectation for Sexual Growth	Disturbance in Sexual Growth
Infancy, birth to age 18 months	Oral sensitivity	Oral deprivation caused by weaning too early
	Need for tactile stimulation: Stimulation of external genitalia by self or others; pleasure from touch	Touch deprivation causes miasma, possible mental retardation, and possible death
	Orgasmic potential in females	
	Erectile potential in males	
	Reinforcement of gender identity	Blurred identity causes later core identity confusion
	Sense of "goodness" or "badness" of body	Disturbance of basic trust
	Gradual capacity to distinguish "self" from "other"	
Toddler period, ages 1–3 years	Gender identification leads to development of core gender identity	Anxiety about acceptable behaviors for boys and girls.
	Anal phase: learns control of bowel and bladder	Strict toilet training leads to shame and doubt, compulsive behavior, or castration anxiety
	Genital fondling and masturbation to produce pleasure; exploration of body parts	Restriction of genital play leads to poor self-image
	Learning sex-role differences and identifying differences between male and female role models	
	Developing vocabulary for genital anatomy, elimination, reproduction	Lack of vocabulary may cause communication problems in later years
	Sensual-erotic activities such as rocking, swinging, hugging people and toys	Difficulty in expressing affection
Preschool period, ages 4–6	Oedipal attachment to opposite-sex parent	Excessive attachment
	Identification with same-sex parent	Seductive behavior of parent toward child
		Lack of identification leads to later gender identity confusion
	Learning about sex roles	Anxiety caused if parents are intolerant of behavior which does not conform to common stereotypes of sex-role behavior
	Sex play: exploration of own body and genitals and those of playmates	Overreaction of parents leads to guilt, feeling that sex is evil.
	Masturbation	Failure to explain cultural expectations leads to inappropriate public behavior
School-age period, ages 6–10	Same-sex friends	
	Curiosity about sex (no "latent period")	Lack of information reinforces fears and may lead to development of negative, rigid views about sexuality
	Sharing of sexual fears and fantasies	Misinformation gained from peers may be confusing or frightening
	Interest in physical and emotional aspects of sexual development: menstruation, nocturnal emissions, secondary sex characteristics, pregnancy, abortion	
	Increasing self-consciousness and self-awareness	
	Using "dirty words" for shock value	Overreaction of parents may cause increased usage

(Continued.)

Table 23-1 Continued

Stage of Development	Expectation for Sexual Growth	Disturbance in Sexual Growth
Preadolescence: puberty, ages 10–13	Concerns about body image (acne, genital size, sexual development)	Lack of positive experiences leads to poor self-image
	Menarche Seminal emissions	Fears relating to onset of puberty before receiving any information or from receiving no information
	Learning self-control Testing behavior limits	Overly rigid limits or overprotective parents may prevent the development of self-confidence. No limits may delay the development of an internal sexual value system
	Homosexual experiences as part of same-sex friendships	Overreaction of parents may lead to fear, guilt
Early adolescence, ages 13–15	Testing of self as primary source of behavior control	Conflicts with parents and society over testing of limits and controls
	Beginning opposite-sex friendships Learning heterosexuality Dating, "puppy love," and crushes	Failure of parents to take feelings seriously leads to lack of trust and loss of communication
	Awkwardness in first sexual encounters	Anxiety over inadequacy, lack of partner, or lack of orgasm
	One-half of teenage population will not have intercourse	Anxiety over whether virginity is "normal"
	Masturbation and mutual masturbation (petting) Sexual thoughts and fantasies	Compulsive, mechanical masturbation which is used as an escape from everyday problems
Late adolescence, ages 16–19	Learning intimacy in a heterosexual relationship	Inability to trust or to succesfully participate in close relationships
	Taking responsibility for sexual activity	Unplanned pregnancy and precipitate marriage Sexually transmitted diseases
	Exploration of sex-role behaviors and sexual lifestyles	Transsexualism: error or confusion in core gender identity. May begin in childhood. Transvestism: cross-dressing for sexual gratification Fetishism: compulsive sexual attraction for an object as a substitute for a person
	More than half of teenagers will not have sexual intercourse until they are in their twenties.	
Young adulthood, ages 20–35	Learning to give and receive pleasure	Inability to communicate with partner about sexual needs
	Knowledge of sexual response cycle enhances sexual relationship	Sexual dysfunction, premature ejaculation, inorgasmia, dyspareunia
	Long-term commitment to sexual relationship (heterosexual or homosexual; possibly bisexual)	Promiscuity or irresponsible behavior involving coercion or nonconsent Homosexual panic caused by feeling "trapped" in this sexual preference
	Experimentation and curiosity about sexual positions and expressions	Stereotypical sexual behavior Fear of experimentation
	Elaboration of sexual techniques	Boredom
	Responsible reproductive health	Spread of sexually transmitted diseases; failure to have yearly Pap smear
	Decisions about childbearing	Unwanted pregnancy; multiple abortions; child abuse or child neglect
	Development of sexual value system and tolerance for values of others	Sexual amorality; rigid, inflexible beliefs about sex

(Continued.)

Table 23-1 Continued

Stage of Development	Expectation for Sexual Growth	Disturbance in Sexual Growth
Middle adulthood, ages 30–55	Understanding and acceptance of body-image changes relating to menopause and male climacteric	Anxiety, relationship problems caused by changes in sexual performance or sexual interest
	Mastery of consequences of lower hormone production (vaginal atrophy, slower erections) which may affect sexual intercourse	Panic about losing sexual prowess Depression and denial
	Focus on quality rather than quantity of sexual encounters	Sexual dysfunction: secondary impotence, secondary inorgasmia
	Relinquishing control of children's sexual behaviors and sexual preferences	Attempts to control sexual behaviors of adult offspring
	Menopause	Crisis of dealing with loss of reproductive ability
Late adulthood, over age 55	Development of new ways to achieve sexual satisfaction or sexual intimacy after loss or illness of partner	Withdrawal, bitterness, guilt, or sexual dysfunction
	Understanding and acceptance of own sexual needs and needs of others	Coercion or lack of self-control leading to voyeurism, exhibitionism, molesting
	Acceptance of slowed sexual response cycle without necessarily stopping sexual relationship	Conformity to cultural stereotypes regarding sexuality and aging

SOURCE: Fern H. Mims and Melinda Swenson, *Sexuality: A Nursing Perspective*, McGraw-Hill, New York, 1980.

Development of Gender Role and Identity

Terms used in discussing psychosexual development are *gender identity* and *gender role*. *Gender identity* is most often used to describe how one perceives one's gender: a person can have a masculine or feminine self-perception or can be ambivalent about his or her gender. Gender identity is relative to time and place in a given society. While *gender identity* refers to self-perception, *gender role* usually refers to the behavioral expression of that perception. The beginning development of one's gender identity is dependent upon sex assignment at birth and is based on the appearance of external genitalia. Gender identity is usually well established by 3 years of age if interaction with the child is consistent.[3] Ambivalent behavior is expressed when gender identity is not well established.

Exactly how a child develops in a masculine or feminine direction is not totally understood. Some of the more important theories of sexual development are: (1) psychoanalytic, or Freudian, (2) social-learning, (3) role-modeling, and (4) cognitive-development theories. It should be remembered that none of these theories explains all aspects of gender development. A few brief highlights of each theory are presented below.

PSYCHOANALYTIC THEORY. Freud describes the *libido* as the force that expresses sexual instinct. This instinct develops gradually during the oral stage, with both sexes focusing on the mouth and lips. In the anal stage, the central concern is the anus and the elimination or retention of feces. Males and females diverge in their development in the phallic stage, which occurs at approximately 4 years of age. The boy is concerned with love of his mother, is jealous of his father, and has castration anxiety (Oedipus complex). The girl comes to terms with her penis envy, renounces her mother, and loves her father (Electra complex). The libido continues to serve males through the phallic, oedipal, and genital stages and is expected to be repressed by females.

One of the major points of Freudian theory is the biological inferiority of the female, based on the lack of a penis and female envy of male anatomy. Other later psychoanalytic theorists moved from this view to a more romantic, idealized, and maternal view of women.

SOCIAL-LEARNING THEORY. A few early psychologists rejected Freudian theory and attempted to explain gender role and identity from a social-learning approach. This theory views sex-role behavior as being maintained by external, social motives rather than internal forces. Social-learning theorists do not believe that internal motives cause the child to adopt sex-role behavior. Rather, sex roles are acquired through reinforcement. Children make sex-appropriate responses because they receive direct social and physical rewards for such behavior; they avoid sex-inappropiate behavior because they are punished for it.[4]

Recent studies comparing the ways parents treat their preschool sons and daughters have produced inconsistent findings about the importance of reinforcement in determining sex-role behaviors.[4] However, pressure from parents, peers, teachers, and other adults may increase as children get older, and that reinforcement may account for some sex-role behaviors.

ROLE-MODELING THEORY. Mechanisms such as observational learning and imitation, called *modeling,* may account for the acquiring of some behaviors. Modeling occurs when a person imitates or copies the behavior of another person. For modeling to occur, children first learn the behavior through observation and then are motivated to imitate it. Neither social-learning theory nor role-modeling theory places much emphasis on the control the child has over behavior.

COGNITIVE-DEVELOPMENT THEORY. Cognitive-development theory considers children to be active learners, and their intellectual development is considered the key to gender identity. Cognitive-development theorists believe that children are motivated by a desire for competence and mastery over the world. Children are thought to seek out information that will improve their responses to their physical and social world.

Both social-learning theory and cognitive-development theory hold that the child wants to be a particular gender, but they differ dramatically in their understanding of what motivates the child. Social-learning theorists believe that the child is motivated by rewards acquired by doing things which others in society consider appropriate for males or females. Cognitive-development theorists emphasize the child rather than the socializing agents or culture. They propose that children imitate same-sex models because they are motivated to maintain a competent, positive self-image and to master the behaviors which they themselves consider important. The basis for gender identity is believed to be formed by the child's cognitive processing, or schematization, of incoming information, and by subsequent generalization of these schemata to new situations.

There is an interaction of the culture with cognitive development in the course of sex-role acquisition. If specific sex roles are obvious and important to a culture or family, then the child is likely to acquire definite sex-role schemata early. If sex role is not important, the child will most likely take longer to develop the sex-role schemata. Research data seem to suggest that concepts of masculinity and femininity have been more clearly identified by working-class families than by the middle class. As sex discrimination in the workplace is corrected, these differences may be expected to be less obvious throughout our society. Stereotypes and values regarding the sexes, however, will probably continue to have a major impact on sex-role identity.[5]

Spiritual Aspects of Sexuality

Sexual identity as male or female provides a person with the capacity for sexual expression of love. The call to love and to intimacy with another person is a prime human characteristic, and a person's sexuality offers the promise of loving unity.[6]

The spiritual dimension of sexuality frees people to differentiate lust from love and to make choices regarding involvement in meaningful relationships and sexual intimacy. Values regarding sexuality, love, and intimacy will be discussed as components of the spiritual dimension of sexuality.

Sexuality and Values

A *value* is a moral principle or quality that a person decides is true or good. When people behave in ways that are congruent with their values, their self-esteem is enhanced. Values and behavior must be congruent if a person is to be free of guilt.

The area of values and sexuality is complex, and sexual terms mean different things to different people. For example, if you ask three people to define *love,* you will probably get three different answers. Researchers are just beginning to study some of the religious, cultural, and family influences on attitudes, values, and norms regarding different aspects of sexuality. Researchers are likely to find incongruent values and behaviors in the various aspects of sexuality in all levels of our society. Since there has been very little scientific study of this subject, the area of values in sexuality has been plagued by irrationality and dogma.

A nurse's sexuality is influenced by religious, cultural, and family norms. Self-assessment in the area of sexuality will help nurses to remain objective and not impose their value systems on clients. Change and intervention in the area of sexuality must be consistent with clients' value systems.

Rights and *responsibilities* are simple words that have complex meanings. Rights and responsibilities are interwoven with values and are communicated to the young by peers, parents, church, school, and the media. Young people often feel they are receiving conflicting messages about sexual standards.[7] Recently, one young woman related the following thoughts about this conflict:

> I guess I had sex with lots of guys because I was trying to prove it was my right. All my friends kept telling me it was my right and that I was missing out on something very special. They kept talking about a meaningful or intimate relationship. So I began to have sex with good-looking guys and hoped each time that it would be good and develop into an intimate relationship. Something went wrong; it did not feel good, nor did it develop into any type of relationship. Each time I felt sad, depressed, and ashamed. I felt so bad about myself and I couldn't talk to my friends, parents, or sexual partners and expect them to understand what I was feeling. I still do not know if my feelings came from my old-fashioned upbringing or if they came from the feedback I was receiving from my sexual partners. I know I have rights and responsibilities. I am just beginning to feel good enough about myself and to understand exactly what I will include in an intimate relationship.

Another young woman related a very different experience:

> I was taught to wait until marriage to have sex. At the ages of 13 to 18, these expectations were comforting. I could say, "No," easily. At 20, I met that special guy who was very handsome, intelligent, and kind. We enjoyed biking, running, tennis, music, camping, cooking, and even studying together. On one special night we started kissing and caressing each other. We had been into some heavy petting before, and each of us had an idea of what the other liked, but that night neither of us wanted to stop and we didn't. After that night I was no longer a virgin, and I could be sad for only a moment. This sexual experience made us even closer and brought such joy to our lives. I have been able to discuss this experience with my parents, since it was so right.

Self-awareness and a high level of self-esteem seem to be prerequisites of the ability to satisfy the need for intimacy. As people age, they are expected to achieve thoughtful self-understanding and to develop realistic expectations for relationships. Actions become more internally generated rather than being responses to the expectations of significant others.

Intimacy

Intimacy describes a special quality of emotional closeness between two people. It is an affectionate bond composed of mutual caring, responsibility, trust, open communication of feelings and sensations, and the nondefensive interchange of information about significant emotional events. Intimacy may include the joys of being touched, feeling the warmth of another person's body, being close to someone, and trusting and being trusted.

It appears that intimacy can be best achieved after one has a sense of one's own identity and feels good enough about oneself to feel worthy of being loved. A negative self-image sets many limits on the capacity to develop an intimate relationship.

Intimacy is a learned behavior. Infants learn intimacy and trust by being held, being cuddled, kissing, and other nonverbal communication that they interpret as feeling good. As the child grows into young adulthood, many of the "feeling good" nonverbal communications are monitored. Touching becomes less acceptable and is replaced by an emphasis on body boundaries. Too often, body boundaries are developed to serve as barriers to meaningful interactions.

The following questions will help nurses assess self-boundaries of clients.

What is close?

Who is allowed to touch?

What parts of the body is it permissible to touch?

Is massaging allowed? If so, by whom? Stranger? Lover? Friend? Family?

What feels good about the relationship?

What feels bad?

What feels good at the time but feels bad afterward?

What in the environment promotes comfort?

People who believe that they are worthy of love, praise, and "special handling" usually do not have problems with interdependence, which is an important ingredient of intimacy. *Interdependence* is the simultaneous interaction that exists between two people who help each other fulfill basic needs. The ability to establish an interdependent relationship has two dimensions. First, one must feel good enough about oneself to know and ask for what is wanted from an intimate relationship. One does not fear being rejected. Second, one must take responsibility for oneself, know oneself, and respect one's own rights and the rights of others.

According to H. Singer Kaplan, fear of intimacy is highly prevalent and may produce problems that extend beyond sexual dysfunction:

> It sometimes seems that people are more afraid of intimacy than they are of sex. They find it easier to masturbate than to make love, to buy impersonal sex than to share love with a lover, to blot out the partner with drugs than to experience him/her fully. Some couples stay together and engage in a movement toward closeness and warmth to a certain point; then the distancing behaviors are employed.[8]

Thus, when relationships become too close, one person will characteristically provoke a fight, or another will become absorbed in golf, business, or politics. Another will become ill, gain weight, or drink, and still another will act destructively with money, focus on a business crisis, or even have an extramarital affair. Typically, neither partner is aware of the actual dynamics of such a situation. Partners often blame each other for their turbulent life together.

Some couples do not develop an intimate relationship until after child rearing is completed. Then they finally take time out for the understanding, companionship, and support that had taken second place to work, child rearing, and housekeeping. Other couples never develop anything that resembles a love relationship; rather, they stay together for financial reasons, out of a need for safety, out of habit, or for other reasons that are unclear. Others discard partners almost as easily as outdated items of clothing. Some people never attempt an intimate relationship, or they consistently choose partners who are incapable of sharing love and intimacy.

Love

The word *love* has many meanings. Love as it relates to sex is referred to as *erotic love.* H. Sullivan states that when the satisfaction or security of another person becomes as significant as one's own satisfaction or security, love exists.[9] Love has also been defined as a sustained emotional response to a known source of pleasure.

A love relationship has three major components—the sexual, the magical, and the sensual. They are in balance, and they are constantly interweaving. The *sexual* component of love is the desire for shared orgasmic release. The *magical* component is the belief that the love object is powerful and wise enough to provide care and security, much as one's parents did in childhood. Finally, the *sensual* component is an appreciation of the physical attractions of a loved one and an idealization of him or her on a highly subjective level.[10]

Intimacy is seen as fundamental to love. Time and privacy are basic requirements for the development of the five components of intimacy: choice, mutuality, reciprocity, trust, and delight. Each of these components develops from the previous one. In intimacy, two people delight in each other as whole persons and express this delight in various ways. One of the most meaningful of these—because it is one of the most delightful—is sexual expression.

Love is usually defined differently by each couple. However, love usually includes mutual respect, mutual responsibility or commitment, and some element of permanence.

Sexual fulfillment and love satisfy human needs of significant importance in the formation of the self. The complex relationship between love and sex is often controversial. Some say that sex is empty and animalistic without love, while others argue that sex can be fun and enjoyable without love. Some say that those who insist upon imposing love on a sexual relationship are guilty about sex and are trying to convince themselves that the act can somehow be made acceptable.[7]

THE SEXUAL ACT: SEXUAL INTERCOURSE

Another component of sexuality is sexual intercourse. *Sexual intercourse* is physical sexual contact between two people that involves the genitalia of at least one person. Intercourse may include genital-genital, oral-genital, or anal-genital stimulation. While intercourse is a physical act, it is not a simple one; it involves all the complexities of two people's present behaviors, previous experience, motivations, and real or fantasized goals. For most people, at least some degree of relationship is required before they will engage in sexual intercourse; for some others, consent requires deep and committed love.

Motivations for the Sexual Act

It is possible to love without having sex and to have sex without love. Both will satisfy needs. Difficulty arises when partners do not agree on the meaning of their sexual relationship or when self-awareness is minimal. For some, the primary purpose of having sex may be to express love. For others, it may be to discharge physical energy or tension. For still others the search for intimacy and feelings of closeness may be primary.

When sexual intercourse is used consistently to fulfill a nonsexual need, it is sometimes classified as neurotic behavior. Some of these nonsexual needs are described below:

- Having sex as a *defense against loneliness* may be thought of as selling one's body for companionship. Many people who use sex to obtain contact with another person have low self-esteem and believe it is the most effective way for them to obtain attention and time from another person. The probable outcome of this type of contact is to lower an already poor self-image.
- Some people use sex as a *means of manipulating another person.* In the exercise of control or power within a relationship, one person emerges victorious and the other is defeated or victimized. This type of relationship can continue in a sadomasochistic vein, with each partner having needs met for many years. In other power struggles, one partner may drop the other immediately after seduction; the conquest is over.
- Some obsessive health faddists indulge in sexual intercourse because it is believed to be an *essential activity for good health.* At certain intervals, such people engage in sex to promote health. The "ritual" of intercourse is thereby used for health or other obsessive needs.
- Intercourse may become a *dutiful chore* which is often routine and lacks tenderness and sensitivity.
- *Nurturing of another* may be a motivating factor. The outcome of nurturing in a sexual encounter is usually not intense pleasure accompanying orgasm but a feeling of "getting" or of "giving" on the part of the two people involved.

Motivation for sexual intercourse is varied; it may or may not be for sexual pleasure. One partner may be in a one-sided emotional relationship and never be aware of this reality.[5]

Arousal and Response

Variations of sexual behavior include many positions and techniques. The concept of consenting adults experimenting and doing what pleases them in private seems to have been accepted. Neither partner should be hurt physically or psychologically. Both people can become aware of their own and their partner's erogenous zones and know how certain stimuli affect the degree of response. With trust, flexibility, and open communication, each person's preferences for stimulation at any given time can be the adopted practice. A superlative technique in one situation may prove to be inappropriate at another time. The most erogenous areas for most people include the genitals, lips, breasts, thighs, and anus. Oral-genital, anal-genital, and hand-genital contact are alternatives used by some couples as variations of coitus.

The reactions during the sexual response cycle are summarized in Table 23-2.

Manual Stimulation: Masturbation

Autoerotic and reciprocal genital manipulation are often used as foreplay or may be used to reach orgasm. Self-manipulation or self-pleasuring cen-

Table 23-2 Reactions During Sexual Response Cycle

Male	Female
Excitement phase	
Penile erection (within 3–8 seconds)	Vaginal lubrication (within 10–30 seconds)
Thickening, flattening, and elevation of scrotal sac	Thickening of vaginal walls and labia
Partial testicular elevation and size increase	Expansion of inner two-thirds of vagina and elevation of cervix and corpus
Nipple erection (25%)	Tumescence of clitoris
	Nipple erection (consistent)
	Sex-tension flush
Plateau phase	
Increase in penile circumference and testicular tumescence (50–100% enlarged)	Orgasmic platform in outer one-third of vagina
Full testicular elevation and rotation (orgasm inevitable)	Full expansion of two-thirds of vagina; uterine and cervical elevation
Purple hue on corona of penis (inconsistent, even if orgasm is to ensue)	"Sex skin," or discoloration of minor labia (consistent if orgasm is to ensue)
Mucoid secretion from Cowper's gland	Mucoid secretion from Bartholin's gland
Sex-tension flush (25%)	Withdrawal of clitoris
Generalized skeletal muscle tension	Sex-tension flush (75%)
Hyperventilation	Hyperventilation
Tachycardia (110–170 beats per minute)	Tachycardia (100–160 beats per minute)
Orgasmic phase	
Ejaculation	Pelvic response (vasocongestion)
Contractions of accessory organs of reproduction (vas deferens, seminal vesicles, ejaculatory duct, prostate)	Contractions of uterus from fundus toward lower uterine segment
Relaxation of external bladder sphincter	Minimal relaxation of external cervical opening
Contractions of penile urethra	Contractions of orgasmic platform
Anal sphincter contractions	External rectal sphincter contractions
Specific skeletal muscle contractions	Specific skeletal muscle contractions
Hyperventilation, tachycardia (100–180 beats per minute)	Hyperventilation, tachycardia (100–180 beats per minute)
Resolution phase	
Refractory period with rapid loss of pelvic vasocongestion	Ready return to orgasm with retarded loss of pelvic vasocongestion
Loss of penile erection in primary (rapid) and secondary (slow) stages	Loss of sex-skin color and orgasmic platform in primary (rapid) stage
Sweating reaction (30–40%)	Loss of remainder of pelvic vasocongestion in secondary (slow) stage
Hyperventilation, tachycardia (150–180 beats per minute)	Loss of clitoral tumescence and return to position
	Sweating reaction (30–40%)
	Hyperventilation, tachycardia (150–180 beats per minute)

NOTES: (1) % = percent of general population of men or women experiencing the reaction.
(2) "Consistent" means that a reaction continues throughout all phases.

SOURCE: Adapted from Herant Katchadourian and Donald T. Lunde, *Fundamentals of Human Sexuality*, Holt, New York, 1972; after Frank A. Beach, ed., *Sex and Behavior*, Krieger, Huntington, N.Y., 1974; and William H. Masters and Virginia E. Johnson, *Human Sexual Response*, Little Brown, Boston, 1966.

ters on an erogenous zone and is sometimes called *masturbation.*

The term *masturbation* is generally used to refer to manual self-stimulation; however, manual stimulation by another person can also be considered masturbation. For both men and women, hand manipulation is the most common method of manual stimulation; however, other objects such as pillows, towels, bedclothes, and vibrators may be used to produce orgasm.

Masturbation provides a safe, convenient, solitary form of sexual pleasure and a means of learning more about one's body and sexual responses. Males are more likely to masturbate than females are, and they begin at an earlier age. Masturbation is used as a treatment technique for teaching women to have an orgasm and for teaching males to control ejaculation.[8] It should be noted, however, that myths about masturbation and disapproval of masturbation still persist in conservative areas of our society.

Oral-Genital Stimulation

There are three types of oral-genital stimulation practiced by a sizable number of adults: cunnilingus, fellatio, and cunnilingus and fellatio in combination ("69"). *Cunnilingus* comes from the Latin for "vulva" (*cunnus*) and "to lick" (*linguere*). *Fellatio* is derived from the Latin for "to suck" (*fellare*). *Soixante-neuf,* the French word for 69, refers to the combined methods of cunnilingus and fellatio between two people.

In cunnilingus, there is kissing, sucking, licking, and tongue exploration of the minor vaginal lips, the clitoral shaft, and the opening of the vagina. Women vary in their opinions of what feels good. What is sexually stimulating may vary from day to day with each woman. According to the *Hite Report,* 42 percent of the study population of 3019 women reached orgasm regularly during oral stimulation.

In fellatio, the oral-genital activity has many variations. Sucking, licking, and movements of the tongue in a circular fashion around the glans, the shaft of the penis, and sometimes the testicles, are used in the excitement stage. A thrusting, up-and-down motion is used in the plateau and orgasmic phases.

The combined methods of fellatio and cunnilingus allow both persons to be stimulated at the same time.

Anal-Genital Stimulation

Some people find the anus particularly sensitive and prefer anal stimulation over all other types of sexual practices. The anus is not as elastic as the vagina, and it therefore requires gentleness, gradual entry, and the application of extra lubrication.

Genital-Genital Stimulation

COITUS. *Coitus* is generally thought to mean a coming together of the male and female sexual organs—the penis and vagina. Coitus may be described as having a wide variety of purposes in addition to reproduction. It is commonly described as a method of expressing a reciprocal love relationship; and, according to some women respondents in the *Hite Report,* "I love it; to me nothing else is really sex."

COITAL POSITIONS. Human beings are known to employ hundreds of coital positions. Variations maintain the novelty of the sex act, although most people tend to settle on the use of a few preferred techniques. The most important consideration is that the flow of sexual activity be mutually acceptable and that the couple feel free to speak openly with one another about their thoughts and feelings regarding sexual activity.[11] Nurses should be familiar with the various coital approaches in order to be able to offer clients alternatives when this is warranted because of medical or surgical disabilities. Table 23-3 lists the various coital positions and the advantages and disadvantages of each.

SEX-ROLE BEHAVIOR

The term *sex role* is ubiquitous but has seldom been clearly defined. The confusion about the definition comes from the factors that have been subsumed under the term. Work, relationships, and psychological characteristics are but a few factors considered in descriptions of sex-role behaviors. The core properties conceptualized in most research into sex roles include a "sense of communion," labeled as *feminine,* and a "sense of agency," labeled as *masculine.*[12] Other properties, such as "rationality" (masculine) and "emotionality" (feminine) have been ascribed to sex-role behaviors in a relationship.

Androgyny is a term used to describe a model that includes both masculine and feminine characteristics. In this model feelings and behaviors inherent in all persons, male and female, are blended and freed from restrictions imposed by the mores and values of society. Psychologically androgynous women and men are expected to be flexible in role performance, while sex-typed people are more comfortable with the behaviors conventionally defined as appropriate for their sex.[12]

Traditionally in our society, women have been expected to be physically attractive and sexually

Table 23-3 Coital Positions

Position	Advantages and Disadvantages
Face to face (man on top)	Opportunity for direct interaction (kissing, etc.)
	Numerous alternatives for woman's legs
	Maximum friction
	Little likelihood that penis will slip out of vagina
	Most acceptable to many people because woman is accommodated effortlessly
	Most likely to lead to pregnancy
	Man's weight may be a problem
	Man's hands not free for stimulation of partner
	Restriction of woman's movements
	Expresses male psychological supremacy
Face to face (woman on top)	Opportunity for direct interaction
	Many variations possible
	Weight of man less a problem
	Woman less immobilized
	Woman has opportunity to express herself fully
	Some men feel threatened
	Mutual stimulation is possible
Side by side	Penetration difficult—woman must lift upper leg
	Maximum play possible
	Eliminates weight on either partner
	Prolonged and leisurely
Rear entry	Great variety (sitting, standing, kneeling)
	Easy for man to fondle woman's breasts and stimulate genitals manually
	Isolates partners, who cannot conveniently see each other
	Penetration not deep
	May be impossible for obese people

SOURCE: From Anita M. Leach, "Sexual Theory and Application," in the first edition of this book.

appealing. Women have been aware of the importance of their attractiveness and have learned how to use this aspect of sexuality to get things they want. They have been encouraged to achieve status through the social activities of their husbands and their children. These traditional sex-role behaviors are beginning to change with the increase of women in the labor force. Economic necessity for some women and self-fulfillment goals for others have altered values regarding working outside the home.

The women's liberation movement has emphasized the changing roles of women and has focused attention on such inequities as the stereotyping of jobs by gender, unequal pay for equivalent work, and the barriers to entry into traditionally male professions.

In recent years much attention has been given to the changing role of women. Men have received far less attention but have nonetheless been involved in the evolution of roles. Men are beginning to be socialized into nurturing and forming significant affectionate relationships with their newborns and young children. A father no longer needs to wait until it is time to learn to throw a ball or go camping to build a significant relationship with his children. Paternal bonding has taken its place with the powerful concept of maternal bonding. Apparently, pockets of society are subscribing to and practicing the blending and freeing concepts of androgyny, while others are advocating a move away from liberation and putting energy into maintaining traditional models.

LIFESTYLES AND SEXUALITY

People's lifestyles—whether they are single or married, heterosexual or homosexual—will determine the way in which they express themselves sexually. A lifestyle is a personal choice. A person chooses to marry, to live in a commune, to remain single and live with a sexual partner, or to remain single and live alone. However, choices are not always simple where sexual expression is concerned. Sexual activity, regardless of lifestyle, can range from celibacy (that is, no sexual activity) at one end of the continuum to a great variety of sexual behavior at the other extreme. The lifestyles discussed here include being single, formerly married, married, homosexual, or a member of a commune or group.

The Single Lifestyle

Being single is increasing as a long-term lifestyle. Some of the realities of being single may be seen as either advantages or disadvantages depending upon a host of factors such as age, place, need for commitment, personality, and need for intimacy.

Previously, males were more likely than females never to marry; however, in the last decade, this trend has changed. With more educational and occupational opportunities, women have gained the freedom to make more choices about their lifestyles. Higher levels of intelligence and education and a greater number of professional choices are associated with being single. At present, however, only about 6 to 7 percent of all Americans go through life without marriage, and they tend to experience this as an evolving process rather than a set of firm beliefs against marriage.[1]

Never-married single adults who choose a single lifestyle are more frequently also choosing celibacy. A lack of sexual activity is a free choice and may represent a commitment rather than simply an accidental result of being single. Celibacy is often experienced as a viable, creative, and healthy expression of individuality and not as a restriction to be endured because of a lack of a sexual partner.[13] Commitment to celibacy need not mean that a person is less sexual; in fact, the person can be more free to love others and to be creative. People who are celibate can remain as masculine or feminine as their sexually active counterparts.

On the other hand, for single people who are sexually active, there is more freedom and less societal restriction about meeting heterosexual needs. Young people are experiencing less parental pressure to marry or to remain virgins. Career choices and sexual facilitation may make the single lifestyle more appealing than marriage for a select group of both men and women. Some people remain single until professional goals are met and then marry in their late thirties or forties.

The Lifestyle of the Formerly Married

Single people who have previously been married represent another lifestyle. Divorced people tend to remarry, on an average, 3 years following divorce. This means that for them, the period of being single is relatively short. These people are more likely to be sexually active while single than those who have never married.

The Married Lifestyle

The traditional marriage is the dominant lifestyle in the United States and the context within which most people express their sexuality. The dominant cultural value remains serial monogamy, and marriage continues to be seen as permanent. The number of marriages over a person's life will be influenced by length of life, lifestyle, and spiritual and moral views of marriage.

Marriage is a collaborative agreement between two parties. It is a partnership between a man and a woman. Traditionally, marriage was a patriarchal system in which the man's surname was adopted and he was designated as the head of the household and sole breadwinner. Women had few legal rights. Now, with new career opportunities, women are increasingly likely to be found in equal income brackets, to have equal professional opportunities, and to continue to use their birth surnames. However, upon marrying, the couple still enters a partnership in which the law and the greater part of our society deem the woman to be the subservient partner.

According to D. Read, two people come together in a healthy marriage because they:

Feel a sense of joy and excitement in being together

Feel a sense of shared experience

Are good friends and enjoy each other's company

Desire each other as sexual partners

Feel a sense of completeness when together[14]

The sexual practices of married couples are as varied as all other activities in a relationship. Some couples desire each other exclusively as sexual partners and meet each other's sexual needs completely. With others, one or both partners have sexual relationships outside the marriage relationship. In the sexually *open marriage,* both partners may become involved in comarital sex separately. *Swinging* usually involves sexual activity with another couple or in a threesome. Whether extramarital sex or comarital sex is a positive or negative alternative depends on the people involved. It may detract from the psychological dependency that some couples desire in the marriage relationship. Other couples like to keep extramarital and consensual sex as a viable option to keep them from feeling smothered or living with traditional rules that they feel are outdated.[5]

The Homosexual Lifestyle

The terms *gay, homogenic love, contrasexuality,* and *homoeroticism* all apply to homosexuality. The homosexual culture has received increasing attention in the media during the past few years. Current psychiatric thinking holds that homosexuality is a sexual orientation or lifestyle preferred by some and that many homosexuals and lesbians have long-term, loving relationships. However, the attitudes of Americans in general have a long way to go in allowing homosexuals to come out of their "closets," perhaps because the homosexual confronts the latent tendencies of those whose sexual orientation is "straight," or heterosexual. Some believe that male homosexuality is a greater threat to men than female homosexuality is to women, because men have a greater underlying fear of their own homosexual tendencies which frequently makes them abusive in their attacks on homosexuality. Those who have dealt with their own homosexual feelings are most understanding and relaxed in their relationships with people of homosexual orientation.

Recent thinking has definitely rejected the concept that homosexuality is an illness. *Ego-syntonic homosexuality* is not considered dysfunctional behavior. Ego-syntonic homosexuals are people who are comfortable with their homosexuality. Ego-syntonic homosexuality is usually internally recognized by individuals before the onset of adolescence. When homosexual behavior becomes troublesome to the individual, it is said to be *ego-dystonic.*

There are a multitude of theories regarding the dynamics of homosexuality; but it should be remembered that those who seek treatment provide the information which forms the basis of these theories and that many of these people are dysfunctional in a general way and not specifically because of their sexual orientation. The theories seem to fall into four broad categories: (1) those based on hereditary tendencies, (2) those based on environmental influences, (3) those based on imbalance of the sex hormones, and (4) combinations of these. That multiple causes have been suggested should not be surprising, since homosexuals, like heterosexuals, have widely varying character traits, personalities, and family histories.

According to research, genetic or hereditary theories should be rejected. Hormonal theories, like those based on genetics, are also generally rejected by most psychologists. The learning and psychodynamic theories describe the psychological basis of homosexual behavior, but these also fail to explain the origins of homosexuality.[1]

Sociologically, another causative factor may be unsatisfactory and threatening early relationships with members of the opposite sex. A sensitive girl may be rejected by a boy she loves and therefore decide not to run the risk of another rejection. Labeling is another factor. A parent or teacher may call a child "queer" as the result of some experimentation that is quite common and normal. Guilt and the belief that they are truly homosexual can cause such children to act out this sexual orientation. Strong castration fears and sexual (oedipal) attachment to the mother is the classical psychoanalytic explanation for male homosexuality.[1]

Recently the term *gay* has been used in an effort to combat the negative connotation that has plagued homosexuality. In 1973 the National Gay Task Force was established, and by 1975, gay-rights networks provided an avenue of communication that focused on legal changes regarding rights and liberation for homosexuals. The gay-rights movement has been successful in lobbying for laws to prevent discrimination against homosexuals and in changing public attitudes in many areas.[1] However, new laws and attitudes have not spread to all parts of the country.

It is important for all nurses, heterosexual and homosexual, to look closely at their attitudes about gay men and women. Gay couples experience the same joys and conflicts in their relationships and their sexuality as heterosexual couples. The diversity of sexual practices among gays is as great as that among heterosexuals. As attitudes toward homosexuality shift, serious concerns are raised by health care professionals. There has been widespread agitation for recognition of homosexuality as a valid way of life; the reclassification of homosexuality by the American Psychiatric Association (APA) has helped legitimize this view and fostered acceptance of the right to choose homosexuality as a means of sexual expression.

Traditionally, "differentness" has been the special defense of the homosexual. Homosexual clients may take great pains to cultivate the illusion that they are different. They may attempt to use society's disapproval of their lifestyle to avoid meaningful relationships, to persist in self-destructive behavior, or to avoid productive employment. (This is not, of course, the case with all homosexual clients.) Because "differentness" is such a subtle defense, nurses need to be aware that it may be present, in the same way that people from minority cultures may use their status as a "minority" defensively. Some homosexuals cling to the chauvinism of the gay culture. If ego-dystonic homosexuals wish to reorient their sexual preference, they must revise patterns which have become established and ingrained. This is a long and often painful psychoanalytic process. If, on the other hand, psychotherapy is aimed at other goals, the defense of "differentness" first has to be challenged and replaced.

Commune or Group Living

Variations of group living extend from sharing living quarters and raising children together but working outside, to having all work and living options determined by the group's needs and goals. Rules regarding sex vary greatly among communes. There may be somewhat monogamous relationships, where couples are in traditional sex relationships while the group takes on the responsibility of raising the children. In other communes, monogamous relationships are avoided and the aim is to have everyone married to everyone else. Read gives an example of the latter:

> The Oneida Commune has a system in which each member has sexual access to every other member, with each member's consent and under the supervision of community leaders. If two people are interested in a liaison and show an excess of special love, they are forced into relationships with others so that a one-to-one relationship will not develop. If a male is interested in a particular female, he must go through a third party. The female with whom sex relations are desired has the right to accept or refuse them.[14]

NURSING PROCESS

An unbiased and professional attitude about others' sexuality is an important component of the nurse's approach to clients; and in the interactive therapeutic process, there is a need for nurse and client to uphold each other's sexual rights. Client and nurse have the right to express themselves as sexual beings and to be self-directed in regard to sexuality. They have the right to select and be with partners of their own choice, whether of the same or opposite sex. Awareness of self as an interacting sexual being who influences others and support of peers as sexual persons are rights and responsibilities of both client and nurse. Acceptance and tolerance of another's sexual attitudes and preferences is another responsibility. A list of sexual rights concludes by stating that people have the right to "assist men and women of all ages to recognize their sexuality as an integral part of their personality, inherited at conception, molded and tempered by environment, sustained by health, threatened by disease and reversed by choice."[2]

Mims and Swenson's Self-Assessment Model

The model of sexual health developed by Mims and Swenson provides a means of self-assessment for practicing nurses and students, a framework for assessing clients and intervening to help them, an organizational structure for learning experiences, and a theoretical framework for research.[2]

Figure 23-1 shows the model, which consists of four ascending levels: (1) life experience, (2) basic, (3) intermediate, and (4) advanced. The *life experience level* includes those intuitively helpful and destructive behaviors that result from family and societal experiences and influences. Destructive behaviors originate from and are supported by irrational fears, myths, stereotypes, and taboos that promote inaccurate, inadequate, or biased information regarding sexuality. Intuitively helpful behaviors include those positive attitudes, feelings, and behaviors that facilitate sexual health. These behaviors appear to originate from and be promoted by feelings of self-worth and the ability to express and receive feelings of affection from others in appropriate and fulfilling ways. Verbal and nonverbal communication patterns foster security, self-esteem, understanding, and comfort with one's own and others' sexuality.

At the *basic level,* awareness is created from the interplay of sexual perceptions, attitudes, and cognitions. It is important that awareness be recognized as a fluid process, as something that changes as human and societal values, needs, and behaviors change. Awareness promotes the identification of problems and concerns which interfere with sexual health. Awareness involves keeping current with increased knowledge and research about sexuality,

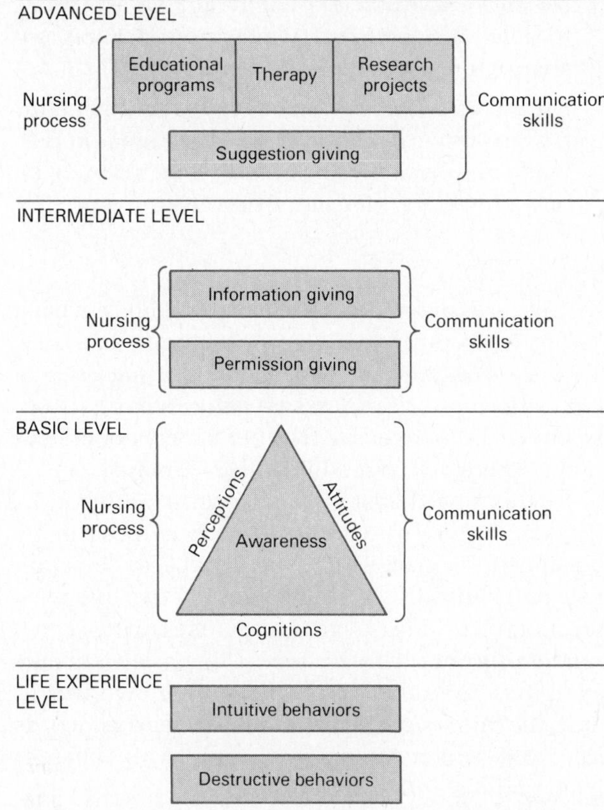

Figure 23-1 Model of levels of sexual health.
(SOURCE: From Fern H. Mims and Melinda Swenson, *Sexuality: A Nursing Perspective*, McGraw Hill, New York, 1980).

identifying one's own and others' attitudes, and sharing and accepting one's own and others' perceptions.

The *intermediate level* includes the processes of granting "permission" and giving information. Granting permission acknowledges a person's sexual rights, concerns, thoughts, fantasies, and responsibilities. Giving information utilizes skills of assessment, counseling, and teaching to impart accurate and desired information.

The *advanced level* includes suggestions, therapy, educational programs, and research projects. Research is needed to generate knowledge that can then be assimilated through therapy and educational programs to benefit both clients and students.

In the past, nurses have needed help in determining what they were prepared to do in the promotion of sexual health. Mims and Swenson's model is helpful in defining and communicating various levels of expertise of nurses on the basis of their knowledge, attitudes, and teaching skills in nursing practice. Experiences with implementation indicate that nurses and students are able to relate and apply the nursing process to activities appropriate to one of the four levels of the model.[2]

Assessment

Both nurse and client have had life experiences that include destructive and constructive behaviors. These are products of past learning and living experiences that will influence the sexual health care of the client.

Aspects of Assessment

Five important aspects of sexuality that will influence the needs and nursing care of a client with general concerns about sexuality are *body image, sex role, relationships, attitudes,* and *knowledge.* Each of these will be discussed briefly.

BODY IMAGE. Nurses must be aware of any of their own prejudices or biases about body image as well as those of their clients. A nurse who has major problems regarding his or her body image is not the best person to play a major role in assessing a client's body image or intervening to help a client improve body image.

Body image can be assessed by asking questions regarding "ideal" body image and how a client's own body measures up to the ideal. Asking clients to make a rough sketch of their sexual self gives much information about how they view their bodies. What do they consider assets? Liabilities?

SEX ROLE. What are early childhood memories of father, mother, and self? What does a client remember about his or her sex-role model's behavior? Associations can be tested by using words such as *tender, sensual, loving, nurturing,* or *cold, nonattentive,* and *castrating.*

Can a client challenge stereotypes of masculine and feminine roles, or does he or she reinforce them? Descriptions of sex roles can be given orally or be written down, depending on the verbal skills of a client.

RELATIONSHIPS. Verbal and nonverbal behaviors are questioned and observed to find out if a client is able to develop an intimate relationship or has ever developed one in the past. Does a client use touches, words of love, gestures, and expressions to convey to others that they are valuable, worthwhile people?

One exercise is having clients write about a fantasy of being shipwrecked on an island with only one other person, answering questions regarding what kind of person they would like him or her to be. This exercise will reveal the major expectations and desires of a client; these responses are then compared with realistic expectations and desires.

ATTITUDES. Nurses need to explore their own attitudes, knowledge, and perceptions about sexuality. Some helpful self-assessment questions are: Does the nurse believe that sexual disorders are health conditions that need further study and development and can improve with care? Or does the nurse believe that concern with sexuality is a fad and prefer to spend time with really "sick" people? Hostile mannerisms on the part of the nurse will communicate a disapproving or unconcerned attitude to a client. Does the nurse believe that sexuality can be an important aspect of health disorders? If so, sex and sexuality will be given the attention they deserve. If not, this aspect of health care will be denied by both nurse and client—and denial will most likely exacerbate problems.

After assessing their own attitudes, nurses should determine the dominating attitudes of a client regarding sexuality. A short sexual-attitude scale or questionnaire will usually provide some important data about the areas in which the client is having difficulty. Responses concerning beautiful bodies, the "ideal self," and the women's movement provide information about sexual attitudes. Consistencies and inconsistencies in attitudes need to be considered in the assessment process.

KNOWLEDGE. Inquiry about and observation of a client's sexual health should be based on knowledge about sexuality. Knowledge about the relationship between particular disorders and sexuality will change as more research is completed. However, the following questions should be helpful in assessing a more general knowledge base:

What is the client's knowledge level?

Does the client's basic distrust of others play a major role in indifference to sex?

Do failure at sexual intercourse and orgasm relate to difficulties with intimate communication and sharing one's emotions?

Do inconsistencies appear in communication? (For instance, does the client place great importance on physical appearance while insisting on being loved for himself or herself?)

Sexual History

In any assessment of a person's sexuality, a sexual history is needed to establish an accurate data base. Table 23-4 outlines the data obtained using a sexual history format. The process of taking a sexual history is similar in many ways to other aspects of assessment. There are some differences, however.

In the sexual history, unlike other interviews, the comfort of the interviewer becomes highly significant for establishing the data base. The comfort and attitudes of clients during the interview are noted as clues to overall comfort with sexual matters. Privacy is necessary. Clients are encouraged to express their concerns in their own words, and the nurse keeps in mind that sexual words have different meanings to people with different backgrounds and experiences.

A physical examination is an extension of the history-taking process and is essential to arriving at a diagnosis where sexual dysfunction is a concern. The terms *sexological examination* indicates that portion of the physical examination concerned with the genitalia and pelvic structures and the other areas of the body associated with physiological sexual responsiveness. Degrees of pleasure or discomfort are ascertained. The effects of surgery, other disease processes, and congenital anomalies are assessed. Loss of muscle tone, skin turgor, and evidence of circulatory problems are also noted.

When the sexological examination is the introduction to sex therapy, the sexual partners are examined in each other's presence and the therapist uses the experience to educate clients and to illustrate a variety of arousal techniques.

Diagnosis

In almost every medical or surgical nursing care plan, at least one nursing diagnosis should relate to the client's sexuality. Many of these diagnoses will relate to psychosocial stressors included in DSM III, such as marital difficulty, ineffective rela-

Table 23-4 Sexual History

Data

Identification and background
(Usually obtained from client's chart)

Socioeconomic data
(Age, date of birth, social status, economic status, sibling position, marital status, education)

Physiological data
(Laboratory tests, drugs, x-rays, medical history)

Physical examination
(Particular emphasis on genitalia, breasts)

Psychological data
(Mental status, affect, counseling, self-concept, parental and family information, religious background, state of marriage)

Male's history

Do you have problems with erection? ______

Are you able to control ejaculation? ______

Have you ever had urinary tract infections? ______

Have you ever had urinary frequency? ______

Have you ever had urinary urgency? ______

Have you ever had urinary burning? ______

Have you experienced trauma to the testicles? ______

Have you ever been treated for venereal disease? ______

Female's history

Menstruation

Length of cycle ______

Duration of flow ______

Discomfort ______

Emotional changes ______

Arousal fluctuations during cycle ______

Age at onset ______

Female's history

When was your last Pap smear? ______

Have you ever been pregnant? ______

Number of pregnancies ______

Number of live births ______

Number of miscarriages ______

Have you ever had gynecological surgery? ______

Have you ever had an abortion? ______

Have you ever had a dilation and curettage? ______

Have you ever had other surgery? ______

Do you have problems with vaginal discharge? ______

Have you ever had infected tubes or ovaries? ______

Have you ever had venereal disease? ______

Both partners' history

	Sex education and information		
	Source of knowledge	**Parental attitudes**	**Age at time information received**
Pregnancy	______	______	______
Sexual intercourse	______	______	______
Menstruation	______	______	______
Contraception	______	______	______
Male erection (females)	______	______	______
Formal sex education	______	______	______
Books read	______	______	______

Contraception

Are you currently using a form of contraception? ______

Does it interfere with sexual pleasure? ______

Are you concerned that it endangers your health or will interfere with future fertility? ______

(Continued.)

Table 23-4 Continued

Data	Data
Current typical sexual behavior with partner	**Current typical sexual behavior with partner**
Who initiates sexual activity? ______	Behaviors and feelings after orgasm or intercourse ______
How does initiation occur? ______	Are you currently satisfied with your sexual responsiveness? ______
What are the consequences of refusal? ______	Are you satisfied with your partner's response? ______
Feelings about nudity ______	Do you think you have a sexual problem? ______
Preference for situation (place, lighting, devices, oils, lotions, etc.) ______	Do you have difficulty with or is there a family history of any of the following?
Frequency of and attitude toward noncoital contact ______	**Male** **Female**
Orgasm: male (frequency, techniques) ______	Alcoholism ______ ______
	Diabetes ______ ______
Orgasm: female (frequency, techniques) ______	Hypertension ______ ______
	Thyroid disease ______ ______

tionships with the opposite sex, discomfort with the female role, lack of information, preoccupation with physical appearance, and difficulty in control. Selected nursing diagnoses follow:

> Lack of comfort about sexuality related to body-image disturbance.
>
> Ineffective sexual relationships associated with retarded psychosexual development.
>
> Lack of sexual satisfaction associated with impotence.
>
> Discomfort with female role related to absence of significant female role models.
>
> Lack of knowledge about sexuality related to restrictive cultural background.
>
> Healthy sexual patterns associated with successful postmastectomy grieving.

Outcome Criteria

Outcome criteria are measurable statements about what one expects to achieve as a result of specific nursing interventions. At the basic nursing level, students will work with clients to promote sexual health and maintain optimum levels of functioning. The achievement of partly and wholly compensatory goals is left to advanced practitioners. Basic nursing-level intervention generally aims at supportive and educative goals. Several examples of such outcome criteria follow:

> Client will verbalize increased comfort with her femininity after four therapy sessions.
>
> Client will verbalize knowledge about female anatomy and function following 2 days of instruction.
>
> Client will permit family members to express affection by hugging after 2 weeks of therapy.
>
> Client will acknowledge sexual concerns after assessment session with the nurse.
>
> Client will telephone sex therapy clinic 1 week after referral by the nurse.

Intervention

At the basic level, communication with clients about their sexuality is a primary intervention.

For many reasons, sex is difficult to discuss seriously. People may find it easier to make jokes about sex than to discuss their real concerns. Nurses are no exception and may frequently feel they should not talk about sex with clients. Some nurses feel that discussing sex is "too personal," "too embarrassing," or "nosy." These comments reflect the nurse's own discomfort.

Often it is necessary for nurses to increase their level of comfort with sexuality through a desensitization-resensitization process. Awareness can then be enhanced by increasing knowledge. When a nurse is able to balance cognitive awareness with an awareness of personal values and attitudes, nursing intervention in the area of sexuality will become easier.

In talking with clients about sexual concerns, nurses may find the following guidelines to be helpful:

1. Approach the situation with an attitude of acceptance and honesty about your own level of expertise.
2. Provide a quiet, private place to talk.
3. Provide a relaxed and unhurried atmosphere; it may take a long time for clients to say what they want to say. Listen without impulsively rushing in to supply an answer.
4. Use direct eye contact as much as possible.
5. Do not write during the interview; notes should be written later. (A possible exception is when you are writing the problem list. The client should participate in formulating the list).
6. Sit as close to the client as is comfortable for both of you. Do not sit behind a desk or across the room.
7. Ask open-ended questions rather than questions requiring merely "yes" or "no" responses.
8. If the client does not bring up sexual concerns, use a *review* statement ("As you probably already know, . . .") or a *universality* statement ("Most people who have had this surgery wonder when they can safely resume sexual relations . . .").
9. If the client has no questions or concerns, it is usually not appropriate to press for a lengthy discussion. The client may be more willing to discuss sexuality at a later time or may actually have no concerns.
10. Communication clues can come from content of discussion, perceptions, and thoughts. It is helpful to think about the central themes coming from the client and the thoughts and perceptions about these themes.
11. Nonverbal clues include appearance and behaviors during an interview. Assess whether or not the client is demonstrating evidence of disequilibrium by anxiety, inability to concentrate, unrealistic perceptions, and disorganization in work and social situations.
12. Understanding a client's sexuality requires observation of not only what the client does and says, but what the client repeatedly avoids. It takes time and skill to make an accurate assessment based on observations.
13. Exploration of covert messages with direct feedback can be useful for some clients. Gestures and actions can reinforce what is being said and make it more meaningful; however, gestures can communicate a meaning different from the words that are spoken. Therefore, the nurse needs to clarify the meaning of gestures, tone of voice, and other behaviors that do not seem to correspond with the oral communication. This can be done by a statement such as, "You say you are comfortable with homosexuality, but I seem to be getting messages to the contrary. What does that mean?" Or, "You say you feel OK about being impotent, but it seems to me that you are really upset about it. Help me to understand which is correct."

The nurse will need to be comfortable with most topics of sexuality before the last four suggestions are followed.

Basic needs must be met before underlying psychological, developmental, and sexual issues are addressed. Giving permission for and encouraging communication about feelings will help the client trust the nurse. The incorporation and discussion of sexual history and a questionnaire on sexual attitudes and knowledge can be used to give permission and also to provide information. Books, videotapes, and movies about sexual, physical, and psychological development add information about sexual activity, sex role, body image, and such issues as menarche, menstruation, and masturbation. Self-image and self-esteem questionnaires provide vehicles for clients to discuss feelings about their bodies, body image, and self-esteem.

Clients and nurses need to identify strengths of clients that can serve as foundations for building self-esteem and self-worth. Suggestions and contracts can concentrate on learning how to be sexual and how to enjoy one's body through touch, smell, taste, and movement. Sex-role behaviors such as nurturing, giving, loving, and comforting the opposite sex are modeled by the nurse.

If the above types of nursing interventions are not successful when a client expresses concerns about sexuality, then a referral for psychotherapy, family therapy, or sexual therapy is usually appropriate.

Evaluation

If the assessment, diagnoses, and interventions are completed in a systematic manner, evaluation and research about nursing outcomes will provide the basis for new knowledge about nursing practice. Following is a case study which utilizes the nursing process in a systematic manner.

Brian is a 57-year-old divorced man who was recently retired from his job as a construction worker. He was admitted to the medical unit for treatment of dehydration and cardiac problems. He is overweight. He has not been active sexually since his divorce, although he has a steady relationship with a widowed woman whom he states he loves. He has minimal contact with his grown children.

ASSESSMENT

What are Brian's attitudes about sexuality?
What does Brian consider his physical assets? Liabilities?
What are his childhood memories of father, mother, and self?
How does he see his role as a man?
Has Brian been able to develop an intimate relationship with anyone? Is he married? Widowed? Divorced?
What are his fantasies about the ideal sexual relationship?
What attitudes does he have toward sexuality? Toward women?
What does Brian know about his illness? About its connection to sexuality?

DIAGNOSES

Lack of comfort about sexuality related to body-image disturbance.
Impotence related to fears about cardiac problems.
Feelings of sexual inadequacy related to absence of consistent sexual partner.

OUTCOME CRITERIA

Brian will lose 3 pounds weekly for 2 months.
Brian will participate in planning his menus.
Brian will verbally acknowledge improved perception of his physical features.
Brian will agree to attend therapy sessions with his partner twice a week while he is hospitalized.
Brian will give verbal feedback to his primary nurse about his knowledge of male anatomy and physiology.

INTERVENTIONS

Involve Brian in the planning of a low-calorie diet.
Have the staff develop a consistent plan for monitoring his meals.
Establish a routine of biweekly weight checks.
Involve woman friend in therapy with his consent.
Discuss attendance at sex-education classes.
Refer for individual therapy sessions twice weekly.
Encourage attendance at men's group and divorce-mediation classes.
Involve his grown children in his treatment with his consent.

EVALUATION

Brian lost 8 pounds after 2 weeks.
Brian verbalized perception of improved body image after nine sessions with his nurse.
Brian has refused to attend family therapy sessions. His children have been attending. Brian's son will be coached to encourage Brian to attend the next two sessions only.
Brian has been attending sex-education sessions. To date he has not verbalized any positive feedback. Sessions will continue with his primary nurse.

SUMMARY

Increased knowledge, revision of attitudes, and the changing role of women in American society have contributed to the sexual health of individuals, influenced sexual behavior, and updated state statutes affecting sexual activities and mores.

Sexuality is an integral part of the self, and it includes physical, mental, and spiritual dimensions. Sexual terms mean different things to different people. Sexual expression may have a self-focus, may be motivated by love, or may emphasize the sensous aspects of sex.

One cannot fully understand sexuality unless one has a solid understanding of the sexual anatomy and physiology of the male and female. External male genitalia include the penis, scrotum, gonads (testes), epididymis, and parts of the vas deferens. Internal male genitalia consist of other parts of the vas deferens, the seminal vesicles, ejaculatory ducts, and the prostate and Cowper's glands. External female genitalia include the mons veneris, labia minora, labia majora, clitoris, and vaginal orifice. Internal female genitalia consist of gonads (ovaries), fallopian tubes, uterus, and vagina. The homologous nature of male and female anatomy brings forth similarities in male and female sexual response.

Psychosexual development occurs throughout the life span and results in a person's sexual self-perception. The term *gender identity* is used to describe how one perceives one's gender. One can have a masculine, feminine, or ambivalent gender identity. Gender identity is relative to time and place in a given society. The term *gender role* usually refers to the behavioral expression of gender identity.

The term *intimacy* describes a special quality of emotional closeness between two people and is characterized by mutual caring, responsibility, trust, and open communication of feelings and sensations, as well as nondefensive interchange of information about significant emotional events. Intimacy is an integral component of love. *Love* includes mutual respect, mutual responsibility or commitment, and some element of permanence. There are three major components of a love relationship: the sexual, the magical, and the sensual.

The sex act, or sexual intercourse, may be enjoyed by couples with or without love relationships. The sexual act may be motivated by nonsexual needs. Arousal and response patterns are individual and occur in response to manual, oral-genital, anal-genital, or genital-genital stimulation. Many coital positions are possible, although most couples settle on a few preferred techniques.

Sex-role behavior includes components of gender role and identity but has seldom been clearly defined. Androgyny is the abandonment of a bipolar sex-role model and the blending of masculinity and femininity. The freeing of feelings and behaviors has influenced the mores and values regarding sex-role behaviors. Flexibility in role performance has been enhanced by economic necessity and self-fulfillment of women working outside the home.

Sexuality finds expression in single, married, homosexual, and communal lifestyles.

Nurses are involved in the promotion of sexual health at various levels of expertise based on their knowledge, attitudes, and teaching skills. Nurses need specific communication skills when discussing sexual concerns with clients. Mims and Swenson's sexual health model provides a framework for assessment of self and client and intervention at basic, intermediate, and advanced levels. Systematic assessment, intervention, and evaluation will provide descriptive data about clients with different sexual health problems. These data can generate new knowledge from clinical nursing practice.

REFERENCES

1. E. R. Mahoney, *Human Sexuality,* McGraw-Hill, New York, 1983.
2. Fern H. Mims and Melinda Swenson, *Sexuality: A Nursing Perspective,* McGraw-Hill, New York, 1980.
3. W. L. Witters and P. Jones-Witters, *Human Sexuality: A Biological Perspective,* Van Nostrand, New York, 1980.
4. I. H. Frieze et al., *Women and Health,* Norton, New York, 1980.
5. J. Hyde, *Understanding Human Sexuality,* McGraw-Hill, New York, 1979.
6. D. G. McCarthy and E. J. Bayer, *Handbook on Critical Sexual Issues,* Doubleday, New York, 1984.
7. Fern H. Mims and A. Chang, "Unwanted Sexual Experiences of Young Women," *Journal of Psychosocial Nursing,* vol. 22, no. 6, June 22, 1984, pp. 6–16.
8. H. Singer Kaplan, *Disorders of Sexual Desire,* Brunner Mazel, New York, 1979.
9. H. Sullivan, *Conceptions of Modern Psychiatry,* Norton, New York, 1953.
10. D. Tennov, *Love and Limerence,* Stein and Day, New York, 1979.
11. Herant Katchadourian and Donald T. Lunde, *Fundamentals of Human Sexuality,* Holt, New York, 1972.
12. J. T. Spence and M. A. Helmreich, *Masculinity and Femininity,* University of Texas Press, Austin, 1978.
13. K. Clark, *An Experience of Celibacy,* Ave Maria Press, Notre Dame, Ind., 1982.
14. D. Read, *Healthy Sexuality,* Macmillan, New York, 1979.

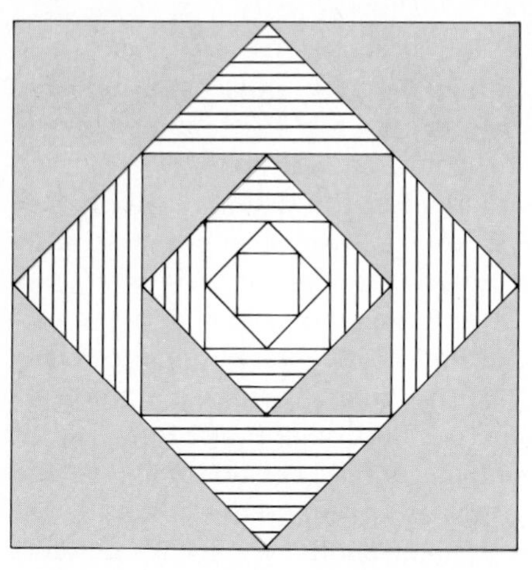

CHAPTER 24
Behavioral and Cognitive Theory and Application

Sandra Jaffe-Johnson

LEARNING OBJECTIVES

After studying this chapter, the student should be able to:

1. Compare the underlying assumptions and approaches of behavioral and traditional therapies.
2. Describe premises and goals of assertiveness training.
3. Discuss ways in which the nurse may help clients to construct assertive plans for change.
4. Describe premises and goals of cognitive theory and therapy.
5. Apply knowledge of the characteristics of a learner in the teaching-learning process.
6. Describe how clients' readiness to learn can be assessed and how it can influence the teaching-learning process.
7. Discuss the use of behavioral objectives in the teaching-learning process.
8. Discuss ways in which nurses help clients to manage their own behavior and direct their courses of action toward valued goals.
9. Develop a nurse-client contract for individual counseling sessions and for behavioral change.

Most people want to be happy and healthy. They are able to think creatively, set certain meaningful goals for themselves, and learn from life experiences the kinds of behaviors that are productive and healthful in their day-to-day interaction with the environment. They appreciate the importance of the quality of life and have an interest in improving their lives. Nurses can help their clients achieve high levels of wellness by promoting synchronous patterns of interaction among mind, body, spirit, and environment.

Nurses try to mobilize clients' innate capacity for self-healing and growth by emphasizing each client's unique personality and patterns of interaction. Because many behavior patterns are learned early and repeated throughout life, they sometimes seem automatic, even when they are not in synchrony with chosen life purposes. The nurse's belief that clients can change patterns of behavior at any age helps create an environment in which concepts of teaching and learning through the various roles and phases of a therapeutic relationship can be reinforced.

Education of clients is an inherent part of nursing. Today, hospital stays tend to be shorter, partly because of diagnostic related groupings (DRGs), and so the nurse needs to prepare clients for discharge as soon as possible.

There are three *domains* (as they are called) of learning: cognitive, affective, and psychomotor. Promotion, restoration, or rehabilitation of health may require clients to learn in all three domains. For example, it may be necessary for clients to understand their health problems (cognitive), alter their attitudes and emotional responses (affective), and follow their treatment regimens (psychomotor). In addition, there is a spiritual dimension to all three domains of learning; thoughts, feelings, and behavior are influenced by beliefs and values. When clients' behaviors, fears, and doubts interfere with their ability to change and develop effective ways of coping, nurses need to recognize what is happening and use various techniques to help them reprogram their negative responses into positive ones.

For the purposes of analysis, this chapter is divided into two main sections: behavioral theory and cognitive theory; social-learning theory is discussed under cognitive theory. As you study this material, you will see many ways in which the behavioral and cognitive theories overlap, and concepts that integrate the two approaches will be discussed. Integrative ways of helping clients in various psychiatric–mental health settings alter dysynchronous patterns of interaction with the environment are explored.

BEHAVIORAL THEORY*

Behavioral theorists hold that the difficulties people have are neither intrapsychic nor interpersonal but behavioral. They believe that all behavior is learned and, therefore, can be unlearned and replaced with more adequate, appropriate behavior.

Behavior patterns and ways of perceiving situations are products of learning and can be unlearned through the patterning of more healthful responses. All behavior has meaning, but behaviors vary in their usefulness for maintenance of health. Dysrhythmic patterns of behavior that are not useful, because they interfere with healthy living, can be extinguished through various deconditioning methods which minimize anxiety and permit clients to learn more healthful responses. Theorists whose work contributed to behavioral theory include Wolpe and Miller and Dollard.

Wolpe

Wolpe's theories[1] state that behavior is what is observable, that all behavior has meaning, and that maladaptive behavior is itself the problem. (Therapists using other modalities would consider maladaptive behavior as symptomatic of underlying problems.) Wolpe holds that maladaptive behaviors do not always disappear as underlying problems are treated. These behaviors are the realm of behavioral therapy. Wolpe considers psychosis to be organically based and deals only with neurotic behaviors.

Wolpe's Definition of Behavior

According to Wolpe, *behavior* is a *conditioned response,* that is, a response which has been rewarded. Many behaviors become habits, which are established, long-standing patterns of response to

* This section from Pamela Price Hoskins, "Theoretical Models," in the second edition of this book.

stimuli. Maladaptive behaviors are thought to have begun in response to uncomfortable levels of anxiety and to have been rewarded by decreased anxiety.

Wolpe's Approach to Behavioral Therapy

The behavioral therapist, in contrast to practitioners using other therapeutic approaches, takes total responsibility for the cure of the client. The client exhibits maladaptive behavior, and the therapist has the tools to correct it. The goals of treatment are to decondition anxiety and to alter maladaptive behavior. Each person has an individually designed program which is based on a clinical history. The behavioral therapist is interested in the history of maladaptive behavior, since it is unique to each client. (Therapists using other modalities, as was noted above, consider behavior symptomatic and are interested in the underlying motivation.)

Deconditioning of anxiety is central to behavioral therapy. Four methods are used:

1. *Assertive behavior* is the expression of emotion appropriate to the current situation rather than an expression of anxiety. Expressions of normal emotions are rewarded. However, clients are warned not to act assertively when doing so is likely to evoke punishment from the environment.
2. *Systematic desensitization* is a step-by-step use of a counteracting emotion to overcome an undesirable emotional habit. This technique occurs in four steps: (a) training in deep muscle relaxation, (b) use of a scale of subjective anxiety, (c) construction of anxiety hierarchies, and (d) use of relaxation techniques in conjunction with anxiety hierarchies. Imagery is often used in conjunction with desensitization.
3. *Evoking strong anxiety* is used as another way to decondition anxiety. Two techniques are used: (a) *Flooding* uses real or imaginary situations to evoke strong anxiety responses. (For example, a girl with a phobia about automobiles was kept in the back seat of a moving automobile for 4 hours. Her fear soon became panic but then gradually subsided. At the end of the ride she was comfortable and henceforth was free from this phobia.) (b) *Abreaction* is the process of stirring up distressing memories to evoke anxiety. These techniques are used repeatedly until the client no longer responds with fear or anxiety. The ability of the situation to elicit fear or anxiety is diminished and finally exhausted.
4. *Operant conditioning* is a method that deals with conditioned motor and cognitive behaviors rather than autonomic behavior. The point of operant conditioning is to elicit adaptive motor and cognitive behaviors. There are five operant techniques: positive reinforcement; negative reinforcement; differential reinforcement; extinction; and punishment or aversion. The techniques are listed in Table 24-1.

Three learning principles underlie Wolpe's[1] behavioral therapy:

1. *Reciprocal inhibition.* When a response that inhibits anxiety occurs in the presence of a stimulus that provokes anxiety, the bond between the anxiety-provoking stimulus and the anxiety weakens. (For example, a child being held by the mother will be less frightened by a barking dog than would be the case if he or she were facing the dog alone.)
2. *Positive reconditioning.* The undesired behavior is not rewarded. The behavior that is to replace the undesired behavior is rewarded every time it is exhibited.
3. *Experimental extinction.* Undesired behavior is evoked but never rewarded; therefore, it becomes progressively weaker. Mechanisms of experimental extinction are still being developed by behavioral therapists.

The major criticism of Wolpe's therapy is that since it treats only the symptom and not the underlying problem, *symptom substitution* will occur—that is, another maladaptive behavior will replace the extinguished behavior. Wolpe, however, holds that the behavior is the problem, and not a symptom. In his clinical experience, there have been no symptom substitutions.

Miller and Dollard

Neal Miller and John Dollard[2] combined the Freudian outlook with Pavlov's learning theories to develop their behavioral theory. Like Freudians, they think that behavior is symptomatic of underlying personality problems, but like behaviorists, they hold that behavior is learned and can be unlearned.

Table 24-1 Operant Conditioning Techniques

Technique	Definition	Example
Positive reinforcement	Use of reward to increase the rate of desired response	When a client makes an effort to control ritualistic behavior and arrives on time for breakfast, the nurse praises the client's effort and promptness.
Negative reinforcement	Removal of tension or pain to increase the rate of desired response	Nurse involves client in strenuous exercise following a tense and upsetting family meeting.
Differential reinforcement	Combination of positive and negative reinforcement	Nurse helps client to imagine a pleasant experience following a relaxation exercise as a means of controlling anxiety related to discharge.
Extinction	Lack of reinforcement of behavior patterns to decrease the rate of undesired response	Client talks constantly about somatic complaints, and the nurse responds by waiting and then changing the subject.
Punishment	Giving an obnoxious reinforcement to inhibit an undesired response	Adolescent client is restricted to his or her room and not allowed to attend the unit Halloween party after punching walls and breaking furniture.

They accept Freud's description of neurosis, defense mechanisms, and treatment. They advocate the use of learning theories as the basis for treatment.

Miller and Dollard's Definition of Behavior

According to Miller and Dollard, behavior reflects a way of coping with conflict and its associated anxiety. There are two kinds of conflicts. An *avoidance-avoidance conflict* occurs when one must choose between two undesirable alternatives. (For instance, a person may not want to suffer with cholecystitis but may not want surgical intervention either.) An *approach-avoidance conflict* occurs when one has ambivalent feelings about an object: one wishes, simultaneously, to approach and avoid it. (For example, a nurse may want the prestige of an administrative position but may not want the responsibility that goes with it.) Conflict theory revolves around the assumption that fear and anxiety are two of the strongest sources of avoidance.

In this view, people are seen as learners. When rewarded, people learn adaptive as well as maladaptive behaviors. *Neurosis* is defined by behaviorists as the result of having learned maladaptive behaviors. It is characterized by manifest differences between the opportunity for enjoyment and the capacity for it. Conflict, stupidity, and misery characterize the neurotic's behavior. Behavior is motivated by primary and secondary drives, including the drive to reduce fear and anxiety.

Miller and Dollard's Approach to Behavioral Therapy

There are four fundamentals of learning: drive, cue, response, and reinforcement. *Drive* is motivation; it can be primary (biological) or secondary (learned). A *cue* is a stimulus, a push to respond. A *response* is a thought, feeling, or action caused by the cue. *Reinforcement* is a reward for a response. Miller and Dollard consider a decrease in fear and anxiety to be the major reinforcement in neurotic behavior. The fear of an object is repressed and is called *anxiety.* Four principles of learning are based on these fundamentals.

1. *Extinction* is a decrease in the rate of neurotic behavior when the behavior is not reinforced.
2. *Spontaneous recovery* is the tendency for neurotic behavior to recur periodically, even in the absence of reinforcement.
3. *Generalization* is the tendency to transfer the learning in one situation to similar situations.
4. *Discrimination* is the ability to notice the similarities and differences in like situations.

Miller and Dollard state that one sign of neurosis is an inability to solve one's own emotional problems. This occurs primarily because of *repression,* a defense mechanism that makes it difficult or impossible to remember thoughts, feelings, actions, and perceptions. Miller and Dollard hypothesize that in order to repress anxiety-provoking situations, a person must either unlabel or mislabel them. As a consequence of unlabeling or mislabeling situations, the person is unable to recall them. Since the problem is unconscious or undefined, the client is unable to use problem-solving processes.

Miller and Dollard submit that conflict is the basis of neurosis. Drives—like the drive for water (a primary drive) or for money (a secondary drive)—build up; but if the way to decrease a drive generates fear, the behavior is blocked. When such a conflict between drive and fear occurs, the result is neurotic behavior that slightly decreases the drive and avoids fear and anxiety.

The behavioral therapist is seen as a teacher, who listens and accepts and does not punish or condemn. The therapist should: (1) be free from repressions and fears, (2) empathize with the client's fears, (3) refrain from talking too much or giving too many rewards, and (4) believe in the client's capacity to learn and unlearn.

The goals of therapy are to remove repressions and restore the use of higher mental processes for problem solving. The processes of therapy are primarily analytic. The therapist creates an atmosphere conducive to openness and trust, one that decreases fear and anxiety. Free association to uncover repressed material is a primary technique. Principles of learning are also used. The therapist helps the client to discriminate between old and new situations and to recognize childhood behaviors that have been generalized to adult situations. The therapist rewards only attempts at constructive new behaviors and encourages the client to seek major rewards essentially outside the therapy situation. The therapist also attempts to construct graded social situations that will help the client overcome fear and anxiety and develop constructive new behavior.

There are two aspects to treatment: talking with the therapist and changing behavior in the real world. The client is encouraged to take risks, to develop connections between plans and actions. If behavior does not change, the therapy has failed. For instance, a person may develop insight into the reasons for distrust of others; however, if relationships based on trust are not developed after insight has been gained, the therapy has failed.

Application of Behavioral Theory

How Nurses Use Behavioral Principles

The principle of discrimination is used to help clients describe cognitive, physiological, and psychomotor changes. For instance, a nurse can encourage a client to describe thoughts, feelings, and actions associated with a new situation (such as beginning a new job); to describe a situation in childhood when these same thoughts, feelings, and actions were elicited; to identify aspects of the present situation that are similar to the past situation and have elicited the childhood responses; and, finally, to identify aspects of the present situation that are different from the past situation. The principle of generalization is used to transfer learning from therapeutic relationships to situations in the real world.

Graduated learning experiences are helpful in teaching clients about procedures that may generate fear and anxiety. For example, expanding teaching to deal with the procedures of preadmission, presurgery, and postdischarge helps the client handle anxieties associated with them. Having the client identify what aspects of a specific technique or procedure generate anxiety—in rank order, from least to most—helps the nurse set priorities. The nurse will not move on to the next aspect of learning until the client is comfortable with what has already been learned.

The concept of labeling encourages nurses to share information about anatomy, body functions, and emotions with their clients. Understanding the dynamics of conflicts in these areas increases nurses' understanding of clients' ambivalence and the very real misery clients often feel.

Assertiveness Training

Assertiveness training, also called *assertive behavioral therapy,* is one way that nurses can help clients to acquire accurate knowledge about the values and beliefs they employ in defining their behavior. The verb *assert* means "state or affirm positively, assuredly, plainly, or strongly." Assertiveness training is a process that helps people develop socially appropriate expression of feelings, attitudes, wishes, opinions, and rights.[3,4]

Verbal and nonverbal assertive behaviors can be learned and practiced by clients. Clients are taught to make "I" statements and encouraged to be less defensive, to exert control, and to take responsibility for their emotions. They are also taught to use descriptive terms, rather than judgmental or value-laden terms, when giving feedback.

Reduction of anxiety may occur indirectly as a positive outcome of such training. When conflicts evoke emotionally painful memories, assertiveness training can help clients to become aware of how these memories influence behavior and to learn new ways of interacting. Table 24-2 outlines assertiveness strategies nurses use to help clients with social anxiety.

Negative attitudes, values, and beliefs that inhibit the ability to be assertive are altered through positive reinforcement of new ways of behaving. Negative self-evaluations are altered as clients recognize their positive assets and begin to interact with the environment in assertive ways.

People exhibit patterns of assertiveness, nonassertiveness, or aggressiveness that were learned in childhood and have been reinforced since then. Along with these patterns of interaction, they learn feelings about the use of the patterns. (For example, a client may have learned to be passive, to feel comfortable behaving passively, and to feel guilty or anxious when behaving assertively or aggressively.) Behavior patterns and associated feelings about modes of interacting become a *script* which is followed regardless of circumstances or consequences. Assertiveness training helps people write new scripts for themselves that allow flexibility and thoughtfulness in interactions with others and promote assertiveness.[5] Examples of items in such a script include the following:

- I can judge my own behavior and learn to revise it if it causes me problems.
- I can take responsibility for my behavior and not blame others when I encounter problems.
- I do not have to give others excuses or reasons for what I think or do.
- I can allow others to find solutions for their own problems and not feel guilty about not finding solutions for them.
- I can change my mind.
- I can say, "I don't understand," rather than pretend that I do.
- I can make mistakes and accept responsibility for them rather than try to cover them up or blame others.
- I can accept that some people will like me and approve of what I do and others will not.
- I can say, "I don't care," when something does not matter to me.

Table 24-2 Assertive Strategies for Dealing with Social Anxiety

Skill	Technique
Recognize area of physical tension	Clients are taught not to overreact to signs of physical tension as if they were being attacked. They are taught to tell themselves, "Feelings are not facts; sensations of discomfort will pass."
Recognize fear and begin to offset feelings of being overwhelmed	Clients are taught to: Keep focus on the present and breathe slowly. Substitute imagery of pleasurable people, places, or things. Practice progressive muscular relaxation exercises. Acknowledge feelings and tell themselves, "This is not the worst thing that can happen."
Reinterpret the situation so it is not as frightening	Clients are taught to tell themselves, "I got through it. I did it. I can control my fear. I am feeling better this time."

Examples of nonassertive, aggressive, and assertive behaviors are provided with descriptions of each in Table 24-3 (page 472).

When clients first begin to change their behavior so that they become more assertive, there is a tendency to behave either more aggressively or more passively, depending on the previous style of interacting. Clients are insecure about their new behavior and unsure of how to act. The nurse helps clients monitor their behavior, practice new behavior in role-playing situations, and analyze situations in which they have attempted to be assertive. The nurse also gives clients positive feedback when they are successful in acting assertively and constructive suggestions when they provide examples of aggressiveness or nonassertiveness. A client's former behavior may have certain rewards that assertive behavior lacks; in addition, defense patterns and personality may be more congruent with the old

Table 24-3 Nonassertive, Aggressive, and Assertive Behavior

Description	Example
Nonassertiveness	
Failing to express honest feelings, thoughts, and beliefs. Permiting others to violate the self. Expressing thoughts and feelings in a self-effacing manner	Client agrees with another's perception of his or her problem even though it has no basis in reality. Client states that it is all right if another client borrows clothes and jewelry without asking or reads his or her personal mail.
Aggressiveness	
Directly standing up for personal rights, but expressing thoughts, feelings, and beliefs in a way which is often dishonest and inappropriate and which violates the rights of others, particularly those with less power. Feeling powerless because of inability to monitor behavior. Being nonassertive with those who are powerful	Client shouts at another client to get off the telephone because he or she wants to use it. Client orders roommate out of their shared bedroom because he or she wants to be alone.
Assertiveness	
Being able to communicate with people on all levels in an open, direct, honest and appropriate manner. Having an active orientation to life and a positive outlook on situations. Taking responsibility for making things happen. Maintaining self-respect by an awareness and acceptance of others' limitations	Client asks the nurse to discuss an upsetting phone call. Client tells another client that he or she does not understand the point of the description of a particular conversation between client and spouse.

behavior pattern than the new one. As a result, anxiety may be generated. For these reasons clients need support throughout the learning process as they work on integrating assertiveness with the environment.[6,7]

COGNITIVE THEORY

Cognitive theorists seek to help clients understand how negative and conflicting thought patterns influence their appraisals of certain situations, with the result that their emotional reactions to these situations—such as anger, depression, and fear—are exaggerated or inappropriate. Nursing intervention has the potential to change clients' negative judgments of themselves and to help clients establish healthful patterns of interaction with the environment. The interactive relationship between people and their environments makes it important to emphasize the clients' active participation in the process of change: defining problems, selecting behavioral objectives, and evaluating outcomes.

Principles of cognitive learning can be used by nurses in the teaching-learning process. The cognitive area includes thinking, reasoning, understanding, and remembering. Thought and memory enter into every cognitive action.

Stages of Cognitive Learning

There are four hierarchical stages of thought development: instinctual (preobject), semantic, space-dependent, and symbolic. Table 24-4 summarizes these stages, with descriptions and examples.

People do not often test the validity of their thoughts but instead tend to regard them as universal truths. One aspect of the therapeutic relationship is educating clients about how to acquire accurate knowledge necessary for handling difficulties in their lives. When nurses attempt to understand clients' cognitive appraisals of situations, they are better able to appreciate each client's unique emotional reactions, such as exaggerated anger, anxiety, or depression. Cognitive therapy offers a way of effecting behavioral and emotional change through analysis and revision of the client's thinking and perception.

Social-Learning Theory

The theory of social learning is discussed here as it relates to cognitive theory; at the same time, it offers a framework that helps nurses apply behavioral as well as cognitive theories to clients' patterns of maladaptive behavior. Social-learning theory views psychological functioning as a continuous reciprocal relationship among personal, behavioral, and environmental factors. Table 24-5 gives an example of this reciprocity.

According to social-learning theory, people are able to learn and acquire integrated behavior patterns by observation. Through the use of symbols,

Table 24-4 Stages of Thought Development

Stages	Description	Example
Instinctual	Thoughts are direct, global, and immediate.	A mother leaves the room. Her child feels that mother will be gone forever. The child has no sense of temporal-spatial perspectives.
Semantic	Thoughts are more selective and concrete. There is attainment of object representation and an ability to perceive. Paradoxical reasoning occurs.	A nurse asks, "How are you feeling today, Larry?" Larry responds, "I feel with my hands." A client with a schizophrenic thought disorder says, "Mary is a virgin. I am a virgin. Therefore, I am the Virgin Mary."
Space-dependent	Thoughts can be perceived as part of a space-field relationship. Thoughts move from general to specific. There is some degree of abstraction.	A nursing-home resident arranges personal mementos on a bedside table and becomes upset if anyone rearranges them. A client participates in body-movement (dance) therapy and afterward shares his or her negative feelings about body image and self-worth.
Symbolic	Use of language establishes a mental sphere, enlarges thinking, adds content to semantic fields of objects. Introspection and volition are present.	A client imitates the nurse's emphatic response in an interaction with another client.

Table 24-5 Social Learning as a Reciprocal Phenomenon

Before Intervention	
Personal factor	Person perceives event as threatening and anxiety-producing. Fears disapproval.
Behavioral factor	Person exhibits avoidance behavior pattern in relation to situation.
Environmental factor	Person lacks social support, but environment is not dangerous.
After Intervention	
Personal factor	Person learns how to operate without direct approval or praise.
Behavioral factor	Person initiates involvement in the situation.
Environmental factor	Person continues to lack support until he or she introduces ways the environment can be supportive.

people are able to preserve experiences in representational forms, which then serve as guides for future behavior. People are also seen as having the ability to regulate themselves; they are able to exercise some measure of control over their behavior through selective use of potential influences in the environment.[8] The potential environment is seen as the same for all people; the actual environment depends upon individual behavior.[9] To illustrate this, consider the following example:

> Two men have moved recently into a retirement apartment complex that has a large lounge area with tables, chairs, and couches. One man sees this area as part of the complex but doesn't recognize how it could help him resolve the loneliness he has experienced since moving to his new home. The other man sees the lounge as a community room, where residents can gather and join in recreational activities. The first man fails to recognize the potential of the environment. The second man recognizes its potential, and he may begin to organize the residents and plan community activities for the lounge.

Social Learning and Role Prescriptions

Role prescriptions serve as ways of structuring behavior. By following their role prescriptions, people set up situations that affect other people's behavior and, therefore, find themselves in negative or positive social climates. In the example of the two men residents in the apartment complex, the role prescription of the first man—a single, self-sufficient resident, not a member of a community—has influenced his behavior pattern: he stays within the confines of his own apartment. The role prescription of the second man—a resident in an apartment community—has had a different influence: his behavior pattern is characterized by reaching out to others and organizing community activities. In analyzing how counterreactions influence behavior, one needs to consider the following: the long-term mutual consequences, predictive clues, and socially structured constraints on behavior, roles, and circumstances.[8]

Nurses help people to interact effectively with the environment by helping them recognize environmental potentials, assess the ways they interact with the environment, and activate environmental potentials for their own benefit.

Social Learning and Cognitive Control

Motivations for behavior are related to the capacity to form mental images of future consequences. Motivation can lead people to develop competence for future interactions by using self-regulated reinforcement: setting up performance standards or goals that can be accomplished within brief periods of time. Sometimes there is a discrepancy between the goals people set for themselves and what they accomplish. This dysynchrony between what people do and what they seek to achieve can serve as a motivational stimulus for change, or it can promote feelings of hopelessness and failure. The nurse helps clients to establish realistic, feasible personal goals and to evaluate their own accomplishments. The anticipation of satisfaction, realistic appraisal of progress, and constructive feedback on how to progress further toward goals can serve as incentives for people to persist in their efforts until their performance matches what they want to achieve.[8]

Goals need to be stated as specific, discrete, measurable, and incremental behaviors. Clients need concrete evidence of progress to sustain their efforts to change behavior. Proximity of goals is also important; the sooner a client is able to recognize progress, the greater the incentive to continue. Immediate attainment of at least one goal establishes motivation to pursue further goals. Even if early successes are short-lived rewards, they provide a motivation to work toward higher goals.

Application of Cognitive Theory: The Teaching-Learning Process

There are five main principles of cognitive therapy,[10] which closely parallel aspects of the teaching-learning process:

1. Focus is on the here and now. Concepts are within clients' awareness. Unconscious meanings and hidden thoughts are not explored.
2. Inferences, connections, and generalizations by the therapist are readily comprehensible to the client.
3. Clients are able to generalize directly from conscious experience.
4. Clients test, refine, and accept or reject data in experiences outside therapy.
5. Teachable concepts are assimilated, and dysrhythmic patterns of behavior are changed to more healthful ones.

People have two concurrent streams of thought that are basically in conflict.[10] One stream consists of critical and hostile thoughts about others; the second stream consists of critical thoughts about the self for daring to have critical and hostile thoughts about others in the first place. For example:

> Mr. J., a client on the psychiatric inpatient unit, is encouraged by the nurse, Ms. W., to express anger when he experiences it. He has gained enough trust in the relationship with the nurse to be able to comment one morning, "I was angry with you when you were late last Thursday for our appointment." At the same time, Mr. J. may be saying to himself, "I am not worthy of the nurse's time. I am boring to be with. I am wrong to criticize her. I should be grateful that she even wants to talk to me. I'm bad—sick."

Self-critical thoughts lead to anxiety and have an effect on many teaching-learning situations. It is important to recognize that self-monitoring of thoughts, feelings, and actions may interfere with a therapeutic relationship. Clients need to have opportunities to discuss their perceptions of particular situations, especially since some perceptions are illogical or significantly distort reality. Discussing thoughts with the nurse makes it more likely that they can be clarified and revised. For example:

> A depressed client, Ms. R., says, "I have lost my ability to drive, read, or go shopping." This is a recognizable distortion of reality. Ms. R. is absorbed with the negative aspects of her life and inattentive to positive aspects. The nurse alters this by having Ms. R. write down positive experiences and bring them to the session for discussion. Through this cognitive learning experience Ms. R. revises her perception and becomes able to perform the tasks she felt unable to deal with.

Illogical thinking occurs when people are unable to make correct inferences from their observations.[10] For example:

> Upon discharge from the hospital, Mr. Q. discovers a water leak in his apartment and overgeneralizes the problem. "The whole apartment is deteriorating. Everything is ruined. If I had not been away in the hospital, this would not have happened." The nurse helps Mr. Q. to focus on the specific event, see the actual cause of the leak and the actual related circumstances, take action to have the leak repaired, and recognize that one problem can be resolved and not become an overall disaster.

Through the collaborative nurse-client relationship, the nurse can help clients express their distorted ideas, then help clients explore and revise them so that they are more realistic. Accurate perceiving and thinking are needed for effective coping.

Cognitive and behavioral therapies differ in some important aspects, but they also have aspects in common. Table 24-6 summarizes the similarities and differences between the two. Cognitive and behavioral approaches can be integrated, using the social-learning concept as a framework. As you study the rest of this section, which deals with the teaching-learning process, you will see areas in which an integration of the two approaches is possible.

Teaching-learning is a process through which change occurs as a result of planned input. It is a major component of the role of psychiatric nurses. Teaching-learning recognizes the holistic, dynamic, and collaborative relationship among nurse, client, family members, and significant others. It is based on the belief of psychiatric–mental health nursing professionals that people can change their behavior within specified periods of time.

Belief in positive change is communicated through interactions between nurse and client that are based on the nurse's therapeutic use of self as well as on planned teaching activities. *Client teaching* is defined as the part of the nursing process that offers opportunities to clients to engage in activities which influence their behavior and produce change in knowledge, attitudes, and skills required to maintain and promote health. Thus it is an interpersonal process in which clients play an active role.

Perhaps the single most important form of expertise necessary for nurses in the teaching-learning process is the ability to impart hope to clients through feedback. Clients are capable of directing themselves and making their own decisions, and they need to be perceived this way by the nurse. Nurses give clients hope that they can change and motivate clients to continue the change process by encouraging them to make their own decisions, take responsibility for the consequences of their decisions, and manage their own lives (even when their chosen life purposes are visionary or unrealistic).[11,12]

The mental attitude of the nurse is vital. Nurses must remain open to their clients' viewpoints. The teaching process requires respect for clients' frames of reference, an understanding of the difficulty clients have in tolerating anxiety and delaying gratification, and an awareness and appreciation of clients' readiness for change.

Table 24-6 A Comparison of Cognitive Therapy and Behavioral Therapy

Cognitive Therapy	Behavioral Therapy
Similarities	
Formulate symptoms in behavioral terms, and design specific set of operations to alter maladaptive behavior.	Same
Collaborate with and coach client regarding reactive responses.	
Seek to alleviate overt symptoms or behavioral problems directly.	Same
Stress here and now, not the past.	Same
Differences	
Use induced and spontaneous images to identify misconceptions and test distorted views against reality.	Apply techniques of systematic desensitization by inducing a predetermined sequence of images alternating with periods of relaxation.
Modify attitudes, beliefs, or modes of thinking that influence behavior.	Modify behavior directly (through reciprocal inhibition, systematic desensitization, and so on).
Modify ideational content (for example, irrational premises and inferences) to aid change in behavior.	Modify behavior directly.
Work with internally experienced cognitive structures (schemas) that influence client's perceptions, interpretations, and images.	Work with observable behavior.

Some important aspects of the teaching-learning process are discussed below.

Readiness to Learn

Readiness to learn is related to developmental tasks and social roles: that is, a learning task must be relevant to a person's roles and needs. Recognition of the many roles a person assumes (for example, student, friend, spouse, child, parent, worker) and the need to feel successful in these roles is important to the learning process because most clients derive self-esteem from roles.[13]

People vary in their educational backgrounds, intellectual abilities, and attitudes toward responsibility. Readiness to learn is influenced by a person's stage of development; life experience, which can be either a resource or a barrier; social roles; and immediate problems. It is useful to the nurse to understand the characteristics of each client when initiating client-teaching activities. For example:

> A nurse, Mrs. T., recognizes that if clients faithfully take prescribed antipsychotic medication as ordered, they will be able to remain out of the hospital and adequately perform daily living activities. She places a high value on keeping people functioning in the community and on the use of medications to accomplish this. Consequently, she is invested in teaching the clients about their medications, the importance of the medications to their health, and the correct ways to follow prescriptions. A particular client, Mrs. V., may have no problems related to taking medications, be willing to take it in the hospital, but not wish to leave the hospital. (In the community Mrs. V. may be lonely and may have substandard living arrangements. She therefore may prefer to remain in the hospital to enjoy the companionship of other clients and a relatively pleasant environment.) In this instance, the client may not be ready for or receptive to the teaching-learning process related to medication, because she believes that it will lead to discharge into the community. Therefore, the nurse must address how the client can overcome loneliness, meet the need for companionship, and find agreeable living arrangements before initiating the teaching-learning process.

The learner's perspective is characterized by an orientation toward particular problems rather than general subjects and by a sense of immediacy: the learner is most concerned about dealing with problems at hand and with gaining knowledge and skills that can be applied directly and immediately to those problems. People are particularly motivated to learn at times of crisis; they need and are receptive to practical problem-solving approaches. Learning activities need to be prioritized on the basis of urgency of the problem and the client's perception of it.[13] Material that is more meaningful to the client is learned more rapidly. For example:

> Miss N. is a client who wishes to be discharged to a particular halfway house and has an admission interview scheduled for next week. She will be more receptive and motivated to engage in a teaching-learning process related to how to behave during the interview than Mr. P., who does not want to be placed in a halfway house and in any case is not scheduled for discharge until next month. Miss N., anticipating her discharge to a halfway house, will experience some degree of anxiety. If her anxiety is moderate, it will motivate her to learn; but if it is severe, it will detract from learning and retention of information. Mr. P.—who is not approaching discharge and does not want to go to a halfway house—will probably experience a low level of anxiety and will lack the motivation to learn or retain information.

Throughout interactions with clients, there are opportunities to nurture readiness to learn. Sometimes, however, a client's apparent lack of motivation may be the result of differences between the nurse's and the client's value systems. For example:

> A particular nurse may place a high value on productivity as a contributing member of society through membership in the work force. The nurse may also value working as a means of avoiding loneliness. If the nurse's client is a depressed, socially isolated woman who perceives entry into the work force as evidence of failure in her roles as wife and homemaker, a conflict of values exists. The client will not be receptive to teaching-learning activities directed toward assessing or acquiring job skills or job-seeking skills.

Nurses should be aware of possible conflicts of values.

Learning Objectives

Stating an objective clearly is an important component of the teaching-learning process. A clearly stated objective addresses the concept to be taught, the specific content to be learned, the sequence of that content, and the desired outcome. (The learning objectives at the beginning of each chapter in this book illustrate the form such objectives should take.)

A major purpose of stating objectives is to help the client understand expected outcomes and become more self-directive. Therefore, objectives are stated in measurable terms such as, "Client will self-administer medications correctly." Subobjectives, which further delineate behaviors to be learned, are also stated. In this case the main objective would end with a phrase like *as evidenced by* and would be followed by the subobjectives:

Taking haloperidol (Haldol), 10 milligrams (two pills) with breakfast

Taking benzotropine (Cogentin), 2 milligrams (one pill) with breakfast

Taking haloperidol (Haldol), 20 milligrams (four pills) at bedtime

Taking benzotropine (Cogentin), 4 milligrams (two pills) at bedtime

The subobjectives are the behavioral evidence that the main objective has been met satisfactorily.[6]

Teaching Activity

In planning teaching activities, the nurse should remember that clients must be able to express their thoughts and fears without shame, particularly if they are feeling ambivalent about taking responsibility for managing their lives. People are more motivated to learn when the information taught is relevant, so that they perceive the need to learn. Life experiences may enhance learning, or they may pose significant barriers to acquiring new information. Each client has unique life experiences. Therefore, it is important to assess clients' beliefs, attitudes, and values related to the problem as well as their learning experiences. Questions for such an assessment might include the following:

- What are the client's perceptions and feelings related to the problem the nurse wishes to resolve through a teaching-learning process that will result in a change in thinking, feeling, or behaving?
- What are the client's perceptions and feelings related to the proposed changes in thinking, feeling, or behaving?
- How does the client describe previous teaching-learning experiences that required changes in thinking, feeling, or behaving? Negatively? Positively?
- How important does the client consider the need for change?

Table 24-7 Teaching-Learning Process

Steps in Preparation
1. Prepare the client by developing the conditions for learning.
a. Motivate the client by stressing how and why the knowledge is needed.
b. Provide feedback to help the client see logical relationships between new material and previously obtained information.
c. Develop a reinforcement system.
2. Organize the materials for learning.
a. Categorize material by grouping it into clusters.
b. Arrange material in a logical or ordered sequence, building on previous knowledge.
c. Use mnemonic devices such as stories, sentences, words, jingles, and mental images to facilitate recall.
3. Plan distribution of time to maximize learning.
a. Plan short sessions, since learning is affected by attention span and fatigue.
b. Provide a pleasant environment.
c. Remember individuals will recall recent and primary factors more easily.
4. Plan a multisensory approach to learning.
a. Incorporate as many of the five senses as possible.
b. Use an acceptable study method.

SOURCE: R. E. Doyle, "Counseling Strategies: The Management of Learning," unpublished manuscript, St. John's University, New York, Division of Human Services, Counseling, 1984.

Before the teaching-learning process begins, the nurse needs to prepare thoroughly.[14] The steps of preparation are presented in Table 24-7.

Behavioral theory predicts that when healthful behaviors are rewarded with recognition, they are repeated. Continual reinforcement of healthful behavior patterns requires positive feedback as soon as possible after the behavior is observed.[15] Mastery of simple tasks helps people master higher or more complex tasks.[16] (For example, a teaching-learning process to help an alcoholic give up destructive drinking patterns will be more manageable and easier to master if it promotes abstinence for one day at a time than if it promotes lifetime abstinence. As more and more days of successful abstinence go by, the person is better able to engage in learning more effective complex ways of dealing with problems and to imagine life without alcohol.)

Learning Activity

Hildegard Peplau's[17] definition of learning as a concept and a process provides nurses with a step-by-step guide to collecting relevant clinical data. It also serves as a method for engaging clients in learning about themselves and gives the nurse guidelines for performing the following three major activities:

1. Imparting new knowledge to explain events
2. Facilitating change in the client
3. Solving problems presented by the client

The learning process is outlined in Table 24-8 in terms of steps, operations, and statements.

Table 24-8 Learning Process

Learning	Operations of the Nurse	Statements by Nurse
Steps in learning as a concept and as a process	Operations, performances, behaviors, separate skills associated with each step in learning	Examples of statements by the nurse to facilitate development of each step in a client in the total sequence of the process of learning:
1. **To observe:** The ability to notice what went on or what goes on now	Major use of the perceptual process—seeing, hearing, smelling, touching, etc.: To see To hear To feel using empathic observation To feel using tactile senses	What do you see? What is that noise? Are you uncomfortable? Do you have something to say to me? Could I share the thought with you, or is it private? Tell me about yourself. What happened? I don't follow. Tell me, what did you notice? You noticed what? Did you see this happen? Who was with you? When did this occur? What is the color? Where were you? Tell me. Then what? Go on. Give me a blow-by-blow description. Tell me every detail from the start.
2. **To describe:** The ability to recall and tell the details and circumstances of a particular event or experience	Increased verbalization Greater recall Enumeration of details Focus on details of one event	Tell me about the feeling. What name would you give to your feeling? Tell me more. Then what? Go on. . . . Give me an example. Who are they? What about that? For instance? Describe that further. Give me a blow-by-blow account of that. What did you feel at the time? What happened just before? Which was it? Who was the person? What did you say? What did your comment evoke in the other?

(Continued.)

Table 24-8 Continued

Learning	Operations of the Nurse	Statements by Nurse
3. **To analyze:** The ability to review and to work over the raw data with another person (Step 3 may occur simultaneously with step 4.)	Identifying needs Decoding key symbols Distinguishing literal and figurative Sorting and classifying: 1 Impressions 2 Speculations 3 Thematic abstractions 4 Generalizations Comparing Summarizing Sequence Application of concepts Application of personality theory as a frame of reference Formulating relations resulting from the foregoing: 1 Cause and effect 2 Temporal 3 Thematic 4 Spatial	Explain. Help me to understand that. What do you mean? What do you see as the reason? What was the significance of that event? What are the common elements in these two situations? What is the connection? Boil this down to the one important aspect. What caused this? What was your part in it? In what way did you participate? In what way did you reach this decision? What caused this feeling? I expected you at 8:30; you were late; that caused my anger. Have you had this feeling before? Is there anything similar in this situation to your previous experience?
4. **To formulate:** The ability to give form and structure to the connections resulting from step 3 and to restate them in a clear, direct way	Restatement of data in light of step 3 Verbal or written result of analysis of data	State the essence of this situation in a sentence or so. What did you feel? What did you think? What did you do? Tell it to me in a sentence or so. Tell me again. Was there a discrepancy between what you felt, thought, and did? What would you say was the problem? What name would you give to the patterns of your behavior as you interacted with the other person?
5. **To validate** (by consensus): The ability to check with another person and to reach agreement as to the result of step 4 (formulation) or to state the issue clearly if there is divergence in the formulations of the two persons	Checking with, comparing notes of, two or more people	Is this what you mean? Let me restate. Is this what you were saying? Do you go along with this? Is this what you believe? Is this the way it appears to you? Is it that you feel angry when people tell you what to do? Am I correct in concluding that . . . ? Are you saying . . . ?

(Continued.)

Table 24-8 Continued

Learning	Operations of the Nurse	Statements by Nurse
6. **To test:** The ability to try out the result of step 4 (formulation) in situations with people, things, etc., for utility, completeness		(Set up situations where patient can try out new behavior patterns.) Now that you have thought about this and come to this conclusion, why don't you try it out? What would you do if a situation like this came up again? In what way can you use this conclusion to prevent repeating this mistake? In what way will this conclusion help you in the future? What difference will it make now that you know this?
7. **To integrate:** The ability to see the new in relation to or as an integral part of the old; to add to previously acquired usable knowledge for active use by the person	Enmeshing the new with the old	
8. **To utilize:** The ability to use the result of step 3 (formulation) as foresight		(Set up situations where patient can use new behavior patterns.)

SOURCE: Adapted from Hildegard Peplau, "Process and Concept of Learning," in Shirley Burd and Margaret Marshall, eds., *Some Clinical Approaches to Psychiatric Nursing*, Macmillan, New York, 1963, pp. 333–336.

Evaluation of Interventions

As part of the teaching-learning process, it is necessary to evaluate—to determine if a desired behavioral change has occurred or if there is need for further intervention. The original learning objectives are used as criteria in the evaluation.

Table 24-9 lists factors to be considered and questions which may be helpful in determining which teaching-learning interventions have been effective in helping clients achieve their goals, gain knowledge, change attitudes, and acquire new skills.[13]

Feedback

An important aspect of the evaluation process is giving feedback to the client. However, clients often feel that they are being judged when the results of their involvement in teaching-learning processes are evaluated; and therefore feedback can be of value only if it is given with sensitivity and offered as a constructive and helpful opportunity to share perceptions of how goals are being met.

Feedback may be either positive or negative. *Positive feedback* is valued by most people, since it is complimentary in nature. It is of especially high value to a client when it is given by a person who is able to individualize the appraisal through knowledge of the client and that client's particular needs. Positive feedback leads to self-enhancement and positive feelings about self; it also acts as a primary motivation for change—anticipation of praise and success maintains clients' interest in continuing the process of change.

Negative feedback communicates how goals or expectations have *not* been met. In order for negative feedback to be helpful, (1) it should be solicited by the client, (2) it should specify what can be done to remedy the situation, and (3) it should be given to the client *after* positive feedback.[11] It is important to give feedback as soon as possible after a client has attempted to implement what has been learned. Negative feedback should focus on the here-and-now performance and should include practical suggestions that will help the client accomplish predetermined goals in the future. The nurse needs to offer the client an opportunity to respond to feedback and must be attentive to both verbal and nonverbal messages of the client.

The nurse must use the process of "consensual validation" to be sure that the client understands

Table 24-9 Evaluating the Teaching-Learning Process

Factor	Definition	Questions
Style	Shape, size, format, and organization of content	Was manner of presentation appropriate for client's biopsychosocial status and learning style?
Content	Actual facts and data	Did client receive necessary facts and practice opportunities to learn desired behaviors? Was content too complex or too simple?
Environment	All that is external to the individual	Did client complain of noise? Was the temperature of the room comfortable? What other distractions were present? Was there adequate space?
Activities	Measurable behaviors performed by the client	Was there time for immediate application of what was learned? Did the client participate actively in the process (for example, asking questions)? What was the quality of the client's participation?
Media	Audiovisuals, graphics, and printed materials	Did media convey intended messages? Were media understandable, legible, easy to read, and stimulating? Were media appropriate to the subject matter?
Feedback	Level of attentiveness observed in client and family. Verbalized comments about content	What materials did client and family find most helpful? Did they appear stimulated, bored, interested? Did they report interest?
Resources	Materials used to develop content	Was material appropriate to the client's level of education, learning style, cultural background?
Revision	Recommendations for changes in content or process	Did the client desire or need any additional content? What suggestions were made by the client for improvement? What parts of the process were effectively implemented?

the messages on a cognitive level. Teaching-learning is a mutual process. The nurse engages in a teaching-learning interaction with clients to understand them and their problems. The client engages in a teaching-learning interaction to get feedback that increases self-understanding and recognition of problems and to use the nurse as a resource in solving problems. (For example, the nurse might say in response to feedback from a client, "Are you saying that the material was interesting but the medical jargon confused you? I appreciate your telling me this, since I take the jargon for granted and did not recognize that it did not help your understanding.")

Learning through Modeling

According to social-learning theory, modeling serves an informative function. Clients acquire new ways of behaving through observation of modeled activities, which serve as guides for appropriate behaviors.[8] For example, nurses model effective communication for their clients through the words they choose to express ideas or feelings, the way they listen, their observational skills, their body language, and their nonverbal gestures.

The processes involved in modeling, for both nurse and client, include attention to the model, retention of the characteristics and behaviors of the model, and motor reproduction of those behaviors. For the nurse, there is the additional step of motivating the client to incorporate the behavior.

Locus of Control

The concept of locus of control explains people's perceptions of who or what is in control of their lives and their environment. A sense of an *internal locus of control* is based on a belief that outcomes are determined by one's own actions and are therefore under one's personal control. A sense of an *external locus of control* is based on a belief that outcomes of behavior and situations are determined by fate, chance, or authority figures and are thus beyond one's control.[18]

If people develop an *internal* locus of control, they tend to assume responsibility for themselves, their actions, their successes, their predicaments, their health, and sometimes their environment as well. From a social-learning perspective, these people are motivated to change because they believe that learning new ways of behaving, thinking, or feeling will alter the ways they interact with and influence the environment.

People who develop an *external* locus of control tend to assume that their lives are influenced by others and by external events. They do not take responsibility for their actions, they blame others for their predicaments, and they view success and good health as matters of luck. From a social-learning perspective, these people may not be as motivated to change as those with an internal locus of control. Since they believe that their lives are controlled by outside forces, they may not see how changing their ways of behaving, thinking, or feeling will make a difference.

Knowledge about clients' locus of control provides information about how they make decisions, their sense of personal power and control over their lives, and their styles of coping under stress.

Locus-of-control theory assumes that whether a behavior can or will occur is a function of the expectation that it will lead to positive reinforcement or reward. The reward becomes a cue: it notifies the client that the behavior is desirable. When people perceive two situations as similar, according to social-learning theory, their expectations are that if reinforcement or reward occurs in one situation it will also occur in the other—it will generalize from one situation to another.[18] For example, if assertiveness is rewarded (reinforced positively) in nurse-client relationships, then clients will expect to be rewarded in real-life situations if they behave assertively. If clients are rewarded by their families when they are nonassertive, then they will expect to be rewarded in social situations when they act nonassertively. It is important, therefore, for nurses to identify what reinforcements exist for current behavior patterns and what reinforcements are needed to motivate new behavior. Unless the reinforcements for new behavior patterns are perceived by clients as more rewarding than the reinforcements for old behavior patterns, they will not become motivators.

Contracts

An important aspect of the teaching-learning process is clarification of the roles, responsibilities, expectations, goals, and time limitations of the helping relationship. A *contract* is an oral or written agreement between nurse and client that makes them equal participants in the therapeutic process. A contract takes the general form of a statement that the nurse-client relationship will be a vehicle for the client to work on problems and seek solutions. Nurses enter into two types of contracts with their clients: informal and formal.

An *informal contract* takes the form of a promise or oral agreement about what can be expected of the client or the nurse. Such a promise usually addresses daily living within a therapeutic milieu. If a promise made in an informal contract is kept, it can provide a foundation of trust; if it is not kept, it can have negative consequences. For example, a nurse may promise to return in 15 minutes to spend time with a client who appeared distressed during nursing rounds. If the nurse fails to honor this contract by forgetting to return to the client in the specified time, then the client may perceive that he or she is unimportant or unworthy—or that the nurse is not trustworthy. Such perceptions may set up a pattern that is generalized to a global distrust of all health professionals and a self-evaluation of worthlessness.

A *formal contract* is an agreement negotiated between nurse and client; it may or may not be set down in writing and signed by both. The contract specifies what the nurse and client will do in specific circumstances and what each expects of the other. For example, the nurse makes a contract with an adolescent client specifying that they will be able to talk together whenever the adolescent experiences the tension associated with destructive impulses and behaviors. The adolescent's part of this agreement is to seek out the nurse and to talk about feelings rather than act them out in a destructive way. Another example would be a contract specifying that nurse and client will meet several times to collaborate on resolving the client's problems. This type of contract notes the purposes, times, places, and ground rules of the meetings.[19] A model for a written formal contract between a nurse and hospitalized client is presented in Table 24-10.

Table 24-10 Contract for Individual Counseling Sessions

Client: Annie S.	_______________ (signature)
Nurse: Susan M., RN	_______________ (signature)
Activity:	Regularly scheduled counseling meetings at which both nurse and client are present.
Purpose:	To reduce the stress of being discharged back into the community after hospitalization. To discuss issues related to discharge such as, "Where is home? What do I need to know about medications? What type of follow-up care is available for health maintenance? What help will be needed to perform activities of daily living? What can be done to reduce loneliness and isolation? How do I approach reestablishing communication with family? How do I find friends? How do I interact with neighbors?"
Time:	Tuesdays and Thursdays from 9 to 9:30 A.M.
Place:	Kepper Building, room 267.
Duration:	Twelve sessions from September 8 to October 15.
Ground rules:	All information is kept confidential except when there is an indication that withholding information from the treatment team would be harmful to the client. The client is expected to be on time and attend all sessions. Smoking will be permitted. If the nurse is unable to attend a session, she will notify the client by phone at least one day before the meeting. If the client is unable to attend a session, she will notify the nurse by phone at least one day before the meeting. The client agrees to refrain from the use of illicit drugs and alcohol while on passes. At the end of the twelve sessions, the nurse and client agree to evaluate whether the purposes of the meetings have been adequately addressed.

SUMMARY

Behavioral theorists hold that people have neither intrapsychic nor interpersonal difficulties; rather, they have behavioral problems. All behaviors are learned and are responses to stimuli. Rewarded responses can become habits, which are long-standing patterns of interaction. According to Wolpe, behavior is a conditioned response, and the goal of behavioral therapy is to decondition and consequently alter maladaptive behavior. There are four deconditioning methods: assertive behavior, systematic desensitization, evocation of strong anxiety, and operant conditioning. Three learning principles underlie Wolpe's behavioral therapy: reciprocal inhibition, positive reconditioning, and experimental extinction.

Miller and Dollard combine the Freudian outlook and Pavlov's learning theories in their behavioral theory. They identify two kinds of conflict: avoidance-avoidance conflict and approach-avoidance conflict. The four learning principles of Miller and Dollard are extinction, spontaneous recovery, generalization, and discrimination. Nurses can use these principles in treating clients.

Assertiveness training teaches people to affirm themselves positively and assuredly. It is a process that teaches people socially appropriate behavior for expression of thoughts, feelings, attitudes, wishes, opinions, and rights. Skills training, reduction of anxiety, restructuring of cognition, and assertiveness scripts are techniques used in assertiveness training.

The area of cognition includes the abilities to think, reason, understand, and remember. Cognitive theorists seek to help clients understand how their negative and conflicting thought patterns influence their appraisal of certain situations and their exaggerated or inappropriate emotional reactions.

The concept of social learning helps integrate behavioral and cognitive theories. In social-learning theory, psychological functioning is seen as a reciprocal relationship among personal, behavioral, and environmental factors. People are able to interact with their environment in healthy ways when they can recognize environmental potentials, assess their role prescriptions, and gain better control of their cognitive processes.

Cognitive therapy makes use of five principles: (1) focusing on the here and now; (2) making inferences, connections, and generalizations that are comprehensible to the client; (3) teaching clients to generalize directly from conscious experiences; (4) helping clients to test, refine, and accept or reject data in experiences outside of therapy; and (5) changing dysrhythmic patterns of behavior to rhythmic patterns through the educational process. These five principles closely parallel aspects of the teaching-learning process, which is a major component of the role of psychiatric nurses.

Teaching-learning is an interpersonal process through which change occurs as a result of planned input. It offers clients opportunities to engage in activities that influence their behavior and produce change in the knowledge, attitudes, and skills required to maintain and improve health. Adult and adolescent learners are capable of self-direction. Their life experience may be a resource or a barrier to learning. The learner's perspective is problem-centered and characterized by a sense of immediacy. Learning objectives are helpful in guiding and evaluating progress when stated clearly, specifically, and incrementally. The teaching-learning process involves therapeutic interactions between client and nurse. Feedback is an important component of teaching-learning process. Modeling serves an informative function in the process. The concept of locus of control, which explains people's perceptions of who or what is in control of their lives and their environment, can assist nurses in their treatment of clients. Contracts are verbal or written agreements between nurse and client that facilitate mutual participation in the process of change.

REFERENCES

1. J. Wolpe, *The Practice of Behavior Therapy,* 2d ed., Pergamon, New York, 1973.
2. Neal Miller and John Dollard, *Social Learning and Imitation,* Yale University Press, New Haven, Conn., 1941.
3. R. E. Alberti and M. L. Emmons, *Your Perfect Right,* Impact, St. Louis, 1978.
4. S. A. Bower and G. H. Bower, *Asserting Yourself,* Addison-Wesley, Reading, Mass., 1976.
5. M. Smith, *When I Say No I Feel Guilty,* Bantam, New York, 1975.
6. K. McQuade, "Assertiveness Training," in S. Lego, ed., *Handbook of Psychiatric Nursing,* Lippincott, Philadelphia, 1984, pp. 349–355.
7. H. Fensterheim and J. Baer, *Don't Say Yes When You Want to Say No,* Dell, New York, 1975.
8. A. Bandura, *Social Learning Theory,* Prentice-Hall, Englewood Cliffs, N. J., 1977.
9. I. M. Ahammer, "Social Learning as a Framework for the Study of Adult Personality," in P. Boltes and W. Shore, eds., *Lifespan Developmental Psychology,* Academic Press, New York, 1973.
10. A. T. Beck, *Cognitive Therapy and Emotional Disorders,* New American Library, New York, 1976.
11. B. K. Redman, *The Process of Patient Teaching in Nursing,* 5th ed., Mosby, St. Louis, 1984.
12. M. S. Knowles, *The Modern Practice of Adult Education,* Association Press, New York, 1970.
13. S. H. Rankin and K. L. Duffy, *Patient Education: Issues, Principles and Guidelines,* Lippincott, Philadelphia, 1983.
14. R. E. Doyle, "Counseling Strategies: The Management of Learning," unpublished manuscript, St. John's University, New York, Division of Human Services, Counseling, 1984.
15. B. F. Skinner, *Science and Human Behavior,* Free Press, New York, 1953.
16. J. S. Brunner, *Toward a Theory of Instruction,* Norton, New York, 1966.
17. Hildegard Peplau, "Process and Concept of Learning," in S. Burd and M. Marshall, eds., *Clinical Approaches to Psychiatric Nursing,* Macmillan, New York, 1963.
18. J. B. Rotter, "Generalized Expectancies for Internal Versus External Control of Reinforcement," *Psychological Monographs: General and Applied,* vol. 80, no. 609, 1966, pp. 1–78.
19. M. Zingiri and P. Duffy, "Contracting with Patients in Day to Day Practice," *American Journal of Nursing,* vol. 80, no. 3, 1980, pp. 451–455.

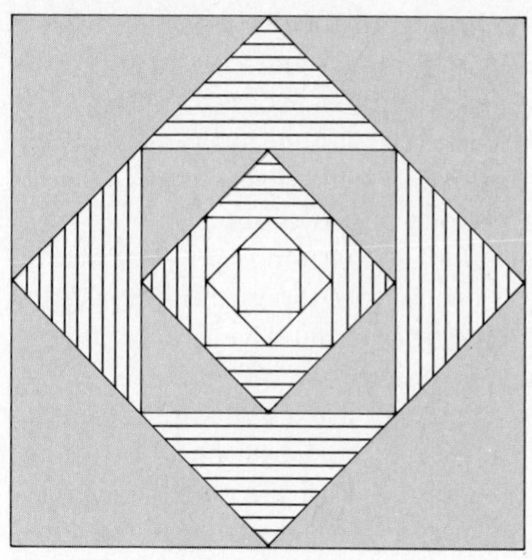

CHAPTER 25
Alternative Therapies

Joy A. Feldman

LEARNING OBJECTIVES

After studying this chapter, the student should be able to:

1. Differentiate between the underlying assumptions of traditional and alternative therapies.
2. Discuss the premises and expected outcomes of using leisure arts as approaches to therapeutic intervention.
3. Identify leisure arts utilized in the treatment of emotionally dysfunctional clients.
4. Evaluate leisure arts activities appropriate for clients in psychiatric–mental health settings.
5. Describe the role of rehabilitative skills in restorative nursing care of chronically impaired clients.
6. Identify rehabilitative resources available to clients.
7. Describe the premises and expected outcomes of selected psychological growth therapies.
8. Describe the premises and expected outcomes of selected mind-body awareness therapies.
9. Discuss the premises and expected outcomes of consciousness-development therapies.
10. Identify the alternative therapies that are appropriate for nurses to use in the promotion, maintenance, restoration, and rehabilitation of their clients' mental health.

Historically, *deviance*—inappropriate behavior or impaired functioning—has been considered the primary indicator that psychiatric treatment is necessary. It has been presumed that deviance is caused by underlying mental pathology. The term *alternative therapies* refers to treatment modalities which have come into use largely out of dissatisfaction with the medical model both as a way of viewing human functioning and as a basis for treatment.

The heart of the distinction between traditional and untraditional, or alternative, approaches is found in the focus of each. Traditional therapies focus on treating the impaired functioning of a client (defined traditionally as "illness"). Alternative therapies focus on helping a client to attain wholeness, growth, and self-realization. In general, the alternative therapies do not seek to address developmental issues underlying a person's behavior or affect; instead, they tend to deal with clients' immediate problems of living and with presently available solutions.

Basic tenets of life have changed, unavoidably reshaping sources of both satisfaction and stress. While the widespread increase of leisure time and the growth of material comforts are positively valued, the overriding milieu of ongoing and rapid social change is in and of itself highly stressful, and the toll it exacts is well-documented.[1]

Emerging from this milieu, the human potential movement grew, combining the evolving scientific understanding of the human being as a complex but unitary whole with the growing recognition of the need for meaning and self-actualization in a potentially meaningless—albeit comfortable—existence. Clinical evidence of existential distress in the face of apparent success illuminated the significance of the spiritual dimension for a person's well-being and wholeness. The human potential movement recognized that each person's unique potential for creativity and growth is derived from the interaction of the person's spiritual, mental, and physical capacities. It is believed that few people ever realize their full potential.

Healing of any sort is an interactional process of influence between the "sufferer" and the "healer" and is always a product of the ideological system in which it is embedded. A healer's perceptions of people and conceptions of what constitutes wellness, what represents illness or dysfunction, and what causes suffering provide foundation for ideas about how to intervene with dysfunction, correct it, or stimulate change and healing.

The purpose of this chapter is to deal with a range of untraditional treatment modalities that have emerged from somewhat divergent concepts of human behavior, health, and growth.

Leisure arts therapies are most often used as adjuncts to some other form of psychotherapy, traditional or alternative, and are used in a wide variety of treatment facilities. Leisure arts therapies considered in this chapter include art therapy, music therapy, dance and movement therapy, poetry and literature therapy, pet therapy, and plant therapy.

Institutionalized clients must develop rehabilitative skills to facilitate their transition to living situations characterized by increased independence. Socialization therapy, occupational therapy, and vocational rehabilitation will be included here in the discussion of rehabilitative skills therapies.

The alternative psychotherapeutic approaches discussed in this chapter also include nine examples of psychological growth therapies and several mind-body awareness therapies and consciousness-development therapies.

LEISURE ARTS THERAPIES

Leisure arts therapies—also called *recreational therapies, expressive arts therapies,* or *creative arts therapies*—share the assumption that nonverbal expression of feelings is valuable because many dimensions of the self are inaccessible to (or at least restricted by) verbal expression: conflict resolution and growth are believed to follow self-expression. These therapies, therefore, have broad and versatile applicability for clients suffering any sort of dysfunction, as well as for those who are unimpaired but want a fuller exploration and realization of their potential.

Frequently clients who enter the mental health care system are found to have few (if any) interests and activities with which to structure and occupy their leisure time. This results in idle passing of time, most often through watching television, eating

Portions of this chapter from Anita M. Leach, "Alternative and Environmental Therapies," in the second edition of this book.

or drinking to excess, or simply sitting and doing nothing. In the presence of affective or cognitive disturbance, such empty time may serve to intensify a person's preoccupation with perceived difficulties. Certainly, it perpetuates an assumption of uselessness and poor self-esteem, through a somatic lethargy that is self-perpetuating. Constructive recreational activities, by contrast, provide avenues for developing competence at those activities, a common ground on which to interact with others, and consequent stimulation and interest in living.

One does not have to be impaired to benefit from constructive use of leisure time. Many humanists endorse leisure arts therapy for every member of society to facilitate growth toward self-improvement and realization of unique potential.

When used in mental health treatment settings, leisure arts or recreational therapy is most often designed and lead by a therapist who has a master's degree. However, use of leisure time may fall into the domain of nursing as a dimension of milieu therapy (see Chapter 17). Attention must be given to the ages, capabilities, and interests of clients in planning activities to be engaged in and taught.

The leisure arts therapies discussed here include art therapy, music therapy, dance and movement therapy, poetry and literature therapy, pet therapy, and plant therapy. Each of these uses a creative means of self-expression to promote wellness.

Use of creative arts, whether for healing, self-actualization, or therapy, stems from recognition of the unitary yet multidimensional nature of the human being and the wealth of communication and self-expression which occurs naturally in nonverbal realms. Feelings, experiences, thoughts, and spiritual aspects of the self which do not lend themselves to being captured and conveyed in words become constricted, untapped, or distorted if the therapeutic process is confined to exclusively verbal interaction. Some clients who are unresponsive to talking therapies may be reached through nonverbal approaches. There are some, isolated in a world of silence, for whom the arts may be the only bridge to others. Expressive arts combined with verbal exchange and therapeutic guidance can promote insight; greatly increase self-awareness; and provide activity which is absorbing, self-expressive, creative, and satisfying.

Leisure arts may be used directly as adjuncts to traditional psychotherapy or as techniques in the context of psychotherapy, or they may be available simply as therapeutic aspects of the milieu. Specialized graduate-level education is required to prepare therapists for these treatment modalities. Nurses may participate with clients in these health-promoting activities, or they may simply help and encourage clients to engage in them. People for whom verbal communication is particularly difficult—whether because of psychosocial dysfunction, physical handicap, or cultural or age barriers—are particularly good candidates for these therapies.

Art Therapy

The field of art therapy is a young, developing one, replete with diverse philosophies and theoretical orientations. The practice of art therapy requires a master's degree. A professional organization, American Art Therapy Association, defined art therapy in its 1977 directory in terms that reflect both psychoanalytic and humanist orientations. The definition acknowledged two major approaches in art therapy: one uses the creative process to reconcile internal conflicts and foster personal development, and the other uses it to gain access to the inner world in order to achieve insight. The predominant orientation of art therapists seems to be psychoanalytic; most rely heavily on symbolism and place a high value on self-expression for the sake of catharsis.[2]

The central utility of art as a therapeutic medium is its rich, multidimensional symbolism. Drawing and painting are the predominant media. A client's feelings, perceptions, and underlying thought processes are thought to be revealed through such aspects of the created work as content, position and relative sizes of drawn objects and people, and use of color. Images produced frequently reveal what may not be recognized consciously by the client, providing clues for assessment and material for discussion in therapeutic sessions.

Children, in particular, can convey through art perceptions of their world well beyond what they could find words for, much less recognize the importance of. For example:

> It was through drawing and painting that a breakthrough finally occurred with a 5-year-old girl. Two years after her parents' divorce, she was still trying terribly hard to be an ideal child, yet she was given to sudden outbursts of tears and night terrors. She

painted a picture of her family—daddy, Ann (dad's wife), and herself—happily at home; off in the lower corner of the page lay a tiny female figure. "Oh, that," she explained "is my mommy. She must be dead." Her biological mother had never explained her absence, was in fact highly unpredictable in her rare visits, and was unavailable to the child overall. Clarification of the child's reality allowed the nurse to stimulate greater understanding from her custodial parents in supporting her through grieving over the loss of her mother.

Art therapy has also found a place in facilitating family therapy. Family members may be asked to draw the family as each sees it or to share in developing a collective family portrait; individual and collective portraits provide significant assessment information and stimulate meaningful communication. "The way we perceive visually is directly related to the way we think and feel."[2] Drawn images have both diagnostic and therapeutic value.

Many art therapists value highly the cathartic function art serves. It enables nonverbal, unreachable clients to communicate, and it provides nondestructive, nondirective, and nonthreatening means of expressing aggression, anger, tension, energy, and sexuality. Art therapists with a humanist orientation believe that the value of a creative act transcends mere catharsis. They see it as a way of reaching out and creating new beauty from the wellspring of the inner self. Uniting the field is agreement that art therapy promotes self-expression and creative impulses and, therefore, functions as both a diagnostic tool and a way to promote growth. Art therapy is broadly applicable as a modality for use with individuals or groups and is used in various treatment settings, such as inpatient units, day care facilities, nursing homes, outpatient clinics, and private offices.

Music Therapy

While it has been recognized over the ages that music is able to calm as well as stimulate the emotions, it was not until World War II that music came into widespread use as a therapeutic modality. Faced with numbers of clients well beyond what could be dealt with in traditional psychotherapy, American veterans' hospitals pioneered *music therapy,* the use of music to provide activity and support for mentally disturbed patients. Research through the 1940s and 1950s explored the relationship of music to physiology, mood changes, and behavior. Researchers found measurable changes in mood and general activity among schizophrenics listening to music. Listening to or playing music also reduced depression.[2] The comprehensive music therapy programs that were developed as a result of these findings were staffed largely by music teachers. By the 1960s university programs in music therapy were well-established, and a master's degree in music therapy is now the usual preparation for a therapist.[3]

Music therapy aims to bring about behavioral change by stimulating motivation, enjoyment, and relaxation. More than the other expressive arts therapies, music therapy adheres to behavioral objectives, and it differs from music education only in that the focus is not on the learners' *musical* behavior but on their general, nonmusical behavior.

Instruments used frequently in music therapy are those in common use in early-childhood music education, such as tambourines, triangles, woodtone instruments, bells, cymbals, and some of the wind and string instruments. These instruments can be learned quickly and easily. In music-making groups, each client makes his or her own unique sound, which promotes individual identity, and at the same time, each collaborates with the others in a prosocial way to create harmonious music which is, indeed, greater than the sum of the individual sounds.

Music therapy also takes the form of a client working individually with a therapist to develop musical skill and knowledge. This is a very effective way to enhance self-esteem and provide a client with a social asset as well as a constructive leisure activity.

Another form of music therapy is listening to music selected purposefully to affect mood, activity, or self-expression; this may occur in dyadic or group therapy sessions. Music therapists point out the essentially social implications of music. Music is shared, and it invites response and reaction, whether one is interacting with others in order to make music or listening in silence while others are playing. Music can be a most effective and nonthreatening means of luring a withdrawn person out of his or her closed world. It is universal in the human experience, touches one's innermost soul, is easily accessible, and is widely applicable to clients of any sort.

Dance and Movement Therapy

The use of dance and movement for therapeutic purposes is called *dance and movement therapy.* Like music therapy, it emerged during World War II in response to the large number of people needing treatment, which exceeded the number of therapists available to give traditional, one-to-one, psychoanalytic treatment. Marian Chase, credited as the founder of dance therapy, began a dance program in 1941 at St. Elizabeth's Hospital for the purpose of fostering communication and expression among clients.

Through the early years dance and movement therapy was used predominantly for cathartic purposes, providing a medium for safely and creatively expressing or acting out tensions, anger, and anxiety. This was found to be particularly helpful for people whose ability to communicate their feelings verbally was very limited. The release of emotions is seen by many practitioners as, in and of itself, healing. Others, including dance therapists of psychoanalytic orientation, see cathartic release as temporary relief rather than facilitative of any change in the underlying problem: movement can help enormously to stimulate recognition of a problem or conflict, but it is naive to presume that awareness of a problem is the same as learning to cope with it. A therapist must actively help a client to translate awareness into learning how to cope better.

Another valuable application of dance and movement therapy derives from the *reciprocal inhibition principle,* which posits that relief in one aspect of a problem will interrupt another aspect. Relaxation training springs from this principle. It demonstrates the validity of using deep breathing or progressive relaxation to counteract the increase of physical signs of mounting tension once the onset has been recognized. Dance and movement can be used to the same effect. For example, dance or other nonverbal expressions of anger can be used to interrupt a pattern of blocking expression of such feelings and then, as a result, needing to seek relief through destructive alternatives, such as impulsive acting out or drinking.

Poetry and Literature Therapy

Change—whether cognitive, affective, or behavioral—is the purpose of therapy. When clients' problems suggest the need for conceptual and cognitive or attitudinal and affective growth, poetry or other literature may be used to achieve therapeutic goals. This is called *poetry and literature therapy* or *bibliotherapy.*

The diversity and availability of literature renders it a rich resource. An appropriate book may be selected and recommended to a client. Objectives may be to broaden knowledge and awareness of alternative solutions to problems in living; to develop understanding of personalities, behaviors, and values demonstrated by the book's characters; and to broaden a client's experience vicariously. Discussion of thoughts, reactions, and feelings stimulated by their reading is important, as it clarifies and enhances clients' understanding of their own experiences in comparison with what has been read. Poetry, in particular, is useful in stimulating thought and discussion about one's own perceptions and feelings. Exploration of the symbolism and meaning poetry may have for clients can effectively touch the spiritual realm while promoting new insights into the self and enlarging a therapist's understanding of clients.

Poetry and literature therapy and related discussions may occur individually with clients or in a group in which everyone participates in reading and sharing responses. These activities are frequently led by nurses. They have enormous potential for addressing a range of clients' learning needs and are particularly applicable with literate clients who are already comfortable about reading.

Pet Therapy

Pets have been found highly beneficial to clients in a variety of situations—astonishingly so in comparison with the slight cost and effort of maintaining them. People who have little to occupy their time and attention—for example, elderly people with impaired mobility and energy—may derive great pleasure from the company and attention of pets and from the need to care for them. Clients for whom human relationships are threatening and seen as unreliable may respond to and invest in a pet as an ever-present source of companionship, unconditional affection, and loyalty.

The use of animals to achieve therapeutic measures in health care facilities is sometimes called *pet therapy.* In addition to the nonthreatening yet comforting relationships pets can offer, their natural dependence on humans can elicit responsibility and nurturing from a client who lacks a role complement or is impaired in these dimensions on the human level. In this regard, pets may be used as a means of teaching healthy relational patterns of behavior.

Nurses may introduce pets into a facility to serve both therapeutic and recreational functions. Animals which are easy to care for yet give a high degree of satisfaction include the range of common domestic pets: cats, dogs, birds, and tropical fish or amphibians housed in aquariums. Such pets may be shared by the client population or individually owned, depending on the nature of the facility.

Plant Therapy

In *plant therapy*, plants are used to achieve therapeutic goals. Inexpensive to acquire and maintain, plants are an ideal vehicle for teaching clients care of nonthreatening yet living things. Many plants are easily propagated, allowing the client satisfaction from the experience of nurturing a growing thing while at the same time beautifying the surroundings.

Plant therapy is in many respects similar to pet therapy. It may be carried out with clients as a group or individually. When a group is involved, plants offer a focus and stimulate cooperation and discussion. In sharing responsibility for and ideas about plant care, clients can be encouraged to make connections between plant growth and human relationships and growth. Plant therapy can be used to foster rapport between individuals. Clients can find analogies between the growth of their plants and the growth of trust and caring in human relationships, noting the need for patience and nurturing. Plants may be seen as tangible and lovely symbols of the experience the client has gone through and may be left as expressions of gratitude to the staff and other clients.

RELEVANCE TO NURSING

While nurses are not leisure arts therapists, as "architects" and round-the-clock managers of the milieu, they can initiate and promote the use of adjunctive therapeutic activities in the treatment setting. In particular, pets, plants, literature, and supplies for art and music are materials within the purview of nursing responsibilities, and the support of nurses is necessary in order to maintain them in the milieu. With nursing's expanded understanding of humans as multidimensional beings, the relevance and importance of these diverse therapeutic agents and activities becomes apparent.

As primary care givers, nurses are in an optimal position to observe and assess clients' potential for and responses to creative, nurturing, and leisure activities. They also collaborate with clients and therapists in planning and evaluating treatment. Encouragement of clients' participation in such activities needs to be tailored to each client and incorporated into individualized care plans. Nurses' familiarity with and participation in leisure arts and recreational therapies can foster clients' willingness and motivation toward involvement. Nursing leadership and participation in such activities is particularly important in combating the low motivation, anergia, and withdrawal which characterize many of the clients in treatment settings and in promoting skill development in social interaction, communication, and collaboration.

REHABILITATIVE SKILLS THERAPIES

Rehabilitative skills therapies assume that basic skills necessary for daily living are therapeutic priorities in caring for dysfunctional clients. Behavioral improvement is the goal of rehabilitative therapies, and insight, self-awareness, and emotional growth are not seen as prerequisites to this. Rehabilitative skills therapies include socialization therapy, occupational therapy, and vocational rehabilitation.

Rehabilitative skills therapies aim to promote competence in the full range of behaviors necessary for daily living, satisfying use of leisure time, and the accomplishment of some form of work. The focus of rehabilitation is on outcome behaviors and learned competencies. Pragmatic approaches to practical problems in daily living are emphasized, with the recognition that successful adjustment to living outside of institutional care rests as heavily on a client's ability to cope with daily needs as on the stability of the client's thought processes and moods.

Skills training may begin with personal grooming skills and very basic social skills. At a higher level, rehabilitative group activities commonly include planning meals, choosing representatives to purchase the necessary items, preparing meals, and cleaning up afterwards; maintenance of surroundings; leisure time activities such as picnicking, sports, sewing, crafts, sharing newspapers, and playing games. Inherent in these activities is the need for interpersonal communication, negotiation, and socialization. Development of these skills is especially valuable, since loneliness is a major problem for many clients. Rehabilitative therapies are implemented in settings such as hospitals, day treatment centers, halfway houses, sheltered workshops, extended-care facilities, supervised apartments, and boarding houses.

Socialization Therapy

Socialization therapy addresses an aspect of rehabilitation by involving clients in informal groups or clubs to promote the development of social skills. The goal is acquisition of social skills which will both improve clients' subjective satisfaction and smooth their transition from living in protective environments to living in the community. These groups or clubs are frequently part of the halfway house setting. Mental health facilities and community organizations may maintain groups for ex-clients. Club activities may involve cooking, attending forms of entertainment together, picnicking, or any generally enjoyable activity. Nurses may be involved as facilitators of these informal social groups.

Occupational Therapy

Occupational therapy, which was formally established as a distinct modality in 1917, is defined as the art and science of directing a person's participation in selected, meaningful, occupation-oriented activities. The expressed aim of occupational therapy is to help the physically and mentally disabled to develop and maintain capabilities that aid self-mastery and role fulfillment in productive living. This aim is achieved by directing clients in goal-oriented activities which promote productivity, social performance, and health, while they diminish or correct pathology.

"Occupational therapy emphasizes learning by doing and is based on the belief that physical accomplishment is an essential source of satisfaction."[4] Learned or relearned skills, whether they are recreational or potentially remunerative, enhance self-esteem, self-confidence, and satisfaction through purposeful and productive use of time. Nurses are well-positioned to promote clients' participation in occupational therapy and may serve clients best by understanding and supporting the multiple benefits to be derived from engaging in such planned activities. Nurses share close working relationships with occupational therapists. Frequently nurses carry out the plans developed by occupational therapists when it is advantageous or necessary for those activities to occur directly on the unit. When a client is acutely ill, when mobility is impaired or restricted for purposes of behavior modification, or when the familiarity and safety of the unit is needed, occupational therapy projects can be brought to a client and facilitated by the nurse.

Vocational Rehabilitation

Vocational rehabilitation aims to establish and maintain clients in jobs through:

1. Evaluation of their interests and abilities
2. Services designed to reduce their handicaps
3. Job training
4. Job placement
5. Personal counseling through the entire period to facilitate successful transition and adjustment

Federal legislation in 1943 (Barden–La Follette amendment) instructed state rehabilitation bureaus to extend remedial services to include job placement of mentally and physically handicapped persons; thus each psychiatrically impaired client is entitled to such services. In each state, there is an agency or a division of an agency that provides vocational rehabilitation.

Vocational rehabilitation is based on the belief that work is a natural component of life and intimately related to one's self-esteem and sense of worth. Work provides an opportunity to express creativity, apply one's abilities, accomplish things and take pride in one's accomplishments, and form satisfying relationships with coworkers. The work one is trained for and accomplishes is a significant dimension of the definition of self.

Equal to the qualitative benefits of working is the pragmatic reality that a means of economic support is essential if one is to maintain an adequate lifestyle outside an institution. Motivating a client and helping the person make the transition from being a cared-for, dependent client to being a person who is employed is among the greatest challenges of working with chronic clients. The successful meeting of this challenge is of major significance in delaying or preventing a client's return to the institution.

RELEVANCE TO NURSING

Most psychiatric nurses are working in secondary and tertiary treatment settings. In such settings, a primary goal of nursing care is to influence the client toward greater self-reliance. Nursing action must strive to enhance self-esteem, self-confidence, and motivation, and these qualities are derived largely from interpersonal relationships. Yet self-esteem, self-confidence, and motivation are not ends in themselves but means to developing or restoring impaired clients to levels of self-reliance and interpersonal skills appropriate to chronological age. Acquisition of skills and knowledge, constructive use of physical and creative capacities, and preparation for assuming a vocational role are central to such restorative goals.

Rehabilitative skills therapies are vital components in secondary and tertiary care, in which the nurse is involved in initiating referrals, facilitating clients' involvement, reinforcing clients' gains, and evaluating progress. As managers of the treatment milieu, nurses are in the most advantageous position to support and monitor clients' progress in acquiring skills, and frequently they function as treatment coordinators with the allied health care professionals.

PSYCHOLOGICAL GROWTH THERAPIES

Psychological growth therapies share assumptions about the dominance of cognitive perspectives over emotional or behavioral functioning. Limitations, conflicts, or signs of distress are seen as products of people's systems of belief and expectations about themselves in relation to others. The goal of psychological growth therapies is to alter clients' belief systems and thereby expand their awareness of potential for greater self-reliance and personal responsibility. These therapies aim toward reaching higher levels of maturity and overcoming inhibitions against fully experiencing feelings, opportunities, and constructive activities.

Psychological growth therapies expand awareness of the holistic nature of human functioning and readily offer implications for nursing practice. The therapies selected for a brief discussion here are gestalt therapy, psychodrama, play therapy, social network therapy, videotherapy, encounter marathon groups, reality therapy, rational-emotive therapy, and Morita therapy.

Gestalt Therapy

Gestalt therapy, one of the best known of the humanist schools, was founded by Frederick S. Perls, M.D., Ph.D., during the 1960s. *Gestalt therapy* emphasizes conceptualization and treatment of people as biopsychosocial wholes. Gestalt therapy is theoretically based in modern psychology and psychotherapy, but Perls stressed the simplicity of the basic gestalt principle: while the organism is naturally developing and growing, one's continuum of awareness works to organize experience and perceptions into wholes, or gestalts. *Gestalts* are patterns involving all levels of one's functioning in interaction with the environment; they follow the laws of nature in tending toward harmony and dynamic growth, creativity and expression. Distress results from incomplete gestalts, an unnatural splitting in dynamic processes, and is manifested in one's awareness of the here-and-now gestalt. Gestalt therapy maintains that "unfinished business" emerges in one's awareness as something requiring resolution. Usually, incomplete gestalts emerge in behavior in the form of avoidance: Perls emphasized pain as nature's signal of distress and pointed out that humans tend to avoid pain. Gestalt therapy, therefore, focuses on the here and now rather than seeking to elicit recollections of the past or expectations of the future.

Gestalt therapists act as catalysts to stimulate clients to work through their sources of anxiety by mobilizing their internal resources, thus restoring growth. They do not offer their clients unconditional positive regard; instead, they deal directly with clients' resistance.

This therapy requires some degree of self-awareness and motivation toward increased emotional experience and interpersonal relationships; thus it is unlikely to be suitable as an approach to chronically psychotic clients. Best-suited to the gestalt approach are intellectual clients who tend to be restricted and constricted in their relationships with others and who feel stultified, unsatisfied, and alienated in their day-to-day lives.

Gestalt therapy can be used in individual treatment, but group treatment is more common. Frequently, gestalt therapy achieves its ends through creating rather intense emotional experiences in group therapy. The approach requires clients to identify *personal* changes they desire, strives to help them recognize ways in which they defeat themselves, and helps them to experiment with change—here and now. Perls identifies the aims of gestalt therapy as follows: to grow up; to mature; to be personally responsible for one's self; and to become whole, fully alive, responsive, creative, flexible, and expressive.[5]

Psychodrama

Psychodrama is the dramatization of clients' personal and interactional problems. In psychodrama, theatrical media such as a stage and lights are used; there is a director; and dramatic techniques such as role playing, role reversal, and soliloquies are used to develop and portray clients' reality.

J. L. Moreno, a Viennese psychiatrist who was the first to use the term *group psychotherapy* in discussing his approach to treatment, originated psychodrama as a specialized form of group therapy.

Moreno recognized the importance of role and social context as determinants of behavior. He explored the potential for conflict arising from the multiplicity of roles each person must assume in the increasingly complex social world. While role prescriptions may not account for the vastness of human psychic functioning, they nonetheless give structure and meaning to the process of daily living.

The psychodrama process involves each group member. Each member in turn acts out with the other participants the "role dilemmas" that are involved in his or her conflicts. The therapist, called the *director* in psychodrama, facilitates the enactment of these roles, eliciting accompanying feelings and thoughts, illuminating and correcting maladaptive patterns, while interacting therapeutically with all members of the group. Most practitioners of psychodrama have a group session following a dramatization in order to complete exploration of the feelings and recognitions evoked in the drama and to relate these gains to real-life situations.[6]

The goals of psychodrama are improved role adjustment and increased interpersonal awareness, empathic understanding, spontaneity, and accurate understanding of reality. This is a highly complex treatment modality requiring training and supervision at the postgraduate level. Nurses may be involved in supportive or facilitative roles for the group.

Play Therapy

Play therapy is a predominantly nonverbal, activity-oriented form of psychotherapy. Clients are encouraged to act out imaginative play with toys, puppets, art materials, or other items furnished by therapists. Clients may explain what they are doing, and the therapist may make observations about the meaning of the play or give explanations and interpretations as needed by clients.

The goal of play therapy is to allow and promote communication in a nonthreatening manner with people for whom verbal communication is limited. Clients such as young children; regressed, aged adults; or regressed psychotic clients are often good candidates for this technique. Pediatric and psychiatric nurses are among those who may become skilled in the use of play therapy. It is a treatment modality heavily relied upon by mental health professionals who specialize in working with children.

Social Network Therapy

Social network therapy is a modification of family therapy and reflects a systems-theory approach to facilitating successful adjustment in the community. A client's system is seen to include all the people with whom he or she comes into contact in daily life, such as immediate and extended family, neighbors, coworkers, community agency personnel, and tradespeople. All the people who constitute a client's social network come together to meet in group sessions with the client. This is used as a means of assessing the client's interactions with others in various roles, facilitating role performance with others, clarifying the extent of social support, and planning reentry into the community.

A disadvantage of social network therapy is certainly the unwieldy task of communicating with and coordinating meetings of diverse groups of people. Those who see themselves as uninvolved with a client (or wish they were so) are unlikely to cooperate. There are cases, however, for which this is an ideal solution to confusion and inability to plan adequately because of a history of fragmented and sporadic involvement by various care givers.

Videotherapy

Videotape-recorded playback (VTRP) emerged in the mid-1960s as a widely applicable tool for mental health practitioners. The use of video technology to evoke accurate awareness and to promote therapeutic interaction is called *videotherapy*. Video playback can be used as an adjunct to other treatment modalities in order to provide information to clients or to confront them with certain aspects of their thinking, behaving, or emoting. It can also be used to train clients in social skills through modeling and even to train clients in the occupational skills involved in the use of video equipment.

When VTRP is used as a tool in therapy sessions, segments of interaction between client and therapist are played back for specific purposes. Playback may be scheduled, with time reserved for this activity, or it may be situation-dependent, that is, used from time to time in the course of treatment to call attention to nonverbal levels of communication. Guided exploration of clients' reactions and the implications of what is observed on tape are critical in promoting therapeutic goals. At its most basic, objective viewing of problematic behavior can help clients move toward eliminating such behavior—since recognition must precede efforts to change. VTRP has also been combined successfully with guidance in teaching chronic schizophrenic clients basic social skills while also promoting interaction among the clients.[7]

VTRP increases anxiety (this has been documented with measurements of increased galvanic skin responses). Presumably, this anxiety is secondary to the anxiety caused by the stripping away of defenses which occurs with objective viewing of the self.[7] This heightened anxiety can be positive in that it can motivate clients to change. Additionally, such objective feedback is likely to alter self-concepts. The direction of changes which occur is dependent on the content played back in combination with therapists' handling of situations.

Clearly this treatment modality requires a high level of competence and adequate training in specialized skills; it is not appropriate for use by inexperienced professionals. Care must be taken not only in managing clients' exploration but also in selecting clients for this therapy. Those who are actively delusional and those who are severely paranoid are generally considered inappropriate candidates for this approach.

Another potential benefit of the use of videotape in therapy is the expansion of opportunities for evaluation and supervision of the therapeutic relationship and process. Therapists will view themselves with fresh eyes, even though the client is the focus of the setting. The ability to "see again" segments of complex communication enables confirmation of recollections or correction of them, suggesting need for further exploration. The use of videotape affords therapists more flexibility; as a result, it can lead to greatly improved objectivity in the supervisory process.

Confidentiality becomes an important concern with use of video technology; another concern is the client's comfort in front of video cameras. These two issues are critical in determining the usefulness of videotherapy. Full explanation must precede any use of VTRP. Clients must be given information explicitly detailing how tapes will be used before they sign the required legal consent forms. Videotapes may be used for therapeutic purposes in sessions with clients, for learning purposes in the supervision of therapists, and for general teaching purposes. Clients have the right to preview tapes before consenting to their use outside the sessions.

Video technology has been employed successfully in inpatient, outpatient, group, marital, family, and individual therapies. Nurses may facilitate the use of video techniques or be involved directly as videotherapists. In either role the prime goals of nursing care are the comfort and care of clients and the preservation of clients' rights to privacy.

Encounter Marathon Groups

The encounter group movement sprang from the recognition of group psychotherapy as a powerful treatment approach and rapidly grew to a peak within the decade of the 1960s. The proliferation of encounter groups drew widespread attention as a social phenomenon. The encounter group movement was unchecked by standards or professional requirements for group leaders and unsupported by a theoretical base that could offer unifying goals or intermediate strategies to achieve those goals. The popularity of the movement has not continued unabated, yet encounter groups remain among the therapeutic modalities in use by many therapists in private practice who represent a spectrum of theoretical persuasions.

Unlike other forms of group therapy, *encounter marathon groups,* once convened, are held for a continuous period of time, usually beginning on a Friday evening and continuing through midday Sunday—hence the name *marathon.* They are held at specific times and places—often at a scenic retreat. The essential aspects of the encounter are intense personal and interpersonal involvement and openness. The focus is on achieving greater authenticity, openness, and intimacy, which for many is the purpose of the experience. For others the goals include resolving conflicts and identifying and developing necessary skills. People who seek encounter group experiences are generally not in deep distress but are basically well and are seeking more personal depth, spontaneity, sensitivity, and happiness in their lives.

Underlying the encounter group movement are the following assumptions: people are capable of exercising decisions and choices about their own behavior; emotional distress is a product of interactive patterns; and increased awareness of one's self and the way others experience one will provide useful information from which alternative behaviors and patterns can be chosen. At its best, the encounter group is a resource in which the group members and the therapist are therapeutic agents in an intensive experience intended to generate growth and personal development. At its worst, it can be unbridled group process marked by destructive confrontation and gratification of basic impulses. Traditionally oriented critics have observed the process as a brief and encapsulated attempt to counteract the boredom and alienation rampant in contemporary American society, noting the low risk involved in buying intensive human contact for a weekend's duration.

Responsible encounter group practitioners carefully screen interested participants, selecting those with adequate ego strength who can both tolerate and benefit from the closeness in the encounter group. Effective termination from the experience requires that the practitioner help the participants connect the encounter experience with their daily lives, thus underscoring the psychosocial lessons available from the marathon encounter.

Reality Therapy

William Glasser, a psychiatrist and the founder of *reality therapy,* contends that the primary psychological needs are to love and be loved, and to feel worthwhile to oneself and others. Inability to satisfy these psychological needs results in irresponsible behavior and failures at living, rather than "mental illness." Glasser does not deal with the development of problems; instead, he offers a here-and-now, behaviorally oriented approach to helping clients adjust successfully or at least learn what is interfering with their adjustment, allowing another approach to be tried.

The underlying assumption of reality therapy is that people are responsible for their own behavior and can change it if motivated to do so. Feelings are acknowledged, but recognition of how behavior contributes to creating feelings is emphasized.

In the context of therapeutic dyadic relationships, reality therapists offer clients high-quality attention, which Glasser calls *involvement,* and guide clients through objective assessment of their current behavior and development of plans for more responsible behavior in the future. Clients must then commit themselves to their plans. Commitment enhances motivation to fulfill plans. No excuses are accepted for failure to follow plans, but neither is any punishment imposed. Glasser sees this process as vital to stimulating change. He believes that punishment weakens the involvement necessary for clients to succeed. Praise for achieving responsible behavior and following plans, on the other hand, is given generously and promotes success.

Reality therapy has been used as a treatment modality with significant numbers of delinquent adolescent girls and psychotic inpatients at a veterans' hospital. Glasser reports a success rate of at least 80 percent with both groups. Proponents of reality therapy see it as a pragmatic and easily learned approach appropriate for use by people in authoritative roles in religious organizations, law enforcement agencies, health care systems, and educational facilities.

Rational-Emotive Therapy

Developed by the American psychologist Albert Ellis, *rational-emotive therapy* is based on the assumption that one's system of values and beliefs has defined certain experiences negatively and therefore produces emotional distress. If one changes negative beliefs about events or negative perceptions of the self or others by relabeling or reevaluating, then one's feelings are altered and are no longer troublesome.

This theoretical framework emphasizes the role of values interacting with cognitive processes in determining behavior and emotional well-being. A therapist takes a directive role to illuminate the negative or irrational nature of a client's beliefs (seen to have been learned from parents and the larger culture) and to persuade a client to adopt more constructive ideas.

Ellis sees this approach as particularly appropriate for relatively bright clients without significant impairment in their functioning, and he employs the encounter group as a medium for this therapy.

Morita Therapy

First developed in 1917 by the Japanese psychiatrist Morita, this treatment approach grew out of its originator's cure for his own heart palpitations, gastrointestinal disturbances, anxiety about death, and difficulty concentrating. Morita was struck by the self-absorption and obsession with excellence (including an obsession with feeling and being all that one wishes to feel and be) which are characteristics of this symptom complex. He noted that these characteristics actually obstruct the attainment of goals.

Central to *Morita therapy* is the assumption that states of feeling are not controllable, but "given" as part of the human condition. Therefore, it is a mistake to be so preoccupied with, for instance, an internal state of sadness, timidity, worry, joy, anticipation, or panic that daily tasks are neglected.

Second, Morita holds that each person is morally, socially, and personally responsible for what he or she does and is able to control behavior regardless of (uncontrollable) underlying feelings. This therapeutic expectation is based on the principle that productive and responsible behavior builds self-trust, which in turn positively influences one's states of feeling. For example, as one transcends a feeling state to attend constructively to life's tasks, one is no longer attending to, say, depression or anxiety. The feeling state has at best dissipated and at least been attenuated.

These first two principles are given direction by a third, the importance of purpose. Each person must recognize a purpose, control his or her behavior to fulfill that purpose, and accept whatever feelings are experienced as natural components of life. Morita therapists are directive; they teach clients, giving very explicit advice in the context of caring dyadic relationships.

RELEVANCE TO NURSING

While techniques, beliefs, and strategies differ among these psychological growth therapies, several commonalities unite them and suggest constructive beliefs and strategies applicable in nursing practice. The unifying beliefs in the dynamic nature of life; in the ability to learn and grow throughout the life cycle; and in freedom, with corresponding personal responsibility for one's biological, psychological, and social self frame a hopeful view of illness or dysfunction as impermanent and open to change. Communication of this hopefulness through the manner in which nurses approach and work with clients is essential for any positive change to occur.

While specialized training is required in order to function as a therapist in each of the above modalities (except, perhaps, reality therapy), the beliefs, goals, and some of the techniques used in these therapies can be incorporated into nursing care plans. Regardless of the treatment setting, nurses' potential to influence clients can be enhanced by giving unconditional positive regard, by facilitating goal setting by clients, by assisting clients toward desired behaviors, by supporting their efforts through praise and recognition of achievements, and by carefully redefining obstacles as either challenges to be conquered or valueless elements which can be avoided. All are strategies that are learned from these therapies.

Psychological growth therapies stress the importance to the client of having a caring—not just knowing—guide to help them change and grow. This has particular relevance to nursing. Probably more than any other professionals, nurses are expected by the public to provide giving, nurturing care. The demanding nature of this care is identified as one of the primary reasons for professional burnout. Nurses need to navigate wisely in order to fulfill the essential therapeutic dimension of caring in a way that enriches rather than depletes them. Psychological growth therapies offer an assumption that can help nurses in this regard. The assumption that each person is responsible for feelings, choices, and behavior reframes the basic premises on which the nurse-client relationship proceeds: this is not a relationship of undirectional giving and nurturing but a reciprocal one of two people working together for mutual learning, growth, and achievement. The way a client acts and the choices a client makes are the client's responsibility; the nurse's responsibility is to demonstrate the potential for positive behavior and choices in a hopeful, valuing, and caring manner.

MIND-BODY AWARENESS THERAPIES

Mind-body awareness therapies have evolved from conceptions of the body as the physical form of the dynamic energy which is the person. As such, the body records psychic pain and trauma with physical pain, rigidity, or malfunction. Eastern philosophies have long seen the person as a mind-body-spirit energy field, and their notions of illness and the means to promote wellness reflect this belief. (Acupuncture is one of the best known interventions associated with this conceptual approach.) Mind-body therapies bridge eastern thought and western approaches to human physiology, with particular attention to neurological, neuromuscular, myofascial, and skeletostructural systems. They seek to free the intrinsically harmonious (mind-body-spirit) essence of clients by resolving physically recorded trauma through the use of biofeedback, physical manipulations, movement awareness exercises, techniques to facilitate emotional release, and techniques to balance energy flow.

Biofeedback

Biofeedback emerged in the 1960s as a result of advances in the fields of electrical engineering, learning theory, and psychophysiology. The major finding which gave birth to biofeedback was the discovery that dimensions of autonomic nervous system functioning, previously thought to be outside the realm of conscious control, were amenable to voluntary influence. Functions such as heart rate, respiration rate, blood pressure, and skin temperature, for example, were found to be alterable by a person through biofeedback training (BFT). Table 25-1 (page 498) lists the physiological processes influenced by biofeedback.

The process of BFT includes (1) acquiring sensitive awareness of the target function, (2) learning to recognize internal operations associated with fluctuations in that function, (3) learning to alter those operations voluntarily, and (4) being motivated to do so. Acquiring sensitivity to a physiological function is facilitated through electronic instruments which visually or audibly "tell," or *feed back,* the activity level to the individual.

The purpose of engaging in BFT originally stemmed from a need for relief of some primary symptom of bodily imbalance. It continues to be a technique with useful clinical application for treating certain cardiovascular disorders, controlling spasticity, and treating psychosomatic disorders.[8]

The ability to objectively measure reciprocal interaction between mind and body through biofeedback represents a giant leap forward in understanding the human being as a complex unitary whole. The emergence of biofeedback provided validation of mind-body-spirit integration, applications for practice, and implications for further research in psychophysiological processes.

Use of biofeedback in the context of psychotherapy takes varied forms and continues to develop, with less emphasis being placed on why clinical applications work than on their usefulness. As an adjunct to therapy, biofeedback is used to help a client achieve a significant level of relaxation. This facilitates a variety of therapeutic

Table 25-1 Physiological Processes Influenced by Biofeedback

Monitoring Device	Health Problem	Application
Electroencephalogram (EEG)	Anxiety and general tension Stuttering Insomnia Chronic pain	Recognition and self-regulation of brain waves associated with states of tranquility, relaxation, and heightened awareness (alpha, delta, theta)
Thermistor (measures skin temperature)	Migraines	Controlled vasodilation of the hands to shift blood volume from central to peripheral sites
Electromyogram (EMG)	Bruxism (teeth grinding) Spasticity	Production of profound levels of muscle relaxation to inhibit undesired motor activity
Electrocardiogram (ECG)	Premature ventricular contractions Decreased pulse rate	Regulation of heart and rhythm
Galvanic skin response (GSR)	Anxiety	Recognition of unconscious emotional states

SOURCE: B. Sideleau, "Stress-Related Illness," in the second edition of this book.

processes by setting the psychological stage for introspection, guided exploration, and resultant self-awareness.

Monosymptomatic clients with complaints such as frequent severe headaches are most responsive to the relatively simple approach of BFT. The more complex and severe the dysfuncton is, the more comprehensive the treatment approach needs to be. Biofeedback may be used to increase relaxation and thereby decrease defenses against and resistance to greater self-awareness; but for more seriously impaired clients, progress in personality integration and responsible behavior must be stimulated by additional interventions.[9]

Relaxation Training

Relaxation training is closely related to biofeedback training through a large body of research based on the theory that relocation training also reduces arousal level. The field of psychology has produced several intervention techniques involving deliberate tensing and then relaxing of successive muscle groups. These techniques are used either to achieve general relaxation or to combat specific states of heightened anxiety. Comprehensive relaxation training (CRT), developed by Turin, involves brief relaxation exercises, audiotapes for home use to aid relaxation, and avoidance of food substances such as caffeine. Foods avoided are those demonstrated to dramatically increase the levels in the body of epinephrine and norepinephrine, which produce physiological effects indistinguishable from responses to external stressors and anxiety.

Clients trained in CRT have been able to lower their general arousal level either for short-term relief (to deal with specific stressful situations) or for daily maintenance. Turin reports that the entire CRT system can be taught by health care professionals to inexperienced clients within 4 to 6 hours. CRT is appropriate for people troubled with chronic anxiety and its physical corollaries, such as tension, migraine headaches, insomnia, or other stress-related illnesses.[10]

Bioenergetics

Bioenergetics was developed by the American psychiatrist Lowen, who holds that "bioenergy"—the basic life force—manifests itself on both the emotional and the muscular planes. Therefore, distress in one plane will manifest itself in the other. While well-functioning people are emotionally responsive and fully alive—allowing their bioenergy to flow freely—others block expression of feelings, which then get trapped and transformed into rigid musculature. Releasing physical tensions is the key to unlocking repressed feelings and allowing resolution to occur. Techniques include direct body contact between therapist and client; exercises which stretch muscles in order to highlight tension-filled areas, thus stimulating feelings in need of open expression; and the acting out of emotional responses through body language. The goal is to move the client to open expression of feelings, which will restore the free flow of bioenergy, release muscle tension, and enhance a sense of autonomy and aliveness.

Therapeutic Touch

Therapeutic touch, or "laying on of hands," is an act of voluntary transfer of some undefined energy from a well person to one who is ill. It involves touching another person with a strong intent to help or heal. The touching must be deeply motivated in the best interests of the person to be touched if it is to be therapeutic.

The person using therapeutic touch must be able to recognize clues to subtle levels of consciousness so that they may be used intelligently. The person must be aware of the processes, both conscious and unconscious, that may be set in motion. The healer must be able to develop the insight to recognize whose needs are being met by using this mode of therapy: the client's needs or the healer's own ego needs.

Laying on of hands is an ancient tradition. Religious writings, mythology, and oral traditions of primitive tribes provide many descriptions. Evidence of people's use of therapeutic touch has been found in the hieroglyphics of early Egypt, the Bible, church histories, and ancient Assyrian and eastern writings.

Explanations of the value of therapeutic touch lie in philosophy and physics, which have always been interactive. Belief systems of both eastern and western philosophies are intertwined and are becoming further defined in the language of physics and other natural sciences.[11]

Dolores Kreiger has pioneered the use of therapeutic touch by nurses. Kreiger's therapeutic touch is congruous with eastern thought and founded on the idea of "energy-field essence" in humans. It seeks to channel or balance energy, using the energy system of the healer. The healer lays hands on the places where the client feels pain; restoring the balance and flow of energy is held to relieve the pain.

Kreiger describes three steps to the healing process: centering, assessing, and rebalancing. *Centering,* which initiates the process, is the step in which a healer integrates energies and recognizes where he or she is and where the client is. It is done in a manner similar to the way one prepares for meditation or prayer. In the centering phase of the process, the person engages in a healing meditation in which he or she focuses on the client and excludes other thoughts from the mind. *Assessing* involves examining the client's energy field and determining where it is imbalanced. The healer moves his or her hands over the client's body from head to feet. The healer tunes into sensory clues received from the client through the hands. The sensory clues become assessment data. When imbalances are found, the healer moves into the *rebalancing* phase to restore balance. The healer uses sweeping hand motions over the body to redirect areas of accumulated tension. This is called *unruffling the field.* These movements release the flow of energy that has been *bound* or *congested* in the client's body. The healer also uses the hands to direct energy to the client. These activities are based on the following principles:

- There is interaction between people: both healer and client are vibrating fields of energy, and they exchange energy.
- The human body is an electrical energy field.
- Energy can become bound or congested.
- When the flow of energy is bound or congested, dysfunction occurs.
- The healer can influence the client's energy field and rebalance it for the purpose of promoting effective functioning.
- Rebalancing is producing a harmonious flow of energy.[11]

Rolfing

Ida Rolf maintains that psychological conflicts are recorded and perpetuated in the body and that resolution of conflicts requires structural reintegration. She views postural distortions as indicative of psychological conflict. *Rolfing* consists of deep manipulation and massage of the musculature and connective tissue to achieve proper alignment of the whole body. The goal of rolfing therapy is emotional release and physical healing.[12]

Primal Therapy

Primal therapy holds that early life traumas become trapped within a person and cannot be resolved in the present without reliving those early experiences and releasing the primal pain. A *primal* is an emotionally intense experience which varies in nature among people and may include screaming, writhing, sobbing, or trembling.

Janov, the psychologist who originated this approach, believes that neurosis is a defense against primal pain. He sees primals as the only way to release the pain of the past and come to terms with the present.

RELEVANCE TO NURSING

In order to practice the mind-body awareness therapies, specialized training in addition to graduate-level preparation is required. The one exception to this is relaxation training, for which basic professional nursing preparation and specialized training are sufficient. This is fortunate, as relaxation training has wide applicability in nursing practice because anxiety is always a part of distressing conditions for which clients have sought care. Unlike pharmacological substances, the traditionally prescribed remedies for anxiety, relaxation training has no untoward side effects or long-term costs, only preventive qualities.

The mind-body awareness therapies are accepted—and available—to varying degrees in the mainstream of western health care. The therapies discussed here are no longer perceived as witchcraft, and they have had an impact in the geographic areas where they predominate: the west, the northeast, or the Great Lakes area. Largely available through the private practices of specially trained professionals or through private institutes, these therapies are generally unavailable in traditional health care institutions or settings. This is unfortunate, as their absence suggests illegitimacy and lack of scientific basis and also results in economic and geographic selection of clients who can avail themselves of these approaches.

Some familiarity with the mind-body awareness therapies can be useful to nurses, for several reasons. First, the intervention techniques are consistent with the holistic nature of the human being and thereby expand the possibilities for treating dysfunction in nontoxic, nonhazardous, and growth-promoting ways. Second, these therapies have the potential to safely enhance well-being and prevent stress-related illnesses. Third, in nursing practice one may encounter clients who have tried such therapies or clients who would like to try them; these clients may seek nurses' opinion about the therapies.

CONSCIOUSNESS-DEVELOPMENT THERAPIES

Consciousness-development therapies reflect approaches to enhance one's general well-being through spiritual growth and attainment of altered or higher levels of consciousness. The effects of some of these therapies are closely related to the effects of psychological growth and mind-body awareness therapies; for example, the deep relaxation attainable through biofeedback and relaxation training is sometimes barely distinguishable from the subjective and objective states reached in meditation or hypnosis. The classification offered here is meant to reflect the fact that these therapies emphasize the spiritual dimension; it does not imply that the other biopsychosocial dimensions are not involved.

Hypnotherapy

Hypnotherapy involves therapeutic use of the human potential to achieve a trancelike state. Although hypnotic states have been reported throughout history, Erikson is credited with legitimizing use of hypnosis in modern-day therapy, on the basis of a belief that the conscious mind can distort and inhibit the spontaneous healing powers of the unconscious.

In a hypnotic trance or altered state of consciousness, a person relinquishes rational control and becomes highly suggestible both physically and mentally. The condition that results allows for fuller recall of troublesome experiences or inner realities and permits the unconscious to work through these experiences or realities to develop desired changes in thinking, feeling, or behaving.

It is believed that nothing can be done with hypnosis that cannot be done without it: neither a therapist's nor a client's conscious mind can control unconscious processes; it can only offer suggestions. Further, people vary in their capacity to respond to hypnotic induction. Clients who are candidates for hypnosis must have the capacity for aroused concentration which can be elicited and guided by the hypnotherapist. Hypnosis is, therefore, generally facilitative to therapy, an adjunct or tool rather than a treatment modality in and of itself.

Hypnotherapists are trained and certified professionals, usually physicians or psychologists. Training and qualification are very important because a therapist using hypnosis must assume a high degree of responsibility for the client. The hypnotic trance is a regressed, disassociated condition of temporary dependency. The therapist must be highly competent and ethical in managing such vulnerability.

Transcendental Meditation

In 1958 Maharishi-Mahesh Yogi left an ascetic life in the Himalayas to take his message of spiritual development through *transcendental meditation* (TM) to the people of India, Europe, and the United States. His vision was for humanity to progress from being preoccupied with material things to valuing pure consciousness. His goal of raising humanity's level of consciousness was to bring about a new world in which pressing social problems (including crime and group hostilities) would be eliminated.

Becoming involved in TM usually requires a course of instruction, which typically follows these steps:

1. An introductory lecture explains the benefits of TM.
2. A second lecture describes the mechanisms of meditation.
3. An interview allows the client to ask questions.
4. Personal instruction is given.
5. A suitable *mantra,* or sound that is meaningless and is to be repeated hypnotically, is taught to the client.
6. Three checking meetings are held to monitor progress and to answer questions.

After learning the technique, the person using TM generally meditates daily for at least 20 minutes. It is believed that the longer one meditates, the more one is able to experience a state of pure consciousness.[13]

Silva Mind Control

Silva mind control, named for its originator, J. Silva, was developed in the 1940s. Silva teaches that the ordinary form of mental activity is *beta consciousness;* achieving *alpha consciousness* improves powers of concentration, memory, and imagination. The inherent benefits of reaching alpha consciousness include fuller, more harmonious functioning and improved coping skills.

Generally, Silva mind control is learned at one of the Silva "growth centers." The program consists of lectures; instruction in relaxation techniques, including those used in relaxation therapy; and the assigning of a mantra, which is also used with other forms of meditation. Once in a state of deep relaxation or a mild hypnotic trance, as the case may be, the client is encouraged to repeat positive expressions of his or her worth, coping skills, or level of well-being.

Effective sensory projection is a technique of this therapy in which clients are taught to project themselves into other beings. Successfully learned, this technique is claimed to enable one to both diagnose illness and transmit positive energy needed to cure it. Adherents to this modality report such cures to have occurred in cases of cancer, deafness, and blindness.[14]

Zen Meditation

While TM and Silva mind control are the two most popular orientations to meditation, Zen is gaining popularity as a treatment modality. Zen has time-tested roots in eastern religion, which required one to retreat from the social order into isolation with an accomplished Zen master to study the technique. It is believed still that to practice Zen effectively, one must learn it from a teacher who has progressed in spiritual development. Students of *Zen meditation* are taught to focus their minds while sitting in a "full lotus" position with the body in proper balance. Concentration is focused on clearing the mind and on breathing correctly, thus moving toward harmony of the mind and body.

Erhard Seminars Training

Erhard Seminars Training (est), named for the American salesman who changed his name to Werner Erhard and founded this modality, originated in 1971. Within 4 years, est reportedly grossed over $9 million, reflecting its rapid growth and popularity. It continues to be a successful program, consisting of techniques used in gestalt and Zen built into a structured format of two consecutive weekends of training.

Beliefs promoted in est are essentially holistic, with the primary message being that each person is responsible for his or her own life. Rationality is seen as preventing people from living fully in the present and is discouraged to the point of ignoring "whys" and "hows." The client is encouraged simply to assume responsibility for each moment as it evolves and to live. The major goal of est is to alter the client's consciousness in relation to daily life. It is a packaged experience contained in 60 hours. Many who have experienced it say that it changed their lives; but others point out that internal acceptance of responsibility must be followed by behavioral change, which is a more difficult matter. Participants are challenged to perceive the world and themselves in new ways by taking total responsibility for their own lives in the here and now. Est teaches that reasonableness or looking for the causes of things prevents people from living wholly in the present and from succeeding. People are taught that they are the creators of their own realities, their own meaning, and their own importance, and they are encouraged to accept this responsibility and act accordingly.

RELEVANCE TO NURSING

Consciousness-development therapies offer yet other approaches to relieving distress. Other therapies use problem solving or removal of symptoms to achieve this, but consciousness-development therapies encourage spiritual development, through which a person can transcend the suffering inherent in lower levels of consciousness. Adherents of these therapies argue that contemporary science (including psychology) underestimates human potential in the spiritual realm. Convincing evidence is lent to this argument by psychophysiological research on the "placebo effect." Other clinical findings demonstrate the influence of hope and the will to live (or to die) on the body's ability to cope with illness. The power of the mind is central to health.

Application of concepts of consciousness development to nursing practice raises numerous possibilities. The value of rest and rejuvenation obtained through deep relaxation and meditation is proved to exceed the value of ordinary sleep. Being in an altered state of consciousness has been shown to diminish pain or even relieve it completely. Use of hypnosis, meditation, and guided imagery with clients who are in pain has been corollated with relief of pain and reduction of symptoms.

For those in psychological and emotional distress, consciousness-development therapies offer nonintrusive, natural, and holistic treatment. The effect of this is perhaps not unlike the effect of a religion in which followers find refuge and comfort. For the client who is not attracted by talking therapies or mind-body awareness therapies but is interested in self-help, consciousness-development therapies offer effective interventions which are inexpensive and quickly learned.

SUMMARY

Several distinctions exist between traditional and alternative therapies. Traditional therapies focus treatment on impaired functioning, defined as "illness," and regard the client as the victim of etiological, intrapsychic, interpersonal, or developmental adversity. Traditionally minded professionals choose therapeutic interventions believed to relieve either the causes or the manifestations of illness. Alternative approaches conceive of wellness as a state of harmony among mind, body, and spirit that is necessary if one is to be fully alive and growing. Wellness is more than the absence of illness. Wellness is a dynamic manifestation of a balanced life characterized by authentic self-expression and relationships, work, purpose, activity, leisure, and creativity. It is each person's responsibility to live in a health-promoting way. Failure to do so results in distress or pain, which may manifest itself psychologically, emotionally, somatically, or spiritually.

Two noteworthy implications of this shift away from the medical model are that since health management is each person's responsibility, it is not under the ownership of medical professionals; and that the consumer of services is a decision-making client, not a dependent patient.

Holistic understanding of human nature encourages recognition of a broad spectrum of experiences as therapeutic and as promoting and restoring physical, mental, and spiritual health. Leisure arts therapies facilitate expression of spiritual and psychological dimensions of the self. These consist of art, dance, music, literature, pet, and plant therapies. Pet and plant therapies offer reflections of one's effort and responses to one's behaviors. Engaging in recreational therapies offers self-expression, constructive use of time, satisfaction from activities and outcomes, and enhanced well-being.

The rehabilitative skills therapies are socialization therapy, occupational therapy, and vocational rehabilitation. These therapies aim for competence at skills necessary for daily living and, ultimately, for self-reliance. Vocational rehabilitation aims to establish and maintain clients in employment and is provided by law to people labeled as *psychiatrically impaired.*

Psychological growth therapies—such as gestalt, psychodrama, play therapy, social network therapy, videotherapy, encounter marathon groups, reality therapy, rational-emotive therapy, and Morita therapy—see wellness as dynamic and see distress as amenable to change. Strategies for effecting positive changes vary among the therapies but generally consist of using new interpersonal experiences to alter people's beliefs, values, and behaviors. The desired consequences of this are reduction of anxiety-provoking aspects of one's life and development of mature and responsible ways of being more fully alive. Social network therapy and encounter marathon groups are forums which allow full communication among participants, in order to provide the people involved with information that can lead to more successful behavior.

Mind-body awareness therapies seek to relieve physical manifestations of psychological and spiritual distress, on the assumption that resolution of distress follows physical relief. Rolfing, bioenergetics, and primal therapy seek emotional release through physical manipulation and expression. Biofeedback and relaxation training offer techniques through which one can learn conscious sensitivity to physical signs of distress and learn to offset these signs. Therapeutic touch employs a healer, who seeks to rebalance a client's energy through the "laying on of hands."

Consciousness-development therapies aim for spiritual growth through episodic use of techniques which alter consciousness. Transcendental and Zen meditation and Silva mind control entail meditation with deep relaxation and altered states of consciousness. These therapies value spiritual growth and devalue material comforts and self-consciousness. Erhard Seminars Training (est) is offered in a normal state of consciousness, discourages intellectualizing, and aims to alter one's thinking (consciousness) regarding aspects of daily living. Hypnosis is a therapeutic tool which uses the altered state of consciousness to facilitate resolution and self-healing. Each of the consciousness-development therapies recognizes the power of the mind to transcend the conditions of the body.

REFERENCES

1. K. R. Pelletier, *Mind as Healer, Mind as Slayer: A Holistic Approach to Preventing Stress Disorders,* Dell, New York, 1977.
2. E. Feder and B. Feder, *The Expressive Arts Therapies,* Prentice-Hall, Englewood Cliffs, N.J., 1981.
3. E. T. Gaston, ed., *Music in Therapy,* Macmillan, New York, 1968.
4. Special Task Force of the Council on Standards and Executive Board for Occupational Therapists, "Occupational Therapy: Its Definition and Functions," *American Journal of Occupational Therapy,* vol. 26, May–June 1972, pp. 204–205.
5. Frederick S. Perls, *Gestalt Therapy Verbatim,* Real People Press, Moab, Utah, 1969.
6. J. Kovel, *A Complete Guide to Therapy,* Pantheon, New York, 1976.
7. J. L. Fryrear and B. Fleshman, *Videotherapy in Mental Health,* Thomas, Springfield, Ill., 1981.
8. J.V. Basmajian, ed., *Biofeedback—Principles and Practice for Clinicians,* Williams and Wilkins, Baltimore, 1979.
9. Henry H. Grayson and Clemens Loew, *Changing Approaches to the Psychotherapies,* Spectrum, New York, 1978.
10. R. Corsini, ed., *Handbook of Innovative Psychotherapies,* Wiley, New York, 1981.
11. D. Krieger, *Foundations for Holistic Nursing Practices: The Renaissance Nurse,* Lippincott, Philadelphia, 1981.
12. Ida Rolf, *Ida Rolf Talks About Rolfing and Physical Reality,* Harper and Row, New York, 1978.
13. R. Shader, ed., *Manual of Psychiatric Therapeutics,* Little, Brown, Boston, 1975.
14. J. Silva and P. Miele, *The Silva Mind Control Method,* Simon and Schuster, New York, 1977.

BIBLIOGRAPHY

J. T. Barter, J. F. Queirolo, and S. P. Ekstrom, "A Psychoeducational Approach to Educating Chronic Mental Patients for Community Living," *Hospital and Community Psychiatry*, vol. 35, August 1984, pp. 793–797.

V. Binder, A. Binder, and B. Rimland, eds., *Modern Therapies*, Prentice-Hall, Englewood Cliffs, N.J., 1976.

R. Carkhuff, *The Art of Helping*, 5th ed., Human Resources Development Press, Amherst, Mass., 1983.

C. Garfield, ed., *Rediscovery of the Body: A Psychosomatic View of Life and Death*, Dell, New York, 1977.

K. Keyes, *Handbook to Higher Consciousness*, 5th ed., Living Love Consciousness Center, St. Mary, Ky., 1977.

H. Q. Kivnick and J. M. Erikson, "The Arts as Healing," *American Journal of Orthopsychiatry*, vol. 53, October 1983, pp. 602–618.

I. W. Rohr, "Biofeedback Applications in Psychotherapy," in Henry H. Grayson, and Clemens Loew, eds., *Changing Approaches to the Psychotherapies*, Spectrum, New York, 1978.

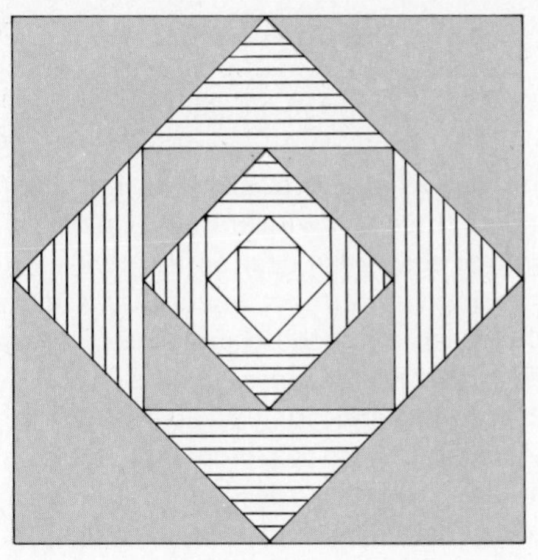

CHAPTER 26
Somatic Therapy

Anita M. Leach

LEARNING OBJECTIVES

After studying this chapter, the student should be able to:

1. Define *somatic therapy.*
2. Discuss the usefulness of having a historical perspective on somatic therapies.
3. Identify the theories, uses, and side effects of electroconvulsive therapy (ECT).
4. Develop a nursing care plan for a client scheduled to be treated with ECT.
5. Discuss the psychopharmacological treatment of mental illness.
6. Identify the actions, clinical uses, and side effects of antipsychotic, antidepressant, and antianxiety agents; identify contraindications for their use and nursing considerations when they are used.
7. Explain the use of antiparkinsonian agents in the treatment of mentally ill clients.
8. Discuss the biogenic amine hypothesis.
9. Discuss the use of lithium carbonate in the treatment of manic-depressive illness.
10. Describe the symptoms and treatment of lithium toxicity.
11. Analyze the issues of food interaction, tolerance, dependence, compliance, the law, ethics, and restraint as they are involved in the administration of psychopharmacological agents.
12. Apply the nursing process to drug administration.

The treatment of clients with physiological agents or physical methods is known as *somatic* therapy. The root of the word, *soma,* means "of the body." Throughout history, healers have recognized the integration of a person's body, mind, and spirit. It has been taken for granted that the cure of the body relieves the mind and spirit and that the relief of mental and spiritual pain leads to healing of the body. Assumptions about the integration of body, mind, and spirit have given rise to the somatic treatment of emotional and spiritual illnesses. Accidental curative responses, often occurring without any scientific explanation of the exact physiological mechanisms, have led some to a deeper belief in the theories of genetic and biological causes of psychiatric illness.

One of the most significant developments in the history of biophysiological treatment of mental illness has been the introduction of pharmacological agents. Until the late 1950s, somatic treatment of psychiatric symptoms was limited to hydrotherapy; electroshock or insulin shock treatments; the selective use of older drugs, such as barbiturates, chloral hydrate, and paraldehyde; megavitamin therapy; and psychosurgery. The advent of psychotropic medication provided the breakthrough necessary for humane, pragmatic, and scientifically accurate biological treatment of clients' disturbed behavioral patterns.

Psychopharmacological therapy and other somatic therapies are rarely used alone; generally they are used as adjuncts to individual, group, family, or milieu therapy. The purpose of this chapter is to familiarize the student with the historical and current use of somatic therapies. The chapter will discuss earlier somatic treatments, but the major emphasis will be on current uses of ECT and psychopharmacological agents.

Drugs will be discussed in terms of their uses and therapeutic effects, side effects, dosages, routes of administration, duration of effect, and contraindications for use. The major focus will be on nursing roles, the nursing process, and the teaching and educating of clients. Nursing responsibility for administering and observing the effects of drugs will be emphasized.

The author gratefully acknowledges Patricia Campion O'Neill for her contribution to this chapter in the second edition.

EARLIER SOMATIC THERAPIES

Insulin coma therapy, orthomolecular therapy, psychosurgery, and hydrotherapy have historical significance. The use of these treatments has been sharply curtailed since the widespread use of psychopharmacological agents began in the 1950s, but nurses in a variety of settings encounter clients treated in the past with these methods. These clients need intervention more because of the sequelae to the treatments they received than because of any acute illness. In psychiatric settings, clients may relate "horror stories" of "shock treatments" without anesthesia and muscle relaxants, exhibit resulting signs of posttraumatic arthritis, or have endocrine disorders as a result of insulin coma therapy. Still others speak of their experiences in ways that make them their "badge of courage." A client might be heard to say, "I'm the only one here who knows what it used to be like. Those 'wet packs' were especially terrible." Nurses need to be alert to the histories of their clients, especially those clients who have been labeled *chronic.* Empathy, genuine understanding, supportive care, and, at times, confrontation by nurses facilitate optimal levels of wellness in clients old enough to have experienced unusual somatic treatments.[1]

Insulin Coma Therapy

Insulin coma therapy involved injecting a fasting client with increasing amounts of insulin in order to induce seizures. Sokel developed the original process. Advocates of insulin coma treatment believed that the sleeplike state of coma rested the brain and cured the symptoms of schizophrenia.[2] Numerous complications, the need for highly specialized equipment and personnel, and the development of safer, more effective treatment modalities led to discontinuance of insulin coma therapy in the treatment of mental illness.

Psychosurgery

In 1935, Moniz received the Nobel prize for his pioneering work in the field of psychosurgery. In the 1930s frontal-lobe surgery for the treatment of schizophrenia was the treatment of choice for chronically psychotic clients and those prone to violence. Some research settings are experimenting with refined versions of psychosurgery to treat frontal-lobe epilepsy, refractory chronic clients, and clients with severe tension stemming from fear, worry, depression, anxiety, or agitation. Generally, psychosurgery is recommended only after all other methods of treatment have failed.

Orthomolecular Therapy

The use of large doses of vitamins to treat mental illness is known as *orthomolecular therapy;* it is also known as *megavitamin therapy* and *niacin therapy*. Orthomolecular therapy is a natural and "popular," or "lay," approach to the treatment of mental illness. Orthomolecular therapy represents an early attempt to deal with the theories supporting a biogenetic basis of mental illness.

Pauling, the founder of orthomolecular treatment, believed that mental illness was caused by excessively low concentrations of specific vitamins in the brain. He believed that this condition was due to genetic makeup and diet.

Orthomolecular therapy can be combined with psychotherapy or electroconvulsive therapy, or it can be used as the sole treatment method. Massive doses of vitamins and minerals are given to clients either alone or as supplements to psychotropic drugs. Extremely large doses of vitamins B_3 and B_6, nicotinic acid, vitamin C, trace metals, and vitamin E are used. Megadoses of vitamins are usually combined with an antihypoglycemic diet or other diet of the physician's choice.[3]

Hydrotherapy

Hydrotherapy is defined as the use of water in the treatment of emotional illness. Historically, it involved the use of "wet packs" and cold sheets. In some cases, specially constructed tubs were used to restrain clients in either hot or cold water over periods of time. Often, hydrotherapy is used by the media to exemplify the "insane asylum"—the punitive stage of mental health treatment.

ELECTROCONVULSIVE THERAPY

Electroconvulsive therapy (ECT) is the only convulsive treatment currently used for clients with emotional problems. *Convulsive therapy* is the artificial induction of a seizure under controlled circumstances. In *electroconvulsive therapy,* a grand mal seizure is artificially induced by passing an electric current through the brain.

Convulsive therapy was introduced by Medura in 1935; he observed that clients who had spontaneous convulsions no longer showed evidence of psychotic symptoms and that epilepsy and schizophrenia rarely occurred in the same client. The widespread and controversial use of convulsive therapy evolved from the repeated observations that convulsions and coma caused remission of symptoms in clients with depression and psychotic behaviors. Cerletti and Bini first used electrodes to induce convulsions in 1973.

Historically, ECT was used indiscriminately to treat all symptoms of mental disorders. Clients were fully conscious during the induction of seizures and frequently sustained broken limbs or developed posttraumatic arthritis as a result of injuries sustained during convulsions.[3]

Over time, there has been scientific validation that clients experiencing feelings of worthlessness, helplessness, and hopelessness; anorexia; weight loss; constipation; and sleep disturbances respond positively with diminished symptoms following convulsive therapy. Its most effective use is with carefully selected depressed clients.

Theories of Action

There are many theories about how ECT works. One psychological interpretation is that the treatment serves as a symbolic punishment for clients who feel guilty and worthless. Another theory proposes that ECT is seen by clients as a life-threatening experience and they therefore mobilize all their bodily defenses to deal with the "attack." It has also been suggested that clients are able to release their inner aggressive impulses through the convulsions associated with the treatment. Still another theory holds that electric shock produces minimal brain damage which destroys the specific area containing memories related to the events surrounding the development of a psychotic condition. Another, more complex physiological theory views the brain as consisting of multiple electric circuits and sees mental illness as stemming from a malfunction of the circuits. An internal self-corrective system assisted by ECT is thought to clear the brain of whatever material has interfered with proper functioning.

The psychobiological theories are most commonly supported by recent research. Fraser states that the therapeutic effect of ECT is most likely due to an alteration in the postsynaptic response to the neurotransmitters in the central nervous system. ECT stimulates synaptic remodeling, causing an increase in synaptic protein. It is the increased synaptic protein that is thought to enhance positive behavior and result in the relief of depressive symptoms.

Uses for ECT

Currently, treatment with ECT is humane and relatively safe. In most hospital settings, treatments are administered in 1-day surgical units because of the use of anesthesia. ECT is rarely the first treatment of choice. It is used only when clients have had exhaustive trials and poor response to psychotropic drugs, when they are known to be highly allergic to psychotropic drugs, or when drugs are contraindicated (for example, during pregnancy or when the client has serious heart disease). Clients for whom electroconvulsive therapy has been successful in the past, those who are severely depressed and those who are violently psychotic are others for whom the use of ECT treatment may be appropriate. ECT is a generally successful and safe treatment for older adults, particularly those unable to tolerate therapeutic dosages of psychotropic drugs.[4]

Clients are generally given a series of treatments. The number varies with the severity of symptoms, the prescribing physician's theoretical orientation, and the individual client's responsiveness. An average series ranges from 6 to 10 treatments. From 20 to 30 treatments have been known to be experienced by some clients, but this practice has diminished in recent years. ECT treatments are generally given on alternating days, three or four times each week. Recent developments support the use of multiple ECT treatments and the induction of several convulsions during a single therapeutic session; however, research into this method of administration has not yet proved conclusive. Still, those who advocate the multiple-convulsion procedure claim that it provides greater therapeutic effectiveness with no increase in confusion or untoward responses in clients.

Complications of ECT

Historically, compression fractures of the vertebrae and long bones of the arms and legs were common complications of ECT. The use of muscle relaxants has virtually eliminated these problems. Today, the two most common side effects of ECT are confusion and loss of memory. The intensity and duration of these effects are related to the number of treatments, the type of stimulation used (unilateral or bilateral), the voltage needed to induce a seizure, and the age and mental status of the client before treatment. Generally, a client's short-term memory and orientation to time and place return within a brief period of time. However, there are clients who have never recovered long-term memory; most of these people were treated before the use of anesthesia or were treated with bilateral electrodes. Confusion and loss of memory are essentially eliminated when unilateral electrodes are used and are placed over the frontoparietal area.[5]

Transient bradycardia may occur because of vagal stimulation. Epinephrine and norepinephrine levels are known to rise immediately following treatment, causing transient hypertension and tachycardia. Because of the latter, there is a risk of stroke or coronary thrombosis. The death rate following ECT is less than 0.03 percent. The most common causes of death following ECT are complications of the anesthesia and ventricular arrhythmias that result in cardiac arrest.[5]

Ethical and Legal Considerations

The legal controversy over ECT as a treatment of psychiatric clients is extensive. It is generally held that if a client is competent, the administering psychiatrist and responsible staff members fulfill their legal and ethical responsibilities by involving the client in the process of informed consent. The legal problem in the administration of ECT involves, first, the fact that it is generally prescribed for clients who are seriously depressed and whose ability to consent might, therefore, be open to question. Second, ECT is held by some to be an intrusive physical technique which has unacceptable risks and is, therefore, beyond the range of rational choice. These two problems are used to argue that "informed consent" to ECT and the current practice of employing ECT on the basis of a client's consent are of questionable validity.[4] Some institutions in states where ECT is administered protect themselves by obtaining a judgment from the courts.

The benefits and risks of ECT must be explained to clients and their families. A detailed consent form that includes a statement informing clients of the risk of death and severe loss of memory should be signed, witnessed, and included in the record. Clients must also be informed of the current lack of precise knowledge about the treatment. When these legal and ethical steps are carried out and appropriate documentation is available in the record, there is little likelihood of legal risk to the practitioner, and the client's rights have been protected.

Nursing Process with ECT

Assessment

The decision to initiate ECT is generally a collaborative one made by the client and the family with significant input from the treatment team or primary therapist. Because of the increasing tendency to look at ECT as a subspecialty of psychiatry, decisions are often made by persons other than those who will actually be involved in its administration. Nurses assisting with ECT ask the following questions in order to formulate a data base:

1. What is the client's level of anxiety?
2. Are client and family fully informed about the procedure and its beneficial and possible untoward effects?
3. What are the attitudes of the client and the family about ECT in general and the successful outcome of treatment in particular?
4. Is the preliminary workup complete?
5. Are the proper consents signed and in the client's record?
6. What medications is the client taking?

In addition to assessing the client and the family, nurses need to look at their own attitudes toward ECT. If they view the treatment as barbaric or primitive, this will be conveyed to the client. If nurses are unable to assume the supportive, educative role that is necessary, they should excuse themselves from involvement in ECT.

Diagnosis and Outcome Criteria

Formulating nursing diagnoses related to treatment with ECT involves consideration of the client's physiological, mental, and spiritual state before, during, and after treatment. Table 26-1 suggests selected appropriate diagnoses with corresponding outcomes.

Table 26-1 ECT: Nursing Diagnoses and Expected Outcomes

Nursing Diagnoses	Expected Outcomes
Hand twitching related to increased anxiety about treatment	Client will verbalize less anxiety after supportive educational input from nurse and physician.
Noncooperative family correlated with lack of information about the procedure	The family will support the client's decision about ECT treatment after receiving educational input.
Prolonged unconscious state related to seizure activity	Client will regain consciousness within 2 hours after treatment.

Intervention

Before treatment, informed consent must be obtained from the client and a thorough physical examination—including complete blood count, urinalysis, electrocardiogram, and x-rays of the chest and the lateral aspects of the spine—must be completed and recorded on the client's chart.

Like any anesthesia-assisted treatment, ECT generally is given in the morning. The client should have an empty stomach. Verbal preparation and reassurance are given as necessary to allay anxiety. The client should void, dress in sleepwear or loose-fitting clothing, and remove any dentures. Atropine sulfate IM is generally given to decrease secretions and to interrupt the vagal stimulation effects of ECT.

Once in the actual treatment room, the client lies in a supine position on a stretcher. An anesthesiologist or nurse anesthetist intravenously administers a short-acting barbiturate. This is followed by an intravenous injection of a muscle relaxant such as succinylcholine (Anectine). Drugs are administered in separate syringes generally in a 5 percent dextrose and water IV solution. The client is preoxygenated with 95 to 100 percent oxygen and posturally supported to maintain an effective airway. Sometimes a soft mouth-bite is used. Once the client is unconscious, electrodes are put in place. Electrojelly or saline solution is used to moisten the electrodes and ensure maximum electrical conductivity. The client is then immobilized to minimize movement and prevent dislocation or breaking of bones.

A psychiatrist specifically educated to administer ECT initiates treatment. It is a *medical* responsibility to adjust the amount of voltage used to induce seizures and to actually activate the electric charge. The more sophisticated ECT machines have built-in electrocardiogram- and electroencephalogram-recording devices. Nurses specifically certified to do so may initiate this cardiac and brain monitoring.

Once the electric charge is passed through the brain, a tonic seizure lasting 5 to 15 seconds occurs; this is followed by clonic movements lasting 10 to 60 seconds. Visual assessment of movement is often the responsibility of the nurse. At times an effective seizure occurs with only minimal or subtle visual movements, so careful observation is essential. Oxygen is administered throughout the treatment; suctioning occurs as necessary. The monitoring of the client's respiratory status is the responsibility of the anesthesiologist or nurse anesthetist.

Table 26-2 is an assessment checklist that includes space for recording nursing observations and interventions that occur before, during, and after treatments with ECT.

Most clients awaken almost immediately after treatment. However, since they are extremely confused and lightheaded at this time, very careful nursing supervision is necessary. Some clients become extremely restless and agitated during this period of confusion and can, if not watched, injure themselves by thrashing about or attempting to get out of bed too soon. The client should remain lying down for at least a half-hour. Often, but not always, the client will sleep soundly for an hour or more. During this time, careful monitoring of vital signs, maintenance of adequate respiration, and reassurance and orientation to surroundings are necessary. Clients do not experience physical pain, nor are they aware of the actual seizure, but they are often very upset by temporary memory loss. A supportive attitude on the part of the staff encourages the client to participate in interpersonal activities. Orientation to reality is particularly important once the actual treatment is over.

Evaluation

Proper documentation of a data base and observations made throughout a treatment is essential.

Table 26-2 ECT Checklist

Client's name: ________ Date of treatment: ________
Physician: ________ Anesthesiologist: ________

Nursing Responsibility	**Date**	**Initials**
1. Workup completed and reports in record		
CBC		
Urinalysis		
Electrocardiogram		
Chest x-rays		
Spinal x-rays		
2. Consent signed and in record		
3. Client teaching completed		
4. Family teaching completed		
5. Vital signs		
T		
P		
R		
BP		
6. Preparation completed		
Voided Time: ________		
Dentures removed		
Hospital gown		
Jewelry removed		
NPO since ________		
7. Medications administered		
Atropine 1/150 IM Time: ________		
8. Medications administered by anesthesiologist		
________ Time: ________		
________ Time: ________		
________ Time: ________		
9. Vital signs: Pretreatment		
P		
R		
BP		
10. Time of administration of shock: ________		
11. Tonic seizure Time: ________ Duration: ________		
12. Clonic seizure Time: ________ Duration: ________		
13. Vital signs: Posttreatment		
P		
R		
BP		
14. Time of return to consciousness: ________		
15. Time of ambulation: ________		
16. Vital signs | at 15 min | 30 min		
P		
R		
BP		
17. Other observations		

Signature: ________ Date: ____ Time: ________

SOURCE: Developed by Anita M. Leach for use at Danbury Hospital, Danbury, Conn.

The client's expressed subjective experience, including attitude and level of anxiety, and significant objectively observed behavioral changes need to be recorded before, during, and after treatments. These evaluations supplement the observations noted on the checklist (Table 26-2).

Ongoing observation of the behavioral effects of treatment usually determines the number of treatments necessary to achieve a therapeutic effect. Whether or not a treatment series needs to be repeated is evaluated periodically.

PSYCHOPHARMACOLOGICAL THERAPY

Drugs used to treat psychiatric symptoms are classified according to their effect on the central nervous system (CNS). The classifications include antipsychotics, antianxiety drugs, tricyclic antidepressants, MAO inhibitors, antimania drugs, and antiparkinsonian drugs. Table 26-3 lists the major classifications of drugs used to treat mental illness, the common nomenclature, and the subgroups of each class. These classes of drugs are known as *psychopharmacological agents*. They are also known as *psychotropic drugs* (that is, pharmacological agents which will affect mood and behavior).

Table 26-3 Major Classification of Drugs Used in the Treatment of Mental Illness

Class	Other Nomenclature	Subgroups
Antipsychotic agents	Major tranquilizers Phenothiazines Neuroleptics Ataractic agents	Aliphatic Piperidine Piperazine Thioxanthene derivatives Butyrophenone derivative Dibenzoxazipines
Antianxiety agents	Minor tranquilizers	Barbiturates Antihistamines Propanediol dicarbamates Beta-adrenergic blockers Benzodiazepines
Antidepressant agents	Mood elevators Energizers	Tricyclics Monoamine oxidase inhibitors
Antimania agent		Lithium carbonate
Antiparkinsonian agents	Antiextra-pyramidal effect agents	Tropine derivatives Piperidine compounds Ethanolamine antihistamines

Psychotropic drugs are among the most commonly used agents on the market today. This does not mean that mental illness is widespread, but rather that those who prescribe the drugs do not fully understand their appropriate use. The symptoms of mental illness are often vague, ill-defined, or misunderstood. While psychotropic drugs have revolutionized the care of mentally ill clients, they remain abused and misused, or not used at all. For example, wealthy clients, who can afford long-term psychotherapy, may not receive drugs that would facilitate their recovery, while clients with limited financial resources may receive unnecessary medication. The appropriate management of a mentally ill client with psychotropic drugs involves a clear differential diagnosis of the client's behavior, objective assessment of the needs of the client, and familiarity with clinical pharmacokinetics.

Pharmacokinetics is defined as the study of the interactions between a drug and the body as the drug is absorbed, distributed, metabolized, and excreted. Clinical pharmacokinetics involves the safe and effective management of individual clients as they move through the phases of drug treatment. An understanding of the anatomy and physiology of the nervous system and neurochemistry is essential for psychiatric nurses administering psychopharmacological agents. Several medical and surgical nursing texts contain excellent presentations of this information. Sufficient to the scope of this chapter is a reminder to the reader that the psychotropic drugs discussed here have therapeutic value because of their direct and indirect effects on the central nervous system (brain and spinal cord), the peripheral nervous system (cranial and spinal nerves), and the autonomic nervous system (sympathetic and parasympathetic nerves). Understanding the physiological effects of a specific drug is helpful in assessing its side effects.

Rational prescription of drugs and selection and adjustment of dosages are as much an art born of experience and observation of individual clients as a therapeutic science.

A nurse performs a vital role when medication is the treatment of choice for a client. It is often

Table 26-4 Selected Antipsychotic Drugs: Potencies, Doses, and Side Effects

Class and Nonproprietary Name	Trade Name†	Relative Potency‡	Dose: Antipsychotic Dose Range—Daily Dosage, mg		Dose: Single Intramuscular Dose¶	Adverse Effects*: Sedative Effects	Adverse Effects*: Extrapyramidal Effects	Adverse Effects*: Hypotensive Effects
			Usual	Extreme‡				
Phenothiazines								
Aliphatic								
Chlorpromazine	Thorazine	100	200–800	25–2000	25–50	+ + +	+ +	IM + + +
Triflupromazine	Vesprin	25–50	50–200	50–400	20–50	+ +	+ + +	+ +
Piperidine								
Thioridazine	Mellaril	100	100–600	50–800		+ + +	+	+ +
Piperazine								
Perphenazine	Trilafon	8	8–32	4–64	5–10	+ +	+ + +	+
Prochlorperazine edisylate	Compazine (edisylate and maleate)	25	75–100	15–150	5–10	+ +	+ + +	+
Prochlorperazine maleate								
Fluphenazine hydrochloride	Permitil, Prolixin (hydrochloride, enanthate, and decanoate)	4	2–10	1–60	1.25–4 (decanoate or enanthate 25–50 every 2 weeks)	+	+ + +	+
Fluphenazine enanthate								
Fluphenazine decanoate								
Acetophenazine	Tindal	20	40–80	20–150	—	+ +	+ +	+
Trifluoperazine	Stelazine	5	4–15	2–64	1–2	+	+ + +	+
Nonphenothiazines								
Thioxanthenes								
Chlorprothixene	Taractan	100	50–400	30–600	25–50	+ + +	+ +	+ +
Thiothixene	Navane	5	6–60	6–60	2–6	+ to + +	+ +	+ +
Butyrophenones								
Haloperidol	Haldol	5	2–6	1–100	3–5	+	+ + +	+
Dihydroindolones								
Molindone	Moban	10	15–40	60–400		+ to + +	+ + +	+
Dibenzoxazepines								
Loxapine	Loxitane	10	20–50	60–400		+ to + +	+ +	+ +

*Less intense +, + +, + + +, more intense.
†Only representatives from the various groups are presented; the trade name list is noninclusive.
‡Dosage (in mg) which gives efficacy comparable to 100 mg chlorpromazine.
§Extreme dosage ranges should not be exceeded except when all other appropriate measures have failed.
¶Except for the enanthate and decanoate forms of fluphenazine, dosage is given IM every 4 to 6 h for agitated patients.
SOURCE: From M. B. Wiener and C. A. Pepper, *Clinical Pharmacology and Therapeutics in Nursing*, McGraw-Hill, New York, 1985.

the nurse's taking of a history, observation, administration, and recommendations that contribute significantly to the selection of an appropriate drug to relieve a client's symptoms.

Administration of a psychotropic drug occurs in several phases:

1. *Initiation phase:* The dose is initiated at a low level and is titrated upward until symptoms are controlled.
2. *Stabilization phase:* Ideally, within 3 to 6 weeks symptoms are eliminated or relieved.
3. *Maintenance phase:* Following remission of target symptoms, the drug is slowly reduced to a minimum dose.
4. *Drug-free phase:* With a newly diagnosed client, the drug is not discontinued until after 6 to 8 months of treatment. A chronically ill client may have to be given medication indefinitely, or with brief periods of discontinuance to reassess drug-free behavior and to reduce the incidence of long-range side effects.

Antipsychotic Drugs

Treatment of psychotic symptoms makes use of *antipsychotics,* which were previously called *major tranquilizers, neuroleptics,* or *ataractics.* There are numerous antipsychotic drugs available for use today. Chlorpromazine was the original antipsychotic; currently, there are seven major groups of antipsychotics. The specific drug prescribed may be chosen because it is preferred by the treating physician, it has fewer side effects than other drugs, the client has been successfully treated with it in the past, or the client believes that it works. There is no evidence that any one drug is superior to the others in reducing psychotic symptoms.[6] Table 26-4 lists selected antipsychotic drugs, noting group, subgroup, trade name, method of administration, usual psychiatric and intramuscular dosages, and relative adverse effects for each drug.

Action

The exact action of the antipsychotic drugs is not known. They affect not only the central nervous system but most organ systems of the body. The drugs are believed to act by affecting neurotransmitters, dopamine, norepinephrine, and serotonin. On the basis of observations of psychotic symptoms, researchers speculate that antipsychotic agents act on anatomic sites in the midbrain and affect the adrenergic blocking and anticholinergic actions of the nervous system. This might help to explain some of the unwanted side effects of these drugs. Table 26-5 lists the effects of antipsychotics in terms of their actions on the nervous system and the results of these actions.

Table 26-5 Effects of Antipsychotics

Action of Antipsychotics	Result of Action
Affect the reticular activating system of the midbrain	Alteration of the monitoring of sensory input
Affect the structures of the amygdala, hippocampus, and limbic system	Alteration of the emotional coloring of incoming messages
Affect the hypothalamus	Alteration of peripheral responses to sensory information
Affect the globus pallidus and corpus striatum	Elicitation of extrapyramidal symptoms
Alpha-adrenergic blockage (anticholinergic activity)	Sedation of central nervous system
	Decrease of seizure threshold
	Alteration of temperature regulation
Alpha-adrenergic blockage of vasculature	Postural hypotension
Blockage of dopamine receptors in the hypothalamus pituitary-adrenal axis	Rise in prolactin, resulting in endocrine abnormalities
Dopamine blockage in the nigrostriatal structures of the brain	Regulates or causes extrapyramidal effects
Dopamine blockage in the hypothalamus	Alteration of temperature regulation, resulting in hyper- or hypothermia

It is known that antipsychotic drugs normalize unacceptable psychotic behaviors such as hallucinations and delusions and decrease agitation, anxiety, irritability, and apprehensions. The ideal antipsychotic drug would be one that clouds consciousness without causing sedation. While research to date has not produced the ideal drug, the goal comes closer to realization as the action of psychopharmacological agents becomes more specific.

Antipsychotics are metabolized in the liver. For the most part, the onset of metabolism is within 2 to 3 hours; total detoxification is extremely slow.

This slow release from the body accounts for the fact that clients remain stable for long periods of time (often for months) after discontinuing use of the drug. For this reason, a client may say to the prescriber, "But I was doing fine without my medication."

Research findings indicate that there is little correlation between blood levels of a drug and the dosage. It is known that absorption is from the gastrointestinal (GI) tract; depending upon how quick an onset one wishes, antipsychotic drugs should be given with or immediately following meals. Concentrations of the drugs have been found in the brain, whereas lesser amounts are found in vital organs.[6]

Clinical Uses

The primary use of antipsychotic drugs is the control of psychotic behaviors such as those exhibited by schizophrenic clients. They are also used to control behavior by sedation during the manic phase of manic-depressive illness. In addition, they are helpful in the treatment of selected clinical syndromes. They are sometimes used as an antihistamine. Hiccups and pruritis are known to respond well to their use. They are used to potentiate the effects of narcotics used for analgesia and for sedation. The specific drug of choice for excessive shivering and the limited treatment of organic brain syndrome is chlorpromazine hydrochloride (Thorazine). Prochlorperazine (Compazine) is used as an antiemetic (that is, an antivomiting agent). Drugs with higher sedative potency are useful to control severe anxiety of long duration.

Great caution should be exercised in using antipsychotic drugs with persons who have known seizure disorders, since the drugs lower the seizure threshold. One of the more common side effects of haloperidol (Haldol) is the sudden onset of seizures.

It should be noted that this group of drugs does not cause physiological dependency and is not physically addicting. Clients, however, may become psychologically dependent upon their medications, a factor which may contribute to abuse.[6]

Side Effects

Antipsychotic drugs produce many troublesome but predictable side effects. Table 26-6 lists side effects, discomforts, and appropriate nursing inter-

Table 26-6 Side Effects of Psychotropic Drugs and Nursing Interventions

Assessment (Side Effect or Discomfort)	Nursing Intervention
Blurred vision	Reassurance (generally subsides in 2–6 weeks)
Dry mouth and lips	Frequent rinsing of mouth Lozenges Lip balm
Constipation	Mild laxative Roughage in diet Exercises Fluids
Nasal congestion	Nose drops Moisturizer
Decreased libido and inhibition of ejaculation	Prepare client for effect Reassurance (reversible) Ask physician about change to less potent antiadrenergic drug
Postural hypotension	Frequent monitoring of blood pressure during dosage-adjustment period Advise client to get up slowly Elastic stockings if necessary
Photosensitivity	Protective clothing Dark glasses Use of sunscreen
Dermatitis	Stop medication Request physician to change order and prescribe systemic antihistamine Initiate comfort measures
Impaired psychomotor functions	Advise client to avoid dangerous tasks
Drowsiness	Give single daily dose at bedtime
Weight gain	Caloric control; exercise-diet teaching
Edema	Reassurance Request physician to prescribe diuretic
Irregular menstruation and decreased sex drive	Reassurance (reversible) Have phsycian change class of drugs
Amenorrhea	Reassurance and counseling (does not indicate lack of ovulation) Instruct client to continue birth control
Sedation	Instruct client not to drive or operate potentially dangerous equipment Ask physician about change to less sedating drug Provide quiet and decrease stimulation when sedation is desired

SOURCE: Adapted from Loretta Guise, "Therapeutic Modalities—Somatic," in the first edition of this book.

ventions. When prescribing antipsychotics, doctors must consider the relative advantages and disadvantages of different drugs in relation to the likelihood of their producing unwanted and uncomfortable side effects. For example, certain drugs cause more sedation than others and may be chosen because of the degree of sedation desired for a particular client.

SEDATION. One of the troublesome side effects of the antipsychotic group of drugs is sedation. Although sedation may have advantages in the treatment of highly agitated or belligerent clients, the antipsychotics are not effective in the treatment of clients who must remain alert and awake in order to function outside the institutional setting. Trifluoperazine dihydrochloride (Stelazine), fluphenazine dihydrochloride (Prolixin), and thiothixene (Navane) produce relatively minor sedative effects while chlorpromazine hydrochloride (Thorazine), chlorprothixene (Taractan) and thioridazine (Mellaril) cause more pronounced sedation.

Haloperidol (Haldol) is frequently used in maintenance doses without any major sedative effect; however, because it is quick-acting and (when given in larger doses) produces sedation, it is the drug of choice for managing highly agitated clients. Loxapine succinate (Loxitane) has intermediate sedating action, and molindone hydrochloride (Moban) has recently been shown to have little sedating potential and some stimulant properties.[6]

HYPOTENSION. *Hypotension,* or a drop in blood pressure from the baseline, is a common side effect of the antipsychotic group. The effect generally occurs following two to three doses. Chlorpromazine hydrochloride (Thorazine) is the most potent drug when considering hypotensive reactions of clinical significance. Trifluoperazine dihydrochloride (Stelazine) and fluphenazine hydrochloride (Prolixin) cause less hypotensive effects.[6]

ANTICHOLINERGIC EFFECTS. The drug with the most pronounced anticholinergic activity is thioridazine (Mellaril). It is the most likely to induce blurred vision, dry mouth, constipation, urinary retention, decreased perspiration, and increased heart rate. Chlorpromazine hydrochloride (Thorazine) and chlorprothixene (Taractan) possess relatively high degrees of anticholinergic action, and trifluoperazine dihydrochloride (Stelazine), fluphenazine dihydrochloride (Prolixin), and haloperidol (Haldol) produce lesser symptoms.

The antiparkinsonian agents also have anticholinergic properties and when used in conjunction with the antipsychotic agents, further accentuate anticholinergic side effects.[6]

EXTRAPYRAMIDAL SIDE EFFECTS. Extrapyramidal side effects occur because of the effect of antipsychotic drugs on the parasympathetic nervous system. The different drugs have varying incidences of these effects. For example, haloperidol (Haldol), fluphenazine dihydrochloride (Prolixin), trifluoperazine dihydrochloride (Stelazine), and perphenazine (Trilafon) have a high incidence, and thioridazine (Mellaril) has a relatively low incidence of extrapyramidal side effects.[6]

Extrapyramidal side effects include the following:

1. *Pseudoparkinsonism.* Pseudoparkinsonism mimics symptoms of Parkinson's disease. Symptoms include tremor, shuffling gait, drooling, rigidity, and looseness of arm movements.
2. *Akathisia* Akathisia is continuous restlessness, fidgeting, and pacing beyond the conscious control of the client. Clients will say things such as, "I didn't realize I was so active," or "I can't stop; I have to keep going."
3. *Akinesia.* Akinesia is muscular weakness and fatiguelike symptoms. Clients will complain of "rubber" legs.
4. *Dystonia.* Dystonia includes involuntary muscular movements of the face, arms, legs, and neck. Clients experiencing dystonia often have difficulty talking or salivate excessively.
5. *Oculogyric crisis.* An oculogyric crisis is a syndrome characterized by sudden onset of uncontrolled rolling back of the eyes. Usually such a crisis is preceded by dystonia and akinesia. The side effects become a psychiatric emergency because of the speed with which they can lead to complete muscular and respiratory collapse. The rolling of the eyes in itself is not dangerous. The treatment of choice for an oculogyric crisis is immediate intravenous (IV) injection of benztropine mesylate (Cogentin methanesulfonate).
6. *Tardive dyskinesia.* Tardive dyskinesia is char-

acterized by bizarre facial and tongue movements, a stiff neck, and difficulty swallowing. The onset of these symptoms is often slow and subtle to the point that clients often "incorporate them into their person" and pay little attention to them. This side effect may occur either after one dose of a particular drug or after long-term use. When the onset is acute, the drug should be withheld and treatment of the side effect should be immediate. In most acute situations the symptom is reversible. However, long-term duration of tardive dyskinesia is irreversible.[7,8]

Recent research on tardive dyskinesia suggests that well-organized screening programs and careful observation in the early phase of drug treatment may help identify clients who will develop long-term irreversible symptoms.[9]

Extrapyramidal symptoms may be treated conservatively with nursing measures such as those suggested in Table 26-6. When megadoses of antipsychotic drugs are used, antiparkinsonian drugs such as benztropine mesylate (Cogentin methanesulfonate) trihexyphenidyl hydrochloride (Artane), biperiden hydrochloride (Akineton), and procyclidine hydrochloride (Kemadrin) may be prescribed. At one time it was common practice to prescribe these drugs routinely. However, newer findings indicate that they potentiate anticholinergic effects. They are therefore used very selectively and only when extrapyramidal effects are serious or life-threatening, as in the case of oculogyric crisis.

Contraindications

Antipsychotic drugs are contraindicated and are generally not prescribed for clients with narrow-angle glaucoma, prostate problems, or cardiac problems. A client with a pacemaker, convulsive disorder, bone marrow depression, or liver disease should not be given antipsychotic drugs.

The antipsychotic group of drugs has a tendency to potentiate the effects of other drugs such as hypnotics, analgesics, and anesthetics. Clients should be cautioned not to use other drugs or alcohol while on antipsychotic therapy, since they may have the effect of further depressing the CNS.[10] Safety of use during pregnancy is not established. Secretion of the drug in breast milk is not well-established.

RELEVANCE TO NURSING

The drug treatment of psychosis may be divided into three phases: the initial, or symptom-control, phase; the second, or stabilization, phase; and the third, or maintenance, phase.

PHASE 1: CONTROL OF SYMPTOMS. In the initial phase the goal is to control psychotic symptoms such as hallucinations, delusions, agitation, and disordered thinking. During this *symptom-control phase* of drug treatment of the acutely psychotic client, medication is administered in gradually increasing dosages until the symptoms subside. The client's clinical response and behavior and the side effects the client experiences will determine whether or not a dosage is adjusted upward or downward. Nursing observations of side effects and overall reactions to medication are critical during the initial phase of drug treatment.

Frequently, the route used to administer these medications is left to the discretion of the nurse. PO (per os, that is, oral) medications may be given in pill or liquid form. It should be remembered that oral concentrated liquid medication frequently leaves a burning anesthetized feeling in the mouth. Clients should be advised to rinse their mouths after administration of drugs in liquid form. A large number of these drugs double their potency when given intramuscularly (IM) or intraveneously (IV). (See Table 26-4 for IM dosage equivalents.) Nurses need to be mindful of this when they are given, by policy, freedom of choice for route of administration. The nursing staff should see to it that orders are written appropriately. For example, an appropriate order is, "Give chlorpromazine hydrochloride 100 milligrams PO. If refused, give chlorpromazine hydrochloride 50 milligrams IM."

PHASE 2: STABILIZATION. The second phase of treatment with antipsychotic drugs is called the *stabilization phase.* During this phase the medication dosage is gradually reduced. Generally, this occurs during the second to fourth week of treatment. The goal during the stabilization phase is to maintain control of symptoms and to minimize unwanted and uncomfortable drug side effects. Generally, the dosage of an antipsychotic drug is stabilized at about one-half the maximum dosage previously required. Physicians rely heavily on nurses to report clients' behaviors and level of comfort as doses are reduced. It is during this phase that information about the side effects and appropriate interventions for them is shared with the client.

PHASE 3: MAINTENANCE. The third phase of antipsychotic drug treatment of the psychotic client is called the *maintenance phase.* The dosage of the drug is reduced to the lowest level necessary to relieve symptoms and minimize side effects. When psychotic symptoms recur during dosage reduction, a temporary increase in the dosage of the medication may be necessary. "Drug holidays" are employed during the maintenance phase; the drug is discontinued temporarily, usually for 24 hours, in order to ascertain continuing clinical need and to minimize the risk of long-term complications such as tardive dyskinesia.

During the maintenance phase, clients begin the real work of psychotherapy. Education of clients is the essential work of nurses during this phase. Family counseling may be necessary in order to ensure compliance by clients. The family and client need to understand the drug, the dosage, symptoms of the disease, and what side effects to expect and report. A schedule for drug holidays should be part of the teaching plan.

When compliance is an issue, either fluphenazine decanoate (Prolixin Decanoate) or fluphenazine enanthate (Prolixin Enanthate) is generally prescribed. These drugs are long-acting antipsychotics and may be given by injection at biweekly or bimonthly intervals. Clients generally experience an exacerbation of side effects for 24 hours following administration and need to be closely monitored during this time interval. Clients are titrated on oral forms of drugs to determine effectiveness before they are given long-action dosage forms.

As a general rule, the simultaneous use of two or more antipsychotic drugs would be considered polypharmacy and is to be avoided. The use of multiple antipsychotic drugs is less likely to facilitate a therapeutic response and more likely to induce the development of side effects and complications.[8] In order to obtain optimal clinical response with minimal complications and side effects, it is important that clients avoid the use of more than two drugs. Nurses play important roles as advocates for clients and educators, since large numbers of clients on a particular medication may simultaneously and without appropriate information seek additional drugs, without the physician's knowledge, in an effort to alleviate unpleasant or frightening symptoms.

Antiparkinsonian Agents

There are many medications used in psychiatry to control the parkinsonianlike side effects of antipsychotic drugs. Table 26-7 outlines parasympathetic blocking agents that are considered *antiparkinsonian drugs.* Their trade names and dosage ranges

Table 26-7 Antiparkinsonian Drugs Used in Psychiatry

Drug	Trade Name	Method of Administration	Usual Daily Psychiatric Dose, mg
Tropine derivatives			
Benztropine mesylate	Cogentin methanesulfonate	PO (tablets)	1
		IM (ampules)	1–2
Piperidine compounds			
Biperiden	Akineton	PO (tablets)	1–2
		IM (ampules)	2
Procyclidine hydrochloride	Kemadrin	PO (tablets)	2–5
Trihexyphenidyl	Artane	PO (tablets)	1–2
	Pipanol	PO (elixir)	1–2
	Tremin	PO (sustained release)	
Ethanolamine antihistamines			
Diphenhydramine hydrochloride	Benadryl	PO (capsules, elixir)	25–100
		IM	50–200

are listed. These drugs are often referred to as *anticholinergic agents.* At present there is no evidence that any one antiparkinsonian drug is more effective than the others. Side effects include blurred vision, mental confusion, dry mouth, constipation, and urinary retention. Antipsychotic drugs have similar side effects. It is therefore important to assess clients before compounding their problems with one of the anticholinergic agents. Historically the antiparkinsonian agents were given routinely whenever an antipsychotic drug was administered. Current practice is to prescribe antiparkinsonian drugs only when clients experience troublesome extrapyramidal side effects and large doses of the antipsychotic drugs remain a necessity.

Benztropine mesylate (Cogentin), a quick-acting antiparkinsonian drug, is used for the acute phase of oculogyric crisis and should be kept in its injectable form on the nursing unit or anywhere antipsychotic drugs are administered. Diphenhydramine hydrochloride (Benadryl) is another drug that should be kept for emergency treatment of extrapyramidal side effects.[10]

Antianxiety Agents

Drugs used to relieve mild or moderate anxiety or to treat psychoneurotic and psychosomatic conditions are known as *antianxiety agents* or *minor tranquilizers.* Barbiturates, benzodiazepines, beta-adrenergic blockers, drugs from the propanediol group, and antihistamines are used as antianxiety agents. Table 26-8 lists selected antianxiety drugs, their generic names, routes of administration, and dosage ranges. Antianxiety drugs are the most widely prescribed class in the United States. They are palliative and relieve the symptoms of anxiety but do not cure the underlying problems.

While there is a considerable amount of ongoing research, the exact mechanism of action of antianxiety agents is not known. As a group they depress the central nervous system, causing sedation and relaxation of muscle tension. There are specific actions theorized about each subgroup.

Older Drugs and Drugs of Second Choice

BARBITURATES. The use of barbiturates in the treatment of anxiety has only historical significance. Studies comparing barbiturates and placebos have shown that they have little or no effect on levels of anxiety. They cause sedation and are very likely to cause addiction. Depressive symptoms are common, and the possibility of suicide is greater than with other agents. They accelerate the metabolism of other drugs metabolized in the liver and tightly bind to plasma proteins, displacing other drugs. They significantly alter rapid-eye-movement (REM) sleep. These actions account for the lethality of

Table 26-8 Antianxiety Drugs

Drug	Trade Name	Initial Single Dose, mg	Method of Administration	Usual Daily Psychiatric Dose, mg
Barbiturates				
Phenobarbital sodium	Luminal	15	PO (tablets), IM, IV (for convulsions only)	45–200
Amobarbital sodium	Amytal	65	PO (capsules), IM, IV (for convulsions only)	45–200
Antihistamines				
Hydroxyzine hydrochloride	Atarax	25	PO (tablets, syrup)	25–150
Hydroxyzine pamoate	Vistaril	25	PO (capsules, syrup)	25–150
Hydroxyzine hydrochloride	Vistaril	25	IM (vial)	25–150
Propanediol dicarbamates				
Meprobamate	Equanil	600	PO (tablets, capsules, suspension)	200–1200
	Miltown	600	PO (tablets)	200–1200
	Meprospan	600	PO (time-released capsules)	200–1200
Tybamate	Solacin	500	PO (capsules)	500–1500
	Tybatran	500	PO (capsules)	500–1500
Beta-adrenergic blockers				
Propranolol hydrochloride	Inderal	10	PO (tablets) IM (ampule)	30–120

barbiturates when combined with other drugs such as alcohol, and the "hung over" feeling that results from long-term use.[6]

PROPANEDIOL DICARBAMATES. Propanediol dicarbamates, or meprobamates, such as Equanil and Miltown were the first nonbarbiturate agents used to treat anxiety; from a historical perspective they deserve mention.

The use of benzodiazepines has rendered these agents obsolete, and newer research findings have questioned their efficacy as antianxiety agents. As a group they are known to impair learning and affect motor coordination and reaction time. Suppressed REM sleep leads to symptoms like those of a hangover, increased anxiety, and depression. Because of side effects of sleepiness, hypotension, and ataxia, these drugs are rarely prescribed.

ANTIHISTAMINES. Antihistamines should be reserved as a second choice of drugs for the treatment of anxiety. However, they are useful in the treatment of anxiety associated with pruritus or other dermatological conditions. They may also be considered for the treatment of clients predisposed to physical dependence, because tolerance to and physical dependence on antihistamines occur infrequently. Anticholinergic side effects, however, are prominent. Hydroxyzine hydrochloride (Atarax) and hydroxyzine pamoate (Vistaril), by oral administration produce fewer anticholinergic side effects but have more sedative properties than other drugs in this group.[11]

BETA-ADRENERGIC BLOCKING AGENTS. Propranolol hydrochloride (Inderal) is a specific beta-adrenergic blocking agent used for the treatment of the peripheral somatic manifestations of anxiety such as tachycardia, palpitations, tremors, and hyperventilation. The drug acts as a beta-adrenergic antagonist and is primarily a cardiac drug perceived by laypeople as "powerful." Rapid withdrawal from the drug has been associated with cardiac arrhythmias and sudden death. Its use in the treatment of anxiety remains experimental, although many studies document its usefulness in the treatment of the somatic symptoms of anxiety.[11]

Benzodiazepines

The barbiturates, propanediol dicarbamates, antihistamines, and beta-adrenergic blocking agents have been replaced by the benzodiazepine agents as the drugs of choice for the treatment of anxiety. The benzodiazepines are the true antianxiety agents. Table 26-9 lists commonly used benzodiazepines by their generic names and gives for each the trade name, dosage range, half-life, and time required to reach peak blood levels. In addition to being used as antianxiety agents, the benzodiazepines are used as muscle relaxants, anticonvulsants, and hypnotics and in the treatment of alcohol withdrawal.

ACTION. As is true with many of the other psychotropic drugs, the exact mechanism of action of benzodiazepines is not known. Research findings suggest that such drugs work by enhancing gamma-aminobutyric acid (GABA) activity at pre- and post-

Table 26-9 Benzodiazepine Agents

Drug	Trade Name	Initial Adult Dose, mg	Dosage Range, mg	Elimination Half-Life, h	Peak Blood Level Reached, h
Alprazolam	Xanax	0.5	0.5–1.5	12–15	1
Chlordiazepoxide	Librium	10	20–60	5–30	2–4
Clorazepate dipotassium	Tranxene	7.5	15–60	24–200	1
Diazepam	Valium	5	5–40	20–50	1
Flurazepam	Dalmane	15	15–30	50–100	1
Halazepam	Paxipam	60	80–160	14	2
Lorazepam	Ativan	1	20–60	10–20	3
Oxazepam	Serax	10	30–90	5–20	4
Prazepam	Centrax, Verstran	20	20–60	24–200	1
Temazepam	Restoril	15	15–30	10–15	2–3
Triazolam	Halcion	0.25	0.125–0.5	2.7–4.5	1–1.5

synaptic nerve endings, indirectly affecting the catecholamine-activating center in the cerebral cortex of the brain. They do not affect REM sleep. In small doses they produce a calming effect and relieve nervousness and anxiety. Larger doses produce drowsiness and sedation. Benzodiazepines increase the seizure threshold and have anticonvulsant action. They are known to cause muscle relaxation.[6]

Physical and psychological dependence on and tolerance to these drugs may develop. They potentiate the CNS-depressive action of alcohol, barbiturates, narcotics, sedatives, and tricyclic antidepressants. When benzodiazepines are used with phenytoin (Dilantin), there is a possible enhancement of toxic effects. They also alter laboratory results. Blood serum, bilirubin, aspartate transferase (AST; formerly serum glutamic oxaloacetic transaminase, SGOT), alanine transferase (ALT; formerly glutamic pyruvic transaminase, SGPT), and alkaline phosphatase levels are increased. Effects on blood creatinine and results of the 17-ketosteroid urine tests are equivocal.[12] The half-lives of the drugs should be noted, since some, particularly cholorazepate dipotassium (Tranxene), remain active in the body for several days after therapy has been discontinued. Sudden withdrawal from any of these agents may cause weakness, nausea, vomiting, and seizures.[13]

SIDE EFFECTS. The therapeutic dose of a benzodiazepine is reached when the client experiences relief without being oversedated. Minimal sedation is an expected side effect of the antianxiety group of drugs. Work or activity requiring mental alertness should be avoided by clients taking these drugs.

Most common among the other side effects of the antianxiety drugs are dizziness, dry mouth, headaches, and sedation. Gastrointestinal (GI) complaints, urinary hesitancy or retention, nervousness, blurred vision, and mental confusion have also been noted in some clients. Although they are rare, rashes, fatigue, ataxia, diplopia, palpitations, irritability, slurred speech, depression, and decreased blood pressure have been reported.

Autonomic side effects sometimes occur in malnourished or debilitated clients. These side effects include mild hypotension, dry mouth, constipation, retarded ejaculation, and sexual impotence. Amenorrhea is common with the use of benzodiazepines. The sedative and euphoric side effects tend to cause physical dependence on the drug.

The withdrawal syndrome for benzodiazepines generally occurs 1 week after cessation of therapy. Reduction of the dose generally alleviates side effects. Nursing interventions for side effects are the same as those listed in Table 26-6.

CONTRAINDICATIONS. The benzodiazepines are contraindicated in clients with histories of hypersensitivity to the drugs. They should be used with great caution when clients have histories of alcoholism or addiction. Safety of use during pregnancy has not been established. It is known that chlordiazepoxide (Librium) is secreted in breast milk; therefore, it should be avoided by nursing mothers.[10] Elderly clients and those with histories of liver disease require lower dosages and careful monitoring to prevent untoward effects.

RELEVANCE TO NURSING

When antianxiety drugs are administered, observation of the effects the drugs are having on a given client are important. Monitoring and observation may result in dosage adjustment. The goal of therapy is to give the minimum amount of a drug with the least sedation and the maximum antianxiety effects. Clients need to be cautioned about the sedating qualities and the CNS-depressant effect of these medications.

Clients and their families need to be advised of the danger involved in taking barbiturates with alcohol or other CNS depressants. Overdose with any drug in this group may be life-threatening. Gastric lavage and administration of a stimulant are generally the treatments of choice when overdose occurs. PRN ("as needed") use of antianxiety drugs generally does not reduce anxiety, since blood levels need to be maintained for optimal therapeutic effect. Clients who experience intermittent anxiety attacks should be educated about alternative ways of dealing with anxiety.

Antidepressant Agents

Drugs used to treat depression are known as *antidepressants*. These include the tricyclic, tetracyclic, and triazolopyridine groups (TCAD) as well as the

Table 26-10 Antidepressant Drugs

Drug	Trade Name	Initial Adult Dose, mg	Available Preparations	Maintenance Dosage Range, mg
Tricyclics				
Imipramine hydrochloride	Tofranil Presamine	50–100	PO (tablets), IM (ampules)	75–300
Imipramine pamoate	Tofranil PM	75–150 (bedtime only)	PO (tablets)	75–150
Amitriptyline hydrochloride	Elavil	50–100	PO (tablets), IM (vial)	75–300
Desipramine hydrochloride	Norpramin Pertofrane	50–150	PO (tablets, capsules)	75–300
Nortriptyline hydrochloride	Aventyl	25–50	PO (capsules, suspension)	50–100
Protriptyline hydrochloride	Vivactil	10–30	PO (tablets)	15–60
Doxepin hydrochloride	Sinequan Adapin	50–100	PO (capsules)	75–300
Amoxapine hydrochloride	Asendin	50–150	PO (tablets)	150–600
Trimipramine hydrochloride	Surmontil	50–100	PO (tablets)	75–300
Tetracyclics				
Maprotiline hydrochloride	Ludiomil	75–150	PO (capsules)	75–300
Triazolopyridines				
Trazodone hydrochloride	Desyrel	50–150	PO (tablets)	800–1600

SOURCE: M. B. Wiener and C. A. Pepper, *Clinical Pharmacology and Therapeutics in Nursing*, 2d ed., McGraw-Hill, New York, 1985.

monoamine oxidase (MAO) inhibitors. Table 26-10 lists commonly used antidepressants by their generic names and gives their trade names, modes of administration, and dosages. It should be noted that clients with endogenous depression may be treated successfully with antidepressants, while clients with exogenous, or reactive, depression derive very little benefit from drug therapy. In either case, researchers have found that there is little or no effect when psychopharmacological agents are used without individual, group, or family psychotherapy.

The choice of a specific drug to treat depression is generally based on three factors: (1) the client's ability to tolerate the side effects, (2) the results of previous exposure to a particular drug, and (3) the outcome of a clinical trial of the chosen drug.[6]

Tricyclic antidepressants may be used to treat anxiety, phobic anxiety, and enuresis as well as depression.

The Amine Hypothesis

To understand the action of antidepressant drugs, one must understand the biogenic amine hypothesis. It states that a deficiency of one or another type of neurotransmitter results in manifestations of depression. There are neurotransmitters thought to be directly involved with the production of depression, mania, and schizophrenia. The neurotransmitters, also known as *monoamines*, are serotonin (5-hydroxytryptamine, or 5-HT), norepinephrine, and dopamine. Norepinephrine is thought to be more involved with the production of depression or mania, whereas dopamine and 5-HT are thought to be involved with schizophrenia.

It is hypothesized that neurotransmitters are substances that occur naturally in the brain and are released by the nerve cells when they are stimulated. Neurotransmitters may also be released spontaneously. Each nerve cell, or neuron, has each of the three neurotransmitters. These are stored in little granules or vesicles near the end membrane of the nerve cell. When the cell is activated, it releases the neurotransmitters from the vesicles into the cytoplasm and from there across the synaptic cleft onto receptor cells. The space between the nerve cell and the receptor cell is known as the *synaptic cleft*. The whole complex—nerve cell, synaptic cleft, and receptor cell—is known as a *synapse*. It is postulated that the enzyme catechol-o-methyltransferase (COMT) inactivates norepinephrine and dopamine at the synpatic cleft, and that MAO is inactivated in the receptor cell. It is also believed that some of the neurotransmitters of the activating cell are inhibited by MAO. The process can be thought of as a cyclic one.[14]

Some antidepressant drugs prevent the activating mechanism of the neuron. Others prevent the action of MAO, causing an increased supply of neurotransmitters. MAO inhibitors prevent metabolism of neurotransmitters, causing more neurotransmitters to be stored; therefore, more are available for release. Tricyclic drugs block the reuptake of neurotransmitters. Simultaneously, new neurotransmitters are synthesized and stored. They are available in the synaptic cleft to act upon receptor sites, thus correcting hypothesized deficiencies. Some tricyclics block the reuptake of norepinephrine, and others specifically inhibit serotonin; this, explains why some clients do well with some drugs and not with others.

The symptoms of depression but not the underlying causes are treated. The antidepressant drugs in effect correct the physiological defects of depression but do not heal the whole person. Treatment with tricyclics or MAO inhibitors generally results in elevation of mood; improved appetite and sleep patterns; increased physical activity; improved mental functioning; a decrease in a client's feelings of inadequacy, worthlessness, guilt, and ambivalence; and possibly a decrease in delusional preoccupation. Antidepressants have also been known to increase tension, cause agitated behavior, intensify a psychotic state, or cause clients to become disoriented and possibly to hallucinate. Decreasing the dosage usually controls these situations.

The selection of specific medications to treat depression is dependent on the symptoms and behaviors observed in clients.[15] Table 26-11 lists the various types of depression and gives the corresponding drugs of choice for their treatment.

Table 26-11 Antidepressants: Classification by Symptoms

Presenting Depressive Behaviors	Antidepressant Medication (Drug of Choice)
Unipolar depression	Tricyclic
Insidious onset	
Anorexia	
Weight loss	
Insomnia (early morning awakening)	
Motor retardation	
Agitation	
Bipolar depression	Lithium
Elation	
Grandiosity	
Weight gain	
Inability to sleep	
Labile mood (depression alternating with elation)	
Family history of bipolar depression	
Atypical depression	MAO inhibitors
Premorbidly well-adjusted	
Known precipitant	
Mild variable depression	
Phobic anxiety	
Hysteria	
Somatic complaints	
Increased eating	
Excessive sleeping	
Insomnia	
Fatigue	
Irritability	
Hysteria	MAO inhibitors
Shallow, labile moods	
Histrionic	
Flamboyant	
Seductive	
Dependent	
Other	MAO inhibitors
Rejection sensitivity	
Self-pity	
Loss of anticipatory pleasure	
Craving for sweets	

SOURCE: Adapted from R. J. Bielski and R. O. Friedel, "Depressive Subtypes Defined by Response to Pharmacotherapy," *Psychiatric Clinics of North America*, vol. 2, no. 3, 1979, p. 484.

Tricyclics

ACTION. Tricyclics are absorbed from the GI tract. Maximum effect occurs in 14 to 21 days after the onset of administration. Some physicians are experimenting with thyroid preparations to shorten the lag period. The results of these experiments, however, have been extremely erratic. Metabolism of tricyclics occurs in the liver, and excretion is primarily via the kidneys. Tricyclic medication may cause cardiac arrhythmias. For this reason dosages should begin gradually. Most physicians currently prefer to titrate the medication while the client is hospitalized. Once a maintenance dose has been established, the client may continue treatment as an outpatient.[10]

Clients should also be withdrawn slowly from the drugs. A lag period of 2 to 3 weeks occurs;

therefore a 2-week drug holiday should be given between administration of tricyclic medication and the initiation of treatment with the MAO inhibitors because of the serious untoward effects that may occur.

Anorexia, nausea, vomiting, diarrhea, and cramps are sometimes experienced by clients receiving tricyclic medication. It should be noted that the absorption of tricyclic medication may be inhibited if antidiarrheals or antacids are administered.

Some clients may be allergic to the tricyclic group of medications. Allergies manifest themselves with photosensitivity, rashes, urticaria, edema, and fever. A complete blood count (CBC) should be done before administration of the drug. Periodic follow-up testing should be done to rule out the possibility of blood dyscrasias caused by the drug.

Extrapyramidal symptoms occur most frequently in the young and the elderly. Tardive dyskinesia usually results from prolonged use of amitriptyline hydrochloride (Elavil).[10] Occasionally, clients being treated with tricyclics experience CNS stimulation. Symptoms such as tremor, psychomotor excitement, insomnia, delusions, and hallucinations may occur. Careful observation and taking the client's history become necessary to ascertain whether behavior is a side effect of medication or symptomatic of a psychotic depression.

SIDE EFFECTS. The anticholinergic side effects of tricyclics are similar to those occurring with the administration of antipsychotic drugs. Dry mouth, blurred vision, tachycardia, palpitations, constipation, and urinary retention are all anticholinergic side effects. Anticholinergic action varies among the tricyclics. Table 26-12 lists the relative degree of expected anticholinergic side effects in selected drugs.

Drowsiness is the most common CNS effect. For this reason, tricyclic antidepressants are frequently given at the hour before sleep. However, REM sleep is affected, and in some cases nocturnal auditory and tactile hallucinations have been noticed with large bedtime dosages. Tricyclics have relative sedating properties. Highly agitated or hypomanic clients may respond to a more sedating tricyclic, and those overly sensitive to sedative properties may respond better to a drug that causes less sedation or no sedation. Table 26-13 lists selected tricyclics showing their relative degrees of sedation. Clients taking tricyclics do not experience impotence, breast engorgement, decreased libido, or weight gain as frequently as those taking antipsychotic drugs. Tricyclic medication should not be given to pregnant women or to women who are breast-feeding.

Administration of tricyclic medication can cause abnormalities on an electroencephalogram (EEG). The most common and most serious side effects are on the cardiovascular system. Tachycardia, brachycardia, ventricular extrasystoles, congestive heart failure, myocardial infarction, AV block, and bundle branch block have been noted in clients receiving tricyclic medication.[13] Clients with known cardiovascular problems should not receive these medications. An electrocardiogram (ECG) should be done before the administration of any of these agents.

CONTRAINDICATIONS. Tricyclic drugs are contraindicated for clients with known cardiac disease. Hypersensitivity to tricyclics is another reason for not using these medications. Clients taking MAO inhibitors require a detoxification period of 14 to 21 days before beginning use of tricyclics. Safety of use during pregnancy is not established.

The use of the tricyclic group of drugs should be discontinued 1 week before elective surgery and is not recommended during electroconvulsive therapy. Tricyclic drugs may activate psychotic symptoms in schizophrenic clients.[13]

Table 26-12 Tricyclics: Degree of Anticholinergic Effects

Degree of Side Effect	Tricyclic	Trade Name
More ↑	Amitriptyline	Elavil
	Doxepin	Sinequan
	Imipramine	Tofranil
↓	Nortriptyline	Aventyl
Less	Desipramine	Norpramin

Table 26-13 Tricyclics: Relative Degrees of Sedation

Degree of Side Effect	Tricyclic	Trade Name
More ↑	Doxepin	Sinequan
	Amitriptyline	Elavil
	Imipramine	Tofranil
↓	Nortriptyline	Aventyl
Less	Desipramine	Norpramin
None	Protriptyline	Vivactil

Table 26-14 Monoamine Oxidase Inhibitors

Drug	Trade Name	Initial Dosage Range, mg	Method of Administration	Maintenance Dosage Range, mg
Isocarboxazid	Marplan	10–30	PO (tablets)	10–50
Phenelzine sulfate	Nardil	30–45	PO (tablets)	45–90
Tranylcypromine sulfate	Parnate	20–30	PO (tablets)	20–60

Monoamine Oxidase (MAO) Inhibitors

MAO inhibitors carry a greater risk than tricyclics and are therefore not considered to be a practitioner's first choice for the treatment of depression. They are generally used for the treatment of atypical depression, depression with a hysterical component, and depression resulting from severe loss. Clients who do not respond well to tricyclic medication, those who have cardiovascular disease, and those who have responded well to MAO inhibitors in the past are also candidates for treatment. A client with a tendency to manipulate others is not a good candidate for the drug. The need to conform to a restrictive diet provides a manipulative client with too much potential to act out around the issue of adherence to the diet. The generic names of commonly used MAO inhibitors are listed in Table 26-14 (above) along with their dosages and trade names.

Some therapeutic effect from the MAO inhibitors is seen within 24 hours, although it is believed that their maximum effect is reached in 3 weeks to 4 weeks.

ACTION. Theoretically, depressed persons have an excess of monoamine oxidase. MAO inhibitors affect norepinephrine and other biogenic amines. They are believed to block the action of a number of enzymes, particularly MAO, which causes the breakdown of biogenic amines. The drugs block or inhibit the action of MAO, causing an increase of biogenic amines at neuroreceptor sites and a subsequent lift in the mood of the client.

SIDE EFFECTS. Hypertensive crisis is the most serious adverse effect of MAO inhibitors. Hypertensive crisis is produced when the medication is taken in combination with tyramine-rich foods. Table 26-15 lists foods and medications that produce hypertensive crisis in clients taking MAO inhibitors. Hypertensive crisis is commonly referred to as a *parnate-cheese reaction. Parnate* is the name of one drug in this class. Its interaction with aged cheese was a common cause of the crisis.

Table 26-15 Agents Contraindicated during Treatment with MAO Inhibitors

Foods and Beverages
Meat tenderizers
Strong or aged cheeses (cheddar cheese)
Sour cream
Yogurt
Pickles
Pickled herring and other canned fish
Chopped liver and chicken livers
Avocados
Bananas
Raisins
Canned figs
Citrus fruits
Pineapple
Broad beans and their pods
Soy sauce
Any product made with yeast or by bacterial action
Beer and wine (particularly chianti and sherry)
Coffee
Chocolate
Chicken
Medications
Narcotic analgesics
Amphetamines
L-dopa
Methyldopa
Phenylpropanolamine (in over-the-counter cold remedies)
Tricyclic antidepressants

SOURCE: M. B. Wiener and C. A. Pepper, *Clinical Pharmacology and Therapeutics in Nursing*, 2d ed., McGraw-Hill, New York, 1985.

Hypertensive reaction is signaled by the presence of a generalized or occipital headache, diaphoresis, increased restlessness, palpitations, pallor, chills, stiff neck, nausea, vomiting, muscle twitching, and chest pains. Hypertensive crisis is considered a medical emergency, since it may lead to intracranial hemorrhage and possibly death. Nursing action involves discontinuing the medication and notifying the physician immediately. Treatment is symptomatic and includes maintenance of hydration and electrolyte balance. Slow administration of 5 milligrams of phentolamine mesylate (Regitine), which is the drug of choice in hypertensive crisis, is initiated. External cooling measures for the fever are common.[14]

Hypotension, headache without blood-pressure elevation, tachycardia, edema, palpitations, blurred vision, and impotence sometimes occur. Other side effects include anorexia, dry mouth, nausea, diarrhea, abdominal pain, and constipation. Restlessness, insomnia, drowsiness, and dizziness have been noted in some clients.[10]

CONTRAINDICATIONS. MAO inhibitors are contraindicated for clients who are unable to conform to the restrictive diet required and those who have cerebrovascular defects or cardiovascular disorders. Clients over 60 years of age, those with liver disease, or those with histories of hypersensitivity to MAO inhibitors should not be given these drugs. Safety of use during pregnancy is not established. Serious drug interactions occur if MAO inhibitors are given in combination with tricyclics, narcotics, alcohol, anticholinergics, antidiabetic agents, barbiturates, reserpine, sympathomimetics, and dibenzazepine derivatives.[10]

RELEVANCE TO NURSING

PHASE 1: CONTROL OF SYMPTOMS. One of the most essential nursing responsibilities with a client who is to begin antidepressant medication is the establishment of an accurate and complete data base. Baseline data include assessment of the physical, emotional, and spiritual dimensions of self. An accurate data base is essential in order to evaluate the effectiveness of a drug. Ideally, clients should be withdrawn from any other medication they may be taking before starting antidepressant agents. This is done because some drugs are known to cause depressive side effects while others interact unfavorably with antidepressants. Evaluation of and stabilization on antidepressant medication are ideally performed in an inpatient setting where diagnostic testing is readily available and observations are consistent and reliable.

Once a data base is established, the nurse monitors and reports improvement. Assessment of side effects and intervention (when appropriate) are essential during this phase of treatment. Clients and nurses need to remain cognizant of the lag period that exists before improvement is expected.

Expected outcomes after 2 to 3 weeks of drug therapy include improvement in appetite, sleep, and other physical functions. Gradually, energy, mobilization, and, finally, mood and attitude improve. Because of this pattern, the nurse may notice improvement before the client does. When such signs of improvement are noted, it is important to point them out to the client. This encourages the client and helps enhance compliance.

Mobilization can be monitored by having clients describe their schedule of daily activities. A resumption of normal activities, such as getting out of the house more often, returning to a normal work schedule, performing chores previously neglected, and resuming hobbies all represent improvement in mobilization.

PHASE 2: STABILIZATION. Doses of antidepressant drugs are increased gradually until therapeutic dosages are achieved. Clients must be educated about this process and the side effects of their medication. Encouraging clients to report side effects immediately is a nursing function. Taking medication exactly as prescribed is another point that needs emphasis during the teaching process.

The potential for dependency and the dangers of overdose are discussed once the client begins to show improvement. It is generally at this point in the treatment process that a severely depressed and suicidal client mobilizes the energy to carry out a suicide attempt. Increased vigilance is necessary, and ongoing assessment of suicide potential is an essential part of the nursing process. The dietary restrictions for clients on MAO inhibitors need to be taught. Clients and their families can be taught to prepare foods without high amounts of tyramine.

PHASE 3: MAINTENANCE. Generally a therapeutic and maintenance dose of an antidepressant is established in 3 to 4 weeks. Antidepressant therapy is only one factor in the treatment of depression. Ongoing psychotherapy should be encouraged. The importance of keeping appointments for periodic review of the medication regimen and blood sampling should be pointed out. Teaching needs to include the signs of hypertensive crisis for clients taking MAO inhibitors. Clients and their families need to be cautioned not to discontinue the medication because of feelings of increased well-being. Ongoing consultation with the physician and primary therapist needs to be encouraged.

Antimania Drug: Lithium Carbonate

Lithium carbonate is a drug that has been used for many years in the treatment of manic-depressive illness (bipolar depression). It is used to prevent the recurrence of cyclic attacks of mania. It is more effective for the prevention and treatment of mania than for the prevention of depression. Clients who have experienced a manic episode begin to show improvement after 2 to 3 weeks of treatment with lithium carbonate.[16]

Action and Uses

While the exact mode of action of lithium carbonate is not clearly understood, studies indicate that it interferes with norepinephrine and serotonin metabolism and affects the electrolyte balance within the brain. It is thought to replace intracellular sodium. Lithium itself is a naturally occurring agent found in minerals, sea water, plants, and animals. Its use as a drug is generally restricted to manic-depressive illness, although it is used in a limited way for the treatment of atypical depressions. Its actual clinical effects can be correlated with effects observed in the laboratory.

Lithium does not bind to plasma protein, and it is excreted exclusively through the kidneys; therefore, the renal function of a client is of primary concern before beginning drug therapy. Peak plasma levels are reached in 1 to 3 hours. In order to maintain a constant plasma level of the drug, doses of lithium carbonate should be taken over a 24-hour period, usually in three or four doses. Lithium carbonate is marketed under a number of trade names. Lithane, Eskalith, and Lithonate are those most commonly used. Standard dosage size is 300 milligrams.

A lag period of from 7 to 10 days exists between the initiation of lithium carbonate treatment and the alleviation of manic symptoms. During this time, manic behavior may be controlled by concurrent administration of antipsychotic drugs or with electroconvulsive treatment. Long-term use of lithium carbonate may lead to thyroid disturbances, fine motor disturbance, and a decrease in glucose tolerance. Use of lithium carbonate during pregnancy is not advised.[16]

Lithium Carbonate Levels

Serum lithium levels are used to regulate the dosage. Therapeutic serum lithium levels range from 1.0 to 1.5 milliequivalents (meq) per liter. At no time should serum lithium levels exceed 2.0 meq per liter. Clients on maintenance doses of lithium carbonate should maintain a serum lithium range between 0.6 and 1.2 meq per liter and should not exceed 1.5 meq per liter. Blood should be drawn 10 to 12 hours after the last dose of the drug.[10]

Lithium Toxicity

Lithium toxicity is an infrequent but possibly fatal side effect. Toxicity occurs when the lithium ingested cannot be detoxified and excreted by the kidneys. Toxicity occurs when serum lithium levels are greater than 2.0 meq per liter. When toxicity occurs, treatment is mainly supportive and is aimed at the prevention of complications. The goal of treatment is to remove lithium from the system as quickly as possible.[16]

The first signs of lithium toxicity are blurred vision, ataxia, tinnitus, increased urination, and diarrhea. Clients should be instructed to stop their medication and to advise the physician immediately if these symptoms occur. It is the responsibility of the nurse to educate clients about these signs and symptoms. Lithium intoxication may last for several weeks but is generally reversible. The prevention of toxicity is the best way to deal with it. Individualized dosage regulation, serum lithium screening, and education of clients are ways in which the health practitioner helps clients prevent lithium toxicity.

Side Effects

Lithium carbonate produces a wide range of side effects. The major effects of the drug are on the central nervous system, the cardiovascular system, the neuromuscular system, and the gastrointestinal system. In addition to the physical effects of the drugs, emotional and spiritual effects are also observed. Table 26-16 outlines the physical symptoms that may occur when clients are treated with lithium and when toxicity may be occurring. Other side effects may include somnolence, confusion, restlessness, and stupor. In extreme toxic situations, mental retardation and coma may occur. Some of the less troublesome side effects may need to be tolerated by clients in order for them to maintain functional status in their communities. If symptoms occur, they should be reported without delay to the prescribing physician. Generalized fatigue, dehydration, lethargy, and a tendency toward sleepiness may appear early in treatment with lithium carbonate but gradually disappear. For some clients side effects may continue for months or years. Clients who are motivated to maintain themselves on lithium carbonate learn to adapt to the side effects, but others periodically sabotage drug regimens.

Table 26-16 Lithium

Side Effects and Toxicity
Cardiovascular system
Pulse irregularities
Fall in blood pressure
ECG changes
Peripheral circulatory failure
Circulatory collapse
Central nervous system
Anesthesia of skin
Incontinence of urine and feces
Slurred speech
Blurring of vision
Dizziness
Vertigo
Epileptiform seizures
Neuromuscular system
General muscle weakness
Ataxia
Muscle hyperirritability
Fasciculation (increased by tapping muscle)
Twitching (especially of facial muscles)
Clonic movements of whole limbs
Choreoathetoid movements
Hyperactive deep tendon reflexes
Gastrointestinal system
Anorexia
Nausea
Vomiting
Diarrhea
Thirst
Dryness of mouth
Weight Loss
Miscellaneous
Polyuria
Glycosuria
General fatigue
Lethargy and tendency to sleep
Dehydration

Phases of Treatment

The stabilization phase takes from 7 to 14 days. The goal of the stabilization phase is to control manic symptoms by reducing the client's extreme hyperactivity, which may otherwise lead to extreme weight loss, physical injuries, and loss of sleep. During this phase, concomitant therapy with sedating antipsychotic drugs is common. Blood samples for serum lithium levels are drawn on a daily basis. Levels should not exceed 2.0 meq per liter. Clients must be observed carefully for signs of lithium toxicity.[17]

The maintenance stage of therapy begins when a client reaches an adequate serum lithium level and manic symptoms have subsided. The usual daily maintenance dose is 1200 milligrams per day, generally given in four divided doses. While a client is on a maintenance dose of lithium carbonate, serum lithium levels should be monitored monthly. Clients may remain on lithium prophylactically for indefinite periods of time. Monitoring of lithium levels will help determine compliance and therapeutic effects. Prevention of toxicity should be one of the prime goals of maintenance therapy.

Despite control of symptoms, many clients dislike their lack of "highs." They will tell nurses that the leveling of their feelings is not as pleasant as the manic state. Failure to comply with the medication regimen often results.

RELEVANCE TO NURSING

The nurse needs to keep several factors in mind when intervening with clients in either the maintenance or the stabilization phase of treatment with lithium carbonate. A complete history and physical examination are necessary for each client before beginning lithium carbonate administration. The examination would include blood pressure determination and blood studies such as hematocrit hemoglobin, white blood cell count, blood differential, blood urea nitrogen, serum creatinine, and electrolyte levels. Urinalysis, serum thyroid function tests, and an electrocardiogram are also necessary. Because lithium is contraindicated in clients with cardiovascular disease, renal disease, decreased sodium intake, or fever, a careful history is essential. Clients who are pregnant should not take lithium. Clients with any condition that involves either sodium or water depletion may experience lithium toxicity if they receive the drug. Lithium should be used with caution by the elderly.

If mood swings start to occur during lithium maintenance therapy, clients should be advised to see their physician immediately. Families should be included in this education. Clients also need to understand and be educated about the signs of lithium toxicity. Toxicity can be prevented if clients understand that the maintenance lithium levels should be monitored monthly. Clients should be encouraged to maintain their usual diet and salt intake with adequate fluids (2000 to 3000 milliliters per day).[16] Change in salt intake will change serum lithium levels and thus be a potential cause of lithium toxicity. Mild, adverse side effects generally diminish as treatment continues. Teaching clients to identify and report severe effects is an important function of the nurse monitoring lithium administration.

By giving careful information to clients and their families, nurses help encourage compliance. The primary function of the nurse is to be an educator. Several teaching points follow:

1. Tell the clients about the side effects factually and without overemphasis.
2. Teach clients how to detect and prevent lithium toxicity.
3. Explain to clients and their families the lag period of up to 3 weeks.
4. Inform clients that alcohol may potentiate adverse effects of lithium.
5. Caution clients not to stop taking lithium abruptly but rather to taper off the dosage.
6. Advise clients not to adjust dosages without consultation with their physicians.
7. Encourage appropriate exercise and diet to prevent weight gain. Weight gain is common for clients on lithium therapy.
8. Advise clients to avoid conditions that cause profuse sweating.
9. Advise clients not to take medications, including over-the-counter products, without consulting their physicians.

Psychopharmacological Therapy: Issues of Concern to Nurses

Many ethical and legal issues are involved in the use of psychopharmacological agents to treat mental illness. Drug tolerance, physiological and psychological dependence, long-range side effects, drug interactions, compliance, and medications used as restraints are issues that concern nurses.

Tolerance and Dependence

A decreased responsiveness to a drug after a period of use is called *tolerance*. A client's tolerance to a drug generally requires increased dosages in order to maintain therapeutic effectiveness. The term *physical dependence* refers to a client's physiological need for a drug. When physical dependence occurs, increasing amounts of the drug are needed to maintain normal functioning, and withdrawal symptoms occur when the drug is discontinued. *Psychological dependence* is a term used to describe craving or emotional need or addiction to a chemical substance. Chapter 33 discusses the dynamics of dependence in detail.

Some clients develop tolerance to psychotropic drugs, although this is relatively rare with the antipsychotic and antidepressant groups. More commonly, clients develop psychological dependence on antianxiety agents, particularly the barbiturates and benzodiazepines.

Intelligent and Rational Selection of Drugs

Most knowledge of the behavioral effects of psychotropic substances in common use has been gained through observation of responses of clients. Although such knowledge is obviously necessary for responsible treatment, one should remember that behavioral effects in a client are qualified in substantial measure by the client's condition and perception of the disorder.[18]

Selecting the drug to be used is a very individual process and should be tailored to the needs of the client. Target symptoms that the physician is attempting to bring under control need to be considered as well as the person's overall environment, including job and family constellation. With the development of specific drugs with very specific actions, the practitioner is able to prescribe more for specific behavior, thereby tailoring and individualizing the drug regimen. As knowledge of psychopharmacology improves, multiple drug therapy has become less common; rather, the trend is to seek one drug that will have the maximum effect.

Interactions between certain drugs may cause long-range side effects. One drug may cancel out the effect of another. As various groups and subgroups within the overall classification of psychotherapeutics have become more refined, drugs are being prescribed more specifically. For example, some drugs cause more sedation than others. From a legal and ethical standpoint it then becomes important that a person who is actively engaged in employment have a drug that is less sedating, even though the person may experience some of the other, more uncomfortable side effects of the drug. A client who must work with machinery should not take an antidepressant or a tricyclic but rather should be given an MAO inhibitor, with its less sedating effects. The client then has to worry about the very restricted diet prescribed when a person is on an MAO inhibitor. A client being evaluated for possible use of an MAO inhibitor must have a relatively high degree of intelligence and must be motivated to take the drug, since it can be dangerous if taken in conjunction with certain foods.

The obligation of the practitioner to be aware of current trends is an ethical one. As legal decisions proliferate and the number of states requiring mandatory continuing education increases, rational and safe prescription of drugs is becoming a legal issue.

Long-Range Side Effects

Currently, one ethical issue that occurs over and over is whether or not the long-range effects of psychotropic drugs warrant their long-range use. This is the same issue as that raised by using insulin with diabetics or phenytoin with epileptics. One has to weigh relief of symptoms, with its consequent long-range effects, against a relatively high level of functioning.

Results of research on long-range effects have recently become available; they suggest that tardive dyskinesia is a long-range side effect of antipsychotic drugs. Clients must be informed about this effect and decide whether or not they want to accept the risk. Informing clients about the complications of treatment with psychotropic drugs is part of the ethical responsibility of the physician prescribing the drug and the nurse who must then teach clients about these long-range side effects and their treatment.

Interactions with Food and Other Drugs

Interactions among drugs or between specific drugs and foods are of increasing concern to nurses. Legal and ethical responsibility requires that nurses be knowledgeable about the possible interactions of drugs. Some interactions interfere with how a specific drug acts. For example, antipsychotic agents may enhance the effect of some pain medications. This may be a desired effect when one wishes to use less medication to achieve a goal.

Other interactions interfere with drug absorption. For example, antacids may prevent the absorption of some drugs. Conversely, the nutrient value of foods may be affected by a drug. For instance, folic acid, necessary for the manufacture of red blood cells, is not absorbed by clients taking some psychotropic medications. Other drugs, particularly those affecting the autonomic nervous system, alter taste and appetite. Toxic reactions occur when tyramine-rich foods are eaten by clients who are on MAO inhibitors. Nutritional guidance and education go hand in hand with responsible drug therapy.

Restraint

Among the legal and ethical issues facing the nurse dealing with mentally ill clients are the issue of restraint by use of psychotropic medication and the issue of behavioral control with drugs. Health care practitioners are aware of the beneficial effect of psychotropic medication. Clients, however, are sometimes more skeptical and therefore less compliant. Questions such as, "When may a nurse force medication?" and, "When is the nurse ethically required to inform clients about the behavioral changes that result from use of psychotropic drugs?" are concerns of those overseeing drug administration. One must also ask whether or not the health care practitioner has the right to impose "expertise" on the so-called incompetent client. Another issue arises around the forcible use of sedating drugs when clients are a danger to themselves or others. What parameters should be used to assess the danger?

There are no simple answers to any of these questions. Nurses need to clarify their own values about the issues (see Chapter 9). Awareness of state legislation is also essential. Most states require specific written criteria and protocols for use of medication for restraint purposes. Generally, danger to oneself or to others is the criterion used to initiate forcible administration of a drug. Some states have defined what behaviors constitute this danger. A nurse becomes an advocate for a client when medicating for purposes of restraint does not seem justified or when values of the nurse and the client differ from those of the prescribing physician or other team members.[19]

Compliance

Clients refuse to take psychotropic medications for a number of reasons. Some of the reasons for noncompliance stated in a recent survey of clients by the *American Journal of Nursing* include the following:

1. Unpleasant side effects of medication
2. Confusion about the drug regimen
3. Drug-drug and drug-food interactions
4. Cost of the drugs
5. Religious reasons
6. Feelings that the drugs are no longer needed
7. Difficulty opening drug containers
8. Difficulty swallowing the drugs
9. Fears about drug addiction
10. Self-consciousness about the need to take medication
11. Fear of losing control or taking too many chemicals[20]

Clients who refuse medication fall into categories referred to in one study as *situational refusers, stereotypical refusers, and symptomatic refusers.* Situational refusers are a diverse group of clients who on occasion refuse medication for short periods of time and for one of a variety of reasons. Stereotypical refusers are chronically ill clients with paranoid traits who habitually and predictably respond to a variety of stresses with brief refusals to take medication. Symptomatic refusers are relatively young, acutely ill clients whose refusal, often based on delusional premises, is sustained over long periods of time. The nurse's attitude toward the issues is frequently reflected back by the client when refusal of medication is an issue.[21]

Other compliance issues are raised when clients take more medication than was prescribed and when clients give their medications to others with similar complaints. In rarer situations, clients sell their medications for profit. In still other cases, clients simply forget to take their medications.

Nurses play a major role in improving compliance with drug regimens. A mutually gratifying relationship between a skilled nurse and client is a primary factor in continuance of a drug. Other interventions found to improve compliance include careful teaching of the client and a supportive family member, weekly follow-up sessions, simplified and clear drug therapy regimens, and inpatient trials of self-medication. Other ways to improve compliance include reducing the number of daily doses and asking pharmacists to simplify directions by clearly labeling drug vials.[22] On a broader scale, nurses may choose to lobby drug companies to reduce costs and simplify product information inserts.[20] Improved compliance with drug regimens is a cooperative venture among clients, their families, nurses, prescribing physicians, pharmacists, and drug companies.

Nursing Process with Psychopharmacological Therapy

The ideal framework for nurses involved in psychopharmacological therapy with clients is the nursing process. Drug therapy is only one aspect of a treatment plan. The needs of clients related to their medication regimens are essential components of their total care.

Assessment

Ideally, drug therapy begins after an intensive investigation of a client's physical, emotional, spiritual, and social functioning has been completed.

The data base upon which subsequent judgments are made about psychopharmacological treatment begins with the completion of a thorough physical examination, including a complete blood chemistry and liver profile. A mental status examination is used to establish emotional and cognitive levels of functioning. Observations should note a client's ability to relate to other clients and the staff, as well as an assessment of the client's sense of hope. A drug history is also obtained.

It is best to discuss the drug history directly with the client; however, it may be necessary to get additional information from family members, friends, or previous medical records.

The following questions can be adapted to a particular client and situation:

- What prescribed drugs are you currently taking? What nonprescribed drugs?
- What prescribed drugs have you taken in the past? What nonprescribed drugs?

  How long have you been taking these drugs?
  How many pills do you take a day?
  What time of day do you take them?
  Do you ever forget to take prescribed drugs?
  What do you do if you miss a dose?
- Do you take drugs exactly as the doctor prescribed them?

  Do you adjust dosage according to the way you feel?
  Do you feel that the drugs have helped you?
  What reactions have you had from the drugs?
  Are there any drugs that you are allergic to?
  Do you use alcohol or marijuana?
- Do you purchase and use over-the-counter drugs such as aspirin or cold remedies?
- Which medications that you have taken in the past have helped you the most?
- Have you ever felt worse after taking medication? Which medications made you feel this way?

Diagnosis

Nursing diagnoses that focus on a client's treatment with psychopharmacological agents usually center on issues of compliance or restraint. At times they are statements about the observed side effects of a particular drug. The following are some diagnoses that may be made when clients are being treated with psychotropic drugs.

- Dry mouth related to therapy with chlorpromazine (Thorazine)
- Tardive dyskinesia associated with 7-year use of amitriptyline (Elavil)
- History of noncompliance related to client's confusion about previous multiple-drug regimens
- History of agitation related to use of haloperidol (Haldol)
- Refusal to take prescribed medication associated with upset about side effects

Outcome Criteria

When an adequate assessment has been completed and specific nursing diagnoses have been formulated, goals or outcomes can be planned for clients. Ideally, the goal or outcome for every client is to take the least amount of a drug that will produce the maximum therapeutic effect. The following are desired outcomes of every drug treatment regimen:

- Clients will name the medications that have been prescribed.
- Clients and their families will verbalize therapeutic effects desired and the side effects of medications.
- Clients and their families will verbalize dosages, times the medications are to be taken, and precautions necessary when taking specific drugs.
- Clients will ask questions that clarify their concerns about drug regimens.
- Clients will periodically make appointments to review their therapy regimens.
- Clients will list foods and other drugs that are incompatible with their prescribed medications.
- Clients will store medications in safe places.
- Clients will verbalize routines for taking medication that are congruent with daily schedules.

Intervention

The nurse's positive attitude toward the use of psychopharmacological agents is an important component in implementing an effective drug treatment program. Clients and family members have a number of realistic concerns about drugs that must be responded to by the nurse. Adequate time should be given to address any new or continued problem that has to be resolved. If the client's concerns are ignored, medication will be refused or compliance may be sporadic.

The following interventions are necessary to ensure success of a drug treatment plan:

- Nurses must have a thorough, current knowledge of psychopharmacological agents, including routes of drug absorption, distribution, biotransformation, and excretion.
- Drugs should be administered so that the minimum effective concentration level is maintained. This is best achieved by strict adherence to recommended times of medication and dosage.
- Nurses or clients should administer medication according to established safety standards. When medication is self-administered, clients or family members should demonstrate knowledgeable awareness of the prescribed drug.

As a part of therapy in a psychiatric milieu, the client is encouraged to maintain as much independent functioning as possible. The drug treatment program is explained to the client, who is then expected to come for medication at the scheduled time.

The following procedure for actual administration is recommended:

1. Check the physician's written order; if there is any doubt about the drug order, check with the physician.
2. Medications should be prepared in a room that is free of distractions for both clients and staff members.
3. Clearly establish the identity of the client. If there is any doubt concerning the identity of the client, seek confirmation from another staff member. Address the client by name to confirm identity and to foster self-respect.
4. Perform necessary preparatory interventions. (Take blood pressure of clients receiving phenothiazines; check most recent lithium level of clients receiving lithium.)
5. Allow the client to ventilate his or her feelings regarding medications. Answer questions honestly and simply.
6. Use only paper or plastic medication cups.
7. Place the medication tray out of reach of clients.
8. Administer medication to only one client at a time. Observe the client closely to be sure that the medication has been swallowed. If a client is suspected of not swallowing the medication, offer additional fluids. Liquid preparations are preferable if resistance to medications is encountered.
9. Chart all medications and include significant information regarding refusal, side effects, unusual behavior, or the client's complaints.
10. Carefully observe the client for drug reactions. Keep a record of vital signs and weight.

Individuals have a wide range of responses to psychopharmacological therapy. Close observations and reporting of behavior and physical reactions to these agents are essential in determining the adequacy of the treatment plan.

Whether a psychiatric client is receiving drug therapy at home or in the hospital, there is always the possibility that the medication may not be taken. Compliance is frequently a treatment issue. It is not unusual for psychotic clients to palm, "cheek," or deliberately vomit medication. Clients at home sometimes "forget" to take their prescribed drugs. Whenever the nurse suspects that this may be the case, it is advisable to recommend an injectable form of medication. At the same time it is important to attempt to find out why the client is averse to taking medication. It should be realized that even the most solicitous nurse cannot always convince a delusional or reluctant client to accept drug treatment.

Planned drug education programs are becoming available in psychiatric inpatient settings, day hospitals, aftercare clinics, and private practitioners' offices. Learning opportunities can be informally and formally offered to the client, both individually and in a group setting.[23] The natural climate for learning presents itself whenever the client first has contact with the nurse administering medications. Basic information concerning the drugs is offered. When initiating drug administration, the nurse discusses the following issues with the client:

Reasons for giving the drug: "Thorazine will calm you down, and you won't be so tense or anxious."

Route of administration: "The doctor would like you to take this medication by injection for the first few doses; after that you can take it by mouth."

How long the drug will be given: "The team is not sure how long you will be given this medication. The team will be evaluating you to see how you appear to be doing on it."

Client's reactions to the drug: "If you have any concerns about this medication, you can talk it over with me, your doctor, or your therapist."

It is important to realize that when first admitted to inpatient services, a client is often so frightened, angry, confused, or depressed that explanations are not really heard or understood. The condition of the client determines the depth and extent of the drug information given.

Reinforcement of oral instruction with written information is an important factor in preventing the "revolving door" syndrome. Some useful guidelines in initiating and maintaining an effective group drug education program include the following:

Keep an updated file on psychopharmacological information.

Develop records, on cards, of instructions to be given to clients about medication.

Keep classes small (six to ten members). Include family members when appropriate.

Remember that group classes are a supplement to individual instruction.

Keep records and charts of instructions given to a client and of client's attendance at classes.

Offer a general overview of psychotherapeutic drugs.

Keep information basic.

Encourage active group participation. Elicit information from clients regarding drugs that they are currently taking.

Have clients refer to their medications by name.

Use printed handouts, audiovisual aids, and charts to reinforce identification of the medication and the specific principles that need reinforcement.

Suggest practical ways to deal with side effects.

Emphasize the importance of taking drugs only as instructed. Make sure that clients understand not to stop or start medication, or alter a regimen, without the doctor's permission.

Reinforce dietary restrictions, limitations on activity or need for exercise, other relevant instructions, and the importance of regular clinic visits.

Answer all questions honestly.

Encourage clients to discuss any unresolved personal concerns or issues.

Compliance with the drug regimen is dependent upon the client's understanding of the medication. For the client to perceive the medication as helpful is another key factor. Ideally, psychiatric clients should know what they are taking into their bodies. From philosophical, legal, and humanistic points of view, nurses certainly must be willing and prepared to assist psychiatric clients to learn as much as possible about the medications that they will be taking. Clients respond positively to honest explanations which suggest that what is being offered is beneficial. This approach means that the nurse must be willing to risk the consequence that a particular client may refuse to take medication.

Evaluation

Decisions to alter or discontinue a drug program for a specific client will be based on the ongoing evaluation of the person's response to drug treatment. Evaluation of drug therapy is a continuing process that occurs throughout the client's treatment. When the client is receiving psychotropic agents, written observations include the overall response to medication, length of treatment, general progress, unresolved problems, and other pertinent data along with recommendations for further intervention.

Much of the evaluation of the effectiveness of a drug treatment regimen is based on the subjective sense of clients that they have improved, feel better, and behave more appropriately. The nurse's objective observations are also integral to the evaluation process. In the symptom-control stage, daily evaluation focuses on whether or not behaviors have improved. As stabilization on a particular drug occurs, education of a client can begin and evaluation becomes focused on minimizing unwanted and uncomfortable side effects. Evaluation in the maintenance stage is less frequent and is focused on compliance issues and assessment of long-range side effects.

SUMMARY

Somatic therapy is the treatment of clients with physiological agents or physical methods. Some older somatic therapies are insulin coma therapy, psychosurgery, orthomolecular therapy, and hydrotherapy. Insulin coma therapy involves the injection of a fasting client with increasing amounts of insulin in order to induce seizures. Psychosurgery involves brain surgery to alter behavior. Orthomolecular therapy uses large doses of vitamins to treat mental illness. It is also known as *megavitamin* or *niacin therapy.* Hydrotherapy involves the use of water in the treatment of mental illness. Historically, wet packs and cold sheets were used to calm or energize clients. Chronically ill clients treated with these therapies in the past can still be found in the health care system today.

Two somatic therapies in use today are electroconvulsive therapy and psychopharmacological therapy. *Electroconvulsive therapy* (ECT) is the artificial induction by electric current of a grand mal seizure under controlled circumstances. *Psychopharmacological therapy* is the use of drugs to treat psychiatric symptoms. Drugs used include antipsychotics, antianxiety agents, tricyclic antidepressants, MAO inhibitors, the antimania agent, lithium carbonate, and antiparkinsonian agents.

Antipsychotic drugs are used to control psychotic behavior. While producing the desired therapeutic effects, this group of drugs has a high incidence of troublesome but expected side effects. Sedation, hypotension, anticholinergic effects, and extrapyramidal side effects are common. The extrapyramidal side effects include pseudoparkinsonism, akathisia, akinesia, dystonia, oculogyric crisis, and tardive dyskinesia.

Antiparkinsonian drugs are used to control the parkinsonianlike side effects of the antipsychotics.

Antianxiety agents are used to relieve mild or moderate anxiety or to treat psychoneurotic and psychosomatic conditions. Subgroups include the barbiturates, propanediol dicarbamates, antihistamines, beta-adrenergic blocking agents, and benzodiazepines.

Antidepressant drugs are used to treat depression. Tricyclics and MAO inhibitors are two groups of antidepressant drugs. The biogenic amine hypothesis states that a deficiency of one or another type of neurotransmitter results in manifestations of depression.

Lithium carbonate is the antimania drug of choice for clients with manic-depressive symptoms.

The nursing process is used by nurses working with clients receiving psychopharmacological agents. Planned drug education programs specify for a client the reasons the drug is needed, the route of administration, the dosage, the frequency with which the drug is to be taken, and the length of time the client is required to take the drug. The client is given an opportunity to discuss reactivity and feelings about being on medication.

The nursing process may be applied in each of the phases of drug treatment. During the symptom-control phase, the drug is introduced and the client is observed until relief of symptoms occurs. The stabilization phase lasts from 3 to 6 weeks and is the time when side effects are eliminated and ongoing relief is achieved. During the maintenance phase, the drug is slowly reduced to a minimum dose. Some clients may eventually achieve a drug-free phase.

There are many nursing issues involved in the administration of psychotropic drugs. Legal and ethical issues include tolerance and dependence, drug selection, long-range side effects, restraint, and compliance.

REFERENCES

1. P. Y. Adelson, "The Back Ward Dilemma," *American Journal of Nursing*, vol. 80, no. 3, March 1980, pp. 422–425.
2. R. J. Corsini, ed., *Current Psychotherapies*, 2d ed., Peacock, Ithaca, Ill., 1978.
3. H. I. Kaplan and B. J. Sadack, eds., *Comprehensive Textbook of Psychiatry*, 3d ed., Williams and Wilkins, Baltimore, 1981.
4. M. Culver, B. Ferrell, and M. Green, "ECT and Special Problems of Informed Consent," *American Journal of Psychiatry*, vol. 137, no. 5, May 1980, pp. 586–591.
5. R. M. Fraser, *ECT: A Clinical Guide*, Wiley, New York, 1982.
6. M. B. Wiener and C. A. Pepper, *Clinical Pharmacology and Therapeutics in Nursing*, 2d ed., McGraw-Hill, New York, 1985.
7. E. Harris, "Extrapyramidal Side Effects of Antipsychotic Medication," *American Journal of Nursing*, vol. 81, no. 7, July 1981, pp. 1324–1328.
8. V. L. Rosal-Greif, "Drug Induced Dyskinesias," *American Journal of Nursing*, vol. 82, no. 1, January 1982, pp. 66–69.
9. A. L. Whall, V. Engle, A. Edwards, L. Bobel, and C. Haberland, "Development of a Screening Program for Tardive Dyskinesia: Feasibility Issues," *Nursing Research*, vol. 32, no. 3, May–June 1983, pp. 151–156.
10. A. Albanese, *Nurses Drug Reference*, McGraw-Hill, New York, 1979.

11. R. Michaels and G. R. Brown, *Drug Consultant 1985–86: The Pocket Clinical Guide,* Wiley, New York, 1985.
12. J. White and K. Williamson, "What to Watch for with Minor Tranquilizers," *RN,* November 1979, pp. 57–59.
13. J. Burton, "Intoxication by Centrally Acting Substances," *Critical Care Update,* vol. 10, no. 9, September 1983, pp. 34–35 and 45.
14. S. Stern, J. Rush, and J. Mendels, "Toward a Rational Pharmacotherapy of Depression," *American Journal of Psychiatry,* vol. 137, no. 5, May 1980, pp. 545–552.
15. R. J. Bielski and R. O. Friedal, "Depressive Subtypes Defined by Response to Pharmacotherapy," *Psychiatric Clinics of North America,* vol. 2, no. 3, 1979, pp. 483–497.
16. F. Prien, M. Coffey, and C. Klett, *Lithium Carbonate in Psychiatry,* American Psychiatric Association, Washington, 1970.
17. R. I. Shader, *Manual of Psychiatric Therapeutics: Practical Psychopharmacology and Psychiatry,* Little, Brown, Boston, 1975.
18. J. R. Wittenborn, "Behavioral Toxicity of Psychotropic Drugs," *Journal of Nervous and Mental Disease,* vol. 168, no. 3, 1980, pp. 171–175.
19. L. Vicherman, "Involuntary Medication: Your Patient Advocacy on the Line," *Canadian Nurse,* vol. 80, no. 5, May 1984, pp. 32–34.
20. N. A. Moree, "Nurses Speak Out on Patients and Drug Regimens," *American Journal of Nursing,* vol. 85, no. 1, January 1985, pp. 51–54.
21. S. Reiser, "Refusing Treatment for Mental Illness: Historical and Ethical Dimensions," *American Journal of Psychiatry,* vol. 137, no. 3, 1980, pp. 329–345.
22. C. Ecock-Connelly, "Patient Compliance: A Review of the Research with Implication for Psychiatric Mental Health Nursing," *Journal of Mental Health and Psychiatric Nursing,* vol. 16, no. 10, October 1978, pp. 15–18.
23. M. Cohen and M. A. Amdur, "Medication Group for Psychiatric Patients," *American Journal of Nursing,* vol. 81, no. 2, February 1982, pp. 343–345.

PART FIVE

Health: Psychosocial Patterns

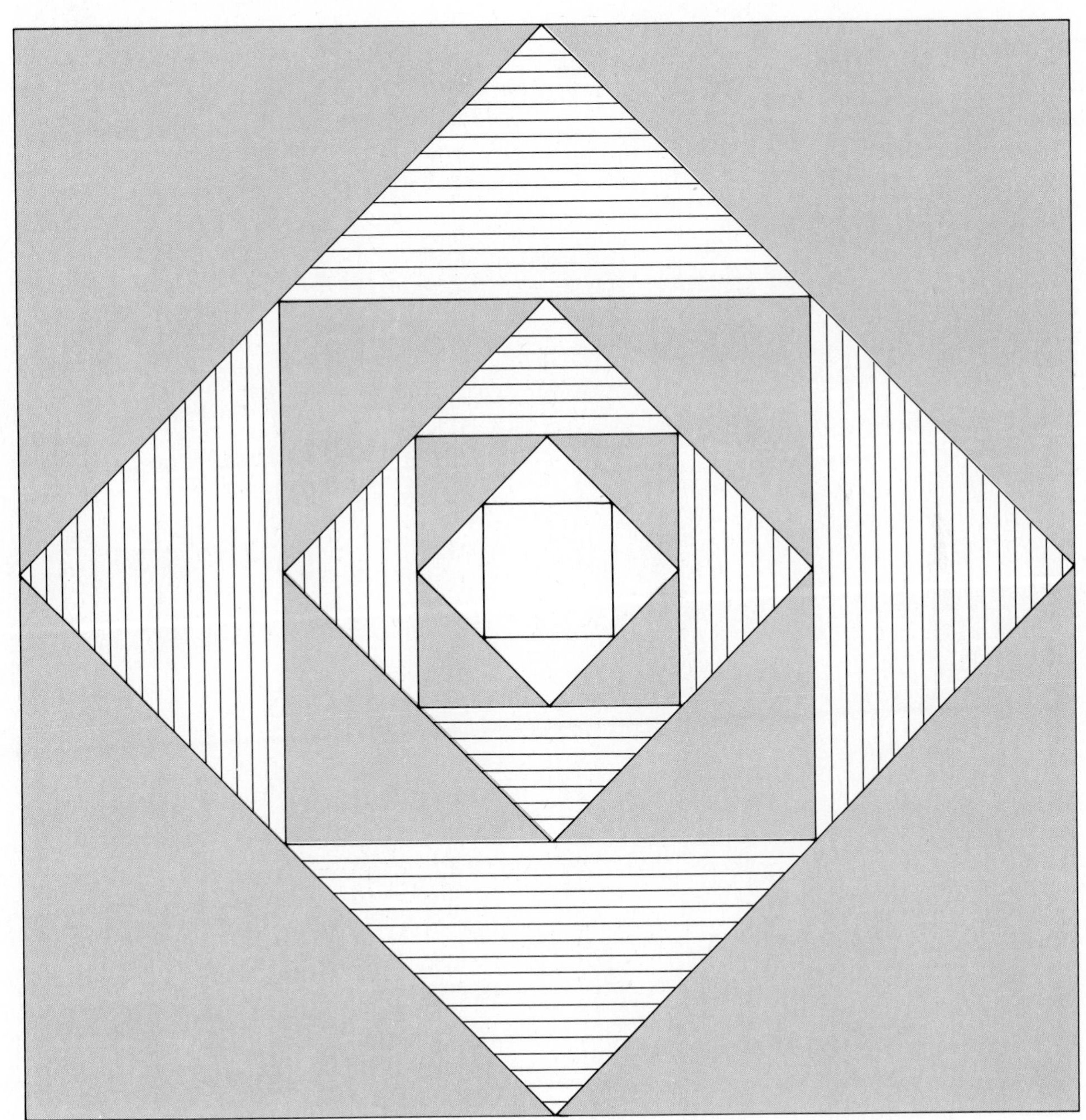

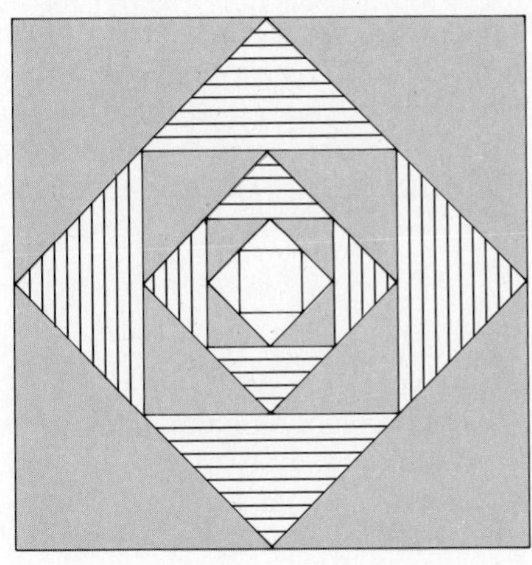

CHAPTER 27
Defining Health

Judith Haber
Pamela Price Hoskins
Anita M. Leach
Barbara Flynn Sideleau

LEARNING OBJECTIVES

After studying this chapter, the student should be able to:

1. Elaborate on the definitions of *health* and *health status.*
2. Recognize the client's needs to which promotion, maintenance, restoration, and rehabilitation of health are addressed.
3. Relate the definition of *health* to psychosocial and biopsychosocial phenomena.

Health is the central concern of nursing. Society has entrusted much of research on and development of health to the nursing profession. The goal of health and the way nursing defines and facilitates health are unique aspects of nursing.

The purpose of this chapter is to expand on the definition of *health,* including its psychosocial and biopsychosocial aspects. The chapter also describes the four approaches to health used in nursing and gives a rationale for the organization of Parts Five and Six.

THE CONCEPT OF HEALTH

Two definitions are important in the concept of health: *health* itself and *health status.* Both are presented and discussed in the following sections.

Health

Health is defined as synchronous patterns of interaction between the client and the environment—or, to put it another way, within the client-environment system. Health is a reflection of a dynamic, positive state which must be actively pursued. Clients pursue health because it is a factor in attaining the goals of life. In order to understand this definition of health, two phrases need to be examined in some detail.

Client-environment system refers to a higher-order system created from the stable relationship that develops between two smaller systems: the client and the client's environment. Three client systems are defined as recipients of nursing services: person, family or group, and community. Each of these is related to systems in its environment. For instance, an individual client, John, identifies his family, in-laws, job, church, and baseball team as his environment. A family client, the Smiths, identify their neighborhood, therapist, parents' places of employment, and day care center as their environment. A community client, Washita County, identifies its state, water and sewage treatment plants, federal block grants, and Big River Dam as its environment.

Synchronous patterns of interaction refers to stable, enduring rhythms that develop over time and facilitate the growth and development of the client system. In contrast, dysynchronous patterns of interaction are chaotic, disruptive, disturbing factors that hinder the client's growth and development. Synchronous patterns may lose their patterning, become dysynchronous, and express themselves in illness.

Health Status

Health status is an expression of life processes, a synthesis of all the patterns of interaction between client and environment, measured on a continuum from functional to dysfunctional patterns of interaction. Health status is a dynamic, changing state, determined by changing patterns of interaction. Health status may be described and measured. Two terms in this definition also need to be explained further.

The term *life processes* refers to all the dynamics that characterize and maintain life in a client; these dynamics come together in patterned wholes. *Expression of life processes* refers to the unique way in which these dynamics are reflected in the client's life; these dynamics are determined by the patterns of interaction within the client-environment system.

Health status exists on a *continuum* from functional to dysfunctional. *Health* implies ability to function, and illness implies inability to function, or functioning poorly. (Other disciplines have different definitions of health; ability to function is the concern of nursing.) A client's health status varies considerably because of the dynamic nature of patterns of interaction. The client and the environment are open systems, influencing and influenced by each other. This view is hopeful, since health status can change if patterns of interaction change. Nurses improve health status by altering interactions between client and environment.

Nursing goals include promotion, maintenance, restoration, and rehabilitation of health. When clients' health status is functional but they are threatened by change, nurses' interventions are geared to promotion and maintenance of health. *Promotion* of health actually improves the client's health status; *maintenance* of health helps the client keep the same level of functioning. When the client's health status is threatened, new, less healthy patterns of interaction may begin to form; nurses aim at *restoration* of health status to the former level. When patterns of interaction are enduring and dysfunctional patterns are well established, *rehabilitation* occurs over a long period of time.

RATIONALE FOR THE ORGANIZATION OF PARTS FIVE AND SIX

Psychiatric–mental health nursing is concerned with the level of functioning of the person, family, and community in the psychosocial and biopsychosocial realms. Psychiatric–mental health nursing looks at the whole person in a unique way, which is reflected in Parts Five and Six. Part Five consists of 12 chapters that explore dysfunctional psychosocial patterns of interaction between person and environment. The patterns explored are psychosocial expressions of an unhealthy integration of physical, mental, and spiritual dimensions of the person with the environment. Part Six is composed of six chapters exploring psychosocial patterns of interaction that also have a strong physical expression—patterns that are not themselves dysfunctional but can produce dysfunctional outcomes. Each of these parts has an introduction that describes the concepts of psychosocial and biopsychosocial phenomena. The nursing process is described in terms of how nurses intervene to promote, maintain, restore, and rehabilitate functional patterns of interaction.

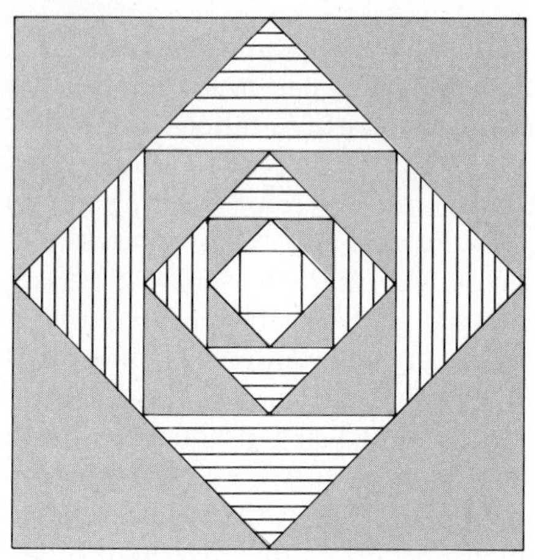

CHAPTER 28
Psychosocial Health

Judith Haber
Pamela Price Hoskins
Anita M. Leach
Barbara Flynn Sideleau

LEARNING OBJECTIVES

After studying this chapter, the student should be able to:

1. Elaborate on the definitions of *psychosocial health* and *dysfunction.*
2. Relate the definitions of psychosocial health and dysfunctions to patterns of overt and avoidant anxiety, borderline behavior, violence, substance abuse, depression, elation, self-destructiveness, impaired reality testing and orientation, sexual dysfunction, and dysfunction in adolescence.

The purpose of this chapter is to explore how patterns of psychosocial health and dysfunction develop and are manifested through interaction with the environment. It also provides an overview of Part Five. Dimensions of psychosocial health and dysfunction will be discussed from a holistic perspective. Several problematic psychosocial patterns will be noted: overt and avoidant anxiety, borderline behavior, violence, substance abuse, depression, elation, self-destructiveness, impaired reality testing and orientation, dysfunctional reality orientation, sexual dysfunction, and dysfunction in adolescence.

PSYCHOSOCIAL HEALTH

Psychosocial health is a dynamic process in which a person's mental, emotional, social, and spiritual patterns of functioning interact synchronously with each other and with environmental patterns. Healthy psychosocial patterns of interaction foster effective and appropriate satisfaction of needs and, in general, a productive and gratifying life. From a holistic perspective, synchronous patterns of interaction among person, family, and environment promote health and growth.

Psychosocial patterns reflect an ability to perceive reality accurately; modulate the ways emotions are experienced; think clearly and logically; communicate thoughts, emotions, feelings, needs, and desires effectively; anticipate events and solve problems; initiate and maintain meaningful relationships; establish and maintain boundaries; use resources appropriately; develop a positive self-concept; and, in general, behave in ways that facilitate personal growth and development.

Interacting family patterns that facilitate psychosocial health include those that foster a positive self-concept, respect for personal boundaries, appropriate separation, effective conflict management, and reasonable use of power. The family that functions effectively enhances psychosocial health by providing for the satisfaction of some needs. It also facilitates development of members' abilities to engage in satisfying relationships and use of resources outside the family.

An environment that is safe and provides opportunities to acquire what is needed interacts in a supportive way with individuals and families. Maximization of personal potential depends in part on the number and scope of occasions for interactions that promote growth. Resources that contribute to psychosocial health not only meet basic survival and motivational needs but also enrich life and foster advancement toward family members' personal goals and chosen life purposes.

PSYCHOSOCIAL DYSFUNCTION

Psychosocial dysfunction is patterns of physical, mental, emotional, perceptual, and spiritual functioning that interact dysynchronously with the environment. Dysynchronous patterns of interaction make it difficult to satisfy needs and pursue a productive and gratifying life. From a holistic perspective, patterns of interaction among person, family, and environment significantly influence the development and maintenance of psychosocial dysfunction and the establishment or restoration of healthy patterns of interaction.

Psychosocial dysfunction is a person-environment phenomenon. To understand its development, its manifestations, and approaches to its resolution, a holistic perspective is needed. This perspective encompasses mental, bodily, and spiritual interactions as well as interactions with family and the environment. When psychosocial dysfunction occurs, it is likely to be manifested primarily in person-environment interactions and emotional distress.

RATIONALE FOR THE ORGANIZATION OF PART FIVE

There are 11 chapters in Part Five, each of which contributes to the understanding of psychosocial dysfunction.

In Chapter 29, "Patterns of Overt Anxiety," anxiety, which can be acute, delayed, or chronic, is introduced as the foundation for understanding psychosocial dysfunction. Mental, bodily, and spiritual aspects of the person are affected by the experience of anxiety.

In Chapter 30, "Patterns of Avoidant Anxiety," psychosocial dysfunction related to management of anxiety is addressed through an exploration of avoidance that is characterized by somatization, ritualistic behavior, amnesia, irrational fears, and compulsive thoughts and actions.

In Chapter 31, "Patterns of Borderline Behavior," the understanding of psychosocial dysfunction is furthered through exploration of how flight from inner turmoil and mismanagement of anxiety generate ways of thinking and behaving that compound emotional pain.

In Chapter 32, "Patterns of Violence," the expression of psychosocial dysfunction through violence toward the environment provides insight into the development and manifestation of anxiety as anger and hostility.

In Chapter 33, "Patterns of Substance Abuse," antisocial interactions and the flight from anxiety through use of mind-altering and emotion-deadening chemicals expand the understanding of the many ways people exhibit psychosocial dysfunction.

In Chapter 34, "Patterns of Depression," the reader learns to understand the feelings of helplessness, hopelessness, and worthlessness that can occur when psychosocial dysfunction is present. The immobilizing impact of mismanaged anxiety and the flight from anxiety which results in withdrawal into self are explored.

In Chapter 35, "Patterns of Elation," psychosocial dysfunction is considered in terms of mismanaged anxiety that is characterized by elation and euphoria, mood alteration, a facade of self-sufficiency, and the use of interpersonal situations to undermine and expose the vulnerabilities of others. The flight from anxiety is evidenced by grandiosity and hyperactivity, and by an exaggerated, labile, emotionally charged overfriendliness that quickly and unexpectedly turns to hostility.

In Chapter 36, "Patterns of Self-Destructive Behavior," mismanagement of anxiety and psychosocial dysfunction are reflected in flight from emotional pain through the self-infliction of physical pain and, in extreme cases, through suicide.

In Chapter 37, "Patterns of Dysfunctional Reality Orientation," the concept of psychosocial dysfunction is expanded to include clients who flee from reality into a fragmented world in which they live a solitary, frightening existence.

In Chapter 38, "Patterns of Sexual Dysfunction," psychosocial dysfunction is illustrated through the development of problematic sexual behavior and failure to experience intimacy and love in a sexual relationship.

In Chapter 39, "Patterns of Dysfunction in Adolescence," an understanding of the interaction between achievement of developmental tasks and psychosocial dysfunction is provided through the examination of dysfunctional behavior patterns in adolescence and parent-adolescent separation dynamics.

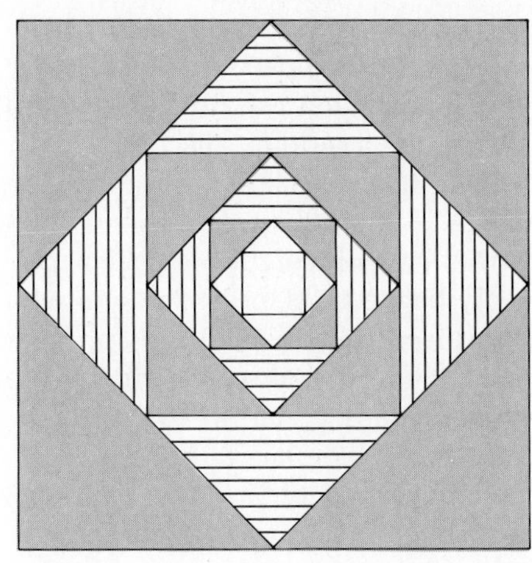

CHAPTER 29
Patterns of Overt Anxiety

Suzanne Sayle Jimerson

LEARNING OBJECTIVES

After studying this chapter, the student should be able to:

1. Describe the history of the concept of anxiety.
2. Define *posttraumatic stress disorder*.
3. Describe behaviors that indicate anxiety.
4. Assess the anxious client, the family, and the community.
5. State nursing diagnoses for anxious clients.
6. Formulate realistic short- and long-term outcomes for an anxious client.
7. Select appropriate nursing interventions for clients with different levels of anxiety.
8. Evaluate attainment of outcomes for the anxious client.

Since scientists first began studying and analyzing the human condition, anxiety has been recognized and written about under a variety of aliases. Although the concept of anxiety has always been with us, only in the past 100 years has its significance to human behavior, in terms of both survival and death, been studied in depth.

The study of anxiety closely parallels the development of psychiatry and has become recognized by students of human behavior and personality theory as a major internal stimulus to perception of self and the environment. Anxiety is present in our everyday lives and is a component of every dysfunctional behavior.

The recognition of anxiety in this country accompanied the turmoil created by the wars of the nineteenth century. Anxiety was initially recognized as a physiological rather than an emotional aspect of self. Those working with soldiers during and after the wars began describing a common problem which was called *irritable heart,* or *Da Costa's syndrome.* J. M. Da Costa believed that the rigors of war, disease, and death caused a disorder in the heart which created pain in the cardiac region and palpitations—with the result that the affected person was unable to function, as the slightest exertion stimulated the irritable heart.[1]

Meanwhile, in Vienna, Freud began to study the importance of anxiety and to formulate the view that anxiety, a psychological rather than a physiological disorder, was responsible for the irritable heart seen among soldiers. Freud viewed anxiety as the major motivator of behavior. He described anxiety as an experience of tension or dread arising from within the self that seemed to have no purpose or object. Freud thought that the source of anxiety was loss of self-image and that anxiety was an unconscious process.[2] His ideas, however, were slow to catch on. In World War I, anxiety was widely termed *disordered action of the heart* (DAH). The cardiac symptoms were the focus of study and treatment, and a basic underlying structural defect in the cardiac region continued to be the hypothesized cause.

Following World War I, Harry Stack Sullivan studied anxiety. He viewed anxiety as an interpersonal phenomenon originating in the mother-infant relationship, generated by threats to self-esteem from a significant other such as the mother. Adult experiences of anxiety occurred in situations in which prestige and dignity were threatened by others from whom the person could not escape. Sullivan viewed all behavior as directed toward avoiding anxiety and its attendant discomfort.[3]

During World War II, as psychiatry began to gain prominence as a field of study backed by research and knowledge, the viewpoint of the medical profession about anxiety began to change. Soldiers who complained of cardiac problems with no apparent organic cause were viewed as anxious and sent to a military psychiatrist rather than to an internist.

In the 1950s, Hildegard Peplau, a nurse theorist, developed a concept of anxiety based on Sullivan's work. She believed that anxiety is a potent force in interpersonal relationships: a response to unknown danger that arises when barriers to need fulfillment, as perceived by the individual, are encountered.[4]

Thus, it took almost 100 years for anxiety to become recognized as such. Interestingly, awareness of anxiety is now so prevalent that the twentieth century has been called the *age of anxiety.*

The purpose of this chapter is to explore problematic patterns of anxiety that develop both within the person and in relation to the person's family and community. This chapter builds on the theoretical foundation of anxiety presented in Chapter 3, and will propose nursing diagnoses, outcomes, and interventions useful with people displaying patterns of overt anxiety. The chapter will also examine the influences of family and community factors on problematic patterns of anxiety.

DYSYNCHRONOUS HEALTH PATTERNS

There are four basic patterns of overt anxiety: acute anxiety, panic, chronic anxiety, and posttraumatic stress disorder. Table 29-1 summarizes the usual manifestations for each of the patterns.

DSM III

The *Diagnostic and Statistical Manual of Mental Disorders* (DSM III) labels panic as *panic disorder* and acute and chronic anxiety as *generalized anxiety disorder.* It also has a third category, *atypical anxiety disorder,* or anxiety that does not fall under the other definitions. *Posttraumatic stress disorder* (PTSD) is also included in the anxiety disorders.[5]

Table 29-1 Manifestations of the Four Basic Patterns of Overt Anxiety

Pattern	Behavior	Affect	Thought
Acute anxiety	Dyspnea Tachycardia Chest pain Palpitations Hyperventilation Faintness Dizziness Blurred vision Trembling Diarrhea Headaches Insomnia Nausea Frequent urination Jumpiness Sweating Vigilance Distractibility Impatience	Irritability, anger Crying Feelings of low self-esteem Feelings of inadequacy Feelings of powerlessness Feelings of insecurity	Preoccupied Distractible Inattentive Attends to only a specific detail Critical of self and others Worrying Anticipation of misfortune
Panic	Acute anxiety behaviors plus: Choking or smothering sensations Hot and cold flashes Aimless running and shouting or inability to move and inability to speak	Feelings of dread Feelings of impending death Terror Feelings of eeriness Feelings of being unreal Feeling out of control Fear of going crazy	Delusional thinking Hallucinations Poor reality testing
Chronic anxiety	Jumpiness Fatigue during day Difficulty sleeping at night Heartburn Belching Muscular tensions Sweaty palms Flushing face Dryness of mouth "Frog" in throat Frequent sighing	Nervousness Irritability Loneliness	Ruminating Worrying Attends only to details, immediate task
Posttraumatic stress disorder	Reexperience of the trauma in a nonstressful environment Recurrent dreams and nightmares Acting as if one is reliving the traumatic event Social numbness, withdrawal, or both Sleep disturbance Avoidance of activities perceived to arouse recollection of the event Intensification of symptoms by exposure to similar events Hyperalertness or "startle response"	Feeling as if one is reliving the traumatic event Guilt about the traumatic event	Recurrent intrusive memories Memory impairment Trouble concentrating

To be diagnosed as having panic disorder, the client must be an adolescent or adult, must experience at least three attacks within a 3-week period, and must experience at least four symptoms of panic listed in Table 29-1.

To be diagnosed as having generalized anxiety disorder, the client must be at least 18 years old, must have been anxious for at least 1 month, and must experience at least three of the symptoms of acute or chronic anxiety listed in Table 29-1.

Posttraumatic stress disorder may be acute, chronic, or delayed. A client may suffer from this disorder at any age. A massive stressful event must have occurred, and at least two symptoms of anxiety must be present that were not present before the event.

DSM III, while developed to provide continuity to medical diagnoses, offers valuable information about anxiety patterns. In addition, DSM III emphasizes other factors that may be responsible for anxiety, such as withdrawal from an abused substance, hyperthyroidism, and hypoglycemia. Because anxiety is expressed physically, it is important that the initial contact with the anxious person include physical assessment data. For instance, people with acute myocardial infarction will experience trembling, chest pain, and overall feelings of dread, as will people experiencing acute anxiety. An assessment of smoking patterns and fluid intake is also important, as both nicotine and caffeine may induce and or escalate symptoms similar to anxiety.

Epidemiology

Descriptions of the population afflicted with patterns of overt anxiety are difficult to obtain. Those who suffer acute anxiety generally are in the midst of developmental or situational crises. Many of these are effectively helped and do not develop patterns of overt anxiety. Chronic anxiety is suffered by people who have unresolved crises with residual anxiety.

Panic disorder affects 2 to 5 percent of the general population, and two-thirds of those affected are women. Men tend to interpret anxiety symptoms as cardiac problems; 10 to 14 percent of patients seen by cardiologists suffer from anxiety disorders.[6] Treatment of patterns of overt anxiety does decrease the impact on functioning; however, depression is the most frequent and serious complication.[7] Sufferers of panic disorder also have a high mortality rate caused by death from unnatural causes; suicide accounts for 20 percent of the excess mortality rate.[8]

Posttraumatic stress disorder afflicts at least 500,000 to 700,000 veterans of the Vietnamese war; according to some figures, as many as 1.5 million veterans suffer from this disorder.[9] Other traumas, such as terrorist attacks, airplane crashes, and rape, can also leave the survivors suffering from PTSD.

PATTERNS OF INTERACTION: PERSON

Anxiety is experienced by everyone and serves as an important measure of general well-being. As anxiety increases, spiritual well-being decreases and a sense of inner discomfort is felt. The spiritual self feels cut off, unloved, and unable to identify with a value system that is supportive and gives meaning to existence. The mind perceives the self as weak and in danger of extinction. The body's response to the threats of extinction and emptiness is almost like a purging—it speeds up its functioning as it tries to rid of feelings of discomfort. Unfortunately, this purging usually increases anxiety by decreasing one's sense of self-control, thereby decreasing trust in self. Thus, anxiety touches all spheres of being.

People who develop patterns of overt anxiety defend themselves from this dreadful feeling by overusing defense mechanisms, described in Chapter 3. Anxious persons spend much or all of their energy defending themselves from the assault of anxiety, and consequently live rigid, stagnant, miserable lives.

Avoidance of anxiety becomes the center of the person's life, and pervades every aspect of living. The feelings of inadequacy and low self-esteem that accompany the four overt anxiety patterns discussed below cause further immobilization.

Acute Anxiety

Acute anxiety is defined as severe anxiety of sudden onset and short duration. Acute anxiety may appear suddenly with no forewarning and may occur in a person who is usually calm and untroubled. It is commonly triggered by an abrupt or unexpected loss or change, such as death of a significant other, a geographic move, or loss of a job, that presents a threat to the person's self-integrity.

Panic

Panic is defined as the most severe level of anxiety, accompanied by feelings of utter dread and a certainty that death is imminent, and by personality disorganization and dysfunction. A person experiencing panic is immobilized and may attempt suicide to relieve the distress.

Preoccupation with the bodily symptoms and feelings of terror severely disrupts normal mental functioning, and people in a panic may experience sensations of eeriness and unreality. The person may experience for a brief period of time some delusional thinking, hallucinations, and an overall decreased ability to test reality. The perceptual field is so severely limited that the person is unable to interact effectively with the environment. Panic does not extend over long periods of time, because it is so overwhelming that people cannot tolerate it for very long. They either seek help in decreasing it or resort to extensive use of dysfunctional coping mechanisms such as projection to distance from it.

Chronic Anxiety

Chronic anxiety is defined as moderate anxiety which is constantly present over months or years. It is relatively stable and unchanging. It is maintained by situations or feelings which continue to be perceived as threatening to self-integrity. It may also be maintained by a personality organization that predisposes one to experience more anxiety than other people. Chronic anxiety encompasses signal, trait, and state anxiety (discussed below).

Chronic anxiety differs from acute anxiety in that the behavioral symptoms are much less severe and longer-lasting, and clients usually learn to live with them. Clients with chronic anxiety complain of feeling nervous, jumpy, and irritable most of the time. Over long periods of time, the physical symptoms of chronic anxiety may actually be manifested as psychosomatic health problems (see Chapter 42).

The most common feature among chronically anxious people is the constant feeling of jumpiness and irritability. In environments where there are a lot of people, not much space, and a lot of noise, these symptoms are intensified. Chronically anxious people will make efforts to decrease stimuli by isolating themselves, remaining aloof from others, and interacting with the outside world only when absolutely necessary. Thus, chronically anxious people often experience their nervousness alone and become lonely; they often develop a pattern of rumination and worry. Because of their decreased functioning, they are unable to resolve the underlying anxiety. Although they can relate to the environment, they are limited to immediate tasks.

Posttraumatic Stress Disorder

Posttraumatic stress disorder is considered a pattern of overt anxiety because the symptoms that force the person to seek help are all anxiety-related. With exploration, the underlying source, an earlier trauma, is discovered. *Posttraumatic stress disorder* is defined as a reliving of a very stressful experience, with accompanying guilt and personal dysfunction. The disorder may be experienced as moderate or severe anxiety, or panic.

The symptoms of posttraumatic stress disorder may occur immediately after the traumatic event (acute), or not until months or years after the event (delayed). The disorder is considered a chronic condition if the symptoms, once experienced, continue for longer than 6 months.

Posttraumatic stress disorder was recognized during World War II but became a prominent concern only later, with veterans returning from the Vietnamese war. The disorder occurs after massive stress, which may be experienced only once (as with a terrorist attack, a rape, or a natural disaster) or over a period of time (as in combat, a totalitarian regime, or imprisonment).[10]

The relation of each of the dysynchronous patterns to the levels of anxiety is shown in Figure 29-1. The ability to perceive the environment appropriately influences anxiety and thus has implications for nursing interventions.

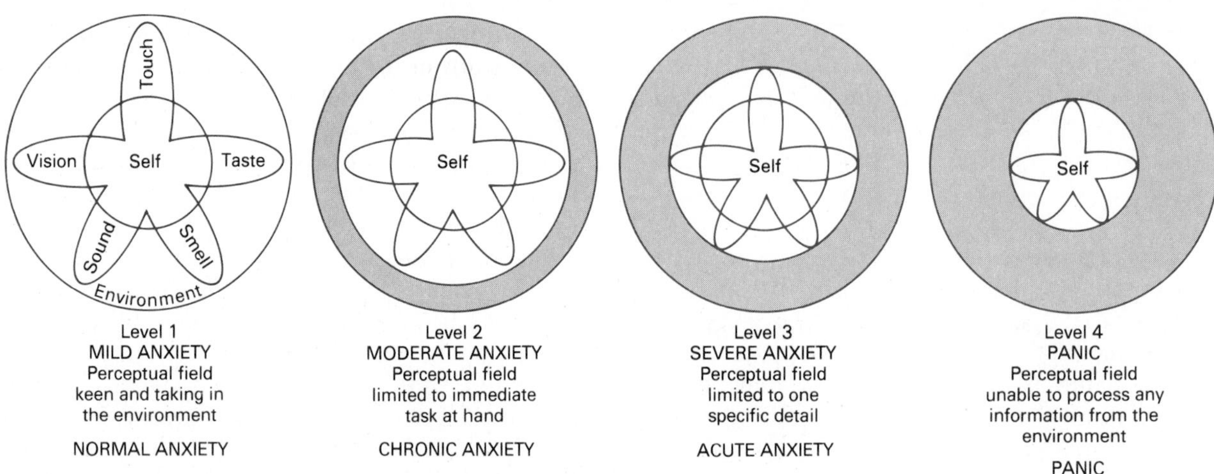

Figure 29-1 Levels of anxiety and the perceptual field.
Shaded area indicates amount of environmental stimuli to which the client cannot attend.

PATTERNS OF INTERACTION: FAMILY

Anxiety is contagious. It is readily communicated between individuals as well as within families, groups, and the community. Much can be learned about characteristic patterns of anxiety by studying family interactions.

Trait anxiety is defined as the overall amount of anxiety a person characteristically experiences. *Signal anxiety* is defined as feelings of dread brought on by the anticipation of danger or threat. *State anxiety* is brought on by a situation that is perceived as stressful and conflictual, and over which the person feels he or she has no control. Much research has been done on kinds of anxiety, and there are several excellent tools for measuring levels of anxiety.

Trait and signal anxiety are largely a result of early family relationships. There are several ways in which these kinds of anxiety are developed.

Parents who have high levels of trait anxiety will rapidly transfer that anxiety to their children.[11] For example, if a mother responds to a child's increased mobility with agitation and alarm that the child will be harmed, her anxiety will quickly be "picked up" by the child, who may express the anxiety through crying, lack of appetite, and fretfulness.

Trait and signal anxiety are passed down through generations of a family in the *multigenerational transmission process* (see Chapter 19).[11] Each family has its own characteristic anxiety level that may fluctuate somewhat around different issues and situations depending on their importance and emotional meaning in the family. For example, money, death, achievement, loyalty, and parenting are topics which have more or less intensity for different families. The family's anxiety level will be related to the intensity of that issue for that family, and each member of the family will carry the resulting anxious feelings into other interpersonal relationships. In general, the family's anxiety level is lower during periods of emotional calm and higher during periods of emotional upset. Each family member may express anxiety in a specific way, or one family member may express anxiety for the whole family and serve as a relief valve for other family members. For example:

Mr. and Mrs. Thomas have lived in one geographic area all their lives. They are now planning to move because of Mr. Thomas's unexpected job relocation. They are upset about the move, because stability is an important value to them. However, they have made plans to move in 3 months when school is out. Their 8-year-old son, John, who had always been healthy, outgoing, and involved with many friends, has suddenly developed stomachaches and leg pains and refuses to go to school. They have consulted several doctors who have found no organic reason for the problem.

In this case, John's somatic symptoms express the family's anxiety about the move and reflect his parents' lack of desire to leave their present home. Since the parents are essentially symptom-free, one can assume that their anxiety is filtering down to John, who is expressing it for the whole family. His anxious behavior allows them to rally around his problems and ignore their own anxiety.

The greater the family anxiety concerning these issues, the greater the potential for conflict. For example, if a mother has been told by family members that children should be toilet-trained by age 2 and her 2-year-old will not cooperate, she may become anxious because the child is not meeting her expectations. Her perception of herself as a good mother is threatened. The child will sense her anxious feelings and become anxious too. The discrepancy between her value about toilet training and the child's wish to continue soiling is the potential point of conflict. Thus, the way in which the family handles the complex socialization process is passed down through the generations and in a real way will influence the anxiety level of the mother as well as how she handles her child's socialization.

Often, anxious feelings are so unpleasant that they are repressed and therefore become unconscious. However, whenever a similar situation arises, such as when a child, now grown, in turn has a child, the anxiety will be triggered by the current situation. Thus the pattern of passing anxiety down through the generations is established.

In addition to the parent's level of anxiety, another way in which anxiety is engendered in a child's life is through inadequate or misinformed parenting. Problems with parenting which generate high levels of signal or trait anxiety, or both, because of inconsistency or uncertainty, include the following:

1. Inconsistently setting limits so that the child does not know what is expected. What may be OK on one day is not OK the next.
2. Expecting performance above the child's intellectual or developmental level. The child fails to please the parents.
3. Giving directions that are incomplete—for example, asking a child to get something, but not explaining where it is, so that the task cannot be completed.
4. Giving conflicting messages—for example, telling the child that he or she is loved and at the same time pushing the child away. Confusion about the truth of the two messages leaves the child not knowing how to respond.
5. Punishing a child for failures without explanation; or giving inappropriate and heavy punishment. This kind of punishment discourages the child from trying again or believing that it will be possible to succeed at another time.

Inadequate parenting abilities can severely damage a child's sense of identity and ability to develop self. Children who grow up in environments which create high levels of signal and trait anxiety will be unsure of their own identities and have inadequate adaptive resources for coping with anxiety in a healthy, growth-promoting way.

Families also informally teach family members how to deal with anxiety by means of coping styles. For example, if a child observes that when dad gets upset he takes a walk, works out at the gym, or says he needs to be by himself for a while, and then returns in a less anxious state, the child will learn to associate those activities with anxiety reduction. While they are growing up, children observe how others cope with anxiety and then develop their own repertoire of coping skills to use when they encounter anxiety in life situations.

PATTERNS OF INTERACTION: ENVIRONMENT

Community factors play an important role in the development and prevalence of trait and state anxiety. Rapid technological development and geographic mobility combine to create stress and tension in people and their communities.

In the past 100 years, technological development and change have occurred at an unprecedented and ever-increasing pace. Rapid societal change has accompanied the technological change. Technology, which continues to mushroom at accelerated rates, has created communities where change rather than stability is the rule. Several potential problems of rapid technological development can be identified.

First, constant change caused by increasingly sophisicated technology makes yesterday's product obsolete and creates a situation in which constant adaptation is necessary; whatever is familiar is left behind and people have little with which to identify in a secure, lasting way. Anxiety is the result.

Second, technological development has decreased the need for the human skills, know-how, and relationships that were formerly required for problem-solving cooperation. Computers now arrange dates, answer questions, predict results of action, and provide formulas for alternative solutions to problems. Anxiety emerges out of technological complexity because people feel unnecessary, unimportant, and not in control of the forces that guide their lives and the development of their communities.

Third, wastes that are the by-products of technological activity have created changes in communities. Air, noise, water, and land pollution create concern about the health not only of humans but of all life forms.

Fourth, the threat of nuclear war looms even larger. Anxiety revolves around the possibility that the nuclear threat will get out of hand and destroy the earth. Technology, representing both survival and death, is intimately associated with anxiety.

Rapid developments in communication and travel as well as changes in people's values about permanence and stability have led to decreased emphasis on job and community stability. The result has been more frequent job changes, transfers, and community relocations. Outcomes of this phenomenon include the following:

1. Geographic distance from extended family and friends. Husbands and wives may even live apart, visiting only on weekends, because of job-related travel requirements.
2. Isolation from the extended family and a stable friendship network, which produces an overall lack of identity with the community.[11]
3. Loneliness or emptiness, which evolves out of an absence of enduring, intimate relationships. People feel a lack of identity with life and cannot accept the fact that everyone is ultimately "alone" in the world. Human intimacy is a universal need throughout life. Inability to satisfy this need represents potential or actual loss of relatedness.[12] The impact of loneliness is profound, perhaps because in our culture people are now taught to rely so heavily on others for their self-orientation. If relationships are less enduring because of our mobile society, the possibility of loneliness increases. Everyone experiences loneliness from time to time. However, the person who experiences loneliness most of the time will experience lack of relatedness and a sense of nothingness; life will seem like a void.[12]
4. A breakdown in traditional values, morals, and beliefs that have been passed down through many generations. These traditional values and beliefs are being challenged by ever-present change. This has led to a search for new values and moral codes which will work in a constantly changing world. Lack of consistent values and beliefs creates confusion as people attempt to find guidelines that will enable them to live their lives effectively.
5. Experimentation with different values, lifestyles, and relationship patterns that will provide rules with which people can identify and pattern their behavior.

People may become increasingly adaptable and better able to cope with uncertainty and novel situations. Anxiety will, however, still be a problem to the degree that people are unable to adapt, that they perceive resources within themselves as inadequate, and that they feel powerless. Frustration will develop, creating a decreased ability to cope and an overall anxious response.

NURSING PROCESS

Assessment

People who cannot keep their anxious feelings under control seek relief from health professionals in a variety of settings. They may go to the emergency room, the outpatient psychiatric clinic, or their family physician. The nurse in an emergency room may identify anxiety in a person who goes there because of somatic complaints such as palpitations, shortness of breath, chest tightness, and persistent headaches or stomachaches. The nurse in a mental health clinic may identify anxiety in a person who arrives for an initial appointment stating, "I cry at the drop of a hat. I'm so jittery and irritable. I'm having trouble sleeping, and I can't stop shaking. Look at my hand; I can't make it stop." The person then goes on to state, "I separated from my wife just 2 weeks ago." The community health nurse may identify anxiety in the school, home, or health department setting. Nurses may also identify anxiety in clients with whom they are already working who develop anxiety during their relationship with the nurse. For example:

> A 35-year-old man who has had a heart attack may exhibit signs of anxiety as discharge from the hospital comes closer. He disregards orders about his activity level, makes seductive remarks to the nurses, is critical of the care they provide, and has difficulty getting to sleep at night. Threats to his biological integrity and his self-concept abound as he wonders about his health and his ability to resume his role as a husband, father, and breadwinner.

It is important that the nurse immediately provide a relaxed, calm environment so that reduction of anxiety can begin. The assessment process should then be initiated as quickly as possible so that formulation of a care plan can follow without delay. This is important because anxious clients are usually in acute distress by the time they seek professional assistance. Their coping skills and problem-solving resources have usually been exhausted. While keeping the need for an immediate assessment in mind, the nurse should at the same time remember that some clients may be fearful about disclosing personal information and may rudely leave the room or respond to questions with "I don't know" or "That's personal; I don't want to discuss it," thus making it difficult to complete an assessment. Other clients will be experiencing such high levels of anxiety that an immediate assessment will be impossible to obtain. When severe or panic levels of anxiety are being experienced, an assessment often has to wait until the anxiety level is reduced. Such clients are unable to make sense of or respond to assessment questions because their perceptual field is so limited. Family, friends, and the police are often valuable informants when a client is unable to provide subjective data. The nurse will have a variety of objective data with which to begin formulation of the initial care plan.

The Person

After ensuring that the anxiety is not related to a physical cause, the nurse will want to determine what the client is experiencing now and whether any events can be identified which may have precipitated the anxious feelings. In doing this the nurse will assist the client in sorting out recent feelings and events. Questions are directed toward eliciting information about family, friends, job, community relations, overall state of health, and manner of coping with anxiety in the past. In completing the assessment of the client, the nurse keeps the following questions in mind:

1. What behaviors (gestures, tone of voice, twitching, etc.) is the client exhibiting? Do these behaviors get more severe as he or she describes a specific experience or aspect of self?
2. What is identified as anxiety-provoking?
3. What does the client deny having anxious feelings about?
4. What questions is the client not able to answer or describe fully, thereby indicating anxiety about that area?
5. What is the client's level of anxiety?
6. What type of anxiety is the client experiencing? What is the relative severity of the anxiety?
7. Does the client describe himself or herself as having been anxious in the past?
8. How does the client use the environment to decrease anxiety? For example, through sports or a favorite pastime?
9. Why are the client's normal ways of dealing with anxiety not working now?
10. Whom did the client go to in the past when feeling anxious?
11. What does the client think the outcome of the anxiety will be?
12. What values are important to the client? Are these values being threatened, thereby increasing anxiety?
13. What is the client afraid of?
14. What does the client think he or she can do to relieve the anxiety?

The Family

If the family is present during the interview, the nurse should also direct questions to them in order to validate information, gather further family data about the problem, and see how much agreement exists between the client and family members. It is important to know if the family views the problem differently from the client and to explore each family member's perception of the problem. In addition, the nurse should carefully observe patterns of relationships among the family members. The following are guidelines for assessing the family.

1. Who is anxious, calm, etc., in the family?
2. What is the family's anxiety level?
3. How do family members handle anxious feelings?
4. Has a recent loss or addition in the family contributed to anxiety?
5. Which family issues generate the most anxiety in family members? Death? Divorce? Money? Parenting? Success? Family secrets? Loyalty conflicts?
6. Which member of the family seems to be most affected by the client's anxiety?
7. Which other members of the family seem to handle anxiety much as the client does?
8. Which member of the family do the family members see as having contributed to the client's anxiety?
9. What do family members do together to reduce their anxious feelings?
10. Who identifies the anxiety in the client?
11. How does each family member relate to the client's anxiety?
12. Is the client more anxious with one family member than with others? What does this family member do to maintain the client's anxiety?

The Community

In addition to assessing anxiety in the client and family, assessing the community is also important.

1. Has the family moved recently? How far?
2. Has a family member changed jobs? Schools?
3. What kind of community does the family live in? Rural, urban, or inner city?
4. Do the family members know the neighbors? Do they socialize with neighbors or other friends?
5. What events in the community do they consider stressful? How many stressful events are there?
6. Does the family consider the community adequate?

The skill with which the initial interview is done is important in terms of gathering baseline data and establishing rapport with client and family. The assessment process continues throughout the relationship as new data emerge and the client changes and moves toward optimal health.

Nursing Diagnosis

Nursing diagnoses for clients with overt patterns of anxiety focus on the level of anxiety experienced, the environmental correlates of the anxiety, and the strengths and challenges of coping with anxiety. Nursing diagnoses appropriate for patterns of overt anxiety are presented in Table 29-2.

Table 29-2 Diagnoses, Outcomes, and Interventions for Patterns of Overt Anxiety

Diagnosis	Outcome	Categories of Intervention
Acute anxiety associated with too few coping strategies	Fewer episodes of restlessness and palpitations, evidenced by decrease to 2 PRN medications for anxiety per 24 hours	Reducing anxiety Repatterning the environment Somatic interventions
Fatigue; inability to concentrate associated with unresolved feelings about husband's leaving	Adequate energy to do a day's work and ability to complete normal tasks at one time, evidenced by client and employer report	Interpersonal contact Identification of feelings
Inability to perceive events clearly, associated with high trait anxiety	Perceive events as an interaction between self and others, showing insight into own behavior	Learning to cope Physical activity and exercise

Outcome Criteria

Outcome criteria for clients with overt patterns of anxiety focus on more effective functioning while anxious, and on a wider variety of more effective coping strategies. The following case study will illustrate the process of nursing diagnosis, derivation of client outcomes, and nursing intervention.

Ms. P., a 34-year-old high school English teacher who commutes 40 miles to work, has come to the walk-in mental health clinic of the community hospital. She states that she is married but separated. Her husband moved out of their apartment 8 months ago and left town 2 weeks ago. Ms. P. describes a close relationship with her family; however, she rarely sees them because they live 250 miles away. She has few friends in her community.

She describes her problems as a pounding heart that has kept her from sleeping for the past 2 nights and restlessness that has kept her driving around in the car for the past 2 hours in order to "have something to do." She states that nothing seems to make sense, that she is receiving complaints from peers at work about lateness and inconsistent behavior, and that she feels very lonely. Her speech is tense during the interview; she chain-smokes, jiggles her legs, and often breaks out crying in the middle of a sentence, which makes it difficult to follow what she is saying. An appointment is made for Ms. P. with a nurse-therapist in the clinic for the next morning. In the meantime, Ms. P. is also interviewed by a physician on the mental health team who prescribes a tranquilizer to decrease her anxiety. A coworker picks Ms. P. up at the clinic, sleeps at her apartment, and brings her back the next morning.

The nursing diagnoses, client outcomes, and nursing interventions suggested for Ms. P are found in Table 29-2. The interventions suggested in the table are expanded upon below. Long-term outcomes for Ms. P. would address development of support systems, clarification of her life purpose, and continuing development of better coping strategies.

Intervention

Nursing intervention with anxious clients takes place in both inpatient and outpatient settings. Clients who experience anxiety have great potential for growth and change with therapeutic intervention, particularly if the family is involved in the treatment process. Most anxious clients are treated on an outpatient basis unless their anxiety is severe enough to interfere with safe functioning in their normal environment. In that case, they are admitted to a short-term inpatient unit for treatment.

Interventions with the Person

Interventions for patterns of overt anxiety include specific techniques for relieving acute anxiety, panic, chronic anxiety, and PTSD. Other goals are reducing levels of anxiety, providing interpersonal contact, and helping clients to learn better ways of coping with anxiety. Criteria for evaluation of the interventions are also discussed below.

INTERVENTIONS FOR ACUTE ANXIETY. People suffering from acute anxiety have difficulty looking beyond specific details and are unable to figure out what is happening to them or why. Interventions focus on reducing anxiety and on preventing it from escalating into panic. An acutely anxious inpatient should be moved to a calm, quiet environment to reduce stimulation. The nurse helps clients to use coping mechanisms that will reduce the anxiety. Clients who experience acute anxiety are feeling too much, thinking too little, and perceiving themselves as vulnerable. By asking questions and making observations about the immediate situation, a nurse can help such a client use the cognitive dimension. For instance, "What are you thinking now, Mrs. Jones?" helps the client to think. "You are safe in this room, Mr. Smith," helps the client to be aware of his safe situation. Nurses must control their own anxiety while working with anxious clients in order to avoid "feeding the anxiety back" to the client. In talking with acutely anxious clients, sensitivity to the stimulation of talking is important; insensitive verbal input may escalate anxiety into panic.

INTERVENTIONS FOR PANIC. Panic requires immediate intervention. The client is in severe distress and is either immobilized or engaging in random, disorganized, and sometimes aggressive activity. The perceptual field narrows to the point where the client is unable to process outside information. Inner thoughts, feelings, and actions are chaotic and make no sense. Clients may experience intense awe, dread, or terror, or may feel that they are losing their minds or going crazy. Since learning cannot take place at this level of anxiety, interventions are directed toward reducing the immediate anxiety to more moderate, manageable levels. The following guidelines should be followed when intervening with a client in a state of panic.[13,14]

1. Remain with the client regardless of whether your presence is acknowledged. The client's feelings of isolation and estrangement may be increased by being left alone.
2. Allow the person to cry or ventilate the array of feelings and thoughts that are experienced. Listening combined with understanding and realistic demands provides a climate of acceptance that is soothing and thus anxiety-reducing.
3. Maintain a calm manner, in order to avoid communicating anxiety to the client. Since clients readily communicate anxiety also, nurses must

use effective coping strategies to decrease their own anxiety.

4. Use short, simple sentences and a firm, authoritative voice when speaking. This conveys that the nurse can provide external controls for the person who is unable to exercise self-control.
5. Minimize environmental stimuli by moving the client to a smaller, quieter place such as the client's room or a quiet room. This is important because the client is already overwhelmed by stimuli.
6. Provide large motor activities, such as sweeping or moving furniture, to channel the client's energy and release tension.
7. If appropriate, administer an antianxiety medication.

INTERVENTIONS FOR CHRONIC ANXIETY. The major goal for clients with chronic anxiety is to help them realize that one may choose a less anxious, freer lifestyle. A decision to grapple with anxiety rather than to avoid it opens the door to effective intervention. The following guidelines may be used in interventions with a person who suffers from chronic anxiety.

1. Help the person to become aware of the high level of the chronic anxiety. For example, say, "You are very anxious. Are you usually this anxious?"
2. Show the person that life could be different. For example, say, "You have a real talent for discerning the heart of the matter. Just imagine really being able to use that gift."
3. Influence the person to consider alternative lifestyles. For example, say, "What would you do with the extra energy if you weren't anxious all the time?"
4. Help the person to identify the source of the anxiety, and to see the source in perspective.

Following is an example of use of these guidelines. Nurse A is talking with nurse B, a colleague on the unit who is chronically anxious, difficult to work with, and prone to make mistakes.

A: What makes you so anxious?

B: I'm afraid I'll fail.

A: What would happen if you failed?

B: I don't know. I think everything would come to an end. I'd lose my job, my family, my license, everything.

A: If I thought I'd lose everything and my life would end, I guess I'd be very anxious too. But I don't think all those things would happen to me if I failed.

B: What would happen to you if you failed?

A: Well, I guess I have already failed. And nothing bad happened. In fact, I became more relaxed, and I have made fewer mistakes.

B: I wonder if I'd have the same experience.

INTERVENTIONS FOR POSTTRAUMATIC STRESS DISORDER. Reduction of anxiety related to PTSD focuses first on the severity of anxiety. The client may be experiencing acute or chronic anxiety, or panic, on initial assessment. The interventions noted above are used as appropriate. The unique feature of working with clients who have PTSD is making the connection between the trauma, the current feelings of stress and anxiety, and the guilt over survival. Often, the PTSD sufferer does not realize that today's feelings relate to a trauma which may have occurred years ago. That link must be made and the feelings reinvested in the trauma before healing can begin. For survivors of a traumatic event such as an airplane crash, the issue of guilt over survival is spiritual in nature. The issue of life's purpose and meaning is different for these people; they must resolve the meaning of the trauma and its implications before they can get on with life.

REDUCTION OF ANXIETY. Strategies for reducing anxiety are appropriate for all clients who express overt anxiety patterns. Once the person is no longer experiencing panic, reduction of anxiety may be further accomplished through physical activity and exercise, environmental repatterning, and medication.

Physical activity. Physical activity such as walking, jogging, swimming, calisthenics, raking leaves, and pulling weeds involves the use of large motor muscles; provides for safe, acceptable discharge of excess tension and energy; and allows clients to focus on simple, concrete tasks. These activities can be done alone or with others and pose no threat to safety because skilled use of machinery is not involved. In addition to reducing anxiety, these activities are constructive for the individual or the community.

Relaxation and meditation. Relaxation exercises and meditation provide another way to decrease anxiety. Relaxation exercises are taught as a self-initiated strategy. The client begins the relaxation process by taking deep, slow, cleansing breaths. The client is then instructed to tense each major muscle group for 10 seconds and then relax, and to systematically rotate tensing and relaxing of each major muscle group until the whole body is relaxed. Once relaxation exercises are learned, they can be initiated independently whenever anxiety and tension begin to rise.[15]

After doing the relaxation exercises, the client is usually relaxed enough to be able to meditate, or concentrate on a visual image. This is when the nurse can encourage the client to visualize something positive, such as the ocean, a sunset, a color, a wavelike pattern, a loved one, or a passage of scripture. The client is to concentrate on the positive visual image for 10 to 15 minutes, which further releases tension and becomes emotionally soothing.

Repatterning the environment. The physical environment can be rearranged to reduce anxiety. It needs to be as calm as possible. External stimuli need to be reduced. Therefore lighting, sound, odor, and color need to be restful. Lighting should be soft, but not shadowy, to reduce the chance of visual distortion. Sound and color should also be soft; blue, green, and beige are colors that don't increase excitation. Bright-colored paintings, murals, or posters can be too stimulating for the anxious client. The number of people in the environment should also be reduced in order to decrease noise and distractions that might increase tension. If hospitalization is necessary, the anxious client should be assigned to a room that is away from the noise and bustle of the hospital unit, but not isolated from others. The client will need a roommate who is not manic, loud, interfering, or disruptive.

Medication. Administration of antianxiety medications can be a valuable intervention, particularly when anxiety is severe. A brief course of an antianxiety agent may reduce anxiety enough to make the client less restless, and able to sleep and think more clearly. It is important, however, not to medicate the person so heavily as to erase all anxious feelings, because the discomfort of anxiety serves as a motivation for changes in behavior.

Headaches, diarrhea, dizziness, or other manifestations of anxiety should be treated as they would be for any client. These problems are usually resolved as the anxious feelings subside.

INTERPERSONAL CONTACT. Severely anxious persons need an accepting person who will be with them, listen, and help them to distinguish facts from perceptions, perceived threats from reality. The nurse must be available not just physically but emotionally, mentally, and spiritually as well. Therapeutic use of self is required. The anxious person needs someone who will refuse to "catch" the free-floating anxiety and who will listen. Anxious clients suffer from a fundamental sense that they are unacceptable as they are; they therefore have a need to be understood and accepted.

LEARNING TO COPE WITH ANXIETY. When anxiety has been reduced to a manageable level, clients can use it to learn about themselves and their coping skills. This is of particular value for clients who experience chronic anxiety and wish to repattern their anxious behavior. Clients must endure their anxiety while searching out factors that contribute to it. They must then develop more effective and satisfying coping skills to replace former ineffective ones. An effective model for assisting clients with this process is the teaching-learning model (see Chapter 24). The case study of Ms. P., presented above, will provide examples to illustrate the teaching-learning approach discussed below.

Observation involves verbalizations by the nurse that help the client recognize and identify an experience as anxiety. Initially, the client may not be able to do this and the nurse will have to act as a role model. For example:

> Ms. P. told the nurse that she had received a telephone call from her husband the night before, and found herself pacing her apartment later in the evening and had difficulty falling asleep. As she was relating the episode, she got up and began pacing around the nurse's office.

In such a situation, the nurse can ask, "Did talking with your husband upset you? You seem uncomfortable. I haven't seen you pacing for a while now." By verbalizing to the client what the nurse is observing, the nurse is helping the client recognize that she is anxious and that her anxiety is related to an event. The nurse is also offering herself to the client as a source of support. If the client is not able to recognize and discuss her anxiety, the nurse should move the discussion toward another, less threatening topic. Stronger confrontation will only increase the anxiety, and the client may attribute her increasing feelings of discomfort to the nurse rather than to her response to the telephone call. When the client is able to recognize the anxiety, then the nurse can move to the next step in the teaching-learning model.

Description involves developing the client's ability to recall and verbalize details surrounding anxious events. The client is encouraged to recall and describe the anxious feeling rather than the symptoms. Allowing the client to recite a list of symptoms becomes unproductive and tedious, and prevents him or her from dealing with the anxiety. The client is helped to recall the events leading up to the anxiety and to connect the anxiety with relief behavior such as anger, depression, or somatic symptoms. For example, the nurse might help Ms. P. to describe the events and how she felt on the days leading up to her anxiety attack and ask her questions such as, "What had been happening? What were you thinking? What were you feeling? How were you acting? How were others behaving toward you?"

To facilitate description, the nurse should be concrete, that is, use terminology consistent with the client's awareness and understanding. If the client describes anxiety as feeling "uncomfortable," then this is the word the nurse should use. For example, the nurse may say, "Tell me, Ms. P., what are some of the things you've done in the past to deal with that uncomfortable feeling?"

Analysis involves making relevant connections between life events and the anxiety they generate. The client must recognize and verbalize the relationship between the feeling and the precipitating event. The client should realize the significance of the event in his or her life experience. The client is asked to identify commonalities between situations and relate current events to past experiences. The client is encouraged to identify his or her part in initiating or maintaining the process. For example:

> Ms. P. was asked if she could identify the event that precipitated her anxious feelings. She said, "It began even before my husband left. It was when he started going on business trips a lot and I was alone so much that I began to feel jittery. His leaving just made me go off the wall." The nurse asked her if she could make any connection between what had happened and the way she felt. Ms. P. said, "Yes, in thinking about it, I think I felt abandoned and unable to manage or feel like a whole person when I was alone." The nurse asked her if she had ever had that feeling before, "Yes," she said, "I can remember having it in school when my boyfriend broke up with me. I felt lost and jittery about how I would be without a steady boyfriend!"

During this analysis phase, the client's relationships with family, friends, and colleagues are explored in a manner that will allow the client to see patterns between relationships, life events, and the development of anxiety.

Formulation can be an extension of analysis. It helps the client examine anxious feelings and events in a crystal-clear way. The nurse assists the client in summarizing what has been talked about. The client states how the anxiety is a problem and how anxiety has influenced behavior and lifestyle. The client is encouraged to examine discrepancies and inconsistencies in feelings, thoughts, behavior, or information, and to consider his or her role in initiating or maintaining interaction patterns that generate anxiety. For example:

> The nurse said to Ms. P., "If you had to boil it down to one sentence, how would you describe your feelings after your husband moved to another town?" Ms. P. responded, "I felt abandoned, unloved, unlovable, and unable to function on my own." The nurse then asked, "Could you identify anything that you yourself did that made you feel that way?" Ms. P. said, "Well, . . . I guess that maybe I never tried to see if I could be on my own and survive. I guess I got that attitude about myself from my family."

Validation occurs as the nurse and client check out perceptions about what has been discussed during the steps of analysis and formulation. This is to make sure, to validate, that each has a clear understanding of what the other means. For example, the nurse might say to Ms. P., "Am I correct in thinking that you feel very insecure and of little value when you consider yourself as an individual?" Ms. P. might validate her perceptions with the nurse to see if she is viewing events in a clear or distorted way.

Through the three steps of analysis, formulation, and validation, the client eventually becomes able to recognize and perhaps alter patterns of handling anxiety.

Testing and *integration* are the final two steps of the teaching-learning process. The nurse helps the client to identify and test alternative behaviors and their consequences. The nurse also helps the client to identify *realistic* methods for handling anxiety-producing situations. The client identifies alternative coping strategies and then seeks out opportunities to test them, first within the nurse-client relationship and then in appropriate life situations. In a subsequent therapy session, the nurse and the client examine the outcome and consequences of these new coping patterns. The client learns that anxiety is a necessary part of everyday living and that effective ways of working through the anxiety are what produce growth and a heightened sense of identity and self-esteem. For example:

> During one session Ms. P. was complaining that her husband seemed to call at the worst times, and for that reason she didn't answer the telephone one Sunday while at home. She stated that at one point during the day she began to feel anxious while searching for her keys. She said she was able to calm herself by doing some relaxation exercises. While thinking about and focusing on the keys, she realized that she was anxious because she had never changed the lock on her apartment. Her husband could walk in at any time! She subsequently had her lock changed. This decreased her sense of helplessness and proved to her that she could experience anxiety and work through the anxiety by doing something helpful for herself.

Testing also involves realistically assessing the extent to which the social support system can be utilized. If a strong support system is available, the client should be taught how to enlist the support and assistance of significant others in working through the anxiety. This is particularly important for a client who lives in the community and thus does not have the protection and support of the hospital setting. Some clients have difficulty in asking for help, and the nurse can assist them in learning to use the available support systems in a meaningful way. Such support systems can include family, friends, community, church, and organization groups. Clients need to learn how to use them not only for support and assistance but also for a feeling of relatedness and stimulation.

As the testing process progresses, the new behavior learned in the therapeutic process is tested and then used in an anticipatory problem-solving manner, independent of the guidance and support of the professional. Ms. P., for example, found herself less and less in need of the nurse's suggestions; instead she enjoyed using her time with the nurse to describe and critically evaluate her successes and failures. She was able to anticipate potentially anxiety-provoking events and list alternative approaches that she could have ready to deal with such an event.

The step just described, integration, provides greater flexibility in approaching potentially anxious situations. In the case of Ms. P., integration will serve an important function as she begins to make decisions about how to resolve her relationship with her husband.

The teaching-learning method has the potential for expanding awareness and promoting growth. It seeks to develop a degree of self-awareness by dealing constructively with the anxiety and by confronting the problems directly. Such learning can take place only in the presence of mild to moderate anxiety and is not useful when the client is experiencing overwhelming, severe anxiety or panic. In such instances, as mentioned above, the anxiety level must be reduced before learning can take place.

Interventions with the Family

Intervention with a family in an anxiety-provoking situation involves promotion, maintenance, restoration, and rehabilitation of health.

Promotion and maintenance of health in relation to anxiety can be accomplished in parent education classes or when providing anticipatory guidance to families. In such situations nurses can identify developmental milestones that present potentially problematic child-rearing issues, and can suggest alternative ways in which they can be handled by parents. For example, when discussing toilet training, nurses can (1) point out why it is an inherently conflictual parent-child encounter; (2) help parents explore attitudes, expectations, and feelings that they have incorporated from their families and that might facilitate or inhibit a smooth toilet-training experience; (3) assist them to look at their particular parent-child relationship for factors that would help or hinder the process; and (4) suggest realistic strategies for dealing with toilet training that would minimize conflict and anxiety for both parent and child. Such an approach would provide opportunities for both parent and child to explore, grow, and develop.

Nurses can also help parents to recognize and identify their level of trait anxiety as well as the triggers that increase anxiety as they relate to their children. For instance, nurses can ask parents to keep a journal in which they note the times at which they felt anxious, the events that were occurring at that time, and their responses to what was happening. This type of journal will help parents identify the source of their anxiety and provide a concrete task for them to focus on during anxious moments. They will be involved in writing about the anxiety rather than spreading it to their child. With the assistance of the nurse they may later gain more understanding of the anxiety-provoking situation and identify alternative approaches in anticipation of future situations.

In addition to promoting and maintaining health, nurses need to intervene to restore and rehabilitate health when they work with families in which anxiety presents an actual rather than a potential problem. In such cases, the nurse needs to understand and to convey to clients that anxiety is a family problem; that is, that families have a characteristic anxiety level and the client's pattern of anxiety was developed within the family milieu.

In the D. family, economic security was an important issue. Many of the men in the family had not been good financial providers. Over the generations, several of them had left secure jobs for new, risky business ventures that did not prove to be successful. At such times money was scarce and not regularly available for rent, food, and other necessities. Anxiety escalated at those times because of the family's loss of prestige, self-esteem, and security. Family members became sensitized to any situations in which financial security was threatened. Whenever a similar situation arose, anxiety would rise and people in the family would begin exhibiting anxiety symptoms.

Frank and Joan D's daughter, Anne, was married to Mike L., who worked for the state civil service as an accountant. Mike came home one day and told Anne that he had an opportunity to begin an accounting firm with a friend who had several good connections for accounts. As Anne listened to what Mike was saying, she could feel her stomach churn, her heart race, and her head ache. She said, "I don't want to hear it. You can't do that; you have to stay at your job," ran into the bedroom and slammed the door. During the next week Anne cried at the drop of a hat and felt ill and tired. She and Mike argued frequently about his career decision. They decided to go for counseling because Anne was prepared to leave him if he decided to leave his present job for the uncertainty of a new business venture.

Table 29-3 gives nursing interventions for family anxiety and applies the interventions to the D. family.

Involvement of nuclear and extended family members helps to expand the knowledge base about anxiety as a family phenomenon. The "triggers" of anxiety are different for each family; the way in which the anxiety is communicated and manifested is also variable. The nurse can help a family understand and modify anxiety as a dysfunctional force by observing the family and discovering how anxiety is initiated, maintained, and enlarged by the family system.

Interventions with the Community

Stressful life events that generate anxiety are often situations which involve change or loss. As discussed above, geographic and occupational mobility; distance from family and friends; and rapid social, economic, and technological change have led theorists to say that we live in an age of anxiety. The interventions listed below address this phenomenon in a constructive way.

1. Increase community support systems to provide a social and resource network for individuals and families—for example, newcomers' clubs, social and activity clubs sponsored by religious and community organizations, and Welcome Wagon services that inform newcomers about community resources and activities.
2. Establish relocation counseling sponsored by industrial concerns to provide individuals and families with support and with guidance about specific issues during relocation. This will help people make changes in more functional ways.
3. Encourage families to find ways of maintaining family and friendship ties through visiting, letters, telephone calls, personal tape recordings, and pictures. Where contact with the extended family in person is impossible to achieve, it is important to encourage surrogate family connections in the form of friend or peer networks, particularly around holidays and other important annual events.

Table 29-3 Nursing Interventions for the Anxious Family

Intervention	Application to the D. Family
1. Identify the anxious behavior.	Anne D. was experiencing fatigue, headache, palpitations, upset stomach, crying, irritability.
2. Identify the source of the anxiety.	Mike D.'s contemplated plans for starting a new business venture and leaving the security of a government job threatened Anne's sense of security.
3. Identify and explore the family anxiety level around the issue of economic security. Explore sources of family anxiety. Explore how family members handle anxiety and adversity.	Family anxiety level was high around this issue because many males in Anne's family had not succeeded at independent business ventures. Anne learned from family members that economic security was very important.
4. Encourage them to verbally communicate their thoughts and feelings about this issue with each other.	Anne was reluctant to explain why she was acting this way; Mike had no idea why she was so upset. He thought that she would be delighted about this opportunity. She had never told him about this family issue.
5. Encourage them to realistically examine the advantages and disadvantages of the opportunity.	Objectifying the pros and cons of the situation helped put it into perspective for both partners. Anne was able to identify long-term benefits of the job change if it was successful.
6. Demonstrate how each partner can take a position regarding a decision about the issue based on individual and couple needs.	Anne saw more positive aspects of the venture once she heard what it was all about. She decided she would try not to overgeneralize and automatically be pessimistic about the venture. She would take the risk with Mike, knowing that he could try out his new business for 1 year and still return to his government job.
7. Explore triggers of anxiety as well as ways of coping with and reducing anxiety when it occurs.	Discussions of events related to threats to security, prestige, and self-esteem. Relaxation exercises, meditation, physical activity.
8. Explore whether one particular family member displays anxiety for the rest of the family.	Anne, the oldest sibling in her generation, was the one who was most anxious of all her siblings and cousins about this family issue.
9. Redistribute the worry to more than one family member.	Mike identified and said he would assume responsibility for several realistic concerns relating to the job change.
10. Explore expectations of self and other family members around this issue. Help family members to modify expectations to more realistic levels.	Anne acknowledged that it was unrealistic to expect that she would always be totally secure and that her husband would cooperate in meeting this expectation.

4. Encourage use or development of organizations that provide social groups, activity groups, transportation, and other outreach programs that involve lonely and isolated people in a community. Examples are Dial-a-Ride services, Meals on Wheels, day care centers for the elderly, and Big Brother–Big Sister programs.
5. Provide adequate education and health services to the underserved of the community. Examples are well-child clinics, neighborhood nursing centers, parent-child nutrition programs, home-visit health supervision by community health nurses, and special education services in schools.
6. Encourage parent-child discussion groups to facilitate cross-generational communication about values, norms, lifestyles, and decision making.
7. Encourage participation in local government, civic activities, and citizens' associations which promote a feeling of active participation in the community. This decreases feelings of estrangement, distance, and powerlessness.

The above interventions help people to deal in a constructive way with community forces that generate anxiety. Most of these interventions are designed to minimize or prevent the occurrence of anxiety through the use of community resources.

Evaluation

Care planned and provided for individuals with overt patterns of anxiety, as well as families and communities, must be evaluated. Evaluation includes the outcomes expected by the client and the nurse as well as the interventions used to bring

Table 29-4 Nursing Care Plan for Ms. P.

Assessment	Diagnosis	Outcome	Intervention	Evaluation
Ms. P. is coping with the finality of the loss of her marriage. She has very few friends, rarely sees her family, works 40 miles from home, and describes no coping strategies. She drives, smokes, and cries to deal with anxiety. Signs of anxiety: pounding heart, restlessness, feeling that nothing makes sense, lateness to work, inconsistent behavior, feeling lonely.	Acute anxiety associated with too few coping strategies.	Fewer episodes of restlessness and palpitations, evidenced by decrease to 2 PRN medications for anxiety per 24 hours.	Repatterning the environment: 1. Have someone stay with Ms. P. at night, primarily as a precaution against suicide. 2. Have her play soft, uplifting music. 3. Medication: Valium 10 milligrams PO every 4 hours as needed.	Outcome: She is now sleeping all night and taking 3 doses of medication per 24 hours. Process: 1. Ms. P. has continued to have someone be with her in the evenings but no longer needs someone overnight. 2. She is playing uplifting rather than melancholy music; she has begun to buy records and tapes that help her to relax. 3. Medication as reported above; but long-range, the Valium may add to her depressive feelings. As soon as possible, Ms. P.'s medication should be reevaluated.

about the outcomes. In other words, the process and outcomes of client care must be evaluated.

The evaluation process should begin soon after goals are established and ideally should be reviewed with the client and the family. This will allow for early modification of outcomes and nursing actions if some of the criteria are not being met. Including clients themselves in the evaluation process is helpful because it teaches them to analyze all aspects of their own behavior. Finally, evaluation allows nurses to analyze the adequacy of their interventions and their own behavior, and to make modifications when needed.

The care provided to Ms. P., described earlier in the chapter, illustrates an appropriate evaluation. It is documented in Table 29-4.

SUMMARY

The purpose of this chapter has been to explore problematic patterns of anxiety that develop within the person, and in relation to the family and the community. There are four basic patterns of overt anxiety: acute anxiety, panic, chronic anxiety, and posttraumatic stress disorder (PTSD); these are related to diagnostic categories in DSM III. Approximately 2 to 5 percent of the general population are affected by panic disorders and as many as 1.5 million may be afflicted with PTSD.

Anxiety is experienced by everyone and serves as an important measure of general well-being. People who develop patterns of overt anxiety defend themselves by overusing defense mechanisms. *Acute anxiety* is severe anxiety of sudden onset and short duration. *Panic,* the most severe level of anxiety, is accompanied by feelings of utter dread, by certainty that death is imminent, by personality disorganization, and by dysfunction. *Chronic anxiety* is moderate anxiety which is constantly present in a person's life over months or years. *PTSD* is a reliving of a very stressful experience, with accompanying guilt and personal dysfunction.

Anxiety is contagious and may be learned in the family and in the community. Families transfer anxiety patterns through the multigenerational transmission process. Community variables that generate anxiety are technological change and sophistication, pollution, the nuclear threat, and geographic mobility.

The nursing process is used to provide care for people who cannot cope well with their anxious feelings. Assessment of the individual, family, and community focuses specifically on causes and effects of uncontrolled anxiety. Nursing diagnoses, outcome criteria, and interventions focus on helping clients to develop strategies for controlling anxiety, increasing their ability to function while anxious, and helping them to discover life's meaning and purpose for themselves. Initial strategies the nurse uses in dealing with an anxious client include remaining with the client, maintaining a calm manner, minimizing environmental stimuli, encouraging large motor activities, and administering medication. Strategies for helping the client to learn more effective ways to manage anxiety include providing physical activity, repatterning the environment, giving medication, maintaining interpersonal contact, and teaching new ways to cope. Criteria for effectiveness of interventions with the person are adequacy, appropriateness, effectiveness, and efficiency. Interventions with the family include giving anticipatory guidance; identifying trait anxiety and triggers of anxiety; and facilitating recognition of anxiety as a family, rather than an individual, problem. Community interventions include increasing community support systems, providing relocation counselling, encouraging clients to maintain contact with family and friends, developing programs that assist the lonely and isolated in a community, providing adequate health and education services, encouraging parent-child discussion groups, and encouraging participation in government and civic activities.

REFERENCES

1. J. M. DaCosta, "On Irritable Heart: A Clinical Study of a Form of Functional Cardiac Disorder and Its Consequences," *American Journal of the Medical Sciences,* vol. 61, no. 17, 1871.
2. Sigmund Freud, *The Problem of Anxiety,* Norton, New York, 1936.
3. Harry Stack Sullivan, "The Meaning of Anxiety in Psychiatry and Life," *Psychiatry,* vol. 11, 1948, pp. 1–13.
4. Hildegard E. Peplau, *Interpersonal Relations in Nursing,* Putnam, New York, 1952.
5. American Psychiatric Association, *Diagnostic and Statistical Manual of Mental Disorders,* 3d ed., APA, Washington, D.C., 1980.
6. R. G. Petersdorf et al., eds., *Harrison's Principles of Internal Medicine,* 10th ed., McGraw-Hill, New York, 1983.
7. R. Noyes et al., "The Prognosis of Anxiety Neurosis," *Archives of General Psychiatry,* vol. 37, February 1980, pp. 173–178.
8. William Coryell et al., "Excess Mortality in Panic Disorder," *Archives of General Psychiatry,* vol. 39, June 1982, pp. 701–703.
9. J. O. Cavenar et al., *Critical Problems in Psychiatry,* Lippincott, Philadelphia, 1982.
10. J. T. Brown et al., "The Anxiety Disorders," *Annals of Internal Medicine,* vol. 100, April 1984, pp. 558–564.
11. Murray Bowen, "Intra Family Dynamics in Emotional Illness," in *Family Therapy in Clinical Practice,* Aronson, New York, 1978.
12. Joseph J. Hartog, J. Ralph Audy, and Yehudi A. Cohen, eds., *The Anatomy of Loneliness,* International Universities Press, New York, 1980.
13. S. F. Burd: "Effects of Nursing Intervention in Anxiety of Patients," in S. F. Burd and M. A. Marshall, eds., *Some Clinical Approaches to Psychiatric Nursing,* Macmillan, New York, 1963, pp. 307–321.
14. Jean W. D. Motto, "Relaxation," *American Journal of Nursing,* vol. 84, 1984, pp. 754–758.
15. Samuel M. Turner, ed., *Behavioral Theories and Treatment of Anxiety,* Plenum, New York, 1984.

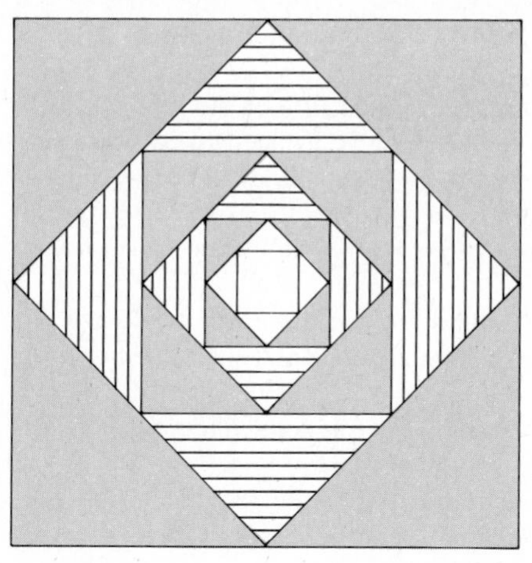

CHAPTER 30
Patterns of Avoidant Anxiety

Hope Fox

LEARNING OBJECTIVES

After studying this chapter, the student should be able to:

1. Describe behaviors associated with somatoform, dissociative, phobic, and obsessive-compulsive disorders.
2. Describe individual, family, and environmental dynamics associated with patterns of avoidant anxiety.
3. Identify the defense mechanisms utilized in these disorders.
4. Distinguish between functional personality traits and the behaviors associated with somatoform, dissociative, phobic, and obsessive-compulsive disorders.
5. Identify assessment factors for the client, the family, and the environment.
6. Formulate nursing diagnoses for clients with somatoform, dissociative, phobic, or obsessive-compulsive disorders.
7. Differentiate nurses' own personal needs from their clients' needs when establishing short- and long-term goals.
8. Describe nursing interventions appropriate to each of these disorders.
9. Construct nursing-care plans for clients with patterns of avoidant anxiety.
10. Evaluate nursing interventions for these clients.

Avoidant anxiety is manifested in ritualistic, avoidant, clinging, distancing, and overly dramatic behavior. Clients with avoidant anxiety may also display somatic symptoms that have no physical basis, or they may have episodes of amnesia or exhibit multiple personalities.

Inherent in the behavior of such clients are specific modes of functioning that are identifiable by patterns of characteristic actions.[1] Such actions represent attempts to cope with or avoid intolerable levels of anxiety. Patterns of perception and thought, emotion, and actions combine to create dysynchronous health patterns.

Development of avoidant anxiety patterns seems to be influenced by the person's underlying personality structure, and the symptoms seem to fit the lifestyle.[2] For example, a woman with a somatoform problem who frequently exhibits inauthentic emotional outbursts may earn a living as a performing artist in the theater. A meticulous accountant is more apt, under intolerable stress, to exaggerate already ingrained ritualistic behavioral patterns and exhibit ritualistic and compulsive behavior. A phobic housekeeper may tell others that she really wants to get out of the house and do things in the community but is unable to do so because of a fear of being outdoors.

The behaviors of such clients often appear, to the onlooker, to be irrational and readily within the clients' control, if only they would exert a little willpower. In many cases their behavior seems to be only an exaggeration of behavior commonly seen in most people. It is easy to be deluded into thinking that such behavior is within their conscious control.

The purposes of this chapter are to describe the modes of functioning evident in clients who exhibit somatoform, dissociative, ritualistic, and phobic patterns of interaction; to explore the individual, family, and environmental patterns that combine to generate and maintain the dysfunctional patterns; and to discuss the nursing process as a vehicle for promoting and restoring synchronous health patterns.

DYSYNCHRONOUS HEALTH PATTERNS

The original clinical studies of most of the behavior patterns described in this chapter were carried out by Sigmund Freud. His earliest manuscripts were concerned with the study of neuroses generally and hysteria specifically, as well as his attempts to cure these emotional disorders. Out of these studies arose the science of psychoanalysis and its many present-day offshoots, which formed as investigators devised new theories.

Freud concluded that *neurotics*, as these clients are sometimes called, are people who experience opposing wishes called *mental conflicts*. These conflicts exist as a result of the id's urges relating to sexuality and aggression and the ego's attempts to repress them. Freud believed there would be no neuroses without psychological conflicts between the id, ego, and superego. The symptoms which neurotics present are substitutions for satisfaction of the id's impulses.[2] They afford a temporary and partial resolution of the conflict.

All clients who demonstrate these behaviors experience a primary gain from their symptoms. *Primary gain* is the reduction of anxiety and conflict through dysfunctional behavior patterns. Many clients also experience *secondary gains*—that is, the advantages or "fringe benefits" the person derives from being dysfunctional. Secondary gains often take the form of gaining attention, being relieved of appropriate responsibilities, and assuming a dependent role.[3] Secondary gains are commonly noted in somatoform disorders in which clients exhibit multiple physical symptoms that have no physiological basis.

> Mrs. P. is a married woman in her fifties. Her children have all grown up, married, and established their own homes. Some of the appropriate developmental tasks to be accomplished by Mrs. P. are to reevaluate her own life goals, revitalize her relationship with her husband, and plan for their retirement years. Instead, Mrs. P. develops multiple physical symptoms which appear and disappear sporadically, making her intermittently incapacitated. She then states that she cannot think about returning to school, finding a job, or planning vacations with her husband because of her many physical problems. She also manipulates her husband into "waiting on her" because of her many disabilities, for which no organic basis can be found.

Neurotics also generally experience chronically low self-esteem. They feel that their efforts are unappreciated by others. In addition, they have a low level of self-acceptance and therefore feel of little value to themselves or others.

Somatoform Disorders

Somatoform disorder is a term applied to various sensory, motor, or psychic disturbances.[3] The term *somatization disorder,* used to describe one type of somatoform disorder, refers to clients who have multiple and recurrent physical complaints, not apparently related to any physical illness.[4] Complaints are presented in a vague but dramatic way and are part of an extensive medical history in which many diagnoses have been considered. It is not unusual for such clients to consult a number of doctors, often simultaneously, for their physical complaints. They are chronically worried about their health and are often called *hypochondriacs.* Their complaints may involve various systems: gastrointestinal (abdominal pain), genitourinary (painful menstruation), cardiopulmonary (dizziness), or musculoskeletal (back pain) systems. Numerous medical evaluations are undergone, both in and out of the hospital. Such clients often have unnecessary back and gynecological surgery. They may be incapacitated for long periods of time even though there is no underlying physical problem.

A *conversion disorder,* another somatoform disorder, is sometimes referred to as *hysteria.* It includes motor disturbances such as tics, tremors, convulsive movements, and paralysis. It also includes sensory disturbances such as numbness, blindness, and deafness.[4] Nurses will most commonly see these clients when they have had a sudden onset of dramatic physical symptoms that have no underlying organic basis. However, the impairment usually has a symbolic meaning for the client. For example:

> A client whose boyfriend broke up with her one night woke up completely deaf the next morning. A medical evaluation revealed no underlying cause for the deafness. It was as if she did not want to have heard what her boyfriend had said to her.

Often clients have a bland attitude toward the conversion symptom and the disability produced by it. They tend to display little anxiety or concern. The classic term for describing this lack of concern is *la belle indifference.*

Another form of conversion disorder which is commonly seen is *convulsive behavior.*[3] In this condition, the presenting symptom is a convulsive seizure closely resembling epilepsy. It is often difficult to differentiate between idiopathic epilepsy and convulsive conversion symptoms. Conversion symptoms may be suspected when the following characteristics are in evidence during the seizure:

1. There is no full loss of consciousness.
2. The episode occurs only in the presence of others.
3. No dangerous falls occur.
4. Pupillary and deep reflexes are present.
5. There is no tongue biting.
6. Bladder and bowel control are not lost.
7. Facial flushing is present, but no cyanosis or pallor.
8. Others' attempts to open the patient's eyes are resisted.
9. Pressure on the supraorbital notch causes withdrawal of the head.[4]

Clients with either somatization or conversion disorder are classified in the *Diagnostic and Statistical Manual of Mental Disorders* (DSM III) as having a somatoform disorder. Somatoform disorders are predominantly[3,4] a disorder of females, often beginning in adolescence or early adulthood. Their course is sporadic and intermittent, depending on the stress being experienced by the client. Because these disorders often take the form of somatic complaints that lead the client to a nonpsychiatric health care setting, documenting their actual incidence and prevalence is difficult.

Dissociative Disorders

The term *dissociative disorders* refers to those reactions in which there is a sudden, temporary alteration in the normally integrated functions of consciousness, identity, or motor behavior.[4] Such clients block off part of their lives from conscious recognition because of the threat of overwhelming anxiety. The mildest dissociative reaction is *sleepwalking* (somnambulism), an alteration in motor behavior. Another possible symptom, *amnesia,* involves an alteration in consciousness that may include either a loss of memory for a specific period of time or a loss of all past memories. The forgotten material is still present beneath the level of consciousness and is accessible to recall at a later time. Alterations in identity are referred to as *fugue states.* In such cases, the person's customary identity may be temporarily or permanently forgotten and a new identity assumed, a feeling of unreality may develop, or both these conditions may occur together. A more unusual dissociative reaction is the occurrence of *multiple personalities,* in which two or more distinct and dramatically different personalities exist within an individual, each dominant at a particular time. This disorder has received a great deal of attention in the media in recent years because of the publication of *Three Faces of Eve* and *Sybil.*[5,6]

DSM III classifies amnesia, fugue states, and multiple personality as dissociative disorders. Dissociative disorders (particularly multiple personality) are much rarer today than they were several decades ago. They most commonly occur during wartime or natural disasters.

Phobic Disorders

In *phobic disorders* there is a persistent fear of some object or situation that presents no real danger, or a danger is magnified out of proportion to its actual seriousness.[3,4] Phobias are fairly common phenomena not unfamiliar to most of us and often compatible with normal functioning. However, when a phobia becomes so severe that it immobilizes the person and normal, routine functioning ceases, then a phobic disorder is present.[1]

Although a phobia tends to be specific and object-oriented and therefore quite circumscribed, it may present profound problems to the client who suffers from it. Phobias which are initially circumscribed often expand and become more pervasive. The resulting limitations on the client's lifestyle can be extreme, depending upon the nature and extent of the phobia. Fear of the outdoors, for instance, can be far more immobilizing to a city dweller's daily activities than fear of rabbits.

Usually, the phobic client has had a specific fear since childhood and as an adult is fairly well adjusted and free of other dysfunctional behavior. Referral usually occurs because of an intensification of fear and a recent change in the environment which transforms a simple phobia into a more paralyzing condition. Phobias also commonly occur in conjunction with other psychiatric syndromes such as depression and obsessive-compulsive disorder.

Many clinicians describe the types of phobias in everyday language. However, clinical names are also used for specific phobias. The following list of common phobias reflects the wide variety of feared objects and situations:

Acrophobia (heights)
Agoraphobia (outdoors)
Astraphobia (thunder and lightning)
Claustrophobia (closed spaces)
Glossophobia (speaking)
Hematophobia (blood)
Hydrophobia (water)
Monophobia (being alone)
Mysophobia (germs and contamination)
Nyctophobia (night and darkness)
Pyrophobia (fire)
Sitophobia (eating)
Zoophobia (animals)

The three main types of phobic disorders are (1) agoraphobia, (2) social phobias, and (3) specific phobias. All three types can occur with or without panic attacks. A panic attack is characterized by rapid heartbeat, increased respiration, weakness of the knees, and other symptoms of the fight-flight reaction. The severity of symptoms will vary according to the phobic experience (see Chapter 29).

The most common phobia is *agoraphobia,* or the fear of going out, especially alone. People who are severely affected are unable to leave home alone. It is obvious that this malady becomes extremely disabling for the client and burdensome to family and friends. Milder forms may be restricted to specific activities like shopping or traveling by bus or train. The symptoms may be relieved when the client is accompanied by a companion.

> One young woman was unable to go out alone but had an infant with a blood disorder which required weekly trips to the pediatrician. Friends and neighbors had to provide transportation and companionship for these medical visits. The young woman also feared traveling on buses.

This example also illustrates how the phobic person manipulates the environment and compounds dependency needs.

In *social phobia* there is a fear of eating, drinking, speaking, writing, blushing, or vomiting in the presence of others. General anxiety and depression may occur as well. The client who has a social phobia is likely to come for help voluntarily as daily functioning becomes more restricted. Social phobias may present management problems for the family of the phobic person or for the staff in residential settings. Sometimes the phobia makes it necessary for clients to have meals in their rooms away from the rest of the community. This special arrangement can be misconstrued by siblings, other clients, or staff as preferential treatment, causing further interpersonal stresses.

A *specific phobia,* as the name implies, is a fear of one special object. In all phobias of this type, factors such as size, movement, distance, and color may play important parts in generating the fear. A moving insect may elicit more fear than a stationary one. Large dogs may activate the phobic reaction, while small ones may not.

DSM III classifies phobic disorders under the broader category of *anxiety disorders.* Statistics indicate that approximately 5 percent of the population have experienced phobic disorders. They appear to occur slightly more frequently in women than in men,[4] except for social phobias, which affect both sexes equally. Although phobic disorders can be quite incapacitating, many people who experience them never seek professional help, which makes it difficult to arrive at accurate figures regarding their incidence and prevalence.

Obsessive-Compulsive Disorders

An *obsessive-compulsive disorder* is characterized by a number of symptoms that often occur together. An *obsession* is a repetitive thought which a person is unable to control or exclude from consciousness. Obsessive thoughts might involve a variety of topics from suicide to changing school or jobs.[3,4] Anyone who has ever had some ridiculous little tune (usually a commercial jingle) repeating in his or her head for a portion of the day will understand, to a mild degree, what an obsession is.

A *compulsion* is a recurring irresistable impulse to perform some act. Examples of mildly compulsive acts that all people can identify with include placing articles in a specific way on a desk or dresser, twirling one's hair, rubbing one's eyes, and jingling change in one's pocket. Often, however, a compulsion is serious enough to disrupt a person's normal lifestyle; an example would be a man who feels compelled to wash his hands 25 times a day. Clients who perform compulsive acts often recognize the irrationality of the compulsion, yet feel unable to stop the ritualistic performance of the act. For example:

> A client, Mrs. N., who feels compelled to shower and change clothing 10 times a day, recognizes the absurdity of what she is doing but is unable to stop, despite the disruption the ritual creates in her daily life. If interrupted while carrying out her ritual, she must begin it all over again.

Obsessions and compulsions may be combined in an obsessive-compulsive reaction. For example, a person who compulsively cleans the house may also experience obsessive thoughts about dirt and germs. A number of other dysynchronous health patterns, such as alcoholism, drug addiction, and eating disorders, have compulsive features. The most important and distinguishing feature of obsessive-compulsive disorders is that the person involved does not want to repeat the thought or act but feels compelled to do so. The recurring thoughts and acts are not enjoyed and are viewed by the person as inappropriate and dysfunctional.

Obsessive-compulsive disorders are classified as *anxiety disorders* in DSM III.[4] Obsessive-compulsive disorder seems to be relatively uncommon in the general population, although its actual prevalence is unknown. No significant difference exists in the incidence with regard to sex. It is interesting to note that a large number of persons in this classification remain unmarried,[4] 50 percent in some surveys.[3] This disorder is more frequently seen in the upper middle class and in people with higher intellectual functioning. The symptoms tend to appear in the mid-twenties, though it is not uncommon to see them under the age of 10. Some theorists indicate that a first onset rarely appears as late as age 40. An acute attack is often precipitated by a stressful environmental incident.

SOMATOFORM AND DISSOCIATIVE DISORDERS

Patterns of Interaction: Person

For clients who develop conversion and somatization patterns, the primary mode of cognition is repression. This adaptive process results in a tendency toward forgetfulness. Memory is impressionistic, global, and lacking in sharpness.[1] As a result, the client lives in a fairly nonfactual world and is often remarkably deficient in knowledge. This is often seen by others as naiveté. In addition, the client is incapable of sustaining intense intellectual concentration and is easily distracted. Conversion patterns are thought to originate from a fixation in early psychosexual development at the Oedipal level,[7] when the person fails to give up the incestuous tie to the loved parent. This leads to anxiety and to conflict regarding sexual drives in adult life. The incestuous wishes and attendant anxiety are repressed. The tension which arises from the forbidden sexual drive is literally converted into a physical symptom. The manifestation of the symptom provides a symbolic expression of the drive, protection from conscious awareness, and reduction of anxiety. It is especially important to be aware that the symptom has symbolic meaning. For example:

> Jane D., during her childhood, had deep unconscious guilt feelings due to early masturbatory experiences. Later, in adult life after her first sexual experience, she developed paralysis of the right arm. It was discovered during treatment that this arm had been actively used in both the early and the later sexual experiences. The hysterical paralysis expressed Jane D.'s deep feelings of sexual guilt.

Along with the symptoms, the client exhibits a noticeable lack of affect in proportion to the apparent severity of the symptoms. This is so characteristic of conversion manifestations that Pierre Janet[8] gave it the name *la belle indifference,* describing the patient's marked complacency in the presence of gross objective disability. For example:

> A middle-aged man experienced total blindness. All organic causes were ruled out. When the nurse spoke with the client, he did not deny the blindness but rather seemed calm and unconcerned about his loss of sight. He asked no questions and expressed no anxiety about his condition, nor did he ask about the medical team's estimate of his prognosis.

This is typical of the behavior of someone experiencing blindness due to a conversion disorder. The nurse's expectation that the client will be frightened, anxious, or depressed about the sensory loss is not met. The client's complacency occurs because anxiety is not manifested but rather has been completely invested in the symptom, bringing psychological relief.

A conversion pattern does, of course, accomplish other things as well. It usually places the client in a regressive "sick role," which calls forth the expected nurturing responses from significant others in the environment. This extra attention satisfies dependency needs, which usually are also repressed, and results in secondary gains. Thus there is a real danger that an acute episode will become chronic. This is a significant factor to be taken into account when planning nursing care.

When clients have pseudoseizures as a form of conversion disorder, the conversion serves as a symbolic rage reaction or temper tantrum for the client and has its origin in frustration or fear of genital sexual wishes. Differentiating between idiopathic epilepsy and the conversion symptom is often difficult. However, unlike epilepsy, the pseudoseizure convulsive episode is unaccompanied by abnormal paroxysmal electrical discharges from the brain.[9]

Because the occurrence of symptoms seems to be related to the amount of anxiety the client with somatization disorder is experiencing, remissions and exacerbations are common. The anxiety is not discharged outwardly but, rather, is unconsciously channeled through the visceral organs and indirectly expressed as physical symptoms. Which organ system is affected will depend on the symbolic nature of the conflict as well as the person's constitutional makeup. For example, a woman who is experiencing conflict and anxiety about a sexual relationship may develop psychosomatic complaints related to the genitourinary system in the form of a spastic bladder and pelvic congestion that have no organic basis.

A dissociative disorder such as amnesia, fugue, or multiple personality involves repression or dissociation of anxiety-laden experiences, conflicts, aspects of self, or traumatic experiences. The onset is often precipitated by severe psychosocial stress such as marital conflict, personal rejections, natural disasters, a threat of physical injury, or death. In such cases, what is repressed or dissociated is usually an unacceptable impulse, action, or part of the self, or an intolerable life situation. For example:

> A young couple had just learned that their 4-year-old son had entered the terminal stage of acute leukemia.

The next morning the husband got up, kissed his wife and son goodbye, took the train to work, and never returned. His behavior probably evolved out of the severe psychosocial stress related to his son's illness and perhaps to unacceptable feelings he was having about this situation.

It is evident that the dissociative disorders protect people from emotional pain. These states tend to begin and end abruptly.

Patterns of Interactions: Family

Family dynamics can contribute to initiating, reinforcing, and perpetuating both conversion and somatization behavior patterns. The family may overtly or covertly teach family members that physical complaints or symptoms are acceptable ways of coping with stress or obtaining attention, care, and gratification of dependency needs. Consequently, when stress escalates for an individual or within the family system, one or more family members may use somatic complaints or symptoms as an acceptable vehicle for escaping the demands and responsibility of the stressful situation. Similarly, when emotional needs are unmet, somatic symptoms may enable the individual to obtain attention, care, and concern in a way that would not be possible with more functional behavior.

Physical illness often, if only temporarily, puts people at the center of others' concern. People with somatization or conversion disorders enjoy being the center of attention and use their symptoms as a way of meeting this need. In addition, they are then in a semilegitimate position to make demands on, manipulate, and control other family members. How family members respond will influence the degree to which this behavior is reinforced and perpetuated. Families may derive unconscious benefits from having an underfunctioning member. Another member may appear stronger by contrast and gain apparent strength from the situation. Consequently, the overfunctioning family member may in subtle ways reinforce and perpetuate the somatic symptoms, encouraging them to become an entrenched pattern. In addition, the individual's symptom provides an organizing focus. The family may unrealistically view each illness as a catastrophe. This mobilizes the entire family into cohesive action, promoting overclose fusional forces within the family.

The S.'s had been married for 10 years. Mr. S. had always had many interests, such as woodworking, gardening, golf, and sailing, that kept him busy when he was not at work. He frequently spent his evenings and weekends in his basement workshop, while his wife put the children to bed and did other chores. Soon after the youngest child started school, Mrs. S. began to have multiple physical complaints: vague backaches, headaches, and muscle aches. She went from doctor to doctor trying to obtain relief. Her husband, who had not previously spent much time with her, took time off from work to go to the doctor with her and massaged her back during the evening. The more dramatic her symptoms, the more concerned he became. After two back operations which brought no relief, the family's schedule and lifestyle came to revolve around how Mrs. S. was feeling during a particular day or week. She had not had that kind of attention from her husband or anyone else since she was a little girl.

In families where repression is the primary mode of dealing with or avoiding overwhelming anxiety, dissociative reactions may be manifested by a family member. In such cases, an individual who has learned to "block off" painful life experiences may repress a traumatic event or experience. The person may develop amnesia—may have no memory of the event and no sense of identity, and may become totally cut off from the family of origin. Sometimes such a person moves to another state or another part of the country and lives under a fabricated identity.

Patterns of Interaction: Environment

Clients exhibiting conversion and somatization disorders are usually well known within the health care system. Their tendency to dramatize and overreact to life situations is highlighted when they come into contact with providers of health care in doctors' offices, clinics, emergency rooms, and hospital units. Nurses, who often have the most sustained contact with such clients, are often struck by the inauthentic quality of their emotional displays. Because of the frequency and intensity of the physical complaints of such clients, which reveal no organic cause, health care professionals eventually come to disbelieve their complaints. The clients are viewed as having "cried wolf" once too often, and providers of health care tend eventually to ignore them. This is unfortunate because the anxiety that underlies the symptoms does not disappear and may only be exacerbated if the symptom does not provide relief. In a health care system conditioned to disbelieve such clients, a vicious circle of symptom presentation and avoidance may occur. Such clients also contribute to increased medical costs because they are frequently in one health care facility or another. Alternative ways of dealing with clients who have somatization and conversion disorders should be developed by the health care system.

PHOBIC DISORDERS

Patterns of Interactions: Person

Present knowledge of phobias is based primarily on principles formulated by Freud.[2] The chief experience of the client is intolerable anxiety characterized by feelings of apprehension, uncertainty, and helplessness. The roots of these feelings are thought to lie in anxiety experienced during the oral phase of development, caused by a loss of love and support from the nurturing figure. These dynamics place the foundation of this disorder in the area of dependency, and the symptom serves to increase the client's dependency requirements. The primary coping mechanism is displacement.[1] The person combats the diffuse anxiety by displacing it onto a particular object or situation. The specificity of the fear makes it manageable. Thus, normal anxiety present in one situation is heightened and then displaced onto another situation or object in the environment. Binding of fear to the external object occurs. This can also be a learned response as a result of early conditioning experiences, in which the parent or care giver communicated inappropriate fear and displaced it onto something in the environment. For example:

> Mrs. R. has had extremely poor eyesight from a very early age. Now, in late middle age, she has developed agoraphobia. She never ventures out of her home unaccompanied, and even going out in company causes her moderate to severe anxiety. The nurse-therapist sees Mrs. R. in the client's home because of her reluctance to go out. In the course of therapy, it becomes obvious that the agoraphobia is a displacement of anxiety related to the near blindness which Mrs. R. experiences but has never dealt with realistically.[10]

It is important to differentiate between normal fear and phobia. Normal fear has an object; it is adaptive, and is therefore a healthy response to danger or threat. The feeling of fear, with its attendant fight-flight reaction, helps the person to take quick protective action to avoid an object or situation which can be potentially harmful. A phobia has an object, but it is maladaptive. For example:

> A teenager was unable to enjoy swimming in the ocean with his peers because of a fear (which he labeled ridiculous) that his body would suddenly fold in two, like some inflated object cleaved in the middle, if he were to float on the water. In all other respects he appeared to be a normal adolescent.

This phobia, rather than being adaptive, was inhibiting normal development and peer relationships.

There are three major components to phobic disorders: (1) subjective experiences of fear and anxiety accompanying contact with a specific object or situation, (2) physiological changes associated with such contact, and (3) behavioral steps taken to avoid or escape the contact.[11]

Phobias often have a symbolic quality. The type of phobia a person develops is often symbolically related to a traumatic and anxiety-laden experience, an unconscious conflict, or an unmet need. The symbolic meaning of the phobia can often be determined by listening to the client's associations. Recall of childhood experiences closely associated with the present fear often can lead to clarification of the phobia.[12]

> A 9-year-old girl, small for her age, was frequently left in the care of her 14-year-old brother, who was instructed by their single working parent to take his sister wherever he went. The young girl was thus led to participate reluctantly in activities which were not age-appropriate and were frightening for her. One of these activities involved sneaking into the local movie house by climbing to the third-story top of an open-stair fire escape and entering a fire-exit door which led to the balcony inside. In adult life, while on a camping trip with her family, the woman attempted to climb an open-stair fire tower which was a popular tourist attraction in a state forest. She experienced no discomfort initially, but upon reaching the third landing, she was seized by a sudden, profound, and paralyzing fear and was unable to continue.

This is a good example of phobia manifested many years after the initial feared experience. The relationship to the earlier childhood situation was subsequently brought out in therapy.

Psychosocial theories provide the most widely accepted explanations of phobic disorders. However, there is recent evidence that a different point of view may have some validity: the fact that panic disorders and certain phobias can be treated effectively with antidepressants suggests a biological basis for specific phobias.[3] These data also raise questions about the relationship between depression and anxiety disorders.

Patterns of Interaction: Family

Within the family system, phobic behavior may be a learned response to stress and conflict that is transmitted from generation to generation. It may range from general fearfulness in threatening situations to exaggerated fear and avoidance of specific situations.

Jane L. would drive from town to town only on local streets. The mere thought of driving on the parkway would make her tremble, perspire, and feel faint. She could also drive only to certain places, or the same feeling would occur. Her mother, Lillian, had followed a similar pattern and had frequently told terrible stories of misfortunes that happened to people who took long trips on parkways. Jane stated that she knew her behavior was absurd and influenced by her mother, but she felt powerless to change it.

"Phobic partners" may develop within the family. These are convenient "helpers" who stand by and help to maintain the phobic behavior. They protect the phobic person from acute panic and anxiety and may actually participate in the phobia.

Mrs. G. had a germ phobia. She would not go out because she was afraid she would be contaminated by germs. In addition, she was afraid that family members would bring germs into the house. Her husband, going along with this behavior, had a special entryway with a sealed door built onto the back of the house. As Mrs. G.'s phobia became more pervasive, the special door became insufficient to keep her anxiety at manageable levels. She soon demanded that Mr. G. undress before entering the house so that he would be less contaminated. Mr. G. felt that his wife was being ridiculous but nevertheless complied with her demands.

The participation of such a partner usually serves to further the secondary gains of the phobic by fulfilling an unconscious wish to be taken care of and to be in control. In addition, the protective maintenance of symptoms perpetuates the phobic person's underfunctioning. This causes the partner to emerge as the stronger-looking family member, a position that might not be available if the affected member were more functional. The question also arises whether the partner could function well and deal effectively with a more functional family member.

Patterns of Interaction: Environment

Societal forces, particularly role expectations, may contribute to development of phobias in women. For example, most agoraphobics are women. Their symptoms range in severity from those who will go out within a limited geographic area or when accompanied by a trusted friend or family member to those who are housebound for months or years. It has been proposed that agoraphobia highlights the conflicting role expectations women face in society. Contemporary women are encouraged to be autonomous, independent, and assertive. This directly conflicts with the traditional expectations that women and wives will be submissive and compliant. In this light, agoraphobia can be viewed as a "declaration of dependence"—one in which women dysfunctionally manage conflictual societal role expectations by unconsciously placing severe phobic limitations on themselves.[13]

The community in which a phobic person lives is often affected by the phobic behavior. For example, agoraphobics require an extensive support system to compensate for their inability to leave home. School personnel, medical personnel, and retail establishments make special adjustments to accommodate agoraphobics. Neighbors are often eager to assist with transportation, shopping, and household errands, until the assistance becomes an ongoing job. In large-scale crises, such as fire, crime, or acute illness, agoraphobics are difficult to move out of the home, and community workers are required to have much patience and great understanding. Other phobias affect the community to varying degrees, depending upon their nature.

OBSESSIVE-COMPULSIVE DISORDERS

Patterns of Interaction: Person

Freud[2] placed the origin of obsessive and compulsive characteristics in the anal stage of development, when holding back (of feces) and learning to let go is a significant developmental task. Children gain pleasure from controlling their own bodies and, indirectly, the actions of significant others.

Erikson[14] defines the second stage of development as autonomy versus shame and doubt. Children at this level have the option of giving up excretions as required by the parent or holding onto them if childish perversity prevails. To be neat and tidy brings parental approval as a reward. To be messy, which the child longs for, brings criticism and rejection. In other words, to be good is to be neat and controlled. To be bad is to obey impulses to be dirty and aggressive.

The obsessional character develops out of the need to obtain approval by being excessively tidy and controlled. At this time of development, the child is reacting to standards set by the parents. These standards are not uncommonly excessively high and in conflict with normal developmental tasks necessary for healthy personality growth. In such cases, frustration continually exists between the child's normal developmental tendencies and the parents' taboos. This type of experience often contributes to the incidence of obsessive-compulsive behavior.

It is important to differentiate between obsessional or compulsive character traits and obsessive-compulsive disorder. All too often, students of psychology, medicine, and nursing judge themselves and their acquaintances too harshly and tend to see gross pathology in what is, in fact, normal behavior. Actually, some typical obsessive-compulsive traits can be helpful in moderation: tidiness, orderliness, precision, punctuality, concern for detail, perseverance, caution. These are helpful in many professions and are frequently associated with intelligence. Such traits differ radically from slavery to ritual. Obsessive-compulsive disorder exists when the behaviors are protective ways of acting that occupy the whole day and create a totally destructive and nonproductive pattern.[1] Thus within normal limits a few compulsive traits are helpful in getting the work of the world done. The crucial difference between mental health and mental illness lies in the ability to function and to control these traits rather than being controlled by them.

Obsessive-compulsive behaviors are an unconscious attempt to reduce an intolerable level of anxiety; the more anxiety there is, the more attention the client will devote to the elaboration and maintenance of a rigid routine. Symptom formation occurs on the basis of several coping mechanisms. First, the client's handling of feelings and thoughts through ritualistic behavior represents a return to earlier, *regressive* methods of dealing with anxiety. Second, clients' obsessive thoughts are either devoid of feeling or attached only to anxiety. When ideas become detached from emotions, *isolation* is being used. Third, the client's overt attitude toward others is usually the opposite of unconscious feelings. Thus, *reaction formation* is exhibited. Fourth, compulsive rituals are a symbolic way of *undoing* or resolving underlying conflict. When critical life events occur, the symptoms, which are defensive attempts to deal with anxiety, may become worse. For example, a client who feels responsibility and guilt about the death of a spouse may engage in excessive hand washing to deal with feelings of guilt and responsibility.

Patterns of Interaction: Family

In the family, obsessive-compulsive behavior frequently acts as an organizing focus. It is often so disruptive that it provides concrete behavior for the family to pay attention to, worry about, talk about, and rally about in an immediate way. Its presence can be so time-consuming that the family cannot focus on other matters of concern. Thus, the dysfunctional behavior can serve a diversionary function in a family, enabling it to shift away, even if only temporarily, from other problems such as marital conflict, drinking, and school failure.

Since neatness and cleanliness are considered next to godliness in our society, the early behavior of some obsessive-compulsive people may be unconsciously encouraged and reinforced, making it difficult for families to assess this behavior as dysfunctional. Obsessive-compulsives tend to develop in overcontrolling families. Parents may encourage obsessive-compulsive behavior by establishing rigid standards to which family members must adhere; and since parents are proud of a child, adolescent, or young adult who is scrupulously clean and keeps an immaculate room, awareness of dysfunction may emerge only when the symptoms become dramatic.

Such families display a need to maintain rigid and purposive activity with continuous self-imposed pressure to "measure up" rather than "go with the flow." The "shoulds" of their lifestyle are extensive, making relaxation impossible. They are overcontrolled by rigid expectations, and consequently they feel that nonpurposive, nondirected activity is bad. Pleasurable activities bring discomfort. Clients who develop obsessive-compulsive reactions extend this ritualistic behavior pattern to dysfunctional proportions by using it to control and avoid anxiety.

Patterns of Interaction: Environment

Contemporary life is extremely fast-paced and sometimes chaotic. Ritualistic behavior is one means of coping with and reducing the anxiety that is integral to a rapidly changing, highly technological society. However, in a fast-paced society, the rituals of the obsessive-compulsive, which are often painfully slow and deliberate, can lead to profound impatience on the part of others, including health professionals. This may contribute to stalls in the relationship between care giver and care receiver. The client's solution to a feeling that life is chaotic is to introduce more rigidity and more ritual, in an attempt to regain a sense of control. The solution, however, becomes a larger problem as the obsessive-compulsive pattern becomes more pervasive. The client and nurse need to work toward a better balance between rigidity and flexibility and toward more functional ways of coping with anxiety.

NURSING PROCESS

Assessment

There are many ways in which nurses may come into contact with clients who exhibit avoidant anxiety patterns. Such clients may have been already diagnosed and may be receiving treatment in a community health facility on an inpatient or outpatient basis, or they may be undergoing treatment at home, where they are periodically seen by a community health nurse. In situations such as these, the nurse is part of an established health team and the nursing care plan encompasses the range of services being offered to the client and family by all members of the team. Or a nurse may be an independent practitioner in the community, in which case clients may seek help on a one-to-one, group, or family basis. In such instances, the nurse may make an assessment alone or in consultation with others.

Nurses play a major role in case finding, recognizing behavioral deviations, and assisting clients to obtain help in an appropriate treatment setting. Some deviations may be observed as behavioral clues signaling the presence of one or more problems. The assessment process should consider factors which include the client, the family, and the environment. Table 30-1 identifies assessment factors for these three areas.

Diagnosis

Nursing diagnoses for clients with avoidant anxiety patterns focus on the client's problematic behavior pattern and the associated rationale for the behavior. Since clients vary so widely in their dysfunctional behavior patterns, the nursing diagnosis will potentially include a wide range of problems. Examples of nursing diagnoses for such clients, based on the more common behaviors identified as avoidant anxiety patterns, are outlined in Table 30-2 (page 576).

Outcome Criteria

The ongoing evaluation of nursing actions is measured against the goals established for the individual client. In general, goals involve outcome behavior that the client will exhibit while moving in the direction of healthier behavior patterns. Some potential outcomes for the clients discussed in this chapter are as follows. The client will be able to:

1. Verbalize feelings of anxiety as they are occurring.
2. Identify methods of coping with anxiety without resorting to avoidance or to ritualistic or somatic behavior.
3. Identify authentic feelings.
4. Express feelings openly and directly.
5. Identify realistic strengths and weaknesses.
6. Evaluate relationships more realistically.
7. Describe ways in which he or she contributes to the behavior pattern.
8. Identify functional ways of exercising control over his or her life.
9. Identify ways in which nurturing needs can be met without using manipulation.

Table 30-1 Assessment Factors for Patterns of Avoidant Anxiety

Client

1. Identify the event that precipitated the behavior and determine its symbolic meaning to the client.
2. Evaluate how the client deals with feelings, thoughts, and actions.
   a. **Somatoform.** Global responses, use of superlatives, dramatic, multiple physical complaints, behavioral responses represent polar extremes. (For example—Interviewer: "How was your vacation?" Client: "Great!" "Fabulous!" Or, "Oh, it was awful, it couldn't have been worse! My back never stopped hurting for a minute.")
   b. **Obsessive-compulsive.** Detailed responses that provide numerous facts but have no affective quality. (For example—Interviewer: "How was your vacation?" Client: "I did Paris in 48 hours. I got to see all the museums, cafes, and nightclubs. Saturday morning I awoke at 7 A.M. to get an early start . . .")
   c. **Phobic.** Describes experiences in terms of personal fearfulness. (For example—Interviewer: "How was your vacation?" Client: "I couldn't go to the observation tower because I'm afraid of heights. There were so many people—mobs of them. I couldn't catch my breath. I had to stay in my room, and the rest of the group went on the tour without me."
3. Evaluate the client's personal appearance and style of dress.
   a. Showy and extreme
   b. Rigidly neat, nothing whatsoever out of place
   c. Inconsistent manner of dress
   d. Appropriate
4. Evaluate the client's level of anxiety.
   a. Mild
   b. Moderate
   c. Severe
   d. Panic
5. Evaluate defensive patterns or security operations utilized to reduce anxiety.
   a. Repression
   b. Conversion
   c. Intellectualization
   d. Regression
   e. Displacement
   f. Isolation
   g. Undoing
   h. Reaction formation
6. Identify the secondary gains of the dysfunctional behavior.
   a. Attention
   b. Nurturing-dependency

Client

6. c. Lack of responsibility
   d. Affection
   e. Control
   f. Manipulation
7. What is the client's decision-making and problem-solving ability?
8. How does the client explain the dysfunctional behavior?

Family

1. Is there a family history of any of the following?
   a. Overcontrolling parenting in early childhood
   b. Obsessive-compulsive or phobic behavior patterns
   c. Somatization patterns that have no physical basis
2. How do family interaction patterns:
   a. Initiate, reinforce and maintain the dysfunctional behavior?
   b. Decrease the dysfunctional behavior?
3. What function does this behavior serve for the family?
4. How do family members characteristically cope with stress?
5. In what way does this behavior provide an organizing focus for this family?
6. What other problems does this behavior divert the family from confronting?

Environment

1. What is the client's current lifestyle like? What would a desirable lifestyle be like?
2. Does the client's lifestyle reinforce the dysfunctional behavior? If so, in what ways?
3. To what extent does the dysfunctional behavior limit the client's lifestyle?
4. How does the client cope with the lifestyle limitations imposed by the dysfunctional behavior?
5. How does the client function in a work setting?
6. Does the client have a social network?
7. How does the client's social network reinforce or maintain the dysfunctional behavior?
8. What are the client's social relationships like?
9. Have any psychosocial stressors occurred recently? If so, what are they?
   a. Internal stressors
   b. External stressors
10. To what extent has the client been involved with health care providers and the health care system?

Table 30-2 Nursing Diagnoses for Patterns of Avoidant Anxiety

Conversion and Somatization Disorders
Paralysis of legs related to dependence-independence conflict
Chronic low back pain related to inability to verbally express anxiety
Complacency regarding blindness associated with secondary gains from assumption of sick role
Sudden outbursts of dramatic emotionality related to control needs
Dissociative Disorders
Inability to recall events pertaining to a fire in the home, related to guilt about the death of a son in the fire
Assumption of an alternate identity and disappearance from family associated with severe anxiety related to the diagnosis of cancer in a young daughter
Sleepwalking related to escalating marital conflict
Phobic Disorders
Fear of leaving the house related to social role conflict
Constriction of social life associated with fears of rejection and abandonment
Fear of heights related to loss of control
Selective fear of driving on highways related to dependence-independence conflict
Obsessive-Compulsive Disorders
Repetitive handwashing and recurring thoughts of dirt and germs related to sexual conflict
Rigid adherence to work schedule related to fear of loss of control
Ritualistic housekeeping related to need for approval
Hostile verbal reaction to unscheduled changes related to loss of order and security

10. Evaluate past and present family relationships more realistically.
11. Define a functional lifestyle.
12. Identify relevant social role conflicts.

It is very difficult for clients to give up firmly established behavior patterns even when they are aware that the patterns are dysfunctional and self-defeating. Consequently, nurses should be careful not to impose their goals on clients. The nurse's goals and the client's readiness for change do not necessarily coincide. The client's readiness to risk change must be established before goals such as the ones described above begin to become realistic. At that point the nurse and the client may collaborate on formulating goals that are appropriate to the needs of that particular client. (For example, if the client has a phobia, the nurse and client may formulate a series of short-term goals that lead toward the long-term goal of desensitization.) Otherwise, this process may appear to the client to be a repetition of the controlling parental relationship that was experienced in childhood.

Intervention

Intervention with the Client

The behavior patterns described in this chapter develop over extended periods of time; therefore, the treatment may also be long and slow. Most clients come for help only after they have unsuccessfully tried remedies suggested by well-meaning family members and friends. Clients who manifest these behaviors have developed them as defenses against anxiety. Therefore, if clients are urged to approach that which they fear, or if they are forced to relinquish their symptoms, their anxiety levels rise. If the clients do comply and the particular symptoms do disappear, other symptoms that are equally if not more frustrating and debilitating may appear in their place. Simply extinguishing the problematic behavior, then, prevents the client from seeking the underlying reason for the development of the symptom.

Intervention with clients who exhibit avoidant anxiety patterns begins with the care giver. The attitude of the nurse affects the client immediately. Nurses must be aware of their own feelings in response to the client as a prerequisite for understanding the client's behavior. Nurses who do not understand the client's need to behave as he or she does may directly or indirectly indicate to the client that the behavior is unacceptable and must be modified. This attitude arises from the nurse's discomfort with the behavior and inability to examine its meaning and purpose for the client.

The nurse needs to have the capacity to empathize with the client, the ability to understand the client's motives, and the willingness to listen to the client's expressions of thoughts and feelings. An attitude of calm reassurance coupled with warmth and recognition of the client as a worthwhile person indicates to the client that the staff members are not merely trying to eradicate symptoms for their own convenience but are interested in helping the client understand behaviors and feelings and develop more satisfying patterns of interaction. The nurse-client relationship allows the client to experience feelings and satisfactions that lead to the development of more mature needs. This is particularly important for clients who have exhausted the patience of relatives and friends with years of complaints and anxieties. The disapproval and rejection they experience confirm the feelings of low self-esteem and fear which originally led to the development of their neurotic responses.

Most clients do not understand or know why they behave as they do; to ask them, "What is wrong?" or "Why are you acting this way?" is an exercise in futility. Rather, nurses need to label the emotion that they sense the client is expressing through behavior. This forces the client to consider a specific feeling, which can then be expressed. If an accurate interpretation of feelings has been made, the client will verbally validate it or respond with an appropriate change in behavior. The excessive repression of feelings by clients who exhibit obsessive-compulsive behavior makes it most appropriate for the nurse to operate on a "feelings" level. The nurse acts as a role model, demonstrating that feelings need not be threatening and that verbal expression is an appropriate way of dealing with them.

LOW SELF-ESTEEM. Many of these clients have low self-esteem, are indecisive, and avoid contact with others in the inpatient setting. Then too, their behavior may be so frustrating that mutual withdrawal occurs. When initiating social or sports activities, nurses should avoid making direct requests that these clients attend, since they are inclined to flatly refuse or to spend prolonged periods of time deciding what they will do. Instead, a more positive approach should be utilized to make clients feel wanted and needed and help them initiate movement toward the group. For example, the nurse may say, "We are going to play (Ping-Pong, shuffleboard, etc.) and we need you to complete the team," at the same time placing the appropriate playing equipment in the client's hand and gently guiding him or her toward the group.[12]

Another important approach is to provide opportunities for the client to succeed. (It helps no one to ask clients to participate in activities beyond their capacity.) Activities and expectations should be structured in an incremental way, since small successes usually precede larger ones. Goal setting must be geared to this slow pace and related to the client, not to the nurse's need for success.

CONVERSION BEHAVIOR. Clients with conversion reactions are usually admitted to the medical-surgical unit of a general hospital for diagnostic evaluation of their physical symptoms. A thorough physical examination and medical history must be completed and tests carried out in order to make a valid differential diagnosis. When the outcome of the tests is negative, staff members are often frustrated and begin blaming and criticizing the client for laziness, malingering, and childishness.

Intervention then is directed at learning how the client's emotional distress is converted into physical symptoms and discovering the meaning and purpose of the behavior. Nurses need to plan their intervention on the basis of the current level of need fulfillment; that is, existing needs must be met before more mature needs can emerge. The client's behavior is not consciously motivated and is an attempt to relieve anxiety and stress in a personally and socially acceptable way. The symptoms are real to the client; the pain, if present, is real; and the need for intervention is real. The staff must share observations and feelings about the client so that effective intervention can proceed without interference from stereotyped images and feelings. Conversion symptoms usually have symbolic meaning which covers repressed feelings. The goal of intervention is to help clients become aware of what they are feeling, achieve greater acceptance of their feelings, and learn to deal with these feelings more effectively. Emphasis is on minimizing the sick role and behavior and on identifying and supporting the client's strengths and areas for growth. For example:

> Gloria M., age 45, was admitted to the general hospital for treatment of paralysis of the lower extremities. The paralysis had appeared during the night before admission. Two days before that, Gloria's husband had entered the same hospital with a myocardial infarction. The couple had no children, and Gloria's mother, when interviewed, stated, "Gloria's husband treats her like a little doll. Now that he's sick, I would have been surprised if she had risen to the occasion to take care of him." A complete physical examination revealed no organic basis for the paralysis.

Gloria seemed submissive and talked very little when her mother was present. She did not ask about her husband, but she dramatically complained about her inability to move and was often irritable and demanding.

Liz B., the nurse, recognized that Gloria enjoyed being the center of attention and being cared for. She sensed a constant undercurrent of anger in Gloria. One day, after visiting her husband in his unit, Gloria was observed curled up in bed, weeping and rubbing her legs. When Liz asked if her legs hurt, she threw a book across the room and yelled loudly, saying, "He's practically dying, and he's still treating me like a baby." Liz listened quietly and, when Gloria had quieted down, helped her to talk about her feelings. She told Gloria that it was normal to feel anger when others did not seem to understand what she was feeling or treated her as she may not have wanted to be treated. They discussed the role binds that people get into and do not know how to get out of because of an inability to communicate their feelings. Gloria stated that she feared that if she told her husband that she wanted to change, he would not understand, and that at this time it would be too much of a shock for him. Also, she was not sure that she knew how to change at this point in her life.

The nurse said, "Strong emotions and the need to change are often frightening feelings that a person may not be willing to acknowledge, much less communicate." As Gloria listened, she relaxed visibly. She said she had become convinced that she was stuck being a "middle-aged doll" and that neither she nor her husband would be able to cope with a change. Liz said, "Your husband's heart attack will necessitate some changes anyway, so this may be a realistic time to start."

During subsequent sessions with a psychiatrist and the nurse, Gloria became more aware of her feelings and the connection between her husband's illness, her loss of dependency, her anger, and the subsequent paralysis. During her recovery, Gloria experimented with new feelings and behaviors, using the nurse as a role model and testing ground.

RITUALISTIC BEHAVIOR. Clients who engage in ritualistic behavior must never have direct limits set on their ritualistic acts unless such intervention is specifically indicated. To forbid such behavior is to eliminate a defense which serves as a security operation for the client and possibly to precipitate panic levels of anxiety. Instead, these guidelines should be followed in interventions with the ritualistic client:

1. Use a quiet manner with the client, keeping the environment calm.
2. Reassure the client of your interest in him or her as an individual.
3. Don't be judgmental or verbalize disapproval of the client's behavior.
4. Do not pressure the client to change.
5. Do not confront the client about the ritualistic behavior. Instead, give reflective feedback, such as "I see you undress three times every morning. That must be tiring for you." This statement communicates empathy and understanding of the client's experience and may serve to lower the client's anxiety level, thus reducing the intensity of the ritualistic behavior.
6. Ritualistic clients have a low tolerance for change. Make only reasonable requests and always explain them. Logic and argument have no place here but only increase the client's anxiety, intensify the ritualistic behavior, and heighten the frustration of the nurse.
7. Engage the client in constructive activities which will leave less time for compulsive behavior. In ritualistic speech, for instance, it becomes obvious to the observant nurse that the client is ensnared in an exhausting compulsion to repeat the same litany over and over again. Nursing action involves planning situations—such as object-oriented activities, rather than interpersonal ones which require conversation—to help the client avoid constant verbal repetition. Examples of such activities are quiet games which require concentration, such as checkers and chess, as well as arts and crafts such as needlework, woodwork, ceramics, and painting.
8. Give positive reinforcement for nonritualistic behavior. Avoid reinforcing ritualistic behavior, so that there are no secondary gains, such as attention and nurturing, for maladaptive behavior. For example:

Mrs. S., a client who compulsively cleaned and recleaned her room many times a day, enjoyed talking with the staff about home decorating. Ms. D., a nurse on the unit, observed this pattern, and the staff decided that Ms. D. would spend time with Mrs. S., during her nonritualistic periods, talking about decorating. When she was performing her cleaning and recleaning, Ms. D. would spend time with her if necessary but without engaging her in talk about decorating. Thus the nurse would not be giving positive reinforcement for an inappropriate activity.

9. Help the clients to find ways of setting limits on their own behavior.
10. Support clients' efforts to explore the meaning and purpose of their behavior. Let them know that you understand and are willing to help them explore their feelings so as to become more comfortable with them. For example:

John was eating well unless someone approached his table, had a change of mind, and then sat elsewhere at another table in the dining room. When this happened, John would stop eating and ritualistically polish and repolish each eating utensil with his napkin. The nurse might say to him, "John, you were eating your dinner, but you seemed upset when David turned away and sat with somebody else. Can you tell me what that feeling was like?"

In managing ritualistic behavior, allow time in the day's routine for the rituals. The attempt to reduce them by not providing the necessary time only leads to the law of diminishing returns. As the client becomes more pressured and anxious, the probability of error within the ritual increases and the client will be more likely to have to start the ritual over again. On the other hand, when the nurse sets aside the necessary time needed for the ritual, the client is given to understand that the nurse accepts the client as a person along with the dysfunctional behavior. For example:

Mr. K., the night nurse in a residential psychiatric unit, is in charge of Mr. L., an obsessive-compulsive client with ritualistic behavior involving repetition of the morning toilet. Mr. K. awakens Mr. L. one-half hour earlier than the rest of the unit population. In planning his nursing care, Mr. K. informed Mr. L. that he would awaken him earlier "to give you plenty of time to finish dressing so that you won't be late for breakfast."

Some success has also been achieved in reducing ritualistic behavior through use of paradoxical injunction; that is, the removal of a symptom by prescribing that the client not change or actually do more of the symptomatic behavior (see Chapter 19). The theoretical premise of this intervention is that clients will instinctively resist the therapist's request for change. Therefore, if the client is told not to change, the suggestion will be resisted and the client will begin to change.[15] This intervention, prescribing the symptom, is illustrated in the following example:

Kate is a 32-year-old mother and housewife with a germ phobia resulting in hand-washing rituals that take up a great deal of her time. She comes to the nurse-therapist for relief from these rituals. In the course of therapy, she is asked to keep a diary of her daily hand-washing rituals, and is subsequently requested to wash her hands more than the usual 25 times per day. She is compliant about keeping the diary, but when asked to wash her hands more, she exclaims, "More? Do I have to?" At the next session she reports that she has been unable to comply with the nurse's request and that the hand-washing ritual has, in fact, diminished to normal proportions.

The client turned against her own symptom, which means that, in this instance, paradoxical injunction was useful in extinguishing the ritualistic behavior.

Because of the extremely resistant nature of the symptoms of obsessive-compulsive disorder, the goal of therapy often is to confine the symptoms rather than eradicate them. Nurses play a significant role in supportive psychotherapy by helping the client to limit the undesired behaviors. There are no drugs currently known which alleviate the symptoms of obsessive-compulsive neurosis. Tranquilizers, in conjunction with psychotherapy, may afford the client some relief from the underlying anxiety.

AVOIDANCE BEHAVIOR. Clients who displace their anxiety onto a particular object or situation will have varying degrees of restriction in their lifestyles. In the past, successful intervention with such clients has been limited when traditional psychotherapeutic interventions have been utilized. Today, phobias are often viewed as responses to anxiety which have been learned and therefore can be unlearned. Behavioral modification strategies such as desensitization may be utilized by nurses working with phobic clients.[16]

Desensitization refers to the gradual systematic exposure of the client to the feared situation under controlled conditions. Densitization strategies utilized by nurses include:

1. Relaxation techniques
2. Construction of a hierarchy of fears

3. Gradual exposure to the feared situation while using relaxation techniques[16]

The rationale for this approach lies in the behavioral hypothesis that a client, when exposed to a fear-producing stimulus, fears disorganization and loss of control of his or her body and mind. This fear leads to an avoidance response. Thus, reality is never tested; the phobic person never finds out if what is feared is true. The therapist's role is to elicit the fear in progressively more challenging but attainable steps. This approach enables the client to realize that the dangerous consequences will not occur.[17] The phobic client is serially exposed to a predetermined list of anxiety-provoking stimuli graded in a hierarchy from least frightening to most frightening. Each of the anxiety-provoking stimuli is paired with the arousal of another affect of an opposite quality that is strong enough to suppress the anxiety. The client is either given tranquilizing drugs or taught relaxation exercises to achieve a state of mental and physical relaxation. Once relaxation techniques have been mastered, the client is taught how to use them when confronting an actual anxiety-provoking situation. As the stimuli are presented in a gradual way from least frightening to most frightening, the client becomes desensitized to each stimulus on the scale and moves up to the next. Ultimately, what was previously most anxiety-producing becomes no longer capable of eliciting that anxious response.[16]

Practice sessions teach the client how to deal with phobic anxiety in real-life situations. Clients are taught to set increasingly difficult goals for themselves. Each step forward represents progress. When phobics enter feared situations with a therapist and begin to realize that they are able to accomplish tasks they previously felt unable to do, they develop enough confidence to attempt more challenging situations and eventually confront feared situations without the therapist's support.[17] It is often helpful to encourage clients to measure their anxiety on a rating scale. This helps them to realize that anxiety levels fluctuate and that relaxation techniques help to bring high anxiety levels down[18] (see Chapter 29). The nurse reinforces the idea that clients must practice exposing themselves to the feared situation. A task sheet may be helpful in outlining specific tasks for each day or week. The nurse and the client should jointly review the task sheets at the end of each week. Clients should be told that there will be times when they feel that they cannot confront the fear. The therapist can encourage the client to:[17–20]

1. Accept having the phobia without being embarrassed or upset. It is only when a difficulty is acknowledged that something can be done about it. Expect and allow the fear to arise when a phobic situation is encountered. Physical sensations such as rapid heartbeat, dizziness, weak legs, and butterflies in the stomach are automatically triggered by past phobic experiences. Thoughts about what one imagines is going to happen accelerate the physical responses. It is helpful to suggest that the client substitute positive thoughts for negative ones. A person who tries to eliminate the fear altogether is fighting it and not accepting it. If it is accepted, it will diminish if not disappear. Learning that one can do things to bring one's own fear level down is the first step toward being able to cope in a phobic situation.
2. Share the seemingly irrational thoughts and feelings with others, especially the therapist. Phobic clients are often reluctant to share their thoughts and feelings because they fear being ridiculed or told to ignore their feelings. The therapist's acceptance of the client's fears as real experiences is important to the client's feeling of being understood. Therapists who have been phobic themselves can tell clients about their own experiences with fear. This is often encouraging to the client, who feels, "Here is someone who really understands and who has really overcome what I am struggling with."
3. Stop, wait, and try not to rush out of the feared situation as soon as discomfort is experienced. Phobic people have a fear of the fear itself. If they can wait out the beginnings of anxiety or decrease it with relaxation exercises, they may then be ready to continue confronting it. Phobics who *wait* to be in the right mood when they approach the feared situation may never be ready to approach or remain in a feared situation. Clients gain more self-assurance and satisfaction if they can cope with situations when their fears are greatest.
4. Do things that lower the fear level and keep it

manageable. Each client needs to find ways of handling fears in particular situations. For example, one person sings while driving, another swims in deep water but near the edge of the pool. Another person says, "I'll just let the feelings come; they're only feelings. I'm not going to faint. I haven't fainted yet; and even if I do faint, so what?"

The following case study illustrates the process of contextual desensitization therapy.

Mrs. B. had developed an automobile phobia. She had not driven in 2 years and was also afraid of being a passenger in a car. Mrs. B.'s first goal was to be able to stand beside her husband's car for 5 minutes without having a panic attack or passing out. Mrs. B. said that those reactions had not happened to her, but she feared that they would if she exposed herself to the feared situation. During this early practice session, the therapist had Mrs. B. describe how she felt walking toward, standing next to, and touching the car. When she began to feel "spacy," the therapist instructed her to touch his arm and begin a relaxation exercise. Her anxiety level began to decrease immediately and she was able to accomplish her goal. In a later session when Mrs. B. was practicing sitting in the unstarted car, she became very frightened and wanted to leave the car immediately, because she felt she was losing control of herself. The therapist instructed her to count to 20, and then leave if she still found it necessary. She counted and was surprised that her anxious feelings passed. Each time she became panicky, the therapist suggested that she ask herself the following: "Am I passing out now? Am I making a fool of myself? Am I losing control?" She was also told to repeat, "I had these feelings before and they passed. I know they will pass again." In this way she was helped to substitute positive thoughts for negative ones and focus on simple manageable tasks in the present such as counting backward from 100 by 3s, reciting a poem, or singing a song. As she experienced success, taking each goal and breaking it down one step at a time, her preoccupation with imaginary dangers decreased. She became more willing to risk exposure to the feared situation. After 1 year, Mrs. B. was able to ride in a car as a passenger within a 50-mile radius of home. Her discomfort remained manageable, and she used the techniques she had learned to deal with it.

Phobic and obsessive-compulsive behavior may, at times, overlap. For example, a client may engage in compulsive hand washing related to a phobic aversion to germs. This behavior may also respond to a desensitization approach in which the client is gradually exposed to the feared object, germs, or dirty objects, and is simultaneously asked to resist or reduce the related hand-washing ritual.[20]

Intervention with the Family

Intervention with families of clients who utilize avoidant anxiety patterns presents several potential areas of focus that involve four areas of intervention: increasing open, direct expression of feelings; restructuring relationships and patterns of need fulfillment; sorting family scripts and coping styles; and revising the client's and the family's expectations.

Open, direct expression of honest feelings is often severely restricted, particularly within the families of clients with somatoform disorders. The family often resorts to inauthentic, dramatic expressions of feelings that are conveyed in manipulative, controlling ways. In working with such families the nurse can act as a role model, demonstrating clear, congruent verbal and nonverbal messages. Asking family members to speak to each other rather than about each other is helpful. The nurse can also facilitate discussion of emotionally charged family issues such as power, control, dependency, and abandonment so that hidden issues are opened up for family exploration. When such issues are defused, they are less likely to be acted out in an emotional manner. Use of these techniques helps to decrease the need to express feelings physically or in other disguised ways.

Relationship patterns in a family may be characterized by overfunctioning of the unaffected spouse and underfunctioning of the affected spouse. The nurse needs to explore mutual patterns of protectiveness that initiate and maintain dysfunctional behavior. The nurse can ask both spouses what it would be like for them if each spouse was different—for example, if they switched roles. Many times the client's dysfunctional behavior satisfies an underlying need for the other spouse, who takes on the role of enabler, unconsciously contributing to the maintenance of symptoms in the underfunctioning spouse.[18,21] For example, the role of enabler is often taken on by the husband of a female agoraphobic who has a vested interest in keeping his spouse dysfunctional. The enabler may sabotage treatment by continuing to shop, do the driving, or run errands in a way that enables the agoraphobic to remain housebound.[22] The nurse can explore with each spouse what would make it possible to assume a more balanced role. Very often, the roles of the spouses are symmetrical with their positions in their families of origin, and discovering this provides rich information for exploration. The nurse uses confrontation and feedback to help clients recognize how they project blame for relationship problems onto others and deny their own part in the process.

Working with obsessive-compulsive clients within a family framework is difficult because they tend to ally with the therapist, thus removing themselves from the family process. Additionally, when they are asked to let down their defenses in the presence of others, their anxiety level escalates dramatically.[23]

Phobic, ritualistic, and somatic behavior patterns are often learned ways of coping with anxiety. Generational family coping patterns need to be examined by the client, the family, and the nurse to discover how the family characteristically copes with stress and conflict. Clients may be programmed to enact dysfunctional family scripts in coping with anxiety and conflict. The goal is to help such clients devise alternative ways to handle stress.

Intervention with the Community

Community interventions with avoidant anxiety patterns focus on educational programs that promote and maintain health. Most theorists agree that early child-rearing patterns, along with stressful life events, are the significant etiological factors in the development of these problems. The nurse's role in primary prevention, therefore, is the organization and implementation of programs that will help people become more effective parents by helping them to explore, understand, and accept their feelings; to enhance their ability to communicate; and to develop a sound understanding of normal growth and development. School nurses, community health nurses, and psychiatric liaison nurses work in a variety of settings within the community. Opportunities to plan preventive programs such as parent education classes and community workshops are numerous.

Stress reduction workshops may contribute to more effective stress management for clients whose daily lives include ongoing tension and anxiety. Exploration and identification of stress levels and early dysfunctional coping patterns may prevent significant dysfunction. For example:

> A corporate executive attending a stress management course sponsored by his company describes himself as orderly, meticulous, and always working, especially when anxious. In the course, he may explore the purpose this behavior serves in his life, the factors that maintain the behavior, and the potential pitfalls of the behavior. Adoption of alternative coping styles may prevent this ritualistic pattern from escalating to dysfunctional proportions in the face of exposure to severe anxiety in the future.

Other aspects of community intervention are educating the community and arranging for media coverage of available treatment programs. All too often, clients and their families are unaware of community resources that effectively treat problems like phobias, hypochondriasis, and obsessive-compulsive disorders. Clients and families alike may seek out available treatment if they know about treatment programs and their theoretical premises. Recent media coverage of behavioral treatment of phobias, for example, has provided hope, relief from feeling alone with phobic problems, and concrete treatment options for phobic people and their families.

Evaluation

Nursing intervention that has been planned and provided for individuals, families, and communities with avoidant anxiety patterns must be evaluated. Evaluation includes the outcomes expected by both nurse and client. The following clinical example and Table 30-3 illustrate the documentation of care for Mrs. R.:

> Mrs. R is a 32-year-old woman who had her second child 4 months ago. She is a fastidious housekeeper who washes her hands as often as 100 times a day. Her hands are reddened and cracked. Unable to sleep, she spends hours at night cleaning the bathroom, scrubbing the walls and floors. Now that she is coping with the needs and demands of her two small children, she has less time for her rituals. During the last month she has become increasingly confused, has developed difficulty in remembering the proper order of her cleaning routines, and has been experiencing suicidal thoughts. She is admitted to the psychiatric unit of the general hospital.

Table 30-3 Evaluation for Patterns of Avoidant Anxiety (Mrs. R.)

Assessment	Diagnosis	Outcomes	Intervention	Evaluation
Mrs. R. engages in ritualistic handwashing as often as 100 times per day. Her hands are red and cracked. She is a fastidious housekeeper who spends much of the night cleaning. She has an irregular sleep pattern. Caring for her two small children disrupts her ritualistic behavior.	Repetitive hand washing and cleaning related to feelings of guilt.	Hand washing will diminish to 25 times per day within 2 weeks. Room will be cleaned once per day.	1. Initially, do not call attention to or interfere with the client's compulsive behavior. 2. Encourage the client to verbalize feelings of guilt and self-blame. 3. Provide activities that will distract her attention from her rituals. 4. Allow specific time periods (5 minutes per hour) for performance of hand-washing ritual. 5. Allow client to clean room for ½ hour daily. 6. Explore the connection between the guilt feelings and the ritualistic behavior. 7. Explore alternative behaviors for coping with anxiety. 8. Positively reinforce nonritualistic behavior. 9. Maintain a regular nighttime sleep pattern.	On admission, Mrs. R. washed her hands 75 times per day and wanted to clean her room constantly. Within 1 week, she was sleeping at night, cleaning her room twice a day for ½ hour, and washing her hands only 40 times per day. At the end of 2 weeks, she was washing her hands only 30 times per day and cleaning her room once a day, and was able to verbalize her guilt feelings about inadequate mothering.

SUMMARY

Clients with avoidant anxiety may exhibit ritualistic, avoidant, clinging, distancing, and overly dramatic behavior. They may also display somatic symptoms that have no physical basis, and they may have episodes of amnesia or exhibit multiple personalities.

Such clients have developed their specific modes of functioning in an attempt to cope with or avoid the intolerable levels of anxiety that they are experiencing.

Patterns of perception, thought, emotions, and actions combine to create the dysynchronous health patterns of clients who have somatoform, dissociative, phobic, and obsessive-compulsive disorders. The primary gain for clients with such dysynchronous health patterns is the reduction of anxiety. The secondary gains are the advantages the person derives from being dysfunctional.

Clients with somatoform disorders convert anxiety into multiple physical complaints or specific sensory or motor dysfunctions. Clients with obsessive-compulsive behavior exhibit repetitive thoughts and actions that persist despite conscious attempts to resist them. Clients with phobic behavior displace their anxiety onto a specific object, converting the anxiety into fear.

In assessing the client, the nurse considers differences in how the client deals with thoughts, feelings, and actions and also identifies primary and secondary gains, defense mechanisms, behaviors, and relationship patterns. In assessing the family, the nurse evaluates ways of dealing with stress, patterns of interaction, and relationship patterns. Environmental assessment factors include the client's lifestyle, work patterns, and recent psychosocial stressors.

Formation of goals must be realistic because it is difficult for the client to give up firmly established behavior patterns, even if they are viewed as self-defeating. Intervention is directed at dealing with low self-esteem and ritualistic and conversion behavior. It is also directed at dealing with avoidance behavior through desensitization and describes the stages of therapy. Family intervention involves increasing open, direct expression of feelings; restructuring relationships and patterns of need fulfillment; sorting out family scripts; and revising clients' expectations of themselves and others. Community intervention includes community education programs such as parenting and stress management. Evaluation provides documentation on the outcomes of nursing intervention.

REFERENCES

1. David Shapiro, *Neurotic Styles,* Basic Books, New York, 1968.
2. Sigmund Freud, *A General Introduction to Psychoanalysis,* Garden City Publishing, Garden City, N. Y., 1943.
3. John Nemiah, "Neurotic Disorders," in H. I. Kaplan, A. M. Friedman, and B. Saddock, eds., *Comprehensive Textbook of Psychiatry,* 4th ed., Williams and Wilkins, Baltimore, 1985.
4. American Psychiatric Association, *Diagnostic and Statistical Manual of Mental Disorders,* 3d ed., APA, Washington, D.C., 1980.
5. C. H. Thingpen and H. M. Cleckley, *The Three Faces of Eve,* McGraw-Hill, New York, 1957.
6. Flora Rheta Screiber, *Sybil,* Regnery, Chicago, 1973.
7. Josef Breuer and Sigmund Freud, *Studies on Hysteria* (1893–1895), J. Strachey, trans., Basic Books, New York, 1957.
8. Pierre Janet, *The Major Symptoms of Hysteria,* Macmillan, New York, 1920.
9. Nancy Konikow, "Hysterical Seizures or Pseudoseizures?" *Journal of Neurosurgical Nursing,* vol. 15, no. 1, February 1983, pp. 22–26.
10. Lynn R. Bernstein, unpublished case history from South Shore Mental Health Services, Wantagh, N. Y.
11. J. P. Watson, "Phobic Disorders, Part I: Clinical Aspects," *Nursing Mirror,* Mar. 3, 1972, pp. 22–23.
12. Gladys Lipkin and Roberta Cohen, *Effective Approaches to Patients' Behavior,* Springer, New York, 1973.
13. Alexandra Symonds, "Declaration of Dependence," *American Journal of Psychoanalysis,* Feb. 2, 1979, pp. 144–152.
14. Erik Erikson, *Childhood and Society,* 2d ed., Norton, New York, 1963.
15. Jay Haley, *Problem Solving Therapy,* Harper Colophon, New York, 1979.
16. Susan Llewelyn and Guy Fielding, "Scope in Psychiatry," *Nursing Mirror,* Jan. 23, 1983, pp. 42–43.
17. Jerilym Ross, "The Use of Former Phobics in the Treatment of Phobias," *American Journal of Psychiatry,* vol. 137, no. 6, 1980, pp. 715–717.
18. M. D. Zane, "Contextual Analysis and Treatment of Phobic Behavior as It Changes," *American Journal of Psychotherapy,* vol. 32, 1978, pp. 338–356.
19. Doreen Powell, *Phobias,* White Plains Hospital Phobia Clinic, White Plains, N. Y., 1974.
20. Andy Farrington, "Obsessive-Compulsive Disorder," *Nursing Mirror,* Aug. 17, 1983, pp. vii–viii.
21. Daniel Lim, "Behind Closed Doors," *Nursing Mirror,* Apr. 21, 1982, pp. 50–51.
22. Cloe Madanes, *Behind the One-Way Mirror,* Jossey-Bass, San Francisco, Calif., 1984.
23. Maurizio Andolfi, Claudio Angelo, Paolo Menghi, and Anna Maria Nicolo-Corigliano, *Behind the Family Mask,* Brunner-Mazel, New York, 1983.

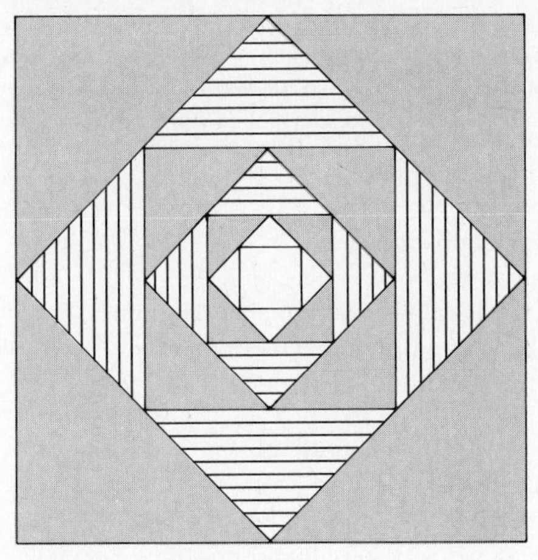

CHAPTER 31
Patterns of Interaction with Borderline Clients

Norine J. Kerr

Learning Objectives

After studying this chapter, the student should be able to:

1. Describe the characteristic behavior patterns and features seen in clients with borderline disorders.
2. Identify the impact of the person's interactional patterns on the clinical picture of borderline disorders.
3. Explain what dynamics give rise to abandonment depression.
4. Discuss these clients' characteristic patterns of interactions within the family and the community.
5. Recognize the significance of the patterns of interaction for the clients themselves.
6. Identify the kinds of information that should be elicited in a comprehensive assessment.
7. Give examples of nursing diagnoses and goals that might be used in working with borderline clients.
8. Provide an appropriate rationale for nursing interventions formulated to deal with borderline clients.
9. Name the criteria by which the nurse can determine whether the nursing interventions have been successful.

Clients with a borderline personality disorder are in flight from an inner world that is so frightening and overwhelming that they will go to almost any lengths, including the most destructive of behaviors, to avoid it. To be freed from their turmoil, they must face this internal world, one in which there are neither demons nor gods, as they suppose, but simply memories of human interactions that caused them pain and pleasure. Freedom from the inner turmoil is difficult to attain because many mental health professionals are deficient in their understanding of the borderline syndrome, and the clients themselves are loath to put aside the chaotic flurry of their lives long enough to focus within.

The purpose of this chapter is to provide a framework for nursing intervention for borderline personality disorder. Patterns of interaction of the person, the family, and the environment are explored. Each step of the nursing process is described for the person with borderline personality disorder.

DYSYNCHRONOUS HEALTH PATTERNS

Borderline clients may look normal or neurotic at times, and may show psychotic symptoms at other times. But the borderline condition does not simply occupy a transitory state of fluctuation between neurosis and psychosis. Rather it is characterized by a specific and stable form of ego pathology, forming an overall symptomatic picture, which is neither typically neurotic nor typically psychotic.[1] A summary of the characteristic patterns of the person, the family, and the community is given in Table 31-1.

Table 31-1 Characteristic Behavior Patterns and Features of Borderline Clients

Person
1. Uncertainty about personal identity
2. Inner feelings of rage
3. Chronic, free-floating anxiety
4. Marked mood shifts
5. Intolerance for aloneness (fear of abandonment)
6. Chronic feelings of emptiness, boredom
7. Self-destructive behavior (accidents, suicidal gestures, fights)
8. Feelings of being phony, inauthentic
9. Unstable attitudes and feelings
10. Pervasive underlying or overt depression
11. Paranoid oversensitivity to real and imagined slights
Family
1. Frequent angry or hostile outbursts at family members or others
2. Impulsive and unpredictable actions
3. Manipulation of family members or others
4. Idealization or deevaluation of family and others
5. Interpersonal pattern of clinging or distancing, both within and outside the family structure
6. Use of intimidation to get one's own way
7. Lack of real concern for family members and others
Community
1. Unstable occupational history
2. Habitual abuse of drugs or addiction
3. Sexual promiscuity or inactivity
4. Shifting and shallow relationships
5. Interpersonal pattern of clinging or distancing, both within and outside the family structure

DSM III

According to the *Diagnostic and Statistical Manual of Mental Disorders* (DSM III) classification of mental disorders, at least five of the following characteristics must be present before a medical diagnosis of borderline disorder can be appropriately made.[2]

1. Impulsivity or unpredictability in at least two areas that are potentially self-damaging, such as spending, sex, gambling, substance use, shoplifting, overeating, and physically self-damaging acts.
2. A pattern of unstable and intense interpersonal relationships, marked by shifts of attitude, idealization, devaluation, and manipulation (consistently using others for one's own ends).
3. Inappropriate, intense anger or lack of control of anger.
4. Identity disturbance manifested by uncertainty about issues, self-image, gender identity, long-term goals or career choice, friendship patterns, values, and loyalties.
5. Affective instability; marked shifts from normal mood to depression, irritability, or anxiety, usually lasting a few hours and only rarely more than a few days, with a return to normal mood.
6. Intolerance of being alone.

7. Physically self-damaging acts, such as suicidal gestures, self-mutilation, recurrent accidents, or physical fights.
8. Chronic feelings of emptiness or boredom.

These characteristics reflect instability in a variety of areas. In addition, this disorder is frequently accompanied by features of other personality disorders manifested in behaviors such as withdrawal, hysteria, narcissism, and antisocial behavior. Transient psychotic symptoms may occur during extreme stress, but the symptoms are of insufficient severity or duration to warrant an additional diagnosis of psychosis.[2]

Epidemiology

The medical diagnosis of borderline personality disorder was first recognized in 1980, in the third edition of *Diagnostic and Statistical Manual of Mental Disorders*. Thus, very little is known about the prevalence of the disorder in the population.[2] As clinicians gain experience with this diagnostic classification, many more diagnoses of borderline disorders are being made. This probably indicates that more people are being correctly diagnosed, rather than that the actual number of people with borderline patterns of interaction is increasing. When people are accurately diagnosed, their treatment is more appropriate and definitive; thus, a greater impact on their health is likely.

PATTERNS OF INTERACTION: PERSON

People who develop borderline patterns of interaction exhibit five characteristic behaviors: (1) splitting, (2) abandonment depression, (3) persistence of feelings of abandonment, (4) projection, and (5) poor reality testing. Abandonment depression consists of a group of interwoven emotions: depression, rage, fear, guilt, passivity, and emptiness.

Splitting

The borderline client separates self and others into two major categories, "all good" and "all bad." Polar opposite affect states such as love and hate are actively separated from each other so that the client feels only love toward one group of people and hate toward another. The use of splitting as a defense precludes awareness that good and bad can coexist in the same object (or self), and obscures the possibility that love and hate can be felt toward the same person. Like people who are color-blind, borderline clients fail to perceive the subtly different shades that lead to a full range of color. Theirs is a world of black and white only.

In the early stage of child development the ego is unable to integrate good and bad; the child perceives goodness as coming from one object and badness from another. This normal phase-specific splitting actually serves the function of preserving a positive relationship with the mother by preventing the "good" image from being contaminated by the aggressive feelings linked with the "bad" one. It is employed as an adaptive measure to protect and avoid exceeding the ego's capacity to manage opposing affect states until the child has matured enough to do so.[3]

For a variety of reasons, the borderline client does not mature beyond this stage, so that splitting persists as a defense, and the integration of good and bad does not occur as it should. As a consequence the child sees others not as "whole objects" with both good and bad features, but as "part objects" in which only good *or* bad can reside. In essence, the child has constructed a world view populated by "synthetic objects," for no human being is altogether devoid of either goodness or badness. Borderline clients view themselves in a similar manner—as either entirely good or entirely bad. The view of self and others may shift in rapid succession from good to bad, but because of splitting the borderline client fails to register the contradictions. The positive aspects of the good object (or self) are exaggerated through idealization, and the negative aspects of the "bad object" (or self) are exaggerated through devaluation. Within the hospital setting the client typically idealizes some staff members while devaluing others, creating special challenges for the nursing staff.

Abandonment Depression

Masterson emphasizes the role that abandonment depression plays in borderline pathology.[4] He proposes that such feelings originate at the separation-individuation stage of development. This phase follows the symbiotic stage (3 to 18 months) and parallels the development of the child's capacity to walk and therefore physically separate from the mother. As toddlers become adept at moving about under their own steam, their attempts to become self-governing independent persons predominate. They realize that they are not just extensions of the mother, but separate human beings with unique potential for gaining control over body and environment. Consumed by the quest for mastery and autonomy, they practice newly found skills with abandonment. They do not seem to mind their mothers' short departures from sight, and return to them only occasionally for reassurance that they are still there. Eventually, *object constancy* is obtained, that is, the ability to evoke a stable, consistent mental image of the mother whether she is there or not.

For a variety of reasons, the child who becomes borderline does not progress through the phases of separation and individuation adequately enough to obtain object constancy. One may be that the mother is unable to support her child's efforts at becoming a separate person. While she immensely enjoys the symbiotic phase and the infant's helplessness, she feels threatened when the child begins to move away from her. Her own fears of being abandoned render her unable to deal with the infant's emerging individuality, and therefore, she clings to the child to prevent separation.[4] She actively thwarts the child's moves toward individuation by withdrawing her emotional support when the child asserts an emerging individuality.

Children discover that the quest for expansion is the very thing that precipitates this loss of mother and support. Their curiosity, explorations, attempts at mastery, and assertiveness—all those intrinsic parts of self in which the desire for growth reside—become associated with the pain of loss. They assert their will, and mother withdraws. They pronounce their newly discovered word "no," and she turns to stone. This withdrawal of emotional availability is a powerful weapon in enforcing conformity, for in so doing the mother deprives the child of what is most needed—a sense of connectedness with her. When she withdraws and withholds her emotional availability—her warmth, interest, approval, support, smile, care, attention—she severs the lifeline that ensures the very survival of the child.

Unlike the schizophrenic mother, who may genuinely lack the capacity to be emotionally available, the borderline mother has given and is capable of giving much that is good to her child. Her withdrawal traumatizes deeply, for it elicits the sense of being banished from all that is good; the child's sense of isolation cannot long be endured.

Thus, between the ages of 18 and 36 months a conflict develops in children of borderline mothers: a conflict between their own developmental push for individuation and autonomy, and their fear that the mother will withdraw the emotional support required for this growth. The conflict cannot be resolved, and the overriding fear of abandonment may have lifelong consequences.

To *abandon* means to withdraw protection, support, or help from another, or to break a close association. It also suggests a complete lack of interest in the fate of the person given up. Abandonment involves an active withdrawal by one person of something that is needed by another, and gives rise to a complex of six interacting emotions: depression, rage, fear, guilt, passivity, and emptiness.[4]

Depression

Depression is one of the most striking components of the abandonment feelings, and has qualities similar to an emotion that has been described as *anaclitic depression*.[5] Bowlby[6] studied the effects of a sequence of responses that occur in children who are separated from their mothers because of hospitalization. The responses begin with active protest which typically lasts from a few hours to several days or longer. The children may struggle violently, become extremely negative, refuse food, become overactive, and cry incessantly. Unless desperately ill, they will watch for the mother unceasingly except when they fall asleep from sheer exhaustion. They use continued crying and all their other powers in an attempt to retrieve the mother.

The second phase is one of increasing hopelessness characterized by subdued moans, a perpetually sad countenance, and declining activity. During this phase the children make few or no demands on their environment; they are anorectic, listless, and withdrawn. Cessation of crying and overt protest does not mean that they have recovered from their loss. Although the need and longing for the mother are still very conscious, this may not be apparent, because the children are in a state of deep mourning.

The third phase is often erroneously interpreted as recovery, for the children begin to show more active interest in the ward, welcome food, begin to play, and accept nursing care more comfortably. However, these signs are misleading: they represent a suppression of all feeling for the mother. This behavior says, in effect: "I don't want to see the person who has disappointed and angered me. If I think of her, I won't be satisfied with the care others provide. I don't need her anyway. There are many other people who will take care of me." It is this quality of profound loss that characterizes the depression in the constellation of abandonment feelings.

Rage

The rage that the borderline client feels stems directly from the conflict experienced with the mother, although the true source of it is seldom conscious until therapy has progressed substantially. Autonomy and potential for growth have been sacrificed for the sake of not being abandoned. These clients have been punished for being strong and rewarded for being weak. As they enter adulthood, they encounter increasing difficulties with life because of their avoidance of individuation. More and more they are faced with their own inadequacies, repeated failures, unfulfilled dreams, loneliness, and fears. Their pervasive rage stems from feeling excluded from life in general; and with all their conflicts, they actually are excluded from those things that make life worth living—joy, happiness, love, creativeness, and growth.

Rage is often projected on the immediate situation. Underlying it are homicidal fantasies and impulses aimed at the mother.[4] Rage may also be turned inward and produce the self-mutilating behavior often seen in the borderline client.

Fear

A third component of the abandonment feelings is fear, which may be expressed as fear of being helpless, facing death, or being killed. Masterson believes that two psychosomatic manifestations of this fear are asthma and peptic ulcer. It is likely that fear exists to the degree that the mother used the threat of abandonment as a disciplinary tactic. The fear of being abandoned may sometimes reach panic proportions, and may explain why the client flees treatment when the source of the fear begins to emerge into conscious awareness.

Guilt

The mother's attitude of disapproval toward the child's wish to individuate now becomes clients' attitude toward themselves. They feel guilty about any part of themselves which is separate and independent of the mother—their own thoughts, wishes, feelings, and actions. To avoid guilt they suppress all aspects of the actual self. But by so doing they sabotage their own autonomy and must resort to a clinging style of relating to others. Such dependency, in turn, generates further guilt, for these clients do sense, on some level, the parasitic nature of their relations with others.

Passivity

Borderline clients are truly in a double bind: by becoming themselves, they lose the mother; by losing themselves, they gain assurance of her continued support. Therefore they associate the fear of abandonment with their own capacity for assertion. When they suppress self-assertiveness to avoid abandonment, they lose the only tool that might give them mastery. Entanglement in this situation generates ever-increasing passivity and helplessness, which in turn feed and reinforce depression and rage.

Emptiness

Since all that they think, feel, want, desire, and believe must be silenced, these clients' internal experience is one of emptiness. Without an internal sense of self there is a terrifying inner void or numbness. In addition, because of excessive projection, the client lacks internal objects, and this increases the sense of inner emptiness. For example:

> Bob described himself as empty; he indicated that no matter what he did he couldn't fill himself up. When he tried to "look inside himself" he was terrified because of the darkness and void.

Persistence of Abandonment Feelings

As the child's world expands and significant others enter the interpersonal sphere, the potential develops for healthier kinds of interactions. The father, an older sibling, a teacher, a family friend, an aunt, or an uncle may encourage and support the child's attempts at mastery. But the intrapsychic structure has been laid down so that the child interprets the external world in light of the original pattern of interaction with the mother. In other words, the pattern no longer requires reinforcement in the external world; the punishing mother and the rewarding mother have become part of the intrapsychic structure of the ego.

Since the split object units have become internalized, subsequent efforts at separation and individuation activate the intrapsychic punishing mother, calling forth abandonment depression. To avoid this, borderline clients are compelled to "call forth" the rewarding mother by behaving in a regressed, clinging, passive fashion. Although that is contrary to their best interests, it serves to ward off abandonment depression and to make them "feel good." In addition, as long as the punishing mother resides within the intrapsychic structure of the ego, it cannot be escaped except by virtue of the primitive defenses that are used to defend against it.

Projection

Projection is one of the major defenses against the internalized punishing mother and abandonment depression. Projection is a psychological defense mechanism in which feelings, thoughts, impulses, or desires which originate from within are disavowed and perceived as originating in the external world. For example, if anger is projected, it is not perceived as originating within the self; rather, an object (person) in the external world is perceived as being angry. Almost any emotion, impulse, or desire can be projected. A man who has an impulse to cheat and outwit others may complain bitterly about how others take advantage of him. A woman teeming with envy may insist that others dislike her because they envy her good looks or achievements. In each case others are seen as the source of an emotion which in fact arises in oneself.

The internalized punishing mother is thus removed from the person's internal world through the mechanism of projection. Although the attacking, critical mother resides within, it is projected onto others, who then become the "bad objects" that the client must attack or flee from.

Likewise, the rewarding mother is projected. It may be projected onto staff members whom clients cling to, and with whom they symbolically act out a wish for reunion with the "good object." The clients will unconsciously perceive the "good object" as approving regressive, self-destructive behavior, and will seek closeness with the object through pathological behavior. This, of course, has profound implications for the planning of nursing care.

Poor Reality Testing

It should be clear by now that all the mechanisms previously described make it impossible for borderline clients to interpret reality with any kind of accuracy. Their perception of others as "all good" or "all bad," their inability to differentiate their inner world from the outer world, their incapacity to relate to others as whole objects—all serve to distort their perception of themselves and the world. In addition, the self-perpetuating nature of their conflicts ensures that ever greater anxiety is generated, calling forth the need for greater defenses which then further distort reality.

PATTERNS OF INTERACTION: FAMILY

The typical family pattern of the borderline client involves a mother who is overinvested in the child, and a father who is essentially unavailable to support the child's efforts to separate from her. The father's influence tends to reinforce the clinging relationship, rather than help the child disentangle from it. The unspoken marital contract seems to be that the father can distance himself physically or emotionally from the home as long as he gives the mother exclusive control of the child.[4] As long as that contract is upheld, there will be a conspicuous lack of complaint from the mother about the father's absence.

PATTERNS OF INTERACTION: ENVIRONMENT

The community must deal specifically with two patterns of interaction displayed by borderline clients: acting out and clinging or distancing.

Acting Out

These clients' intrapsychic conflicts are acted out in the interpersonal realm within the community, and can have particularly negative consequences for the individual and the society. Acting out, in essence, represents an attempt to flee the feelings of abandonment and depression by discharging them through some kind of action. Acting out serves to obscure internal distress, because as soon as uncomfortable feelings, thoughts, and impulses become dimly perceptible, action is taken to dispel them.

Since acting out is a protection from internal signals of emotional pain, a highly compelling and habitual response to escape through action becomes a characteristic pattern of borderline clients. The incapacity to tolerate internal discomfort leaves them with little capacity for reflection or introspection. Often hospitalization is needed for this very reason, to curb destructive acting out through the provision of structure and boundaries. As the nursing staff sets limits on clients' behavior, their internal feelings of discomfort will increase. The nurse then must help them express in words, rather than behavior, what is going on in their internal world.

Borderline clients act out in many ways. On the hospital unit, self-mutilation may be common. Anger may be acted out directly through violent attacks on staff members or other clients, or indirectly by manipulation of clients to rebel against the unit structure. Feelings of hopelessness may be acted out by sabotaging progression to more liberal privileges. For instance, after the first weekend pass a borderline client may return late or come back to the unit drunk.

The use of chemicals to alter mood or state of consciousness is a common form of acting out. In more classical drug abuse, one drug or type of drug is usually preferred; the borderline client, however, often seeks a variety of drugs to produce a variety of highs. Heavy use of marijuana and alcohol is common with these clients.

Another common arena for acting out behavior is sexuality. To escape feelings of abandonment, borderline clients often seek contact with others through sexual promiscuity. Since one of their major difficulties is their inability to maintain intimacy, they find in sexual partners the human contact they seek, but they are unable to sustain a relationship. If they are not promiscuous, they may exhibit a pattern of entry into partial relationships. For instance, a woman may repeatedly involve herself with married men with whom she cannot have a committed relationship. Often the female borderline client is sexually comfortable only with men she considers "losers"; she becomes terrified or frigid when a man she respects shows interest. In addition, homosexuality or bisexuality, especially when characterized by promiscuity, is not infrequent in borderline clients.

Depression may be acted out through suicide attempts that range from primarily dramatic to entirely serious. Masterson believes that the risk of suicide actually increases as treatment progresses because as defenses are successfully countered, abandonment depression comes more to the forefront.[4] Even when suicidal remarks or gestures appear manipulative, they should be taken seriously. Given the propensity toward acting out and the reality of abandonment depression, suicide remains a real risk with these clients.

Although the function of acting-out behavior is to escape from the internal world of pain and chaos, the result is an external world of pain and chaos. By "interpersonalizing" intrapsychic conflicts, the borderline client seeks to gain some sense of control. But acting out distracts these clients from the real source of their difficulties and thwarts any potential for change. Aside from the fact that acting out may pose a serious physical threat to self and others, it must be interrupted if any insight into the real nature of the clients' problems is to be gained.

Clinging and Distancing

As with other aspects of the borderline syndrome, clients relate to others in two diametrically opposing styles; that is, they either cling or distance.

When in a clinging mode, clients behave in a helpless, dependent, and regressive manner. In the hospital community they may, for instance, attach themselves to a particular nurse who will be approached frequently with urgent requests to talk, give advice, reassure, grant special privileges, and protect them from other staff members. The primary wish or fantasy is to be the exclusive center of attention, and to receive undiluted and constant approval from the chosen person. Frustration of this wish or separations caused by days off may precipitate acting-out behavior.

Clinging behavior is simply a reenactment of the original pattern set up with the mother; it represents an avoidance of individuated, self-assertive behavior in favor of entering into a magical reunion with the "good mother."

Avoidance of self-assertive behavior makes it difficult for borderline clients to function in employment situations where a mature level of behavior, thought, and productiveness is required. For this reason borderline clients often have unstable occupational histories. Unless they can find employment situations where clinging "matches" the need of the employer, frequent changes in jobs are common. The propensity for clinging may also keep the borderline client in relationships that are clearly destructive.

When in a distancing mode, these clients avoid or flee from contact with others that might reawaken their fear of being pulled back into the symbiotic whirlpool or being abandoned. Either clinging or distancing can be used alone, but more commonly both are used at different times; the client may be clinging at one time and distancing at others.

Some common distancing defenses are the following:[4]

1. Having no relationships—being isolated
2. Picking a mate who is also anxious about closeness and blaming the conflict in the relationship on the mate
3. Keeping relationships (either one at a time or many at a time) superficial and breaking off when involvement threatens
4. Having deep relationships with two people at one time but avoiding commitment to either of them
5. Relating only to men or women who are involved with others—having partial relationships.

NURSING PROCESS

Assessment

The Client

A theoretical framework is necessary for understanding the complex and often chaotic clinical nature of borderline disorders and absolutely essential if the nurse is to have a positive impact on treatment. Borderline clients can be helped when a skilled and unified nursing approach is effected in collaboration with the overall treatment effort. The therapeutic road is rocky and dangerous but rich in potential. Borderline clients can emerge from treatment with a new capacity for interpersonal patterns; or they may have so successfully provoked rejection and hopelessness in the staff that their pathological patterns have become more deeply entrenched. These clients can be successfully treated within the hospital milieu only if the nursing staff understands how health can be promoted through a skilled and intelligent repatterning of human interaction. The competence of the nursing staff can truly make the difference between success and failure. If the staff is inadequately equipped, the treatment turns to trauma for both client and nurse.

To have a positive impact, the nursing assessment must encompass the particular ways in which the clients are attempting to defend against emotional pain, and the effects these attempts have on their lives. The questions outlined in Table 31-2 can help guide the nurse in the assessment.

The Family

Family dynamics that interact to maintain the clients' patterns of interaction need to be assessed. Table 31-2 offers some questions that will help the nurse explore relevant dynamics.

The Community

The impact of the client's patterns of interaction with the community need to be assessed. The community's response to the client is also important. Questions that will provide an adequate assessment of the community are given in Table 31-2.

Diagnosis

Ongoing assessment becomes possible as the client replays specific features of dysynchronous patterns

Table 31-2 Assessment Questions for Use with Borderline Clients

Client

1. What is the client's potential for acting out? Has physical violence toward self or others occurred in the past? Have there been any suicide attempts recently or earlier?
2. What is the client's drug history? What is the pattern of alcohol use? How much marijuana does the client smoke? What drugs are used regularly? What drugs have been used experimentally? What reactions did the client have to the various drugs (such as becoming paranoid)?
3. How impulsive is the client? To what degree is he or she able to reflect on or verbalize feelings before taking action?
4. How aware is the client of feelings of depression and fears of being abandoned? Does there tend to be a general denial of depressive affect? Are psychosomatic complaints common? Is there a history of ulcers or asthma?
5. To what degree can the client differentiate between inner and outer stimuli? Does the client tend to project easily? What is the nature of the projections?
6. What is the client's capacity to sublimate? Does he or she have any special interests, talents, or hobbies? How can these be supported?
7. What level of control does the client have over aggression or anger? What events seem to precipitate intense anger? How is the anger manifested?
8. To what degree is an identity disturbance evident? How clear is the client's sense of self? What circumstances seem to trigger feeling bad, evil, worthless, etc.? What circumstances trigger feeling good, gratified, compliant, etc.?

Family

1. Does the client live at home with his or her parents beyond the age when most young adults are out on their own? In what ways do the client and the family create distance in their relationships?
2. To what degree is aggressive affect expressed or acted out toward family members?
3. Does the client overtly cling to the mother or a mother figure? Is the relationship characterized by rage or distancing? Or do both rage and distancing occur?
4. How does the client relate to siblings? Does he or she tend to idealize or devalue them or to idealize one (or several) while devaluing another (or others)?
5. To what degree is the father supportive of the client's autonomy?

Community

1. Has the client ever been arrested? In trouble with the law? Has he or she committed antisocial acts without being caught? Has he or she been involved in drug trafficking? Shoplifting? Writing bad checks?
2. Has the client been sexually promiscuous? Has the client been involved in a homosexual lifestyle? Prostitution? What has been the general pattern of sexual relatedness? If married, has the client been sexually active outside marriage?
3. Has the client been able to establish and maintain any ongoing interpersonal relationships? Does he or she report having any close friends?
4. Are there relationships marked by both emotional and sexual intimacy? If married, how satisfied is the client with the marital partner?
5. Has the client become physically abusive or assaultive toward another? What were the circumstances?
6. Does the client report any membership in groups, clubs, churches, etc.? Are these perceived as supportive?
7. Does the client employ a predominant interpersonal style of clinging or distancing, or are the two used generally to the same degree?
8. What is the client's occupational history? Has he or she been able to stay with one job for any length of time? If the client is employed, does the job seem to reflect his or her capabilities or potential?

of interaction within the hospital milieu. On the basis of these assessments, the nursing diagnosis and goals are formulated. Since the nursing diagnosis is a way of attributing meaning to the information gained in the assessment, it provides a link with a theoretical frame of reference. In Masterson's model certain nursing diagnoses are fairly common; these are summarized in Table 31-3 (page 594).

Client Outcomes

Outcomes for clients suffering from borderline personality disorder are developed for the short term as well as the long term. These clients progress slowly, and meeting short-term goals is encouraging to them as well as to the nurse. Table 31-3 gives some long-term outcomes and nursing diagnoses. Outcomes must be tailored to individual clients; this is accomplished by adding measurement criteria. In Table 31-3 client outcomes are not individualized.

Intervention

Intervention with the Client

Nursing interventions are the specific actions taken by the nurse to facilitate the conditions necessary

Table 31-3 Diagnoses and Outcomes for Borderline Clients

Diagnoses	Outcomes
	Client will:
1. Avoidance of autonomous behavior related to fear of abandonment by significant others	1. Learn that healthy, mature behavior does not lead to abandonment by significant others.
2. Acting-out behavior related to inability to tolerate, contain, or reflect upon internal sources of emotional pain	2. Put feelings into words rather than into actions.
3. Self-destructive behavior related to defense against abandonment depression	3. Express discomfort with self-destructive behavior.
4. Perception of the staff (or a particular staff member) as "all good" or "all bad" as a result of the splitting mechanism	4. Describe others as having both good and bad qualities.
5. Suicidal thoughts or behavior related to activation of abandonment depression	5. Verbalize and sublimate feelings of depression.
6. Assaultive behavior related to excessive aggression and poor impulse control	6. Refrain from hurting self and others.
7. Clinging, regressive, and helpless behavior related to earlier learned patterns of interaction	7. Recognize cause and effect.
8. Nonadherence to milieu structure related to self-view as being special and exempt from rules and expectations	8. Hold self accountable for consequences of violation of structure and expectations.
9. Loneliness and emptiness related to conflicts that impede interpersonal closeness and intimacy	9. Retain a consistent degree of relatedness with selected others in spite of emotional conflicts and upheaval.
10. Poorly formulated self identity related to incomplete separation-individuation from maternal object.	10. Client will continually clarify own thoughts, goals, values, and feelings with staff.
11. Frequent and intense mood shifts related to client's feelings of being reunited with the "good mother" or abandoned by the "bad mother."	11. Client will relate fluctuation in moods to internal processes rather than perceiving them as environmentally induced.
12. Disruptive, manipulative, negative impact on ward milieu related to covert acting out of aggression and rage.	12. Client will relate disruptive and manipulative behavior to negative reactions from others that are contrary to client's self-interest.
13. Perception of others as hostile and dangerous related to projection of aggressive impulses.	13. Client will seek validation from others to determine if they are genuinely angry. Client will discriminate between real anger and projected anger.

for a goal to be met. A well-thought-out plan must be designed before action is taken in order to avoid "flying by the seat of one's pants." When the nurse is faced with the confusing and disjointed clinical picture seen in borderline disorders, knowledge of four well-grounded principles can bring clarity and precision to the actions that need to be taken.

PRINCIPLE 1. By providing auxiliary ego functions for the client who has deficits in ego structure, the nurse can help the client to internalize these functions. The auxiliary ego functions may include:

1. Impulse control
2. Judgment
3. Object relatedness
4. Ability to sublimate
5. Sense of self-identity

PRINCIPLE 2. Support, encouragement, approval, and positive reinforcement of mature, autonomous behavior can facilitate development of a more healthy ego structure,[7] as represented in Table 31-4.

Table 31-4 Healthy Object Relations

Object Representation	Affect	Self
(Parental) image of the nurse who approves, encourages, and rewards effective and realistic planning and coping behavior (such as efforts toward mastery)	Gratification (good feeling) in the wake of achievement	Self-image of a successful, coping, achieving person

PRINCIPLE 3. Nonapproval, nonreinforcement, and the application of consequences for regressive, destructive, and self-defeating behaviors can render the behaviors increasingly ego-dystonic.

PRINCIPLE 4. Ongoing assessment, processing, and management of the nurse's emotional response to the borderline client must occur, both individually and in a staff group, if the nurse's efforts are to have a positive impact on the treatment outcome.

Some specific interventions related to deficits in ego functioning are summarized in Table 31-5.

Intervention with the Family

Since borderline clients have been unsupported in their efforts to separate from the family of origin,

Table 31-5 Ego Deficits and the Aims and Rationales for Specific Strategies

Ego Deficit	Aim of Intervention	Specific Strategies	Rationale
Poor impulse control; tendency toward acting-out, destructive behaviors toward self and others	The prevention of destruction to self, others, and property	1. Although it seems self-evident, inform the client from the beginning that harm to self, others, and property is unacceptable. Obtain a written contract from the client, as you would a "no-suicide pact" from a depressed client.	This will not necessarily prevent destructive acting out, but it conveys in the strongest possible terms the staff's stand against destructive behavior. Because of the internalized rewarding mother, the client unconsciously believes staff will approve destructive behavior. If the staff take a consistent stand against it, without becoming punitive, the behavior should be rendered ego-dystonic.
		2. Assist the client to reflect on internal feeling states; to describe what he or she is feeling rather than act on it.	Acting out is a means of discharging feelings to avoid having to experience them. To the degree that the feelings can be experienced in the supportive presence of the nurse, acting out becomes unnecessary.
		3. If the client cannot respond to "talking it out" and shows intent to continue destructive behavior, act immediately to interrupt it by whatever appropriate means is available—seclusion, restraint, etc.	Inaction or delayed action reinforces the client's unconscious idea that destructive behavior is tolerable to staff and may elicit their approval.
		4. Formulate a unified plan for response to destructive behavior, and have it carried out consistently by all nursing staff on each shift.	A principle of learning theory is that intermittent reinforcement keeps the behavior active. The client is unconsciously testing the staff to see how they will respond to destructiveness. The client has also split the staff members into "all good" and "all bad" categories. If some nurses respond passively and others firmly, the splitting is reinforced. When both "good" and "bad" objects respond in the same way, the client will initially become enraged, but the destructive behavior will come under greater control and the splitting defense will be undermined.

(Continued.)

Table 31-5 Continued

Ego Deficit	Aim of Intervention	Specific Strategies	Rationale
Poor impulse control (continued)		5. When it is necessary to restrain or seclude the client, explain the rationale for doing so, and if possible have a staff member who is not very angry with the client (perhaps the nurse who has been idealized) carry out the decision to restrain or seclude.	Although the client will perceive limit setting as punitive and hostile, the intent is not to punish but to control and contain destructive behavior. "We are putting you in restraints because we can see you are intent on hurting yourself and that's not OK with us." This message will be conveyed more strongly if staff members who are directly involved are not unduly angry with the client. Placing the idealized nurse in charge can also help undermine splitting; however, the nurse's idealized status may be lost.
Failure to comprehend laws of cause and effect, to anticipate or perceive consequences of one's behavior (poor judgment)	The provision of insight into the relationship between behavior and consequences	1. Make sure the client understands the unit policies, structure, expectations, requirements for privileges, etc. Obtain written contracts when appropriate.	The client will invariably test these factors. The point is not so much to enforce compliance as it is to assist the client in understanding the meaning of the staff's expectations. Unless the expectations are clearly understood, learning cannot take place.
		2. Anticipate with the client what consequences will follow certain behaviors.	The client often feels like a victim and unfairly picked on, and may tend to deny the possible consequences of behaviors. This intervention helps to undermine the denial.
		3. Enforce consequences consistently and fairly.	Helps build trust and undermine splitting.
Relates to others as part objects rather than whole objects, thus splitting perception of others as "all good" and "all bad"	The integration of "all-good" and "all-bad" self and object images into a realistic whole self and object image	1. Identify the nursing staff members who are being idealized and those who are being devalued.	This allows changes to be noted, keeps the staff conscious of the process, and provides a potential source of feedback to the client.
		2. The nurse who is the object of idealization should anticipate with the client that there may be times when he or she will feel differently. "I'm glad you feel that I am able to understand your problems. There may be a time in the future when I don't seem to understand as well."	When shifts in feelings are predicted, the client is more likely to register that there has indeed been a dramatic change and can begin to gain insight into the splitting defense.
		3. Point out contradictions in the client's perception: "Have you noticed that yesterday you felt I could do no wrong and today you feel I can do no right?"	Helps to facilitate a more integrated perception of others.

(Continued.)

Table 31-5 Continued

Ego Deficit	Aim of Intervention	Specific Strategies	Rationale
Relates to others as part objects (continued)		4. Redirect the client to deal with anger directly. Do not allow the client to simply discharge anger without attempting to discover constructive ways of dealing with the negative feelings.	Complaining to the "good object" simply reinforces splitting. This intervention helps redefine the problem from "That person is bad" to "I have bad feelings about that person."
		5. If the split persists, have the "good" and "bad" staff members meet with the client to clarify that both have the same expectations. (This split may occur between shifts, and if so, arrangements for the meeting should be made.)	Having both people meet together with the client dilutes the power of the splitting mechanism.
		6. The nurse who is cast into the role of "bad object" should not withdraw from the client, but instead should offer supportive, consistent contact at noncrisis times.	If the "bad object" avoids the client except at crisis times or when needing to set limits, the client's perception of badness is reinforced.
		7. Have regular staff meetings to process feelings generated by the good-bad split and to develop strategies to cope. Call in a nursing consultant when indicated.	Unless the staff's feelings are processed and understood, they will be acted out with the client. The "good object" will feel unduly responsible—become overinvolved—and the "bad object" may go through defensiveness, counterattack, rejection, and appeasement of the client.
Lack of sublimatory channels; lack of ability to redirect into constructive outlets energy arising from conflicts or fear	Release of dormant talents, skills, and capacities requiring autonomy	1. Refer client to a psychodrama group if available. Borderline clients can often make productive use of this resource to discharge emotions and work through conflicts.	This provides a safe structure in which strong affect states can be safely discharged, and allows for expression of the dramatic component of the personality.
		2. Obtain a detailed history of special interests, hobbies, skills, talents, both past and present. Often such interests have been pursued in childhood and then abandoned.	The borderline client often is a gifted individual whose talents lie dormant because of the conflict in the personality structure. These gifts may be overlooked if not actively explored.
		3. Place the client in groups or activities that allow creative potential to be expressed.	This can serve to drain off much of the energy put in the service of destructive acting out.
Lack of a clear sense of self-identity; confused and unformulated self-view; feelings of phoniness, inauthenticity, unreality	Strengthening of self-knowledge	1. Solicit the client's opinions on various topics whenever possible *without* giving counteropinions	An opinion is a belief that falls somewhere between an impression and positive knowledge. Asking an opinion helps the client focus on beliefs and helps clarify who he or she is as a person.

(Continued.)

Table 31-5 Continued

Ego Deficit	Aim of Intervention	Specific Strategies	Rationale
Lack of self-identity (continued)		2. Place the client in a values clarification group if available.	Values require an even deeper assessment of who one is and what one believes.
		3. Encourage physical activities that strengthen the sense of body boundaries.	A vague body image is common in identity problems. Activities that facilitate greater body awareness can give the client a greater sense of being grounded in reality.
		4. Provide the client with opportunities to receive feedback about how others perceive him or her.	The client projects a great deal and often distorts others' views. Opportunities for realistic feedback can help.
		5. Encourage the client to keep a written journal of feelings, thoughts, and experiences throughout a day.	Writing is an excellent way to get in touch with what one thinks, feels, and believes.

interventions in the family context center on helping each member accept the appropriateness of clients' becoming autonomous adults. When the family is the unit of treatment, as in family therapy, Murray Bowen's model of family therapy becomes an especially effective approach[8] (see Chapter 19). This approach emphasizes that each family member must accept and develop his or her own individuality. In either case, interventions would include clarifying:

1. How the client is like and different from other family members
2. How to determine appropriate levels of closeness and separateness within the family structure
3. How to decrease emotional reactivity and use one's thinking capacity to solve problems
4. How to achieve appropriate levels of autonomy and self-sufficiency while retaining ties to family members

Intervention with the Community

Because borderline clients have failed to mature in important areas, they encounter difficulties with employers, teachers, friends, legal authorities, spouses, and even casual acquaintances. These clients tend to place the blame on others, disavowing their own role in creating these difficulties. Interventions must begin to penetrate the client's denial of cause and effect without being punitive or preaching (for instance, missing work 3 days in a row without calling in relates directly to being fired). Confrontations should always have a theme: how a particular behavior evokes natural consequences and how it undermines the client's best interests. If interventions are successful, clients identify with the nurse's perceptions, integrate them, begin to use them, and stop acting destructively.[9]

Evaluation

When interventions have been successful and goals accomplished, it is possible to witness concrete changes in borderline clients and their relationships with others. Acting-out behavior diminishes or ceases. Anxiety is better tolerated, so that there is an increased capacity to reflect on internal states. Affects are toned down and integrated as the client decreases use of splitting as a defense. There is a better capacity to tolerate depression and to discharge it through verbalization. A clearer sense of self-identity evolves, as autonomous, individuated behaviors are tested and met with support by significant others. An increased capacity for closeness with others brings with it an emerging gentleness, and brittle anger recedes into the background. These results show that the interventions have been successful in accomplishing the desired goals. Documentation of evaluation for one diagnosis, one

Table 31-6 Evaluation of Care Plan for a Borderline Client

Diagnosis	Outcome	Interventions	Evaluation
Assaultive behavior related to excessive aggression and poor impulse control	Client will refrain from destroying self, others, and property as evidenced by discharging aggression through verbalization and sublimation.	1. Inform the client from the beginning that harm to self, others, and property is unacceptable. 2. Obtain a written contract from the client, as you would a "no-suicide pact" from a depressed client. 3. Assist the client to reflect on internal feelings rather than act on them. 4. If the client cannot respond to "talking it out" and shows intent to continue destructive behavior, act immediately to interrupt it by whatever appropriate means is available—seclusion, restraint, etc. 5. Formulate a unified plan for response to destructive behavior, and have it carried out consistently by all nursing staff on each shift. 6. When it is necessary to restrain or seclude the client, explain the rationale for doing so, and if possible have a staff member who is not very angry with the client (perhaps the nurse who has been idealized) carry out the decision to restrain or seclude.	*Documentation of outcome:* Mr. G. has had one episode of assaultive behavior in 2 weeks, a decrease by 12 episodes from the 2-week period immediately preceding. *Documentation of process:* 1. Mr. G. was oriented to expected unit behavior. Part of the nursing care plan is to orient him each shift. 2. Mr. G. did write a no-assault–no-aggression contract. 3. Mr. G. has verbalized very little about feelings; he is extremely uncomfortable about discussing his feelings of emptiness. He is able to discuss anger, fear, and passivity after the feelings are resolved. He claims no feelings of guilt or depression. 4. Mr. G. responds well to suggestions that he go to his room or terminate conversations. Once he separated himself when he was enraged, without prompting. 5. The staff protocol for response to destructive behavior has worked well. All students will need to be oriented to the protocol. 6. Mr. G. has not been restrained or secluded.

client outcome, and several interventions is presented in Table 31-6.

SUMMARY

The inner worlds of clients with borderline personality disorders are frightening and overwhelming, with the result that they develop a variety of behaviors, including self-destructive acts, to avoid facing their own feelings and fears. Borderline clients sometimes look normal or neurotic; at other times they show psychotic symptoms. The borderline diagnosis has become more clearly delineated in the recent past, and the diagnosis is seen with increasing regularity in both inpatient and outpatient settings.

Persons who develop borderline patterns of interaction exhibit five characteristic behaviors: splitting, abandonment depression, persistence of abandonment feelings, projection, and poor reality testing. Abandonment depression consists of interwoven emotions: depression, rage, fear, guilt, passivity, and emptiness.

A typical family pattern of the borderline client involves a mother who is overinvested in the child, and a father who is essentially unavailable to support the child's efforts to separate from her. The client's intrapsychic conflicts are acted out in interpersonal relationships, and can have negative consequences for both the individual and the larger society. The community must deal specifically with two patterns displayed by the borderline client: acting out and clinging or distancing.

The nursing process begins with an assessment of the individual, family, and community. Assessment of ego deficits assists the nurse to focus on areas of functioning that are amenable to nursing intervention.

Nursing interventions are derived from four principles: (1) By providing auxiliary ego functions, the nurse can assist the client to internalize these functions. (2) Support, encouragement, approval, and positive reinforcement of autonomous behavior facilitate healthy ego structure. (3) Nonapproval, nonreinforcement, and the application of consequences for inappropriate behaviors render the behaviors increasingly ego-dystonic. (4) Ongoing assessment, processing, and management of staff members' emotional responses to the borderline client must occur, both individually and as a staff group, if the nurse's efforts are to have a positive impact on the treatment outcome.

Interventions in the family context center on helping each member to accept that it is appropriate for the client to become an autonomous adult. Interventions on the community level focus on confronting the client with the consequences of acting out inappropriate behavior in the community. Both the dynamics of the illness and the client's potential for health must be understood if the nurse is to help a struggling human being to overcome personal adversity and emerge with a greater measure of wholeness.

REFERENCES

1. Otto Kernberg, *Borderline Conditions and Pathological Narcissism,* Aronson, New York, 1975.
2. American Psychiatric Association, *Diagnostic and Statistical Manual of Mental Disorders,* 3d ed., APA, Washington, D.C., 1980.
3. Norine Kerr, "The Destruction of Goodness in Borderline Character Pathology," *Perspectives in Psychiatric Care,* vol. 17, January–February, 1975, p. 42.
4. James Masterson, *Psychotherapy of the Borderline Adult,* Brunner/Mazel, New York, 1976.
5. Norine J. Kerr, "The Effect of Hospitalization on the Developmental Tasks of Childhood," *Nursing Forum,* vol. 18, 1979, pp. 110–112.
6. John Bowlby, "Childhood Mourning and Its Implications for Psychiatry," *American Journal of Psychology,* vol. 128, no. 6, December 1961.
7. James Masterson, *The Narcissistic and Borderline Condition,* Human Science Press, New York, 1977.
8. Murray Bowen, *Family Therapy in Clinical Practice,* Aronsen, New York, 1978.
9. James Masterson, *Countertransference and Psychotherapeutic Technique,* Brunner/Mazel, New York, 1983.

BIBLIOGRAPHY

G. Adler, "Hospital Treatment of Borderline Patients," *American Journal of Psychiatry,* vol. 130, 1973, p. 1.

John Gunderson and M. Singer, "Defining Borderline Patients: An Overview," *The American Journal of Psychiatry,* vol. 131, 1975.

P. Hartocollis, *Borderline Personality Disorders,* International Universities Press, New York, 1967.

Otto Kernberg, "Early Ego Integration," *Annals New York Academy of Science,* vol. 193, August 1972.

B. Mark, "Hospital Treatment of Borderline Patients: Towards a Better Understanding of Problematic Issues," *Journal of Psychiatric Nursing,* vol. 18, 1980, p. 25.

James Masterson, *Psychotherapy of the Borderline Adolescent,* Brunner/Mazel, New York, 1974.

T. Nadelson, "Borderline Rage and the Therapeutic Response," *American Journal of Psychiatry,* vol. 134, 1977, p. 748.

J. C. Perry and G. Klerman, "The Borderline Patient," *Archives of General Psychiatry,* vol. 35, 1978.

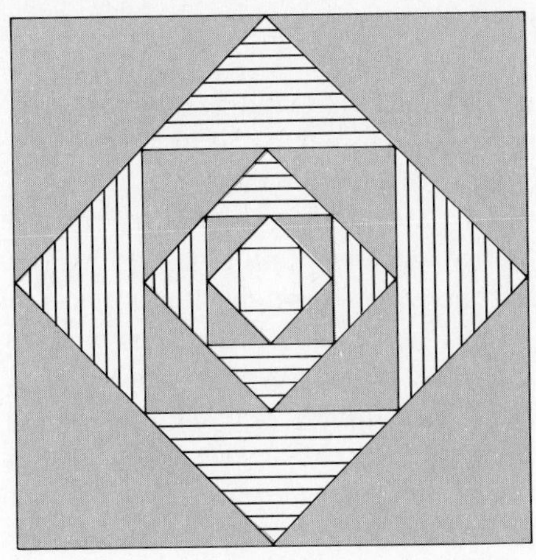

CHAPTER 32
Patterns of Violence

Eugenia McAuliffe Kelly

LEARNING OBJECTIVES

After studying this chapter, the student should be able to:

1. Discuss the mental, physical, and spiritual components of people who express aggressive feelings with assaultive or violent behavior.
2. List precursive signals of violent and assaultive behavior.
3. List family and environmental factors that perpetuate violence.
4. Describe assaultive and homicidal behavior of people who are psychotic, have an organic condition, are depressed, or experience one of the disorders of impulse control.
5. Identify criteria for assessing assaultive behavior.
6. Design a plan of intervention for assaultive or potentially violent clients.
7. Formulate nursing diagnoses and outcome criteria for clients who manifest violent or potentially violent behavior.
8. Evaluate the effectiveness of the nursing process in the care of violent or potentially violent clients.

Violence is defined as a physical or moral force, unjust strength, or power applied to any purpose. Violence does not occur in a vacuum but rather results in serious consequences for perpetrators as well as victims. Safety or its lack has a major impact on the psychosocial health of a society, particularly on individuals' levels of fear and anxiety. People can arouse fear in others through assaultive or homicidal behavior or merely by threatening violence. They can generate fear whether the assaultive or homicidal behavior is deliberate and calculated or results from the loss of control. Besides fear, violence creates anxieties in its victims. Human beings are afraid of many things. The extent to which they are fearful depends on what fears they innately have as people and on what they perceive as fear-inspiring in others.

When people are assaultive or homicidal, or when they "act out" in a violent, unpredictable, dissonant, or incongruent fashion, they pose a threat to the persons, places, and objects in their environment. The threat to personal safety results in dysynchronous patterns of behavior in the victims. The dysynchronous emotional patterns observed in victims are generally fear and increased levels of anxiety, as well as bodily injury. The trauma remains vivid in the imagination, dreams, and thoughts of victims long after the assault. Assault often undermines a spiritual sense of safety, trust, and belief (see Chapter 52).

The violent behavioral patterns of the assaultive person are dysynchronous or unhealthy. Violent acts may be deliberate, as in premeditated homicide, or they may occur because a person loses control over aggressive impulses. Violence may be symptomatic of disordered thought processes that misinterpret reality as threatening, causing the assaultive person to strike out at other people, objects, or places in the environment. Intense emotions of hatred and rage characterize the spiritual dimension of assaultive people and periodically threaten to overwhelm them.

The purpose of this chapter is to relate the nursing process to the care of clients who behave in an assaultive manner. The causes of assaultive behavior are explored. Constructive ways to prevent and manage violent behavior, including appropriate uses of physical and chemical restraints, are described.

DYSYNCHRONOUS HEALTH PATTERNS

It is important to distinguish violence from aggression, to discuss violence as a lifestyle, and to explore the fears it generates in its victims.

Aggression is a natural drive which, under the direction of the ego, can be channeled into higher-level productive activity (through the process of *sublimation*) which helps people to master other animal species, control the environment, and achieve goals in industry, commerce, science, and other fields. In response to threat, aggressive instincts directed by the ego enable self-protection even to the point of killing others. The aggressive drive is both a motivating force and an enabling power, but when aggressive instincts are not sublimated, molded, and controlled in the service of life and growth, they are used to do harm and wreak destruction. The aggressive drive can be used deliberately in the service of violence. For example, it can be used to kill, injure, plunder, rape, assault, and abuse other human beings. All people are born with a natural instinct for aggression, but learning and socialization turn this instinct toward either constructive or destructive goals.

How feelings of aggression are expressed, then, is a learned reaction. In acts of violence, the aggressive drive is expressed destructively. This destructive expression is learned, just as constructive use of aggression is learned. Violence can be learned directly through exposure and imitation or indirectly when children are not taught to channel aggressive impulses constructively.

Human beings must be socialized to identify aggressive impulses as angry feelings, to think about the consequences of unchecked aggression, and then to direct those feelings in a rational, ego-serving way. Some people who learn violent ways of acting feel guilty about their behavior; others do not. Working against the violent use of aggression is a personal and evolutionary struggle—one which is thought to be pivotal in striving for mental health.

In recent decades, individuals, families, and the community have become increasingly preoccupied with violence—a preoccupation that sometimes borders on paranoia, particularly in urban areas. The current wave of vigilantism in cities is a protective reaction against unchecked violence. People consider carrying guns or become obsessed with locks, window bars, and security systems for their homes in an attempt to feel secure. Some violence is criminal and is clearly different from the assaultive or violent behaviors symptomatic of illness that are observed in mental health settings.

For some people violence is a way of life. Violence as a lifestyle or way of coping can be divided into two main types: explosive and acting-out. An *explosive lifestyle* is defined as follows: the person impulsively acts out rage, frustration, and hatred in an assaultive way on others because of an inability to think before acting. Such a person does experience guilt after a violent act and may say things like, "I don't know what came over me," and "I saw red, and the next thing I knew, I was punching him."[1]

An *acting-out lifestyle* is defined as a lifestyle in which actions tend to be impulsive and not adapted to reality. Actions are aimed at relieving unconscious tensions without consideration of the effect on others and without guilt over the consequences. A person with this style is usually considered criminal in our society.[1]

Although a psychotic or organic condition may cause violence, the violence is considered deliberate and destructive. Violence stems from the person's perception of real or imagined threats. People who act out use violence as a way of meeting their needs immediately. Assault or killing is the most expedient way of meeting a need, and the conscience or superego is not strong enough to restrain the violent behavior. Many people who act out aggressive impulses are considered criminals, and thus caretakers in correctional facilities may see them more often than nurses in health care settings do.

Violent or assaultive and homicidal behaviors occur in some acute psychotic or organic states when a threat is imagined; a medical condition makes it difficult or impossible to perceive reality correctly. People whose violence arises in this way are usually not held legally responsible for their actions. However, there are others for whom assaultive and homicidal behavior is part of a lifelong pattern characterized by a disorder of impulse control. Such a disorder is caused either by faulty superego development or by incomplete or poorly organized ego development. People whose violence is of this nature usually are held responsible for their behavior.

DSM III

There are no explicit DSM III categories that label behavior as *violent*. Violence is a crime, not a mental illness. However, several indirect categories describe dysynchronous assaultive behaviors. *Undersocialized and socialized aggressive disorders, intoxication associated with substance abuse, atypical or mixed organic brain syndrome, disorders of impulse control, specifically intermittent and isolated explosive disorders*, and *atypical impulse control disorders* are some of the diagnoses used to label the behaviors of clients who behave in an assaultive manner.[1]

Epidemiology

The incidence of violent behavior has risen dramatically in the last decade. This is explained only in part by improved mechanisms for reporting domestic abuse of children and the elderly.[2] Reported violence includes grabbing, shoving, slapping, kicking, hitting with fists, beating up, threatening, and assaulting with weapons. While the incidence of violent behavior is on the increase in the population as a whole, only 2 percent of psychiatric clients act out in an assaultive manner in psychiatric settings. However, much more than 2 percent of health professionals' time is spent in coping with the threat of danger from these clients. Assaultive clients are also seen in nonpsychiatric health care settings such as emergency rooms or medical-surgical units, especially when the behavior is precipitated by alcohol, drugs, or organic brain syndrome.

PATTERNS OF INTERACTION: PERSON

People use assaultive behavior primarily to protect themselves or their significant others from real or imagined dangers. Where the threat is objectively real, assaultiveness is understandable. However, there are four patterns of violence that are not understandable and not acceptable. These patterns are the result of (1) psychotic conditions, (2) organic conditions, (3) depressive states, and (4) disorders of impulse control.

Psychotic Conditions

The thought processes of psychotics are so disordered that thoughts, feelings, and behaviors are not connected in a logical fashion, making it difficult to understand their assaultiveness. Professionals interacting with psychotic clients cannot validate their subjective reality or predict the associated behavior. Such clients' need to protect themselves is based on a personal or autistic perception of danger which is often difficult to understand.

Acute attacks of paranoia are psychotic episodes which can result from a functional mental disorder or from an organic brain syndrome. These clients present the greatest danger to others. The pattern of thought is projective and leads to the development of delusions which are usually persecutory in nature. In this disorder, reality testing is impaired; as long as this condition remains uncorrected, the delusions persist, causing the client to perceive the environment as hostile and destructive. The client then becomes assaultive in an effort to protect the self. In episodes of acute paranoia, there are often visual and auditory hallucinations; these are confusing and frightening to the client, who is unable to test external reality. Hallucinations that are bizarre, cruel, or commanding cause clients to see reality as dangerous; thus they feel forced to use assaultive acts to protect themselves.

Since psychotic clients are often unable to communicate their uniquely personal perceptions of danger, health personnel may have only vague hints of the impending violent behavior. The most reliable clues are (1) increase in psychomotor activity and rapidly expanding "body space" which communicate a need for distance; (2) intensity of affect; (3) verbalization of delusional thinking, especially that which is threatening; (4) hallucinations that are threatening, new, commanding in nature, or in any way upsetting; (5) history of violent behavior under stress.

Organic Conditions

Clients may also suffer from distorted thinking and impaired reality testing caused by an organic or toxic physical state called an *organic brain syndrome*. Like psychotics, these clients may resort to violent behavior in an effort to protect themselves. In people with organic conditions, there are the added problems of disorientation of time, place, or person; loss of recent memory; and a much higher incidence of visual hallucinations. Organic states are particularly dangerous because they may cause violence without warning. Often there is no history of either organicity or assaultive behavior. Intervention must be immediate. Clients with organic conditions, in particular, may not be able to communicate either their fear of being harmed or the impending loss of control. Organic conditions that may be manifested in aggressive behavior include seizure disorders, metabolic and endocrine imbalances, space-occupying lesions, and alcohol and drug withdrawal syndromes.

Seizure Disorders

People who have epilepsy may suddenly become violent at the beginning of a seizure. However, these violent episodes tend to be less dangerous than attacks made by clients who are not diagnosed as epileptic but who have "seizure equivalents," that is, disorganized discharges of energy leading to unprovoked fights. One epileptic condition that causes violence is temporal lobe epilepsy, which is often misdiagnosed as a rage reaction. Here the client does not show any physical manifestations of an epileptic seizure but rather has a history of getting into vicious and violent fights with little or no provocation. The client may complain of a sense of "inner pressure" before the fight and often does not remember what occurred during the fight. Such a person understandably has difficulties in relationships with others and often takes to drinking. To complicate matters, the fights are usually viewed by family, friends, coworkers, and health professionals as a complication of use of alcohol, and the primary causal factors remain unknown. If the client is carefully checked by a physician, however, the sleep-derived EEG record shows abnormality in the temporal lobe area.[3]

Metabolic or Endocrine Imbalances

Clients with metabolic or endocrine imbalances, including high fevers, may be so toxic that the physiology required for logical thinking is impaired. Some of these clients (especially those with a history of violence under stress) may become assaultive. Health professionals should be especially watchful in such situations.

Space-Occupying Lesions

Clients with *space-occupying lesions,* including brain tumors, may have violent episodes. These episodes may be difficult to understand, especially if the brain tumor's growth has been insidious. If such a client has had a lifelong tendency to be explosive as well as a history of unexplained violence, the current, organically based explosive behavior may be misunderstood. Keep in mind that any organic brain syndrome causes, among other things, an extension or magnification of preexisting behavior trends.

Withdrawal from Alcohol or Drugs

A person with either impending or full-blown *delirium tremens* (alcohol withdrawal syndrome) is always assaultive and belligerent. Clients in *drug withdrawal* or those who are coming out of a *drug overdose* (especially barbiturates) also can be violent and assaultive because of the irritability of their central nervous systems. In general, anyone who uses alcohol or drugs is prone to become violent when under stress.

Depressive States

Clients who have depressive states may become violent and assaultive or, on occasion, homicidal in an attempt to release some of their pent-up rage and thus relieve their depression. Such situations are more unpredictable and hence more dangerous if the depression is associated with psychosis. Depressed people may abuse alcohol and addictive drugs. Their defenses against rage are temporarily lowered by these substances, especially alcohol; this causes them to develop violent behaviors that may include belligerence, assault, homicide, or suicide.

Disorders of Impulse Control

Clients with disorders of impulse control also behave violently. A *disorder of impulse control* is typified by a lifelong pattern of either assaultive acting-out or explosive behavior.

Acting Out

In clients whose disorders of impulse control are exhibited by acting out, transference is extraordinarily strong. They repeatedly undergo experiences similar to or identical with old conflicts such as rage at a parent. The person seeks to find belated gratification of repressed impulses or to find relief from inner tensions.[4]

For these clients the environment is an arena in which to stage their internal conflicts. Common to all acting out is an impulsive haste to meet needs and a lack of guilt feelings for the consequences of the behavior. Clients with disorders of impulse control have strong security and dependency needs along with an inadequately developed conscience or superego. They often aggressively take what they want or discharge rage and frustration in assaultive and murderous ways. It is theorized that early childhood deprivation or trauma causes arrested development, making the establishment of superego or conscience impossible. Thus no controls against aggressive impulses are developed. As children, these people never internalized the wrongness of the destructive use of aggression; hence they either do not experience guilt or displace the guilt onto something other than themselves.

Explosiveness

The client whose disorder of impulse control is explosive, in contrast to the acting-out client, does experience remorse for behavior that has harmed others. This client has enough intact superego function to experience guilt following violent behavior. The problem here is poor control of impulses, especially aggressive impulses. This can be caused by inadequate socialization: the child was not taught to subjugate angry feelings to the direction of the ego, or to use alternative outlets for aggressive energies, such as a workout at a gym. As children, these aggressive people lacked healthful role models for ways to handle angry feelings. For example, a child who saw the father come home angry from his job, get drunk, and beat his wife has a poor role model for control of aggressive impulses. As an adult, such a person is at the mercy of angry feelings. It should also be noted that some clients classified as explosive may actually have temporal lobe epilepsy or another organic condition.

Violence-Prone Children

Some children of grammar and junior high school age may be categorized as *juveniles* but are nevertheless capable of inflicting severe physical harm or even committing murder. There is generally a childhood history characterized by (1) frequent changes of milieu; (2) a loveless or inconsistent environment; and (3) a disorganized, weak, and inconsistent role identity process. Some of these young people simply have never learned to develop object relationships.[5]

PATTERNS OF INTERACTION: FAMILY

Four family patterns of interaction are conducive to violence: (1) dysfunctional family systems, (2) disturbed roles, (3) disturbed marital relationships, and (4) violent expressions of anger.

Dysfunctional Family Systems

Rage and violence in one or more members of a family can indicate a dysfunctional family system in which the balance in the family is maintained by periodic violent discharges of aggressive energies.[6] Tension builds in the family system, threatens the balance, and is temporarily restored when one or more of the members act out in a violent fashion, thus reducing the family tension level. Typically, when violent behavior dominates, learning does not take place, and consequently the violence recurs because (1) it is not seen as dysfunctional, (2) factors that precipitated the incident are not identified, and (3) basic problems are not resolved.

Disturbed Roles

Violent discharges of tension also occur in families where the roles are disturbed. If the roles are fixed, no growth or change is permitted, frustration builds up, and violent acting out may occur. These dynamics are frequently seen in dysfunctional attempts by adolescents to assume different roles in their families.

In some families, roles are fused and there is no sense of separateness among individual family members. For example, a fused, overclose relationship between a mother and daughter may cause frustration and feelings of rejection to build up in the father, who is outside that overclose relationship. Because the fusion may not be understood by the rejected father, and because typically there is little or no family communication about problems, the father may resort to an outburst of violence which is usually directed at the child. The violence is often an inappropriate attempt to achieve some kind of connectedness with the fused pair, especially the child.

Disturbed Marital Relationships

Violence is also a possibility in families where there is a disturbance in the marital relationship. Some marriages are characterized by frequent quarreling or rage that is repressed and left unexpressed. An acting-out child may express these tensions. Not only is a child's security threatened by marital tension, but the child may feel responsible for the unexpressed conflict.

Violent Expressions of Anger

In some family systems, anger may be expressed violently rather than being channeled in socially acceptable ways. Uncontrolled expressions of rage become the family's way of life. This is typical in families where alcohol or drugs are used excessively to cope with problems. Use of alcohol significantly reduces the ability of the ego to monitor angry feelings.[7] In studying these families it has been found that violent expression of anger is learned behavior that is repeated in succeeding generations. Chapter 51 discusses domestic violence in detail.

PATTERNS OF INTERACTION: ENVIRONMENT

The nurse's role includes keeping clients from becoming assaultive and intervening when there is violent behavior. Nurses carry out these roles in clearly defined mental health settings as well as in the community. They teach parents to socialize small children in nonviolent ways, and they are also concerned about the safety of society at the hands of violent and potentially violent criminals. Nurses work in correctional facilities and residential treatment settings to teach clients new ways of coping that replace impulsive, violent, and homicidal acting-out behaviors.

In mental health environments nurses monitor the "pulse" of the particular setting and use strategies designed to prevent violence. They provide outlets for aggression such as punching bags or quiet rooms, and they set limits. The protective environment of the inpatient setting can be a deterrent to violent acting out, but admission of a potentially assaultive client will also change the "atmosphere" of a therapeutic environment (see Chapter 17).

During treatment of any client—child or adult, in prison or out—the community must be considered. The environment often condones and supports rage and violence, and creates breeding grounds for continued assaultive behavior. Frustration about environmental stresses may build up, and people either may lack outlets for discharging their aggressive energy or may have never learned how to channel it in constructive ways. This buildup of frustration with either no outlets or unacceptable outlets for constructive expression of aggression serves to perpetuate violent behavior. Drug and alcohol abuse, and abuse of children and the elderly are but a few of the symptoms of poor impulse control and its resulting violence.

Victims of child abuse or neglect in turn become abusive adults.[8] The extent to which violence on television affects the behavior of children is still being studied by the Surgeon General's Office. An increase in violent behavior is noted in *aggression-prone children*—children with known abusive parents, as well as those from broken homes and high-crime areas.

Current inflation and economic instability throughout the world have heightened feelings of tension and insecurity. There has been a corresponding increase in crime, probably because of a mistaken belief that violence is necessary for survival. The feeling is that shooting, stealing from, fighting, and overpowering others will prevent the assailant from being killed, robbed, assaulted, or starved. The ever-present threat of nuclear war and world devastation has further fostered a "live for today" and "take while you can" mentality. Frustration leads to aggression, and exploitation leads to fruitless rage in an environment devoid of meaning and purpose.

NURSING PROCESS

With potentially violent or assaultive clients, assessment, diagnosis, formulation of outcome criteria, and intervention are based on nurses' perceptions, thoughts, and feelings as they interact with the clients and the environment. Nurses perceive threats of violence through modes such as eyes, ears, skin, and "gut reactions." When a client suddenly begins to pace and to mumble angrily, the nurse senses that the client is behaving strangely, that people nearby may be in danger, or that the client may be self-destructive. Nurses will assess the potential danger not only on the basis of perceived external reality, but also in terms of their experience and how their "insides" feel. Thus, nurses who have seen these warning signs before will sense danger more quickly than those who are inexperienced.

Nurses need to attend to their own reactions to violence if their interventions are to be therapeutic. Being comfortable with oneself and avoiding overreactive fear in the presence of assaultive clients are necessary for success in dealing with these clients. The following self-assessment questions can assist the nurse in recognizing responses to an assaultive client:

1. Do I have a constant sense of fear around this client?
2. Do I feel comfortable turning my back on the client?
3. Do I avoid the client?
4. Do I take sides with either the client or the family?
5. Do I feel capable of handling this client's violent, assaultive behavior if it occurs?
6. Do I feel judgmental about the client's behavior?
7. Do I want to punish the client for the behavior?

Assessment

The Person

It is important for nurses to know how to intervene in a client's violent behavior when it is already in progress. It is equally important to be able to predict that a client is about to act violently and to take steps to prevent the violence. Making a nursing diagnosis of violent and assaultive behavior that is already going on is not difficult, but it takes skill to assess clients who may lose control and to intervene before they do so. With clients who have a history of violent outbursts, it takes skill to predict at which point and under what conditions they will lose control.

In order to diagnose impending dangerous behavior, the nurse needs to have an array of assessment tools, some derived from a variety of theories and some developed from experience. One invaluable tool that is not to be underestimated is the nurse's perception of signals of impending violence, many of which come from gut feelings or intuitions. The nurses who have greatest success in dealing with assaultive clients are those whose antennae for picking up signs of impending danger are highly developed. Various observations may impinge on one's gut feelings before they are integrated by the brain, and thus gut feelings should be given the utmost attention. Examples are the feeling that a client has a hair-trigger temper or a chip on the shoulder, that the nurse has to "walk on eggshells" around the client, or that the client has to be "handled with kid gloves."

After the nurse has intuitively assessed potential violence in a client, the degree of potential violence in that person at a given moment must be assessed in order to prevent the outburst, restore control, or both. Table 32-1 identifies six criteria or "cues" which can help nurses predict when assaultive behavior may occur in a particular client. If any of these six "cues" is present, the client can be diag-

Table 32-1 Criteria for Assessing Assaultive Behavior

Criterion	Behavior	Comment
Increase in motor agitation	Pacing Inability to sit still	These are attempts to discharge aggression via large muscle activity.
	Sudden cessation of motor activity	The stillness is uncomfortable, like the "calm before a storm."
Threatening verbalizations or gestures toward real or imagined objects	Retaliation toward actual persons who are seen as threats	
	Aggressiveness in response to threatening visual or auditory hallucinations	Such hallucinations are bizarre, threatening, unfamiliar, or confusing. Many psychotics do live comfortably with an entourage of *familiar* "voices."
	Aggressiveness in response to expansion of delusional thinking	The degree of violence is related to how desperately the client perceives the need to protect the self.
Intensification of affect	Very tense expression Jumpiness Elated expression	Such intensification indicates loss of control, especially if accompanied by laughing.
History of assaultive behavior	Has acted assaultively in the past Has been violent under stress in the past	One who has used violence in the past is likely to do so again.
	Has never been assaultive in the past	One who has never been violent and suddenly becomes so may be suffering from organic illness.
Use of alcohol or addictive drugs	Intoxication with drugs or alcohol	Client can act out rage with inhibitions dissolved.
	Withdrawal from drugs or alcohol	Violence is due to irritability of the central nervous system.
Presence of acute organic brain syndrome	Sudden rise or fall in level of consciousness	
	Disorientation as to time, place, person	Sense of time is lost first.
	Impairment of recent memory	Especially significant where no memory impairment existed before.
	Auditory hallucinations within the psychic horizon (i.e., within earshot)	Such are heard coming from under the bed or outside the door. "Voices" out of earshot, as the voice of God or sounds from another planet, indicate functional mental disorder.
	Visual hallucinations	These rarely occur in our culture except in religious people.
	Abnormal muscle movements such as tics, jerks, tremors, akinesia	These are significant only where none existed before.

nosed as potentially assaultive. The next step is to determine how dangerous the client is or may become. The more sudden the change in behavior and the more signs present, the more out of control the client is or may become. Once the situation becomes violent or potentially violent, health personnel must take steps to return the client to control and to prevent further loss of control. To ensure safety, they must be one step ahead of the client. The following case is an example of loss of control:

> A 42-year-old woman became belligerent on a medical ward, heard doctors "plotting" outside the door "to get rid of me," and refused to eat because "the food was poisoned." Her daughter denied any previous similar behavior. Soon after, laboratory studies revealed a blood urea nitrogen (BUN) of 54, which would account for the increasing confusion and belligerence.

The Family

Violence occurs more in certain family systems than in others. Following is a guide for assessing the potential for assaultive behavior in a family.

1. Violent behavior as a way of handling problems, including using excessive corporal punishment in disciplining children and routinely beating domestic animals
2. History of past or present violent abuse of children or spouse
3. Excessive use of alcohol, hard drugs such as heroin, or both
4. Acute paranoid episodes in a family member who acts out by retaliating against imagined threats
5. A family system in which roles are fixed or egos fused, thus frustrating attempts at growth and individuation

Families that show any of these characteristics have a high potential for violent behavior under stress. How a family deals with violent episodes of a client is also assessed. Some families reject violent members, while others want to punish them. In some cases family members appease a client or even join in the violent or assaultive behavior. Family patterns of dealing with violent behavior are an essential component of the assessment process.

The Community

The incidence of violent behavior is higher in some settings than in others. Areas where violence is more common include emergency rooms of general hospitals; intensive-care units; scenes of accidents, natural disasters, and warfare; scenes of crimes; bars and taverns; jails and prisons; and acute inpatient psychiatric units. In these settings there is a greater risk of violence because of the higher incidence of stress, disordered thinking, abnormal organic states, and opportunities for acting out.

The possibility of violence should be kept in mind and anticipated. Four immediate causes of violent behavior have been suggested:[9]

1. Alcohol or drug intoxication
2. Criminal activity related to the desire to obtain addictive drugs
3. Acute episodes of functional mental disorders such as paranoia or agitated depression
4. Acute physical illness or brain injury, including delirium tremens

Diagnosis

Nursing diagnoses that involve violent behavior of clients focus on whether the behavior is impending, in progress, or part of a lifestyle used by the client as an everyday way of coping. Diagnoses are therefore very closely connected to the nurse's assessment of the potential for violent behavior or actual violent behavior. When violent or assaultive behavior is impending, diagnoses will reflect a need to prevent the actual occurrence of violence. Specific preventive diagnoses include the following:

- Inability to sit still correlated with impending assaultive behavior
- Sudden cessation of motor activity related to impending acting-out behavior
- Pacing related to impending assaultive behavior

Other diagnoses will relate to assaultive or aggressive behavior that is already in progress. Because of the potential danger involved, these diagnoses point out the need for immediate action to prevent further harm or restore equilibrium. Diagnoses appropriate for a violent behavior crisis include the following examples:

- Verbal threats related to delusional thinking
- Agitated behavior related to a recent visit from a spouse
- Assaultive behavior associated with alcohol intoxication
- Tense, angry affect correlated with visual hallucinations

When assaultive or violent behaviors such as those listed below are part of a client's lifestyle, diagnoses will need to set the stage for long-term reeducative interventions:

- Aggressive speech related to coping style
- Assaultive behavior associated with inadequate coping style
- Retaliative behavior correlated with dysfunctional expression of anger
- Destructive behavior associated with maladaptive expression of frustration

Outcome Criteria

When nurses are working with clients who exhibit violent, assaultive behavior, they need to be specific about what changes in clients' behavior they are working to achieve. Table 32-2 identifies measurable outcomes applicable to violent and assaultive clients. The immediate goals of nursing interventions with assaultive or homicidal clients are (1) to prevent further loss of control and (2) to restore control in clients already behaving in a violent or assaultive manner.

Intervention

Nursing interventions with clients who are actually or potentially violent involve use of strategies that are supportive, educative, and partly or wholly compensatory. Interventions are carried out not only with clients, but with clients' families and the environment.

Table 32-2 Outcome Criteria for Violent and Assaultive Clients

Client Will Be Able To
1. Verbalize to the nurse that violent behavior is impending.
2. Seek help from staff.
a. Report command hallucinations to staff.
b. Ask to talk to a staff member.
c. Ask for help in avoiding situations or persons who have provoked violent behavior.
d. Ask for assistance in restoring equilibrium.
3. Accept limits set by staff.
4. Identify violence and impulsivity as a major component of personal lifestyle.
5. Think before acting impulsively.
6. Identify alternative ways of dealing with angry feelings.
7. Identify factors in the environment which contribute to an acting-out lifestyle.

Intervention with the Person

Strategies that prevent potentially violent episodes are the essence of nursing intervention with violent clients. Early diagnosis and treatment of problems includes early identification and treatment of assaultive and violent behavior. Early diagnosis and treatment of functional mental disorders, especially the paranoid states, prevents clients from acting out their delusions and hallucinations. Identification of violence-prone clients is necessary so that they can get both behavioral and chemical treatment. Early repatterning of behavior prevents an acute problem from becoming entrenched and chronic (repetitive).

PENDING VIOLENCE. Once a nurse has determined that a client is potentially violent, the following recommendations for intervention apply:[10]

1. Be aware of precursive signs—especially agitation, threatening verbalizations and gestures, sudden signs of organicity, and the presence of drugs or alcohol—and use them as an index to monitor whether the client is regaining or further losing control. For example, a client on a medical ward may at first express general suspicion of all hospital personnel and gradually, with treatment, complain only about those not wearing white. There is still potential for violence, but it is diluted.
2. Reduce stimuli by removing from the environment objects or people that appear to frighten the client. Remove the client to an area where there is less stimulation—for example, a place with fewer people and less noise, light, and activity.
3. Provide distance between the client and the health care professionals involved.
4. Professionals should explain who they are by giving their names and positions. It is helpful for the health professional to be further identified by a name tag. The client should normally be called by last name with a title (Mr. Smith, Mrs. Jones), but first names may be used with clients who appear frightened. Nicknames are to be avoided.

5. Usually a nurse in uniform can get closer to a violent client than a physician in street clothes can.
6. Clients who tend to use paranoid coping mechanisms relate better to staff members of the opposite sex, especially where physical contact must be made. This is because people suffering from paranoia fear attack or intrusion from outside, often in the form of a homosexual attack. Physical contact by a staff member of the same sex can be interpreted by the client as a homosexual overture, and this heightens the potential for homosexual panic. Such panic, in turn, increases the risk of violent acting out. If a female nurse must give an injection to a paranoid female client, a male staff member should be in attendance to communicate protection; similarly, a male nurse should not give an injection to a male client unless a female staff member is present.
7. Give assurance to clients by explaining what is happening, telling them that they will be safe, and asking them whether they have any questions. Express an attitude of helpfulness and calm.
8. Try not to allow a power struggle to develop between the client and the staff. If such a conflict does develop, make every effort to do what the client wants, provided that it is safe. For example, either sitting in a chair or lying in bed may be OK, provided that the client stays in a safe area. If the client's demands pose risks, however, explain these risks to the client and do not give in to them.
9. Like people who threaten suicide, those who threaten violence must be taken seriously. If a client expresses fear of committing a violent act, assess the seriousness of the danger and initiate steps to avert it; for example, remove weapons or objects that could be used in a destructive fashion.
10. Respect for the client's confidentiality does not extend to situations where the client may be dangerous to others. If a nurse learns that a client has a gun at home and has been having impulses to kill someone, it is the nurse's responsibility to notify the psychiatrist and the appropriate legal authorities.
11. Whenever a client shows signs of impending assaultive behavior, every effort should be made to find the cause and correct it. However, while this search is taking place, the potentially violent client should be prevented from becoming overtly violent. The nurse provides vehicles for discharge of tension, talks with the client, and removes the client to a less stimulating environment.
12. Sedation should also be considered. For example:

A 72-year-old woman was escalating to a potentially violent state. She had become suspicious of the staff on the medical floor and was verbally abusive to anyone who came near her. It was discovered that she was experiencing cerebral anoxia due to a hemoglobin count of 6 grams of hemoglobin per 100 milliliters blood. In order to correct the low hemoglobin with a blood transfusion, she had to be sedated with chlorpromazine until the transfusion could be started and the cause of the agitation corrected.

VIOLENCE CRISIS. When a client is overtly violent, immediate and stringent intervention is recommended. Four stages of this process are discussed below.

First, a health professional who is alone with a violent client should never attempt contact. Get immediate emergency help, preferably from people trained in the techniques of restraint, such as trained psychiatric attendants or police. Staff members who are not trained in the use of restraint should keep away from the client and supervise the emergency help from the sidelines. No one should approach an overtly violent client alone, not even a psychiatric attendant or police officer. If professionals need to stop the violence and make an impact on the client before the police or security personnel arrive, three or more can work together, making a "show of force."

The nurse should never hesitate to ask police to restrain a violent client. Since the need to act assaultively comes from a real or imagined loss of inner control, the client often calms down just at the sight of several blue uniforms representing external control. In fact, to a confused client, a blue uniform is often more understandable and reassuring than a white one.

It is sometimes necessary for nurses to use physical or chemical restraints, to manage the violent behavior of a client, to prevent injury to another, or to prevent a client from harming himself

Table 32-3 Nursing Care Checklist for the Patient in Restraints

Client's Name ______
Physician's Order for Restraints (specify date and time) ______ **Physician's signature** ______

Reason for restraint (please check and write explanatory note):
- Other approaches have failed ___
- Sustained assaultive or aggressive behavior ___
- Risk to self or others ___
- Self-control absent ___
- Other ___

Procedure explained to client and family.
Record remarks:

	Time	Initials	Time	Initials	Time	Initials
Airway patent						
Vital signs (record every 30 minutes):						
Pulse						
Respiration						
Blood pressure						
Circulation intact (record every 30 minutes):						
Left ankle						
Right ankle						
Left wrist						
Right wrist						

	Amount	Initials	Amount	Initials	Amount	Initials
Elimination:						
Bowel						
Bladder (record amount)						

	Time	Amount	Initials	Time	Amount	Initials	Time	Amount	Initials
Hydration (record amount):									
PO liquids									
IV liquids									

	Dosage	Time	Initials	Dosage	Time	Initials	Dosage	Time	Initials
Medication (record type, dosage, time, and route)									

Physicians's order to continue or release restraints every 2 hours

Physician's signature ______

Nurses' signatures ______
______
______

or herself. The laws in most states are very specific about clients' rights and the guidelines for use of restraints. Most laws stipulate that physical restraints may be applied if a client is a danger to self or others, but the danger must be reevaluated every few hours and physical restraint can be continued only until medication or another treatment becomes effective. The problem is compounded when a client is intoxicated or has taken an overdose of drugs. It usually is not wise to give sedatives until the alcohol or drug has been metabolized; in such instances, physical restraints under continued observation are necessary.

The most common legal form of restraint is the *camisole* (straitjacket) or restraining sheet. The *four-point restraint* (both wrists and both ankles restrained separately) is used only infrequently; when it is used, each extremity must be freed at a specified interval and restraints rotated, much as tourniquets are rotated. Whenever any type of physical restraint is used, *continuous observation* by nurses is mandatory.[11] Table 32-3 shows a model checklist that may be used to record nursing care for a client in restraints. Seclusion, another form of restraint, requires the same standard of care as physical restraint. The use of physical restraint or seclusion is discontinued as soon as the client either becomes somnolent from medication or communicates that self-control has been regained.

Second, if clients do not quickly calm down by their own efforts, medication will probably be necessary. The nurse must make this assessment and call a physician to further evaluate the client and to order sedation. Overtly violent clients respond quickly to intramuscular (IM) doses of major tranquilizers like chlorpromazine and haloperidol. Some clients have been given slow-acting barbiturates (amobarbital, Benital) or diazepam intravenously if they need to be sedated quickly. This route carries a risk of respiratory depression; therefore, the nurse should be sure to have the equipment for intubation available. The IM route for barbiturates and diazepam is slower but less risky. For a client who continues to be agitated, IM or oral paraldehyde can be helpful, until the client is asleep.

When a violent client must be kept sedated, especially over a period of time to permit workup and treatment of an organic condition, the major tranquilizers have been most effective. Chlorpromazine is usually ordered intramuscularly in 25-milligram increments every hour until the client is somnolent but arousable to eat and speak. With geriatric clients, the chlorpromazine is usually ordered in 10-milligram increments. Blood pressure should be checked before and one-half hour after each dose and the medication held if the systolic pressure is below 90 millimeters mercury. When a maintenance dosage has been reached, the amount is doubled and given in oral liquid concentrate form every 4 hours. The side effects of Thorazine are not likely to develop in the average client, and generally not during the emergency. In fact, clients with violent outbursts from hepatic encephalophathy have been satisfactorily sedated with chlorpromazine with no further compromising of the liver condition. In any case, the risk of side effects must be weighed against the risk of harm to self or others.

Third, the nurse who is dealing with an overtly violent client attempts to get the client's history from relatives, police, or anyone else who was a witness to the client's difficulties. The nurse may have to telephone agencies that know the client, as well as the client's landlord or building superintendent. The following questions should be asked: "Has the client taken a hallucinogenic drug? Is he or she on any other type of medication? Is the client physically ill? Has the client ever been treated for mental illness? Has the client ever been in a psychiatric hospital? Is the present behavior like or unlike the client's problem in the past?" The information obtained should be recorded and shared with other concerned professionals.

In obtaining and interpreting the client's history, the nurse should consider possible alternative causes of violent behavior. For example, a chronic schizophrenic who becomes suddenly agitated and paranoid may be going into kidney failure (uremia) rather than having an acute psychotic episode.

Fourth, when stabilization begins, the nurse continues to monitor the client for further violent outbursts using the six criteria listed in Table 32-1. Any hint of another violent episode should cue the nurse to reactivate the plan of intervention.

IMPULSIVE BEHAVIOR. Besides working with clients who are potentially or actually violent because of acute psychotic states or organic conditions, nurses have many opportunities—in schools, hospitals, day hospitals, prisons, and clinics—to work with clients who have character disorders and whose impulsive assaultiveness is part of their repertoire of coping behavior. These people have poor superego controls and habitually act out impulsively in order to meet their needs when frustration builds up.

Criminal charges for assaultive or homicidal behavior are often brought against clients who have character disorders, and although the potential for improvement among clients who have not freely chosen to seek treatment is a topic of debate among both law enforcement and mental health professionals, these clients are often put on probation or parole on the condition that they accept psychiatric treatment.

A team approach is recommended in treating these clients, for two reasons: first, because a constant show of force is an external control for the client; second, because working in a team helps to dilute both transference and countertransference problems. The treatment team can take specific steps to teach clients to recognize the problems that their violent behavior creates and to cope with their hostile feelings in ways that will not inflict trauma on themselves and others. Some of the most rewarding results with violent clients have been obtained in outpatient psychiatric services and day hospitals where the clients come into contact with their home environments every day.[12]

The goal of treatment is to help clients to understand their hostile feelings and to stop acting them out. In general, this is done by helping the client (1) to control or set limits on impulsive and aggressive behavior, (2) to examine the immediate situation which promoted the impulsive reaction, and (3) to learn more acceptable ways of discharging aggressive energies in similar situations.[13]

Until clients become able to respond to the emotional limits set by the treatment team, they need to be in an area where physical protection is built in. They may thus first need to be in seclusion or in a locked inpatient unit secure enough to prevent them from escaping and from harming themselves or others. The next step may be a day hospital, or simply an area where there is no heavy or dangerous equipment or furniture.

Setting limits shows violent clients that external controls have been placed on their behavior. Limits are conveyed by two methods: (1) speaking to the individual client in short, direct commands (such as "Don't hit her!" and "Hold your arms still!"); (2) imposing a set of rules upon everyone at a facility (such as "No alcohol or drugs" and "No physical contact except in sports or games").

Acceptable outlets for aggression—heavy cleaning, competitive games, vigorous walks, calisthenics, sports—are an integral part of the treatment program. Motor activity involving the large muscles is of great value for violent clients. Sports, in particular, are beneficial in channeling aggression, and they also provide additional benefits, such as a reward system, support from others, emotional involvement, and potential for gaining social position.

Intervention with the Family

The family, a major part of the client's environment, is often the arena in which assaultive and violent behavior is learned. Families provide a model for expression of anger and frustration. When a family is known to have a violent or explosive lifestyle, it is essential to involve the members in treatment.

When a client is hospitalized, the family treatment approach should be started in the inpatient unit; after the client is discharged, family treatment should be continued in the day hospital or outpatient department. Sessions include the client, family members, and significant others.

Multiple-family support groups have also been used with success. Sharing strategies for healthy expression of violent impulses helps clients to modify their destructive behavior. Violence has different meanings in different families; levels of tolerance for assaultive, acting-out, and violent behavior vary widely. An essential part of nursing intervention with a violent client's family involves negotiation of healthier expression of violent impulses within the family structure.

In some situations, particularly when clients are being abused or are abusing other family members, intervention involves removing the client from the family. Nurses with advanced education who are skilled in family intervention become involved in the process of placement and working through the separation. When a client who has assaulted others or has been the victim of violence is removed from the family setting, there is a shift in the family's dynamics; other members may assume the role of either abuser or abused. Intensive family therapy over many months is an appropriate strategy for preventing this situation from developing.

Intervention with the Community

In some communities, especially in cities, awareness of and vigilance against crime have become heightened to a degree which in itself increases tension, inhibits cooperative interaction among people at all social levels, and interferes with school, business, professional, and social activities. There is intense concern about the safety of persons and possessions, and much energy is expended on protecting homes and businesses. More and more community members are taking matters into their own hands; they carry weapons, form neighborhood patrols, hire private security guards, and install elaborate alarm systems in their homes.

Many people believe that perpetrators of violence have been given more rights than the citizens they victimize. The inadequate size of many urban police forces, combined with a general perception of urban police officers as indifferent to the needs of the law-abiding public, contributes to further escalation of this already heightened vigilance.

In contrast, vigilance and fear are less apparent in some suburban areas, where a quieter lifestyle, a less dense population, and the availability of adequate numbers of police officers to respond to citizens' needs contribute to a greater sense of security among the population. Unfortunately, however, statistical evidence does not validate the assumption that violent behavior occurs less frequently in suburbs.

Police statistics throughout the country are filled with incidents of homicide, aggravated assault, armed robbery, forcible rape, and many other crimes. The causes of these acts of violence are diverse, as indicated in the following list.

- Acutely disordered mental processes account for a sizable amount of violence in the community, and between 2 and 5 percent of clients in mental hospitals act out in a violent fashion.
- There are significant problems with violence caused by alcohol and drug abuse.
- Abuse of children, women, and the elderly is a problem which is passed along from generation to generation, and which often occurs concurrently with alcohol and drug abuse.
- There is a higher incidence of violent acting out among the deformed, the scarred, and those with other physical defects, as compared with the general population.
- Machismo—a tough, violent stance thought to be necessary for survival in urban ghettos—is responsible for much violence.
- Unstable economic conditions and unemployment contribute to a rise in violent crime.
- There is public disagreement over the possible roles of gun control and prison reform in prevention of crime; these issues need further study and debate.
- Respect for nonviolence is not generally taught in schools; educators at all levels need to develop and promulgate programs designed to help prevent violence.
- The media—including television, movies, magazines, and newspapers—depict violence as acceptable and even glamorous and desirable. The destructive consequences of media saturation have not yet been fully assessed, but what is clear is that equal exposure should be given to alternative ways of handling aggressive energies.

Nurses' intervention with violence in the community takes several forms. Working with police officers, who are frequently involved in initial management of violent behavior, is often part of the nurse's role. Nurses can do much to promote close and friendly relations between mental health emergency services and police departments. Cooperative and open exchange of information between such organizations helps to promote safer communities.

By setting up and running community education programs, nurses can work to prevent future outbreaks of violence. "Rap" sessions are effective in working with young people. Awareness that children learn violence firsthand from parents, guardians, and the environment is essential. Early results of research about this issue indicate that classes on parenting and child abuse, as well as treatment opportunities for abusive parents, help to reduce aggressive and violent behavior. Teaching abused children healthy ways to express aggression helps to prevent them from abusing their own children after they, in turn, become parents. Healthy attitudes and habits related to use of drugs and alcohol can be promoted by nurses who work with young

Table 32-4 Evaluation: Case Study (Alice R.)

Assessment	Diagnosis	Goal	Outcome Criterion	Interventions	Evaluation
The nurse recognizes Alice's behavior as showing that she has the potential to erupt violently.	Agitated behavior related to recent home visit.	Prevent Alice from acting out in an assaultive way.	Alice will choose to express assaultive impulses by using exercise equipment available in the "quiet room" or by jogging.	1. The nurse gives Alice space and allows her to continue pacing. 2. After a time the nurse speaks to Alice calmly, allowing her to verbalize the anger she feels toward her parents. 3. The nurse asks Alice if there is need to offer external controls. 4. When Alice says she would like to "work it out," the nurse suggests Alice spend time outdoors jogging (a strategy that has worked previously).	When Alice returns from jogging, the nurse observes that she is much calmer. The nurse compliments her and suggests discussing the problem further. The nurse notes observations and successful intervention in the record. The care plan is updated to include jogging as a suggested healthy outlet for Alice's assaultive tendencies.

people in community settings such as schools, camps, adolescent health clinics, and youth centers.

Evaluation

Successful intervention with violent clients is achieved when clients no longer exhibit assaultive behavior or when a violent episode has been prevented. A violent episode that does *not* occur shows that the nursing intervention was successful. Table 32-4 provides an example that will help illustrate the effectiveness of the nursing process with Alice R., an assaultive client:

> Alice R. has just returned to the unit after a weekend visit with her family. She is pacing; she is jumpy and agitated; and her facial expression is tense. She has a history of assaultive episodes following visits with her family.

SUMMARY

Violence and assaultive behavior are unhealthy expressions of the aggressive drive, caused by (1) a psychotic state, (2) an organic condition, (3) a depressive state, or (4) acting out. The thought processes of these clients are disordered; thoughts, feelings, and behaviors are not connected in a logical fashion.

A client who is already out of control or violent is easy to diagnose; what is more difficult is assessing criteria to diagnose a potentially assaultive client. The signals of impending violent behavior may be only vague, such as an increase in psychomotor activity and expanding "body space," intensity of affect, verbalization of delusional thinking, and threatening or upsetting hallucinations. A nurse's perceptions of, intuitions about, and "gut feelings" about these signals are an invaluable assessment tool. A client's violent behavior may be diagnosed as in progress, impending, or part of a day-to-day lifestyle, and intervention can be planned accordingly. The goals of intervention with these clients are to impose external control and to restore self-control if violence is already occurring; to anticipate and prevent further loss of self-control; to identify environmental factors, including the client's family, that contribute to or promote violent behavior; and to teach the client alternative reactions to stressful situations. The first step toward health has been taken when a violent client begins to choose nonviolent ways of discharging aggression.

Not all nurses have the qualities or experience needed to work with violent clients. Self-assessment and rational scrutiny of their own feelings about and responses to fear and aggression are necessary before nurses can become effective members of a treatment team.

REFERENCES

1. American Psychiatric Association, *Diagnostic and Statistical Manual of Mental Disorders,* 3d ed., APA, Washington, D.C., 1980.
2. R. J. Gelles, "Violence in the Family: A Review of Research in the Seventies," *Journal of Marriage and the Family,* vol. 42, November 1980, pp. 873–885.
3. E. A. Serafetinides, "Aggressiveness in Temporal Lobe Epileptics and Its Relationship to Cerebral Dysfunction and Environmental Factors," *Epilepsia,* vol. 6, 1965, pp. 33–42.
4. C. H. King, "Counter-Transference and Counter-Experience in the Treatment of Violence Prone Youth," *American Journal of Orthopsychiatry,* vol. 46, January 1976, pp. 43–52.
5. R. E. Umana, S. J. Gross, and M. T. McConville, *Crisis in the Family,* Gardner, New York, 1980.
6. M. Bowen, *Family Therapy in Clinical Practice,* Aronson, New York, 1978.
7. E. Kaufman and P. N. Kaufman, eds., *Family Therapy of Drug and Alcohol Abuse,* Gardner, New York, 1979.
8. J. Haley, *Leaving Home: The Therapy of Disturbed Young People,* McGraw-Hill, New York, 1980.
9. G. Pisarcik, "Facing the Violent Patient," *Nursing 81:* September 1981, pp. 61–66.
10. L. West, "The Violent Patient—Causes and Management," *Practical Psychiatry,* vol. 2, April–May 1974, pp. 1–4.
11. J. M. Roger, A. Coutts, J. Sather, and R. Taylor, "Restraint and Seclusion: A Standard Care Plan," *Journal of Psychosocial Nursing,* vol. 23, no. 6, June 1985, pp. 18–23.
12. R. S. Henschen, "Learning Impulse Control through Day Care," *Perspectives in Psychiatric Care,* vol. 9, May 1971, pp. 218–224.
13. M. E. Loomis, "Nursing Management of Acting-Out Behavior," *Perspectives in Psychiatric Care,* vol. 8, April 1970, pp. 168–175.

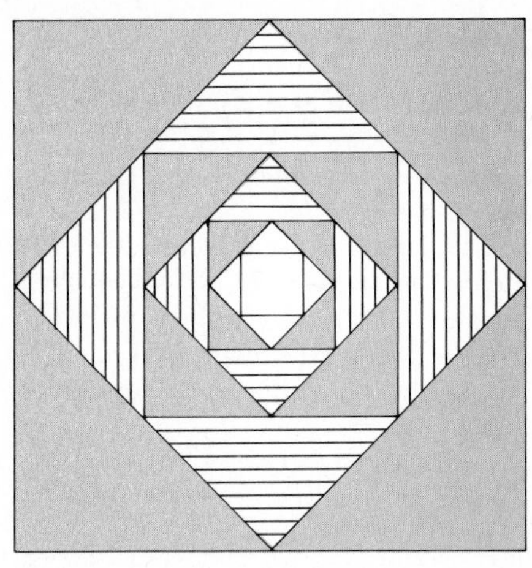

CHAPTER 33
Patterns of Substance Abuse

Laura Coble Zamora

LEARNING OBJECTIVES

After studying this chapter, the student should be able to:

1. Describe the dysynchronous behavioral patterns of substance abusers.
2. Associate the behaviors of alcoholics and other substance abusers with DSM III labels.
3. Operationally define the *manipulative, avoidant, impulsive, angry,* and *grandiose behavioral patterns* of substance abusers.
4. Assess the specific physical, mental, and spiritual problems of clients with acute alcoholism, alcohol withdrawal syndrome, delirium tremens, Wernicke-Korsakoff syndrome, and drug dependency.
5. Describe unanticipated side effects of abuse of cocaine, PCP, and LSD.
6. Construct a nursing care plan for use with substance abusers.
7. Formulate nursing diagnoses and outcome criteria for use with substance abusers.
8. Discuss community services available to alcoholics and other substance abusers.
9. Describe appropriate family interventions in the care of alcoholics and other substance abusers.
10. Describe the evaluation process utilized with clients who abuse drugs or alcohol.

There is no precise agreement on the definition of *substance abuse,* but broadly speaking, it is any use of alcohol or another chemical substance that causes damage to individuals, families, and society. Most definitions refer to the following interrelated clinical features: patterned episodic or continuous heavy abuse of substances; undue preoccupation with intake of substances; loss of control over the pattern of abuse itself; use of alcohol or other substances in a way that impairs social or occupational functioning; use of alcohol or other drugs as a universal solution to problems.

Substance abuse is a pervasive disorder in that it involves the mental, physical, and spiritual dimensions of the person. Mentally, substance abusers defend against their conflicting inner and outer selves with high levels of anger, denial, rationalization, mistrust, and contempt. Physically, they are dominated by a need to eradicate pain and tension through chemical means; but their neglect of physical health often results in malnutrition, physical deterioration, and impairment. Spiritually, substance abusers fail to value the self, lack self-esteem and self-differentiation, and have either no relationship or an overdependent relationship with a power beyond themselves. The patterns of behavior that result from disruptions in all three dimensions include manipulation, impulsivity, grandiosity, dysfunctional anger, and avoidance of responsibility.

The purpose of this chapter is to discuss the dynsynchronous interactional patterns of substance abusers. The nursing process is utilized as the framework for discussing comprehensive inpatient and community interventions with alcoholics and drug abusers.

DYSYNCHRONOUS HEALTH PATTERNS

Since alcohol is itself a drug, *alcoholism* and *drug abuse* are not mutually exclusive terms. Alcoholism and drug abuse may collectively be considered *substance abuse.* Clients who abuse substances experience physical, cognitive, and spiritual changes that alter their effective functioning as whole human beings. The abused substances cause physiological dependency, impair cognitive function, and facilitate development of spiritual dependency. The physiological syndromes associated with alcoholism include alcohol addiction, alcohol withdrawal syndrome, delirium tremens, and Wernicke-Korsakoff syndrome; these are discussed under "The Alcoholic." Drug habituation and drug abuse are discussed under "The Drug Abuser."

The Alcoholic

The alcohol abuser is a person who drinks excessively. The progressive, untreated alcoholic may begin by developing an increasing physical dependence on and tolerance for alcohol. Drinking may then become surreptitious and uncontrollable. Periods of intoxication may become prolonged, with loss of memory for the actual episodes (blackouts). Alcoholics often become guilty and persistently remorseful about drinking, and this, of course, impels them to drink more in order to relieve their feelings. Relationships with others become dominated by feelings of self-pity and unreasonable resentment. Attention span and ability to concentrate are decreased. The client develops tremors, recurrent somatic symptoms, insomnia, and signs of physical withdrawal when alcohol intake stops suddenly.[1]

Though there are characteristic clinical features, the reader should be cautioned against conceptualizing a "universal alcoholic profile." The stereotype of the alcoholic as a skid row bum applies to only 5 percent of the alcoholic population. In reality, there are wide individual variations in patterns of excessive drinking. For example, some people begin to drink excessively during adolescence. Others do not start drinking until late middle age, when they have suffered a loss or losses and life seems empty. Many people who use alcohol excessively drink only on "weekend binges"; but some drink continuously every day, starting with a cocktail at lunch or an afternoon sherry; others drink only during the evening, when work is over for the day; and still others go on a drinking spree a few times a year. A few—the minority—drink to excess constantly. Of particular note is another variation: an increased pattern of multiple substance abuse, that is, the combination of alcohol and one or several drugs. This pattern is especially alarming in light of the known toxic and potentiating interactions of alcohol with other drugs.

Alcohol Abuse and Addiction

Various categories of alcohol abuse have been defined; in practice, however, it is difficult to distinguish between "alcoholics" and "problem drinkers." Broadly speaking, *alcoholism* is any use of alcoholic beverages that causes any damage to the individual, to society, or to both. Most definitions of alcoholism refer to the following clinical features:

- Chronicity as a disease or behavioral disorder
- Undue preoccupation with intake of ethyl alcohol
- Loss of control over the drinking pattern itself
- Use of alcohol in a way that is damaging to the drinker's physical health, interpersonal relations, or economic functions
- Use of alcohol as a universal solution to problems

Alcohol addiction develops when there is a physiological dependence on alcohol and a tolerance for increasing amounts of alcohol. Dependence is demonstrated by the appearance of withdrawal symptoms when the alcohol is abruptly stopped.

Alcohol Withdrawal Syndrome

Alcohol withdrawal syndrome (AWS) occurs when alcohol is abruptly discontinued, and includes the following symptoms:

- Diaphoresis, tachycardia, and elevated blood pressure
- Tremors
- Nausea and vomiting
- Anorexia
- Restlessness
- Hallucinations
- Convulsions
- Delerium tremens (DTs)

Delirium Tremens

Delirium tremens (DTs) is an acute complication of alcoholism that constitutes a medical and nursing emergency. It is one of the manifestations of the alcohol withdrawal syndrome. DTs has a mortality rate of 5 percent when treated and 15 percent when untreated. Nurses are frequently in a position to note the signs of impending alcohol withdrawal or to obtain a history that includes a previous episode of DTs. The signs of impending DTs include increasing tremors, restlessness, irritability, headache, nausea, insomnia, and nightmares. Before full-blown DTs develops, withdrawal signs may include visual and tactile hallucinations without disorientation, and seizures.[1] Clients with impending DTs may be found in any circumstance that has suddenly interrupted the excessive intake of alcohol. For example, a client may enter a general hospital for gallbladder surgery and, 2 to 4 days later, develop beginning signs of DTs. The challenge to the nurse is amplified because lifesaving measures are often necessary at the same time that the mental functioning of clients makes them at best uncooperative and at worst actively resistant to treatment.

Although still not entirely clear, the etiology of DTs is thought to be sudden withdrawal from or significant decrease in the intake of alcohol following a period of chronic intoxication. Other contributing factors include physical trauma, infections, metabolic disorders, and anxiety-provoking stimuli.

DTs is an acute pathological state of consciousness resulting from interference with brain metabolism. It includes the following symptoms: increased psychomotor activity and tremulousness, confusion and disorientation, fearfulness, signs of vasomotor lability, tachycardia, temperature of 37.8 to 40.5°C (100 to 105°F), and illusions and hallucinations. The latter are most commonly visual and tactile, often consisting of terrifying animal images and crawling skin sensations. The onset of DTs is typically quite sudden and dramatic, and the condition usually lasts from 2 or 3 days to a week.[2] Less commonly, it may last for as long as 4 to 5 weeks.

Wernicke-Korsakoff Syndrome

Relatively rare and apparently a result of vitamin B deficiency, Wernicke-Korsakoff syndrome is associated with long-standing use of alcohol and inadequate nutritional intake. The symptoms include disorientation, memory impairment, and fabrication of elaborate stories to fill memory gaps (confabulation). A client may recover from a single episode, but irreversible damage to the cerebral cortex results from continued drinking.

The Drug Abuser

A *drug abuser* is a person who repeatedly uses a chemical substance or substances (other than alcohol) in a way that is harmful to self and society.

Even though drug use does not receive the same overt moral and legal acceptance as drinking, more and more people are turning to chemical means of resolving their life problems and are considered "drug-oriented." The "addiction" phenomenon, seen in every age group, includes abuse of illicit drugs such as marijuana, cocaine, and heroin, as well as legal drugs such as tranquilizers, sleeping pills, analgesics, and laxatives.

The availability of drugs and the frequency with which they are indiscriminately prescribed combine to perpetuate abuse, despite well-publicized warnings.[3] Table 33-1 lists some of the drugs commonly abused.

Traditionally the terms *habituation* and *addiction* have been used by health care professionals to define the nature and extent of drug abuse. In essence, *drug habituation* involves repeated use of a drug to the point of psychological dependence. *Drug addiction* is more compulsive drug use involving craving, psychological dependence, and physical dependence; it includes the development of tolerance for increasing doses and the appearance of withdrawal symptoms. Withdrawal symptoms differ for various substances. Among the most common are the symptoms of withdrawal from heroin, which may include rhinorrhea, lacrimation, sweating, chills, elevated temperature, dilated and sluggish pupils, insomnia, restlessness, and muscle and joint pain. In actual practice, distinctions between habituation and addiction are often meaningless; therefore the World Health Organization's term *drug dependence* has been adopted by many health workers. *Drug dependence* refers to a "psychological and/or physical dependence on a drug that is taken periodically or on a scheduled basis."[2] In treating a given person, this term is further clarified by specifying the drug or drugs involved.

Excessive use of substances crosses all personality and diagnostic categories and therefore should be evaluated in the context of the total person and the environment. Although most drug abusers are still viewed by some as people who are engaging in "criminal" behavior, the conscious attitude of most people is that alcoholism is an illness. For example, in many areas public intoxication has been decriminalized. When police encounter someone behaving in a "drunken" fashion, they sometimes take the person to a local community mental health center or emergency room rather than to the police station. In such an instance, the abuser is being defined as *sick*. In one respect, this is a positive step; it brings the abuser to a treatment center for detoxification and decreases the danger of a withdrawal syndrome going unrecognized in jail. In another respect, the label *sick* can be used by the abuser to excuse irresponsible behavior.[4]

Table 33-1 Drugs of Abuse

Category	Examples
Controlled analgesics	Heroin, morphine, methadone, codeine, propoxyphene (Darvon), oxycodon (Percodan)
Stimulants	Amphetamines, cocaine, "crack," amyl nitrite
Sedatives	Barbiturates, methaqualone (Quaalude), glutethimide (Doriden)
Antianxiety agents	Diazepam (Valium), chlordiazeposide (Librium), clorazepate (Tranxene), hydroxyzine (Vistaril)
Hallucinogens	LSD (lysergic acid diethylamide), marijuana (cannabis), mescaline, phencyclidine (PCP or angel dust)
Volatile substance	Hair sprays, insecticides, model airplane glue, lighter fluid
Over-the-counter drugs	Antihistamines, cough syrups, sleeping medicines, aspirin, acetaminophen

DSM III

The *Diagnostic and Statistical Manual of Mental Disorders* (DSM III) classifies disorders of substance use under *substance abuse* and *substance dependence*. Subcategories provide for medical diagnosis based on the class of substance abused and the course of the abuse. The five classes of substances include alcohol, sedatives or hypnotics, opioids, amphetamines, and cannabis. The course of abuse may be categorized as *continuous, episodic,* or *in remission*. Cocaine abuse and hallucinogen abuse are separate and specific medical diagnoses. Tobacco dependence and caffeine intoxication are also included.

The organic mental disorders associated with substance abuse include intoxication, withdrawal, delirium, and dementia and are discussed in Chapter 44.[5] Also associated with persons who abuse alcohol and other drugs is a medical diagnosis of antisocial personality disorders. One of the characteristics of the antisocial personality is repeated drunkenness or substance abuse. Similarly, elements of the antisocial personality are found in persons who are labeled *drug abusers* or *alcohol abusers*.[5]

Epidemiology

Substance abuse is a major issue for health care. Alcoholism is said to be the third most important health problem in the United States, after heart disease and cancer. Current estimates indicate that at least 9 to 10 million adults in this country are alcoholics or "problem drinkers." Especially alarming is the continuing abuse of alcohol among the young. Eighty percent of 12- to 17-year-olds report having had a drink, and nearly 3 percent drink or use drugs every day. Other reports indicate that 1 in 16 high school seniors drinks alcohol *daily*.[6] Alcohol also figures in 10 percent of all deaths in the United States.

Alcoholics adversely affect the mental health or functioning of about 30 million relatives and friends. Although it has been estimated that 70 percent of alcoholics are male, the number of known female alcoholics is rising. The National Institute on Alcohol Abuse and Alcoholism notes that possibly 50 percent, or some 5 million, of alcoholics in the United States are women.[7]

The actual extent to which drugs are abused in this country has been difficult to document. Burkhalter comments that the available statistics on heroin dependency, drug-related deaths, and the like "point to the existence of a fluctuating, pervasive health problem that is of vital concern to all health professionals."[8]

Abuse of illicit drugs such as marijuana, cocaine, and heroin is also on the increase among all segments of the population. Reported statistics state that use of marijuana is most frequent among males in cities and that the first marijuana use occurs between the ages of 14 and 21.[8] Cocaine is used in various forms by approximately 5 million people between the ages of 18 and 25, and use among teenagers (particularly of a chemically treated form, "crack") is said to be rising. Use of heroin, while less prevalent than it was in the past, continues to be a major health problem.

In addition to human suffering, the economic cost of alcoholism and drug abuse is thought to be upward of $50 billion in medical expenses, lost wages, reduced industrial productivity, motor vehicle accidents, violent crime, fire losses, and social responses.[6] Substance abuse is therefore considered a continuing drain on the nation's health in terms of both human and economic resources.

PATTERNS OF INTERACTION: PERSON

Alcoholics

The forces that prompt alcoholic behavior have been studied from biological, psychological, and sociocultural points of view. At this time there is insufficient evidence to "prove" one causal theory over another. Rather, the evidence supports the argument that human behavior is determined by many factors, and that a variety of biological, psychological, and sociocultural factors interrelate to produce and perpetuate alcoholic behavior. Although the present discussion focuses on psychological and sociocultural factors, it should be noted that the major theories of biological causes have included genetic factors, allergic responses to food and chemicals, biochemical imbalances, central nervous system pathology, nutritional deficiencies, and endocrinological dysfunctions, particularly hyperadrenocorticism.[1]

Psychological explanations of problem drinking vary somewhat, but each generally points to the use of alcohol as a means of escape or relief from anxiety. Some of the more traditional explanations for the existence of severe anxiety incorporate theories of oral and oedipal fixation. *Orally*, what is sought in the bottle and oblivion is a regressive reunion with the all-caring mother figure. *Oedipally*, the fantasized reunion excludes such unwanted interlopers as fathers and siblings. This implies that the roots of alcoholism may lie in anxiety-ridden early relationships with significant others.

Unresolved conflicts in the early phases of development predispose to severe anxiety, confusion, and self-doubt during adolescence. These unresolved conflicts interfere with developmental tasks of adolescence—clarification of sexual identity, movement toward independence, and forming effective relationships with authority figures. If unresolved, these conflicts and uncompleted developmental tasks may continue to be significant areas of conflict that will influence the development and maintenance of substance abuse.

Drug Abusers

It is important not to overgeneralize about personality traits or to oversimplify the complex interplay of forces which may perpetuate drug abuse in any individual. The clinical features present in many drug abusers and their families, however, are similar to some of those mentioned in relation to the alcoholic. For example, drugs are used as a distancing maneuver, which ultimately elicits anger from other family members and shifts the focus of tension from dyadic conflicts to the drama of drug abuse itself.

The drug abuser is often described as an excessively dependent, passive person who has difficulty tolerating frustration and anxiety. Theoretically this occurs when very early emotional needs are not met. For example, Singer[9] notes that the sense of competence and hope essential to emotional maturity derives from a normal progression through phases of symbiosis, individuation, and adolescence. Certain mothering behaviors—such as rigid feeding schedules and the restriction of children's efforts to move and explore—interfere with this normal progression and predispose children to addictive patterns. Furthermore, punishment for normal expressions of anxiety and anger prevents children from learning how to express or cope with these feelings adequately. The development of the trust in self and others that is necessary to tolerate delays in gratification is thwarted. Such persons search instead for immediate ways of escaping rising tension. Drugs become a means of escape through euphoria, oblivion, or both. The euphoria or oblivion that is available through drugs becomes a potent factor in perpetuating drug abuse. For those who are IV abusers, the injection process and resultant high are similar to feelings experienced in sexual orgasm.

Antisocial Personalities

Alcoholics and drug abusers frequently have an accompanying antisocial pattern of behavior. Thus an understanding of the dynamics of this pattern is relevant here.

The antisocial person's interpersonal relations are chiefly characterized by manipulation, shallowness, and lack of duration. Behavior is governed by an overwhelming need for immediate satisfaction of basic needs and desires. Therefore, such a person views others primarily as sources of potential danger or gratification. Because of their underlying feelings of powerlessness, these clients often seek out persons of power and status to manipulate for the fulfillment of their needs. It is as though, in this way, they achieve the power and control they do not themselves possess.

Antisocial personalities seem to have few scruples about how they achieve satisfaction. Thus, their behavior is often in direct conflict with accepted legal, social, and moral codes. They feel little responsibility or remorse for the trouble they cause and seem unconcerned about the lies or self-contradictions that emerge in their glib attempts to smooth over rough situations. Although these clients usually try to avoid punishment, the threat of possible punishment does not serve as an effective deterrent to their behavior. In general, they fail to profit from experience in the sense of learning from their mistakes, although there is nothing amiss with their basic intelligence.

What happens theoretically to these clients' emotional equipment is highly controversial. One view holds that they are unable to feel anxiety and that their behavior is therefore virtually closed to modification. Another interpretation is that they have failed to develop the more common security operations in response to anxiety. For example, such mechanisms as selective inattention, dissociation, and sublimation are not available to the antisocial personality as a means of reducing the impact of tensions or rechanneling them. The antisocial individual, thus, has a peculiarly low tolerance for anxiety or any painful emotion; the slightest hint of pain calls for seemingly drastic action. On the surface, there seems to be little ability or desire to control this pattern. (Chapter 31 elaborates on the behavior of clients with borderline personalities.)

Behavioral Patterns of Substance Abusers

Alcoholics and drug abusers have several dynamics in common. Dysfunctional anger, manipulation, impulsiveness, avoidance, and grandiosity are at the heart of how they are perceived by others and by themselves. These dynamics permeate the personalities of substance abusers, influencing who they are and how they behave.

Dysfunctional Anger

To understand dysfunctional anger, a general discussion of the dynamics of anger is helpful. Anger is an experience of great significance for the mental, spiritual, and physical functioning of clients and nurses. Awareness of anger and related emotions such as hostility, resentment, and rage has been identified as critical to the therapeutic nurse-client relationship.

Anger is a feeling or emotion that is a learned means of neutralizing or avoiding the anxiety which arises in response to an interpersonal threat. Anger is "learned" in the sense that it is absorbed from significant others through empathy during the process of socialization. Anger is an inherent response to the inevitably frustrating issues that arise between parent and child during socialization. Young children notice that when they challenge the authority of significant adults, remarkable degrees of anger can be generated in the adults. Furthermore, children sense that angry people seem to wield much more power than anxious people do. Consequently, they begin to cope with their own anxiety by converting it into the more powerful feeling of anger.

Anger, then, is developed as an important, unrefined tool to be used in situations where people would otherwise feel anxious and powerless.[1] It can be seen from this model that one situation in which anger is typically engendered is when one's sense of authority or perceived right to exercise influence over another is challenged or doubted.

There are three points about anger which must be emphasized as significant for interpersonal relationships:

1. People become angry when their sense of authority or influence is threatened in interpersonal situations.
2. Anger can be more functional than anxiety in that its expression gives a person a sense of power and immediate relief rather than powerlessness and insecurity.
3. Anger can be dysfunctional for interpersonal relationships in that its expression is more conducive to relieving anxiety than to mutual learning or problem solving.

The development of self-esteem and positive self-differentiation rests upon a variety of factors and depends upon the degree of anxiety associated with early interpersonal experiences. Development and use of anger as a response to anxiety has aspects that are unique to each individual's experience. Any of a wide range of behaviors may evoke anger; however, the sense of being unfairly used, which results from manipulation by another, is what most commonly generates it. The interaction is complicated by the passive nature of manipulative behaviors. At times, neither the person who is provoked by the stimulus (the manipulative behavior) nor the person who is behaving manipulatively can identify the true source of the anger.

Dysfunctional anger is manifested when people reenact early conflicts over trust, independence, and identity, during which expressions of anger were forbidden, ignored, or otherwise rendered ineffective as a means of relieving anxiety. Anger then becomes a source of tension rather than a source or relief. Relationships with others become dominated by attempts to rid the self of these tensions in other ways. Clients in such situations often appear to be "asking for it," and yet almost any response elicits from the client either contempt or repeated efforts to test limits. Clients' behaviors become increasingly incomprehensible and exasperating as they continually test and reject others' responses. Eventually, the repeated behaviors make others feel powerless. Anger arises as a means of restoring a sense of power. Inherent in this interpersonal chaos is a profound disruption of spiritual needs, which have little chance to survive or even to emerge.

Long-term problematic behavioral themes relating to dysfunctional anger can be understood in part as cycles of testing, rejecting, and ultimately escaping from relationships with others. Figure 33-1 will help the reader to conceptualize the dysfunctional anger cycle as it applies to substance abusers.

Manipulation

Manipulation is a term frequently used by health workers to label a client's offensive attempts to get something the worker does not want to give. In order to intervene therapeutically, recognition of one's own reactions is necessary. Manipulation can then become an explanatory concept rather than a disparaging label.

The process of manipulation begins with a conflict over needs or goals of the client and the nurse;

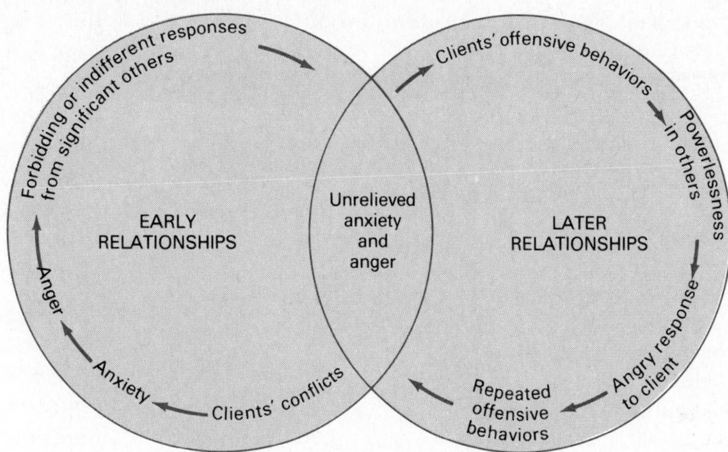

Figure 33-1 Problematic anger cycle.

the client wants something from the nurse, and the nurse cannot or will not give it. Because they have developed little self-esteem and trust, substance abusers are poorly equipped to cope with the tensions of unmet needs. Their interpersonal experiences have arrested the spiritual dimension of their development and severely limited their ability to consider any needs or goals that other people may have. Consequently, instead of engaging in mutual problem-solving processes, these clients increase their attempts to influence others to meet their needs. These attempts almost inevitably include elements of deception—insincerity, fabrication, denial, or rationalization—which make the interpersonal process with these clients uniquely difficult. Although part of the process may remain unconscious, at least part of it is a conscious, deliberate attempt to avoid authentic ways of relating.[10]

A client's aims may range from simply trying to avoid anxiety, to achieving pleasurable ends, to attempting to put something over on another even when there seems to be no real advantage. The result for the health worker is a feeling of having been used, and a diminution in capacity to respond accurately to the client's interpersonal and spiritual needs.

In substance abusers, the manipulative process often revolves around unmet dependency needs. This may appear in the client's deliberate maneuvers to get the forbidden substance itself, or more subtly in demands for time or for physical contact, attention, permission, approval, or disapproval. Substance abusers manipulate others by a sort of "taking-in" process that reflects the infantile nature of their difficulties.

The manipulative behavior of some substance abusers seems related to mistrust and a contemptuous view of the motivations of others. Abusers seem to con others in order to reject them. Faulty identification and learning as well as low tolerance for anxiety contribute to use of manipulation as a survival technique.

Table 33-2 (page 626) outlines an operational definition of manipulation and gives a specific nursing example.

Impulsiveness

Impulsiveness is a predominant theme in the behavior of substance abusers. In fact, *impulsiveness* is the one word that sums up the trying attributes of such clients. *Impulsiveness* here refers to a pattern of behavior that is directed toward immediate gains and gratification, with little time between thought and action.[11] Diminished feelings are the result; guilt, anxiety, and anger as conscious feelings are avoided. The brief time between thought and action prevents clients from "thinking things through" or weighing consequences, particularly in relation to others. Actions appear abrupt and unplanned in a long-term sense, although cleverness and aplomb may be noted in their immediate execution.

Impulsiveness may be active or passive. The antisocial acts of the client often take the form of a dramatically *active* pursuit of some spur-of-the-moment exploit, with blatant disregard for others. The attitude is one of contempt. The substance abuser may behave similarly under the influence

Table 33-2 Operational Definition of Manipulation

Definition	Example
Client wants (needs) something from nurse.	Client: It's so nice out. How about letting me sit outside, on the bench? (Client is on bed rest for infected leg.)
Nurse perceives client's want as pathological or unreasonable.	Nurse: No, Mr. A, you have to stay in bed because of the infection.
Nurse does not fulfill client's want.	
Client's tension increases.	Client gets out of bed.
Client increases attempts to influence nurse by:	Client: Aw, c'mon. Its my leg! This is ridiculous—I'll rest much better outside.
1. Becoming dependent, clinging, demanding, helpless	
2. Denying either the meaning or manifestation of the want	
3. Rationalizing the want by supplying logical reasons for its appearance and fulfillment	
4. Fabricating statements and making promises about behavior	
5. Questioning or defying nurse's competence and authority	Client (to group): That nurse is a stupid bitch. What do you say we all refuse to take our meds until she lets us out?
Nurse feels powerless and angry.	Nurse: I'm calling the doctor. Then we'll see who's boss!

of a chemical, but the basic mode of impulsiveness is then more *passive*, a sort of giving in to temptation. One senses here the helpless, dependent, "I have no control over it" attitude, which is passive-manipulative.

Among alcoholics, impulsiveness that occurs must be atoned for; this differentiates it from the impulsiveness of the antisocial person and, to some extent, that of other substance abusers. The guilt and anxiety associated with forbidden oedipal sexual and aggressive urges are impulsively obliterated through the use of alcohol. The intoxicated state permits even greater impulsiveness, which subsequently lowers self-esteem and gives rise to additional guilt feelings. Alcohol abuse also takes a tremendous toll in physical suffering—hangovers, toxicity, damage to body organs. Thus, in one cycle of impulsiveness, alcoholics achieve momentary release and gratification, feel guilty, and punish themselves. Unfortunately, because of their underlying low self-esteem, the punishment aspect becomes a potent secondary source of gratification, and so the cycle must be repeated.

Substance abusers who encounter serious obstacles to their goals are quite capable of the kind of impulsiveness that generates fear. However, the resultant behaviors are more likely to be viewed as maddeningly erratic, self-serving, thoughtless, and infantile than as rage-filled or frightening.

Table 33-3 presents an operational definition and example of impulsiveness.

Table 33-3 Operational Definition of Impulsiveness

Definition	Example
Client perceives need for gratification in a material or bodily sense.	Client: I need to get out of here—a night on the town!"
Nurse communicates expectation of delay in gratification and focus on interpersonal relatedness.	Nurse: You and I are scheduled to talk for a while now.
Client experiences slight but intolerable rise in tension.	Client feels frustrated.
Client acts abruptly and without reflection by: 1. Actively moving toward gratification 2. Passively submitting to temptation of drugs, food, alcohol	Client walks away from nurse and leaves the unit with a friend, saying to nurse, "We can talk tomorrow sometime."
Client thus avoids anxiety of nurse-client relatedness by 1. Disregarding the nurse's significance and influence 2. Blunting awareness of the nurse's significance and influence	
Client's tension is decreased momentarily.	
Nurse feels rejected, powerless, angry.	Nurse asks to have client assigned to another staff member.

Avoidance

The term *avoidance* refers to an extreme pattern of behavior that facilitates escape from the real or anticipated anxiety of relatedness. Escape through avoidance can occur only to the extent that others participate in the process.[12]

Avoidance can be physical, but in clients with problems of substance abuse, it is more likely to be emotional or spiritual, and its manifestations rarely go unnoticed. The avoidance process is usually provocative and infinitely exasperating; it is by no means a simple "fading into the woodwork."

For example, excessive use of substances such as alcohol and drugs accomplishes "escape" by dulling a client's feelings of guilt, anger, or sexual insecurity. At the same time, the behavior at some point demands, as a response, physical care, punishment, or forgiveness.

Avoidance may also take the form of withholding of emotional involvement, so that relationships are shallow and fleeting. It is as if the client were constantly escaping from feeling and thus always running away from people. The running away, or distancing, is often sensational in its style and hurtful to others.

The process of avoidance involves not only escape but also control. The tragedy for the client is that this often leads to real loneliness. It is not by simple choice that the person is isolated and distant; it is from inability to tolerate the anxiety and anticipated emotional demands of interpersonal relatedness. In effect, the client has been sensitized to threatening or indifferent interpersonal relationships in the past and therefore mistrusts the present experience.

Table 33-4 operationally defines avoidance and illustrates the dynamics with an appropriate example.

Table 33-4 Operational Definition of Avoidance

Definition	Example
Nurse communicates an expectation of interpersonal relatedness.	Nurse asks client to join a client group for discussion of problems.
Client is fearful, mistrustful, or contemptuous of the intentions or actions of the nurse.	
Client escapes from anxiety of interpersonal demands by:	
1. Physically removing self from nurse 2. Blunting awareness of feelings associated with relatedness through drug or alcohol abuse	In middle of nurse's response, client suddenly leaves to attend to something "important."
3. Keeping relatedness at a superficial, pleasant, chitchat level 4. Maintaining an "as-if" involvement in the nurse-client relationship	Client readily goes to discussion group with nurse, smiles pleasantly, comments and looks interested, responds to question about self with: "Oh, I'm working things out, you know; it takes time to develop insight."
Client maintains distance by controlling access to the self.	
Nurse feels rejected, powerless, angry.	Nurse begins to have difficulty focusing on the group process.

Grandiosity

Another common and problematic behavioral theme encountered in substance abusers is grandiosity. According to one author, "grandiosity is the assumption of an exalted, superior state which is beyond realistic possibility of actuality." Such clients manifest remarkable denial and rationalization of, as well as arrogance and irresponsibility toward, the consequences of their behaviors. It is as though the rules that apply to people in general bear no relation to them. In effect, the client maintains a "privileged status."[13]

Substance abusers often reveal grandiosity in their beliefs or fantasies about giving up alcohol or drugs. They may, for example, boast of being able to give up the substance any time they feel like it; or they may refer to elaborate and patently unrealistic plans for becoming functional within society. Grandiosity is also apparent in the suffering of alcoholics: they see their guilt and sins as being much worse than those of ordinary people; nobody else could possibly be so awful.

Grandiosity may be manifested by clients as an unshakable belief in their own cleverness. Such clients are convinced that they can outwit those in authority; they invariably overestimate their own cunning while underestimating the capacities of the police and all others.[13]

Table 33-5 Operational Definition of Grandiosity

Definition	Example
Nurse communicates expectation of relatedness.	Nurse asks client how job interview went.
Clients' tension rises, because of an underlying view of self as worthless, inadequate, powerless (inhuman).	
Client defends against anxiety by adopting a superior and exalted attitude toward nurse.	Client flippantly responds that interview went "right down the drain—right where you'd expect it to go, considering that I'm overqualified!"
Client reacts overtly to nurse's expectations by: 1. Disclaiming knowledge of or responsibility for behavior and its consequences 2. Arrogant, derogatory attitudes toward rules and expectations 3. Exaggerated self-pity and resentment of demands by others	Then: "It was your idea anyway—and obviously a poor one." Then: "I don't need the job anyway, so it doesn't really matter."
Client avoids anxiety at the expense of failing to develop real abilities	Client refuses to discuss incident further.
Nurse feels rejected, powerless, angry.	Nurse reminds client that he'd better get a job soon, as he's up for discharge.

Grandiose spiritual patterns are based on extremely shaky foundations of low self-esteem, powerlessness, and inadequacy. In a sense, clients compensate for their felt powerlessness to influence others by taking the opposite view of their behavior, its motivations, and its consequences. The false view of self in relation to others is doubly unfortunate for such a client in that it obscures and leaves underdeveloped the client's real assets and interpersonal potential.

Table 33-5 provides an operational definition of grandiosity and an example of the dynamics.

PATTERNS OF INTERACTION: FAMILY

The Alcoholic's Family

Alcoholism is viewed as a family disease. Excessive drinking affects not only the client but the entire family. Accordingly, the term *alcoholic family* is common in the field. Coalcoholics (spouses of alcoholics) and para-alcoholics (children of alcoholics) emerge in the family system, and develop dynamics similar to those of the alcoholic.[14,15]

The risk factors that have been researched as predictive of alcohol addiction all involve the family. These include:

- Multigenerational family history of alcoholism
- Family history of total abstinence accompanied by a strong moral atmosphere
- Belonging to a cultural group in which the incidence of alcoholism is higher than among other cultural groups
- Family history of marital discord or conflict, or an absent or rejecting father, or both
- Cross-generational family history of recurrent depression among female relatives[13]

Whether these factors represent genetic predispositions or socially learned behaviors, or a combination of both, remains unclear at this time. However, such patterns do tend to be associated with models of drinking behavior for individuals within a particular familial environment.[4,16]

Alcoholic families operate in a number of ways to foster the development of excessive drinking.

A developing child can be socialized into drinking by role models who use alcohol as a means of relieving anxiety and releasing rage. Children may observe and identify with this behavior in significant adults and then use the same kinds of anxiety-relieving measures in their own lives as they grow up. In contrast, they may be profoundly intimidated by morally condemnatory messages about alcohol. In this instance, social situations where drinking is approved and expected may evoke fear, conflict, and an impaired ability to deal rationally with alcohol.

A more complex process occurs when family members communicate conflicting messages about the acceptability and morality of drinking and indirectly encourage forbidden behavior in the form of alcohol abuse. That is, children may be the recipients of double-bind communications about the use and abuse of alcohol. Parents may overtly forbid the purchase of alcohol or its presence in the home and depict its use as morally reprehensible; on the other hand, they may describe with relish how tipsy everyone was at the last office party. Children thus gradually receive the message that the "forbidden pleasure" is worth seeking even though it is disapproved of by the family.[14]

Steinglass[4] reports that alcohol abuse has several stabilizing and organizing functions in families. First, it allows an alcoholic and nonalcoholic spouse to strike a covert bargain about meeting each other's needs. The alcoholic spouse needs to be nurtured, and the nonalcoholic spouse usually needs to nurture. This need pattern results in reciprocal episodes of underfunctioning and overfunctioning in the spouses. One is covertly permitted to be less responsible because of the other one's need to be more responsible.

Second, alcohol abuse facilitates development and maintenance of emotional distance in relationships, particularly in the marital relationship. For example, if emotional demands in a relationship are too steep and anxiety-provoking for one spouse, that spouse can distance from the demands by drinking too much. The excessive intake of alcohol screens emotional demands and may dull some of the discomfort. Having once experienced relief from anxiety in this way, the person may use alcohol again to relieve discomfort. Distance is maintained by repeated alcohol abuse, and the alcoholic spouse usually becomes emotionally unavailable when drunk. The nonalcoholic spouse is likely to say, "He's no comfort to me" or "All she cares about is her bottle; I may as well not be married."

Third, alcohol abuse provides an organizing focus for the family that distracts attention from underlying conflicts. Frequently, a teenager who abuses alcohol may be attempting to divert attention from the parents' marital conflict. The conflict does not manifest itself as long as the parents are worrying about more important things such as the teenager's drinking problem.

Fourth, alcohol abuse provides an organizing focus for families in conflict. Families that are unable to agree on anything or get together to do anything frequently unite by discussing or helping the problem drinker in some way. One teenage girl described her parents as both distant and conflictual. The only time they stopped fighting and were united was when she came home drunk.

In each of these cases, alcohol abuse is learned from or reinforced by forces within the family system that enable it to be maintained. Often, when excess drinking stops, other problems that have long been covert emerge because the alcohol abuse no longer provides a stabilizing albeit dysfunctional force. Thus, use and abuse of alcohol in a family may be related to the needs of individual members as well as the overall anxiety level in the family.[15]

The Drug Abuser's Family

Although the family dynamics of drug abusers are similar to those of alcoholics, several factors deserve mention.

First, drug abuse by adolescents seems to be related to their parents' use and abuse of drugs, especially alcohol.[15] Parental role modeling becomes a vehicle for adolescents' decision making about the acceptability of drug use and abuse, as well as its value as an anxiety-reducing mechanism. Parents' use of drugs or alcohol reinforces the child's belief that this behavior is permissible and of value.

Second, onset or escalation of drug abuse is likely to coincide with periods of high family anxiety, which often escalates around significant family events. The anxiety, which is felt by all family members to some degree, may be channeled to one "special" member of the family through the projection process. The special family member will act out the family anxiety in a dysfunctional way, that is, by abusing drugs so that the rest of the family will feel calmer and have something beside their own internal upset to focus on. An example will help demonstrate the dynamics of this situation:

> Mark was born without a right hand. He was very close to his mother, who spent a lot of time helping him master his artificial hand. Mark was also very close to his grandfathers, particularly one who was a bilateral lower-extremity amputee. The other grandfather had had a retarded son who was institutionalized against his wishes.
>
> Starting when Mark was 13, a series of family events occurred over 4 years, which seemed to precipitate and then contribute to his drug abuse. First, the family moved to another part of the state. They were separated from both sets of grandparents by a 1-hour drive. Mark's father now had to commute to his two jobs in the old neighborhood and was rarely home. Mark missed his father a lot and also had to make new friends at school, hoping that they would accept him with an artificial hand. Within the next year, one grandfather died, his mother had a back operation, and his younger brother developed a near-fatal kidney disease. The family had to move again because their medical bills were so high that they could not afford a house.

With each event, Mark's mother became more frantic. Mark's worry also increased, and so did his drug abuse. Since his father was not home much, his mother had only Mark, the oldest, to talk to about what was happening. The more she told him, the more anxious he got. The last straw was the death of the second grandfather. For 6 weeks after that, Mark was on a binge of "acid" and amphetamines which ended only when he was caught burglarizing a house and was sent into a residential treatment program.

Looking back, Mark was able to identify his desire for acceptance in a new neighborhood, despite having an artificial hand, and the catastrophic series of family events that shot the family anxiety level sky-high and particularly affected him as the oldest child and the child closest to the mother. The loss of his two grandfathers was the key factor in his escalating drug abuse.

PATTERNS OF INTERACTION: ENVIRONMENT

One way of understanding substance abuse is to see it as learned patterns of behavior and attitudes within a sociocultural context. In assessing alcoholism from this viewpoint, one must look at sociocultural patterns of drinking and at operations that teach, invite, and reinforce substance abuse. For example, in this connection, it should be noted that drinking itself is a typical behavior in the United States. In advertising and other portrayals, the media bombard us with presentations of drinking as pleasurable and socially approved.[17]

The importance of the sociocultural context in the development of addictive behaviors is further emphasized by the risk factors that have been identified from epidemiological and sociological studies, and by the overwhelming predominance of ambivalent, moralistic, and pessimistic attitudes about substance abuse. Cultural values of achievement, profit, competition, and mobility have resulted in attitude shifts and increased stress. This has led to the need for immediate emotional gratification and escape through alcohol and other substances.

Use of "forbidden" drugs or alcohol allows expression of rebellion toward society both through use of the substance itself and through the crime that is often necessary to support its use. Occasionally, an addicted person follows the example of a parent in using substances to escape reality and express rebellion. More often, however, younger substance abusers are following the example of a peer group.

Drug abuse or alcoholism is reinforced by lifestyles in which distinctive language, customs, and mores afford abusers some sense of belonging to a special group. The combination of the effects of drugs or alcohol, preoccupation with securing and administering a substance, and identification with a deviant subculture prevents alcoholics and drug abusers from perceiving and testing alternative solutions to their problems.

Adolescents are a particularly vulnerable population in our society. They are under pressure from peers to engage in at least recreational use of forbidden substances,[16] particularly when the norm is to develop intimacy with contemporaries. To the extent that a shift from intimacy with parents to intimacy with peers is encumbered by parent-child conflict, normal growth needs may be distorted by anger and anxiety. Thus, adolescents and young people become vulnerable to the attraction of escaping, rebelling, and finding a new identity by "doing drugs" or drinking with peers. Moreover, certain drugs, such as cocaine, are glamorized and used openly by celebrities who symbolize youth and wealth. The appeal is almost irresistible, especially when there seems to be official indifference to the use of such substances, as at rock concerts and in some bars and discos where young people gather.

NURSING PROCESS

Substance abusers may be clients in outpatient treatment settings; may be hospitalized in medical, surgical, or acute psychiatric treatment units where their substance abuse is not the primary diagnosis; or may be clients in an alcohol or drug treatment facility. The dynamics of substance abusers make it difficult to implement an effective treatment plan unless all team members are on the same "wavelength." Use of the nursing process in formulating a *written* approach to treatment facilitates objective and successful intervention with alcoholics and drug abusers.

Assessment

Nurses encounter clients and families with problems related to drugs, alcohol, and antisocial behavior in a wide variety of settings in which case finding and assessment take place. Nurses in industry are integrally involved with programs designed to prevent and treat drug abuse by employees. School and community health nurses are also intimately involved with substance abuse and antisocial behavior in schools, homes, and communities; their role includes prevention, education, and referral. A nurse on a medical-surgical unit of a general hospital may suddenly become involved with a client who is going into drug or alcohol withdrawal syndrome. A nurse in an emergency room may regularly encounter clients who are brought in drunk, overdosed, or psychotic from psychedelic drugs, or who have been injured during an episode of antisocial behavior. Nurses who work in the prison system commonly treat the health problems of substance abusers and antisocial personalities whose behavior has landed them in jail. Nurses who work on specialized detoxification units and in long-term rehabilitation centers will be involved with such clients on a regular basis. In many of the settings mentioned above, nurses are in a position to perform case finding, assessment, and referral. The extent to which these three activities are carried out will be determined by the clinical agency. In some instances, assessment and treatment will be carried out in the same agency by the same primary care giver. In other instances, initial assessment will be followed by referral to another more appropriate resource.

In order to make a complete assessment, the client, family, and environment must be considered. The questions listed below serve as an assessment guide.

The Person

1. What function does the substance serve for the client?
2. What substance(s) is (are) being abused? How much is being taken and when?
3. Who has defined the behavior as a problem?
4. What function does the problematic behavior serve for the client at the present time?
5. What factors support or maintain the client's continued drug or alcohol use?
6. In what way and to what extent does the client perceive substance abuse as a problem?
7. What particular circumstances trigger the behavior?
8. What is the client's developmental level?
9. Is the client employed? What is the pattern of employment?
10. How does the behavior affect job or role performance?
11. What are the realistic possibilities of altering the client's behavior in the present environment (home or health facility)?
12. What is the client's physical condition?
13. What are the client's dietary habits?
14. Has the client recently withdrawn from the substance?
15. Has the client ever been arrested because of substance abuse or antisocial behavior?
16. Does the client display angry, manipulative, avoidant, impulsive, or grandiose behavior patterns?

The Family

1. Is there a family history of drug or alcohol abuse?
2. What are the parenting patterns in the family? For example, are limits set? If so, are they consistent? Are moral values taught? Is there role modeling?
3. Who and where are the significant others?
4. Does the client have a special position in the family?
5. How does the client's behavior influence (alter or maintain) family roles and behavior at home?
6. What are the family's attitudes toward use of this substance?
7. What is the family's anxiety level at this time?
8. Did the client's behavior begin in connection with a significant family event?
9. What is the organizing function of the client's behavior in this family?

The Community

1. How available is the substance? How is the source of supply controlled?
2. What are the cultural attitudes toward use of this substance or this behavior?
3. Who in the client's environment also uses or abuses the substance?

4. Who else in the client's environment engages in the antisocial behavior?
5. What is the influences of the peer group?

In addition to the questions noted above, further assessment of the core behaviors of dysfunctional anger, manipulation, grandiosity, impulsiveness, and avoidance is made. Clients are observed for overt expressions of anger, for covert expressions inherent in patterns of manipulation and avoidance, and for impulsive and grandiose behaviors. The goal of observation is to determine when, how, and where the client becomes angry, acts out manipulatively, or withdraws from meaningful interpersonal relationships.

Diagnosis

Clinically, substance abuse and alcoholism overlap. It is rare to meet a "textbook case" of either. Common dynamic elements are mistrust, excessive dependency, faulty identification and learning, and low tolerance for the tensions of anxiety, guilt, and anger. Behavioral expression through patterns of dysfunctional anger, manipulation, impulsiveness, avoidance, and grandiosity form the basis for nursing diagnosis. These behaviors are not in and of themselves pathological or maladaptive; in fact, circumstances may cause such behaviors in almost anyone at one time or another. What concerns nurses is a repetitive pattern which emerges as an obstacle to healthy interpersonal relations. Table 33-6 designates specific nursing diagnoses related to the major dynamics of substance abusers.

Table 33-6 Nursing Diagnoses for Substance Abusers

Pattern	Behavioral Result
Manipulation	Legal difficulties associated with drug abuse
	Failure to honor financial obligations related to excessive use of alcohol
	Deceptive, exploitive behavior associated with manipulative behavior pattern
Impulsiveness	Inconsistent work patterns related to impulsive behavior pattern
	Recklessness associated with alcohol intoxication
	Stupor related to excessive drug ingestion
Dysfunctional anger	Irritability and aggressiveness associated with alcohol intoxication
	Explosive behavior related to alcohol withdrawal syndrome
	Excessive abusive language related to a dysfunctional, angry pattern of behavior
Avoidance	Inability to maintain attachment to a sexual partner associated with an avoidant behavior pattern
	Loss of job associated with alcoholic binge drinking
	Ineffective parenting skills related to excessive distancing through alcohol
	Inconsistency in interpersonal relationship related to avoidant behavior patterns
	Lack of community education programs associated with avoidance and denial by society
Grandiosity	Lack of concern for the feelings of others related to a grandiose behavioral pattern
	Superiority and irresponsibility related to excessive drug use
	Excessive alcohol ingestion associated with denial of physical tolerance

Outcome Criteria

The outcome criteria that are established when preparing a nursing care plan for substance abusers will depend on the client's phase of treatment. The outcome in the acute phase of treatment will be physical detoxification from the alcohol or other abused substance—that is, a safe weaning from the abused substance. The second major outcome is preventing recurrence of substance abuse cycles. Treatment also aims to resolve related health problems such as malnutrition, venereal disease, and endocrine disorders. The final goal is for the client to assume or reassume a functional role in the community. Outcome criteria are measurable behaviors that allow nurses as well as clients to assess and evaluate progress toward wellness. Table 33-7 lists some sample outcome criteria that are realistic for substance abusers.

Intervention

Intervention with substance abusers involves the efforts of several health care professionals. Nurses are integral members of the treatment team and

Table 33-7 Nursing Assessments for Substance Abusers

Outcome Criteria
Client's vital signs will remain stable for 48 hours following detoxication.
Client will verbalize willingness to discontinue use of substance.
Client will submit willingly to periodic blood and urine screening to assess continued abstinence.
Client will attend a vocational rehabilitation workshop for 2 weeks.
Client will report consistent job performance for 1 month (with no absences).
Family members of substance abusers will attend weekly therapy sessions.
Spouses of substance abusers will verbalize willingness to avoid rescuing behavior.
A substance abuse education committee will be established during the first 3 months of the coming fiscal year.

carry out interventions at all levels of care. Following are some of the facilities that cooperate in comprehensive intervention with substance abusers:

- Acute emergency care units
- Crisis intervention units
- Detoxification facilities
- Short- or long-term medical or psychiatric inpatient treatment facilities
- Halfway houses that bridge the transition to the community
- Aftercare in the home or in a day treatment center, clinic, or rehabilitation center

In this section, intervention will be discussed first in terms of current treatment approaches for alcoholics and drug abusers. Then behavioral interventions with individuals, revolving around manipulation, impulsiveness, avoidance, and grandiosity, will be presented. Finally, family and environmental intervention will be discussed.

Current Approaches to Treatment of Alcoholism

Current approaches to treatment of alcoholism encompass five aspects: (1) managing acute episodes of intoxication, (2) managing alcohol withdrawal syndrome, (3) managing Wernicke-Korsakoff syndrome, (4) managing chronic health problems associated with alcoholism, (5) repatterning the long-term behavior of alcoholics, including helping family systems to develop healthier patterns of relating.

MANAGING ACUTE EPISODES OF INTOXICATION. Detoxification entails withdrawing the client from alcohol in a controlled environment by using one of several protocols. Table 33-8 provides guidelines for management of alcohol detoxification. The setting and criteria for detoxification will depend on the institution. Nurses should participate in development as well as implementation of such protocols.

Clients who seek or require detoxification are not necessarily admitted directly to an acute treatment center. They are frequently found in hospital emergency rooms and on the various units of general hospitals. The presenting complaint may be physical trauma as a result of an "accident," another physical illness which has interrupted alcohol ingestion, or an emotional disturbance. Because of the emotional and behavioral aspects of alcohol abuse, clients may be admitted to a psychiatric facility for other emotional problems; such a facility may not be equipped to deal with detoxification. The client may be admitted with a diagnosis of depression or schizophrenia, and the staff may not initially realize that the client also has an active alcohol problem that will evidence itself within a matter of hours. For these reasons, nurses should be alert to a history of alcohol abuse or early signs of impending withdrawal. The potentially life-threatening consequences of withdrawal from excessive use of alcohol necessitate careful assessment and a well-monitored detoxification process.

In general, detoxification is done on a unit specifically set up for this purpose, which has a clearly defined detoxification protocol similar to the one outlined in Table 33-8 (page 634). Detoxification is usually completed within 1 week. During detoxification, the nurse permits the client to rest as comfortably as possible. The client must be protected from injury and observed for signs of psychological or physiological instability which suggest the development of complications such as alcohol withdrawal syndrome. Detoxification is best handled in a quiet environment where lighting is adjusted to reduce shadows and distortions in

Table 33-8 Guidelines for Management of Alcohol Detoxication

Treatment	Rationale
Complete history and physical including: complete blood count, urinalysis, venereal disease reaction level, electrocardiogram, chest x-ray.	Assessment of a client's health status is necessary to obtain data base and to plan safe holistic care.
Bed rest depending on assessment of seizure potential; seizure precautions.	Client who is in impending alcohol withdrawal syndrome has a seizure potential, therefore bed rest and other seizure precautions are indicated.
Anticonvulsant therapy: magnesium sulfate 50% solution, 2 milliliters every 8 hours IM (no more than 6 doses).	Will provide effective anticonvulsant therapy in combination with Librium.
Diet as tolerated including ad lib fluids. Intravenous fluids are not usually necessary.	Prevent dehydration by maintaining fluid balance in body.
Multivitamin supplements throughout detoxification program: Thiamine 1 gram daily IM or PO for 3–5 days.	Clients may have not been eating a balanced diet and may or may not have nervous system involvement; therefore B-complex vitamin therapy is required.
Librium PO as per schedule below. Hour 1 occurs in emergency room (ER), if client enters hospital via ER. Direct unit admissions will commence treatment as quickly as possible.	Chlordiazepoxide is used in decreasing doses for its sedating and anticonvulsant effect during detoxification.

	Hour	Dosage, mg
	1	100
	4	0–100
Day 1	8	50–100
	16	50–100
	24	50–100
Day 2	8	25–75
	16	25–75
	48	25–75
Day 3	8	0–50
	16	0–50
	72	0–50
Day 4	8	0–25
	16	0–25
	96	0–25

Then, discontinue all chlordiazepoxide.

order not to cause the client unnecessary anxiety or panic.

While a client is still intoxicated, the introduction of other chemicals into the body should be avoided if possible. This is primarily because alcohol may potentiate or compound the action of other drugs.[18] Alcohol (ethanol) acts pharmacologically as a central nervous system *depressant*. It acts to block synaptic transmission, retarding or preventing the stimulation of one neuron by another. In very large doses, alcohol apparently interferes directly with oxygen metabolism of cell bodies. Excessive alcohol ingestion often appears to alter behavior in the direction of either hilarity and high spirits or aggression and violence. This "stimulant" effect is more apparent than real. What happens is that alcohol depresses the highest cortical centers first; therefore, such altered behaviors can be understood as caused by decreased cortical inhibition and control of behavior.

Because of the progressively depressant effects of alcohol, sedation during detoxification is difficult. In general, the aim should be to prevent acute withdrawal symptoms without immobilizing the client unduly with additional sedation. Agitation that interferes with rest, sleep, or physical safety should be controlled with sedatives such as paraldehyde or tranquilizers such as chlorpromazine or chlordiazepoxide.

Detoxification is *not* a cure; it is the first step in a treatment process that is often long and arduous for both clients and health professionals. Therefore, one difficult aspect of caring for clients who are acutely intoxicated or undergoing detoxification may be the nurses' task of dealing with their own attitudes toward "drunkenness." Awareness of such attitudes is particularly important for nurses who work in emergency rooms, walk-in clinics, or other facilities where they are likely to encounter the same client repeatedly. Nurses can often use these repeated encounters to encourage and coordinate long-term treatment, but negative or despairing attitudes will prevent nurses from acting effectively in this capacity and will most likely be communicated to the client and family as well.

MANAGING ALCOHOL WITHDRAWAL SYNDROME. The aims of treatment for AWS customarily include rest, restoration of nutritional and metabolic equilibrium, prevention of seizures, reduction of fear and anxiety, and prevention of impulsive acts. Table 33-9 outlines the nursing care for the client in AWS.

One nursing measure that does not appear in Table 33-9 but deserves separate comment is the use of restraints for clients in DTs. If at all possible, the use of restraints *should be avoided* because restraint tends to agitate clients who are confused and disoriented. Clients must, however, be protected from self-injury—in which case restraints may be necessary. (See Chapter 32.)

Another important nursing aim in the care of an alcoholic client is to view the acute organic episode in the context of the client's overall, continuing needs. In other words, instead of allowing care to end with management of the acute episode, the nurse may be able at this critical point to influence the client to accept long-term therapy for the underlying chronic alcoholism. It is well within the nurse's province to take the initiative in discussing this with the client and the rest of the health team.

MANAGING THE WERNICKE-KORSAKOFF SYNDROME. Treatment of Wernicke-Korsakoff syndrome entails enforcing strict abstinence from alcohol and administration of large doses of B-complex and C vitamins. When there is severe brain damage, long-term custodial care may be required. When clients are less severely impaired, family members may be willing to offer supervision. Nurses in the hospital and in the community may be called upon to assist such clients and their families in coping with the responsibility and frustrations of long-term abstinence and care.

MANAGING CHRONIC HEALTH PROBLEMS. Alcoholism has many related physical symptoms and health problems that are associated with both acute

Table 33-9 Care of the Client with Alcohol Withdrawal Syndrome

Nursing Diganoses	Expected Outcome	Nursing Intervention
Sleep disturbance	Restore normal sleep pattern. Decrease agitation.	Assess effectiveness of chemical sedation (paraldehyde, chlordiazepoxide, chlorpromazine, hydroxyzine hydrochloride). Reduce external stimuli by speaking calmly and distinctly, adjusting lighting to prevent shadows and extremes of light and dark, restricting interpersonal contact to as a few people as possible, adjusting room temperature, eliminating extraneous noises.
Metabolic and nutritional disequilibrium	Restore fluid and electrolyte balance. Restore nutritional balance.	Force fluids as ordered. Monitor intake and output and record. Check bladder for distention. Administer high-protein, high-carbohydrate, low-fat diet. Administer vitamins B complex and C.
Potential seizures	Prevent seizures.	Administer anticonvulsant medication as needed (diphenylhydantoin). Observe seizure precautions.
Fear, anxiety, panic; impulsive, self-destructive behaviors	Reduce fear, anxiety. Prevent panic. Prevent impulsive, self-destructive behaviors.	Note signs of anxiety, agitation. Reduce external stimuli (as above). Remain with client and inform him or her of your intent to do this. Repeat as necessary. Orient client to where he or she is and to what is happening. Respond to client's fright by acknowledging client's fearfulness and emphasizing your intent to remain present. Interpret situation and surroundings to client clearly. Respond to client's reports of illusions and hallucinations by saying that these frightening sights, etc., are part of the illness and that, as improvement occurs, they will no longer bother the client. Use side rails. Assess effectiveness of chemical sedation (as above).

Table 33-10 Common Health Problems Associated with Acute and Chronic Alcohol Intoxication

Problem	Nursing Intervention
Acute health problems	
Poor nutritional status	
Loss of appetite	Provide nutritional information.
Imbalanced diet	Vitamins B complex and multivitamins.
Diarrhea Vomiting	Fluids PO: 2000 milliliters per day antiemetic and antidiarrhea medication.
No PO fluids except alcohol	Referral to community nutrition resource (for example, Meals on Wheels).
CNS dysfunction and irritability	
Tremors	Provide quiet, nonstimulating environment.
Seizures	Administer chlordiazepoxide.
Neuritis	Administer thiamine.
Motor restlessness or stupor	Administer magnesium sulfate and take precautions against seizure.
Memory loss	Explain that CNS dysfunction will decrease as alcohol leaves the system.
Sensitivity to light	Soft lighting. Glasses with tinted lenses.
Rambling, incoherent speech	Communicate in simple, direct sentences. Focus client's communications in a concrete way.
Acute health problems	
Susceptibility to recurrent respiratory infections	Administer antibiotics. Culture and sensitivity for sputum. Monitor temperature, pulse, and respiration. Chest x-ray.
Insomnia	Provide a quiet environment. Administer chlordiazepoxide.
Chronic health problems	
Liver dysfunction, cirrhosis Pancreatitis Chronic brain damage and mental deterioration	Refer for appropriate medical treatment.
Malnutrition	Provide nutritional information about foods that are easy to prepare. Refer to community resources for nutritional teaching and supervision.
Poor hygiene habits	Provide hygiene information and supervision. Involve in grooming and hygiene classes. Refer for dental care. Refer to community resource for home hygiene teaching and supervision.

intoxication and prolonged abuse. Table 33-10 summarizes common health problems associated with acute and chronic alcohol abuse and the related nursing interventions.

REPATTERNING BEHAVIOR OF ALCOHOL ABUSERS. Individual, group, and family treatment modalities are used to repattern behavior in alcohol abuse. Such treatments aim for increased self-awareness, enhanced self-esteem, assumption of appropriate roles, and improved interpersonal skills. Nurses may be involved directly in individual, group, or family treatment of alcoholics; or nursing roles may be more concerned with establishing a therapeutic milieu for alcoholic clients.

Behavior modification. In treatment of alcoholism, behavior modification is designed to modify and eliminate drinking behaviors by using basic principles of classical conditioning. The best-known aversive agent used in the treatment of alcoholism is disulfiram (Antabuse). Disulfiram blocks the action of an enzyme required for the metabolism of alcohol. When disulfiram is taken on a regular basis, the result for the client who imbibes even small amounts of alcohol is nausea, vomiting, palpitations, and general prostration. (Large doses of alcohol are highly toxic, however, and can lead to death.) The client is thus conditioned to avoid the use of alcohol. Disulfiram has sometimes been used as an adjunct to other therapeutic approaches, such as individual, group, and family therapy.[19] It is also sometimes used to provide a dry period for someone unable to abstain from alcohol in any other way. At a minimum, it gives the brain a chance to "dry out." It should be noted that the long-term physiological effects of this drug are not thoroughly understood, and its use remains controversial.

In addition to aversion therapy, innovative applications of behavior modification have included use of avoidance procedures as well as positive reinforcement techniques. Although an interpersonal relationship is not the major vehicle of this treatment modality, the accompanying elements of caring, emotional support, and encouragement are generally felt to be important for successful treatment.

Rehabilitation groups. Alcoholics Anonymous (AA) continues to be one of the major traditional approaches to alcoholism, which may or may not be accompanied by participation in other treatment modalities. It has a higher success rate than any other type of treatment program. This group is composed entirely of former alcoholics. Through education, self-help, and supportive fellowship of a strongly spiritual nature, it aims for sobriety through total abstinence from alcohol. As a primary resource for the rehabilitation of alcoholics, AA has been most successful in helping clients who can identify with the socioeconomic background of a particular chapter's membership. Referrals are most effective when contact with AA is established before the client is discharged from an acute treatment setting. The AA program focuses on group meetings at which members acknowledge their alcoholism and share their personal experiences of alcohol abuse and control. These meetings are held throughout the country, in hospitals, churches, and industrial and other community settings.

Other groups such as Al-Anon and Alateen have been formed to assist family members with the problems of alcoholism. Al-Anon is an organization of spouses and Alateen is an organization of teenage children of alcoholics. The emphasis is on education, guidance in relating to the alcoholic family member, and the sharing of problems and experiences.

Current Approaches to Treatment of Drug Abuse: Physical Problems

Treatment for drug abuse includes both inpatient and outpatient approaches. Clients may experience uncontrolled withdrawal as an unexpected acute care problem, or detoxification may occur in accordance with prescribed protocol in specially staffed facilities. Methadone maintenance and other drug-free programs are utilized for rehabilitative care.

Physical problems related to drug abuse warrant nurses' attention in terms of both direct care and health teaching. These problems are inevitably intertwined with clients' psychosocial status and most often emerge from three predisposing conditions: (1) neglect of nutritional needs, (2) administration of drugs by injection under septic conditions, and (3) the properties of the drug themselves. Table 33-11 lists specific physical disruptions associated with drug abuse and nursing interventions for each.

Another health problem includes the unanticipated side effects of several drugs that are in common use today—LSD, PCP (angel dust), and other hallucinogenic drugs. These drugs are popular with dealers because they can be synthetically made at low cost and sold to consumers at a fantastic profit. They are swallowed on sugar cubes,

Table 33-11 Health Problems of Drug Abuse

Physical Problem	Nursing Intervention
Malnutrition, including vitamin deficiencies	Provide nutritional information, particularly about foods of high value that are easily available and require little preparation.
Dental caries and loss of teeth	Explain how the drug habit gives rise to problems.
Respiratory infections	Monitor antibiotic therapy.
Skin abscesses	
Cellulitis	Assess for signs of infection.
Hepatitis	Teach clients to avoid contaminated needles, etc.
Bacterial endocarditis	Refer for appropriate medical and dental treatment.
Constipation	Provide instruction on diet and exercise.
Amenorrhea	Make a referral to a gynecologist.
Impotence	Arrange for a complete medical workup and make a referral to a urologist.
Seizures (in cocaine sniffers and during barbiturate withdrawal)	Utilize seizure precautions.

sniffed, smoked, or taken intravenously. Psychological effects vary and can be influenced by the simultaneous use of alcohol or other drugs. Problematic psychological side effects include a schizophrenic-like syndrome that may last for days or weeks; it includes paranoid delusions, command hallucinations, impulsivity and agitation, or withdrawal. In such cases the client must be protected from impulsive actions that may have fatal outcomes.

The client who has had a "bad trip" on LSD often responds positively to reassurance and can often be "talked down." However, a client who has taken PCP reacts with increased anxiety, agitation, and even violence when this technique is used. Such a client is exquisitely sensitive to auditory and visual stimuli and may vacillate rapidly from being withdrawn to being combative and agitated. The client should be placed in a quiet environment with minimum stimulation. Subsequent treatment for other residual symptoms is very similar to treatment modalities used with clients admitted for acute schizophrenic episodes.[20] Flashbacks which reevoke the visual, auditory, or emotional perceptions of the previous drug experience may reappear at varying intervals, particularly when the person is under stress, and serve to reintensify the anxiety and disorganization of the earlier drug experience.

Associated physical problems that may be life-threatening are: status epilepticus, cerebral hemorrhage, elevated blood pressure, renal failure, fluid and electrolyte imbalance, alterations in level of consciousness, and cognitive dysfunction. Nursing intervention follows traditional measures: maintaining a patent airway, following seizure precautions, monitoring vital signs, and maintaining fluid and electrolyte balance.[20,21]

Intervention with the Person

Intervention with substance abusers includes management of their manipulative, impulsive, avoidant, and grandiose behavior. The following sections suggest applicable interventions.

MANIPULATION. Nursing intervention with clients who engage in manipulative behavior is directed toward defining the relationship in terms of a mutual experience in learning and trust rather than a struggle for power and control. This involves goals that help clients (1) to increase their awareness of manipulative behavior as a problem that *curtails* their experience; (2) to recognize the feelings and thoughts that prompt the behavior; (3) to lessen the need for exploitative, deceptive, and self-destructive maneuvers; and (4) to discover and test alternative ways of relating to their interpersonal environments.

In endeavoring to assist substance abusers, it is well to remember that they are often operating at a "pretrust" level. Early expectations of solid confidence or trust are unrealistic, although on a superficial level it may appear that such a level has been reached. The pretrust nature of the clients' experience means that they cannot deal effectively with other people's expectations. In particular, their manipulative tactics are exacerbated by excessive rigidity or permissiveness, inconsistencies, or ambiguities in environmental expectations. Therefore, nursing actions in response to manipulation often take the form of *setting limits, acting as a role model,* and *providing learning experiences.* The rationale is that what the client needs from a person in authority is a reasonable, consistent, and clearly defined framework within which to learn and grow interpersonally.[22] The nurse operates on the basis of open, clear, self-actualized communication.

Setting limits. In setting limits, the nurse:

1. Defines clear expectations for the client and communicates these positively and firmly.
2. Limits only those behaviors that clearly impinge upon the health of the client, the rights and interests of others, or both. Automatic opposition to all behaviors of clients does not allow them the opportunity to discriminate among various behaviors in themselves or others.
3. Confines the *means* of limiting clients' behavior to actions that feasibly can be carried through. Empty threats or promises only reinforce the clients' idea that others are not to be depended upon.
4. Offers an alternative; often this entails encouraging the client to talk with the nurse about problem episodes.
5. Avoids making a public issue out of manipulative behavior. Bringing it up for discussion in a community meeting, for example, may revive the "contest" and in a sense reward the client for the manipulative behavior.
6. Does *not* engage in accusations, arguments, and demands for justification from the client. Again,

this only exacerbates the power struggle, which is fatiguing and futile.

7. Collaborates with all involved members of the health staff in achieving a consensus about expectations for clients' behavior and the means of approach. Conflicts among staff members about setting limits almost guarantee that the clients' manipulations will thrive; the need is to maximize clear, direct communication.

One complex issue the nurse must confront in setting limits is whether it is clients' initial needs or wants, the manipulative process itself, or both that are truly pathological or unreasonable. In some instances, a little reflection on what has occurred will show that while the want was valid, the method of expressing it was offensive and disruptive.

Common manipulations which these clients present early in a therapeutic relationship are seizing the initiative and focusing on the helper's "flaws." There is an element of role reversal in these behaviors which can easily put the nurse on the defensive.

For example, such a client often will ask nurses how they are feeling or how their day has been. The client may express an interest in the personal life and qualifications of the nurse: "I notice your pin is from ________University," or "I see that you're wearing a wedding band." While on one level these behaviors may seem sociable, they are often attempts on the part of clients to avoid discussing their own difficulties. Beyond that, they may represent efforts to prove that the nurse, like everyone else, is not really concerned about anyone but self; or that the client is not worthy of the nurse's interest or respect.

Setting limits in response to these initial behaviors is an important but delicate issue. If the nurse becomes immediately bogged down in conflicts between the client's possible motivations and how much personal information the nurse should reveal, the chances are that initial steps toward rapport and respect will be impeded by defensiveness. It is probably wise for the nurse to *notice* the client's behavior, to answer questions or comments briefly, and then to refocus on some aspect of the client's day without confronting the manipulation directly at this point. If the client's maneuvers continue, it may help for the nurse to reclarify the purpose of the interaction: "Use the time to talk about yourself," or "I'm here for you to talk with about whatever difficulties *you're* having." In this regard, nurses often state their purposes erroneously by saying, "I'm here to talk with you." Such words convey that the *nurse* will do the talking—the client is provided with a means of avoiding talk.

Role modeling. As a corollary to setting limits, the nurse acts as a role model. First, this means that the nurse is ready to give up the functions of authority when that is appropriate. Second, it implies that in representing rational authority through knowledge and competence, the nurse also has the human capacity to be fallible.

While it is important for nurses not to be naive or gullible in relation to manipulative clients, it is equally important that they demonstrate how to deal with one's own mistakes or imperfections without resorting to manipulative or crazy behavior. Probably the only way to communicate to these clients that such aspects of the self are human—and therefore tolerable—is to admit any obvious errors that may occur in relation to the client. For example, when a client boasts of outwitting the nurse, the nurse might reply casually that indeed the situation was misjudged, but that nevertheless something was learned. The message is that it is neither shameful nor virtuous to admit one's mistakes but rather a sign of mature responsibility. That enables people to learn from their mistakes and use this learning in anticipating future similar situations.

IMPULSIVENESS. Nursing intervention when the client engages in impulsive behavior is directed toward defining a relationship in terms of opportunity for long-term mutual satisfaction rather than as a source of immediate pain or pleasure. The goals involve helping clients (1) to spend time "thinking through" and talking out rather than acting out, (2) to increase awareness of and tolerance for feelings as "danger signals" which precede impulsive acts, (3) to recognize the ways in which impulsive behavior hurts oneself, and (4) to develop self-control and self-responsibility.

Setting limits. One emphasis is on providing concrete external controls while the client learns internal control. For example, the client may require a structured setting such as a residential treatment center or a day hospital where behavioral regulations restrict both substance abuse and harm to others. It also may be necessary to convey limits on impulsive behavior in an authoritative, direct manner. This is because impulsive behavior by its very nature does not permit "thinking through." There may be no opportunity to reason with clients before an impulsive act is carried out, and thus limits are needed to protect the clients and others from the consequences of the act.

Role modeling. Providing substance abusers with regular opportunities to apply problem solving to life experiences is extremely important. It takes a great deal of patience and practice to teach these clients to feel and to think. They have no faith in the validity of talk unless that talk leads to an immediate, concrete gain. The nurse will be confronted repeatedly with evidence of resentment or distrust. Such remarks as, "You're supposed to help me, but I still don't have a job" may reflect this distrust. Such attitudes can easily tempt the nurse to become defensive, too helpful, or disillusioned. If the nurse can overcome such reactions and recognize that the behavior is prompted by the client's tension rather than the nurse's failure to help, it may be possible to elicit more of the client's thoughts and feelings and problem-solving skills. In the above example, the nurse might respond by asking the client to share his or her thinking about their talks leading to a job; or the nurse might comment on the client's frustration with the perceived lack of help. The nurse may ask the client to outline the steps necessary in trying to find a job, and go on to discuss the facets involved in each step. The nurse thus invites the client to learn and at the same time presents a role model as a problem solver.

AVOIDANCE. Nursing intervention when a client uses avoidance is directed toward defining the relationship as an opportunity to experience feelings directly and safely with another person rather than as a signal for escaping feeling. The goals involve helping clients (1) to recognize and label feelings of anxiety, anger, guilt; (2) to tolerate interpersonal contact, with its attendant levels of feeling; and (3) to express thoughts and feelings in ways that are gratifying to the client and productive for interpersonal relatedness.

Providing interpersonal contact. Nursing actions frequently center on providing opportunities for interpersonal contact while at the same time respecting the client's needs for privacy and distance. Attention should not be limited to the client's "bad" moments, moments when the client is physically or emotionally withdrawn. This has the effect of rewarding the withdrawn, withholding, controlling aspects of behavior. Rather, the nurse conveys an expectation that the client will at some point wish to relate in a different way. For example:

> Bill M. was undergoing long-term hospitalization for peripherovascular disease. He had a history of alcohol and drug abuse and a long criminal record. On the unit his behavior shifted between charming concern for other clients; loud, angry demands for improved care and attention; and episodes of avoidance. During one of the avoidant episodes, Mr. M. drew the curtains around his bed, posted signs warning others not to disturb him, and, to all appearances, went to sleep. As a care giver in the situation, the nurse felt concern and yet wondered about the wisdom of intruding on Mr. M.'s territory. The nurse finally spoke to Mr. M., who barely responded, and asked him what the trouble was. When Mr. M. did not reply, the nurse said that she would return in an hour and perhaps Mr. M. would like to share his thoughts then. When the nurse returned, Mr. M was sitting up and talked for a while, although the curtains remained closed.

In this incident, the nurse was primarily concerned with providing contact and communicating some expectation that the client would make use of the contact.

Facilitating recognition and expression of feelings. When nurses observe signs of mood change or avoidance, they should ask clients what they are feeling. Often the response will be noncommittal, a denial of feeling, or a response that does not answer the question. "Try talking about what you're feeling," and "If you're upset, it would be useful to talk about it," suggest that it's human to feel and that verbal expressions of feelings are more comprehensible interpersonally than unverbalized, acted-out feelings.

Setting limits. In maintaining a pattern of avoidance through the use of substances, limits are usually set on access to the substance as well as on behaviors associated with securing and administering the substance. These limits are implemented through milieu controls, such as peer pressures, and rules and regulations of the treatment setting. Such environmental limitations may indeed increase anger and anxiety, but the clients are thereby faced with an opportunity to recognize these feelings and cope in ways other than chemically induced euphoria or oblivion. Structure for clients that specifies regular one-to-one and group interaction sessions calls for adherence to others' expectations and increasing one's levels of tolerance for involvement and anxiety.

GRANDIOSITY. Nursing intervention with the client who is grandiose is directed toward defining a *relationship* as an opportunity for recognizing and developing one's real competence, worth, and responsibilities—not as a situation that allows clients to demonstrate their superiority or unconcern for the real effects of their behavior on themselves and others. The goals involve helping clients (1) to use those attributes within themselves that are positive, (2) to act with an increased sense of responsibility for their own behaviors, and (3) to recognize realistic limitations to their influence over people and situations.

Nursing actions, as with diagnoses of manipulation and impulsiveness, often involve setting limits, role modeling, and providing learning opportunities. These actions are often integrated in actual practice and will be presented in that way.

The tendencies of substance abusers to be unrealistic about their motivations and behaviors, as well as the consequences of their acts, are often manifested in denial, rationalization, arrogance, or irresponsibility. Nurses have to determine to what extent and when they should set limits by "pointing out reality" to such clients. Considerable controversy exists about whether it is wise to confront a client's defenses directly. The ability of these clients to cope with confrontation in relation to their grandiose themes is largely dependent upon the confronter's relationship with that client. This may be so for two reasons. First, the client may have developed some degree of rapport or trust with a given nurse, which allows that client to respect that nurse's judgment. Second, the nurse may have developed a sensitivity that allows for an accurate clinical judgment of a client's ability to cope with confrontation at a given time. At the root of the confrontation decision are the following questions:

> To what extent is the behavior interfering with the client's physical and psychosocial adaptation at this time?
>
> To what extent does the client need this defense at this moment in order to survive?

The nurse does not have to make the decision alone; consulting with colleagues for validation is often valuable.

Denial and rationalization of feelings and behaviors characterize stages that the particular client is going through. Alcoholics, for example, may gradually give up these behaviors as they discover an ability to be trusting and to tolerate anxiety. There is, however, some agreement that substance abusers need to be confronted about their habits of substance abuse.

Another way the grandiose theme manifests itself is in clients' elaborate or vague plans for the future. It is well to question, through a mutual problem-solving process, some of the clients' conclusions about themselves. For example:

> A client, Mr. Y., mentions that he's going to get a job and everything will be OK. The nurse responds by asking Mr. Y. when he began to think about getting a job. The focus is on the thinking aspect; there is no direct attack on the client's capabilities or his real situation.

Clients who abuse substances often demonstrate a blatant lack of concern for the consequences of their actions. The question about confrontation in this instance is not so much whether the client can tolerate it but to what extent confrontation will reinforce the client's familiar "bad me" self-concept and thereby exacerbate irresponsibility and arrogance. Again, to reduce the latter aspect, it is probably better for the nurse to set the necessary limits as directly, quickly, and privately as possible. The more noise, attention, and people involved, the more likely the person is to retain dreams of superior influence.

It is useful for nurses (1) to provide realistic feedback for clients, (2) to set realistic goals, (3) to break problems down into manageable subproblems that can be handled one step at a time, and (4) to demonstrate acceptance of responsibility for their own behavior. If nurses present themselves as nondefensive in the face of errors in judgment and other imperfections, clients may observe that the outcome for the nurses and thus for themselves may not be catastrophic.

Intervention with the Family

As was noted earlier, substance abuse involves the whole family. Nurses work with families of alcoholics and drug abusers which have potential or actual substance-abuse problems. Interventions may be aimed at preventing or repatterning problematic behaviors within the family system.

FAMILY EDUCATION. Nurses practicing in community health settings assess family communication patterns and child-rearing practices. They identify early patterns of parental rejection, indifference, and inconsistency.

Assessment of these family dynamics may lead to early counseling of parents about children's problems. For example, parents who complain that their children are "too dependent" or "unmanageable" may offer the nurse an opportunity to explore developmental behaviors that tend to generate anger in others. Specifically, parents may need assistance in handling such behaviors as tantrums, food fads, hunger strikes, and separation anxiety. It is important to assess problem behaviors before alcoholism, drug abuse, or antisocial behavior becomes chronic and disruptive. Nurses listen for clues to anxiety, depression, frustration, and conflict. When such feelings within the family are elicited, the nurse should encourage clients to tell how they seek relief. If the "relief" is problematic, then nurse and clients can explore alternatives.

Actions and comments by all family members are significant in that they convey information about family problems. For example, one might question why a teenager does not come home at night or why a child spends too much time at home. The stress to which the teenager or the child is responding may be substance abuse by another member of the family.

In addition to working directly with affected families, nurses can refer families to community programs—educative programs and programs established to prevent substance abuse. Mothers Against Drunk Driving (MADD) is only one of many such programs. Clearly, family education entails full-scale community efforts.

FAMILY THERAPY. When a specific problem with alcohol or other drugs is identified, family therapy is indicated where possible. This is particularly true if the substance abuser is an adolescent or a parent. Nurses may decide to work with the nonabusing spouse, the children, or the whole family. When substance abuse is involved, much of the process is educational.

Nurses work with nonabusing *spouses* to help them (1) learn about alcoholism, drug abuse, and antisocial behavior; (2) recognize and alter their own problematic coping behaviors; (3) identify their own part in facilitating the process; (4) stop blaming their partner for the current situation; and (5) reach realistic decisions about their own present and future welfare.[23]

The impact of substance abuse on *children* is complex. Family loyalty becomes important: children wonder if they should love a parent who hurts them and makes them feel ashamed, who doesn't provide money for rent or food, who is absent or unavailable much of the time, who members of the family say is bad, and who makes the other parent unhappy. In an effort to help children sort out such feelings, the nurse tries to help them (1) understand that the affected parent is a human being who has problems, (2) understand the situation as a family problem, (3) identify strengths of the affected parent which they can call on, (4) sort out their own feelings toward the affected parent (as distinguished from the rest of the family's feelings), (5) take a position on their own feelings about the parent, (6) express their positive and negative feelings toward the parent, (7) identify ways of moving closer to the parent in nonthreatening ways, and (8) accept the fact that for now they may not be able to have a relationship with the affected parent.

Children often have ambivalent feelings about parents who abuse substances. On the one hand, they love them and want to be with them, but on the other hand, they feel rage, shame, and hatred because of the impact the parent's behavior has on them. In addition, they may feel guilty about these feelings.[24] Nurses can be most useful when they help children to accept ambivalence as inherent in the situation, without feeling disloyal, and when they teach clients how to reduce the reactive distancing that so commonly occurs. But sometimes the most a nurse can do is help the child find a way to maintain some connection with the parent.

When working with the *whole family,* the nurse deals with the dysfunctional structure, relationship, and communication patterns of the system. The nurse should keep in mind that the family will want to focus on the problem—the drinking, drug taking, stealing, or whatever—because this provides an organizing focus for the family that enables the members to obscure underlying issues. Dynamics and interventions for use with whole families, as outlined in Chapter 19, are applicable to families where substance abuse is the issue.

Intervention with the Community

At the community level, intervention in substance abuse problems involves services to individual clients and large-scale educational programs. The goal is prevention of substance abuse and enforcement of legal constraints to deter the use of illicit substances.

COMMUNITY RESOURCES. Several community treatment programs are available for active treatment of drug and alcohol abuse. Nurses need to be familiar with local agencies so that they can make appropriate referrals. For people who no longer have support systems—such as family or fellow employees—upon whom they can depend, a significant need is rehabilitation resources. Substance abusers succeed so well, through their offensive behaviors, in alienating family and community that they frequently are in need of these comprehensive services. Nurses can also assist clients by referring them for vocational rehabilitation. This type of referral may be done through private programs or through the Division of Vocational Rehabilitation, a public service.

The use of groups is an integral aspect of many treatment approaches to substance abuse. Alcoholics Anonymous and Narcotics Anonymous (NA) are groups that provide support and motivate clients to achieve and maintain sobriety. Community and milieu approaches often call upon such groups to provide lecture presentations and discussions of the problems of substance abuse and addiction.

Halfway houses are an example of resources offering group living, referral for ongoing treatment, and, in some cases, close health supervision. Community nurses may work in the home setting to provide health supervision in the areas of hygiene, nutrition, exercise, living arrangements, and use of community resources.

Groups also provide assistance in breaking through the denial and rationalization that characterize substance abuse and antisocial behavior. Group members are encouraged to confront one another on substance-abusive or antisocial behavior, and to respond directly to confrontation by acknowledging feelings evoked in the process. Emphasis is on facing the "here and now" of interpersonal experience. Group methods are particularly useful with adolescents, with whom the developmental need is to strengthen peer relationships and to separate from significant adults.

INDUSTRIAL RESOURCES. Industrial health programs are receiving increased attention as a major environmental means of identifying and treating substance-abuse problems. Programs developed in industry often involve educating supervisory personnel to recognize early warning signs of alcohol abuse and to overcome prejudices about alcoholism.[19] In addition to providing such training, industrial health personnel—physicians and nurses—are in a position to detect substance abuse directly, particularly during physical examinations. Nurses in industrial health practice can be instrumental in bringing to the attention of employers and union leaders the need for definitive policies on substance abuse. Nurses can be innovative in developing programs that incorporate the family. One thing noted repeatedly in effective industrial health programs is that both management and unions are involved.

RESOURCES FOR CHILDREN. The rise in children's abuse of substances signals a corresponding need for school nurses to implement programs designed to confront this problem. Often school is the first place where changes in a child's behavior are noted.[25] Programs are needed that alert teachers to early signs and help them deal with their own attitudes toward substance abuse and antisocial behavior. The community can also be educated about the problems of substance abuse through lecture presentations to political, social, and religious groups. In addition, a nursing priority should be to support the use of public media to combat rather than encourage these behaviors. Because cocaine, for example, is glamorized in the media, equal time to present its untoward effects is needed.[26,27]

NEED FOR CONTINUING RESEARCH. Finally, nurses can use their expertise to encourage systematic study of the problems of substance abuse and antisocial behavior. Clearly, the nature of these difficulties is not thoroughly understood. Considering the numbers of substance abusers who populate corrections systems and health agencies—and considering as well the human suffering involved—the problems of substance abusers and antisocial personalities deserve continued research.

Evaluation

In order to make judgments about the effectiveness of interventions, nurses need to periodically evaluate person, family, and community interventions. Behavioral changes related to outcome criteria established at the beginning of treatment form the basis for evaluation strategies. Several questions facilitate the process: Has the impulsive client learned to interrupt others' conversations and activities less? Does the client use more time in problem solving? Does he or she carry out the plans that are verbalized during treatment? Has substance abuse stopped, or is it under control? Do family members have the resources to cooperate with the treatment plan? Are the messages between and among family members clearer? What do these changes mean? Nurses analyze behavioral outcomes so that their interventions may be altered appropriately. Table 33-12 illustrates the evaluation of a specific behavior related to a client who is a substance abuser:

> Mr. K. is a 33-year-old man who was admitted 3 weeks ago to an acute psychiatric treatment center. At the time of admission, he was hallucinating and verbalized paranoid delusions about ghosts and cemeteries. An initial diagnosis of schizophrenia was made. Within a few hours the nurses observed several physical symptoms. Mr. K. was diaphoretic, complained of headache, had vomited, and registered unstable vital signs. A new diagnosis of alcohol withdrawal syndrome was made. Mr. K. was transferred to the detoxification center at the same hospital.

Table 33-12 Evaluation: Case Study of Alcohol Abuse (Mr. K.)

Assessment	Diagnosis	Outcome Criteria	Intervention	Evaluation
Is there a family history of alcohol abuse? What particular circumstances trigger Mr. K.'s binge drinking episodes? What are the realistic possibilities of altering Mr. K.'s behavioral patterns? Is a family or community support system available to Mr. K.? What physical problems remain following Mr. K.'s detoxification? Has Mr. K. attended AA? Have family members been involved in Al-Anon or other support groups?	Legal difficulties associated with episodic drinking Inconsistent work patterns related to impulsive behavior pattern Inconsistency in interpersonal relationships related to avoidant behavior patterns Superiority and irresponsibility related to grandiose personality style Periodic excessive alcohol ingestion associated with denial of physical tolerance	Client will contact lawyer to discuss legal difficulties and formulate structured time-bonded solutions. Client will verbalize willingness to meet with vocation counselor. Client will attend and participate in daily meetings while hospitalized. Client will assume responsibility for his personal grooming. Client will contribute to functioning of therapeutic community by assuming responsibility for cleanliness of the dining room while he is hospitalized. Family members will participate in weekly family therapy meetings. Mr. K.'s wife will verbalize a willingness to attend Al-Anon meetings.	High-carbohydrate diet and vitamin supplements. Group therapy five times a week. Encourage plans to attend AA meetings after discharge. Encourage Mr. K. to assume responsibility for personal grooming and job in the therapeutic community. Insight-oriented therapy sessions twice a week. Arrange family therapy meetings and job counseling. Encourage Mr. K. to arrange meeting with his lawyer. Set limits on Mr. K.'s avoidant and inconsistent behavioral patterns.	At the end of 1 week, Mr. K. agreed to cooperate with the treatment plan. The family expressed willingness to cooperate in family treatment meetings. Mr. K. remained sober. Mr. K. gained weight, and his physical condition stabilized. Frequency of client's boasting about binge drinking episodes has decreased. Participation in group has been minimal. He has been absent twice and nonverbal when present. Discuss further involvement in group during individual counseling session. Suspend unit privileges until client is more cooperative.

When detoxification was complete, Mr. K. requested rehabilitative services. He is currently hospitalized at a veterans' hospital, on an alcohol treatment unit. His nurse has noted that he is occasionally irritable and aggressive and brags about his drinking binges and arrests. He reports that he has not held a steady job for the past 5 years.

SUMMARY

Substance abuse is a behavioral pattern that involves the physical, mental, and spiritual dimensions of the client. Abused substances include alcohol and both legal and illicit drugs.

Alcoholism is a major health problem in the United States. It cuts across all personality and diagnostic categories. The physiological syndromes associated with alcoholism are alcohol addiction, alcohol withdrawal syndrome, delirium tremens, and Wernicke-Korsakoff syndrome. A variety of biological, psychological, and sociocultural factors are interrelated in alcoholic behavior.

Drug abuse and alcoholism are not mutually exclusive, but *drug abuse* is defined as repeated use of a chemical substance or substances other than alcohol in a way that is harmful to self and society. Attempts to distinguish between drug habituation and drug addiction are often unsuccessful, and the term *drug dependence* is now commonly used.

Problematic behavioral patterns of substance abusers include dysfunctional anger, manipulation, impulsiveness, avoidance, and grandiosity.

The nursing process facilitates planned care of substance abusers. Assessment, diagnosis, establishing outcome criteria, intervention, and evaluation are functions of nurses involved in the care of substance abusers.

REFERENCES

1. J. W. Woodell, "Alcohol Withdrawal Syndrome," *Family and Community Health,* vol. 2, no. 2, 1979, pp. 23–30.
2. P. K. Burkhalter, *Nursing Care of the Alcoholic and the Drug Abuser,* McGraw-Hill, New York, 1975.
3. R. Hughes and R. Brewin, *The Tranquilizing of America: Pill Popping and the American Way of Life,* Harcourt, Brace, Jovanovich, New York, 1979.
4. P. Steinglass, "Experimenting with Family Treatment Approaches to Alcoholism, 1950–1975," *Family Process,* vol. 15, no. 1, March 1976, pp. 97–123.
5. American Psychiatric Association, *Diagnostic and Statistical Manual of Mental Disorders,* 3d ed., APA, Washington, D.C., 1979.
6. Metropolitan Life Insurance Co., "Alcohol and Other Drug Abuse among Adolescents," *Statistical Bulletin,* vol. 65, no. 1, January–March 1984, p. 4.
7. National Institute on Alcohol Abuse and Alcoholism, *Alcohol Abuse and Women: A Guide to Getting Help,* U.S. Government Printing Office, Washington, D.C., 1978.
8. R. R. Carr and E. J. Mayer, "Marijuana and Cocaine: The Process of Change in Drug Poligy," in Drug Abuse Council, *The Facts about Drug Abuse,* Free Press, New York, 1980, pp. 153–189.
9. A. Singer, "Mothering Practices and Heroin Addiction," *American Journal of Nursing,* vol. 74, no. 1, January 1974, pp. 77–82.
10. W. H. Reid, *The Psychopath: A Comprehensive Study of Antisocial Disorders and Behaviors,* Brunner/Mazel, New York, 1978.
11. R. A. Mackinnon and R. Michels, *The Psychiatric Interview in Clinical Practice,* Saunders, Philadelphia, 1971, pp. 297–338.
12. B. Bersten, *The Manipulator: A Psychoanalytic View,* Yale University Press, New Haven, 1973.
13. N. Krasner, J. S. Madden, and R. J. Walker, *Alcohol Related Problems: Room for Maneuver,* Wiley, New York, 1984.
14. W. P. Arentgen, "Impact of Alcohol Misuse on Family Life," *Alcoholism: Clinical and Experimental Research,* vol. 2, no. 4, 1978, pp. 349–351.
15. K. Brooks, "Adult Children of Alcoholics: Psychosocial Stages of Development," *Focus on Family and Chemical Dependency,* vol. 6, no. 5, September–October 1983.
16. M. Klagsburn and D. Davis, "Substance Abuse and Family Interaction," *Family Process,* July 1977, pp. 149–173.
17. J. Defoe, W. Breed, and L. A. Breed, "Drinking on Television: A Five-Year Study," *Journal of Drug Education,* vol. 13, no. 1, 1983, pp. 25–38.
18. J. Coleman and W. Evans, "Drug Interactions with Alcohol," *Alcohol Health and Research World,* Winter 1975–1976, pp. 16–19.
19. A. Knauert, "The Treatment of Alcoholism in a Community Setting," *Family and Community Health,* vol. 2, no. 1, 1979, pp. 91–102.
20. C. Vourakis and G. Bennett, "Angel Dust: Not Heaven Sent," *American Journal of Nursing,* vol. 79, no. 4, April 1979, pp. 649–653.
21. "The Deadly Delights of Cocaine," *Emergency Medicine,* February 28, 1983, pp. 67–81.

22. G. G. Lyon, "Limit Setting as a Therapeutic Tool," *Journal of Psychiatric Nursing and Mental Health Services,* vol. 8, no. 6, 1970, pp. 17–24.
23. M. Bowen, "Alcoholism," *The Family,* vol. 1, no. 4, November 1973, pp. 18–25.
24. E. Kaufman and P. Kaufman, eds., *Family Therapy of Drug and Alcohol Abuse,* Gardner, New York, 1979.
25. J. E. Clute, "Aiding the 'Other' Victims on the Job," *Occupational Health and Safety,* vol. 49, no. 2, 1980, pp. 34–38.
26. H. S. Mittleman, R. E. Mittleman, and B. Elser, "Cocaine," *American Journal of Nursing,* vol. 84, no. 9, 1984, pp. 1092–1095.
27. Stephanie Brown, *Treating the Alcoholic: A Developmental Model of Recovery,* Wiley, New York, 1985.

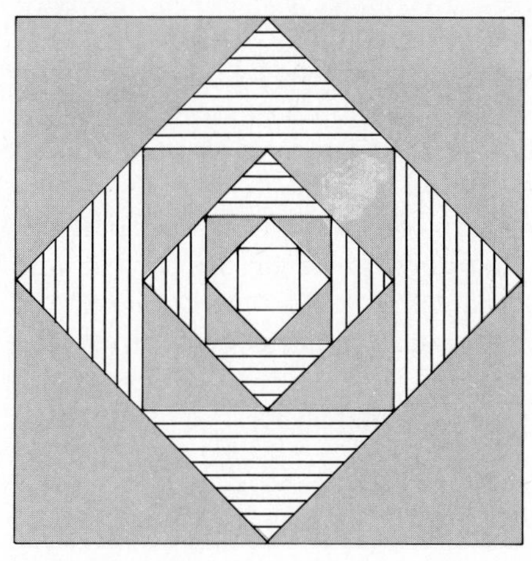

CHAPTER 34
Patterns of Depression

Norine J. Kerr

LEARNING OBJECTIVES

After studying this chapter, the student should be able to:

1. Identify dysynchronous health patterns associated with mild, moderate, and severe levels of depression in terms of:
   a. Affective changes
   b. Cognitive changes
   c. Behavioral changes
   d. Physiological changes
2. Discuss individual, family, and environmental patterns of interaction associated with depression.
3. Discuss depression as a multidimensional syndrome.
4. Identify assessment factors for the client, family, and environment.
5. Formulate nursing diagnoses for depressed clients.
6. Formulate realistic short- and long-term outcome criteria for depressed clients.
7. Differentiate nursing interventions appropriate for clients with mild, moderate, and severe levels of depression.
8. Evaluate the effectiveness of a nursing care plan for a depressed client.

Descriptions of depression are nearly as old as written documents; recognizable accounts of depressive states occur in ancient Egyptian, Greek, and biblical texts. Feelings of sadness, disappointment, and frustration are within the natural context of human experience, and the distinction between such normal moods and depression is not always clear.

The baseline for normal healthy functioning is "feeling good." Healthy people feel good most of the time in the things they do: their relationships, their work, their recreation, and their movement. Occasionally, their pleasure rises to joy and even ecstasy. They also occasionally experience pain, sadness, sorrow, and disappointment. However, they regain their faith and hope when the pain or disappointment is alleviated or heals. A healthy person who feels blue will light up at the prospect of pleasure. But nothing evokes a response from the depressed person; often the promise of a good time or pleasure serves only to deepen the sense of depression. In severe depression, lack of responsiveness is clearly evident. Severely depressed people may sit in a chair and stare at nothing in particular for hours on end. They may lie in bed throughout a good part of the day, unable to find the energy to move into the mainstream of life.

Others who suffer from depression are not so disabled, and may be able to carry on the daily routine of living. They may have jobs they seem to handle adequately. Or they may be housewives and mothers who perform the necessary activities, or college students who manage to get the grades that are needed. But these people may still be depressed in their emotional aliveness or responsiveness. Feeling heavy-hearted and weighed down, they may lack the inner excitement that would add verve to their lives. They carry on, but with a determination that is often grim and with a rigidity that constricts any sense of inner aliveness. The grimness, rigidity, and dullness of their inner life are clearly manifested in their bodies, and directly reflected in their lives.

An interrelatedness between body, mind, and spirit is evident in the depressed person. Depressed people have lost faith in themselves and other people, in life, and in a higher power, whatever they understand that power to be. They are people whose spirits are oppressed, whose minds are filled with despairing thoughts, and whose bodies are sluggish, dull, and unalive. Only when all these interrelated factors are understood can the nurse hope to transform the depressed person's shattered view of life into one which holds a reasonable basis for hope, faith, and freedom from the temptation to despair.

The purpose of this chapter is to explore patterns of depression that develop within the person, and in relation to the family and environment. The section on the nursing process will propose a systematic framework for addressing the health needs of depressed clients.

DYSYNCHRONOUS HEALTH PATTERNS

Depression, as a dysynchronous health pattern, refers to moods and conditions of responsiveness that range from mild and transitory to severe, intense, pervasive, and persistent. Conceptualizing depression on a continuum highlights its dynamic nature; that is, its *duration* may vary from brief to ongoing, sustained episodes, and the *intensity* and *pervasiveness* of symptoms may be mild, moderate, or severe. Depressions may change qualitatively as they deepen or lift. For example, the mood of the moderately depressed person may be one of sadness and pessimism, whereas the mood of the same person with deepening depression may change to hopelessness. However, because of the holistic nature of a person, it is often difficult to sharply define the boundary between two levels of depression.

Levels of Depression

Behaviors associated with depression can be classified into affective, physiological, cognitive, and behavioral manifestations. While not all people exhibit all of them, most people experiencing depression exhibit clusters of behaviors from each category. At each level of depression, the manifestations within each of the categories will vary in occurrence, intensity, pervasiveness, and duration.

Mild Depression

Mild depression is characterized by its transitory nature. It is often precipitated by events in a person's life, but it may occur for no clearly definable reason. Events that may trigger mild depression include disappointments at school or work, such as failure on a test and failure to receive a promotion.

The loss of someone or something highly valued and meaningful, such as a friend, lover, family member, home, or job, ordinarily brings on deep sadness of limited duration. Such an experience is a normal reaction: grief (see Chapter 3).[1] A cross-cultural study of grief and mourning in 78 cultures indicated that the mourning process and the accompanying state of grief are a universal human response,[2] although the specific form of emotional expression varies from culture to culture. Generally, when the loss is acknowledged and the accompanying feelings are expressed and worked through, grief tends to be of limited duration.

Without this adaptive response to loss, the grieving process may be distorted, and a deeper depression may evolve. In other cases, the grief may lie dormant for weeks, months, or years and then be reactivated. Or sadness may persist over time and progressively intensify.

The manifestations of a mild, transitory depression are almost exclusively emotional in nature, as distinguished from those of moderate and severe levels of depression. Mildly depressed people describe themselves as feeling sad, blue, downcast, or down in the dumps. They may feel let down or disappointed. People with mild depression may, however, describe mild physiological changes such as alterations in sleep patterns; they either have difficulty sleeping or can't get enough sleep and continue to feel fatigued.

Even though mild depression is largely characterized by emotional changes, there may be some cognitive effects; people may feel less alert to the environment or describe having difficulty concentrating or thinking logically or productively. There may also be some behavioral manifestations; people may be tearful and cry, may feel inclined to withdraw, may be irritable with others, and may generally seem socially uninterested. They can, however, pull themselves together for a period of time. They may increase their use of alcohol or drugs to try to diminish their low mood.[2]

Moderate Depression

People experiencing a moderate level of depression are more likely to experience their condition as a "change" (they seem unlike themselves) which persists over time, and often leads them to seek help.[3] Moderate affective, cognitive, behavioral, and physiological changes occur.

AFFECTIVE CHANGES. Moderately depressed people describe their mood as one of despondency, dejection, and gloom. Feelings of low self-esteem contribute to feelings of powerlessness, helplessness, and ineffectiveness. Anxiety and anger may or may not be felt; if they are felt, they may be intense. Both depression and anxiety may show diurnal variation; that is, a pattern of changes whereby certain times of the day, such as morning and evening, are consistently better or worse. People who are moderately depressed describe themselves as unable to experience pleasure from activities they ordinarily enjoy; their joie de vivre seems to have vanished.

COGNITIVE CHANGES. These people's thoughts are slowed, and their interests are narrow. Concentration becomes difficult; and indecisiveness and self-doubt are common. Their thoughts tend to be ruminative; they go over and over the same content and issues with no movement forward or recognition of alternatives. Their thoughts have an obsessional quality. A pessimistic outlook that includes self-blame combines to create a hopeless attitude about the possibility of change or the motivation to change. Suicidal thoughts may intrude as an aspect of hopelessness.

BEHAVIORAL CHANGES. Depressed people tend to withdraw socially. Initially, the withdrawal may appear to be simply a reluctance to socialize or interact with others. It may extend to other spheres of life such as school, work, and community involvement. Tears and irritability may be evident, seemingly with no provocation. Changes in personal hygiene may be noted. A formerly meticulous, stylishly dressed person may begin to appear at work with unwashed, uncombed hair and wrinkled, uncoordinated clothes. There may also be a slowing of movement and speech (psychomotor retardation) or agitated, increasing, but aimless activity, such as pacing. Some such people will escalate their normal use of alcohol or drugs in an attempt to anesthetize their depression, anxiety, or anger.

PHYSIOLOGICAL CHANGES. It is very common for people with moderate levels of depression to experience somatic complaints such as headaches, chest or back pains, indigestion, nausea, and vomiting or constipation. Frequently, they will seek medical care for these symptoms without associating them with other affective, cognitive, or behavioral changes. Only after a thorough biopsychosocial assessment does the true nature of their problem emerge. Some depressed people also have anorexia, frequently accompanied by weight loss. Others overeat and gain weight. Menstrual changes such as amenorrhea are common, as is decreased sexual desire and responsiveness. Feelings of fatigue and weakness persist regardless of the amount of rest. Sleep disturbances are common. Sleep is desired but not satisfying. Some depressed people sleep a great deal; others, who are anxious as well, may have difficulty falling asleep (initial insomnia), may wake up during sleep and return to sleep only with difficulty (middle insomnia), or may experience early-morning awakening (terminal insomnia).

Severe Depression

People who experience severe depression have intense, pervasive, and persistent manifestations of depression. Life seems to have come to a standstill, and they may have alterations in their reality orientation. Severe depression may or may not include a psychotic dimension.

AFFECTIVE CHANGES. Despair and hopelessness are the predominant feelings experienced with severe depression. There seems to be no light at the end of the dark tunnel. Upon observation, the person displays *flat affect,* a mood that is unchanging regardless of what occurs. Feelings of worthlessness and guilt are evident. The person feels of no value to self or others and frequently assumes responsibility for real or imagined wrongdoings. A sense of isolation and loneliness pervades the self; the person feels cut off from human connectedness. An overwhelming feeling of bottomless emptiness envelops the severely depressed person.

COGNITIVE CHANGES. Confusion, inability to concentrate, and indecisiveness are evident. Severely depressed people have no interest in mobilizing themselves, and no motivation to do so. Intense self-blame and self-depreciation reinforce their feelings of worthlessness and guilt. Self-destructive thoughts occur as a solution to the hopelessness of their situation, and the wish to die is common. However, because of the severity of the depression they rarely have the energy or clarity of thought to organize and act on such thoughts. Misinterpretations of reality (which may represent a psychotic dimension of depression) may be present, as well as delusional thinking or hallucinations or both. Delusions usually confirm these people's feelings of worthlessness, guilt, and powerlessness. A common delusion is that they are being persecuted because of sinfulness or some inadequacy. They may have delusions of causing personal destruction or even worldwide destruction, somatic delusions (cancer, for example), or delusions of poverty.

BEHAVIORAL CHANGES. Severely depressed people develop psychomotor retardation; that is, their motor activity comes to a near halt. These people can sit immobile for hours on end. Walking is slow and appears to consume great effort. There is such a lack of spontaneity that they often look like robots. Or, in contrast, frantic, aimless, agitated pacing may occur, along with gestures such as pulling the hair and rubbing the skin, hair, or clothing. There may also be outbursts of complaining or shouting. Posture is poor; when resting the person often sits slumped or curled up. There is a markedly decreased amount of speech (an effect sometimes called *poverty of speech*). Speech may be slowed, with increased pauses before answering, or it may be low and monotonous. Such people do not attend to their hygiene needs and have a disheveled, unkempt appearance. Social withdrawal from family and friends is common. What to the observer appears to be a simple task is often viewed by the depressed person as a complex and overwhelming demand.

PHYSIOLOGICAL CHANGES. Just as the behavioral aspects of the person have slowed, so does the physiological domain. Elimination is sluggish; constipation is common. There may be urinary retention, amenorrhea, lack of sexual interest, and impotence. Sometimes there is a marked loss of weight caused both by anorexia and by lack of motivation to prepare food and to eat. Initial, middle, or terminal insomnia may be evident; terminal insomnia is most common, with despondent thoughts occurring on awakening. In contrast, hypersomnia, or excessive sleeping, can also occur. The person often feels worse in the morning but better as the day progresses.[1,4]

DSM III

In the *Diagnostic and Statistical Manual of Mental Disorders* (DSM III) *depression* is categorized as an affective disorder. Mild depression is referred to as a *reactive depression*—that is, depression precipitated by environmental events such as a loss. Moderate depression is classified as a *dysthymic disorder* or *depressive neurosis;* it is characterized by a chronic mood disturbance involving either a depressed mood or loss of pleasure or interest in all or almost all usual activities and pastimes. Associated features are similar to those of major depressive episodes, except that there are no delusions or hallucinations.[5] Severe depression is classified as a *major depressive episode.* It may also be referred to as a *psychotic* or *endogenous depression.* The depressed mood and loss of pleasure and interest are prominent, relatively persistent, and associated with other, previously described symptoms, including delusions and hallucinations that are mood-congruent. Sometimes a major depressive episode will alternate with a manic episode. This is called *bipolar disorder* and is discussed in detail in Chapter 35.

Epidemiology

The prevalence of depression is difficult to estimate. It is thought that approximately 15 percent of the population are experiencing depression at any given time. However, statistics from hospitals, clinics, and other mental health agencies indicate only a fraction of the incidence of depression in the population at large. The difficulty in assessing the actual prevalence of depression stems from problems of definition and diagnosis; that is, depression manifests itself in many ways and appears in varying degrees of intensity and duration. For example, in one person depression may be clearly identifiable; in another person back pain or headaches may be the predominant symptom, although a depressed mood is also present. A person may be given a diagnosis which does not even include the word *depression* and yet be decidedly depressed. A more accurate approach to the collection of epidemiological data would be to conduct a field study surveying the entire population of a specific geographic area for symptoms suggestive of depression (such as tiredness, sadness, sleep difficulties, and lack of interest and pleasure in usual activities) rather than symptoms actually diagnosed and treated as depression.

The epidemiological data that do exist indicate that depression is a major mental health problem. These data reveal that:

1. Some 400,000 clients per year are treated for depression in the United States, most as outpatients or by nonpsychiatric physicians.
2. Between 50 and 80 percent of all suicides are attributed to depression.
3. As many as 75 percent of all psychiatric hospitalizations are related to depressive episodes.
4. There is a high incidence of depression among clients hospitalized for medical illness, and much of this depression is unrecognized and hence untreated by providers of health care. Certain types of health problems have been frequently associated with depression, especially gastrointestinal (35 percent), neurological (21 percent), and respiratory (20 percent).[6]
4. The incidence of depression is 2 times higher among women than among men. However, depression in men is probably higher than reported statistics suggest. Men may feel less free about revealing tiredness, sadness, sleep difficulties, weight problems, and social changes, and thus may be more likely to carry depressions which remain unreported. Depression is often masked by alcohol or drug abuse or somatization.[7]
5. Depression is positively correlated with increasing age in most studies. However, in a recent field study in the United States, young people showed at least as much depression as middle-aged people and possibly more. Symptoms of depression in different age groups are not necessarily similar. For example, depression in adolescence is often characterized by rebellious, acting-out, or delinquent behavior.[7,8]

PATTERNS OF INTERACTION: PERSON

The existence of depression has been explained by numerous theoretical models which identify the dynamics that provide the foundation for the development of depression. Some of the theories conflict with another, some are supported by research and some are not, and certainly not all of them are applicable to any one person. Rather, they represent the range of major theories that propose to explain depression. Selected for presentation in this chapter are theories related to ego functioning, unresolved mourning, object loss, cognitive processes, learned helplessness, entitlement depression, and genetic and biochemical factors.

Ego Functioning

The core function of the ego is to provide a sense of self-identity, a sense of reality, and the adaptive use of defense mechanisms. The dynamic interplay that occurs between existing ego strengths and external factors is relevant in determining whether a depression will be mild, moderate, or severe. Bellak[9] has identified several categories of ego functioning that can be used as a model for understanding levels of depression and their associated behaviors. These include: reality testing; judgment; sense of reality of the world and the self; regulation of drive, affect, and impulses; object relations; thought processes; and stimulus barrier. When ego functions are relatively intact, there is a greater tendency for depression to be mild and transitory. When the ego is less capable of performing its executive functions, depression is more likely to be severe. Each of the categories is described below in terms of optimal functioning. Table 34-1 provides a model for understanding normal ego functioning as well as how ego functioning is affected by each level of depression.

Reality Testing

The term *reality testing* refers to the capacity to distinguish between stimuli that arise from internal sources, such as thoughts, feelings, impulses, and somatic sensations, and stimuli that are based in

Table 34-1 Levels of Depression and Ego Functioning

Ego Function	Characteristics	Examples
	Normal state	
Reality testing	Inner and outer stimuli are well distinguished. Occasional denial of external reality in the service of adaptation.	Accurate perception of external events prevails.
Judgment	Very few errors in anticipation of consequences. Behavior shows good judgment in all areas.	Past errors in judgment are repeated only occasionally, and the person is able to apply past learning to current situations.
Sense of reality of the world and self	Derealization and depersonalization occur only under conditions of extreme environmental alterations. A stable ego identity, a distinct sense of self, and realistic self-esteem are internalized.	Derealization and depersonalization disappear with restoration of average, expectable conditions. Requires only occasional feedback to maintain a solid sense of individuality.
Object relations	Conscious and automatic maintenance of optimal closeness or distance. Object relations tend to be mature, and other people are seen as separate individuals. Empathy is well established without getting "lost" in the other person's feelings. Losses are weathered with little strain.	Flexibility is shown in the choice and mode of relating to others. Object constancy is well developed, as important people are internalized. Thoughts about and respect for others continue whether or not they are physically present.
Thought processes	No substantial lapses in memory, concentration, or attention except when distracted, sick, or upset. Satisfactory use of conceptualization, with thinking which is usually logical and ordered. Typically, communication is clear, precise, and flexible.	Evidence of flexibility in willingness to entertain and explore new ideas. Possible egocentric modes of expression, but no serious peculiarities in language.
Stimulus barrier	Automatic and flexible fluctuations in thresholds to stimuli prevail within a reasonably high range. Coping modes are reasonably flexible, and sleep is not used as a defensive withdrawal from stimuli.	Good "screening mechanisms" permit adequate input and avoid sensory overload.

(Continued.)

Table 34-1 Continued

Ego Function	Characteristics	Examples
	Mild depression	
Reality testing	Confusion about inner and outer states occurs mainly upon awakening or going to sleep.	Relatively minor perceptual inaccuracies. Can correct distortions fairly easily.
Judgment	Awareness of consequences fluctuates from one situation to another. Areas of faulty judgment are fairly encapsulated.	Behavioral manifestations of distorted judgment may take the form of chronic intrusions on others with belief that one is just being friendly, or inappropriate assessment of one's own capabilities.
Sense of reality of the world and self	Occasional signs of derealization or depersonalization, occurring primarily with radical environmental changes or altered ego states. May have unrealistic feelings about the body, such as feeling too fat or thin, although self-identity is somewhat stable.	The person may seem to be role playing an identity, rather than experiencing it from within. Sometimes is dependent on external feedback to maintain identity, although generally the person can sustain a feeling of separateness.
Regulation of drive, affect, and impulses	Drives are experienced and expressed somewhat more or somewhat less than average. Controls are not exerted in an automatic fashion except in conflict-free areas. Impulsivity, irritability, and arousability occur in response to conflict-ridden areas, situational stress, and external provocations.	When controls are not automatic, they can be mustered at the time with moderate effort. Occasional work or social inhibitions may occur. There is some symptomatic acting out of unconscious conflicts, and there may be mild feelings of depression.
Object relations	Disturbed interactions with only a few people, sporadically rather than chronically. Others are perceived as separate and well differentiated from self. Internalization of objects is evident, except under stress. Absences and losses are overreacted to at times.	Repetitions of early patterns of relationships are the exception rather than the rule. Some recurrent difficulties may occur in important relationships. Object choice shows some important degree of flexibility, but under stress may become more compulsive.
Thought processes	Memory, attention, and concentration show periodic lapses, usually in emotionally charged situations or competing distractions. Some flexibility in conceptualization, but thinking may become disordered or illogical under stress. Moderate degrees of looseness and disorganization in speech, with mildly imprecise choice of words at times.	Effort is required to maintain memory, attention, or concentration under stress. There may be rigid or meticulous modes of communicating, or else moderate degrees of looseness and disorganization. Some doubting and blocking, as well as occasional peculiar ideas, are common.
Stimulus barrier	Thresholds to sensory stimuli range from fairly low to average, and a bit above. While occasionally irritable, jumpy, or annoyed by some distressing stimuli, the person is able to contain responses to stimuli fairly adaptively. However, the effort thus expended may lead to fatigue, poor adaptive resilience, or both.	The person may be sensitive to some specific noises but not to others. Adaptive behavior is only moderately disrupted by incidental stimuli. May seek solitude, and then have difficulty returning to a more stimulating environment.
	Moderate depression	
Reality testing	Projection of inner states into external reality more likely than frank hallucinations or delusions.	Reality is distorted to conform to strong need states. The person can often discover distortions when out of situation which precipitated them.
Judgment	Awareness of potential consequences is defective, leading to inappropriate judgments involving moderate dangers to life and limb.	The person takes unnecessary risks, for example, will drive with defective brakes or be negligent with respect to health. Socially, people may be bizarre, provoking others to do them harm.
Sense of reality of the world and self	Marked but only partial derealization and depersonalization. Parts of body may seem somewhat bigger than usual. Self-identity is fragmented, unintegrated, and usually dependent on external feedback.	Self-esteem is quite poor. Insatiable quests for money, status, assurance of sexual attractiveness often dominate. The person may often ruminate, "Who am I?" and when feedback is absent (or negative), the sense of self falters.

(Continued.)

Table 34-1 Continued

Ego Function	Characteristics	Examples
	Moderate depression	
Regulation of drive, affect, and impulses	Strong urges are usually experienced and acted on. Attempts at control are either excessive or ineffective (overcontrol is first seen here). Excessive controls are rigid or brittle, so that periods of overcontrol alternate with flurries of impulsive breakthroughs. There may be sporadic rages, tantrums, or binges, as with alcohol, food, and sex.	Affects and moods may be very labile. The individual may be physically "on the go" all the time. In cases of overcontrol, sexual and aggressive urges are expressed in areas other than overt behavior.
Object relations	Considerable difficulty striking a comfortable balance between distance and closeness. Prefers either very intense or very cool relationships. Other people are not usually perceived as existing in their own right. Representations of significant people are not well internalized, with overreactions to loss or separation common.	Present relationships are quite childlike—expects to be "fed" emotionally. There are inordinate attempts to "change" others, with the belief this will crystalize self-identity. Often exploits others to satisfy own ambitions. Feels unable to live alone, or else prefers isolation from others in living arrangements. Relationships are characterized by either detachment or clinging.
Thought processes	Gaps in memory. Easily distracted when attempting to concentrate. Some trouble with remote and current memory. Periodic failures of abstract reasoning and conceptualization. "All-or-none"-type thinking, with questionable logic. At times thoughts are disorganized and difficult to follow.	Attention and concentration remain relatively unimpaired if there are no competing distractions. Heavy reliance on concrete or overinclusive modes of thinking. Rigid thinking makes it difficult to consider more than one possibility. Frequent disruptions in communication due to intrusion of fantasy and drive-related thoughts.
Stimulus barrier	Thresholds to most sensory stimuli are quite low. Above-average sensitivity to peripheral or incidental stimuli. General irritability, rather than chaotic motor discharge. Attempts to filter stimulation are relatively ineffective. Sleep patterns are irregular.	Cold, heat, noise, bright lights are very bothersome. The person may hear, see, and smell things the average person would not be aware of. Stimulus seeking or stimulus hunger may be present despite hypersensitivity and excitability.
	Severe depression	
Reality testing	Hallucinations and delusions may occur, but do not pervade all areas of functioning. Delusions are more likely than hallucinations.	When delusions or hallucinations occur, confusion and disorientation about time, place, and person may occur.
Judgment	Minimal or no awareness of consequences of behavior. Faulty anticipation of consequences often leads to highly dangerous behaviors.	Behavior may be extremely inappropriate, socially and otherwise. Minimal ability to learn from past mistakes. Infantile feeling of omnipotence is often present.
Sense of reality of the world and self	The world is felt as completely strange and alien. Surroundings, people, and things feel unreal and changed in appearance (extreme derealization). Parts of the body feel strange or disconnected (extreme depersonalization). Near-total loss of boundaries between self and outside world creates gross identity and self-esteem distortions.	Possible oceanic feelings of nothingness. Sensations of being inanimate, selfless, dead. Identity disturbance creates pathological regulation of self-esteem, so that the person either feels worthless or extremely grandiose. These people may experience states of extreme fusion or merging with others, and may believe they possess mystical powers of communication.
Regulation of drive, affect, and impulses	Extreme lack of control of aggression, depression, sexual drives, or all three. Inability to restrain impulse-dominated behavior. Rational thought processes are not used to delay or control impulse expression. Almost nonexistent tolerance for frustration.	Impulses achieve full discharge through direct expression. The individual may have committed or attempted murder, suicide, or rape. Externally imposed restraints are the only effective way to curb urges.
Object relations	Essential lack of object relatedness, with "relationships" being presymbiotic or autistic. Minimal ability to perceive people in their own right. People do not exist when not present, and there is bland withdrawal in response to object loss.	Withdrawal may take the form of a stupor or muteness, or of living an isolated lifestyle. When rudimentary relationships do exist, they may tend to be parasitic, narcissistic, and fraught with turmoil. Relationships are generally not developed enough for separation anxiety.

(Continued.)

Table 34-1 Continued

Ego Function	Characteristics	Examples
	Severe depression	
Thought processes	Memory for only stereotyped content such as name and colors. Attention and concentration poor. Thinking fairly illogical. Blocking and peculiarities in verbal expression common.	Easily distractible. Thinking is excessively concrete or generalized; and there is failure to see relationships between discrete events. Some autistic and peculiar ideas. Thinking may be loose or rigid.
Stimulus barrier	Very low threshold to most sensory stimuli. Chaotic motor discharge patterns are common. Keen awareness of minor body changes. People feel like "jumping out of their skin." Attempts at adaptation are poor because attention and efforts are riveted on the experience of overstimulation. Severe sleep disturbances commonly occur.	Awareness of sensory stimuli is hyper- or hypoacute. Relatively small changes in temperature produce considerable discomfort. Noise may produce a diffuse excitability and too much light may cause agitation. Women may experience high degrees of premenstrual tension and agitation. In contrast, unresponsiveness to environmental stimuli may also occur.

sources external to the self. When an accurate perception of external events prevails, the tendency to project internal perceptions onto others is minimal. For example, perceiving others as angry when the feelings of anger actually reside within the self seldom occurs. When reality testing is intact, people are well in touch with their own feelings and make excellent use of consensual validation to confirm reality, by checking their perceptions against those of others.

Judgment

The term *judgment* refers to the ability to foresee or anticipate the probable consequences of a particular behavior, action, or response. When a behavior has had negative or unfavorable consequences, the person tends to use what he or she has learned to avoid further negative consequences. Thus, judgment involves the capacity to generalize what one has learned in previous situations. A person who is using sound judgment is also able to estimate the time and resources required to complete a task, and demonstrates effective planning and decision making.

Sense of Reality of the World and Self

The term *sense of reality* refers to the extent to which external events are experienced as real, and as occurring within a familiar context. The body and its functioning are also experienced as familiar and unobtrusive, as belonging to or emanating from the self. The person has developed a stable body image and a healthy sense of self-esteem. Other people are distinguished as independent entities, so that self-representations are distinguished from object representations. Ego boundaries are clearly demarcated between the self and the outside world.

Regulation and Control of Drive, Affect, and Impulses

The term *regulation and control* refers to the effectiveness with which a drive, affect, or impulse is controlled or delayed, in healthy adaptation. Control of urges operates calmly and automatically, so that the person is able to respond according to conscious personal choice, rather than responding to internal, uncontrollable pressures. When drives are aggressively or sexually oriented, the person is able to relax or tighten control as appropriate to the situation, or to sublimate or neutralize the drives effectively. Depression and related states are limited to sadness, grief, and mourning in appropriate response to loss.

Object Relations

The term *object relations* refers to the degree and quality of relatedness to others, and the extent to which present relationships are adaptively influenced by, or patterned upon, earlier relationships. The person is able to exercise flexible choice in the degree of closeness or distance that is maintained with others. Others are perceived as independent entities, rather than as mere extensions of self. The ability to obtain object constancy—that is, the ability to evoke a stable, consistent mental image of the object in its absence, and to tolerate frustration or anxiety related to the object—is well developed. The person has internalized stable image representations of significant people in early life, and thus shows adaptive resilience following loss of important objects in the present.

Thought Processes

Thought processes are the characteristic mode of thinking and language expression, as well as the degree to which memory, concentration, and attention are adaptively operationalized. The person is able to use either abstract or concrete modes of thinking appropriate to the situation. Communications reflect shared meanings of words and ideas, and give evidence of ordered and logical thinking. The person is able to focus attention and concentrate well, and both recent and remote memory for all kinds of events are excellent. These functions are automatic and remain intact even under the influence of distractions and intrusions.

Stimulus Barrier

The term *stimulus barrier* refers to the degree to which external and internal stimuli impinge upon various sensory modalities, and the quality of adaptation that occurs in response to sensory stimulation. The person's threshold for, or registration of, sensory stimulation is such as to allow for adaptive responses even in the face of high levels of stimulus input. Coping modes, including motor discharge patterns, are flexible and automatic in response to all degrees of stimulation. There are excellent "screening mechanisms" to avoid sensory overload, so that perceptual integration, sleeping patterns, and overt behavior are not disrupted by sensory impingements.

Unresolved Mourning

Freud studied the depressive reaction in its most severe form, melancholia. He noted similarities between patients who were grieving because of the recent loss of a loved one and patients who were suffering from melancholia (depression) but had no such discrete loss evident in their recent history. He observed that both reactions involved "a profoundly painful dejection, abrogation of interest in the outside world, loss of the capacity to love, and inhibition of all activity."[10] While similarities between depression and mourning unquestionably exist, some of the differences that have been delineated are equally important.

Mourning is an alive and energetically charged activity in which the pain of loss is expressed and discharged with the full support of the person's ego.[11] People who mourn *express* their grief; they cry, wail, and become angry about the loss. Mourning performs a necessary function; it enables the person to withdraw the feelings (libido) invested in the lost love object, so that they are available for other relationships. If this mourning does not occur, if the pain is not released by grieving, the separation is never completely worked through. The ego remains bound to the lost object and inhibited in its ability to establish new relationships. This is what occurs in pathological or unresolved mourning; the mind holds on to the lost object in order to deny the reality of the loss and to avoid the pain of separation. In grief the loss is known and accepted; in depression it is either unknown or unacknowledged.

Feelings and emotions are human responses to events in the environment; the depressed state is a lack of responsiveness. This lack of responsiveness is due to a diminishment of impulses and feelings that normally flow from the vital centers of the body to the periphery. Under normal conditions an internal force, or electrical charge, activates tissues and muscles in its path, giving rise to a sensation or feeling. When it results in action, it is called an *impulse*—a "pulse from within." In the depressed state, impulse formation is sharply reduced, in regard to both the number of impulses and their strength. This diminution produces a loss of feeling on the inside, and a loss of action on the outside. The ability of the organism to respond to environmental events with appropriate impulses is thus greatly diminished. Everything about the depressed person indicates this impoverishment of energy. All major bodily functions are reduced (vegetative signs). There is a noticeable diminution in spontaneous gestures and a visible lack of facial change. The depressed face droops and the skin seems to sag, as if it lacked the energy to do otherwise.

Thus in depression the ego is undermined by the energetic collapse of the body, resulting in an unalive and unresponsive condition. This occurs because feelings of loss are suppressed and unresolved. Depressed people continue to function as if loss had not occurred, and modify their behavior to prevent acknowledging it. The pain of loss is suppressed, but so too are many vital aspects of the person's personality. The whole emotional life becomes impoverished because suppression of any one feeling operates pervasively to suppress a wide range of feelings. Thus, Freud noted that in grief the world becomes poor and empty while in depression the ego itself becomes poor and empty.[12]

Object Loss

The term *object loss* refers to the traumatic separation of the person from significant objects of attachment. Loss of a significant object during childhood is seen as a *predisposing* factor for the occurrence of depression in adulthood; separation in adult life is considered a *precipitating* factor for depression in adulthood.

This psychoanalytic model of object loss suggests that the infant has formed a bond with the mother figure by 6 months of age, and that if that bond is severed, the child experiences separation anxiety and profound grief about the loss of the love object. The loss sustained during these early years and the subsequent mourning process are thought to predispose the child to respond dysfunctionally to losses that occur in later life.[13]

The direct effect on the child of the loss of physical contact with the mother was studied by René Spitz.[14] He studied the behavior of babies separated from their mothers after 6 months of life. In the first month of separation, the babies made vigorous efforts to regain contact with a mother figure. They cried, screamed, and reached out to anyone who was available. As these attempts to restore their lifeline to the mother proved unsuccessful, they gradually withdrew. After 3 months of separation their faces became rigid, their crying was replaced by whimpering, and they grew lethargic. If the separation continued, they became more withdrawn, refused contact with anyone, and lay quietly in their beds.

Studies have shown that both human infants and infant monkeys need physical contact with the mother's body in order to function normally.[15] Eye-to-eye contact of a loving kind between mother and baby is important for the development of children's visual relationship with the world, and by being in touch with the mother's body, children learn to be in touch with their own bodily selves. In the absence of this contact, the children's energy is withdrawn from the periphery of their bodies and from the surrounding world. The children lose full functioning of their bodies and lose their inner aliveness. For an infant, loss of loving contact is loss of world, of self, and potentially of life. How much is lost depends upon the actual degree to which the infant is deprived of loving contact.

Whether this anaclitic depression is caused just by separation or is compounded by the adverse effects of institutionalization is not altogether clear. Recent work by Robertson[12] raises questions about the universality of the mourning response, and suggests that appropriate substitute mothering during the separation period can prevent its occurrence. Although studies indicate that as a group, depressed people have sustained more parental loss than normal or other diagnostic groups, this factor, alone, may not be sufficiently universal to account for all forms of depression.

While people who have experienced loss of a love object in childhood may be sensitized to losses that occur in adult life, other adults who have not sustained a significant childhood loss may also respond to a real or imagined loss with a depressive reaction. Such losses may include loss of love, a person, physical functioning, status, or self-esteem. Since many losses are significant because of their symbolic meaning, the person's response to the loss may appear to be disproportionate. For example, a job change because of an important promotion may involve the person's feelings about the loss of old colleagues and security, as well as fear of loss of self-esteem in a new and challenging position.

Another aspect of object-loss theory views depression as the turning inward of aggression which is not directed at the appropriate object, with accompanying feelings of guilt. The process is initiated by loss of an object toward whom a person feels both love and anger (hatred). Unable to express the angry feelings because they are perceived as irrational or unacceptable, the person directs the anger inward and turns it against the self.[10] Abraham believed that the paralysis of feeling in the depressed person was caused by equal feelings of love and hate blocking any movement. The hatred is repressed and turned toward the inner self, forming a negative layer over the feeling of love, which cannot then be expressed. Self-hatred also contains the wish to destroy the person responsible for the feeling. Freud believed that the self-destructive act of suicide could be regarded as a lashing out against the hated, loved object as well as against the self.

This explanation of depression needs more empirical verification. Some investigators have identified depressed clients who do outwardly express their anger and hostility. Furthermore, redirection of anger to external objects has not always led to clinical improvement of depression. Object-loss theory, like other models, is only one possible explanation for depression.

Cognitive Processes

The cognitive model of depression evolved from systematic clinical observation and experimental testing by Aron Beck.[16] Two specific concepts used to explain depressive illness are the cognitive triad and cognitive errors (faulty information processing).

The Cognitive Triad

The cognitive triad consists of three major cognitive patterns that induce depressed persons to regard themselves, their future, and their experiences in an idiosyncratic manner.

The first component of the triad is a negative view of the self. Depressed people see themselves as defective, inadequate, diseased, or deprived. There is a tendency to attribute unpleasant experiences to a psychological, moral, or physical defect in the self. Such persons also believe that *because* of their presumed defects they are undesirable and worthless, and they tend to underestimate or criticize themselves. In addition, depressed people believe that they lack the attributes necessary to attain happiness and contentment.

The second component of the cognitive triad is depressed peoples' tendency to interpret their ongoing experiences in a negative way. They see the world as making exorbitant demands on them, or as presenting impossible obstacles to reaching their life goals, or both. They misinterpret their interactions with their environment as representing defeat or deprivation. These negative misinterpretations become evident when one observes how the clients negatively construe situations for which more plausible alternative interpretations are available. With help they may come to realize that they have tailored the facts to fit their preformed, negative conclusions.

The third component of the cognitive triad is a negative view of the future. As depressed people make long-range projections, they anticipate that their current difficulties or suffering will continue indefinitely. They expect unremitting hardship, frustration, and deprivation. When they consider undertaking a specific task in the immediate future, they expect to fail.

The cognitive model views the other signs and symptoms of the depression syndrome as consequences of the activation of the negative cognitive patterns. For example, if clients incorrectly *think* that they are being rejected, they react as if they have already been rejected. If they erroneously believe that they are social outcasts, they will feel lonely in spite of the actual circumstances. Suicide can also be explained as a consequence of negative cognitions, for suicidal impulses represent an extreme expression of the desire to escape from *apparently* insoluble problems or an *apparently* unbearable situation. Since depressed people often see themselves as worthless burdens, they may consequently believe that everyone, themselves included, would be better off if they were dead.

Increased dependency is also understandable in cognitive terms. Because such people see themselves as inept and helpless, and because they unrealistically overestimate the difficulty of normal tasks, they expect their undertakings to turn out badly. Thus, clients tend to seek help and reassurance from others whom they consider more competent and capable.

Finally, the cognitive model may also explain the physical symptoms of depression. Apathy and low energy may result from depressed people's belief that they are doomed to failure in all efforts. This negative view of the future, or sense of futility, may lead to the "psychomotor inhibition" that is so typically seen with the depressed client.[16]

Cognitive Errors

Faulty information processing and errors in thinking maintain these clients' belief in the validity of their negative concepts despite the presence of contradictory evidence. Specific errors are presented in Table 34-2.

A way of understanding the thinking disorder seen in depression is to conceptualize it in terms of "primitive" versus "mature" modes of organizing reality.[9] Depressed people are prone to structure experiences in relatively primitive ways. They tend

Table 34-2 Cognitive Errors

Error	Interpretation
Arbitrary inference	The process of drawing a specific conclusion in the absence of evidence to support the conclusion, or when the evidence is contrary to the conclusion.
Selective abstraction	Focusing on a detail taken out of context, ignoring other more salient features of the situation, and conceptualizing the whole experience on the basis of this fragment.
Overgeneralization	Drawing a general rule or conclusion on the basis of one or more isolated incidents, and applying the concept across the board to related and unrelated situations.
Magnification and minimization	Errors in evaluating the significance or magnitude of an event that are so gross as to constitute a distortion.
Personalization	Proclivity to relate external events to oneself when there is no basis for making such a connection.
Absolutist, dichotomous thinking	The tendency to place all experiences in one of two opposite categories; for example, flawless or defective, immaculate or filthy, saint or sinner. In describing themselves, clients select the extreme negative cagetory.

SOURCE: A. Beck, A. J. Rush, B. Shaw, and G. Emergy, *Cognitive Therapy of Depression*, Guilford, New York, 1979.

Table 34-3 Characteristics of Primitive and Mature Forms of Thinking

Primitive Thinking	Mature Thinking
Nondimensional and global: I am fearful.	**Multidimensional:** I am moderately fearful, quite generous, and fairly intelligent.
Absolutistic and moralistic: I am a despicable coward.	**Relativistic and nonjudgmental:** I am more fearful than most people I know.
Invariant: I always have been and always will be a coward.	**Variable:** My fears vary from time to time and situation to situation.
Exemplified by "character diagnosis": I have a defect in my character.	**Exemplified by "behavioral defect":** I avoid situations too much and I have many fears.
Characterized by irreversibility: Since I am basically weak, there's nothing that can be done about it.	**Characterized by reversibility:** I can learn ways of facing situations and fighting my fears.

SOURCE: A. Beck, A. J. Rush, B. Shaw, and G. Emergy, *Cognitive Therapy of Depression*, Guilford, New York, 1979.

to make global judgments about events that impinge on their lives. The meanings that flood their consciousness are likely to be extreme, negative, categorical, absolute, and judgmental. Their emotional responses, thus, tend to be negative and extreme. In contrast to this primitive type of thinking, more mature thinking automatically interprets life experiences in quantitative rather than qualitative terms, and according to relative rather than absolute standards. In primitive thinking, the complexity, variability, and diversity of human experiences and behavior are reduced to a few crude categories.

The characteristics of typical depressive thinking seem analogous to Piaget's descriptions of the thinking of children. The term *primitive* serves to distinguish it from the more adaptive thinking observed in later stages of development. The differentiating characteristics of these forms of thinking are summarized in Table 34-3.

According to this model, depressed clients tend to view their experiences as total deprivations or defeats (nondimensional thinking) and as unchangeable (fixed or invariant thinking). At the same time, they categorize themselves as "losers" (categorical and judgmental thinking) and doomed (thinking that is exemplified by irreversibility and by character diagnosis).

Clinical and experimental studies provide substantial empirical support for the cognitive theory of depression.[15] Thus the cognitive theory provides a theoretical foundation for understanding the depressed person's thought patterns and for structuring nursing interventions.

Learned Helplessness

The learned-helplessness model proposed by Seligman[17] was derived from experiments with dogs. During these experiments, it was observed that when the dogs were repeatedly unable to escape electric shocks, they accepted shock passively without attempting to escape. Over time, the dogs learned that they could not control the shocks, that no response produced relief. The dogs thus "learned" that they were totally "helpless." Laboratory tests suggested that an animal which had once "learned helplessness" had difficulty relearning that there were times when a response would produce relief from shock.

Seligman defines *helplessness* as a belief that no one *will* do anything to aid you, and *hopelessness* as a belief that neither you or anyone else *can* do anything.[17,18] Depression is thought to be rooted in the belief that one has no control over the important outcomes of one's life, and people who hold such a belief refrain from making functional responses. People with such a belief feel a lack of control over the reinforcers in their lives. Their negative expectations result in hopelessness, passivity, and inability to assert themselves.[17] The behavioral manifestations of helplessness and depression parallel each other.

In contrast, people who experience mastery in life appear to be more resilient, better able to resist depression. Life has taught them that their actions have had a positive effect on outcomes; they have been able to produce gratifying results and remove annoying or frustrating forces in their lives.

More recently, Abramson, Seligman, and Teasdale[18,19,20] have reformulated the learned-helplessness model in light of attribution theory. From the perspective of attribution theory, the kinds of causal attributions people make about control influence whether or not their helplessness will include low self-esteem and whether or not it will generalize across situations and times.

Three attributional dimensions are essential to an explanation of helplessness and depression:

Internal-external factors

Stable-unstable factors

Global-specific factors

Table 34-4 identifies the relationship between manifestations of helplessness and each attributional dimension. The helplessness that is manifested may be cognitive, motivational, or emotional in nature. Four premises underlie the attributional model, the occurrence of which is hypothesized to be sufficient for depression to exist:

1. The person expects that desired outcomes are improbable.
2. The person feels that no response in his or her repertoire will change the likelihood of the outcome.
3. The degree to which the attribution style of the person is internal, and the degree to which stable and global attributional factors are perceived to be operating are significant.

Table 34-4 Attributional Dimensions and Manifestations of Helplessness

Attributional Dimension	Manifestations of Helplessness
Internal-external factors	Attributing lack of control to internal factors leads to lowered self-esteem, and hence to helplessness, whereas attributing lack of control to external factors does not lead to helplessness.
Stable-unstable factors	Attributing lack of control to stable factors leads to an expectation of not being able to control future situations, and hence, helplessness behavior extends over time. In contrast, lack of control in relation to unstable factors leads to short-lived situation-specific helplessness.
Global-specific factors	Attributing lack of control to global factors leads to an expectation of not being able to control outcomes of other situations, and hence, helplessness is generalized across situations. In contrast, perceived lack of control in relation to specific factors leads to short-lived situation-specific helplessness.

4. The greater the certainty of uncontrollability, the greater the strength of cognitive deficits (negative expectations) and maturational deficits (passivity). The greater the importance of the uncontrollable event, the greater the effective deficit (low self-esteem).

At present, research studies investigating the relationship between the reformulated attributional learned-helplessness model and depression as well as personality attributes have yielded ambiguous results.[21,22] Methodological problems have been cited as factors plaguing the research studies. However, it must also be noted that while attributional learned helplessness appears conceptually to be a sound explanatory model for the occurrence of depression, it may not be. Finally, this model is proposed as a sufficient but not necessary cause of depression, which means that other physiological and psychological factors can also contribute to the development of depression.[20]

Entitlement Depression

Denial of deprivations and disappointments in early life leaves one open to similar disappointments in later life. When a child has experienced losses or trauma in childhood that undermine self-acceptance, unrealistic expectations may be projected for the future. The mind, in its fantasies and daydreams, may attempt to reverse the unfavorable and unacceptable reality of early life by creating images that exalt the person and inflate the ego. The result is an inflated sense of self that causes vulnerability to what has been termed *entitlement depression.*[23]

The inflated sense of self occurs as the child constructs an "idealized image" to compensate for the painful feelings in the past. The idealized self that emerges has some basis in reality, for it is fashioned from the child's own experience, imagination, needs, and faculties. However, as this idealized version becomes more real to the child than the actual self, he or she goes astray into the realm of the fantastic. Karen Horney points out that as long as this idealized image is perceived as real, the child grows to believe that he or she is *entitled* to be treated by others, or by fate, in accord with grandiose notions about the self. Horney states that the child "tries to assert the exceptional rights to which his uniqueness entitles him whenever and whatever ways he can."[24] Self-inflation thus gives rise to feelings of entitlement.

Originally, the term *entitlement* meant a right to possession, or the provision of title to an estate.[25] It was then generalized to mean a rightful claim to a possession, privilege, designation, or mode of treatment.[26] In a legal sense, *entitlement* means the right to benefits, income, or property which may not be abridged without due process.[27] A person who is entitled in this sense has a legitimate right, which is based in reality, to benefits, privileges, or special treatment.

Narcissistic entitlement, on the other hand, is the *belief* that one has a rightful claim to special privileges when, in fact, one does not. Although the person perceives the claim as legitimate, this perception has no basis in reality. Thus, *narcissistic entitlement* can be defined as an irrational belief, based on an inflated view of self, that one possesses a legitimate right to receive special privileges, modes of treatment, or designations when, in fact, one does not.

Narcissistic entitlement creates a propensity to become depressed for two important reasons. First, people with this outlook are bound to encounter acute disappointment when the world fails to treat them especially well. This creates ongoing "narcissistic injuries" which result in lowered self-esteem (depression), outbursts of rage and frustration (typically seen in manic episodes), or both. Second, the outlook is bound to bring people into painful conflict with others. The beliefs and behaviors that are typical of narcissistic entitlement explain why this is so.

Beliefs Underlying Entitlement Depression

The beliefs characteristic of entitlement depression are unrealistic and irrational. Irrational components of narcissistic entitlement include such ideas as, "Conditions under which I live must get arranged so that I get practically everything I want comfortably, quickly, and easily," and "Things must go the way I would like them to go, because I need what I want." Entitlement is also unrealistic because it presupposes an exemption from the laws that govern "ordinary people." Entitled persons are not exempt from the law, of course; but their fury at, say, receiving a ticket for illegal parking betrays their belief that they should be.

The beliefs of entitlement depression are also egocentric. Narcissistic entitlement is rooted in an assumption of one's own superiority, specialness, or uniqueness. Because of this, what appears clearly egocentric to the observer is not so perceived by entitled people themselves. Without a second thought, a woman who feels entitled not to have to wait may barge in front of others to have her question answered; the man who feels entitled not to make an effort may park in a space reserved for the handicapped. The egocentricity of entitlement is rooted in the underlying conviction that other people's needs may be important, but one's own needs should have absolute priority. The "motto" of the entitled person whose beliefs are egocentric might be summed up as follows:

> "I am special" (idealized image).
> "Therefore, my needs have absolute priority."
> "And therefore, I am entitled to what I need."

A specific belief typical of narcissistic entitlement is that things should come easily and without effort. This irrational belief seems logical to those who hold it. These people have shifted the center of gravity from the actual self to an idealized version. Because they are aliented from their real selves, they cannot self-initiate; thus the belief develops that things should come to them without such initiation. Any reminder that effort is required may stimulate rage: "It should be easy for me!" Effort is disdained because the inflated self believes that everything should be effortless; it does not take kindly to struggle or disequilibrium.

This underlying belief explains how entitlement can lead to depression in a person's life. If, for instance, a child expects learning to require no effort, he or she is likely to give up and become depressed when that doesn't prove to be the case. The same may be true of adults. For example:

> One client requested various psychological and intelligence tests while in therapy. She was convinced that she had failed in college because of a learning disability and was genuinely disappointed when the tests showed her to be of average intelligence. To her, the idea of making an effort to master difficult coursework was abhorrent; she preferred to believe that she had some intrinsic deficit.

Ideas like this, of course, set the stage for depressive reactions.

Another aspect of the beliefs typical of entitlement depression is that they assume a right to be vindictive. Vindictiveness is the desire to cause anguish or injury. People who feel entitled believe that their expectations are legitimate and feel betrayed when they encounter frustration. Depending on how painful the betrayal is perceived to be, the person feels justified in lashing out in return. For instance:

> A woman has an idealized image of herself as always in control in all circumstances. She receives a last-minute cancellation from a man who had accepted her invitation to a dinner party. She becomes enraged; she had expected eight couples, and this cancellation ruins her seating arrangement. She spitefully plans how she will slight this man in the future, never noticing how absurdly out of proportion her reaction is.

The vindictiveness seen in entitlement is attributable to these people's feeling that they may inflict injury on anyone who threatens their idealized image. When vindictiveness is turned against the self, as it often is, it expresses itself in acute depressive symptoms.

Behavioral Manifestations of Entitlement Depression

Entitled persons may vigorously assert their "rights," but sometimes the only evidence that entitlement exists is the fury or emotional upset that follows frustration. The degree of awareness of entitlement varies from person to person, and indignation may not always be conscious. Instead, there may be psychosomatic manifestations or a feeling of depression or irritability, unconnected in the person's mind with the frustrated expectations. Table 34-5 illustrates behaviors that suggest the presence of entitlement.

Table 34-5 Entitlement Depression

Behaviors that Suggest the Presence of Entitlement
1. Direct, verbal assertion that one has a right to expect that circumstances occur as one needs, wants, or desires without regard to reality.
2. Overt, visible, and seemingly irrational emotional reactions ranging from irritation to fury when claims of entitlement are frustrated.
3. Covert reactions of unexplained fatigue, psychosomatic symptoms, or depression when claims of entitlement are frustrated. Usually these reactions become overt only through self-exploration in the context of the psychotherapeutic relationship.
4. Interpersonal vindictiveness and "righteous fury" toward others when claims of entitlement are frustrated.
5. A demonstrated lack of self-initiative and effort in solving problems and acting on the best behalf of one's own personality.

Significance of Entitlement Depression

It would seem that entitlement depression is becoming increasingly common today. It predisposes the person to painful, depressed states because injuries to self-esteem are constantly being perceived. The whole notion of learning to express anger is meaningless if anger is being created daily by frustration of perceived "rights." Anger may be present in other kinds of depression, of course, but it does not tend to have the vindictive quality that characterizes entitlement depression. Since vindictiveness is a desire to cause anguish, when it is turned against the self it is far more intense than in other forms of depression. The cycle of disappointment, injury, rage, and depression generates hopelessness.

Entitlement depression represents another theoretical framework for understanding depression; this new, inductive theoretical perspective has progressed through the stages of theory development, which will now be followed by empirical investigation.[23]

Genetic Factors in Depression

In recent years extensive research in many countries has investigated the relationship of genetic factors to affective disorders. The results of twin studies which compare illness rates in monozygotic and dyzygotic twins suggest a greater concordance rate for depression in monozygotic twins than in dyzygotic twins. Familial aggregation studies, which compare illness rates between and within generations of the same family, indicate an increased frequency of depression among first-degree relatives of the depressed person as compared with the general population.[28] Cross-rearing studies of high-risk children raised in adoptive homes attempt to separate the proportional influence of genetics and environment.[29] These types of family studies indicate a genetic basis for at least an inherent vulnerability to depression, particularly the manic-depressive forms.

Biochemical Factors in Depression

Biochemical alterations in many body systems have been identified in depressed people. Whether these biochemical alterations cause depression or are the result of depression is not yet clearly understood. Alterations in normal biochemical functioning have been proposed in relation to electrolyte disturbances, hormonal disturbances, and neurochemical alterations in the neurotransmitters, especially in the biogenic amines.

Electrolyte metabolism studies indicate that there is an increased sodium level during depression and a lower sodium level following recovery from the depressive episode. Other electrolytes, magnesium, potassium, and calcium have also been examined, but no definite conclusions have been reported as yet.

Studies of the relationship between female sex hormones and depression have been inspired by the higher prevalence of depression in women than in men. It has also been observed that clinical depression tends to occur in association with events in the reproductive cycle, including the menstrual cycle, the use of oral contraceptives, the postpartum period, and menopause. However, research findings have not yet definitively established a link between depression and any specific female hormone.

The amine hypothesis relates depression to a deficit in one or more brain transmitter amines at specific central synapses, and relates mania to an increase of amines. Norepinephrine, dopamine, and serotonin are the neurotransmitter amines that regulate the flow of impulses to the brain areas that control vegetative functioning and affect. Evidence suggests that in depression, a deficiency in norepinephrine at the synaptic junction combines with lowered serotonin levels to inhibit clinical activity at the receptor site.[30]

Another finding relevant in this context is that tricyclic antidepressants, while not directly altering the amine levels in the brain, do block the presynaptic reuptake of the amines so that there is a functional increase in amines at the synaptic junction. This more continuous stimulation is thought to be responsible for the elevation in mood brought on by these drugs. In contrast, Lithium, an effective drug in the treatment of mania, enhances the reuptake of amines at the synapse, thereby lowering the amount of amines at the synaptic junction.

The findings of biochemical research studies do not yield consistent results on the amine hypothesis. No matter how promising the evidence suggesting connections between changes in biogenic amines and the pharmacological mechanisms, it must be remembered that the biochemical interactions and shifts that occur during depression are extremely complex and that more careful research is necessary.

PATTERNS OF INTERACTION: FAMILY*

Family theorists propose that dysfunction in family members can be accounted for on the basis of family relationships.[31] Expectations about the self originate during childhood in the family. People who are predisposed to depression often acquire overly high expectations of themselves and others from early parent-child relationships. They view compliance with parental expectations as a prerequisite for receiving love. Love from significant others becomes internalized as self-worth. Self-worth becomes linked with fulfillment of parental expectations and receipt of parental approval.

This pattern is inevitably carried into adult relationships. Love and approval from others is a major source of self-esteem, and others important to the person are expected to deliver appropriate amounts of love and approval on a regular basis.

* Portions of this section from Ardis Swanson, "The Client Who Generates Depression," in the second edition of this book.

Problems invariably arise from these expectations. It is unrealistic to expect that one will always succeed or that others will be emotionally available in the desired ways. The person has been unavoidably set up for failure, disappointment, low self-esteem, and depression. The person feels deprived and sad, and may feel that if efforts to succeed are doubled, praise will be forthcoming. Unfortunately, it often is not, and the person is caught up in an expectation–achievement–self-esteem cycle from which it is difficult to escape.

Role relationships in a family with a depressed member may be characterized by a reciprocal pattern of overfunctioning and underfunctioning. Decreased activity and thought, sadness of affect, and social withdrawal make a person appear to be underfunctioning. Dependency, demandingness, and lack of physical self-care add to the picture. In a relationship system, this behavior enables another member to appear relatively overfunctioning. The overfunctioning member appears to be more active, responsible, nurturing, and functional, and thus gains temporary strength from the other's dysfunction. The family achieves a kind of balance over a period of time, and the balance may be threatened when the depressed person improves. Dysfunction may appear in other family members, particularly the one who has been overfunctioning. Depression may serve the purpose of keeping a familiar balance within the family system.

Depression may also be a response to a significant, or nodal, event in the family, especially when the event arouses anxiety but is not discussed within the family. Such an event frequently involves significant change or loss which stirs emotions in all family members. When some members do not want, or are unable, to acknowledge these emotions, the depression of one family member may express them. The rest of the family can thus continue to function, without major symptoms. By becoming a focus of concern, the depressed member enables others to divert attention from their own emotional pain.

PATTERNS OF INTERACTION: ENVIRONMENT

Societal forces combine to provide yet another explanation of the causes of depression: that stressful life experiences of an episodic or enduring nature contribute to disturbances of mood. Nodal events, social-role stressors, and lack of social resources are three major factors that are thought to contribute to the occurrence of depression.

Nodal Events

Nodal events are significant additions and subtractions of people, places, or objects in a person's or family's life. Such events inherently involve stress, since they effect a change in the balance of a person or a family (see Chapter 22). Research indicates that, on average, people who become depressed have experienced three times as many nodal events during the 6 months before their depressive episodes as have normal subjects.[32] Categorizing the events as "exit" events, involving separation and loss, and "entrance" events, involving introduction of a new person into the social sphere of the person, the data revealed that exit events (subtractions) were more frequently followed by depression and other symptoms than were entrance events (additions). The concept of exit events in this study contains similarities to the psychoanalytic theory of object loss.

Nodal events include births, deaths, geographic moves, losses of or changes in social roles, physical illnesses, changes in financial status, and changes in self-esteem. Paykel[32] found that events perceived as undesirable most often precipitated depression. Additionally, when multiple nodal events occur within a brief period of time, stress escalates dramatically, and the likelihood of depression as well as other stress-related symptoms increases (see Chapters 3 and 42). However, all people experience nodal events, but not all people become depressed. This suggests that stressful life events alone are not enough to cause development of depression.

Social-Role Stressors

Social-role stressors, most notably role strain, have emerged as significant factors in the development of depression. The term *social-role strain* refers to aspects of a role which are considered problematic or undesirable. The relationship between role strain and depression has been increasingly scrutinized as a result of the women's movement in the United States.[7] Women have higher rates of depression than men, and social-role strain has been proposed as one of the stressors contributing to depression in women.[7]

In a recent research study, Ilfield[33] developed scales to measure nine current social stressors that contribute to role strain: neighborhood, job, financial affairs, homemaking, parenting, marriage, single status, unemployment, and retirement. The scales measure ongoing stressful experiences. The study population was divided into five subgroups, and the relative strength and differential effect of the defined social stressors were examined across each subgroup. Analysis of the data revealed that current social stressors are significantly related to depressive symptoms for each of the five groups.[34] For employed married mothers and fathers as well as unemployed married mothers, marriage emerged as the greatest stressor. Parenting, job, and financial stressors were intermediate stress factors, except for employed single women, for whom financial stressors were of greatest magnitude. For employed single men, single status was the stressor of greatest magnitude. Role strain associated with marriage emerges as a major stressor related to depression for both men and women. However, Gove,[35] in studying the rates of mental illness in men and women, found higher rates of mental illness among married women. In contrast, single, divorced, and widowed women have lower rates than men. Gove concludes that marriage has a protective effect for men but a detrimental effect for women.

Role strain inherent in parenting may be another source of stress, especially for married employed women. Young women with extensive career involvement have been found to have an extreme crisis reaction to the birth of their first child. In contrast, multiparas have been found to have more pregnancy-related problems than principaras. These findings suggest that women may view pregnancy and parenting as sources of conflict and dissatisfaction.

Ilfield found that for married employed women, both marriage and parenting were primary stressors.[34] Literature on dual-career families indicates that a working mother often has to combine and juggle the roles of career person, wife, and mother; further, the roles and responsibilities are additive, contributing to role overload.[36,37,38] While in some families husband and wife make an equitable division of parenting and household responsibilities, in the majority of households the wife is responsible for fulfilling these multiple roles.[36] In untraditional households in which responsibilities were shared, men were found to have higher levels of depressive symptoms than women.[39] This finding gives further support to a sex-role basis for sex differences in depressive symptoms.

Lack of Social Resources

Lack of social resources, such as income, education, occupation, social position, family (extended and nuclear), friends, and community organizations combine to create another stressor for many people. The effects of poverty, discrimination, inadequate housing, and social isolation cannot be underestimated.[7]

Lack of social resources that provide support and amelioration of hardship make it difficult to achieve mastery by direct action and self-assertion, a situation which contributes further to emotional distress. It has been suggested that a real or perceived void in this area leads to feelings of legal, economic, occupational, and social helplessness, dependency on others, chronically low self-esteem, low aspirations, and ultimately, vulnerability to clinical depression.[7] For example, in a study by Brown and Harris,[40] the relationship between psychosocial stress and subsequent affective disorders among women was investigated. They found that working-class women with young children at home had the highest rates of depression. They were 5 times more likely to become depressed than middle-class women, given equal amounts of stress. Four factors were identified as stressful:

1. Having lost the mother in childhood
2. Three or more children under the age of 14, living at home
3. Absence of an intimate or confiding relationship with a husband or boyfriend
4. Lack of full- or part-time employment outside the home

Of primary importance in preventing depression in the presence of stress was the amount of emotional support provided by the husband or boyfriend. Second in importance was employment outside the home, which was seen as alleviating boredom, increasing self-esteem, improving financial position, and increasing social contacts.[40]

While a causal relationship between stressful life experiences and depression has not been established, the presence of significant stressors in a person's life certainly suggests a vulnerability to depression—across the life span, but particularly among specific target populations.

In short, no one theory sufficiently explains depression. Rather, a holistic perspective on depression reflects aspects of individual, family, and environmental theories. Depression is caused by the interaction of these biopsychosocial variables. Alterations in any one variable result in changes in the other two.

NURSING PROCESS

Assessment

Nurses encounter depressed clients in a variety of health care settings. Psychiatric nurses meet such clients in both inpatient and outpatient mental health agencies. Obstetrical nurses encounter women with postpartum depression as well as husbands and wives responding to the nodal event of the birth of a new baby and its accompanying role strain or extra demands for social resources. Nurses working on medical and surgical units, in health maintenance organizations, and in doctor's offices encounter clients whose depression appears in the guise of physical symptoms, or whose depression has evolved out of a physical health problem such as a heart attack, recurring malignancy, or loss of a body function or part. Pediatric nurses deal with the stress of an ill child and its ripple effect on the family system. Community health nurses work with families striving to cope with and master the ongoing effect of physical or mental illness, often without adequate social resources.

Regardless of the setting in which a nurse encounters and works with clients, systematic assessment of depression should be a holistic process that involves evaluation of the person's body, mind, and spirit, as well as family and community assessment factors. Assessment factors for the person, the family, and the community appear in Table 34-6.

In addition to the assessment guide in Table 34-6, nurses should familiarize themselves with some of the most commonly used self-report measures of depression such as the Beck Depression

Table 34-6 Assessment of Person, Family, and Community

Person	Person
Body	**Mind: Ego functions**
1. Does the client report either an increased or a decreased need for sleep? What are the current sleep patterns?	**Reality testing**
2. Is there either depressed appetite with weight loss or increased appetite with weight gain? How much weight has been gained or lost in the last month?	1. Does the client's depression include any delusional ideas? If so, what is the nature of those ideas?
3. Does the client show evidence of physical restlessness? Psychomotor retardation?	2. To what degree does the client tend to use projection as a defense, (for example, projecting feelings of worthlessness onto others? What feelings or impulses tend to be most commonly projected?
4. Does the client report either an increase or a decrease in sexual interest?	3. To what degree does the client deny external reality?
5. Is there evidence of low energy and chronic fatigue? Or does the client report more energy than usual?	4. What is the client's perception of his or her situation? Is the need for treatment of depression recognized?
6. Is the client suffering from constipation? Are there signs of urinary retention?	**Judgment**
7. Is the client able to maintain self-care or self-nurturance?	1. Does the client demonstrate awareness of the consequences of his or her behavior?
8. What is the client's posture like? Is there a tendency to sit slumped or curled up?	2. Is the client's behavior inappropriate socially or otherwise?
9. To what degree does the client show physical signs of responsiveness to the environment?	3. Has the client been involved in behaviors that could be considered dangerous or high-risk?
	4. To what degree is the client able to appraise his or her own capabilities realistically?

(Continued.)

Table 34-6 Continued

Person	Person
Mind: Ego functions **Sense of reality of world and self** 1. Is the client's depression so severe that others or self seem unreal and alien (derealization)? 2. Are there indications that the client has feelings of nothingness, of being inanimate, selfless, dead? 3. How is the depression affecting the client's sense of self-esteem? Are feelings of worthlessness expressed? 4. Does the client express the idea that his or her body feels strange, peculiar, or unfamiliar? Are there any somatic delusions? 5. To what degree is there congruence between the client's self-view and ego ideal? How realistic is the client's sense of self-esteem? 6. Does the client seem to have a stable sense of body boundaries? Or does he or she seem to experience states of extreme fusion or merging with others (extreme dependency)? 7. To what degree is the client dependent on external feedback to maintain a sense of self? 8. Does the client seem to be playing roles rather than experiencing a sense of self that emanates from within? **Regulation of drives, affect, and impulses** 1. Is there evidence of excessive control of drives or impulses (unresponsiveness)? 2. To what degree does the person seem pressured by sexual and aggressive drives? Are there excessive controls? 3. Are aggressive drives evident in the client's verbalization toward self or others? Is there pressure to act on suicidal thoughts? 4. To what degree are irritability and arousability evident? 5. To what degree is the mood despondent (mild, moderate, or severe)? **Object relations** 1. Is the client depressed to the point of withdrawal from contact with others? 2. Does withdrawal take the form of muteness or stupor? 3. To what degree does the client's relationship with others seem to be characterized by conflict and turmoil? 4. What has been the client's typical response to loss and separation from significant others? To what degree is separation anxiety evident? 5. To what degree is the client able to strike a comfortable balance between distance and closeness? Is there evidence of either extreme dependency (clinging) or detachment (distancing)? 6. To what degree is the client able to tolerate being alone? To tolerate being with others? 7. To what degree do current relationships seem to be influenced by infantile and childhood experiences?	**Mind: Ego functions** **Thought processes** 1. Does the client tend to use either overly concrete or overly abstract modes of thinking? 2. To what degree does the client tend to draw a negative conclusion from one or more isolated incidents (overgeneralization)? 3. Is there a tendency to draw a specific conclusion in absence of evidence to support the conclusion (arbitrary inference)? 4. To what degree have the depressive symptoms interfered with concentration, memory, and attention? 5. Does the client tend to demonstrate absolutistic, dichotomous thinking, that is, to place all experiences into one or two opposite categories? 6. Does the client show illogical thinking by focusing on a detail taken out of context and conceptualizing the whole experience on the basis of that fragment (selective abstraction)? 7. To what degree is the client able to consider more than one possibility? 8. How well ordered or disorganized are the thought patterns? 9. To what degree does the client express self in a coherent, understandable way? 10. Does speech reflect ideas of helplessness, hopelessness, and worthlessness? 11. Does the client verbalize suicidal intent or preoccupation? **Stimulus barrier** 1. How responsive is the client to internal and external stimuli? Is there evidence of hyperkinetic or chaotic motor discharge patterns? Or lack of responsiveness to almost all stimuli? 2. Does the client give evidence of being unable to sleep? 3. What are the client's typical responses to noise, light, and groups of people? **Spirit** 1. In what does the client place his or her faith? (The following questions can help determine this.) a. In times of crisis, where do you find comfort and solace? b. What is your source of security? c. What is it that you can do that gives you an inward peace? d. Do you have an inspirational source for when you get to feeling down? e. What or who have you found to be a source of strength in your life? f. What factors in your life help you best to cope with crisis, unpredictable problems, and stress? g. Do you rely most heavily on yourself, others, or a higher power?

(Continued.)

Table 34-6 Continued

Person	Family
Spirit 2. What provides meaning and purpose in the client's life? 3. What is the client's philosophy of life? 4. Does the client express the belief that he or she is being punished for some past sin or transgression? 5. Does the client view a higher power or God as punitive and revengeful? Is there evidence of self-hatred and self-condemnation? Of a total inability to forgive oneself? 6. In what manner does the client attempt to reduce or remove feelings of guilt? 7. Does the client's spiritual belief system seem more characteristic of a punitive "should" system or a healthy moral conscience?	5. What significant family events or changes may be factors in the client's depression? 6. How do various family members seem to respond to feelings of guilt evoked by the depressed person?
Family	**Community**
1. How well does the individual feel that he or she measures up to the expectations of other family members? 2. What degree of openness is there within the family system for expression of negative emotions? 3. How supported or unsupported does the depressed person feel by other family members? 4. To what degree is there evidence of reciprocal patterns of overfunctioning and underfunctioning?	1. Have one or more nodal events occurred in the person's life within the past year? If yes, what is the nature of events and their relationship to the onset of depressive symptoms? 2. Does the person demonstrate evidence of social role strain? If yes, what is the nature of the role strain? 3. What is the person's employment or educational situation? 4. What social networks and support systems exist in the person's life? 5. How do the person's sex, age, race, ethnicity, and financial resources affect coping resources? 6. How contented is the person with his or her lifestyle? 7. What kinds of social relationships does the person have? 8. How does the person spend leisure time? 9. To what extent does the person feel helpless about controlling outcomes in his or her life?

sion Inventory[41] and the Zung Self-Rating Depression Inventory.[42] These may be administered to clients during an intake interview.

Diagnosis

The nursing diagnosis is a way of attributing meaning to the information gained in the assessment, by linking observed behaviors to some frame of reference. Table 34-7 gives examples of nursing diagnoses for depressed clients.

Outcome Criteria

Establishing realistic outcome criteria with depressed clients can be difficult for several reasons. First, these clients often feel unable to control their environment. They perceive themselves negatively, as having no ability or skills, regardless of objective data. They are hopeless about the likelihood that they themselves, their lives, or others will change. Thus, they say, "There's no use." Negativism and resistiveness ("I can't"; "I won't"; "It won't work") destroy or impair motivation. Clients also often have unrealistically high expectations for themselves. This inhibits formulation of goals because these clients—feeling that they can never fulfill their expectations—think, "Why bother? If I can't do it all, I won't settle for second best." Finally, severely depressed clients often have such extensive psychomotor retardation that it is extremely difficult for them to mobilize their thoughts and speech to participate in the formulation of goals.

In light of the above discussion, it is essential that nurses establish realistic goals for depressed clients. Failure to do so will probably lead to further disappointment, evoke feelings of failure, and reinforce these clients' low self-esteem. Nurses should involve clients in the formulation of goals whenever possible. This enables clients to begin assuming self-responsibility and control of their lives. When clients are included in formulation of goals, they also feel listened to and respected for their thoughts and feelings. Above all else, goals should be realistic; that is, they should be expressed in accomplishable, measurable units, the attainment of which will, perhaps, make inroads into the client's negative

Table 34-7 Nursing Diagnoses and Outcome Criteria for Depressed Clients

Nursing Diagnoses	Outcome Criteria
Low self-esteem	
1. Low self-esteem related to internalization of aggressive impulses	Client learns to "own," understand, and appropriately discharge feelings of aggression so that aggression is no longer turned against the self.
2. Low self-esteem related to having absorbed negative feelings and self-blame that arise from not having had one's early needs met	Client ceases to blame self for early deprivation, and comes to realistically view (and forgive) limitations of parents and significant others.
3. Low self-esteem related to repeated narcissistic injuries that arise from unconscious or conscious feelings of entitlement	Client relinquishes claims of entitlement after perceiving the nature of his or her irrational and excessive claims on life.
4. Low self-esteem related to inadequate problem-solving and life mastery competencies	Client assumes responsibility for his or her own life by developing the competencies and skills needed to cope.
Object loss	
1. Feelings of despondency related to losses precipitated in current life	Client fully expresses grief, anger, and emotional pain so that loss is accepted and integrated, and emotional investment in others becomes possible.
2. Feelings of despondency related to unresolved mourning over past losses and deprivations	Client grieves over the extent to which past losses have hindered the full development of potential and aliveness, with the result that capacity for pleasure in the present is released.
3. Feelings of despondency related to faulty cognition which perpetuates negative patterns and expectations	Client recognizes the distortions inherent in certain thought patterns, replaces them with logical patterns of thought, and becomes free of negative thought patterns.
Object loss	
4. Feelings of despondency related to poorly developed object constancy (low functioning on the object relations scale) so that losses are poorly tolerated	Client accepts both positive and negative aspects of early relationships (especially mother) so that internal representations can be evoked and retained.
Stressful life experiences	
1. Role strain associated with new role as parent	Client identifies sources of role strain related to first-time parenthood.
2. Role strain related to multiple role demands as wife, mother, and professional	Client reevaluates self-expectations by prioritizing role demands.
3. Social isolation related to lack of intimate social relationships	Client identifies potential relationship options.
4. Helplessness related to perceived lack of child care and support systems	Client explores available community child care and support systems.
Vegetative signs of depression	
1. Poverty of thought associated with negative cognitions in which efforts to improve situation are perceived as doomed to failure	Client perceives negative cognitions as irrational so that positive expectations of the future release physical energy.
2. Psychomotor retardation related to diminution of energy	Client reverses constructed patterns of bodily function through voluntary engagement in activities that require expenditure of physical energy.
3. Inability to recognize and express negative emotions associated with ambivalent feelings of love and hate	Client recognizes and discharges negative emotions so that the core feelings of love are also freed.
4. Constipation related to psychomotor retardation	Client has regular bowel movements.
5. Initial and terminal insomnia related to severe anxiety	Client sleeps 6 hours at night without waking.

view of self, life, and the future. Table 34-7 illustrates realistic outcome criteria for depressed clients.

Intervention

Intervention with the Person

Nursing intervention with depressed clients can take place at home, in an outpatient setting, or in a hospital. The location will depend on the intensity and duration of the client's symptoms, available support systems, and resources of the treatment center. With depression, as with any other dysfunctional health pattern, nursing intervention must address the physiological, cognitive, emotional, behavioral, spiritual, family, and environmental dimensions of self.

PHYSICAL NEEDS. Depressed clients' physical well-being may be forgotten or ignored because they are not capable of caring for themselves. Clients' physical needs may require interventions that deal with nutrition, elimination, sleep, and hygiene. Safety needs, medication regimens, and electroconvulsive therapy (ECT) are other possible areas of intervention.

Loss of appetite. Clients who have a loss of appetite may need to have their nutritional intake monitored. Recording intake and output and weighing them daily will help in evaluating nutritional needs and ensuring adequate hydration. Staying with clients while they are eating, allowing them to select preferred foods, and encouraging small frequent meals will help to increase caloric intake.

Sleep disturbances. Sleep disturbances are common in depression. Clients who have difficulty falling asleep or who wake during the night and have difficulty returning to sleep may be relaxed by a back rub, a shower, or a short period of quiet companionship. Sometimes a glass of warm milk may prove relaxing. A scheduled rest period during the day may be helpful, but clients should not be encouraged to nap during the day, as it will interfere with their ability to sleep at night. Clients who do not want to face a new day often have difficulty getting out of bed in the morning. The nurse must gently, but firmly, tell them when to get up. If clients are unable to manage this themselves, the nurse should help them get out of bed and assist them with their hygiene needs.

Elimination problems. Depressed clients often have elimination problems. Because of their psychomotor retardation and decreased nutritional intake, they are often constipated and may even have fecal impactions. Interventions that promote fluid intake, a high-fiber diet, and exercise will prevent bowel elimination problems. Clients may also have urinary retention, but adequate fluid intake and exercise will usually prevent this problem. However, catheterization is sometimes necessary.

Neglect of hygiene. Neglect of grooming and hygiene is very common, because of psychomotor slowing of movement, loss of interest, and decreased self-esteem. If clients are unable to take care of their own hygiene needs, the nurse will help them to bathe, dress, and groom themselves—or, if necessary, even do it for them. This help should be given in a matter-of-fact manner, with the explanation that clients who are temporarily unable to take care of themselves routinely receive such help. However, the nurse should not maintain or reinforce the client's helplessness or dependency longer than is necessary, and should always encourage clients to care for themselves whenever possible. Cleanliness and interest in appearance can be noticed and positively reinforced. Even when clients do not have the energy to care for themselves, they may incorporate the nurse's attention and caring.

Risk of suicide. When clients express suicidal thoughts or make suicidal gestures, the nursing staff must intervene by first assessing the risk and then monitoring the clients' safety needs. If a client's symptoms are rapidly progressing and if environmental support systems are not available, hospitalization is usually strongly indicated. When admitted to a psychiatric unit, the client is placed on constant or regular suicide observation. The purpose of this intervention is to help clients manage their self-destructive impulses, which often feel overwhelming. A detailed discussion of nursing intervention with suicidal clients is presented in Chapter 36.

Medication. Clients receiving antidepressant medications—tricyclics, MAO inhibitors, or lithium—must be observed for medication compliance, side effects, toxic effects, and onset of effectiveness. With MAO inhibitors, dietary rules must be taught whether the client is in an inpatient or an outpatient setting. Necessary laboratory tests, particularly for clients on lithium, must be scheduled at regular intervals. ECT is also used with depressed clients, particularly those with recurrent depressions and those who are resistant to drug therapy. It is regarded by some as the treatment of choice for depressed clients who have somatic delusions and delusional guilt accompanied by loss of interest in the world, suicidal ideation, and weight loss. A detailed discussion of antidepressant medications and ECT is presented in Chapter 26.

BEHAVIORAL NEEDS. Vegetative signs of depression reflect that the body physiology has slowed to almost a standstill. The lack of bodily energy causes every physical demand to be perceived as an irritant and an intrusion, since monumental effort is required for the slightest task. Ironically, however, as long as the body physiology remains at a standstill, the emotional state is unlikely to change. A depressed mood is often improved after the body physiology has been speeded up, because strenuous exercise produces chemical substances called *endorphins,* which create a natural "high." The problem is often that depressed people may use their mood as a rationalization for inactivity. They believe, in a rather magical way, that once their depression lifts, they will be productive again. This idea is consistent with feeling helpless to control one's life. Compounding the problem still further are the client's low self-esteem, rigid self-expectations, and perfectionistic "should" system which lead to the commonly heard statement, "There's no use trying. I never do anything well anyway."[43]

Nursing intervention focuses on mobilizing clients to productive activity. Nurse and client collaborate in the formulation of activities or strategies that are congruent with the treatment goals. Involving clients in the planning and assignment of therapeutic tasks places responsibility for change with the client. This implies that the client *can* change and thus instills hope for the future. Therapeutic tasks will also restructure the client's negative perspective and track problem-solving skills by providing experimental learning. They also shift the client's preoccupation with self to interests in the outside world. Additionally, it is hoped that accomplishment of such tasks will generalize beyond the therapeutic setting to the client's life.

Initially, the nurse should judge the client's readiness to participate in activities and should provide opportunities for increasing involvement. A structured daily program of activities can be beneficial. Severely depressed clients will rarely initiate involvement in unit activities. The nurse provides a realistic structure based on the client's tolerance for people and activity, and on the probability of success. Since the client's self-esteem is low, the activities planned should not be too difficult. Success tends to increase self-esteem and hope. Failure tends to reinforce feelings of worthlessness and hopelessness. An activity should also not be too time-consuming. Depressed clients have short attention spans and difficulty concentrating. Tasks that can be completed quickly and successfully will be most therapeutic. Attention should be focused on the task at hand, not what was done in the past or needs to be done in the future. Positive reinforcement should be based on actual performance. A nurse who is truthful with clients will gain their respect and trust.

Other therapeutic activities include exercise. Physical fitness is often associated with a feeling of well-being and reduced anxiety and depression. However, the emotional state of these depressed clients makes it difficult indeed to mobilize their will to become more physically active. By framing the intervention within a teaching model, the nurse may have a greater measure of success. The nurse might say:

> I know that right now you have no energy, and everything seems like a supreme effort. But we have found that physical activity helps people like you feel better in the same way that medication does. As you become more physically active, there will be chemical changes in your body that will help you feel less depressed. Let's just see if this works for you.

Movement therapy, dance therapy, exercise classes, walking, jogging, swimming, and bicycling provide opportunities for body movement and activity that will mobilize physical responsiveness and decrease tension.

As clients begin to feel better, recreational needs become more important. Planning renewal of an activity that they used to enjoy—an outing, movies, dinner out, attending a lecture, a social gathering, playing a sport or game—is heartening for clients. Carrying out such activities also gives clients a sense of accomplishment. For example, a client who has long dreaded social gatherings because of self-perceived social awkwardness might begin to feel hopeful after successfully initiating a conversation with an acquaintance at a church supper.

COGNITIVE NEEDS. As discussed earlier in the chapter, depressed clients have a negative cognitive triad. Cognitive interventions are directed at increasing clients' self-esteem and sense of control over their goals and behaviors, and modifying their negative self-expectations.

Depressed clients often define their problems negatively. This is because their thinking tends to be dominated by negative ideas. As a result, these clients will, despite successful performances, take a pessimistic view of outcomes and their part in them and continue to have low self-esteem. When clients describe their view of their problem, the nurse accepts the client's perceptions, but does not necessarily accept the conclusions that have been drawn. Frequently, negative thinking is an automatic process of which a client is unaware. The nurse can assist the client in exploring the extent to which negative thoughts occur. Once aware of the frequency of this pattern, the client can be taught how to substitute a positive thought for a negative one. For example, a client who absolutely states, "I have been and always will be a coward," might be instructed to substitute a more realistic thought such as "My fears vary from time to time and from situation to situation." Simultaneously, the client is encouraged to increase positive thinking by appraising personal assets, strengths, accomplishments, and opportunities.

Since depressed people tend to interpret experience in a negative way, the accuracy of their perceptions, logic, and conclusions must be examined.[44] People tend to generalize from specific experiences. For example:

> A client who couldn't balance a checkbook properly while in college concludes that he will not be able to manage his financial affairs now that he is living on his own, and that he will soon be in financial ruin. When he examines this pattern of thought with a nurse, the distortions and irrational beliefs become evident, and his self-understanding is enhanced.

Clients are encouraged to modify their perceptions of their experiences and themselves in a more realistic direction.

Clients' negative self-expectations lead them to anticipate failure. A nurse will often hear, "I can't" or "I won't" from a client who envisions failure and would rather not try than fail. Other clients have unrealistically high expectations of themselves that become negative expectation because they can never meet their own standards.[43] For example:

> A severely depressed young woman dreaded going to the supermarket, because even with a shopping list, she feared forgetting items. Nevertheless, she expected herself to remember every household item needed. She became so anxious about not living up to her standards that she would become immobilized when shopping.

Clients should be encouraged to move from unrealistic to realistic goals, and to decrease the importance they attach to unattainable goals.

Clients who have a negative view of current experience and their part in it have a negative view of the future as well. Anticipating failure, they are unable to hope that life will ever be any different, and feel that they are not able to make it any different. "What's the point of going on?" "Why live like this?"—these are questions often asked by depressed clients. Suicidal thoughts are common when the futility of existence is ever-present. Nurses should attempt to limit the amount of time clients spend in negative self-evaluation, for this tends to reinforce their self-criticism. Engaging clients in productive tasks or activities limits the time they spend brooding or criticizing themselves. Then too, such activities in and of themselves provide a sense of mastery, positive reinforcement, and a ray of hope that things can be different.

AFFECTIVE NEEDS. Affective interventions are integral to any nursing care plan for a depressed client. Depressed clients have difficulty expressing their emotions, especially anger, guilt, sadness, hopelessness, and anxiety. They tend to view such feelings as unacceptable, "abnormal," or antithetical to their "should" system. Thus, awareness of such feelings tends to reinforce the client's already low self-esteem.

However, the negative aspects of clients' feelings may be totally unconscious; they may have not the slightest idea that they are angry with, resentful of, or disappointed in others. When a feeling is unconscious, it is because awareness of the feeling would threaten the person in some way. Therefore, the nurse must proceed with great sensitivity, never assuming that direct interpretations will be helpful, let alone effective.

Helping a client become aware of aggressive feelings will be successful when it is done slowly, tentatively, and with genuine patience. Making observations is one way to start, but an observation should always be framed in a tentative way to decrease resistance. "I notice that when you talk about your husband you get a certain look on your face. I may be wrong about this, but it looks to me like a feeling of irritation. Were you aware of feeling that just now as we were talking?" This is very different from saying, "When you talk about your husband you are obviously angry." The latter is disrespectful and presumptuous, creates anxiety, and imparts a sense of threat. The former is respectful of the client's autonomy, leaving the person free to consider the possibility or to reject it. Often, the initial response will be an automatic denial, such as, "Of course I am not angry with my husband." The nurse then retreats for the moment, but over a period of time, with repeated interventions, the client may become trusting enough to view the possibility with more objectivity.

Depressed clients in state hospital settings often seem to improve when they are made to scrub floors or clean toilets. This is probably because their aggressive energy is expressed through activities that eventually become tiresome and create conscious resentment. Activities that allow for physical sublimation of aggressive drives are almost always helpful, even if the client does not become consciously aware of the aggressive feelings.

Another means available to the nurse in moving a client from denial to recognition of a feeling is to model appropriate superego evaluations of feelings. This is not done in a persuasive way, nor even with the expectation of further discussion. Rather, an offhand comment like, "If that happened to me, I think I would have felt angry" or "That seems like a situation which would make many people angry" can be effective. Such comments, when offered in a consistent and kind manner, plant an idea in clients' minds that can be thought about more at a later time. Clients may gradually alter their rigid superego evaluations of their personal feelings.

On the other hand, since aggressive feelings may contain elements of destructive impulses, we cannot simply assure the client that anger is acceptable. Mental health professionals in general tend to do more harm than good when they rush in to assure clients that anger is a perfectly natural feeling, and that it should not be judged as "bad." Appropriate anger is indeed healthy, but a client may be harboring hate, vindictiveness, and wishes for revenge. If these feelings are labeled *OK*, the client will feel that the nurse does not truly understand. People sense, if only intuitively, how destructive such negative feelings can become. Inappropriate reassurance causes them to retreat into isolation and secrecy. Once a client has become willing to share concerns about negative emotions, the nurse must come to understand the full range and content of these emotions before deciding on an intervention.

The following examples illustrate inappropriate and appropriate interventions with a client who expresses negative feelings. Here is an inappropriate intervention:

CLIENT: Yes, you're right. I am angry with my husband.

NURSE: But anger is a natural feeling. You are being too hard on yourself. You shouldn't feel so guilty for being angry.

Here is an appropriate intervention:

CLIENT: Yes, you're right. I am angry with my husband.

NURSE: Could you tell me what this is like for you—to be angry with him?

CLIENT: Oh, I don't know. (Pause.) Sometimes I want to hurt him just as much as he has hurt me.

NURSE: That sense of hurt must be very deep and painful.

CLIENT: (Begins to cry and shares the ways husband has bullied her and made her life miserable.)

NURSE: So you are really in a dilemma with your anger. On one hand, if you let yourself dwell on it, you are really afraid that you will become as mean as he has been to you. On the other hand, the more you hide from your anger, the more depressed you become.

Approaching this client's anger appropriately accomplishes two things. First, the client becomes aware of the feelings beneath the anger—the hurt and pain. Vindictive urges toward the husband are probably reduced to the degree that the hurt is released. Second, the client's true dilemma has been acknowledged, allowing exploration of more constructive ways to deal with the feelings of anger.

When nurses accept clients' anger, despair, or anxiety without criticism, the clients are encouraged to feel that the expression of such feelings need not be destructive or a sign of weakness. Increased emotional responsiveness may, at first, be frightening to clients for whom depression has been a flight from painful emotions, particularly anger. Facilitating expression of feelings by calm acceptance leads clients out of their depression because as emotional responsiveness returns, so does a reasonable basis for hope.

Initially, a nurse must provide hope for a depressed client. While acknowledging the client's pain, the nurse can also provide reassurance that depression is self-limiting and that, although recovery is a slow process, the client will not remain at this level of depression. However, nurses must also realize that clients often resist hopeful attitudes and may try to prove that they, in fact, are hopeless. Statements like "I can't," "I won't," and "It's useless" reflect their tendency to become entrenched in a hopeless position. In this situation, nurses may find that "going with the resistance" is quite effective. For example, a nurse may say to a client who responds negatively to any reassurance or suggestion, "I think it would be helpful for you to go and sit on the couch and stare at the wall for a half hour." Paradoxically, the client may rebel at the directive to "do nothing" and say, "I'm not doing that; that's ridiculous." Instead, he or she may be mobilized by the anger to express a feeling or do something productive.

Finally, nurses who work with depressed clients must of necessity be self-aware. Depression can be contagious. Nurses must be aware of the extent to which their depressed clients trigger their own feelings of sadness, pessimism, and despair, as well as the degree to which their feelings are negatively interacting with clients' similar feelings. Even when nurses have a positive outlook, depressed clients can be frustrating to work with because of their passivity, resistiveness, and pessimism. Nurses need to be aware of when, why, and how the therapeutic relationship is being stalled by the interacting feelings of the nurse and the client. The effectiveness of nurses' interventions will be a function of their own emotional responsiveness, their values about positive and negative feelings, and their ability to offer genuine respect and nonjudgmental acceptance. Nurses must be able to recognize, experience, and express feelings themselves if they expect to help their clients in this important aspect of life.

SPIRITUAL NEEDS. Depressed people have generally lost their faith in whatever previously gave meaning to their lives. Nurses will see this loss of faith expressed in any number of ways. Depressed clients may believe that God has deserted them or takes perverse pleasure in their pain and suffering. Or they may believe that God is the source of their pain and is punishing them for some past sin. People who have tended to put faith in a different source—ethical principles, for example, or other people—may experience a loss and sense of betrayal differently. The important thing is for nurses to assess what beliefs have given their clients' lives a sense of meaning in the past, in order to determine how the loss of faith is interacting with the depression in the present.

A difficult issue that often arises is to determine whether the guilt and self-condemnation that are so typical in depression actually arise because of certain religious beliefs in the first place. A nurse must learn to differentiate feelings that are generated from an unhealthy "should" system from those that characterize a healthy moral conscience. Unhealthy "shoulds" do not help people to grow but rather lead them to aim at the appearance of perfection, and thus lack moral authenticity. Many "shoulds" do not even have a pretense of morality, particularly when they involve such ideas as "I should be able to get away with anything" or "I should always get the better of others." In contrast to genuine moral strivings, these ideas are arrogant and have the goal of enhancing the person's glory and making him or her godlike. Moreover, such "shoulds" have a coercive character. When the person does not measure up, there are quick retributions ranging from severe anxiety and despair to self-condemnation and self-destructive impulses. While a healthy conscience encourages striving toward certain standards, it does not set such harsh tasks. It motivates the person to overcome the difficulties encountered in life through a constructive examination of what is wrong, without magnifying or minimizing the reality of the situation. As a moral agency interested in furthering growth, it uses failure creatively to guide the personality to evolution and growth.

When clients are encouraged to explore their spiritual beliefs, they may feel more hopeful and optimistic. Clarification of values and one's own "should" system contributes to a sense of hopefulness by reducing conflicts. Identifying a meaningful philosophy of life provides meaning and purpose in life; that in itself instills hope. As clients begin to resolve inner conflicts, they are able to grow in hope and to become more authentic human beings. When their inner strengths are identified and maximized, they have a greater sense of self-worth and value. Finally, nurses can arrange for clients to be visited by a member of the clergy, either their own or one affiliated with a hospital, and can also provide opportunities for them to attend religious services when possible. This demonstrates respect for clients' beliefs and can provide an important resource.

Intervention with the Family*

Hospitalization of a depressed client disrupts the family's usual patterns of interaction. Other family members may begin exhibiting symptoms of the family's distress. Group sessions enable nurses to observe the family's patterns of interaction. Family members can be helped to notice and change problematic patterns. In family therapy, the focus is shifted from the client to the family as a unit—a family with whom the depressed person was unable to find a solution other than to be depressed. The family needs help with self-observation and with evolution of new patterns of relating.

When one family member goes to the hospital, another member often needs special help. The family member who has loved the depressed person the most may experience intense pain, frustration, or anger, quickly followed by guilt and confusion. The same pattern also occurs frequently when the depressed client makes progress.

An important prerequisite for being helpful to a family member is familiarity with experiences that the family and the depressed person have in common. It is important to be calmly and knowingly accepting of family members who are undergoing frustration, guilt, and confusion. The presence of a helpful nurse whose knowledge base makes sense out of an otherwise confusing world is comforting. A manner which is neither detached nor overinvolved, and behavior which is neither an attempt to escape nor an expression of alarm, will also have the effect of organizing and role modeling for family members. Some family members may be taught a deeper understanding of the depressed person. Nurses should use the theoretical base most likely to be understandable and useful. For example, for a family member, understanding the psychodynamic origin of depression is likely to be less useful in relating to the depressed person than developing some understanding of the loved one's tenacious but temporary commitment to a poor self-view.

* This section from Ardis Swanson, "The Client Who Generates Depression," in the second edition of this book.

There are certain kinds of family experiences which the nurse needs to become familiar with. For example, frustration and anger may be evoked in family members who make an effort to express love and caring which is seemingly not appreciated. Guilt over the feelings of frustration and anger adds to the burden. The family needs to know that the depressed person often responds negatively to expressions of love—feeling both needing and undeserving, both demanding and unable to receive. A depressed person may try to respond in a reciprocal, loving way but be unable to do so. The caring one thus feels drained and rejected. If the caring person responds totally to the needs of the one who is depressed, to the extent of retreating from day-to-day obligations, another burden will be added to the depressed person's guilt and humiliation. Therefore, those close to depressed persons need to help themselves: they need to grow in self-understanding and to maintain an ongoing life as best they can.

A depressed person needs help in modifying an unrealistic self-view that was, to some extent, derived from the family of origin. A nurse can help such clients to assess both family expectations and their own self-expectations realistically, to sort out the "shoulds" of life from the "wants," and to reappraise their life plans. Family members can be guided by the nurse in reviewing the family's goals, their own individual goals, and the origins of family members' expectations in the family system. Unrealistic expectations and goals may be examined and modified. Alternative options may be identified, tested, and evaluated by each individual as well as by the family as a unit.

Clients may need to spend time relating to family members in order to validate their assumptions about the reasons for the ways in which love is given in their families. A client may discover that love is available even without strict compliance or that relying on others for validation of self-esteem is unrealistic.

A nurse can guide a client in developing a sense of separateness and wholeness as a person that is not dependent on or determined by the family. The nurse can support the client in giving up hope for a "perfect other" and in exploring realistic options for relationships both in and outside the family. For example, the client may discover that the sense of loss following the death of an important family member comes not so much because the person has died as because of the loss of love and approval. The client may initially feel that these resources will not be supplied in any other relationship. The nurse can help such a client to identify other gratifying relationships that will involve less dependency.

Sessions with the family unit also help the nurse to identify overt or covert depression in other family members. Sometimes the "identified patient" is expressing the depression of other family members. If this situation is picked up by the therapist, exploring it with the family may help rechannel the depression to the appropriate people. In this way the client may be freed from the burden of expressing others' depression. Other family members who are then appropriately feeling their own depression may be helped in family sessions or referred to another resource.

Intervention with the Community

Interventions on a community level deal with problems that interfere with clients' ability to meet the social exigencies of life. Many depressed clients lack or perceive themselves to be lacking in interpersonal skills and thus feel uneasy in social situations. Low self-esteem usually accompanies people's appraisal of themselves as socially ineffective, powerless, or helpless.

Self-esteem must ultimately rest on a sense of competence to deal with life's demands. All too often, nurses fail to appreciate that a poor self-image may arise from feeling generally ill-equipped to deal with life. The dependency so often seen in the depressed client may indicate that the person has failed to achieve an adequate level of autonomy, and instead has come to rely on the resources of others. Helping clients develop the concrete skills needed to achieve higher-level autonomy is well within the province of nursing practice and yet is often overlooked. For instance:

> A man who is being released from the hospital may feel overwhelmed at the prospect of setting up an appointment to return to the clinic for outpatient treatment. The nurse who has given the clinic number to the client and instructed him when to call may think the rest is up to the client. But more can be done. The nurse can support the client in making the call from the hospital, in getting the appointment confirmed and in exploring his feelings about the process. Likewise, the nurse can help the client to get a bus schedule and perhaps even accompany him on a "practice run" during a special outing.

Hospitals offer many such opportunities for nurses to lend ego support and to assist clients in practicing the skills that create so much anxiety and that seem so overwhelming until support is given.

Clients may be helped to modify their interpersonal styles or improve their social skills through a sequential learning process that may combine training in assertiveness, social skills, and overcoming shyness. In working directly with clients rather than referring them to such programs, nurses will do the following:

- Assess clients' social skills in terms of strengths, weaknesses, supports, and interests.
- Evaluate existing and potential social resources available to clients.
- Instruct clients about how to develop effective social skills.
- Serve as role models for clients.
- Role-play and rehearse problematic social situations and interactions.
- Provide feedback for and positive reinforcement of effective social and interpersonal skills.
- Encourage participation in expanded areas of social interest and interaction.

As clients feel increasingly competent, they will develop more of a sense of control over their social experience and thus will feel less helpless in social situations.

The final phase of mastery of social skills is to involve clients in social activities. Depressed clients often express difficulty in meeting new people and thus do not readily engage in an active social life.[44,45] Nurses work with clients to identify their social, recreational, religious, cultural, and career interests. Clients can then be directed to resources such as community organizations, groups, and clubs through which these interests can be pursued. Special-interest groups such as women's support groups, single-parent groups, jogging clubs, chess clubs, parenting groups, political clubs, and adult education classes are potential vehicles for expanding one's social network. This may sound like a relatively simple intervention, but the nurse's creativity may be challenged by the combination of clients' self-doubts and the need to find appropriate resources.

Involvement in outpatient group therapy may be another effective method for enhancing interaction, by promoting social support through group relatedness.

Clients who have a great deal of situational stress because of life events, role strain, or inadequate support systems can be helped by nurses to:

- Accept the stressful life events that have occurred.
- Identify functional coping strategies for dealing with stress.
- Modify stressful lifestyles.
- Explore options regarding relationships, when role strain occurs.
- Identify actual or potential physical, emotional, and social support systems and resources.
- Utilize available resources and support systems to ease stress.

When clients perceive themselves as able to control the outcomes of their lives, they feel more powerful and more in command. Experiencing this feeling in just one area of life may help the client to feel hopeful about achieving control in other areas of life.

Evaluation

Evaluation of the nursing care plan is particularly important with depressed people. These clients can be quite unrealistic in their expectations of themselves, tending to expect either too much or too little. Not only is evaluation a tool for nursing accountability, but it also provides a realistic perspective on the accomplishments of the care plan.

The following clinical example shows how evaluation is used to appraise the effectiveness of nursing care for Carrie K., a depressed client who has unrealistically high expectations of herself (see Table 34-8):

Carrie K., a 30-year-old woman, has been increasingly depressed since the birth of her first child 1 year ago.

Table 34-8 Evaluation (Carrie K.)

Assessment	Diagnosis	Outcomes	Interventions	Evaluation
Carrie K. states that she has always expected a lot of herself. Now more than anything, she wants to be a perfect wife and mother. She feels that she has been only inadequate in these roles, accomplishing little or nothing each day. Her husband and mother state that you could eat off the floors, the house is so clean, and that nothing Carrie does is good enough for her. The nurse observes that Carrie and her baby are always neat and clean, although Carrie's personal grooming and style of dress seem to indicate low self-esteem.	Distorted perception of accomplishments related to unrealistic expectations of self.	1. Carrie will complete a day-by-day activity schedule for 1 week, using the prescribed ranking system. 2. Carrie will realistically evaluate the quantity and quality of her accomplishments. 3. She will not call her mother to come over and tell her if her house is clean enough. 4. Carrie will modify her activity and stress level by choosing one thing to eliminate from her schedule each day.	1. Explore client's self-expectations. 2. Nonjudgmentally accept client's self-expectations 3. Provide information about cognitive triad and about negative views of self. 4. Instruct client about purpose of task assignment and how to do it. 5. Review client's weekly level of productivity with her. Request feedback from others. 6. Explore relationship between self-esteem and productivity. 7. Explore options for modifying client's schedule while maintaining self-esteem.	During the therapy session Carrie criticized herself constantly about being totally unproductive, incompetent, and inadequate. At the end of 2 weeks, Carrie acknowledges that she is productive; in fact, she states that she doesn't know how she does so much while feeling as miserable as she does. She has not called her mother for reassurance about her competence. Twice last week she took the baby for a walk rather than wash the floor or vacuum, and she allowed a friend to take her to an aerobics class. At the end of 3 weeks, she has eliminated one chore per day from her schedule and has substituted a "fun" activity.

She berates herself for not being productive enough. She expects herself to care for herself, her child, her husband, and her household in a perfect way. She is not able to perceive that she actually does accomplish that goal even while she is depressed and is undergoing much stress and anxiety. During a therapy session, the nurse and Carrie establish a goal of having Carrie analyze her daily productivity.

SUMMARY

Depression, a universal experience, affects approximately 15 percent of the population at any given time. Depression can be conceptualized as occurring on a continuum from mild to moderate to severe. It involves an alteration in mood that is characterized by feelings of sadness and loss of interest or pleasure in all, or almost all, one's usual activities and pastimes. Affective, cognitive, behavioral, and physiological changes are associated with depression. Symptoms of depression can vary in duration, intensity, and pervasiveness.

Causes of depression can be discussed in terms of psychoanalytic, cognitive, interpersonal, genetic, biochemical, family systems, and social stress theories. Depression is not completely explained by any one theory, but rather may be a result of a complex matrix of interacting forces.

Assessment of individual, family, and community factors is important in identifying factors that are relevant to planning individualized care for depressed clients and their families. Nursing diagnoses and outcome criteria for clients must be realistic and attainable. Intervention with depressed clients considers their physical, safety, behavioral, cognitive, affective, social, spiritual, family, and community dimensions. Evaluation of nursing intervention is accomplished by appraising clients' attainment of projected behaviors.

The overwhelming majority of people who experience depression recover and achieve a higher level of wellness than before the depression, if they use the opportunity to develop a more realistic view of themselves, others, and their world.

REFERENCES

1. G. L. Klerman, M. M. Weissman, B. J. Rounsaville, and E. S. Chevron, *Interpersonal Psychotherapy of Depression,* Basic Books, New York, 1984.
2. P. Rosenblatt, R. Walsh, and D. Jackson, *Grief and Mourning in Cross-Cultured Perspective,* HRAF, New Haven, Conn., 1976.
3. P. Clayton et al., "Mourning and Depression: Their Similarities and Differences," *Canadian Psychiatric Association,* vol. 19, 1974, pp. 309–315.
4. S. Arieti and J. Bemporad, eds., *Severe and Mild Depression,* Basic Books, New York, 1979.
5. American Psychiatric Association, *Diagnostic and Statistical Manual of Mental Disorders,* 3d ed., APA, Washington, D.C., 1980.
6. S. Secunder, ed., *The Depressive Disorders,* Special Report, U.S. Department of Health, Education and Welfare, National Institute of Mental Health, 1973.
7. G. L. Klerman and M. M. Weissman, "Depressions among Women: Their Nature and Causes," in M. Guttenberg, S. Salasin, and D. Belle, eds., *Mental Health of Women,* Academic Press, New York, 1980.
8. M. Scharf, *Unfinished Business,* Ballantine, New York, 1981.
9. Leopold Bellak, *Ego Functions in Schizophrenics, Neurotics, and Normals: A Systematic Study of Conceptual Diagnostics and Therapeutic Aspects,* Wiley, New York, 1973, p. 436.
10. Sigmund Freud, "Mourning and Melancholia," in *Collected Papers,* Hogarth, London, 1953, vol. IV, p. 153.
11. Alexander Lowen, *Depression and the Body,* Coward, McCann and Geoghegan, New York, 1972, p. 129.
12. J. Robertson and J. Robertson, "Young Children in Brief Separation: A Fresh Look," in *The Psychoanalytic Study of the Child,* International Universities Press, New York, 1971.
13. John Bowlby, "Childhood Mourning and Its Implications for Psychiatry," *American Journal of Psychology,* vol. 128, no. 6, December 1961.
14. René Spitz and K. M. Wold, "Anaclitic Depression," in *The Psychoanalytic Study of the Child,* International Universities Press, New York, 1946.
15. A. Beck and A. Rush, "Cognitive Approaches to Depression and Suicide," in G. Servan, ed., *Cognitive Defects in the Development of Mental Illness,* Brunner/Mazel, New York, 1977.
16. A. Beck, A. J. Rush, B. Shaw, and G. Emergy, *Cognitive Therapy of Depression,* Guilford, New York, 1979.
17. M. Seligman, *Helplessness: On Depression, Development and Death,* Freeman, San Francisco, 1975.
18. L. T. Abramson, M. Seligman, and J. D. Teasdale, "Learned Helplessness in Humans: Critique and Reformulation," *Journal of Abnormal Psychology,* vol. 87, 1978, pp. 49–74.
19. J. M. G. Williams, *The Psychological Treatment of Depression,* Free Press, New York, 1984.
20. M. E. Seligman, "A Learned Helplessness Point of View," in L. P. Rehm, ed., *Behavior Therapy for Depression,* Academic Press, New York, 1981.
21. I. R. Hargreaves, "A Test of the Reformulated Learned Helplessness Model of Depression," unpublished M.Sc. dissertation, University of Aberdeen, Scotland.

22. G. I. Metalsky, L. Abramson, M. Seligman, A. Semmel, and C. Peterson, "Attributional Styles and Life Events in the Classroom: Vulnerability and Invulnerability to Depressive Mood Reactions," *Journal of Personality and Social Psychology,* vol. 43, 1982, pp. 612–617.
23. N. J. Kerr, "Behavior Manifestations of Misguided Entitlement," *Perspectives in Psychiatric Care,* vol. 23, no. 1, 1985, pp. 5–15.
24. Karen Horney, *Neurosis and Human Growth,* Norton, New York, 1950, p. 210.
25. H. Bradley, ed., *The New English Dictionary on Historical Principles,* vol. 3, Macmillan, New York, 1888.
26. J. Stein, ed., *The Random House Dictionary of the English Language,* Random House, Boston, 1967.
27. D. Black, ed., *The Law Dictionary,* 5th ed., Weston, St. Paul, Minn. 1979.
28. G. L. Klerman and J. E. Barret, "The Affective Disorders: Clinical and Epidemiological Aspects," in S. Gershon and B. Shopsin, eds., *Lithium: Its Role in Psychiatric Research and Treatment,* Plenum, New York, 1973.
29. S. S. Kety, D. Rosenthal, P. H. Wender, F. Schlusinger, and B. Jacobsen, "Mental Illness in the Biological and Adoptive Families of Adopted Individuals Who Have Become Schizophrenic: A Preliminary Report Based on Psychiatric Interviews," in R. R. Fieve, D. Rosenthal, and H. Brill, eds., *Genetic Research in Psychiatry,* Johns Hopkins University Press, Baltimore, Md., 1975.
30. R. Cancro, "An Overview of Affective Disorders," in A. Freedman, H. Kaplan, and B. Sadock, eds., *Comprehensive Textbook of Psychiatry,* 4th ed., Williams and Wilkins, Baltimore, Md., 1985.
31. M. Bowen, *Family Therapy in Clinical Practice,* Aronson, New York, 1976.
32. E. Paykel, J. Meyres, M. Dieneff, G. Klerman, J. Lindenthal, and M. Pepper, "Life Events and Depression: A Controlled Study," *Archives of General Psychiatry,* vol. 21, 1969, pp. 753–760.
33. F. Ilfeld, "Characteristics of Current Social Stressors," *Psychological Report,* vol. 39, 1976, p. 1231.
34. F. Ilfeld, "Current Social Stressors and Symptoms of Depression," *American Journal of Psychiatry,* vol. 134, 1977, p. 161.
35. W. R. Gove, "The Relationship between Sex Roles, Marital Status, and Mental Illness," *Social Forces,* vol. 51, 1972, pp. 34–44.
36. J. H. Pleck, "The Work Family Role System," *Social Problems,* vol. 24, 1977, pp. 417–427.
37. A. S. Rossi, "A Biosocial Perspective on Parenting," *Daedalus,* vol. 106, 1977, pp. 1–32.
38. L. W. Hoffman, "Changes in Family Roles, Socialization and Sex Differences," *American Psychologist,* vol. 6, 1977, pp. 644–657.
39. S. Rosenfield, "Sex Differences in Depression: Do Women Always Have Higher Rates?" *Journal of Health and Social Behavior,* vol. 21, 1980, p. 33.
40. G. Brown and T. Harris, *Social Origins of Depression,* Tavistock, London, 1978.
41. A. T. Beck, "Depression Causes and Treatment," University of Pennsylvania Press, Philadelphia, 1967.
42. N. Zung, "A Self-Rating Depression Scale," *Archives of General Psychiatry,* vol. 12, 1965, p. 63.
43. N. Kerr, "The Tyranny of the Shoulds," *Perspectives in Psychiatric Care,* vol. 22, 1984, pp. 10–19.
44. S. B. Helm, "Nursing Care of the Depressed Patient: A Cognitive Approach," *Perspectives in Psychiatric Care,* vol. 22, 1984, pp. 100–102.
45. G. W. Stuart and S. J. Sundeen, *Principles and Practice of Psychiatric Nursing,* Mosby, St. Louis, 1983.

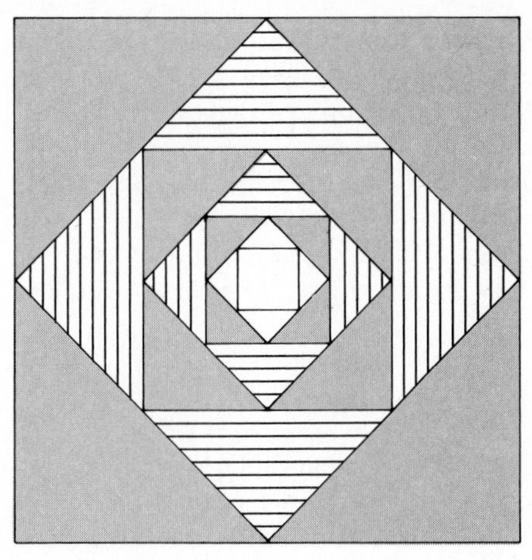

CHAPTER 35
Patterns of Elation

Judith Haber

LEARNING OBJECTIVES

After studying this chapter, the student should be able to:

1. Describe the thoughts, affects, and behaviors associated with mild elation, acute elation, and delirium.
2. Discuss how individual, family, and environmental patterns of interaction are associated with patterns of elation.
3. Identify individual, family, and environmental assessment factors for manic clients.
4. Formulate nursing diagnoses for manic clients.
5. Formulate attainable short- and long-term outcome criteria for manic clients.
6. Differentiate nursing interventions appropriate for clients with mild elation, acute elation, and delirium.
7. Evaluate the effectiveness of a nursing care plan for a manic client.

Patterns of elation are manifested by clients who experience manic episodes. Such episodes occur cyclically with or without alternating episodes of depression. This pattern reflects an alteration in mood that is characterized by elation, euphoria, or both. The alteration in mood is reflected in changes in mind, body, and spirit.

Clients with this health problem appear to be self-sufficient and to "know it all." They frequently take command in an interpersonal situation and are skillful in evoking and utilizing the feelings of others, making them feel exposed, undermined, and vulnerable.[1,2] This process is integral to problems that develop within the client's individual, family, and environmental systems.

The purpose of this chapter is to provide a framework for nursing intervention for clients experiencing manic episodes. Patterns of interaction within the person and with the family and the environment are explored. The nursing process for the client who has manic episodes is developed.

DYSYNCHRONOUS HEALTH PATTERNS

Clients who have manic episodes tend to have affective moods of *elation*, which is a heightened mood of joy, happiness, and pleasure; and *euphoria*, which is an exaggerated feeling of vigor and physical well-being. These people exhibit alterations in affect, thought, and behavior. Affective changes include manifestations of elation and euphoria. Alterations in thinking include distractability, flight of ideas, and delusions of grandeur. Behavior is characterized by increased activity and excitability.[3,4]

Stages of Manic Patterns of Interaction

It is helpful to conceptualize manic patterns of interaction as occurring in three stages ranging from mild elation to delirium. Although each stage is presented below as a discrete entity, in actuality the stages may overlap and interact.

Stage 1: Mild Elation

Mild elation is often difficult to detect. Many people who exhibit behaviors characteristic of this stage never become clients. Some become clients in outpatient treatment settings, and still others enter inpatient settings if the symptoms increase and their behavior becomes dysfunctional. These people are often referred to as *hypomanic*, which means that they have relatively consistent baseline patterns of good mood, increased activity, and sociability. They often lead outwardly successful and productive lives in the community. Perceptions of them will include the following features.

AFFECT. Perceptions with regard to affect include these:

1. Lively, happy, free of worry, unconcerned
2. Extroverted, witty, joking, without concern for reality or the feelings of others
3. Confident, uninhibited
4. Often, indifferent to events that would normally make a person sad
5. Moody, changing easily to irritated and angry, especially when others are critical or do not respond enthusiastically

THOUGHTS. Following are perceptions regarding thoughts:

1. Content of thought often reveals an exalted opinion of self as a great lover, or a person of great wealth and ability, or both.
2. Ideas move quickly from one subject to another, with poor ability to concentrate and pursue an idea to a goal-directed end.
3. The person has the ability to associate ideas rapidly and thereby to grasp aspects of the environment which would otherwise go unnoticed. However, because of increased distractibility, the person is unable to utilize the perceptions in a meaningful way. For example, elaborate business schemes are devised, but they either fail or are never implemented.
4. There is little evidence of introspection.

BEHAVIOR. Following are perceptions regarding behavior:

1. Motor activity is increased. These are people who are always on the go. They talk, tease, and joke excessively. They may sing while walking down the street, dance as they walk, and laugh when others would find laughter inappropriate.
2. They may periodically experience loss of appetite, loss of weight, constipation, insomnia, and

irregular menstrual periods. The sex drive may increase.

3. Activity is not always appropriate for the person's age and the place. These people may engage in a great deal of purposeless activity or in activities aimed at irrelevant goals. For example, they may write numerous unnecessary letters or go on spending sprees to purchase unneeded items. Frequently, rapid changes of activity may be observed.
4. These people engage in superficial relationships and have many acquaintances but few close friends.

Stage 2: Acute Elation

Symptoms, more pronounced during this stage, have either intensified from those manifested in stage 1 or appeared suddenly. At this point most affected people appear as clients in the inpatient treatment setting.

AFFECT. Symptoms with regard to affect include these:

1. The affect is characterized by feelings of exaltation and expansiveness. The client appears to be on a real "high."
2. The expansiveness turns rapidly to anger when attempts are made to control it. The person reacts with fury and may scream, curse, or strike out violently at others or the environment.
3. The affect may be changeable, unstable. A client may be happily talking about the success of a recent business venture, then may suddenly burst into tears and begin dwelling on what a failure he or she has been.

THOUGHTS. Symptoms with regard to thoughts include these:

1. The thought process is characterized by flight of ideas and loquaciousness. *Flight of ideas* is a sudden, continuous, and rapid shift in topics. *Loquaciousness* is often referred to as *pressure of speech*. It is difficult to interrupt the client to get a word in edgewise. Communication patterns also include rhyming, playing on words, and making associations of words having similar sounds but no relationship in meaning.[4] Here is an example of these characteristics:

   NURSE: Mr. D., how do you like it at the hospital?

   CLIENT: Fine, fine, good; . . . good-looking women. I say women because they're different from the men at home. Home is a place to roam; place the food on the table. . . . I want to place first in the stable.

   The ideas and associations seem illogical, but the content and underlying message usually relate to an overvalued idea or egocentric interest of the client's which directs the stream of thought. Clients, not realizing the significance of their statements, often give information about the unconscious motivation of their ideas.[5]
2. The thought content also includes grandiose and persecutory delusions (see Chapter 37). Clients may think that they have x-ray vision or that they must destroy self and family to escape from Satan's wrath.[6]

BEHAVIOR. Behavioral symptoms include these:

1. Dress may be inappropriate. Female clients may dress as if in costume, wearing excessive makeup, too much jewelry, and brightly colored, poorly matching outfits. Their hair may be decorated with beads or flowers. Male clients may also wear bizarre outfits. Clothing may be inappropriate for the weather, and grooming may be poor.
2. Motor activity increases to a constant, urgent rate. Clients continuously meddle with others in ward or family activities. They may suggest numerous ways in which people should conduct themselves. Constant rearrangement of furniture, making and remaking beds, and frequent changing of clothing are also prompted by this activity drive.
3. Despite increased activity, the client has little or no appetite and does not want to stop moving to eat. Sleep patterns are disrupted, and the client may go for days without sleep and without exhibiting signs of exhaustion. Even when objective signs of exhaustion are evident in eyes and body posture, clients continue to move about in random, agitated fashion.
4. Normal inhibitions may decrease, and normally modest clients may engage in sexually indiscreet acts or use profane language.

5. The attention span is disturbed, and the client is easily distracted. Environmental stimuli such as noises, movement, and changes in temperature constantly divert the client's attention. People are sometimes misidentified because they present some slight similarity to persons the client knows well, and the client seizes upon similarities without examining differences. For example:

   When a short, chubby female nurse walked onto the unit, a manic client named Susan ran over to her, shouting, "Mary, Mary, you bitch, why didn't you visit me yesterday?" The nurse identified herself, saying, "Susan, I'm Rhoda Jones, the nurse on the unit." Susan replied, "You are? Yes, I guess you are, but you're short and chubby just like Mary."

Stage 3: Delirium

The client is in a state of extreme excitement at this stage. Feelings, thoughts, and behavior patterns observed are intensifications of those previously described. Clients appear disoriented, incoherent, and agitated. There is a frenetic quality to their behavior. They may injure themselves and others with their increasing, frantic, aimless activity. They exhibit grandiose or religious delusions and sometimes visual or olfactory hallucinations (see Chapter 37).[7] Exhaustion, injury, and death are real possibilities. These clients must be protected against themselves.

DSM III

Manic episodes most commonly occur as one phase of a cyclical pattern that alternates between elation and depression. This is referred to as a *bipolar disorder* and is one of the *major affective disorders*. Another name for this syndrome is *manic-depressive disorder*. When clients are in the manic phase of the cycle, they experience alterations in affect, thoughts, and behavior that range from what is perceived as normal liveliness to intense elation, euphoria, or delirium. In the depressive phase, clients exhibit some of the physical, cognitive, affective, and behavioral changes that are discussed in Chapter 34. Between manic and depressive episodes, clients may exhibit appropriate affect, thinking, and behavior and conduct their lives in a perfectly normal manner. When manic episodes occur without a history of depression, the *Diagnostic and Statistical Manual of Mental Disorders* (DSM III) continues to classify these manic episodes as a *bipolar disorder*. DSM III may also refer to this pattern as *major affective disorder, manic type*.[8]

It is important to remember not to generalize about the form the two mood patterns will take, because each client will manifest a unique pattern and will even exhibit individual variations within a single pattern or cycle.

Epidemiology

Although a large body of data on the epidemiology of affective disorders has been amassed in recent years, it is not easy to interpret. Difficulties in accurately estimating the incidence and prevalence of bipolar disorder occur because of the great variation in the classification systems and measures used, in the control variables studied, and in the reliability of the diagnostic categories. However, in the United States, an estimated 300 persons per 100,000 population, or 0.3 percent of the population, are identified and treated as having bipolar disorder each year. This means that approximately 600,000 bipolar clients are diagnosed and treated annually.[4] Because many manic clients are treated privately as outpatients, the actual incidence of manic clients is underreported.

PATTERNS OF INTERACTION: PERSON

Integral with patterns of interaction in manic people are themes related to loss, superficial relationships, dependency, and anxiety. Genetic and biochemical factors contribute physiological parameters to the occurrence of manic episodes.

Themes

Loss

The manic state is often referred to as a mirror image of depression. It is held that the elation represents a massive denial of underlying depression (see Chapter 34). Clients deny the feelings about actual, threatened, or symbolic loss of love that are seen in depression. These feelings have their roots in a helpless, infantile response to premature separation that occurs around the time that separation-individuation takes place; such a response leads to loss of self-esteem. To counteract this depression, manic clients act out with intense drive the fantasies of strength that enable them to feel liberated from their depression. Heightened activity levels and thought processes enable them to avoid or escape omnipresent depressive thoughts or activities. Joviality is a mask for the client, who is really saying, "I am crying beneath the laughter and jokes." The loss is often not apparent to the onlooker. The client may, for instance, have recently received a promotion. The promotion, however, is perceived by the client as a loss of dependency or as a loss of support from a superior.

Superficial Relationships

Manic clients present themselves defensively to themselves and others as lively, hearty, and friendly. They characteristically have many acquaintances with whom they appear to be on excellent terms. On closer inspection, it becomes apparent that these relationships are very superficial and are not at all suggestive of intimacy, especially since the communication of these clients has little or no depth. These clients carry out stereotyped social performances in which the other person's traits or needs are not considered despite an overt attitude of helpfulness and consideration. Relatedness always remains superficial, so that the manic clients' envy, competitiveness, and fear of rejection will not be accurately perceived and acted upon by others. These clients vacillate between overselling and underselling themselves. Recurring envy of others, underlying competitiveness, and fear of rejection are ever-present, as is sensitivity to the envy of others. This adaptive position protects these persons from ever finding out that others might like and accept them despite transitory lapses in behavior. Never having learned to consider their own feelings in relationships, they are unable to relate to others on an open, empathic level. They have never learned to put themselves in another's place in order to sense what is actually going on. They are afraid that real closeness will lead to rejection; afraid of knowing themselves, they are therefore unwilling to know others.[9]

Dependency

Manic clients project an air of independence in an attempt to mask underlying wishes for dependency. The principal source of anxiety is the *fear of abandonment*. They perceive danger and threat in acknowledging the need to be cared for by others.[10] This evolves from early experiences relating to premature separation and withdrawal of love. To maintain self-esteem and the feeling of power and strength, these clients present a repertoire of behaviors that suggest omnipotent independence. On the surface, the grandiose ideas indicate that these people don't need to be cared for, that they can take care of anyone and everyone. A common remark from such a client is, "I don't need anybody." Such egocentricity is suggestive of narcissism, but the underlying dynamics are those of negative narcissism.

While appearing jovial, outgoing, and friendly, such people are actually self-centered, controlling, and manipulative. They repeatedly attempt to test, manipulate, and overcommit others into involvement with them so that the others will actually be caring for them. Those dependent relationships that do exist are usually of a demanding nature. These relationships provide the praise and approval that such clients need to maintain their fragile self-esteem.[9] The needs of a significant other, usually a spouse, are negated, and the relationship becomes a one-way street. When these clients' demands on significant others are frustrated, they become angry and hostile, thus further jeopardizing the desperately desired ties to others.

Anxiety

Increased physical activity is an attempt to escape the anxiety aroused by a punitive superego. The frenzied activity allows these clients to be selectively inattentive to messages that are unacknowledgeable as components of awareness. Thus feelings of helplessness, worthlessness, and guilt are temporarily avoided.[10]

The psychotic attack occurs when the mask of joviality, manipulativeness, and demandingness no longer serves its defensive purpose. Emptiness is felt, anxiety rises, and behavior becomes more disorganized. The experience of elation may occur in isolation or preceding or following a period of depression.

Genetic Factors

Research findings from family aggregation studies indicate that there is an increased incidence of bipolar disorder in first-degree relatives of clients with this disorder as compared with control groups. The incidence of major depression among first-degree relatives is increased as well. The rates of illness among relatives with bipolar disorder are equal with respect to sex.[11,12,13] The distinction between mild and severe bipolar illness did not discriminate rates of illness in relatives; it was concluded that severity of illness does not predict transmission of illness.

A summary of research on patterns of genetic transmission of bipolar disorder suggests that if there is a genetic component, simple recessive transmission is unlikely to account for the patterns observed. A dominant mode of transmission or transmission by many genes is more likely to explain the transmission process. It is unlikely that one genetic hypothesis will explain the observed familial patterns.

Biochemical Factors

Biochemically, two divergent disorders of neurotransmitter substances have been suggested, catecholamine (norepinephrine) deficiency and indoleamine (serotonin) deficiency. A relationship seems to exist between catecholamine metabolism and the production of norepinephrine. Drugs which stimulate the production of norepinephrine produce behavioral expressions of excitement. Depletion or inactivation of norepinephrine seems to lead to sedation and depression. Therefore, an excess of amines, specifically norepinephrine, at the adrenergic receptor sites in the brain seems to play a significant role in elation.[4]

Both manic and depressed clients appear to have an abnormality in serotonin metabolism, with an enhanced cortisol response to 5-HTP as compared with normal controls. The two hypotheses are not mutually exclusive but rather highlight the potential interactive effect between norepinephrine and cortisol activity in clients with affective disorders. Further research in this area will more clearly define the biochemical factors in affective disorders.[4,14]

Research studies indicate that sodium transport may be another biochemical parameter operating in manic episodes. Research findings suggest that the intracellular distribution of sodium is lowered during manic states and appears to return to normal levels as the manic episode is resolved. Whether lowered levels of sodium are a cause or an effect of the manic episode remains unclear at this time.[15]

In recent years the CAT scan has been used as a tool to investigate possible changes in brain structure associated with manic-depressive as well as other major psychiatric disorders. Such changes, found by CAT scan, include lateral cerebral ventricular enlargement. These findings may result from atrophy or hypoplasia. In a study of 27 bipolar clients and their matched controls, there was a significant difference in the ventricular brain ratio (VBR) of the two groups. The increased ventricular size in the bipolar clients was also significantly associated with greater number of hospitalizations and persistent unemployment, but not with other measures of severity of illness or social deterioration. The meaning of these findings remains uncertain. Increased VBR could represent a risk factor for the disorder, an index of severity, or an etiologic factor. It is to be hoped that further research will provide more meaningful clinical data.[16,17]

PATTERNS OF INTERACTION: FAMILY

Patterns of interaction within the family include early developmental patterns, the family social network, and later developmental patterns.

Early Developmental Patterns

For children who will have manic problems later in life, infancy appears to be a time when they feel loved and accepted. The complete dependence of the infant seems to be pleasurable to the mother. (Schizophrenics and their mothers, on the other hand, perceive all parenting and nurturing experiences as anxiety-provoking.) The infant offers little resistance to her care. The mother is generally described as one who feels "duty-bound" to provide everything the child needs. The image of mother is incorporated by the child as good. As the infant begins to separate from the mother and reach out to explore the environment actively, his or her growing independence and rebelliousness are perceived by the mother as threatening. Unconforming or unconventional behavior on the part of the child is labeled "bad" by the mother, and she makes every effort to eliminate it. Toward the end of the infant's first year of life, the previously loving and tender mother abruptly changes into a harsh, punitive figure.[10]

The small child's ability to integrate a unified object image of the tender mother and the harsh mother is impaired by the anxiety accompanying the conflicting images. Opposing parental images exist to some extent for all children and are normally resolved and incorporated into one coherent image as the ego matures (see Chapter 5). However, children vulnerable to mania wish to maintain only the "good" mother image. They do this through compliance and conformity. The harsh mother is repressed. This dichotomy sets the stage for ambivalence toward others in later life.

During the second year there is a continued change in parenting patterns. Not only is direct care decreased, but demands that the child be independent and self-sufficient are made. The child continues to receive some love and affection if parental expectations, no matter how unrealistic, are accepted and fulfilled. For example:

> One client recalled that as a child she was expected to learn to ride a bicycle at age 3 but was not allowed to fall while learning. The bicycle was taken away when this expectation was not fulfilled.

The attitude that "what is obtained is deserved" evokes an early sense of duty and responsibility.[18]

The child adapts by:

1. Accepting and trying to live up to parental expectations at all costs.
2. Accepting the values and symbols of significant others without attending to his or her own wishes, feelings, and desires.
3. Complying, obeying, and working hard in an effort to recapture the early tenderness from the mother and to maintain the love that does exist.
4. Harboring strong resentment against parents who have made so many demands and have not given enough. This can result in temper tantrums and apparently unprovoked rage, which is an outcome of bottling up feelings until they bubble over. These episodes end quickly because of the fear of loss of love. The feelings are repressed and retained unconsciously. They may reappear in dreams.
5. Acting rebellious and becoming the incorrigible child, exhibiting self-defeating behavior, and fulfilling negative parental perceptions.

Children who conform to the directions and demands of others have several problems which follow them in later life. First, they do not learn to rely on their own problem-solving resources or perceptions of the environment. Second, trust in themselves and others is poorly developed because they have had so little experience of consistent, unconditional caring. Third, anxiety is always present because these children live in fear of losing love and approval from significant others. Fourth, the parents continue to be viewed as good. The child's self-image is that of the "wayward lamb." The parents are seen as attempting to salvage the child through direction and punishment. Unlike the preschizophrenic, this child is felt to be salvageable. Additionally, a preschool child is often dethroned by the birth of a sibling to whom the mother must "give her all."[10]

Family Social Network

The family of origin is often socially, economically, or religiously different from the community in which the family lives. The nuclear and extended family are often unified in a wish to elevate the family prestige within their own social group as well as the larger society. Often, the client was the specially endowed family member in whom all hope of family salvation rested.[10] A child acquires this special position by virtue of possession of a special gift or talent or by being the oldest, the youngest, or the only son or daughter. High family expectations for this child are communicated to him or her; the mission becomes fulfillment of these expectations regardless of individual wishes or goals. One client said this about her special status as a child:

> I was an only child. My mother would not let me go to our neighborhood high school. It was not good enough for me. She obtained special permission for me to go to another school on the other side of town where all the "right" kids went to school. She felt I would have a chance to meet "Mr. Rich" and make the right career connections. This would save my

> family from their genteel poverty. The other kids' lives seemed so effortless to me, who had to struggle for everything. I never felt that I made it, despite all the clothes and things mother worked so hard to give me.

This feeling existed despite the fact that the client graduated with honors, belonged to many clubs, and had many friends.

The client's special position often arouses envy and jealousy in siblings, which is anxiety-provoking because it creates distant or conflictual relationships among the brothers and sisters. The client often feels like a special outsider, which is a lonely position, and remains sensitive to envy and competition while growing up. This sensitivity is often negated through underselling of self and hiding the full extent of abilities—the client does not want to alienate siblings, or eventually friends, because of a perceived specialness. Paradoxically, these clients dislike themselves for not actualizing their abilities and hate others for their demands and envy.[10]

The family is viewed as having a fused and undifferentiated ego mass where the individuating experiences of the separate family members are not considered as important as the common good of the family as a whole (see Chapter 19). A kinship clan of several generations results in role blurring and multiple authority figures. Relinquished by the mother, the child is often unsure who is really significant and to be looked to for sustained support, guidance, and approval. Despite the overt togetherness and apparent closeness among family members, relatedness remains superficial and distant, with a significant lack of one-to-one relationships. Consequently, the child never develops a reliable, intimate relationship, with open, free, and genuine communication. Additionally, stereotyped family rules and myths govern relationships within the clan; this contributes to rigid, formal relationship patterns.[19,20] The pattern of communication learned in the family is perpetuated in limited relationships outside the family. Essentially, the child and other family members are lonely and have few ties outside the family.

Later Developmental Patterns

The communication and relationship patterns previously described as learned in the family of origin continue to be played out in adult life. The client, never having developed a solid sense of self, alternates between positions of hyperindependence and dependence. On one hand, the client feels that it is unsafe to rely on others and unacceptable to want to be cared for. As a result the client projects an image of self-sufficiency and competence. The client is often busily involved with management of his or her own life and the lives of others as well. This behavior often gains the client a reputation as a "busybody," "meddler," "know-it-all," and "whirlwind." The competent self-image and excessive involvement with others protect the client from confronting underlying feelings of vulnerability, helplessness, dependency, and limitations. On the other hand, the client fuses with others in the environment and assumes a dependent role by default; the client resists and fails to acknowledge the loss of self-sufficiency, for that would be a blow to self-esteem. For example, as the client's mood escalates, the hyperactivity, overcommitment, extravagant spending, impulsive decision making, lack of self-care, and exhaustion ultimately *require* that others assume responsibility for the client's care. The client tries to make others, particularly the family, feel responsible for his or her well-being. The behavior communicates the messages, "Take care of me," "Pay attention to me," and "Validate me as a good person."

Superficial relationships abound, even in the family. Within the family context there is no reciprocity to relatedness. The client appears to be searching for the perfect other who will see through his or her charade,[18,21] tolerate demands, and supply controls and meet dependency needs without insisting on reciprocity. The client uses the spouse to meet ungratified dependency needs without consideration of or attention to the needs of others. The narcissistic "I" is all-important.[22] The client will also shift responsibility for behavioral outcomes onto the family. (For example, a client who loses a job after telling the boss off might blame the spouse for encouraging him or her to be assertive.) When the client fails to carry out agreed-upon plans, the spouse feels betrayed. While covertly seeking fulfillment of needs from the spouse, the client is often overtly projecting an image of being the overfunctioning spouse. This is an illusion. The client is drawing temporary strength from the spouse, who may at times appear to be underfunctioning. The illusion shatters when the client crashes into a manic episode and the spouse emerges as the more functional person in the relationship. The seesaw balance of overfunctioning and underfunctioning in the spouses will vary over time depending on the anxiety level in the family.

Manic behavior tends to be *cyclical,* and the client may be highly productive and good company when the problem is not manifest. At these times, the family members are lulled by a feeling that all is well; or else they may feel that they are sitting on a powder keg, waiting for the next explosion. Because of the client's manipulativeness, it is difficult to determine the point at which irrational, unreasonable behavior takes over. As the dysfunctional behavior becomes more evident, marital discord is more frequent. The state of elation is perceived as threatening and exasperating. At some point, the spouse and children often feel that they have "had it," and distance themselves from the client. Then, as normality returns, they are usually tempted to give the client one more chance.

PATTERNS OF INTERACTION: ENVIRONMENT

Manic clients are very sensitive to change, which they often perceive as loss. Consequently, seasonal changes, geographic moves, job changes, leaving home for college, and changes in the social network that add or subtract relationships are potential stressors. Inherent in any change is a possible inability to meet self-expectations and required external demands. Thus, loss of self-esteem remains a constant threat. For example:

> Mike had had a 20-year history of both manic and depressive episodes. His latest episode followed the opening of a new landscaping business. He described the business as thriving, but he was very worried about getting enough help to complete all the work he had contracted to do. He stated that since business was good, his upset didn't make sense. His wife said that whenever he had too much to do, he would get "sick." She said that he didn't know how to moderate his activity; that he immediately became overinvolved in any job, overcommitted himself, and then couldn't handle it. It was apparent that his need to succeed was jeopardized by unrealistic self-expectations and commitments, resulting in potential failure and loss of self-esteem. The escalating manic behavior represented an attempt to get everything done and deny the possibility of a negative outcome.

Clients often minimize the impact of these potential stressors and the conflicts they generate. However, situations in which there is enforced pursuit of an activity that is at odds with the client's own goals and aspirations seem likely to contribute to increased stress. For example:

> Mr. C., a 21-year-old man, was the oldest of four children and, of the four, had the strongest relationship with both parents. His father was an ambitious, successful physician but at times was prone to self-doubt and looked to his oldest son (Mr. C.) for companionship and a sympathetic ear. The father was critical of his son for not being more successful. Mr. C's mother had divorced his father when Mr. C. was in his teens, leaving her son feeling abandoned and angry with her for leaving him to care for the father.
>
> Mr. C. was a premedical student but dropped out of college after his first manic episode, during his freshman year. After that, he held a series of menial jobs with which he was dissatisfied. Lacking job skills, he did not know how to improve his economic position enough to live independently. His father's criticism did not help his self-esteem or motivation. After being fired from his most recent job, Mr. C. had another manic episode. Discharge plans for Mr. C. included living in a halfway house rather than with his father. Referral to vocational rehabilitation resulted in a well-paying job that he enjoyed. During the last 18 months, he has been asymptomatic, has taken his lithium regularly, has obtained increasingly better jobs, has moved into his own apartment, and has found a girlfriend.[20,23]

NURSING PROCESS

Assessment

Nurses encounter manic clients and their families in the home, outpatient clinics, emergency rooms, and short- or long-term inpatient treatment settings. Regardless of the setting, the nursing assessment must encompass client, family, and environmental factors. The data may be collected from the client and the family as well as significant people in the client's life. The nurse can consider the items in Table 35-1 as assessment criteria from which to formulate nursing diagnoses.

Sometimes manic behavior and schizophrenic behavior have the same suspicious, agitated quality. Manic behavior must be differentiated from schizophrenic behavior so that an appropriate therapeutic plan may be formulated. (See Chapter 37.)

Table 35-1 Nursing Process: Assessment for Patterns of Elation

Assessment Questions	Responses of Client (C) and Family (F)
	Assessment of client
Why has the client been hospitalized?	C: Nothing's wrong; ... I'm fine; ... fine a cop a thousand dollars. F: During the last 2 weeks he hasn't slept or eaten, is writing bad checks, is calling the White House collect 3 times a day.
What is the client's mood state?	C: I feel great, I feel like I'm floating on cloud nine! Who could be happier? F: He's happy, lively; jokes all the time; always up for a party.
What factors do you see contributing to this hospitalization? Has there been a change in lifestyle, an upset in structure, or a recent loss, or is this the anniversary of a previous loss?	C: No change; ... change is money; ... when you have money, make the change. F: There hasn't been any real change except for his new promotion. He's had to travel a lot more and work longer hours seeing important clients at night. It was also at this time last year that he refused a promotion and became ill.
What have previous patterns of "highs" been like in terms of intensity, duration, and periodicity?	C: It happens not often enough; I'm at my best; put others to the test. Being singled out from the rest really puts you over the crest. ... F: He's been having these mood swings for about the last 6 years. They started after we got married and come about almost every spring. I can see him getting higher and higher, wanting to party, travel, and buy everything in sight. I take the checkbook and credit cards away or we'd be bankrupt. He's so clever he even ends up charging things where we have no accounts, and then I have to deal with the telephone complaints. As soon as he's hospitalized and medicated, he comes down and seems ready to go home.
How would you describe the way the client relates to people? Testing Manipulation Denial, etc.	C: Problems, I don't have any problems; they just don't have the energy to keep up with me. F: He doesn't listen to anybody when he's like this. He does whatever he pleases and tries to convince you that he's right.
How would you describe the client's overall activity level, sleep patterns, appetite, grooming, and medication compliance? What has it been? How has it changed?	F: Activity! He's off the wall. Now he never stops, up all night roaming around, no food, lost about 18 pounds in the last 2 weeks. And lithium—if he'd only take it, this might stop.
	Assessment of family
Family of origin	
Is there a history of extreme mood swings in the family of origin?	F: His grandmother had mood swings all her adult life. They began coming closer together as she got older. She died in a mental institution.
Who lived in your house when you were growing up?	C: My mother was a cold fish, literally threw us out on our own as tiny kids; ... always expected me to be able to do everything perfectly the first time.
What were your parents like when you were growing up?	C: My grandparents lived with us. There were lots of bosses in the house. My mother was very ambitious. My father was quiet and let her do the bossing around.
Describe your relationships with each of your brothers and sisters.	C: I was the oldest and the one to bring the family fame and fortune. My parents expected more of me than the other kids. My little brother and sister were always jealous of me.
What was your family's social and financial status while you were growing up?	C: We lived on the fringes of the "right" neighborhood. Mom and Dad had very few friends outside the family, and we never quite fit in with the neighbors.

(Continued.)

Table 35-1 Continued

Assessment Questions	Responses of Client (C) and Family (F)
Assessment of family	
Nuclear family	
What is your relationship like with your spouse?	C: She's the perfect soul mate for me, always saving my skin. F: We have no children. He doesn't want any. If he weren't so independent most of the time, I'd say he's my baby. I always end up bailing him out of scrapes, cleaning up his mess, and taking the blame for his misfortunes. Between episodes it's great, but I am getting weary.
What does your spouse do when you start to get high? How does this differ from when you are low?	C: She's too good to me. F: I'm not tough enough on him. After a while you get so used to this craziness that it becomes a normal crazy way of life.
Assessment of environment	
Describe your lifestyle.	C: I winter in Palm Beach with the jet set. I summer in Spain with the best people. You can reach me through my private secretary. F: He likes to live a fast, extravagant way of life, far beyond our means.
What kind of work do you do?	C: I'm the king of the roost. I'm the backbone of the company. F: When he's not "up," he's a terrific salesman. He wins awards for sales records.
What effect does your behavior have on work relationships and performance?	C: I'm the best; they couldn't do without me. F: He's such a supersalesman that they take him back after each hospitalization. They think he's a great guy—funny, witty, and effective.
What is your socioeconomic status?	C: Aristocracy, the top, fine old family, ha, ha, ha! F: We're really middle class. But, we struggle to keep up because of the neighborhood we live in.
How easily does the client make friends? What are these friendships like?	C: Friends, I have a million of them. They all want to be around me. F: We have lots of acquaintances. I have some good friends of my own.
How does the client react to changes or disruptions?	F: Change is very unsettling for him whether it's good or bad. Just a change of season can upset him. The promotion he got should make him happy, but I'm convinced that it set off this episode.
What is the impact of the client's behavior on staff members and other clients in the treatment setting?	The staff avoids the client because he is always telling them that they don't know anything. Turns the place upside down.
What is the probability of effecting change in the client's interpersonal relationships and lifestyle?	Good, if the client's patterns of denial and superficiality can be decreased.

Most manic clients have had fairly successful interpersonal relationships. They relate easily, if dependently—as opposed to schizophrenic clients, who are withdrawn and aloof in relationships.[3,4] Periodicity is another important difference. Manic behavior is characterized by its episodic nature and symptom-free intervals. Schizophrenic reactions either are single experiences or tend to leave a distinct, enduring trace despite a relatively stable reconstitution. Manic client's delusions and pathological communications are similar to those of schizophrenia but do not display the highly symbolic quality that characterizes looseness of associations in schizophrenia.[3]

The emotional response of others to manic clients tends to be warm and humorous, as opposed to the sense of distaste and puzzlement the schizophrenic may evoke in others.

Diagnosis and Outcome Criteria

The nursing diagnosis and outcome criteria are formulated on the basis of data collection and analysis. Table 35-2 gives examples of diagnoses and outcomes applicable to manic clients.

Table 35-2 Nursing Process: Diagnoses and Outcome Criteria for Patterns of Elation

Diagnosis	Outcome Criteria
	The client will:
1. Denial of anxiety, dependency, and worthlessness related to need to maintain perception of personal power	Verbally acknowledge and explore underlying feelings of anxiety, dependency, and low self-esteem.
2. Lack of confidence in own abilities related to low self-esteem	Identify own strengths and weaknesses.
3. Pseudo independence associated with denial of dependency needs	Identify sources of pseudo independence.
4. Superficial relationships related to fear of rejection	Explore real and fantasied sources of rejection.
5. Inconsiderateness of others associated with envy and competitiveness	Identify the needs of self and others in a relationship.
6. Demanding behavior related to dependency needs	Verbalize recognition of demanding behavior and its onset. Set limits on own demanding behavior, and verbally articulate needs in an open, direct manner.
7. Manipulative behavior related to need for control	Verbalize recognition of manipulative patterns of interaction; communicate openly and directly with others.
8. Verbal hostility toward others related to failure to manipulate others	Decrease verbal hostility and express feelings in an appropriate manner.
9. Weight loss of 18 pounds in 2 weeks related to hyperactivity	Increase caloric intake to 4000 calories per day.
10. Dehydration associated with profuse diaphoresis and inadequate fluid intake	Increase fluid intake to 2000 milliliters per day.
11. Difficulty staying asleep associated with manic episode	Sleep 4 to 6 hours without waking.
12. Hyperactivity and distractability related to decreased sensory threshold	Be less distracted by sensory stimuli; sit in a chair without getting up for 30 minutes.

Intervention

Intervention with the Person

The manic client usually arrives at the treatment facility in a highly excited state. Entry into treatment will usually follow a period in which the family has tried to cope with the client at home. The client's boisterous, jovial facade may mask the feelings of anxiety, worthlessness, and isolation that actually are being experienced. This makes it difficult for the staff to decide on appropriate nursing interventions. Understanding the underlying dynamics of the client's behavior is essential to implementing effective nursing intervention. The interventions presented in this section provide a variety of approaches to manic clients' problems: increased physical activity, denial, dependency, hostility and aggression, and manipulative, testing, and acting-out behavior.[24]

INCREASED PHYSICAL ACTIVITY. Hyperactivity on the part of the client requires decisive nursing intervention because uninterrupted activity can be life-threatening. The following interventions are directed toward restoring and maintaining a more functional activity level.

Decreasing environmental stimuli. Environmental stimuli can be decreased by soft lighting, low noise level, and simple room decorations. There should be as few people as possible in the client's environment. The client may need to be removed from the general unit milieu, which may be too stimulating, and spend time in a quiet room. A consistent care giver becomes the agent for supplying external controls on physical activity. Firm, clearly stated instructions will facilitate transitions from one activity to another. Hazardous objects and substances should be removed from the environment to protect the client from impulsive self-harm.

Providing adequate hygiene, nutrition, and rest. The client needs to be provided with flexible opportunities to shower and change clothing. Diaphoresis (perspiring) may be profuse; incontinence may occur. Thus frequent opportunities for washing or showering are necessary. Loose, comfortable clothing is preferable. High-calorie finger foods and drinks that can be consumed easily while standing or moving are suggested. A quiet environment, sedation, and opportunities for frequent short naps will facilitate restoration of a regular sleep pattern.

Involving the client in activities. Activities involving large motor skills provide for appropriate discharge of energy and tension. Initially, the manic client often cannot tolerate activities that are highly structured and confining. Therefore, choice of activities should consider the client's high activity level, short attention span, and easy distractibility. Examples of activities that are effective are walks, housekeeping chores, painting, dance or movement therapy, and exercise.

Monitoring medications. The lithium family of drugs is effective in preventing recurrences of chronic and cyclical manic episodes and in treating manic-depressive episodes.[4,18] Long-term maintenance therapy, if adhered to, helps the client remain a well-functioning member of the community.[16] The medication is administered to the client with dose adjustments until a therapeutic blood level is achieved. Then a maintenance program is instituted. Nursing interventions are directed toward:

1. Administering the medication and making sure the client takes it
2. Assessing the client behaviorally to determine the effectiveness of the medication in decreasing the presenting symptoms
3. Identifying the occurrence of side effects and toxic effects of the medication
4. Coordinating the regular collection of blood samples to monitor lithium levels
5. Checking laboratory values pertaining to lithium levels
6. Sharing observations on medication with other members of the mental health team
7. Teaching the client and family about lithium therapy (see Chapter 26)
8. Dealing with client and family issues regarding noncompliance (see Chapter 26)

Lithium therapy, the associated nursing responsibilities, and issues having to do with clients are discussed in greater detail in Chapter 26.

DENIAL. Manic clients often attempt to deny that they have any problems by presenting a facade of wellness to the staff and other clients. Use of denial represents the client's attempt to avoid confrontation with threatening inner feelings of inadequacy, dependency, and loneliness. Confrontation of these feelings generates anxiety and feelings of vulnerability; the client attempts to distance from them so as to remain emotionally calm. To acknowledge the existence of such feelings would be to expose the parts of the self that the manic client spends each day trying to hide. Clients must face their inner vulnerability if they are to modify dependency and relationship patterns and achieve a realistic, separate sense of self.[10,25]

The first step in intervening to counteract denial is to establish an open nurse-client relationship in which thoughts, feelings, and meanings are discussed.[10] The nurse focuses and comments on themes, nonverbal gestures, and tone of voice rather than verbal content. This facilitates recognition of what is actually occurring rather than what the client would like the nurse to believe is occurring. The client, unable to confront feelings, needs assistance to bring them into awareness and engage in the problem-solving process. Here is an example of this process:

MS. B.: I think I'll leave the hospital; nobody here can help me. You're all just a bunch of no-good do-nothings. I'm going to get the CIA after all of you! (Voice rising, wringing her hands.)

NURSE: You sound upset, Ms. B. Your voice is rising and you're wringing your hands. I sense that you're feeling alone and perhaps unloved.

MS. B.: Alone, alone. . . . I'm never alone. I'm the most loved person around here. (Starts crying and laughing.)

NURSE: You say you're never alone or unloved. Yet you're laughing and crying. Most people feel alone or unloved sometimes. It's all right to feel that way, and it's OK to share the feeling with someone.

Interventions to counteract denial are appropriately initiated when hyperactivity has decreased and the client no longer needs the denial as a self-conservation measure. Once the intensity of the manic episode has diminished, and a nurse-client relationship has been established, more confrontative approaches in relation to denial can be used. One such approach is to introduce "startle experiences" which dislodge the client's stereotyped response patterns. *Startle experiences* are direct, unexpected responses by the therapist that unsettle the client and decrease the likelihood that an entrenched dysfunctional response pattern will be pursued. For example:

> A very witty male client continually entertained other clients on the unit. His jokes persisted even in light of a discussion about death and loss. In an effort to dislodge the facade of humor, the nurse said, "Tom, you were talking about your father's death. Why don't you have a good cry now? It's OK; we can bear your painful feelings."

The client may not cry at this point. However, the bold suggestion may dislodge the denial and create a climate of acceptance that will enable the client to begin talking more directly about the loss.

Role modeling can be a valuable tool for counteracting denial in the nurse-client relationship. The nurse communicates feelings in a direct way, demonstrating that openness and vulnerability need not lead to put-downs and rejection. The client can then see that the real self, which is perceived as terrible, is not in danger of rejection if it is exposed.

A nurse should not assume that a client is finally engaging in meaningful communication when the client's reality orientation is good and data are offered about self. Manic clients have the ability to maintain the flow of information on a superficial level. The nurse will want to decrease the quantity of the client's verbal output and increase its quality. (This is in contrast to the depressed or withdrawn client from whom the nurse initially wants to hear *any* verbalizations that occur, regardless of their quality.) The nurse must frequently reassess the level of denial and the depth of the relationship, in working with manic clients.

DEPENDENCY. Although these clients' dependency needs are strong, the clients think their need to depend on others is unacceptable, and they act independent.[10] The nurse may work with a client who resists therapy by using a variety of methods. The client may state, "I don't need you" and "I don't need therapy." The client may miss appointments, arrive late, or discuss trivialities during the session. In dealing with such resistance, the nurse should clearly state the time and frequency of the therapeutic sessions. The nurse must verbally acknowledge the dynamics of the resistance that is occurring and confront the client about discrepancies in behavior. For example, the nurse might state, "I see that you are having difficulty managing your life right now, yet you seem unwilling to come to sessions to talk about what is bothering you or to work at straightening out any of it." The nurse may go on to indicate that dependency is not such a terrible thing, that people sometimes need others to lean on for a while. It can be helpful to point out that the client can use the therapeutic sessions to learn how to deal with dependency feelings.[26]

Irrational demands should be firmly and consistently refused.[27] The nurse must be careful that in saying "no" to one request, he or she is not agreeing to another. For example:

> One nurse refused permission for a client to go to a friend's house for Christmas day but ended up taking the client to her own home for Christmas dinner.

Demands for advice and answers to problems are common examples of dependency. Manic clients exhibit lack of faith in their ability to work out problems independently or interdependently. As soon as a nurse begins to provide guidance for the client, the client's dependency needs are being met and the stage is set for the client to make more and more demands for direction. The effectiveness of the problem-solving process is thus inhibited and clients are allowed to maintain their dysfunctional dependency needs.

Guidelines for dealing with dependency are as follows:

1. Show awareness when demands are made. For example, "I explained the privilege policies to you this morning. Your request for a pass this afternoon does not fit in with the guidelines I explained to you."
2. Convey acceptance of the client while refusing to comply with excessive, irrational demands. For example, "I hear you repeatedly telling me that it's a nice day out and that you need a pass. However, you are not eligible for a pass. Would you like to sit down and talk for a while?"

3. State observations of and themes characterizing the dynamics of the behavior. For example, "I sense that you are attempting to have me guide your life and take responsibility for mistakes that occur."
4. Provide here-and-now feedback about interpersonal maneuvers that involve dependency or demandingness. For example, "I get annoyed when you continue to ask me to do things for you that you and I agreed you could do on your own."
5. State how behavior can be utilized in the therapeutic process. Help the client to identify feelings, acknowledge them, analyze them, and learn how to develop alternative ways of seeking gratification.[10] For example:

   NURSE: Can you tell me how you felt when you went out to look for your own apartment?

   CLIENT: At first I felt great, but then I began to think about whether I'd like living alone.

   NURSE: What was the feeling that went along with thoughts of living alone?

   CLIENT: Aloneness, utter aloneness.

   NURSE: What's behind these feelings? What sense do you make of them?

6. Reinforce the client's self-esteem. For example, "You have the ability to do it; let's work together."
7. Engage the client in learning how to make decisions and accept responsibility. For example, "What would be the logical decision to make? How would it be for you to stick with the job even though you were uncertain about your ability to succeed?"

HOSTILITY AND AGGRESSION. Hostility and aggression are defensive responses to anxiety, loss of self-esteem, and loss of power. Hostility and aggression are utilized by the client as "as if" behaviors to enhance an illusion of power and control.[9,10] Hostility and aggression protect the client from underlying feelings of low self-esteem and enable him or her to feel "one up" on everyone else. Hostility and aggression also create distance between the client and others, thus eliminating opportunities for more than superficial relatedness. Nursing actions are directed toward:

1. Recognizing the purpose the behavior serves for the client.
2. Nonjudgmentally documenting observations about the behavior.
3. Refraining from any overtly defensive personal response to criticism, physical attack, or profanity.
4. Setting limits on the behavior. For example, "Barbara, I will not allow you to hit the other clients. You'll have to go to the quiet room for 30 minutes."
5. Avoiding positive reinforcement of negative behavior by ignoring it or minimally responding to it.
6. After an episode is over, giving clients an opportunity to discuss feelings experienced before, during, and after the episode. Help them to analyze their participation in the episode. Alternative coping patterns can then be explored.

MANIPULATION, TESTING, AND ACTING OUT. The client, feeling alone and unloved, manipulates and acts out to test the caring and limits that are conveyed by others. Paradoxically, clients perceive that "giving in" to an unacceptable activity is equivalent to rejection. Escalation of manic activity usually follows; it is an attempt to elicit caring and controls from others. Thus, the fear that many care givers have about provoking rage reactions when setting limits is unfounded. Clients really welcome such controls, even though they may protest loudly and violently.

The following guidelines are suggested for helping the staff set limits on manipulation, testing, and acting-out behavior.[27,28]

1. Identify the need for a limit; the client is unable to exercise self-control and needs external controls. For example:

   A client, John, was making 20 collect telephone calls a day. His telephone privileges were therefore restricted for a week.

2. The decision on setting limits and what these are to be must be agreed upon and understood by *all* staff members on *all* shifts. Care plans must be *written* and posted conspicuously so that problems, goals, and interventions are clearly understood by all.

3. Communicate the limits to the client in clear language. (For example, "Mr. Jones, you cannot undress in the dayroom. If you want to remain undressed, you must stay in your room.")
4. Enforce the limits in an unambiguous, firm manner. The eventual relaxation of restrictive rules will depend on what the client is *doing*, not on what he or she is *saying*. Clients' demands for greater freedom are usually connected with a continued need to act out. For example:

   John requested that his telephone privileges be restored. As soon as his request was complied with, he was back to making 20 telephone calls a day to "old friends."

   Clients who are effectively engaged in problem solving will have little time for testing and manipulation.

5. Reevaluate the need for limits at regular intervals, and also review the impact of the inappropriate behavior on others.
6. It is essential to have clear communication channels among team members in order to provide a consistent approach to the client. Sometimes dual therapists are utilized—one as the just disciplinarian and the other as the loving, accepting person. The objective splitting of roles minimizes the ability of the client to divide and conquer the staff.

Limits may have to be set on general meddling and advising to prevent further isolation and decreased self-esteem. For example:

Jean, a manic client, was constantly going over to other unit members, giving directions for a crafts project that she had tossed aside. She also gave them advice about boyfriends and showered them with jewelry from her pocketbook. This behavior was initially received positively by them. Then their reaction turned to annoyance and anger. They said, "Jean, why don't you just get lost?"

Limits may also have to be set on grandiose plans such as business deals and spending sprees.

Intervention with Groups

The use of group therapy with manic clients is sometimes advised and sometimes contraindicated. In general, it is difficult for clients exhibiting full-blown manic behavior to be effective group members. They talk incessantly despite repeated requests that they stop, are insensitive to the needs and feelings of others, and avoid meaningful group discussion by changing the subject, giving advice, or abruptly leaving, thereby disrupting the group process and creating mutual withdrawal.

When group sessions are indicated as an intervention, the leader must understand the potential disruptive maneuvers of the manic client. The leader must provide an effective role model and demonstrate to group members that limits can and will be set, disruptiveness will not be tolerated, and feedback will be given. Each group member must be encouraged to continue participating in the group and to provide feedback to the client about how his or her behavior is affecting that particular person. Peer pressure exerted within the group is sometimes the only thing that makes the manic client cut down on monopolizing and disruptive behavior. For example:

Mark had been admitted to the general hospital psychiatric unit the evening before in a highly agitated state. He talked for hours about his recent business deals, his extensive social life, and his plans for a political career. He slept intermittently, pacing the hall outside his room while he was up. The next morning he had talked with every client on the unit before breakfast was over. When group began, Mark walked in late and interrupted another client who was already talking and began a monologue. "Hi, everybody; how are you this morning? Great day. Hey, nurse, can we go for a walk today? It's a damn shame we don't go for more walks; don't you think so, guys?" When nobody answered, he said, "What's the matter? Everyone tired today?" He displayed complete lack of awareness of the impact of his behavior. The group leader intervened and posed a question to the group: "I wonder if people are tired or whether there is another problem going on right now?" Another client, who had also had a manic episode but was now calmer, said, "I can't get a chance to say a word, and if I can't, I'll bet nobody else can." Two other clients looked at each other and smiled. The group leader asked one of the members if she could explain to Mark how the group worked. She told him that each member had a chance to talk about his or her problems, and that members listened to one another and provided feedback, support, and suggestions. Mark said, "I just made a great suggestion, that we go for a walk." The woman said disgustedly, "Not that kind of suggestion." The group continued to try to point out how Mark's behavior was affecting the group. However, he remained oblivious to what they were saying. After 3 days of much the same behavior in the group, other group members began to follow the example of the leader and collectively began to set limits on Mark's monopolizing behavior. The peer pressure finally began to have an effect on Mark; he quieted down and began to be a more functional group member, using the group as a vehicle for experimenting with new ways of interacting.

If the client does not profit from feedback and limits but continues to use the group as an audience, group sessions may be temporarily or permanently contraindicated.

Intervention with the Family

Intervention with the family can be useful in exploring the family's participation in maintaining the client's symptoms, the family's expectations for the client, and the family's scripts and myths about dependency and intimacy. The client can be helped to use family data to sort out and clarify self-perceptions and expectations and arrive at a more valid self-concept.

The family often participates in maintaining the client's manic behavior when they deny its presence, display increasing tolerance for it, and don't act on the need to rehospitalize a family member until the situation has reached crisis proportions. Although family members may complain about the client's behavior, they don't label it as deviant or "crazy." It is helpful for families to have objective criteria on which to base a decision to seek early in- or outpatient treatment. The following criteria can be given to the family by the community health nurse or by the hospital:

- Noncompliance in taking lithium regularly
- Hyperactivity, insomnia, anorexia, weight loss
- Excessive, impulsive spending
- Impulsive decision making
- Increased alcohol abuse
- Sexual acting out
- Physical aggression directed at others
- Delusions of grandeur

When such criteria are given to the family by a specific resource person, that person may provide a connection which the family will more readily contact when there is a need to seek treatment.

The family may also participate in the escalation of manic behavior when family members don't consistently set limits on "crazy" client behaviors. They may continue to have joint bank and charge accounts with the client, despite his or her extravagant, impulsive spending. They may continue to respond enthusiastically to new business schemes and may not take firm positions about alcohol abuse, sexual promiscuity, or household disruptions. Family members may not feel entitled to take a position on an issue. For example:

One wife had been told by her mother-in-law, "All the men in the family are wheeler-dealers in business and big drinkers; it's just something you learn to live with." Consequently, this woman felt that she had to accept such behavior in her husband regardless of how outrageous it was and felt guilty for wanting to put her foot down. In this case, the nurse helped the wife see how her lack of position taking and seeming acceptance of her husband's "business deals" and drinking only served to perpetuate this behavior. The nurse and the woman explored areas in which she could set limits for her husband and ways in which she could set them without feeling guilty.

As stated earlier in this chapter, manic clients often hold a "special child" position in the family of origin. They feel burdened by unrealistic family expectations. They see themselves as unable to fulfill the family's hopes and dreams. Yet the manic client really doesn't have a clear picture of who and what he or she is as a person separate or different from the family. The nurse can intervene to help clients and families sort out generational expectations, family scripts, and myths. From such a sorting process, clients can begin to realistically examine their self-expectations, needs, and wants and arrive at a less fused, more individual self-concept. Modifications in lifestyle may be necessary following this type of self-evaluation. Changes must be mutually negotiated between family members with the hope that the changes will lead to a more interdependent relationship pattern.[29]

Intervention with the Community

Many manic clients function quite successfully in the community between manic and depressive episodes. However, others repeatedly overinvolve and overextend themselves financially, in business, and in community activities, and may need assistance in developing a lifestyle that is less stressful and more stable. Both client and family may need to be referred to a financial or business consultant, an employment agency if a job has been terminated, or a career counselor or vocational rehabilitation services if new career options need to be explored. Help in realistic, goal-directed planning may be obtained from such resources.

Clients for whom it would be nontherapeutic to return to their family and home, and those without either family or home, will have to have alternative living arrangements. Halfway houses, group homes, rented rooms, and apartments are among the options available, depending on the client's financial resources, needs, and level of functioning.

For manic clients who tend to be unrealistic and grandiose, small goals that can be achieved are of paramount importance. Formulation of a concrete discharge plan will help structure the client's environment in a manageable way. Once clients feel better, they may deny the need for such structure. For this reason, the nurse collaborates with the client in formulating a discharge plan that is not only realistic but also acceptable to the client. A plan that is acceptable to the client has a much greater chance of success. Community health nurses may play a role in monitoring clients' lithium regimes when they return to the community after hospitalization.

Evaluation

Evaluation of nursing care plans for manic clients not only is necessary in order to demonstrate professional accountability but also becomes a tool for assessing the extent to which dysfunctional patterns of behavior have been resolved. Evaluation, in fact, is particularly appropriate for manic clients. Often their grandiosity, manipulation, denial, and physiological problems, to mention just a few patterns, are not systematically addressed and resolved because staff members find them too anxiety-provoking, too exhausting, or too "entertaining" to deal with.

The clinical example below will show how the nursing process is used to appraise the effectiveness of the nursing care plan for Fred D.; the nursing care plan is presented in Table 35-3.

Fred D., a 45-year-old man, has been having cyclical manic and depressive episodes. Fred will feel affectively normal for months or even years but gradually will feel his mood becoming higher and higher. He will find himself spending a lot of money, dressing garishly, and socializing extensively. Eventually, he becomes unable to sleep, eat, bathe, or organize his thoughts, feelings, or behavior. He describes himself as a motor racing at high speed. Fred is admitted to the psychiatric unit of the community hospital. It is observed that he is not sleeping, eating, bathing, or taking care of his personal possessions.

Table 35-3 Evaluation for a Manic Client (Fred D.)

Assessment	Diagnosis	Outcome	Intervention	Evaluation
Problem: Wakefulness				
Fred D. is observed prowling around his room at 1 A.M. He comes out to the nurses' station for a "chat" at 3 A.M. He is dressed, and about to start waking other clients up at 6 A.M. Fred states: "Sleep! Who needs to sleep? Can't waste time doing that—there's too much else to live for."	Fatigue related to difficulty falling asleep.	Within 1 week, client will sleep 4 to 6 hours per night without waking.	1. Establish and enforce a regular but flexible bedtime. 2. Administer a back rub before bedtime. 3. Decrease sensory stimulation 1 hour before bedtime. 4. Provide warm milk 30 minutes before bedtime.	Fred initially refuses to go to bed, stating "Nobody's bossing me around." With repeated limit setting about bedtime disputes, along with other therapeutic measures, client gradually begins to fall asleep with less difficulty. Within 10 days he is sleeping 6 hours per night without waking.

(Continued.)

Table 35-3 Continued

Assessment	Diagnosis	Outcome	Intervention	Evaluation
Problem: Weight loss				
Fred has lost 20 pounds in the past 2 weeks. He paces the dining room, stopping momentarily to give advice to other clients but never sitting down to eat. Oral fluid intake 500 cubic centimeters. Urinary output 1000 cubic centimeters dark amber urine. Profuse diaphoresis noted throughout day. Lips dry and cracked. When approached by the nurse, he says, "Too much to do; too much to do."	Nutritional inadequacy related to hyperactivity. Potential dehydration associated with profuse diaphoresis and inadequate fluid intake.	Nutritional adequacy as evidenced by caloric intake up to 4000 calories per day, with a balanced selection from the basic food groups. Hydration as evidenced by fluid intake to 2000 milliliters per day.	1. Provide high-calorie, nutritious finger foods that client can eat "on the run." 2. Weigh client every 2 days. 3. Provide easy access to nutritious drinks of choice. 4. Provide nutritious high-fluid snacks (milk shakes, custards, ice creams).	1. Fred has gained 8 pounds in 10 days. 2. Fred's urinary output is clear, straw-colored, and 2000 cubic centimeters per day.

SUMMARY

Patterns of elation are manifested by clients who experience manic episodes. Such episodes occur cyclically with or without alternating episodes of depression.

Patterns of elation occur in three stages—mild elation, acute elation, and delirium. Characteristic alterations in affect, thoughts, and behavior occur in each stage.

The person's patterns of interaction revolve around issues of loss, dependency, anxiety, and intimacy in relationships, and are affected by genetic and biochemical factors. Family patterns of interaction include issues relating to expectations, loss, self-concept, communication, and relationship styles. Environmental patterns of interaction focus on environmental stress and change as risk factors that contribute to the onset of manic episodes.

The nursing process addresses the formulation of a treatment plan based on the analysis of individual, family, and environmental assessment data. Interventions are directed at creating a safe and nonstimulating environment, monitoring medications, and resolving interpersonal issues such as denial, dependency, unrealistic expectations of family and self, fused self-concept, and manipulation. Individual, group, and family approaches are used to deal with such issues, as appropriate.

REFERENCES

1. D. M. Janowsky et al., "Playing the Manic Game," *Archives of General Psychiatry*, vol. 22, March 1970, pp. 252–261.
2. Freida Fromm-Reichmann, *Psychoanalysis and Psychotherapy*, D. M. Bullard, ed., University of Chicago Press, Chicago, 1959.
3. S. Tyrer and B. Shopsin, "Symptoms and Assessment of Mania," in E. S. Paykel, ed., *Handbook of Affective Disorders*, Guilford, New York, 1984, pp. 12–21.
4. H. E. Lehman, "Affective Disorders: Clinical Features," in H. I. Kaplan and B. J. Sadock, eds., *Comprehensive Textbook of Psychiatry*, 4th ed., Williams and Wilkins, Baltimore, 1985.
5. E. A. Wolpert, *Manic-Depressive Illness: History of A Syndrome*, International Universities Press, New York, 1977.
6. K. M. Lipkin et al., "The Many Faces of Mania," *Archives of General Psychiatry*, vol. 22, March 1970, pp. 262–267.
7. Gabriel Carlson and F. K. Goodwin, "The Stages of Mania," *Archives of General Psychiatry*, vol. 28, February 1973, pp. 221–228.
8. American Psychiatric Association, *Diagnostic and Statistical Manual of Mental Disorders*, 3d ed., APA, Washington, D.C., 1980.
9. Lawrence C. Kolb, *Modern Clinical Psychiatry*, 9th ed., Saunders, Philadelphia, 1977, pp. 357–386.
10. Mabel B. Cohen et al., "An Intensive Study of Twelve Cases of Manic Depressive Psychosis," in E. A. Wol-

pert, ed., *Manic-Depressive Illness: History of a Syndrome,* International Universities Press, New York, 1977, pp. 291–343.

11. M. Weissman et al., "Psychiatric Disorders in the Relatives of Probands with Affective Disorders," *Archives of General Psychiatry,* vol. 41, no. 1, 1984, pp. 13–21.
12. G. Winokur, M. T. Tsuang, and R. R. Crowe, "The Iowa 500: Affective Disorder in Relatives of Manic and Depressed Patients," *American Journal of Psychiatry,* vol. 139, 1982, pp. 206–212.
13. J. Angst, "The Reliability of Morbidity Risk Figures in Affective Disorders," in J. Mendlewicz and B. Shopsin, eds., *Genetic Aspects of Affective Illness,* Spectrum, New York, 1979, pp. 21–26.
14. A. Y. Meltzer et al., "Effect of 5-Hydroxytryptophan on Serum Cortisol Levels in Major Affective Disorders," *Archives of General Psychiatry,* vol. 41, no. 4, 1984, pp. 366–373.
15. J. A. Egeland et al., "Amish Study; V: Lithium-Sodium Countertransport and Catechol O-Methyltransferase in Pedigrees of Bipolar Probands," *American Journal of Psychiatry,* vol. 141, no. 9, 1984, pp. 1049–1054.
16. G. D. Pearlson et al., "Clinical Correlates of Lateral Ventricular Enlargement in Bipolar Affective Disorder," *American Journal of Psychiatry,* vol. 141, no. 2, 1984, pp. 253–256.
17. G. D. Pearlson and A. E. Veroff, "Computerized Tomographic Scan in Changes in Manic-Depressive Patients," *Lancet,* vol. 2, 1981, pp. 470–472.
18. Silvano Arieti, "Affective Disorders: Manic-Depressive Psychosis and Psychotic Depression," in Silvano Arieti, ed., *American Handbook of Psychiatry,* Basic Books, New York, 1975, chap. 21.
19. Y. B. Davenport et al., "Early Childrearing Practices in Families with a Manic-Depressive Patient," *American Journal of Psychiatry,* vol. 141, no. 2, 1984, pp. 230–235.
20. P. B. Lieberman and J. S. Strauss, "The Recurrence of Mania: Environmental Factors and Medical Treatment," *American Journal of Psychiatry,* vol. 141, no. 1, 1984, pp. 77–79.
21. E. Corker, "Manic-Depression," *Nursing Mirror,* vol. 157, no. 2, July 13, 1983, pp. 43–45.
22. A. L. Lesser, "Hypomania and Marital Conflict," *Canadian Journal of Psychiatry,* vol. 28, no. 5, 1983, pp. 362–366.
23. S. Kennedy, "Life Events Precipitating Mania," *British Journal of Psychiatry,* vol. 142, 1983, pp. 398–403.
24. N. Hosker, "Excitement on the Ward," *Nursing Mirror,* vol. 157, no. 13, September 28, 1983, pp. 39–40.
25. P. Barker et al., "Psychological Therapy in Affective Disorder," *Nursing Mirror,* vol. 160, no. 22, May 29, 1985, pp. 34–36.
26. H. S. Klein, "Transference and Defense in Manic States," *International Journal of Psychoanalysis,* vol. 55, 1974, pp. 261–268.
27. Glee Gamble Lyon, "Limit Setting as a Therapeutic Tool," *Journal of Psychiatric Nursing and Mental Health Services,* vol. 8, no. 6, 1970, pp. 17–24.
28. Maxine E. Loomis, "Nursing Management of Acting-Out Behavior," *Perspectives in Psychiatric Care,* vol. 8, no. 4, 1970, pp. 168–173.
29. Y. B. Davenport et al., "Manic-Depressive Families: Psychodynamic Features of Multigenerational Families," *American Journal of Orthopsychiatry,* vol. 49, 1979, pp. 24–35.

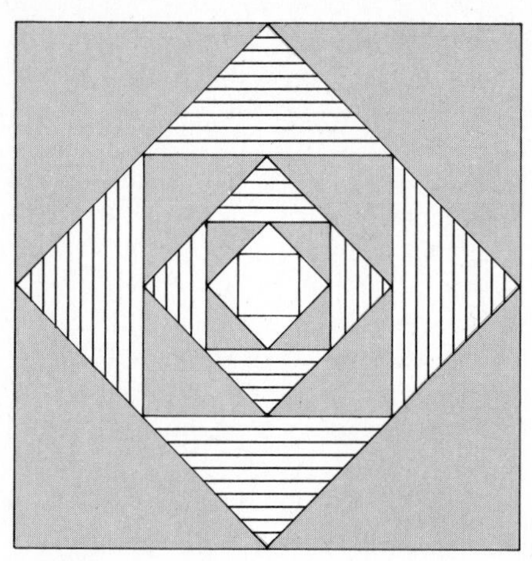

CHAPTER 36
Patterns of Self-Destructive Behavior

Leonora J. McClean

LEARNING OBJECTIVES

After studying this chapter, the student should be able to:

1. Describe myths about suicide, and discuss why they are invalid.
2. Describe the characteristics of indirect and direct self-destructive behavior patterns.
3. Identify stages of a suicidal crisis.
4. Identify populations at a high risk of self-destructive behavior.
5. Discuss individual, family, and environmental patterns of interaction as they pertain to self-destructive behavior.
6. Identify criteria for assessment of a suicidal client.
7. Formulate a nursing care plan for a suicidal client.

Self-destructive behavior is an intrinsic part of the human condition. As people become productive adults, striving to reach life goals, two parts of their personalities come into conflict. Usually, the life-preserving force remains in command of the life-destroying force. If the two forces are not in balance, people are torn by conflict. If such a conflict becomes overwhelming, or if the negative force prevails, the manifestation is often self-destructiveness in a variety of behavioral patterns ranging from subtle to terrifyingly dramatic. Never is despair—bodily, mental, or spiritual—more evident than in overt self-destructive behavior. The purpose of this chapter is to provide an overview of some identifiable indirect and direct patterns of self-destructive behavior as well as guidelines for using the nursing process with self-destructive clients.

MYTHS ABOUT SUICIDE

Myths about suicide have, over the years, perpetuated excuses for avoiding involvement with suicidal clients. Some of the more common myths about suicide follow:

1. Once someone has decided to commit suicide, there is nothing anyone else can do to stop it.
2. If someone is despondent, suicide should not be mentioned: that will give him or her the idea of doing it.
3. People who talk about killing themselves will never do it.
4. People who repeatedly try to commit suicide but don't succeed are only looking for attention.
5. Once a person's depression has lifted, the danger of suicide is over.

Although myths frequently do have an element of truth, the statements above are all untrue. Moreover, they are often embellished with fanciful or uninformed beliefs.

The truth is that, first, in many cases suicide is preventable; crisis hot lines, for example, can identify and prevent self-destructive behavior. Second, not talking about the possibility of suicide is denial. Health care personnel should not let suicide remain a closed, "toxic" issue, but should explore such thoughts even if they have not been verbalized by the client. Third, people who talk about killing themselves or who make repeated suicidal gestures are at high risk of killing themselves on another occasion. Fourth, those who have survived a suicide attempt often indicate that the failure to die has reaffirmed and intensified their feelings of worthlessness: "Look, I can't even commit suicide right." Fifth, when people are so depressed that they decide, on some level of consciousness, to die, there is often an apparent improvement in their condition. A conflict has been resolved, a decision has been made, and therefore they have nothing at stake. Thus a client who has been indecisive about everything may begin making decisions and may gain new stature in a group. The client may sleep better, eat better, work better, and generally venture into activities and relationships that were previously threatening or even immobilizing. For many reasons, it is difficult to prevent such people from committing suicide. It is difficult to know how and when the decision to die was reached if it was made subconsciously. Health care personnel as well as family members, friends, and employers must always suspect a sudden, dramatic improvement in a severely depressed person: it may indicate a decision to commit suicide. In fact, the risk of suicide remains high for about 90 days after discharge for treatment of depression.

DYSYNCHRONOUS HEALTH PATTERNS

At least two types of suicidal behavior, indirect and direct, have been identified by Farberow.[1] *Indirect self-destructive behavior* (ISDB) is defined as any activity that is detrimental to one's physical well-being and might cause death, when the person engaging in it either is unaware of its potential consequences or (if confronted) denies its destructive nature. In other words, the suicidal motivation is subintentional. ISDB is a long-term, repetitive pattern that occurs over a number of years. In contrast, *direct self-destructive behavior* (DSDB) refers to thinking about, talking about, attempting, or actually committing suicide. The intent of the behavior is pain, self-injury, or death, and the person is aware of this. DSDB, an overt behavior, will lead to injury or death if it is not quickly interrupted.

Indirect Self-Destructive Behavior

Indirect self-destructive behavior (ISDB) reflects a physical condition (previously present or absent) and its primary effect on the body or the person. Five groups with a potential for ISDB can be identified.

1. People in whom a physical illness is present and is used against the self by being made worse. The same effect may be achieved if other physical conditions are made worse. (For example, a person with diabetes does not adhere to the diabetic diet; a person with coronary artery disease continues to smoke.)
2. People in whom there is a preexisting physical condition—generally, loss of a body part or function—which requires an extensive change in self-concept or self-image. ISDB is directed against the self: these people lose their self-concept or identity and appear unwilling to redefine themselves in a new and constructive way. (For example, 1 year after a 25-year-old man has had a bilateral above-the-knee amputation following a car accident, he is still unable to perceive himself as a productive, attractive, worthwhile person.)
3. People who have no preexisting physical problem but have incurred injury from self-initiated activities like overeating, smoking, drug and alcohol addiction, and self-mutilation.
4. People who have no preexisting physical problem but are at risk of injury or damage because of self-initiated activities. (Examples include people who commit violent crimes, have many industrial or vehicular accidents, or participate in riots.)
5. People whose pastimes or occupations are inherently risky—involving possible harm as well as excitement, challenge, or mastery. (Examples include mountain climbing, sports parachuting, hang gliding, automobile racing, playing games of risk or chance, and speculating on the stock market.)

There is a great diversity among those who exhibit ISDB which makes it difficult to categorize them distinctly. In fact, people may be identified as belonging to more than one of the five groups.

Direct Self-Destructive Behavior

Direct self-destructive behavior (DSDB) is infliction of pain, self-injury, and death on oneself. An attempt to commit suicide can most often be seen as an appeal, a cry for help. It is a desperate way of saying, "I no longer know of a way to live; therefore I shall die—unless someone can help me." The suicide plan will involve hanging, shooting, taking pills, slashing a major artery; that is, it is genuinely lethal and reflects a genuine intention to die. But the intention may or may not be communicated to others; and so others may or may not be in a position to answer the cry for help. Thus DSDB is in contrast to ISDB; in ISDB, the risk entailed represents an ordeal or a test of ability to survive an extremely dangerous situation. People who have survived such a risk (such as playing "chicken" with automobiles) sometimes feel that they have relieved tension by putting themselves through the ordeal; they feel better able to live afterward. For others, surviving an ordeal may reaffirm a fantasy of immortality which has served as a defense against self-destructive impulses.

Clients who engage in DSDB usually exhibit characteristic alterations in affective, cognitive, and behavior patterns for a variable period preceding the suicidal act. Table 36-1 illustrates alterations in these three dimensions as they relate to the level of intention and lethality (the seriousness of the attempt).

Before a suicide attempt, many people show symptoms of depression. Most noteworthy is their perception that they have exhausted their resources: their ability to cope and their personal, family, or environmental supports. For these people, the future can be viewed only with despair. Often, their family and friends will observe an increasing physical, emotional, and social withdrawal, and feel powerless to reverse it. But in other cases people will go through the motions, acting as if they were involved with others, but inwardly feeling alone, lonely, and permanently estranged. They may also feel either dead or enraged.

Stages of a Suicidal Crisis

A suicidal crisis is precipitated by self-destructive thoughts or actions. The crisis, which usually lasts about 1 to 6 weeks, occurs as a result of four interrelated factors:

- A disastrous event, such as the loss of a loved one
- Threatened loss of a basic source of gratification, as when loneliness reflects a loss of human relatedness.

Table 36-1 Profile of Suicidal Behavior

Level of Intent	Affect	Thoughts	Behavior	Level of Lethality
Gesture	Variable—angry, flat, or depressed	Ambivalence	Dependent upon others Passive Aggressive Manipulative	Low
Aborted attempt	Shocked, angry, or depressed Mood elevates with anxiety reduction	Ambivalence Guilt Helplessness Hopelessness	Aggressive against self; may or may not be socially isolated	Moderate
Successful attempt	Depressed, complacent, or angry	Perseverance of self-destructive ideas Helplessness Hopelessness	Makes lethal suicide plan Obtains means to carry out plan Secretive Socially isolated	High

- Failure to cope with the stress created by these two factors
- Perceived absence of situational support from significant others

There are four phases of a suicidal crisis: onset, impact, recoil, and reorganization. The *onset phase* is characterized by increasing tension; the person attempts to deal with it by using every coping strategy in his or her repertoire. When all efforts to cope are futile, the *impact phase* begins. Disorganization, confusion, frantic activity, and anxiety may be evident. Cognitive functions are impaired; the person cannot think clearly or speak accurately about the cause of the crisis or the precipitating factors. However, catharsis may occur as a jumble of thoughts and feelings are expressed. The *recoil phase* begins as the person pulls away from the pain of open confrontation. Coping mechanisms are mobilized, anxiety diminishes, and logical thinking is restored. But the chaotic state of the client's life is still difficult for him or her to understand. The *reorganization phase* begins as the client starts to organize the chaos and develop alternative ways of coping in similar situations.[2]

DSM III

Indirect and direct self-destructive behaviors are not listed as a separate classification in the *Diagnostic and Statistical Manual of Mental Disorders* (DSM III).[3] However, intentional and subintentional suicidal thoughts, feelings, and behaviors are included under various other categories. For example, suicidal thoughts, wishes, and actions are included under *major affective disorders, major depressive episode.*

Epidemiology

Of those who are known to have directly attempted suicide in the United States in 1980, 12.7 percent succeeded.[4] Among those who commit suicide, about three times as many men die as women; although women more often attempt to kill themselves, they typically choose less effective means. Suicide rates are higher among certain sectors of the population: alcoholics, police officers and physicians, previous attempters, adolescents, the terminally ill, the elderly, minority groups, and psychotic people. Rates also vary by age group. Suicide among adolescents has increased in the past 20 years (see Chapter 39), as it has among people over 50 years of age. With increasing awareness of the connection between fatal accidents and self-destructive feelings experienced by children, statistics may, in the future, reveal a surprising number of suicides among the very young. In general, married people have the lowest rate, those never married are next, and divorced or widowed people have the highest rate, with the exception of older, never

Table 36-2 High-Risk Groups for Indirect and Direct Self-Destructive Behavior

High-Risk Group	Contributing Factors	Dynamics	Example
Alcoholics	Impairment of thinking Impulsivity	Dependency	Client: "I drink only to relax."
Police and physicians	Bombardment of stress from work experience Disruption of life and relationships by work	Isolation from personal resources Personal feelings conflict with societal expectations	A police officer is attacked trying to break up an episode of domestic violence.
Previous attempters	Stress Ineffective coping mechanisms	Cry for help Ordeal to test ability to survive	Client: "I have tried everything; I don't see how I can go on living."
Adolescents	Emotional lability Identity crisis Separation from family Peer pressure	Ambivalence Conflict about dependence versus independence	An 18-year-old on drugs who has overdosed three times.
Terminally ill	Disease Pain Loss of functional ability Disruption of relationships with significant others	Loss of control of life Grief	Client: "This disease has taken over my life. I am only a burden to my family."
Accident repeaters	Stress Ineffective coping mechanisms Unconscious wish to die	Cry for help Ordeal to test ability to survive May fantasize immortality	A person has a series of automobile accidents, each more severe than the last.
Elderly	Disengagement Displacement Loneliness Illness	Diminution of resources as losses occur Struggle to maintain independence and control	A move from a long-time residence to a smaller apartment or house causes depression.
People who reject treatment	Negative previous experiences Loneliness	Defiance of reality Denial of seriousness of problems Fantasy of omnipotence	Client: "I don't need medication; I will overcome this problem alone."
Medically ignored clients	Inability to communicate problems; social and professional barriers to acknowledgment of suicide, influencing physicians and nurses to deemphasize the seriousness of suicidal thoughts and attempts	Feelings of failure (i.e., failed to show the doctor something was wrong)	Client is told, "Go have a few drinks; then you'll feel better."
Minority groups	Social discrimination Displacement Poverty Deprivation	Passive-aggressive to aggressive striking out at society through self	One man murders another, then gives himself up for arrest to be jailed and punished.
Psychotic clients	Impairment of reality testing and problem solving, leading to command hallucinations and heightened impulsivity	Fantasy of omnipotence; denial of underlying feelings of inadequacy	Client stands on window ledge and states, "God is calling me to be an angel," and then jumps.

married white men.[5] Overall, the suicide rate has remained fairly steady in the last few years.

The extent of the human problem represented by suicide is far greater than a count of actual deaths would indicate. Statistics encompass only an incomplete reporting of suicides. High-risk behavior—for example, behavior involving alcoholism and accidents—is also an indicator of self-destructiveness. Table 36-2 identifies some of those at high risk of indirect and direct self-destructive behavior, related factors, dynamics, and examples.

Family members and loved ones are also considered victims of a suicide. Multiply the 28,290 actual reported suicide deaths in 1980 by as few as three family members or close friends for each, and you have 84,870 people who have suffered unusual and terrible grief and whose lives will always be affected by their loss.

PATTERNS OF INTERACTION: PERSON

Recognition of the dynamics underlying cognitive, affective, spiritual, and behavioral patterns is essential in understanding a suicidal person's situation. Ambivalence, guilt, anger, aggression, helplessness, hopelessness, loneliness, and future orientation from a "matrix" for suicide.[6,7,8]

Ambivalence

With DSDB, one of the most common features of suicidal people is that they are ambivalent: they have an inner struggle between self-preserving and self-destructive forces. Their ambivalence is apparent when they threaten or attempt suicide and then try to be rescued. When the possible outcomes of suicide are discussed with these clients, it is remarkable how often they talk of life-related outcomes, such as being relieved of an unhappy situation or getting revenge. Although they consider suicide as an alternative to the way they are living, they may not be considering "not living" as an outcome. For example, it is incongruous for a woman to do her laundry in the morning and then attempt suicide. If she will be dead by evening, what difference does it make if some of her clothes are not clean? It would make a difference only if she survived—if she felt more inclined to wear clothes or if she remained vulnerable to embarrassment or criticism for leaving dirty laundry. This kind of incongruity is so common in the behavior of suicidal persons that it is impossible to assume that suicide is necessarily consciously equated with death.

In contrast, with ISDB, suicidal people are *not* ambivalent. They are not aware that their behavior is self-destructive and would deny anyone's suggestion that it is.[1]

Guilt

A person who feels guilty experiences a pervasive sense of being wrong or of having committed a wrong. Guilt feelings may arise from an awareness of having behaved badly toward another person or of having transgressed one's own moral or ethical principles; or they may entail a feeling of responsibility for wrongs that have occurred or that the person perceives to have occurred. A personal definition of guilt is usually far more severe than a theoretical definition; yet it is the personal definition that professionals who work with suicidal clients must recognize and come to terms with.

Feelings of guilt and remorse are exaggerated and intensified in depressed or suicidal people who engage in DSDB. Clients frequently claim responsibility for all kinds of difficulties and misfortunes—situations and events far beyond the capacity of any one person to generate—in addition to their own personal problems. This exaggeration is so great it can be described as "cosmic guilt," a responsibility for any and all failures and wrongs of oneself and others. It is illogical, of course—omnipotence in reverse. No one human being could be as perverse and destructive as these people believe themselves to be. These clients' guilt feelings may be seen as a subjective explanation for their sorrow or melancholy. Sometimes they include self-perception of sinfulness, stemming from a perceived violation of a personal or religious moral code. Their sense of their own guilt leads to despair, just as, in functional people, a sense of achievement leads to hopefulness.

In contrast, people who engage in ISDB do not have a strong sense of guilt. They are oriented toward themselves and toward self-gratification. The indirect self-destruction that they accomplish is acceptable to them, and thus guilt does not play a prominent part in their lives.[1]

Anger and Aggression

Although people who exhibit DSDB often turn their aggression against themselves rather than other people, there is strong clinical evidence that outward-directed aggression may also be characteristic. Newspaper accounts of combined homicides and suicides are not uncommon. Some people who call suicide crisis centers either threaten to kill or express a fear of killing another person: "I'm going to kill my children"; "I'm afraid I may kill my mother."

Aggression turned outward can also take a more subtle form: manipulative behavior. Some people use threats of suicide to rule the lives of others. The following note was found by a man who was the youngest child in his family and the last to be married:

> "Charles, darling—Tomorrow you will marry the woman you love, and my life is over. I have lived for my children, and you were my last reason to go on.—Love, Mother." It is doubtful that the woman who wrote this note would actually have committed suicide, because she achieved her objective of preventing her son's marriage: Charles and his future wife postponed their wedding. However, they sought counseling because they had realized his mother's motives and wanted to work through their feeling of responsibility toward her and its effect on their own relationship. They did not want their marriage sabotaged by guilt, regardless of what she did. By the time they did marry, Charles's sister had given birth to the first grandchild; the mother was happy about that and had a new "reason to live." However, her earlier note had clearly communicated hostility and aggression toward others.

Suicide is clearly not simply a question of living or dying; it has several components related to oneself and others: a *wish to kill,* stemming from aggression and rage; a *wish to be killed,* stemming from feelings of guilt and worthlessness; and a *wish to die,* stemming from fear and helplessness. People who are suicidal focus their violence on themselves. Murder is an option, but suicide accomplishes at least three objectives that murder does not: it destroys that part of the self which is formed by experience with another person; it destroys the self that is experienced as an identity; and, of course, it results in death and thus gives release from intolerable stress. It is not unusual to see another person implicated or blamed in a suicide note. Such notes document the rage that suicidal people feel toward others but vent on themselves.

One might speculate that ISDB turns anger against the self in the form of physical neglect or taking risks. However, noticeable changes in affect are absent. If emotions such as anger are experienced, it is at a subconscious level.[1]

Helplessness and Hopelessness

Helplessness and despair are characteristic of DSDB. When attempts to cope with problems fail, the problems remain as stressors and may worsen. Moreover, the client is left without the coping mechanisms that previously helped to protect and enhance the self-concept of capability. Diminished self-esteem leaves one less able to develop new coping mechanisms; all this has a snowball effect which eventually causes the client to feel not only that he or she is helpless to change matters but that there is no hope of change or relief. When life is seen as hopeless and the self as helpless, the meaning and purpose of life disappear. The future seems bleak, and the person despairs.

Helplessness and hopelessness are frequently related to the feelings of worthlessness and guilt characteristic of depression (see Chapter 34); it is difficult to tell which of these feelings develops first. In combination, they pose difficult problems for intervention. When clients feel that they have no right to feel better, it is difficult to help them develop new interpersonal behaviors that may relieve some of their stress.

People who exhibit ISDB do not feel helpless or hopeless. They feel that they exercise a moderate amount of power and control over their lives. Also, because of their weak future orientation, they do not tend to dwell on the future at all and thus do not tend to become hopeless even if their future prospects are not good.

Loneliness

Loneliness is often a factor in DSDB. It is a feeling of emptiness—a feeling that one has no investment in others and that others have no investment in oneself. A person can be alone but not lonely; it is possible to feel cared about even in the absence of others. And one can be lonely in the presence of others if one does not feel connected to them or feel them to be part of oneself. Investment in others and by others is a lifeline; without it, suicide (to escape from painful emptiness) becomes an option.

ISDB presents a different picture. The relationships of persons engaging in ISDB tend to be casual, detached, and self-centered. They do not represent a major source of gratification or confirmation of self-worth. Thus the presence or absence of *significant* relationships becomes unimportant, and loneliness is not experienced to the same degree as with DSDB.[1]

Future Orientation

Clients exhibiting DSDB and those exhibiting ISDB both have little future orientation.[1] In directly suicidal clients, this is as a result of someone else's action: through rejection or abandonment, these clients feel deprived of a future they had counted on and therefore see no use in struggling to live. They may also perceive themselves as so inadequate that any future they hope for could never be obtained by their own efforts. While they do envision their own death, they are unable to visualize or care about its long-term consequences. For example.

> A 45-year-old woman who slashed her wrists was concerned only about ending the pain of her everyday existence; she did not consider that if she succeeded, she would not experience her children's marriages and the birth of grandchildren.

People exhibiting ISDB also have little investment in the future, but for a different reason: they are overinvested in the gratifications of the present. They are uninterested in the long-term consequences of their behavior.[1]

Reunion Fantasy

Many clients have thoughts of suicide or even make plans for dying, but they stop short of death itself and being dead forever. Some, however, see death as a means of remaking their lives with other people. The "reunion fantasy" is often related to a belief in life after death. These clients may see themselves as rejoining deceased loved ones and being free of loneliness and hopelessness for all eternity; for them, death is a release of the soul. Such fantasies place clients at an extremely high risk of suicide; giving them reasons to stay alive if they are unhappy will be of no value in intervention.

PATTERNS OF INTERACTION: FAMILY

Family members of a suicidal client may see themselves as victims, bystanders, or precipitators. Richman[9] has observed that a suicidal person may be acting out a family drama. He identified characteristic family dynamics that appeared when a member became suicidal:

1. *Scapegoating.* One member of the family (the suicidal person) becomes the focus of hostility and rejection, and is blamed for the misfortunes or disequilibrium of the family.
2. *Family depression.* The family's style of thinking and interacting suggests a bias against the self. Helplessness and hopelessness are the prevailing attitude.
3. *Intolerance for separation.* Every member seems to be a "captive" of the family; each person's self-image, self-esteem, and coping ability are dependent upon others in the family.
4. *Sadomasochistic relationships.* Some family members behave in hostile, controlling ways, while others are submissive and dependent upon the control of others.
5. *Infantilization of a family member.* Some families "infantilize" one or more members, making them incompetent to deal with the harsh realities of life. These members become aware of their supposed incompetence and feel worthless and hopeless.

Conflict and lack of empathy between parents and suicidal adolescents were also noted by David Lynn.[10] Not all families had the same characteristic features, but it was apparent that the family members were deeply involved in the destructive situation. In some complex way, one family member either chooses or is chosen to act out the family's destructiveness or "bad self." During the crisis of a suicide attempt and a rescue, not only the client but the family members who are available must receive professional attention and assessment. However, a judgmental or hostile attitude toward the family is to be avoided. A family does not "cause" someone to become suicidal; rather, the relationship builds up in an interactive way. In families where suicidal behavior is an established pattern, a way of dealing with aggression, a suicide attempt may be a first option rather than the last desperate effort it looks like to professionals.

The importance of the family in self-destructive behavior can also be seen in the serious implications of the death of a family member for the growth and maturation of survivors. Loss of a parent has long been thought to be a precipitating factor in many suicides. In 1972, T. L. Dorpat[11] reported that children or adolescents who lose a parent through death may be arrested at the stage of psychological development they have reached at that time. This arrest in development may be considered, from a psychoanalytic perspective, a protection against the pain of loss. Later, Solomon and Hersch[12] identified a denial pattern in family dynamics that prevent the normal, time-limited, healing process of grieving. In their research, they found that each family member functioned in some way to deny that a death had occurred and to avoid facing reality.

Following the suicide of a family member, many families develop a denial mechanism and seal themselves off from support they might receive from outsiders. This becomes a self-perpetuating, guilt-generating process in which the social stigma of the death is internalized. The anniversaries of such a death are tantamount to recurrences of it. Thus, the family may deteriorate, and another member may attempt suicide.

PATTERNS OF INTERACTION: ENVIRONMENT

Suicide is a perplexing problem in a culture that teaches the value of life and abhors death. Regardless of one's philosophy and value system, it may be difficult to understand and accept suicidal behavior in a historical, sociological, or psychodynamic context.

Emile Durkheim dismissed the genetic theory of suicide on the ground that if heredity determined suicide, then males and females would kill themselves with equal frequency.[13] (As was noted earlier in the chapter, about three times as many men commit suicide as women.) Durkheim focused on the characteristics of an individual's integration with social forces. Conceptualizing society as an aggregation of forces larger than the number of individuals in the population, he hypothesized that suicide varies inversely with the degree of integration of religious, domestic, and political aspects. In his theory, suicide takes one of four forms:

1. Egoistic suicide, which is brought about by separateness, "excessive individualization," or lack of relatedness to others in society.
2. Altruistic suicide, which may occur when an individual's identity is insufficiently differentiated from the social group. This is the reverse of egoistic suicide.
3. Anomic suicide, which is brought about by abrupt changes in social norms, even though these may be temporary. Durkheim defined *anomie* as "normlessness" or "deregulation."
4. Fatalistic suicide, which is brought about by the imposition (by external forces) of excessive demands or structures on an individual. This is the reverse of anomic suicide.

In contemporary society there are factors that can make people feel unrelated or lead them to overidentify with small peer groups. The rapid technological and industrial development of the twentieth century has brought about social change that in turn has disrupted traditional family lifestyles. Modern transportation has made people geographically mobile. New industry has created jobs, drawing people away from agricultural communities. Individuals who are separated from their extended families by distance and lifestyle may feel that they have lost their roots and find it difficult to adjust to rapidly changing social norms.[14]

NURSING PROCESS

Nurses work with suicidal clients in both inpatient and outpatient settings. The client or family is often encountered initially in a crisis clinic or in the emergency room of a general hospital. Because the client is in an acute crisis, the initial treatment process is compressed into several interventions that occur in the same time frame.

In the initial contact with a suicidal client, the nurse must recognize that there is a clear order of business to be conducted and that it is helpful to get started as soon as possible. Suicidal clients should not be kept waiting, either for an appointment or in emergency rooms or clinics, even if there is no physical or verbal evidence of impending disaster. Only a few people who are suicidal are able to verbalize their discomfort in such a way that others will know they are suicidal, although some people give clues—they may, for example, give away prized possessions or visit the family doctor with vague somatic complaints. (Many people who see a doctor for such somatic problems eventually kill themselves with an overdose of the sedative or tranquilizer prescribed.)

Assessment: Risk Factors

Assessment begins with the first contact between the suicidal client and the helping person; as the assessment process continues, the family of a suicidal person figures prominently in it. The nurse initially collects data from the client about himself or herself. The immediate objective is to determine how likely the client is to die in the immediate future. At best, one can do no more than make an educated guess about the lethality (risk of death) of the client's self-destructive motivations and the relative strength of the will to live. Essentially, such a guess is an assessment of the client's ambivalence.

Assessment also involves identification of risk factors. Immediate risk factors related to lethality are age, sex, marital status, level of intention, the suicide plan, availability of means to carry out the plan, stress factors, and symptoms.[15,16]

Age, Sex, and Marital Status

Mortality data indicate that people between the ages of 15 and 24 and people over 50 have higher suicide rates than other age groups. Thus an adolescent, for example, is at higher risk of committing suicide than a 30-year-old in similar circumstances. In general, as has already been noted, males commit suicide three times more frequently than females (although women attempt suicide more frequently). Those at greatest risk of suicide are divorced or widowed people, with the exception of older, never married white males.

Levels of Intention

Degree of consciousness or willingness to act on wishes or thoughts reflects levels of intention in self-destructive behavior. Suicide is *intentional* when a person takes a direct, conscious part in self-destructive behavior (taking one's own life by hanging is an example). Suicide is *subintentional* when a person plays an indirect role (though this role is nevertheless important) in bringing about death. Subintentional behavior is a way of fulfilling both conscious and unconscious wishes. (For example, many vehicular accidents may be suicide attempts: driving too fast on dangerous roads may result in a fatal accident that is the equivalent of suicide.)

Evidence that self-destructiveness may be present unconsciously is seen in the different ways people experience it. However, it is most common for clients to say that they have been thinking about suicide off and on for some time, but that lately—because of stressful circumstances which they have tried but failed to cope with—they can think of nothing else but their misery and suicide. They are engaged in perseveration, thinking the same thing repetitively.

Suicide Plan and Availability of Means

The suicide plan is an important assessment criterion because it is an index of danger; it may also suggest something about the mental state of the client. Any plan that is straightforward, is easy to carry out, and has little or no margin for error is highly lethal. The difference between planning to put a gun to one's head and pull the trigger and planning to take an overdose of pills is obvious. There is little margin for error with the gun, one gun being about as lethal as another. The margin for error with the pills can be large or small; it depends on (among other things) the type of pills, the number of pills, and the possibility of reflex vomiting while the pills are being swallowed. In complex plans, the outcome may depend on a small detail. Bizarre plans may be evidence of psychosis, but this is also true of many simple, highly lethal plans which are dictated by hallucinated voices. (For instance, a young man who was rescued from the edge of a high roof said that he had been instructed by an "angel of the Lord" to "rise up to meet God.") Plans that are ceremonial may also be the product of psychosis. Psychotic clients in general are a high-risk group because of their impulsivity and distorted thought processes. Finally, a plan may have a special significance or may have been decided upon because the alternative seems repulsive (as in the case of people who, because they can't stand the sight of blood, decide to take pills rather than cut their throats).

The availability of means is crucial if even the simplest of plans is to be carried out. For a person who has a gun but no bullets, there is still an important barrier between life and death. For a person who lives in New York and plans to commit suicide in Chicago, time and space may represent barriers: they may not decrease the lethality of the plan, but they increase the possibility that the client will be rescued before it is carried out.

Stress Factors

Assessment of recent stress factors—physical, social, and emotional events or changes that may increase anxiety, feelings of loss, helplessness, and hopelessness—is critical in identifying factors precipatating suicidal thoughts or actions. For example, environmental factors such as loss of a job, a geographic move, or a change in social or economic status should be identified. Family or marital problems that have created feelings of estrangement, alienation, or futility are also important in assessment. Loss of a loved one through death, separation, or divorce frequently causes an acute grief reaction which may include thoughts of suicide. The anniversary of the death of a significant person may also be a stressor; an "anniversary reaction" can precipitate suicidal thoughts or actions in a client.

Assessment of the client's health history is also important. A client may, for instance, have a chronic, painful illness from which he or she seeks relief by suicide. Detoxified alcoholics, who have lost their old defenses against anxiety and have to confront themselves while they are developing new, healthier defenses, may be at risk for suicide.

A nurse determines the existence and relevance of stress factors by asking the client, "What are your reasons for seeking help now?" or "What has happened in the last 24 hours (week, month)?"

Behavioral Symptoms

Among the behavioral symptoms the nurse assesses are those related to depression, psychosis, extreme anxiety, irritability, and agitation. Characteristics such as guilt and helplessness are common.

An important dimension of behavioral assessment is determining how and to what extent the client's patterns of daily living have changed recently. For example, changes in sleep, eating, hygiene patterns, work, and social habits are often indicators of severe dysfunction. The severity of behavioral symptoms usually has some relationship to the severity of stress.

In summary, a suicide assessment includes evaluating the risk that a client will engage in direct self-destructive behavior. Table 36-3 provides guidelines for assessment of clients who present a constellation of risk factors. High lethality and high intention indicate a need for continued observation in a safe setting. Paykel et al.[17] found that two factors distinguished a high-risk attempt from a low-risk attempt: (1) suicidal history and (2) risk of death posed by the suicide plan. More recently, Beck[18] reported the results of a study of suicidal patients over 14 years. Of the 14 patients in the study who did commit suicide, 13 had scored high on a "hopelessness" scale. If the nurse can assess the depth of a client's hopelessness, it may be considered an indicator of lethality.

Diagnosis

Formulation of the nursing diagnosis involves identifying the client's actual and potential problems. The need to rank problems in order of threat to the client's life is of paramount importance because unless the client's most pressing problems are dealt with immediately, the client may die. For example, if a client has a loaded gun and does not want to give it up, obviously the gun is a greater threat right now than the fact that the client has just lost a job or is without financial resources.

Examples of nursing diagnoses for clients who engage in indirect or direct self-destructive behavior are given in Table 36-4 (page 712).

Outcome Criteria

Establishment of outcome criteria involves developing short- and long-term goals. This can be done by the nurse, by other members of the health team, or by both.

Clients who exhibit DSDB participate minimally in this process at first, because goals imply the future, and at that point clients are unable to visualize a future. Short-term goals established by a care provider, if they are concrete and feasible, often give the suicidal client a sense that not all efforts are doomed or futile and that there may be hope for the future. For clients who have "tunnel

Table 36-3 Assessing Risk of Suicide

	Intensity of Risk		
Behavior or Symptom	**Low**	**Moderate**	**High**
Anxiety	Mild	Moderate	High, or panic state
Depression	Mild	Moderate	Severe
Isolation, withdrawal	Vague feelings of depression, no withdrawal	Some feelings of helplessness, hopelessness, and withdrawal	Hopeless, helpless, withdrawn, and self-deprecating
Daily functioning	Fairly good in most activities	Moderately good in some activities	Not good in any activities
Resources	Several	Some	Few or none
Coping strategies, devices being utilized	Generally constructive	Some that are constructive	Predominantly destructive
Significant others	Several who are available	Few or only one available	Only one or none available
Psychiatric help in past	None, or positive attitude toward	Yes, and moderately satisfied with outcome	Negative view of help received
Lifestyle	Stable	Moderately stable or unstable	Unstable
Alcohol, drug use	Infrequently to excess	Frequently to excess	Continual abuse
Previous suicide attempts	None, or of low lethality	None to one or more of moderate lethality	None to multiple attempts of high lethality
Disorientation, disorganization	None	Some	Marked
Hostility	Little or none	Some	Marked
Suicidal plan	Vague, fleeting thoughts but no plan	Frequent thoughts, occasional ideas about a plan	Frequent or constant thought with a specific plan

SOURCE: C. L. Halten, S. M. Valente, and A. Rink, *Suicide: Assessment and Intervention*, Appleton-Century-Crofts, New York, 1977, p. 56.

vision"—who cannot see any option other than death—observing the establishment and accomplishment of goals may expand their focus. Long-term goals will not be formulated until the suicidal crisis is over. At that time, goals such as establishing a network of friendships, reevaluating job skills, and mending breaches in the family become the outcome criteria for ongoing therapy.

When clients engage in ISDB, it is equally difficult to engage them in formulation of goals such as changing their behavior, their lifestyle, or other patterns of risk. The problem is that they do not consciously see their behavior as dangerous. They are concerned only with immediate gratification, not with the consequences of their behavior, and thus do not perceive any need to change. As a result, nurses or other providers of health care often encounter resistance. Table 36-4 also shows outcome criteria for clients exhibiting direct or indirect self-destructive behavior.

Intervention

Intervention with the Person

Intervention in a suicidal crisis is characterized by (1) authoritativeness, (2) activity, and (3) involvement of others.[15] *Authoritativeness* communicates that the care provider is knowledgeable about suicide and capable of sharing knowledge in a reassuring, helping way. *Activity* communicates that the nurse will do whatever is possible and that the client will be expected to do something as well. *Involvement of others* communicates that the client is not alone, even though he or she may feel that way. The nurse and other care providers will facilitate the mobilization of the client's social support systems.

Table 36-4 Nursing Diagnoses and Outcome Criteria for Self-Destructive Clients

Nursing Diagnosis	Outcome Criteria
1. Suicidal thoughts related to feelings of hopelessness and despair	Client replaces suicidal thoughts with problem solving, as evidenced by: a. Verbalizing understanding of conflicts that have generated hopelessness (unrealistic goals). b. Setting goals that are realistic and obtainable.
2. Intense anxiety related to loneliness	Client decreases anxiety experienced, as evidenced by: a. Identifying family and friendship supports. b. Contacting one family member and one friend.
3. Noncompliance with low-salt, low-fat cardiac diet, related to denial of health problem	Client demonstrates understanding of noncompliant health patterns, as evidenced by: a. Verbally acknowledging health problem b. Examining consequences of noncompliance. c. Examining self-destructive nature of this behavior pattern.
4. Self-destructive behavior related to wish to punish others for their perceived lack of support and love.	Client directly expresses thoughts and feelings, as evidenced by: a. Directly verbalizing resentment to family members. b. Negotiating, with the family, ways to satisfy needs perceived by both client and family.
5. Impulsive suicidal attempt related to command hallucinations	Client will validate actions with others before acting, as evidenced by: Distinguishing inner subjective perceptions from outer objective perceptions.
6. Suicidal wishes related to desire to be free from physical pain and disability	Client will consider a variety of alternatives to dealing with intractable pain, as evidenced by: a. Examining whether dying will accomplish desired goal. b. Evaluating consequences of his or her other actions for significant others.

ESTABLISHING A RELATIONSHIP. The first step in intervention with suicidal clients is to establish a relationship in which the nurse assumes an authoritative role. A client does not want to ask a stranger, who is going to cringe at the word "suicide," for help. The nurse needs to use a matter-of-fact approach and to care about what the client is relating. The relationship is helped if the nurse communicates that the client's complaints are legitimate. Many people still believe that only physical complaints are worthy of attention in health care facilities. Some clients may feel embarrassment at being unable to cope with their problems. A comment from the nurse (such as, "I see you're really upset. You've done the right thing in coming for help.") may lessen the client's embarrassment.

Clients need to know from the outset that the nurse will assist them in seeking every possible solution to problems, but no promises should be made. False assurances are dangerous. The client knows that there are no easy answers, and promising the impossible diminishes the credibility of the nurse. Most clients allow care givers to make some errors in communication, but adolescents are particularly sensitive to unrealistic or condescending messages.[19]

Many clients who have the ego strength to ask for help are still ambivalent about getting it. Crying, profane language, arrogance, and silence are obstacles to effective communication. Clients who are arrogant and condescending are particularly likely to provoke anxiety in the care giver. For example:

> A woman called a suicide prevention center for help, and when a young man answered, she began badgering him with questions, including this: "What are your credentials that you presume to hold this position?" She also said, "My problems are very complex; I need to talk to your best psychiatrist immediately."

It is best to assign such clients to an alternative care giver who more closely meets their needs for self-esteem, even though the nurse may be very capable. Knowing when to refer is important, and failure to refer a difficult client is sometimes related to a nurse's personal feelings of rejection and anger.

A nurse may realize that an adversary relationship is developing when a client asks for help but maintains the right to die. In their zeal to rescue clients, nurses sometimes try to remove the option of suicide immediately. It is not possible and not wise to deny the reality of the client's option. Maintaining this option may be one way for the client to control the situation. Suicide may be a final act of desperation for some people, but it is an act of courage and self-determination for others. In either case, assessment quickly moves beyond lethality to the problems which bring people to that point. Instead of saying, "Don't kill yourself," say, "Wait. Give us some time to understand this and to see if some problems can be solved."

MONITORING THE CLIENT'S SAFETY NEEDS. At some point in the intervention process, it may be necessary for clients exhibiting DSDB to be hospitalized in order to ensure their safety. Criteria for admission that should be observed by community health nurses or emergency room nurses are:

1. What is the likelihood that the client will commit suicide in the near future (on the basis of the total assessment)?
2. What is the likelihood that the client is psychotic, or uses drugs or alcohol?
3. What is the client's ability for self-care?

Clients who are psychotic are more often committed for treatment than clients who realize that they are in danger; the latter may be hospitalized voluntarily. Depending upon the outpatient resources available, a client who is assessed as "low" to "moderately" suicidal may be treated as an outpatient.

The decision to hospitalize is usually made by a physician who determines that the client cannot control his or her destructive impulses without help. The client's safety is the primary reason for hospitalization.

Typically, when a suicidal client is admitted to the hospital, the chart, or clinical record, is clearly labeled "suicide precautions." Included in the treatment orders are some of the following measures, designed to ensure physical safety:

1. Search personal effects for toxic agents (such as drugs and alcohol).
2. Remove sharp instruments (razor blades, knives, letter openers, glass bottles which could be broken, etc.).
3. Remove straps and clothing that could be used for self-destruction (belts, neckties, stockings, pantyhose, etc.).
4. Place the client on one-to-one observation, constant or at regular intervals.

Such measures are intended to reduce obvious opportunities for committing suicide. These physical precautions, however, may have negative implications for the nurse-client relationship. The nurse sees a client admitted who is disconsolate—feeling worthless, hopeless, and guilty. The search of personal effects is an invasion of privacy such as would rarely be imposed on a client with, say, a gallbladder problem. The removal of "sharps and straps" carries the message that the client, if left with them, might use them destructively. One-to-one observation may seem to communicate that the client is being held prisoner. The cumulative effects of hospitalization may add to the humiliation and depersonalization of someone who already has such diminished self-esteem that self-destruction is imminent.[20]

Although this criticism is valid, there is also a rationale for safety measures:

1. The client needs to be in the hospital because danger is apparent.
2. The hospital accepts a legal obligation to provide protection for a client diagnosed as a suicide risk.
3. The nurse has a legal and professional responsibility to provide care which is life- and health-directed.

Until better strategies of protection and intervention are developed, these measures are required. However, the manner in which they are implemented can do much to lessen their negative impact. Clients deserve an explanation of why a search is made and certain articles are removed; they should be told when, in relation to their progress, such personal property will probably be returned. Once clients are established on a service unit, their personal identity, rather than their classification as suicide risks, should be emphasized in introductions to others.

A client's self-destructive behavior should be treated as matter-of-factly as other symptoms or problems. Even a poorly oriented psychiatric client knows that one-to-one observation is a precaution against suicide. No attempt should be made to keep the matter confidential; otherwise, the client's interaction with other clients will be inhibited and the resulting isolation will become a barrier to intervention.

Similarly, nurses need to monitor the safety of clients who engage in ISDB. For example, a nurse might say to a diabetic client, "We will not allow you to kill yourself by eating junk food and not taking your insulin. Either you will follow your diet and administer your insulin, or it will be done by us; but you will be prevented from killing yourself."

ENCOURAGING VERBAL COMMUNICATION. It is common for inexperienced nurses to avoid talking with clients about suicidal thoughts and impulses, for fear that this will make clients more likely to act on them. But usually the opposite is true: people who talk out their self-destructive ideas are less likely to act them out. For one thing, nurses cannot make an adequate assessment if the lethality of impulses is not examined. Appropriate questions to ask include these:

1. Since you have been depressed, have you had thoughts of wanting to die or wanting to hurt yourself?
2. Have you formulated in your mind a specific plan for how you would hurt yourself?
3. How pressured do you feel to act on your suicidal thoughts?
4. What time of the day are you most aware of these thoughts?
5. Has any member of your family ever made a suicide attempt? Was it successful?

Clients often have suicidal thoughts that are never verbalized simply because no one asks about them. By talking about these issues openly the nurse conveys an intention to deal with the client's self-destructive tendencies. One intervention that can be particularly effective is a "no suicide" pact. This is a written agreement between client and nurse that the client will not act on suicidal impulses, but instead will approach the nurse to talk about them. This, of course, cannot be taken as an absolute guarantee that the client will abide by the contract, but often the commitment required to put it in writing provides clients with some needed distance between their thoughts and actions. Clients become aware that other means are available to deal with their impulses, and that other people care about which option they choose.

In these ways, clients gain some measure of assurance that they will be protected from and helped to control their self-destructive impulses. The fact that interventions occur within the context of a relationship reduces the sense of isolation which makes suicide a risk. The concern which is conveyed may provide a spark of hope that things can be different.

ENHANCING SELF-ESTEEM. Self-destructive clients generally have low self-esteem. Nursing intervention is directed toward treating them as people who deserve attention and concern; their positive attributes should be recognized with genuine but realistic praise.

> Mr. J. was a suicidal client who perceived himself as having no value to others. His wife was distressed about his situation and shared with the nurse a description of Mr. J. before he became depressed and suicidal: he had been a fine craftsman who made toys for orphaned children at Christmas time. The nurse arranged to get materials so that Mr. J. could make a few toys for the children on the hospital's oncology unit. Initially Mr. J. agreed only reluctantly, but he put a lot of energy into filing, sanding, and gluing the precut parts, and he also explained his activities to the nurse. He received sincere praise for the completed toys from the other clients on the unit as well as from the sick children, whom he visited to distribute his gifts. The nurse had made this project an effective part of Mr. J.'s therapeutic program.

Nurses should not manufacture reasons to praise a client; clients are sensitive to genuineness and will recognize manufactured comments as artificial. This will lower their self-esteem even more, the message being, "I'm so bad that they have to make up things to praise in me."

MODIFYING COPING PATTERNS. Clients who exhibit direct or indirect self-destructive behavior often have a variety of dysfunctional coping patterns. For example, clients who express their anger through self-mutilation would exhibit healthier ways of coping with anger if, like Mr. J., they hammered, sawed, sanded, and built toys. For clients who are noncompliant, healthy coping would imply the assumption of responsibility for self-care. Interventions must be directed toward understanding the meaning of the illness for the client as well as exploring denial patterns. Finding acceptable and functional ways to deal with a health problem represents a healthier way of coping.

Intervention with the Family

A suicidal crisis of one family member involves the entire family. Family members, who may be upset by the client's behavior, should engage in the treatment process from the beginning. Their guilt or hostility toward the client is a symptom which will be important to deal with in the course of treatment. Also, early engagement of the family gives health professionals an opportunity to make them aware of other resources in the community, such as hot lines, self-help groups, and community health nurses. Family intervention involves exploration of family coping styles. For example, have other family members dealt with stress by expressing suicidal thoughts, making suicidal gestures, attempting suicide, or actually committing suicide? In other words, is suicide a learned coping style? With regard to ISDB, do other family members understand its significance and the consequences of not complying with treatment? Do family members habitually take risks? If so, what purpose does risk serve in the family? Clients may need to be helped to evaluate their own risk taking as it reflects their own needs and style rather than their family's.

Patterns of family relationships need to be explored. Very often, suicidal people perceive themselves as outsiders, physically or emotionally cut off from the nuclear or extended family. This perception intensifies feelings of worthlessness, loneliness, and estrangement from significant others. Forces on the client's as well as the family's side that contribute to that perceived or actual pattern need to be modified. More functional communication patterns and ways of spending relationship time can be modeled and suggested.

When a family member commits suicide, intervention with the family is extremely important. Grief following the loss of a loved one by natural death is a temporary healing process, but grief following a suicide is a self-perpetuating agony of loss from death, rejection, and disillusionment.[12] Moreover, the social rituals and amenities through which bereaved families receive support from friends who share their loss are lacking when a suicide is involved. If a death is self-inflicted, friends sometimes blame the family; even if they do not, they are puzzled and perplexed. They do not know what to do for the family; frequently they do nothing. The resulting isolation of the family confirms the sense of guilt. Families tend to respond to a suicide as a rejection which is attributable to lack of trust or love, or even to hatred. The family sinks into self-recrimination for having been inadequate or blind. A family scapegoat may be identified as the destructive force who "caused" the suicide.

Children are particularly vulnerable to the death of a parent by suicide. Dorpat identified several psychopathological findings in a group of 17 subjects: (1) feelings of guilt for having "caused" the parent's death, (2) depression, (3) preoccupation with suicide, (4) self-destructive behavior, (5) absence of grief, (6) arrest of some aspects of personality development.[11] Apparently, suicidal behavior can be a learned pattern for coping with overwhelming stress; this may explain its frequency across generations and families. Developmental arrest is sometimes related to a family's tendency to try to keep from the child the facts of the parent's death, generally by making up an explanation which is supposedly less traumatic.[21] Even if children know the truth anyway (as they frequently do), or are told by someone else, they are not permitted to deal with the fact of suicide, because their families are seemingly too fragile to allow it.

Because a suicide is such an overwhelming trauma to a family, there is a tendency to relive over and over the events surrounding it. Occasionally, another family member will commit suicide later, near the date of the previous suicide; this is called an *anniversary suicide*. Some family members live for years expecting to die by suicide.

Many families will not permit the intrusion of a helping person following a suicide, but those who do allow it have a greater opportunity to grieve and to lessen the long-term effects of the loss. There is very little clinical expertise with intervention strategies, but it is clear from experience that one should never attempt to help alone: family members are full of hostility and destructiveness, and a stranger is an easy target. Community health nurses may be the least threatening of health professionals for follow-up, since they are not likely to have been associated with the crisis itself.

Intervention with the Community

Community intervention involves identification of health and adjustment needs or risk factors in groups of people. Intervention through health education or counseling strategies can prevent self-destructive behavior.

The nurse assesses the community—the life context of an individual client who lives, works, and functions in an ecological and demographic area. For example, population density is correlated with higher suicide rates. In urban neighborhoods, many people live close together but are emotionally distant; such people may not be resources for each other. Where poverty is pervasive, there will be people who have so few alternatives in coping with problems that suicide is likely. There are also densely populated urban neighborhoods in middle- and upper-income areas where people are alienated from each other by pressures of work and demands for achievement in a complex, competitive world. Here too, suicide is a likely option for many people.

RISK FACTORS. Nurses can use strategies of primary prevention by assessing a community to identify factors related to health problems. But equally important is identifying the strengths and resources of the community. This important information must be communicable to residents. Social "consciousness raising" involves working with people so that they will know how to use existing resources, or obtain more, to reduce the incidence of health problems and improve the quality of life.

GROUPS AT RISK. Community intervention also focuses on identifying those who may be at risk in a given population and who show a degree of disorganization. For example, people with hypertension, diabetes, or vascular disease and people who smoke, drink alcohol excessively, or have had repeated vehicular or occupational accidents are at risk of health problems and indirect self-destructive behavior. Engaging such people in education and treatment programs will maintain their health and limit their self-destructive behavior.

THE BEREAVED COMMUNITY. Finally, community intervention deals with the "community" of a client who has committed suicide while in the hospital or following discharge: the staff and other hospitalized clients. When clients kill themselves despite preventive measures, staff members and other clients have an intense reaction which includes anger, guilt, helplessness, and hopelessness. Clients on the unit may also demonstrate self-destructive behavior or even carry out their own suicides. Staff members tend to go through a process of grieving in addition to experiencing failure, guilt, and helplessness. It is usually helpful to assemble staff members and clients so that they can share and express their feelings of loss. Such feelings may include other clients' anger and fear for their own safety. Surviving clients (like family members) may identify with the person who committed suicide; they may be afraid that they will succumb to their own self-destructive impulses and that staff members will be unable to prevent this. The professionals have the responsibility of supporting and protecting clients as well as working through their own feelings.

Evaluation

Evaluation is an ongoing process that occurs regularly throughout the nursing process with suicidal clients and their families. As the risk of suicide, the stress factors, and the symptoms fluctuate, the goals and plan of intervention will vary. The evaluation will ultimately rest on whether risk factors, stressors, and behavioral symptoms were reduced in a population at risk or for an individual or family.

The case study of John V. illustrates the evaluation process for a suicidal client:

> John V., 23, moved to a large metropolitan area to start his career. He received a big sendoff from his family and friends, who assumed that he would "make it big" in the city. After a few months of job hunting and rejection, John became weary and depressed. Eventually, he had to face reality: he realized that he was competing in a difficult job market and that a low-level job was the best he could hope to start with. A great deal of his self-esteem depended on how the people at home saw him. His problems began to mount as his self-esteem diminished and his self-image as a capable, competitive adventurer was shattered. He believed he should be able to get a good job and send money home. John began to have insomnia; and after several nights with little sleep, he visited the emergency room of a hospital, saying that he felt like hurting himself.

Table 36-5 Evaluation for a Self-Destructive Client: John V.

Assessment	Diagnosis	Outcome Criteria	Intervention	Evaluation
"I hate living in the city." "I have no friends. People in this city are totally unfriendly."	Intense anxiety related to loneliness	Client will manage anxiety effectively, as evidenced by: Identification of potential friendship networks Calling potential social contacts	1. Encourage client to verbalize feelings of loneliness. 2. Explore family and friendship support systems. 3. Contact community resources related to employment counseling and socialization. 4. Identify and provide practice in needed social skills.	John telephones family within 48 hours. John contacts the local Y to find out about a health club membership. John reevaluates his job skills and calls two employment agencies for interviews. John goes to the singles group at a local church.
"Since I haven't been able to land a job in my field, I have not been in touch with my family for 6 months. I know they'll be disappointed in me and think I'm a failure. I could go from one week to the next without talking to anybody." "What's the use? I have to make it here, and I can't go home." "I can't sleep. I pace the floor all night. I'm a wreck."	Emotional cutoff from extended family related to self-perception of failure	Reestablish contact with family, as evidenced by: Verbalizing worst fears about contacting his family Exploring fantasy about family reaction to his joblessness	1. Explore worst-best outcomes related to contacting family. 2. Explore family expectations. 3. Explore self-expectations. 4. Explore realistic nature of self- and family expectations. 5. Formulate a strategy for contacting family.	John telephones his parents within 48 hours, apprising them of his situation. John writes to his family weekly.

Short-term crisis intervention helped John V. to identify his problem and explore options. The evaluation phase of the nursing process (Table 36-5) documents the attainment of the goals set forth in the initial nursing care plan.

SUMMARY

Self-destructive behavior is a part of the human condition; but myths about suicide have perpetuated excuses for avoiding involvement with self-destructive clients. These misconceptions may contribute to an avoidable loss of life.

Two types of suicidal behavior are indirect self-destructive behavior (ISDB) and direct self-destructive behavior (DSDB). ISDB is a subtle, long-term, repetitive pattern; DSDB is overt thinking about, talking about, attempting, or actually committing suicide.

A suicidal crisis usually lasts 1 to 6 weeks. There are three interrelated factors in such a crisis: a disastrous event, threatened loss of a basic source of gratification, and failure to cope with these.

Approximately 12.7 percent of those who attempt suicide succeed. Women attempt suicide more frequently, but men complete suicides three times more often than women.

Patterns of ambivalence, guilt, helplessness, hopelessness, anger, aggression, loneliness, and future orientation provide a basis for understanding self-destructive behavior. Family and environmental patterns of interaction may also influence the development and onset of self-destructive behavior.

The nursing process provides a framework for assessing risk factors: age, sex, level of intention, a suicide plan and the availability of means to carry it out, stress factors, and symptoms. Nursing diagnoses must be realistic; outcome criteria must be short-term and attainable. Intervention with the suicidal person is characterized by authoritativeness, activity, and involvement of others. Intervention with the family and the community includes exploring family and community patterns that support suicide as a way of coping with stress. Intervention may also include "postvention" with clients, staff, and family following a completed suicide. Evaluation, as determined by outcome criteria, examines the degree to which self-destructive behavior has been alleviated and a more functional coping style instituted.

REFERENCES

1. N. L. Farberow, *The Many Faces of Suicide: Indirect Self-Destructive Behavior,* McGraw-Hill, New York, 1980.
2. Lydia Rappoport, "The State of Crisis: Some Theoretical Considerations," in Howard J. Parad, ed., *Crisis Intervention: Selected Readings,* Family Service Association of America, New York, 1965.
3. American Psychiatric Association, *Diagnostic and Statistical Manual of Mental Disorders,* 3d ed., APA, Washington, D.C., 1980.
4. Corrine Loing Hatton and S. McBride Valente, *Suicide: Assessment and Intervention,* 2d ed., Appleton-Century-Crofts, Norwalk, Conn., 1984.
5. L. L. Linden and W. Breed, "The Demographic Epidemiology of Suicide," in Edwin Schneideman, ed., *Suicidology: Contemporary Developments,* Grune and Stratton, New York, 1976.
6. L. Webstein, *Handbook of Suicidology: Principles, Problems,* Brunner/Mazel, New York, 1979.
7. David Lester, *Why People Kill Themselves,* Thomas, Springfield, Mass., 1972.
8. Karl Menninger, *Man against Himself,* Harcourt, Brace, New York, 1938.
9. Joseph Richman, "Family Determinants of Suicide Potential," in Dorothy B. Anderson and Leonora J. McClean, eds., *Identifying Suicide Potential,* Behavioral Publications, New York, 1971.
10. David B. Lynn, *The Father: His Role in Child Development,* Brooks/Cole, Monterey, Calif., 1974.
11. T. L. Dorpat, "Psychological Effects of Parental Suicide on Surviving Children," in Albert C. Cain, ed., *Survivors of Suicide,* Thomas, Springfield, Mass., 1972.
12. Michael Solomon and L. Brian Hersch, "Death in the Family, Implications for Family Development," *Journal of Marital and Family Therapy,* April 1979.
13. Ronald Maris, *Social Forces and Urban Suicide,* Davey, Homewood, Ill., 1969.
14. Irene Goldenberg and Herbert Goldenberg, *Family Therapy: An Overview,* Brooks/Cole, Monterey, Calif., 1980, p. 10.
15. Norman L. Farberow and Edwin Schneideman, *The Cry for Help,* McGraw-Hill, New York, 1961.
16. Edwin Schneideman, "Sleep and Self-Destruction: A Phenomenological Approach," in Edwin Schneideman, ed., *Essays in Self-Destruction,* Science House, New York, 1967.
17. E. Paykel et al., "Treatment of Suicide Attempters," *Archives of General Psychiatry,* vol. 31, 1974, pp. 487–491.
18. Aaron Beck, *American Journal of Psychiatry,* April 1985. (Not yet available.)
19. Jerome Motto, "Treatment and Management of Suicidal Adolescents," *Psychiatric Opinion,* vol. 12, no. 6, 1975.
20. M. M. Blythe and D. R. Pearlmutter, "The Suicide Watch: A Reexamination of Maximum Observation," *Perspectives in Psychiatric Care,* vol. XXI, no. 3, 1983, pp. 90–93.
21. Max Warren, "Some Psychological Sequelae of Parental Suicide in Surviving Children," in Albert C. Cain, ed., *Survivors of Suicide,* Thomas, Springfield, Mass., 1972.

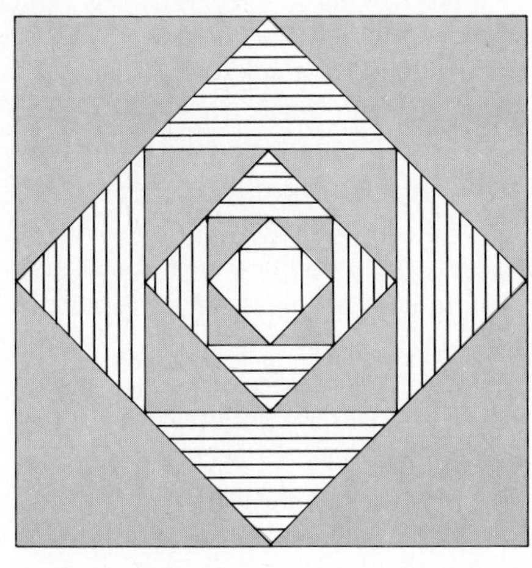

CHAPTER 37
Patterns of Dysfunctional Reality Orientation

Lynn R. Bernstein

LEARNING OBJECTIVES

After studying this chapter, the student should be able to:

1. Define *psychosis*.
2. Discuss cognitive, perceptual, affective, motor, and social changes that occur in schizophrenia.
3. Discuss individual, family, and environmental patterns of interaction associated with schizophrenia.
4. Identify assessment factors for the client, the family, and the environment.
5. Formulate nursing diagnoses for schizophrenic clients.
6. Formulate realistic short- and long-term outcome criteria for schizophrenic clients.
7. Identify nursing interventions for schizophrenic clients.
8. Evaluate the effectiveness of a nursing care plan for a schizophrenic client.

People who experience an overwhelming degree of anxiety and whose coping mechanisms fail to maintain their anxiety at a tolerable level may feel that they have lost control of their perceptions, thoughts, feelings, and behavior. A massive disintegration of ego functioning occurs, causing the person to be unable to deal effectively with self, others, and the environment.[1] Disintegration indicates that the person's perceptions, thoughts, feelings, and behavior are different or altered. There is a profound dysynchrony in the dimensions of self—that is, mind, body and spirit. The person may have difficulty evaluating reality in a consensually validated way; that is, reality may be perceived differently from the way in which the majority of people would view it. This disintegrative process is referred to as *psychosis*, the etiology of which is largely unknown.

When psychosis occurs, people often enter the mental health system for help in dealing with the overwhelming internal and external forces with which they cannot cope. The person may be labeled *psychotic* and display some of or all the behaviors of *schizophrenia*. Others may not enter a mental health system but may endure intense anxiety alone or with the help of outside support systems and ultimately be able to evaluate reality in a more accurate way. Psychosis, and specifically schizophrenia, can occur once in a person's lifetime, or it can be a recurring process characterized by remissions and exacerbations. The goal of treatment is to restore the client's maximum potential for health in terms of a functional lifestyle.

The purpose of this chapter is to explore one of the disintegrative patterns that occur in psychosis, the schizophrenic disorders. The dysynchronous health patterns related to schizophrenia will be presented along with the individual, family, and environmental patterns of interaction. The nursing process will be applied to the care of clients with this health problem.

DYSYNCHRONOUS HEALTH PATTERNS

Schizophrenia is characterized by changes in five areas: cognitive, perceptual, affective, motor, and social.[1] Schizophrenics appear to relinquish control of self in these essential areas of life. The degree to which this happens may vary sharply at critical points in the person's life and from person to person. *Regression*, that is, a return to earlier, more primitive, ways of experiencing self, others, and the environment, provides the basis for changes in cognition, perception, affect, relationships, and behavior. Energy is withdrawn from the exigencies of the environment with which the person cannot cope, an intense self-focus ensues, and customary ways of experiencing self, others, and the environment disintegrate.

These changes rarely occur in only one aspect of the person. Most people demonstrate behavior that overlaps in all five areas.[1,2] However, in order to explain the various manifestations of each category with clarity, each will be discussed separately.

Cognitive Changes

Schizophrenia and Cognition

The term *cognition* refers to the mental processes involved in obtaining knowledge, that is, the use of intellect, reason and judgment. The term *cognition* is often used interchangeably with the term *thought*. One of the major characteristics of schizophrenia is the disruption of normal modes of thought. The person deviates from logical thought patterns that characterize adult thinking and returns to earlier, more primitive, thought patterns. This most commonly occurs at times of stress, anxiety, or fear, times at which all people are vulnerable to becoming unable to think clearly and logically. The schizophrenic has difficulty acting coherently; actions tend to be based on private interpretations of reality which are not consensually validated, that is, understood and accepted by the majority of the population.

Autistic Thinking

A basic aspect of regressive cognitive thought processes is autistic thinking. *Autistic thinking* is a form of subjective thinking that relies on a personal, illogical interpretation of reality. It involves minimal distinction between inner and outer experience, between self and environment. Thoughts and perceptions are not checked out or validated in terms of objective reality. Reality is interpreted on the basis of inner needs, drives, and desires. Fantasy and daydreaming replace objective observation and logical thought patterns. Personal meanings, rather than those generally accepted by the culture, are applied to persons and events.[2] M. Feffer[3] notes that the schizophrenic can be viewed as having returned to an early stage of Piaget's model of cognitive development, the stage of preoperational thought (see Chapter 5).

Autistic thinking is a normal part of cognitive development in childhood. The normal processes in the development of thought are: (1) sensorimotor exploration and free association; (2) autistic-egocentric thinking; (3) refinement of egocentric thinking, along with development of concrete thinking and rudimentary ability to organize and classify information; and (4) abstract reasoning. Autistic thinking should gradually disappear from the foreground of thought as it is replaced by increasingly sophisticated abstract thought patterns that emerge during the elementary school years and are consolidated during adolescence. This evolution is consistent with ego development.

As people develop, they attempt to organize and make sense of stimuli they are receiving from inside and outside the self. However, if this process is disrupted by lack of stimulation, lack of opportunities to validate experience, or repeated experiences with high anxiety that lead to distorted perceptions, the self will be used as a personal frame of reference for making interpretations about reality. A primitive, intrapersonal, autistic system of thought and communication develops. Lacking satisfaction and validation in the outer world, schizophrenics turn to their inner worlds for rewards. This form of thinking is not reality-oriented and consists of distortions of reality. Self-centered thinking fosters fantasy and daydreaming, which become a substitute for reality. People apply their own personal and private meaning to situations and words rather than those that are consensually validated.[2]

Autistic thinking provides the basis for the cognitive changes that are observed in schizophrenia: primitive thinking, looseness of associations, magical thinking, delusions, and linguistic changes. These are described below.

PRIMITIVE THINKING. Primitive thinking is manifested by movement away from abstract, connotative thought which is central to adult thought processes. Concrete, denotative thought, similar to that seen in childhood and among primitive cultures, reflects a lack of conceptual meaning in thoughts and words. Concrete thought is characterized by ignoring situational contexts of words, misunderstanding of nuances and inferences, inappropriate shifts in focus, lack of selectiveness in sorting out the essential components of experience, and an inability to abstract common qualities and forms.[4] The person remains tied to concrete data; this decreases the ability to sort and classify things according to logical categories or generalize from specific examples. The person attends to the discrete details of a thought rather than to the main idea.[2] For example:

> A client who was asked how a coat and a sweater are similar said, "They are both brown," responding to the concrete, denotative color of each. When asked to describe other ways in which they are similar, the client was unable to respond. A more abstract, connotative response would have been, "They are both items of clothing," or "They are both outerwear garments that would be chosen according to the weather."

The schizophrenic, then, lacks the ability to recognize similarities which transform the world from a set of unrelated facts into an ordered pattern of meaningful data. The person is unable to appreciate the abstract nature of humor and consequently feels that jokes have personal meanings. Proverbs cannot be interpreted in any but a concrete, literal way. For example, the proverb "A rolling stone gathers no moss" may be interpreted by a schizophrenic as "A moving object is unsuitable for plant growth."

LOOSENESS OF ASSOCIATIONS. The term *looseness of associations* refers to the inability to organize thoughts into a logical pattern that leads toward an end or a conclusion.[2] Thoughts do not flow from one another in a logical, connected manner. The person expresses successive ideas that appear to be unrelated or only slightly related. The person does not indicate any intention of changing the subject or of explaining unexpected transitions. There is an apparent interruption in the train of thought by the expression of irrelevant ideas. In addition, the logic of the thought pattern is not governed by consensually validated rules of logic. A single concept is not pursued to its logical conclusion. As a result, such a person's language is confusing, bizarre, and difficult to follow. An example follows.

> A client who was asked how he was feeling replied, "I'm alive, I'm feeling, feeling my heart beating, I read about a beating, drums have a peculiar beat, drums give you a real feeling for music."

The term *overinclusiveness* refers to another disturbance in associational thought patterns: a focusing on irrelevant details which results from the loosening of associations. Overinclusiveness may be attributed to a central impairment of the process of filtering incoming stimuli.[5] A client may dwell on a single thought, often seemingly trivial, and allow it to dominate mental and verbal activity. For example, the client may talk at length about one aspect of a person he or she barely knows.

MAGICAL THINKING. Magical thinking is another type of primitive thought process; it is normal for preschool children but is identified as a regressive behavior in adults. The person who engages in magical thinking attaches personal meaning or power to objective events or neutral situations, and believes that he or she has secret powers and can effect change with thoughts alone. This omnipotent view of self makes such people feel that the world is within their control.[2] For example:

> A male client believed that the thoughts he had while asleep were responsible for the messages that were found on the psychiatrist's desk each morning. They were conveyed to each piece of paper via special electronic message circuits.

Magical thinking often stems from a need to be important, needed, loved, and wanted. The thoughts fulfill needs that are not being met in a reality-oriented way. For example:

> A female client claimed that she had developed special radar powers that allowed her to remain in touch with her brother, who had recently been killed in a car accident—a death that left her with no other living family connections.

DELUSIONS. Delusions are another manifestation of regressive thought processes that interfere with a person's ability to test and evaluate reality. A *delusion* is a belief system which is not validated or tested against reality and which is firmly maintained in the face of contradictory information.[6] Delusions develop in the following manner:

1. The person, feeling threatened by others or from within, experiences anxiety and has a sense that something ominous is happening.
2. The person attempts to deny the threat of self-perceptions or objective reality by misinterpreting impressions of events and things.
3. The person projects inner thoughts and feelings onto the environment so that negative or unacceptable feelings, thoughts, and wishes appear to be coming from the outside, rather than from within the self.
4. The person attempts to justify or rationalize personal interpretations of reality to self and others. The delusions may become *systematized;* that is, they are no longer viewed as unrelated beliefs but are rationalized or explained more or less logically in reaction to the rest of the person's life. When the delusion is unshakable, it is referred to as a *fixed delusion.*[2]

Delusions reflect an underlying need to deny unacceptable feelings about the self that may relate to hostility, sexuality, power, control, dependency, and self-esteem. For example, a man may consider himself clumsy and ridiculously inadequate. He develops the impression that people are laughing at him. The impression soon becomes certainty: he is sure that they think he is no good and inadequate. Not only does the man claim that others accuse him of traits he does not like in himself; eventually he ascribes to others the characteristics he cannot accept in himself. Whereas he started by being merely suspicious, he soon becomes convinced that other people conspire or plot against him, and he collects "evidence" that supports this position.[2] Delusions of many types exist. The more common delusions are described (with examples) in Table 37-1.

LINGUISTIC CHANGES. Linguistic changes also reflect a disruption in abstract thought patterns which exemplify the regressive, chaotic, and fragmentary nature of the client's world. The private, and sometimes obscure, meaning of the client's verbalizations reflects an abandonment of conceptually based language patterns. The client's communication has a tendency to identify segments or fragments, which may be the result of an inability to separate a part

Table 37-1 Delusions

Type	Definition	Example
Ideas of reference	A person believes that certain events, situations, or interactions are directly related to himself or herself.	Dick, a 40-year-old man, telephones the police to inform them that he sees two people standing in front of his house who must be talking about him. He requests that a squad car be dispatched to stop the people from loitering in front of his house, which would interfere with their ability to talk about him.
Delusions of persecution	A person believes that he or she is being harassed, threatened, or persecuted under the influence of, or at the mercy of, some powerful force. A person may be driven to act in drastic ways by such persecutory thoughts.	Monica, a 35-year-old unemployed bookkeeper, has always led an isolated life with few friends or recreational interests. She worked for a large corporation, whose clerical staff was about to be unionized. Monica became convinced that the supervisors were harassing the employees, including her, because they had voted to become union members. She believed that she was being singled out and harassed by her supervisor who was giving her the most difficult and heaviest workload of all the bookkeepers. Monica eventually involved the company officers, her family, and childhood teachers in her delusional system, thinking that they were all involved in a conspiracy to punish her because she joined the union. She resigned from her job as a protest against the harassment she felt she was receiving. She did not keep in touch with her friends at work, nor did she return their calls. One day she was spotted by a security guard, hovering outside the building where she had worked. The guard heard her muttering something about a conspiracy as she bent to light a greasy rag with a match. She was hospitalized for attempted arson. She was discharged from the hospital 2 months later, with little change in her delusions of persecution except that she was no longer driven to act on her delusional thoughts.
Delusions of grandeur	A person attaches special significance to his or her position in relation to others or the universe. A person commonly has an exaggerated sense of self-importance that has no basis in reality, thinking either that he or she *is* an important person, either living or dead; is *related* to such a person; or is *influential* in important affairs.	Jane, a 45-year-old unmarried female, walked around carrying a bundle swaddled in a baby blanket. She said that it contained the baby Jesus and that she was his mother, Mary. She refused to put the bundle down because she thought people, envious of her special position, were trying to kidnap her baby.
Somatic delusions	A person believes that his or her body is changing or responding in an unusual way that has no basis in reality.	Joe, age 50, had had gallbladder surgery in a general hospital. Following the surgery, he began to complain to his family that he was convinced that other vital organs had also been removed at the time of the surgery. He claimed that his stomach had definitely been removed and consequently refused to eat for 2 days. Following consultation with the psychiatric liaison nurse, it was discovered that Joe had always been overweight and viewed the "removal" of his stomach as a punishment for not having listened to his physician's advice about losing weight.

or to distinguish any of the parts of a whole. This may progress to the point where a single idea, phrase, or word comes to represent a large context, so that finally the language of the client is impoverished to the point of being reduced to relatively few words or stereotyped expressions. Language can also be used to obscure the exchange of meaningful information between the client and others. This negates communication and any relatedness with another person.[2]

Some of the more common linguistic changes may be observed in the initial phase of a schizophrenic episode or at later points if regressive changes become more firmly entrenched. Examples of these linguistic changes follow.

Echolalia is the purposeless repetition of a word of phrase. The client may repeat the last few words the nurse has said each time the nurse stops talking. For example, a client may repeatedly say, "Feel about that, feel about that, feel about that."

Clang association is the repetition of words or phrases that have similar sound relationships. For example, if the nurse asks the client, "How do you feel about moving closer to Sam?" the client may respond, "Sam, Bam, Cram, Ram," leaving the nurse puzzled. Clang associations can also involve the substitution of words similar in sound to those seemingly intended.[7] For example, the client may say, "The *ghost* ate the can," instead of saying, "The *goat* ate the can."

A *neologism* is a privately coined word or group of words having meaning only for the speaker and not understood by others. For example, the client may say, "Tavotactation, negrum, flailia, spirodactylia." The client under the influence of autistic thought withdraws from using consensually validated language and develops an intensely private language that is directed toward symbolic self-expression rather than communication. Personal linguistic rules are developed that may be difficult for others to understand.

A *word salad* is a form of speech in which ordinary words or phrases are linked in a way that seems meaningless and illogical. The flow of words appears to be disconnected and without linguistic organization. For example, the client may say, "Horses can softly sugar cat. . . ."

The manner in which the client's speech is presented can also be altered. Some clients speak with altered intonation—that is, a high-pitched whine instead of their normal voice. Others may speak rapidly and incessantly, paying little attention to whether anyone is listening. Still others speak haltingly; thoughts either come slowly or are expressed with difficulty. Some clients speak so haltingly that they communicate in monosyllables. Others are completely mute.

Perceptual Changes

The term *perception* refers to the response of sensory receptors to external stimuli. Perception involves not only a response to the stimulus but also a recognition and understanding of a sensation as, say, a person, object, or thought.[2] For example, when seeing a book, people know that they see it and know that it is a book. Perception cannot be completely differentiated from cognition. The cognitive processes would have no incoming stimuli to filter, interpret, and transform into images if they did not receive sensory data. Cognitive interpretations are influenced by the emotional associations connected with perceptions. Perception involves both cognitive and emotional understanding of the perceived object.

Perceptual changes can occur in one or more of the auditory, visual, olfactory, tactile, or gustatory sensory processes. Perceptual changes can be mild and transitory or profound and long-lasting. It is not uncommon for most people to have had an experience in which they felt that a familiar object was not recognized in a familiar way. This phenomenon is often referred to as an *illusion,* which is a misperception or misinterpretation of reality. Visual and auditory illusions are much more common than tactile, gustatory, or olfactory illusions. For example, a cloud in the sky is misperceived as a flying saucer, or a linen sheet on a clothesline is momentarily misperceived as a ghost. People are usually quick to regain their reality orientation, and the transient experience fades as they identify the object in a consensually validated way, that is, in a way that is agreed upon by most people. Profound perceptual changes are most commonly seen in hallucinations and changes in body image.

Hallucinations

Hallucinations are one of the most common perceptual dysfunctions in schizophrenia and reflect a loss of reality testing. *Hallucinations* are sensory perceptions of objects, images, and sensations that occur in the absence of actual external stimuli. Visual and auditory hallucinations are the most common types. Tactile, olfactory, and gustatory hallucinations are more commonly associated with organic conditions such as brain tumors or drug and alcohol toxicity. Hallucinations also may be intertwined with illusions and delusional systems.[2] Table 37-2 defines and gives an example of each type of hallucination.

Hallucinations evolve from the dissociated components of the self-system and have an uncanny,

Table 37-2 Hallucinations

Type	Definition	Example
Auditory	Voices or sounds are heard by the client which are not heard by others and which do not relate to objective reality. The voices, which are often derogatory and berate the client, are projections of the client's unacceptable inner thoughts which are then attributed to outside forces.	A female client, experiencing anxiety and guilt about a recent abortion, heard the voice of God berating her for her sexual promiscuity and abortion.
Visual	Visual images or sensations are experienced by the client that occur in the absence of external stimuli. The client may see images of figures, objects, or events that may be grotesque, frightening, or comforting.	A male client repeatedly sees himself and his family being shot to death by a firing squad for an unknown crime. The scene flashes in front of his eyes as if it were on a movie screen.
Olfactory	Odors are smelled which appear to be emanating from specific or unknown places.	A female client who feels that she has a rotten personality complains that she smells rotten flesh and singed hair emanating from herself and people around her.
Gustatory	Tastes are experienced that have no basis in what is actually happening.	A male client, who feels that his wife is making his life miserable, develops a gustatory hallucination in which every time he eats food prepared by his wife, he experiences a peculiar bitter taste in his mouth.
Tactile	Strange body sensations are felt that may or may not be part of a delusional system. At times tactile hallucinations involve misperceptions about body parts. This type of hallucination is common in alcohol toxicity.	A female client, who has no children and has completed menopause, feels that her reproductive organs have turned to stone. They feel like heavy weights suspended in her lower body. Another client felt that bugs were crawling up his legs when in fact there was nothing there.

real quality for the person experiencing them.[8] They often meet needs that the client feels cannot be met in the real world. Needs involving self-esteem, relatedness, control, and communication are often expressed symbolically in the hallucination, which takes on dynamic significance for the client.[9] For example:

> A nurse walked over to Terry, a female client, to ask her to join a dance therapy group. The nurse noticed that Terry was sitting in her chair with her head tilted as if listening to somebody. Her lips moved constantly as if she were talking silently to herself. She had a frightened look on her face. The nurse said, "You seem to be frightened." Terry said, "It's the voices. They're telling me that I'm a whore and a pervert and that I should stab myself with my knitting needles. I'm praying to keep in touch with God, and that's the way I try to keep the devil quiet. Anytime I do something good, the devil and a whole chorus of voices chant about how bad I am." The nurse asked Terry to join the group. Terry replied, "I can't concentrate or do anything but pray. I guess I must really be as bad as they say; sometimes I feel as though I'm in hell with all of them."

The voices confirmed Terry's feelings of worthlessness, lack of control, and fear of relatedness. Feelings about herself which she was unable to acknowledge or express directly and work through were expressed by the hallucinations.

Hallucinations develop in a characteristic way. Four phases in the development of a hallucination can be identified.[10]

During the first phase, the client experiencing anxiety, stress, feelings of estrangement, and loneliness may daydream or focus on comforting thoughts to relieve the anxiety and stress. However, this provides only temporary relief if anxiety continues to escalate. The person, still retaining control over focal awareness, recognizes these thoughts as part of the self even though perceptual intensity is heightened.

During the second phase, as anxiety connected with the internal and external experience increases, the client puts himself or herself into a "listening state" for the hallucination. Inner thoughts become more accentuated. Hallucinatory images, voices, and sensations may be only vague whispers. However, the client becomes fearful that others will hear, notice, or repeat them and at this point feels ineffective in controlling these thoughts. Terror may occur as anxiety escalates; the client attempts to put distance between the self and the hallucination by projecting the experience outward as if the hallucination were coming from another person or place.

During the third phase, the hallucination becomes more prominent, authoritative, and controlling. The client becomes accustomed to it and "gives in" to it. Often the hallucination is comforting and affords the client a sense of temporary security.

During the fourth phase, the client becomes increasingly preoccupied with the hallucination and feels helpless to free himself or herself from the control it exerts. Not uncommonly, a formerly comforting hallucination becomes menacing, commanding, and berating at this point. The client, increasingly involved with the hallucinatory experience, feels unable to form meaningful relationships with real people. As anxiety continues to rise, the hallucination may become more elaborate and interwoven with a delusional system in an endless, but unsuccessful, effort to satisfy the needs it is partially serving. The client's control over focal awareness diminishes, and withdrawal from consensually validated experience ensues. The client may dwell in a terrifying world, for fleeting moments or for hours on end. This process may become chronic if intervention is not forthcoming.[10]

Changes in Body Image

Regression and the inability to test reality often include not only the loss of a sense of the world and the person's place in it, but also a perceptual distortion of body image and ego boundaries. *Body image* is a person's cognitive and affective picture of his or her own body. It is the changing presentation of the body in one's mind. In schizophrenia, attention becomes focused on the person's own body, and disruption of physical and personal identity occurs. For example:

> A female client described her experience in the following way, "I look in the mirror and it's not really me that I see. I don't have any definite image of myself, but many different ones, all horrible to me. I look like a cracked doll's face."

Ego boundaries—that is, the physical and emotional boundaries that define the person as a separate individual—are not firm enough to form an integrated self separate from the environment.[2,11]

Depersonalization is a disturbance in which there is a feeling of unreality concerning the self or the environment. It results from lack of ego boundaries. Feelings of estrangement or changes in body image are common. Clients may feel that they are machines, that they are dead, or that they are living in a dream. Activity may have a dreamlike quality. Clients may be unable to distinguish inner and outer body parts and may experience a loss of control over the body. Parts of the body may become dissociated from an integrated self-concept. Several examples of depersonalization illustrate this concept:

> "My ability to think and decide and do is torn apart by itself. Instead of my wishing to do things, they are done by something that seems mechanical and frightening ... with the longing to come back and yet without the power to return."
>
> "I feel as if my face has turned to stone. If I smile, it will crack into pieces."
>
> "I feel like an empty shell; there is a black, bottomless pit inside of me, a sea of nothingness."

Clients' ego boundaries may be so fluid that they feel fused with others or with the environment. For example:

> Leah always walked around barefoot. When she was asked if her feet were cold, she replied, "Yes, but I need to have bare feet in order to feel where I stop and the floor begins." Insisting that Leah wear shoes for the sake of cleanliness or comfort would be to demand that she maintain body boundaries which do not exist for her. Her sense of diffuseness would cause her anxiety level to escalate.

Identity confusion is often demonstrated by these clients. For example:

> One client stated, "Gradually I can no longer distinguish how much of myself is in me, and how much is already in others. I am a conglomeration, a monstrosity, modeled anew each day."

Clients with confused identity feel that they are in some way themselves, yet a part of others with no firm, separate sense of identity. They may also lose a sense of their position in space. For example:

A client stated, "When I am ill, I lose the sense of where I am. I feel 'I' can sit in the chair, and yet my body is hurtling out and somersaulting about 3 feet in front of me."

Clients whose ego boundaries are weak and whose body image is distorted may also be unable to recognize their sexual identity. They may become convinced that they look like or have some body parts of the opposite sex and see their bodies as alien, unfriendly, and unpredictable. Such problems evolve from an inability to establish a definite and stable gender identity, and from feeling sexually inadequate. A sense of sexual inadequacy can be reinforced by general feelings of inadequacy and low self-esteem: thus a vicious circle is created. Added to this is a central feeling of being unloved, unlovable, undesired, and undesirable. Persons with these feelings may become terrified about an inability to relate adequately and may become compulsively promiscuous at times in order to reassure themselves that they can be accepted as sexual partners. Active or latent homosexual behavior may also arise from this confusion and often is frightening as well as unacceptable to the person because of real or imagined rejections that may follow.[11]

As the client withdraws interest and energy from others and the environment and assumes an intense self-focus, preoccupation with bodily sensations and functions may increase. *Hypochondriasis* refers to a preoccupation with the body and complaints about a myriad of physical symptoms that have no basis in reality. For example, a client may feel that his intestines have shriveled up and may therefore refuse to eat. Other clients have a sense of impending doom and become convinced that they have cancer and that their vital organs are decaying. Hypochondriacal complaints often evolve into somatic delusions.

Affective Changes

Affect refers to a person's emotions. It includes the internal experience of feelings and the external expression of feelings. It is expressed verbally and nonverbally through the spoken word and body language. Affect is a component of thoughts and ideas. It may be experienced in relation to self, others, and the environment. All people commonly experience emotions such as happiness, sadness, fear, loneliness, and anger.

Affective changes in the schizophrenic evolve from a need to distance from the intensity of feelings that provoke anxiety if they are experienced directly. The affective changes are self-protective because they enable the client to deny the painful emotional impact of the external world.[12] In addition, as a result of cognitive and perceptual changes, in which the client alters the common symbols of thought and perception, he or she will no longer have the usual emotional responses to common life experience. Such clients will replace conventional emotional responses with other emotions that may appear bizarre and inappropriate because they are coming from a different frame of reference.[2] Among recognized affective changes are *blunted affect, flat affect, inappropriate affect, overresponsiveness,* and *ambivalence.*

Blunted affect refers to a decrease in the intensity of appropriate emotional responsiveness to a thought, person, or experience. For example:

A man related a recent experience in which his house and all contents were destroyed in a fire, with no more than mild sadness and regret.

Clients with blunt affect are sometimes described as apathetic or indifferent.

Flat affect is an affective change in which there is an absence of feeling tone. When a verbal message is communicated by the client, no feeling tone is connected to it, either in tone of voice or in body movements. Although all people experience emotional flatness at different points in their life, this behavior is exaggerated in both duration and intensity with the schizophrenic. For example:

Bob, when told that his parents had been killed in an automobile accident on the highway, neither showed nor felt shock or grief.

Inappropriate affect refers to affect that is incongruent with an idea, content of thought, or situation. The expression of emotion seems unrelated to actual experience. For example:

While describing sexual overtures made by her father when she was a young child, Debra could not stop laughing. Later that day, she became enraged when she was asked if she was ready to eat.

Overresponse refers to exhibition of emotions that appear to be an exaggeration of appropriate emotional intensity. An example follows.

John responded to the death of a distant cousin, whom he had never met, with grief so intense that his family became concerned and called the family physician.

Ambivalence refers to opposing feelings that are simultaneously experienced within the self about objects, events, situations, or relationships. These feelings produce the desire to do two opposite things at once. Ambivalent feelings are normally experienced by all people at different times. However, schizophrenics experience excessive ambivalence. It may dominate clients' lives to a point where they are unable to commit themselves to an idea, feeling, relationship, or action.

Clients may exhibit ambivalence in different ways. Some clients will express the opposing feelings verbally. For example:

Larry would express a desire to get his own apartment after being discharged from the hospital but would repeatedly tell the staff how much he needed his parents' protection and supervision.

Other clients express their ambivalence through excessive *compliance* which is characterized by a refusal to act at all unless they are told what to do and how to do it. For example:

Candy waited to get dressed each day until she was told what to wear and was given step-by-step directions on how to get dressed.

Such compliance often reflects the client's attempt to deny a commitment to a specific wish or feeling. This leaves others responsible for what happens. Consequently, conflicting feelings remain unresolved. Ambivalence can also be expressed through *negativism,* in which the client refuses to participate at all. The refusal may be expressed verbally or nonverbally. The refusal to act reflects the client's attempt to avoid confronting any opposing feelings.[2] For example:

Paul was described by the staff as very negativistic. He refused to get out of bed in the morning, get dressed, eat, or participate in ward activities. However, once he was involved in any of these activities, he would usually refuse to stop doing them.

Still other clients' ambivalence will be expressed in *constant, repetitive activity* that may be stereotyped and appear meaningless to those observing it. For example:

Freda unceasingly paced the lounge, patting the furniture and the walls as she paced. She constantly tugged at her hair and the hem of her dress. When the staff attempted to stop her, she would pause momentarily but then resume her pacing and patting.

Ambivalence may result from early communication experiences with double-bind messages and from lack of consistent, consensually validated experiences.[13] The client never learns how to synthesize feelings and identify or commit to a dominant emotional state. This protects the client from feeling positively or negatively about others and decreases the intensity of feelings like love, hate, anger, and rejection. However, the constant indecisiveness creates an internal double-bind feeling state in which the person feels caught in a no-win position.[14] For example:

Tommy, a male client, felt so ambivalent about forming a relationship with a student nurse that he alternated between waiting eagerly for her to arrive and hiding in the bathroom once she got there. Tommy was in conflict about wanting the relationship yet at the same time fearing it, but not wanting to lose it for fear of being isolated once again.

Such a conflict makes any choice difficult or impossible and leads to a feeling that no matter which choice is made, the outcome will be negative. Consequently, the client becomes caught in a way of life which makes denial of feelings seem crucial to survival.

It is important to remember that interpretations of affective behavior must be measured against cultural norms. All cultures have norms about how feelings should be expressed. These norms influence the accuracy with which interpretations are made about this behavior. Judgments about affective behavior are often influenced by a person's cultural interpretation of emotion and how much of it is appropriate in a particular situation.[1]

Motor Changes

Motor behavior is visible physical activity exhibited by the client. *Motor changes* that are observed in the schizophrenic are frequently external manifestations of the cognitive, perceptual, and affective changes occurring simultaneously. Motor changes are manifested in heightened or reduced levels of motor activity, and in impulsivity, mannerisms, automatism, and stereotypy.

Motor activity is generally *reduced* in schizophrenics. The client will walk and talk slowly, as if each step or word requires profound effort. Clients will sometimes sit, as if glued to a chair, for hours on end, without apparent boredom or discomfort. An extreme degree of inaction is illustrated by the catatonic stupor, in which the client appears immobilized. Such inaction may be explained as an attempt to avoid the responsibility of exercising conscious choices and decisions. Fearing criticism or disapproval for whichever choice or decision is made, the client, once again caught in an internal double bind, makes no decision; any movement made might be wrong. Action, connected with motivation and choice, is perceived as a path leading to negative appraisals of the self by significant others. Such clients, never having developed confidence in their own capacities for decision making, hold the real or anticipated appraisal of others as supremely important.[1,2]

However, motor activity may also be heightened. *Motor excitement* is sometimes observed in the agitated, unceasing movements of schizophrenics. Motion may also be awkward or uncoordinated. This behavior may reflect clients' escalating anxiety level. At times, clients who sense that they are sinking into a stupor because they fear to act may try to prevent this by becoming overactive and engage in a sequence of aimless acts, designed to deny concern with responsibility and decision making.[1,2] For example:

> A client, Sal, paced back and forth in the dayroom. He stopped to turn on the water fountain but never took a drink; he kicked furniture as he passed it, interrupted conversations (but never stopped to talk), and finally kicked the medication cart so that it went flying across the room.

Impulsivity is the tendency to act suddenly, without conscious thought. It is observed in the schizophrenic under different circumstances. Sometimes impulsivity occurs in a client who is agitated and engaged in motor excitement. A client whose motor excitement reflects a defiance of responsibility is likely to act without thinking in order to maintain that pattern and avoid sinking into a stupor of inaction. For example:

> Julie moved restlessly around the lounge muttering to herself. She put the television on. Another client shouted, "Turn that noise down!" Julie picked up the television and hurled it across the floor, barely missing another client.

At other times a client acts in an unpredictable way that is not apparently motivated by external events. The person is unable to exert external controls and may be verbally or physically destructive, aggressive, or violent. For example:

> Sandy was found sitting in a corner burning her arms with a lighted cigarette. When a nurse asked her to explain what was happening, she said, "The voices told me to burn myself to get rid of the badness in me."

Mannerisms are noted in speech and movement. Grimaces may be grotesque or ticlike. They often appear as disapproving gestures which may indicate that the client is censoring private thoughts. Imitative behavior may reflect the client's attempt to get close to another person by being like him or her, submerging all individual differences in the process. For example:

> Paula hovered around the nurses' station each day. She would modify her facial expression, posture, gestures, and gait so that they were like those of the nursing staff. Her explanation for this was, "If I act like them, I can be like them."

A sense of weak self-boundaries and identity is reflected in this statement. It is also an example of concrete thinking.

Automatism is seen when clients carry out requests in robotlike fashion, as if to say, "I will satisfy you. Don't bother me; don't ask me to make choices. I can respond only in a programmed way."

Stereotypy refers to the persistent, repetitive movements that are sometimes seen in schizophrenia. For example:

> As Eloise slowly walked about the inpatient unit, her arms and legs constantly moved in a wavelike pattern that began at her head and ended at her feet. She would stop if her arms and hands were restrained, but the ritualistic, stereotyped movements would begin again as soon as the restraints were removed.

Waxy flexibility is exhibited by clients who maintain a limb in a particular fixed position for an extended period of time without apparent discomfort. Many such positions have a stereotyped quality to them.

Social Changes

The self is created by the matrix of social relationships that people maintain with significant others in their lives and the reflected appraisals that are an integral part of such relationships. If these relationships are unhealthy and create an excessive amount of anxiety, the socialization process will be disrupted; the person will experience an internal spiritual emptiness. Consequently, relatedness in adult life and during schizophrenic episodes may be fraught with actual or anticipated unpleasantness and anxiety.[15]

Cameron[16] states that people with socially inadequate development fail to learn and to maintain communication with others. They have a tendency to separate themselves from others and engage in their own private thinking, which does not require conformity to the thinking of others. Social changes occur as the client substitutes personal, highly individual habits for consensually validated communication patterns. Social relatedness becomes difficult to achieve.

Silvano Arieti[2] also suggests that social changes occur in schizophrenics because they relinquish common ways of experiencing the world and rely on their own individualistic modes. Clients retain an intellectual understanding of social experience, but it loses its emotional meaning. Their world, instead, is governed by private, autistic thought processes. As psychosis develops, there is also a tendency to discard social attitudes and roles that were incorporated from others as parts of the self. For example, the critical, nagging attitude of a parent may be incorporated as a critical, condemning attitude toward the self. When the person becomes psychotic, this attitude may be projected onto others who become the condemning persecutors.

The pain associated with relatedness coupled with the retreat into a world of private symbols creates social changes in which the client may experience loneliness, social isolation, relatedness characterized by superficiality, the "need-fear" dilemma, and dependency.

Loneliness

Loneliness as experienced by the schizophrenic is not simply a feeling of aloneness. It includes a sense of isolation and estrangement, an utter sense of emptiness, barrenness, and desperation that makes the client feel totally apart from others and, at times, spiritually barren. Many clients describe the experience of loneliness as a wide chasm, separating them from others, which they cannot bridge, regardless of their attempts to do so. The person may feel lonely and isolated amid a group of people. Loneliness is not a chosen position but one to which the client feels involuntarily committed.[17,18,19] A client may want to be involved in relationships, but when one is offered, be unable to participate because relatedness is perceived as so threatening. Thus, such clients are condemned to their lonely state.

Loneliness evolves from early life experiences in which remoteness, indifference, or emptiness was the major theme that characterized the child's relationships with others.[18] These early experiences influenced the child's feelings of isolation in the world and sense of failure to establish meaningful relationships. Feelings of isolation and lack of meaningful relationships follow the person into adult life and nourish the development of loneliness.

In order to protect themselves from loneliness, clients may:

Develop a rich fantasy life in which they spend a great deal of time daydreaming about imaginary situations.

Engage in intellectual pursuits that eliminate the need for emotional relatedness.

Utilize the coping mechanism of intellectualization which explains experience in a cognitive, but not an emotional, way.

Worship others from afar.

Develop somatic symptoms in an attempt to gain attention and caring from others.

Engage in violent behavior which represents a dysfunctional attempt to connect with people.

Retreat to a private, autistic world of hallucinations and delusions which blame others for the client's loneliness and inability to form relationships.

Totally withdraw from relatedness into a state of psychogenic death which removes the person from intense feelings of anxiety and loneliness.

Social Isolation

Social isolation occurs when the schizophrenic withdraws physically or emotionally from relatedness with others. The degree of withdrawal can range from intense shyness to complete reclusiveness. The extent to which clients isolate themselves will depend on the degree of pain and anxiety that is associated with relatedness and the degree to which they have cognitively retreated into a private, autistic world and discarded the common conventions of society.[2]

Superficial Relationships

Mistrust of relatedness is a core problem in schizophrenia. Previous painful relationships have sensitized the client, who will perceive people in current relationships as inauthentic, unreliable, and dangerous. The client feels vulnerable when in the company of others, who are experienced as controlling, threatening, and abandoning; the client chooses to remain isolated rather than risk the pain of relatedness once again. Some clients may maintain a protective shell by not relating to others at all except when necessary. Others maintain a protective barrier by engaging in transitory, superficial relationships that contain a minimum of threat.

"Need-Fear" Dilemma

Many clients, regardless of their degree of social isolation, experience the "need-fear" dilemma. Burnham[20] describes this situation as one in which the client struggles between overwhelming fears about the inherent threat of relatedness and an insatiable need for relatedness. On one hand, these clients, because they are poorly differentiated and integrated, have an incredibly strong need for external structure and control and require others to provide the organization and regulation that they are unable to provide for themselves. Clients may perceive that their psychological existence depends on maintaining contact with others and may also yearn for the comfort of relatedness. On the other hand, the clients' great need for other people means danger because others can destroy the clients through abandonment. Such a client may attempt to deal with the anxiety surrounding the dilemma by:

1. Overtly denying the need for others, remaining distant and withdrawn.
2. Utilizing approach-avoidance behavior, which is a combination of cautious involvement and then distance when relatedness becomes too intimate or threatening.

For example:

> Tom spent 2 weeks physically distancing from Laurie, the student nurse, each time she approached him to spend time with him. However, he maintained eye contact with her as he paced the dayroom, moving close to the area in which she was sitting and saving a chair for him. Another client approached Laurie and sat down without asking if he could. Before she had a chance to ask him to leave, Tom approached and said, "Don't talk to her. . . . Do you know *what* you're talking to?" The other client replied, "Yes, I know *who* I'm talking to." Tom said, "It's not human; it's dangerous." The other client got up and left. Tom sat down in the chair Laurie had been saving for him, but moved his chair about 4 feet away, saying, "Robot, you'd better not come tomorrow, because if you do I won't be here. Just don't come."

On one hand, Tom did not want to share Laurie's attention, the "need" part of the situation, even though he had formerly given no indication of his desire to interact with her. On the other hand, frightened of committing himself to his need for relatedness with her (the "fear" part of the situation), he physically distanced from her once again and told her not to return the next day. This might have been a way of protecting himself from possible hurt by strengthening his "I don't care" posture.

Other clients, needing the nurse but fearful of eventual separation and loss, may also abruptly terminate a relationship, especially as predictable separation times approach, such as vacations and job changes. These clients defend against potential feelings of abandonment by controlling termination and in this way protecting an already fragile ego from further assault. Acting as their own worst enemy, they take refuge in their isolation.

Dependency

Dependency involves excessive reliance on others to meet physical or emotional needs. This behavior pattern occurs because the ego strength of schizophrenics is very fragile, largely because they have never differentiated from the family ego mass and developed self-confidence about personal capabilities or a separate identity.[21] These clients, feeling inadequate and incapable of self-direction, often manipulate others into providing the kind of direction they feel unable to provide for themselves. The requests may become demands that seem never to end. The nurse must be wary of reinforcing dependency patterns that inhibit clients' movement toward self-direction.

DSM III

The term *schizophrenia* encompasses a group of disorders which may or may not have a common etiology.[22,23] These disorders have certain characteristic features. Table 37-3 summarizes general diagnostic criteria for a schizophrenic disorder in the *Diagnostic and Statistical Manual of Mental Disorders* (DSM III). In DSM III, there are also several types of clinical entities that belong to this

Table 37-3 Diagnosis of Schizophrenic Disorders

Criteria in DSM III	Criteria in DSM III
A. At least one of the following occurs during a phase of illness: 1. Bizarre delusions, such as belief that one is being controlled, thought broadcasting, thought insertion, or thought withdrawal 2. Somatic, grandiose, religious, nihilistic, or other delusions without persecutory or jealous content 3. Delusions with persecutory or jealous content if accompanied by hallucinations of any type 4. Auditory hallucinations in which either a voice keeps up a running commentary on the person's behavior or thoughts, or two or more voices converse with each other 5. Auditory hallucinations on several occasions with content of more than one or two words, having no apparent relation to depression or elation 6. Incoherence, marked loosening of associations, marked lack of logic a. Blunted, flat, or inappropriate affect b. Delusions or hallucinations c. Catatonic or other grossly disorganized behavior B. The client has deteriorated from a previous level of functioning in such areas as work, social relations, and self-care. C. There are continuous signs of illness for at least 6 months at some time during a person's life, with some signs of illness at present. The 6-month period must include an active phase during which there were symptoms from item A, with or without a prodromal or residual phase. The phases of schizophrenia are listed below. 1. *Prodromal phase:* A clear deterioration in functioning which occurs before the active phase of the illness and is not due to a disturbance in mood or a substance use disorder, and which involves at least two of the symptoms noted below. 2. *Residual phase:* Persistence, following the active phase of the illness, of at least two of the symptoms noted below, not due to a disturbance in mood or to a substance use disorder.	C. 3. *Prodromal or residual symptoms:* a. Social isolation or withdrawal b. Marked impairment in role functioning as wage earner, student, or homemaker c. Markedly peculiar behavior (such as collecting garbage, talking to self in public, or hoarding food) d. Marked impairment in personal hygiene and grooming e. Blunted, flat, or inappropriate affect f. Digressive, vague, overelaborate, circumstantial, or metaphorical speech g. Odd or bizarre ideation, or magical thinking, such as superstitiousness; possession of clairvoyance, telepathy, or a "sixth sense"; belief that "Others can feel my feelings"; overvalued ideas; ideas of reference h. Unusual perceptual experiences, such as recurrent illusions, sensing the presence of a force or person not actually present 4. *Examples:* Six months of prodromal symptoms with 1 week of symptoms from A; no prodromal symptoms with 6 months of symptoms from A; no prodromal symptoms with 2 weeks of symptoms from A and 6 months of residual symptoms; 6 months of symptoms from A, apparently followed by several years of complete remission, with 1 week of symptoms in A in current episode. D. The full depressive or manic syndrome (criteria A and B of major depressive or manic episode), if present, developed after any psychotic symptoms, or was brief in duration relative to the duration of the psychotic symptoms in A. E. Onset of the prodromal or active phase of the illness occurred before age 45. F. The illness is not an organic mental disorder or mental retardation.

Table 37-4 Major Clinical Syndromes Associated with Schizophrenia

Type	Characteristics
Disorganized schizophrenia (hebephrenia)	Marked incoherence and flat, incongruous, or silly affect. Delusions and hallucinations, if present, are fragmented and not well organized. Other features include extreme social withdrawal, unpredictable laughter, grimaces, mannerisms, hypochondriacal complaints, and regressive behavior. Social impairment is profound, onset tends to occur at a young age, and a chronic course without significant remission is common.
Catatonic schizophrenia	Psychomotor disturbances. Catatonia is manifested by periods of stupor or excitement, or rapidly alternating periods of both behaviors. Catatonic stupor is associated with generalized inhibition characterized by rigidity, mutism, negativity, waxy flexibility, and posturing. Catatonic excitement is associated with excessive, sometimes violent, motor activity and agitation that appears to be purposeless and not influenced by external stimuli.
Paranoid schizophrenia	Onset tends to occur later in life; features are more stable over a period of time. This type of schizophrenia is associated with persecutory or grandiose delusions, or hallucinations with a persecutory or gandiose content. The coping mechanism most frequently used is projection, which attributes to others characteristics the person cannot accept within the self. Suspiciousness, argumentativeness, jealousy, mistrust of others, and excessive religiosity are frequently observed. The person may display doubts about gender identity or fears of being thought of as a homosexual or of being approached by homosexuals.
Undifferentiated schizophrenia	Includes those diagnostic groups which display mixed characteristics that are not classifiable in any of the more clearly defined diagnostic categories or that meet the criteria of more than one category.
Residual schizophrenia	Included in this type of schizophrenia are those individuals who have had at least one episode, who are currently without overt psychotic features, but for whom other signs of the syndrome still persist. They may display social withdrawal and eccentric behavior, emotional flatness, illogical thinking, and looseness of associations. However, these features do not fully interfere with their ability to function.

group of disorders. A diagnostic label and clinical features are associated with each type. Table 37-4 summarizes the major types of clinical syndromes associated with schizophrenia.

Other diagnostic categories formerly classified under *schizophrenia,* such as *schizoaffective disorder, simple schizophrenia,* and *acute schizophrenic episode,* are now categorized under other diagnostic groups. Schizophrenia is organized not only according to subjective and objective symptoms, but also according to the course of the syndrome. A diagnostic label of *schizophrenia* is not valid unless the syndrome has existed for 6 months or more. Consequently, the terms *subchronic, chronic, subchronic with acute exacerbation,* and *in remission* are used to describe the course of the syndrome. Table 37-5 provides definitions of these terms. It should be noted that this axis of the diagnostic criteria is controversial in that it implies that the condition can never be changed, that a person who was once diagnosed as *schizophrenic* must always retain the label. As such, it has been attacked as a misuse of language.[24]

Table 37-5 Terms That Describe the Course of Schizophrenia

Term	Definition
Subchronic	The time period beginning with the first symptoms of the syndrome, which have been displayed more or less continuously, is less than 2 years but at least 6 months.
Chronic	Symptoms have been present for at least longer than 2 years.
Subchronic with acute exacerbation	Prominent psychotic symptoms reemerge in a person who has followed a subchronic course and has been in the residual phase.
Chronic with acute exacerbation	Prominent psychotic symptoms reemerge in a person with a chronic course who has been in the residual phase.
In remission	A person with a history of schizophrenia is currently free of all signs of the syndrome whether or not he or she is on medication.

SOURCE: American Psychiatric Association, *Diagnostic and Statistical Manual of Mental Disorders,* 3d ed., APA, Washington, D.C., 1980.

Epidemiology

Despite many advances in knowledge of schizophrenia, there is still considerable difficulty in developing valid and reliable estimates of the incidence and prevalence rates of the disorder according to age, sex, race, and other demographic factors. The basic problem is the absence of sensitive and specific diagnostic criteria, uniformly applied within and among countries, for the behaviors involved with schizophrenia.[25] For example, Cooper et al.[26] report that in Britain and the United States different criteria were used in formulating a diagnosis. Currently, the major criterion used to diagnose schizophrenic disorders is DSM III. However, Bleuler's[27] description of primary and secondary behaviors and Schneider's[28] first- and second-rank symptoms provide other descriptive systems for formulating a diagnosis. The International Pilot Study of Schizophrenia (IPSS) was initiated by the World Health Organization (WHO).[29,30] It represents an effort to establish transcultural, standardized diagnostic criteria for epidemiological use in all nine countries participating in the study; these criteria are to have as high a degree of reliability and validity as possible. This study represents a major advance in the epidemiological study of not only schizophrenia but mental illness as a whole.

Another epidemiological problem relates to the fact that statistics rarely reflect an accurate assessment of the incidence rates in the population.[1] Statistics are based on the number of reported cases, not on the total number of actual cases. Many cases, it is suggested, are not diagnosed, not reported, or both, because they never become consumers of public mental health services, may not be receiving any mental health services, or receive services from the private sector, which largely go unreported. Thus the apparent incidence rate is lowered. Moreover, this discrepancy between actual and reported incidence rates reflects the influence of cultural factors, socioeconomic factors, and proximity to treatment facilities and may result in over- and underreporting from certain segments of the population. For example, minority groups and the lower socioeconomic groups tend to utilize public mental health facilities and therefore are more likely to be included in statistical reports.[31] Consequently, statistics may report a higher incidence of schizophrenia among the lower classes. However, it remains unclear whether this is an accurate picture or whether it merely reflects underreporting of similar diagnoses in other classes who do not utilize public mental health facilities to the same extent. The statistical reports concerning incidence are, therefore, somewhat variable and should be examined critically. Incidence statistics range from 0.3 to 1.20 cases per 1000 population.

If a higher incidence of schizophrenia among the lower socioeconomic classes is not simply a bias of a statistical sampling, then two explanations for this phenomenon are possible. (1) According to the "breeder hypothesis," poverty contributes to the development of mental illness. (2) According to the "drift hypothesis," preschizophrenics and schizophrenics follow a path of downward mobility as a result of their marginal functioning and disability and end up clustering in the lower social classes, irrespective of where they began, creating the illusion that a preponderance of such people originate from these social strata.[32] Others have found that living in a community of an ethnic or cultural composition different from one's own increases vulnerability to schizophrenia.[33] If this is true, the stress generated by culture conflict may be a contributing factor.

Babigian[34] finds that the highest vulnerability for onset occurs between the ages of 15 and 35. Age of onset differs for men and women. The average age of onset for men is 15 to 24, for women between 25 and 34.[35] The prevalence rates of schizophrenia are higher than the incidence rates because of the frequent pattern of remission and exacerbation. The approximate figure for the prevalence rate is 2 per 1000 population.[36]

PATTERNS OF INTERACTION: PERSON

Numerous theories have been formulated to explain the development of schizophrenia. Whether schizophrenia represents a single clinical syndrome or whether each clinical subtype represents a distinct and different syndrome remains unclear. At this time, theory and research support the assumption that a variety of forces—biological, social, and psychological—combine to form an interactional matrix that contributes to the development of schizophrenia.[31] While clinical and laboratory studies abound, those presented in this section represent a cross section of the most current and well-known theories and research in schizophrenia.

Biological Theories

Biological theories postulate that schizophrenia is caused by organic dysfunction. This explanation describes a cause-and-effect relationship between a specific biological factor and the development of schizophrenia. The process and outcome of the syndrome depend on finding the cause and correcting the dysfunction. However, a human being is so complex that it is difficult to identify and isolate the single factor, much less correct its dysfunction. Today, genetic and biochemical studies are the major focus of biological research. However, brain structure and brain hemisphere functioning are also being examined.

Genetic Theory

Genetic studies have attempted to clarify the role of heredity in the development of schizophrenia. Early research testing of this question evolved from observations concerning the tendency of schizophrenia to occur in family clusters. Current research indicates that genetic potential for the syndrome is possible. Genetic factors have been explored primarily through twin studies and family studies.

Twin studies identify how often the twin of an identified client is also schizophrenic. These figures are then compared with the prevalence rate of schizophrenia in the population as a whole. Concordance rates—that is, rates of occurrence of similar traits in twins—vary widely. Consequently, it is difficult to make generalizations from these studies. However, numerous twin studies show similar significant trends. The proband concordance rate for monozygotic twins is 3 to 6 times higher than for dizygotic twins.[37,38,39] Concordance rates for dizygotic twins are the same as for other nontwin siblings.

Family studies have also been designed to explore the genetic basis of schizophrenia. Studies of adopted children reared apart from twin and nontwin siblings as well as from the biological family of origin provided the data for family studies.[39,40] The findings indicate several distinct trends. (1) The biological families of adopted children who develop schizophrenia have a higher rate of schizophrenia than the biological families of adopted children who do not develop schizophrenia. (2) Adopted children whose biological parents are schizophrenic are at greater risk of developing schizophrenia, and other problems, than adopted children from nonschizophrenic biological parents.[40] (3) Children of schizophrenic parents are at greater risk of developing schizophrenia than the general population.[41,42]

At this time, genetic studies have not identified the precise nature of the genes involved in the transmission of schizophrenia. Since the concordance rate for schizophrenia is below 100 percent, it seems clear that other factors besides heredity play an essential part in the transmission and development of schizophrenia.

Biochemical Theory

The biochemical processes associated with schizophrenia are not clearly understood. Numerous research efforts are being directed toward discovering a biochemical disorder associated with at least some of the schizophrenic disorders. The findings of such research studies tend to be confusing because various studies frequently contradict each other.

A number of biochemical factors that rely on the neurotransmission process have been identified with the development of schizophrenia. One of the most promising theories speculates about possible biochemical dysfunction of the synaptic receptor or transmitter sites. Imbalances of such chemicals as serotonin, noradrenaline, and dopamine have been associated with schizophrenia. This hypothesis is elaborated on in research studies which find that schizophrenia is associated with overactivity in certain dopamine or norepinephrine tracts of the brain.[43,44] It has also been established that neuroleptic drugs perform their antipsychotic action by blocking dopamine receptors.[45] The presence and effect of enkephalin and neurotensin, which act in the limbic system as neurotransmitters that regulate emotions, are also now being studied.[45]

Another biochemical perspective focuses on the study of monoamine oxidase (MAO) activity.[46] MAO is an enzyme essential to the production of biogenic amines. MAO activity is largely genetically determined, but it is influenced by factors such as diet, certain drugs (especially some antidepressants), hormonal activity, and age. Research has focused on measuring MAO activity in platelets, and the past findings have generally been that MAO activity was lower in people diagnosed as having chronic schizophrenia. People diagnosed as having acute schizophrenia show little, if any, variation from normal MOA activity. However, recent studies have yielded evidence of contradictory findings.

Biochemical studies are thus far from conclusive about a specific biochemical basis for schizophrenia. However, as scientists continue to study both normal and abnormal brain processes, they hope to learn more about the biochemical basis of schizophrenia.

Brain Structure

In recent years use of the computed tomography (CAT) scan has demonstrated ventricular enlargement in schizophrenics, particularly third and fourth ventricular enlargement in chronic schizophrenics, as well as widening of the sylvan fissure. Disturbance in the flow of cerebrospinal fluid contributing to ventricular enlargement has been largely ruled out, as has the presence of hydrocephalus. While this finding appears to be characteristic of the ventricular pattern of many schizophrenics, particularly chronic schizophrenics, there is as yet no general or specific understanding about why this occurs.[47]

Brain Hemisphere Functioning

The prominence of cognitive and language dysfunction in schizophrenia suggests the possibility of abnormalities in brain hemisphere functioning, especially in the left brain hemisphere, which deals with language and analytic processes. Tests for eye dominance, right- or left-handedness, and lateral eye movements are associated with hemispheric dominance and are utilized to assess dysfunction in this area. Although the findings of some studies support the theory of specific left-hemisphere dysfunction in schizophrenia, many others support marked to severe bilateral hemispheric dysfunction.[39,48] The unilateral or diffuse bilateral impairment in cognitive functioning suggests an organic basis for the thought disorder that is seen in schizophrenia. However, further research will have to clarify the nature of that relationship.

Psychosocial Theories

Psychosocial theories relevant to the development of schizophrenia are interpersonal, psychoanalytic, cognitive, and communication theories. No psychosocial theory has yet been developed to provide a definitive explanation of schizophrenia. However, students should be aware of the major psychosocial theoretical formulations.

Interpersonal Theory

Interpersonal theorists propose that the schizophrenic process begins during infancy. Inadequacies and impairment in the parent-child relationship set the stage for behavioral problems in later life.

According to Sullivan, a child's self-concept develops from the appraisals of significant others. Children internalize the appraisals of others into a coordinated image that can be described as "good me," "bad me," or "not me."[15]

The "good me" develops from satisfying and rewarding experiences with a tender, nurturing care giver, usually the mother or a substitute for the mother. Through a positive care-giving experience with this person, the child begins to view others as well as the self in a positive way.

The "bad me" evolves from the repeated anxiety communicated empathically to the child by the care-giving figure, which may or may not be directly related to the child. The relationship is often fraught with tension, ambivalence, and distancing behavior. Children of such mothers develop a picture of others as bad and a picture of themselves as bad.

If anxiety in the parent-child relationship repeatedly becomes intense and is accompanied by conflicting and confusing messages, the child will lack a feeling of consistency and continuity in relationships with significant others. If this occurs before the chid is able to clearly evaluate the meaning of these experiences, the child may be unable to formulate an accurate picture of self or others and instead develop a "not me" self-concept. This consists of a confusing, distorted array of perceptions about the self, others, and the world. The result is that the child may not develop a sense of trust in self or others. The child may feel inadequate, unlovable, and unloved. He or she may have difficulty relating to others in a trusting way, anticipating criticism, hostility, and rejection from all relationships. The child may also distort reality, events, situations, and interactions, because anxiety is an ever-present force.

Sullivan states that all children have opportunities at later stages of their life to modify and strengthen their self-concepts. Fathers, relatives, teachers, friends, and family friends may act as modifying influences that communicate positive appraisals to a youngster whose self-concept is negative or confused. However, often these opportunities go unused or are not sufficient to create a dramatic change in a self-concept that has been damaged in early life. Consequently, these people continue to have interpersonal difficulties throughout their lives.

Adolescence appears to bring many anxiety-provoking experiences to the foreground. It is normally a period of turmoil for young people. However, for the young person with a shaky identity, the demands to develop a firm sense of personal and sexual identity, engage in intimate relationships, and assume increasing responsibility and independence may be overwhelming. This may lead to extreme anxiety and feelings of inadequacy and loneliness. The adolescent is caught between the desire to become a separate person capable of establishing other relationships and fears of being unable to succeed as an independent person and of losing the limited relatedness that he or she currently has. This often happens as the adolescent or young adult moves out of the safety of the home into an independent lifestyle such as school, career, marriage, or parenthood. The coping mechanisms which were adequate for living in a protective home environment become inadequate. The person may be faced with a situation requiring intimate relatedness or academic and work performance, demands which are overwhelming to someone whose ego, self-esteem, and identity are weak. Such demands may create intolerable conflict with which the person is unable to cope.

A schizophrenic episode may be precipitated when dissociated portions of the self system that are threatening, unacceptable parts of the self come into awareness and generate overwhelming anxiety which the person's coping mechanisms are unable to manage effectively. The person develops a pattern of self-protective behaviors, based on a distorted view of reality, that represent an effort to deal with this experience, with which he or she is otherwise unable to cope. The retreat into psychosis, however profound and disorganizing, provides a degree of relief, comfort, and security.

Psychoanalytic Theory

Psychoanalytic theorists state that schizophrenic behavior occurs when the ego can no longer withstand pressure arising from the id and from external reality. The ego of the schizophrenic is fragile and has a limited ability to cope with internal and external stress because of profound disturbances in the symbiotic mother-child relationship. Disturbances in this relationship result either in premature termination of the symbiotic relationship, which leads to feelings of anxiety, rejection, and abandonment, or prolongation of the symbiotic relationship, which leads to lack of separation and individuation. In either case ego development is severely inhibited.[49]

Experiences that threaten a person's self-esteem or security or that generate guilt or an upsurge of erotic or hostile impulses are likely to create stress and increase anxiety.[16] The first response to high levels of anxiety and stress is to utilize ego defense mechanisms in dysfunctional ways in an effort to control unacceptable impulses and thoughts. For example, the person who develops delusions of grandeur dysfunctionally utilizes the defense mechanism of identification when he or she takes on the identity of a powerful figure such as God. A great deal of psychic energy is invested in maintaining repression. Consequently, there is little left over to invest in the conduct of daily living. The person withdraws from the activities of daily living and begins neglecting basic human needs such as nutrition, rest, and grooming. If stress continues and the anxiety level continues to escalate, ego functioning may deteriorate further. When anxiety reaches severe and panic levels, the person has trouble maintaining repression. Unacceptable, frightening, and primitive thoughts and impulses may flood conscious awareness. The person will have difficulty differentiating self from environment as ego identity disintegrates. Communication becomes confused and highly symbolic. The person's capacity for relatedness with others is minimal.

Information-Processing Theory

Research studies focusing on the attentional deficits in schizophrenia suggest an impairment in the cognitive-perceptual filtering mechanism. People can usually focus their attention on several relevant aspects of the environment and are able to filter out extraneous stimuli. Impairment of the cognitive-perceptual filtering mechanism may lead to the person's being bombarded with stimuli that become overwhelming and lead to massive sensory overload and distortion. Attentional problems revolve around selection of focus, maintenance of focus, and shift of focus. Clients often do not know how and to which stimuli they should respond. Impairment in the ability to discriminate and respond selectively to stimuli decreases the clients' ability to anticipate and respond appropriately to the most relevant stimuli in the perceptual field.[50,51,52] This is illustrated in the following passage from McGhie and Chapman:[53]

> Everything seems to grip my attention, although I am not particularly interested in anything. I am speaking to you just now but I can hear noises going on next door and in the corridor. I find it difficult to shut them out and it makes it difficult to concentrate on what I am saying to you.

Communication Theory

Bateson and others[14] identified the double-bind communication pattern that has been linked to the development of schizophrenia. The concept of the double-bind message is based on the premise that considerable ambivalence is present in family relationships. The components of the double-bind message are as follows:

1. Two or more people are involved in an interaction.
2. Two conflicting messages are communicated. The first message is communicated on one level. The second message, which is expressed on a nonverbal, metacommunicative level, contradicts the first message. It is unclear which message is to be obeyed.
3. However, there is an injunction against noticing that the double message exists. As a result, the person is unable to confront the inconsistency to determine which is the real message. The person may feel paralyzed about selecting a course of action and feel that there is no escape from the situation.
4. This pattern is repetitive and becomes the predominant communication pattern in the family or between two people in a particular relationship.

Double-bind communication commonly centers on messages that convey love, hate, anger, disapproval, rejection, or abandonment. For example:

> A mother, smiling, says to her little boy, "Johnny, I love you." Johnny moves toward her and when he reaches out to hug and kiss her, she frowns and moves away from him saying, "How could Mommy love a little boy with such dirty hands?" Johnny, feeling confused, moves away from his mother. As Johnny moves away, she says, "See, you never show me how much you love me. You are an unloving little boy."

Johnny now feels paralyzed—totally confused about which action he should take. He may resolve the confusion by trying to figure out which message is really intended; responding to one message, ignoring the other, and taking the risk of being wrong; or not responding to either message and withdrawing from the situation. The child does not confront the inconsistency of the situation, because the injunction prohibits awareness of the double bind. If this type of communication becomes a pattern, the person may develop a sense of insecurity and confusion which inhibits the ability to relate trustingly to others. Such people may become mistrustful about incoming messages, fearing that they are threatening, rejecting, and impossible to respond to in a satisfactory way. The behavior related to the need-fear dilemma becomes easier to understand in light of double-bind communication.

To some extent, all people send and receive double-bind messages. They are not sent intentionally; and most people, when confronted about such messages, tend to respond defensively. This pattern is not restricted to the mother-child dyad; it appears to reflect a communication pattern of the total family system. For example:

> A father bought his daughter a sheer blouse and then called her a slut for allowing him to buy her such a blouse. The mother, who was present at the time, said nothing. However, she was equally responsible for the double bind because she did nothing about the ambiguous and contradictory communication.

People who develop schizophrenia may come to perceive everyone in their environment as capable of putting them in a double bind. They may eventually choose to pull further and further away from people, withdrawing into a private, autistic world where they feel "safe" from the pain and anxiety that are experienced in relatedness with others.

PATTERNS OF INTERACTION: FAMILY

Bowen[21] explains schizophrenia as a systems phenomenon in which all family members participate. The family is viewed as a single organism, and the schizophrenic member is seen as that part of the family organism through which the overt symptoms of the family's dysfunction are expressed.

The development of schizophrenia in a family member is based on a dysfunctional parent-child relationship which evolves out of low levels of differentiation (see Chapter 19). The child becomes a stabilizing force in a marital relationship that is characterized by emotional distance, conflict, and reciprocal overfunctioning and underfunctioning of the parents. Emotional overinvestment in a particular child enables one parent to feel needed and important by caring for a child more helpless than the parent. The parent who assumes this role is usually the mother. Through her relationship with the child she is able to stabilize her own immaturity and anxiety and function on a less anxious level. When the wife's anxiety is more stabilized, the husband is also less anxious. Their relationship, in general, becomes calmer and more distant. She has a child to overinvest in; he is able to move to a more distant, uninvolved position. The child is, in this case, a cornerstone for the maintenance of calmness in their relationship.

The process becomes one of parental *overattachment* in a particular child which remains unresolved. The overinvolved parent and child *fuse* together in a pattern of intense relatedness. It is not uncommon for the parent and child to say that they can know what the other is thinking or feeling. They sometimes even dream the same dreams. The survival of the relationship is based on the child's ongoing helpless position. The overinvolved parent denies his or her own feelings of helplessness and desire to be babied and instead perceives the child as helpless and wishing to be nurtured. The rest of the family participates in this process by accepting these perceptions as real, not opposing them, and consenting to remain on the periphery of the relationship between the overclose parent and the child. The child responds by complying with the parent's expectation and offering little or no resistance to the demands. Therefore, the child can be viewed as a participant and not a victim.

When the child commits to overcloseness with one parent, the capacity to develop a separate sense of self is lost. The balance of their relationship is threatened when either person changes or when someone else in the system takes a different position. The child is often caught in a double-bind communication pattern in which two levels of messages are received. The verbal-level message may say, "Be mature." The action-emotion-level message says, "Stay helpless." For example:

> The mother of a 23-year-old male schizophrenic had just finished talking to the nurse-therapist about how she hoped her son would get well, find a job, and become independent. Five minutes later she was observed helping her son eat lunch. She cut his meat, buttered his bread, and poured his milk, and then sat down to encourage him to eat.

The ambivalence exhibited in this example makes it difficult to know which message is intended. Many times the action-emotion message represents the real message. Consequently, the child, responding to the real message, remains in a helpless, infantile position.

As the child grows up, periods of change present the greatest threat to the stability of the relationship. To grow and develop a differentiated self means that the relationship may be lost. To comply and remain overattached means that the relationship will continue, but at the expense of personhood. If the pattern of overattachment continues long enough, the child, by this time an adolescent, will usually be poorly equipped to function independently. If the child, acting on the verbal message, "Grow up," makes trips into the world alone, he or she may find it difficult to function effectively in school, in relationships, or in work. The inability to function effectively will reconfirm the notion, "I can't function without my parent to guide me." The anxiety that accompanies this feeling may be sufficient to draw the child back into the intense parent-child relationship. Schizophrenia represents the unsuccessful attempt to deal with the demands of adult functioning. The feeling of helplessness is acted out in the psychosis. Bowen[21] states that improvement in the schizophrenic family member will not occur in a lasting way unless the relationship patterns in the marriage and between both parents and the child are explored and changed.

PATTERNS OF INTERACTION: ENVIRONMENT

Schizophrenia has been described as a cultural creation of modern western civilization, since it was first defined in a western cultural context. There are those who criticize the very concept of schizophrenia. For example, Kubie[54] finds that there are no distinctive features about schizophrenia that allow the syndrome to be described as a distinct entity. A more radical critique is provided by others, among them Foucault and Szasz, who find that the concept of madness, with which schizophrenia is very much intertwined, is a culturally produced definition which is not universally valid or defined as a medical disease.[55,56] Szasz supports the position that psychiatric diagnoses are stigmatizing labels, that one is ill only if one feels ill; he believes that people should not be labeled and treated as ill simply because they demonstrate behavior that has traditionally and culturally been labeled ill. Szasz takes a position that the psychoses, and schizophrenia in particular, were originally conceptualized as "illnesses" by physicians who continue to support this definition because they have a vested interest in protecting and preserving their professional bailiwick. He views emotional problems instead as a study of personal conduct.[56] Like Szasz, Laing[57] states that schizophrenia is not a disease but is defined in that way by the culture. Neither Laing nor Szasz contends that the behavior labeled *psychosis* does not exist. They simply take the position that this behavior is not a disease. Both Szasz and Laing have wide followings among those who agree that psychiatric diagnoses are cultural artifacts. However, their theories are far from being universally accepted. The important point to remember is that they raise questions and provide insights that deserve serious consideration.

Social definitions are a function of the norms and values of the particular culture and reflect the behavior that the family, tribe, or community will accept. It is important to know what the culture or subculture defines and accepts as *normal* and what it defines and labels as *deviant.* For example, what Americans describe as *catatonic rigidity* is regarded by the Eskimos as an effect of the spirits.[58] As long as a person adheres to the standards and norms of the social group, he or she is accepted as normal. Social groups have different norms and standards. Standards also change, as the recent experience of American society demonstrates. For example, dual-career families were at one time accepted only as economic necessity dictated. Today, dual careers and dual parenting are becoming cultural norms and acceptable, irrespective of economic need.

Certain behaviors that are already very prevalent in a culture are often considered normal for that ethnic community. For example, hyperactivity is not considered very deviant in Portuguese cultures, but this same behavior is considered a manifestation of psychosis in Filipino cultures.[33] Because norms and standards vary from culture to culture, they may have to be interpreted differently by observers from outside the culture.

Cultural and social experience may also shape the expression of the psychosis. For example, in an epidemiological study comparing cultural expressions of psychosis, it was found that Japanese subjects demonstrated a high degree of suspiciousness and paranoid ideation as opposed to Hawaiian-Caucasian subjects, who exhibited a high degree of helplessness. The authors hypothesized that this was reflective of dominant cultural themes such as the importance of trust and control over emotions to the Japanese and of independence and productivity to the Caucasians.[33]

NURSING PROCESS

Assessment

Nurses encounter schizophrenic clients and their families in a variety of settings. An acutely disturbed client may be admitted to a short-term acute-care inpatient setting or a long-term residential setting. The client may receive further treatment in a halfway house, day treatment center, community rehabilitation program, or outpatient clinic, or in the home. The nature of the assessment process will vary according to the setting, the goals of the particular facility or agency, and the condition of the client on admission.

Assessment of acutely disturbed clients in an inpatient unit takes place on admission. The nurse is often the person to admit a client to the unit and then complete the initial assessment. Other members of the mental health team, according to their particular areas of expertise, also contribute to the assessment. The ability to gather data may be limited by the client's suspiciousness, confusion, disorientation, anxiety, fearfulness, or inability to communicate. In addition, family members may not be present or available. Consequently, the initial assessment process may extend over time until the client is sufficiently responsive or other informants are available. Because the acutely disturbed client is often frightened by the idea of being interviewed, the nurse should try to ensure that the environment is as calm as possible. Distracting stimuli should be avoided. Lighting should be bright and not shadowy. Privacy should be provided for, but not to the extent that the client feels anxious and threatened by it. Sufficient personal space should be allowed so that the client's boundaries, which may be fragmented or diffuse at this time, are not invaded. The nurse should address the client by name, speak in a clear way, use understandable language, clarify questions that are misunderstood, and use restatement to ensure understanding of the client's response. The nurse's attitude and feeling will be reflected in the approach to the client. A calm, unharried, and competent manner may go a long way toward helping the client respond to the fullest extent possible. Assessment is also an ongoing process. The client's behavior is reassessed on a day-to-day basis so that changes in status can be used in appropriately revising the nursing care plan.

Assessment includes collection of data about the person, the family, and the environment. All three areas provide baseline data which contribute to formulation of a comprehensive treatment plan. The following case study of Cindy L. illustrates the initial assessment process for a schizophrenic client who is acutely disturbed. Table 37-6 contains assessment questions for the client, the family, and

Table 37-6 Assessment of Client and Family

Assessment Question	Responses of Client (C) and Family (F)
Assessment of the person	
How does the client describe the problem she is having right now?	C: I'm so scared. I hear voices telling me I'm bad. I try to be good. . . .
How does the client describe the circumstances that precipitated the behavior?	C: It's hard to concentrate. I couldn't think in school, had to stop, heard noises, they got louder. . . . F: As I think about it, Cindy's behavior has been changing for about the last 6 months. Last night when a man from work called and asked her for a date, Cindy started screaming, hiding, and doing other horrible things. It must have something to do with that.
Does the client present evidence of cognitive or linguistic changes (loss of abstract thinking, delusions, hallucinations, magical thinking, autistic communication)?	C: The devil is out to get me. If he gets me, I'll be saved and redeemed from being a sinner; it's another chance. I guess I'll nelwas a frignunx ungar merrilium. (Cindy appears to look off into space, lips moving, talking to people who are not there.)
Does the client present evidence of perceptual changes (hallucinations, hypochondriasis, depersonalization)?	C: Tramp, whore, kill me! The voices—they're voices now! They were only noises! I have to pray. I feel as though I'm dying; I have a knife searing my belly. If I didn't have that pain, I'd feel empty like a shell. At least if I feel the pain, I know I'm alive.
Describe the client's affect. Are thought and affect congruent?	Cindy's face remains blank when she relates the "scary" experiences of the past week. She giggles suddenly when talking about the devil being after her because she's a tramp. On the unit her mood is unpredictable and changeable.

(Continued.)

Table 37-6 Continued

Assessment Question	Responses of Client (C) and Family (F)
Assessment of the person	
What objective data are the client presenting (gestures, posture, gait, tone of voice, mannerisms)?	Cindy huddles in the corner of the room with her face turned away from family and nurse. Her arms are wrapped tightly around her sides, and she does not maintain eye contact when speaking.
What does the client describe as personal strengths and problems?	C: I have only problems; I can't do anything anymore. F: Cindy is very bright. She is artistic. She is a kind person.
Does the client abuse alcohol or drugs (liquor, beer, heroin, PCP, LSD, marijuana, tranquilizers)?	C: Never. F: Never.
Has the client had any physical illnesses or accidents in the past year?	C: No. F: No.
Assessment of the family	
Who are the client's significant others?	C: I have nobody; nobody understands how it is. . . . F: Cindy lives at home with her mother, father, 15-year-old brother, and 13-year-old sister.
How do the client and the family describe the relationships in their nuclear family?	C: I have no relationship. My mother tries to run my life. She and my father hardly talk. She doesn't depend on my brother or sister as she does on me. F: We're a very close-knit family. My husband travels a lot, so I try to make up for it by being involved with the kids.
How do the parents describe the relationships in their family of origin?	F: I was an only child. My father died when I was 8. My mother and I were very close. When she died, I wanted to die. But I had to live for this baby I was having. My husband was the youngest of five. He's the only boy. He was his mother's favorite. We rarely see his family. They live 1000 miles away. I have no family to speak of. We have only each other to rely on.
What is the client's sibling position in the family?	C: I'm the oldest. I feel so old—the ancient mariner. F: Cindy's the oldest; 22 now. Sometimes you'd never know it. She's more like a frightened baby.
Describe the family communication patterns.	C: Things are never said straight. Mom says she's upset that I don't date or live away from home, but I don't believe her. I'd never tell her that, though; she might get too angry at me. Then what would I do? F: Mother was observed saying to Cindy, "Get dressed, like an adult." When Cindy hesitated, Mother said, "I'll just have to dress you," and proceeded to dress her.
Describe the role relationships in the family.	F: Dad's never home to be the boss. In a funny way, Mom relies on him, but we always think of her as the boss. Dad's not here even now. He's very distant. Mom has no family, so she's always been very close to all of us, especially Cindy.
Are there special events or issues in the client's family that people would find difficult to talk about with one another?	F: I don't think there is anything we can't talk about. C: Oh, Mom, come on. As long as it's clean and pure, it's fine. I think if mothers could be virgins, my mother would be it.
How do family members perceive and deal with independence?	C: Independence, that's scary. I couldn't do that! Who would Mommy have? F: I went from my mother's house to my husband's. Even though he's not home much, I don't know how I'd function alone. I wanted to die when my mother died. I wasn't ready to be a mother without her.
Has anyone in the client's family been hospitalized for mental illness?	F: Nobody at all.

(Continued.)

Table 37-6 Continued

Assessment Question	Responses of Client (C) and Family (F)
Assessment of the environment	
What is the client's educational background?	C: One and one-half years of community college. F: She dropped out. There was too much pressure.
What is the client's employment history (type of job, duration of job, job satisfaction, relationships at work)?	C: I never had a job until this one. I's OK. I work by myself in the stockroom even though I'm supposed to be selling. I don't like to be around all those people. F: It's a nothing job. She's a bright girl, capable of much more than that. They seem to like her at work; after all, that young man called to find out what was wrong with her and asked her for a date.
What is the client's and the family's socioeconomic status?	C: We're middle-class. F: We manage to make ends meet without struggling.
How do the client's and the family's cultural background and beliefs fit with the social system in which they live?	F: We're just like everybody else. You don't think that I believe that Cindy is having a religious vision, or something like that?
Does the client have friends? How easy is it for her to make friends? Has the client ever had a sustained relationship?	C: I've never made friends easily. I am uncomfortable around people. I always think they're better than me. I don't like boys; I don't know what to say. I don't see my old friend from high school. She went away to school, and at my school everyone seemed so unfriendly. F: She's always been shy and a loner.
To what extent is the client or family involved in the community network?	C: I don't do anything. F: My family is my life. I don't have time for things like church or clubs or even friends. With my husband away so much, who would want me by myself?
Does the family have support systems available in the community (family, friends, church, community organizations)?	F: No, we keep to ourselves. (Client agrees.)
How does the client spend leisure time?	C: I've had a lot on my mind. I think a lot. F: Nothing; she daydreams and sleeps.

the environment as well as the corresponding responses to such questions.

Cindy L., age 22, appears disheveled. Her hair looks greasy; her makeup is smeared; she is wearing a crookedly buttoned pajama top, sweat pants, and slippers. She agitatedly paces the emergency room, muttering to herself, suddenly laughing for no apparent reason.

Cindy is admitted to the inpatient unit. She is negativistic, labile, and anxious. Her thoughts are characterized by looseness of associations and suspiciousness. Her speech is sprinkled with neologisms. Her lips constantly move in a repetitive pattern. Cindy refuses to follow the hospital schedule. She does not want to shower, comb her hair, or change her clothes. She sleeps in her clothes if she can. She alternates between agitatedly pacing the hall and huddling in the corner next to her bed. She ignores the requests of others and will not participate in activities. She is noted to mutter to herself under her breath in words that no one can understand and is frequently found hiding in the laundry closet. When asked what she is doing there, she responds, "Praying wasn't enough. I tried to pray. I tried! The devil is coming to get me. He says I'm a whore. I have to hide."

PRECIPITATING EVENTS

Cindy is a former college student who worked part-time as a salesperson in a local variety store. She lived at home with her parents and two younger siblings. Cindy had been attending a local community college until about 6 months ago, at which time she stopped going to classes, complaining that she was having trouble concentrating and that she was too tired to get up and go to class in the morning. At home she was moody and withdrawn and spent a great deal of time sleeping. Her mother often heard her talking to somebody in her room but knew that nobody was there. Cindy's mother brought her to the emergency room on Sunday morning. Cindy had refused to go to work all week, complaining of a burning pain in her stomach. Saturday one of the young men with whom she worked called to find out why she had been absent and asked her to go to a movie that night. Cindy dropped the phone and ran into her room crying. She lay huddled in a corner of her room, shaking, alternately laughing and crying. She seemed to be whispering to herself and refused to go to bed. Cindy's father was out of town on a business trip, so her mother stayed up to make sure that Cindy was safe. Cindy began shouting in her room, 'Whore Devil Tramp! Sinner!" Her mother rushed into her room and found Cindy hiding in her closet, sobbing uncontrollably and saying, "Help, help, they're killing me!" Her mother took Cindy to the emergency room.

When Cindy was interviewed by the nurse who admitted her to the unit, she told the nurse that a man from work had called and asked her for a date. As he was asking her to go to the movies, she began to hear frightening voices shouting, "Whore, slut, devil, no good!" She had been hearing vague, unpleasant voices for about 6 months, especially when she was at school or in a social situation. The voices had now became much more condemning and frightening. She felt that she must be a sinful person.

FAMILY HISTORY

Cindy is the oldest of three children. She has a 15-year-old brother and a 13-year-old sister. Cindy was born 3 months after the unexpected death of her maternal grandmother, with whom Cindy's mother had been very close. She was named after her grandmother and her mother told the nurse, "I was so lucky to have a little girl; it helped to ease the pain of my mother's death. I've also been alone a lot in my marriage because my husband travels so much."

Mrs. L. stated that the birth was normal but she had felt very lonely and sad at the time of the delivery, because her mother was not there to share it with her and she was uncertain whether her husband would arrive at the hospital on time. Cindy was described as a colicky baby who, her mother felt, was difficult to care for. She was also unsure about how to care for her, having counted on her mother for guidance. On one hand she was grateful to have Cindy for comfort and cuddling; but on the other hand Cindy was helpless and demanding, and Mrs. L. often felt overwhelmed by her new responsibility.

The family moved four times during Cindy's childhood, when she was 4, 7, 11, and 14, because of Mr. L.'s job transfers. Although her mastery of developmental tasks was age-appropriate, she became more timid and shy with each move. She was a compliant child, obedient and a good student. She had few friends, seeming to prefer the company of her mother. Cindy's siblings seemed to be much more easygoing and flexible. Mrs. L. said, "I was lonely a lot. Perhaps I gave too much attention and affection to Cindy; maybe I didn't let her grow up. The other children never meant as much to me as she did."

Cindy's shyness and social withdrawal increased in adolescence. In high school her grades began to fall. She dropped out of the few school activities in which she had been active, and she had only one friend with whom she felt comfortable. She stated that her other friends were "boy-crazy" and that she wasn't "into that," and she refused all social invitations. She spent a great deal of time in her room, daydreaming, listening to records, and sleeping. She chose to go to a local community college, even though her parents had hoped she'd go to an out-of-town, 4-year college. Cindy told them that she was afraid to go so far away from home and felt that she could not handle the academic demands. She received passing grades at the local community college until she stopped

Throughout the treatment process, the nurse must constantly assess the client's behavior in order to (1) identify the behaviors the client is exhibiting; (2) understand the meaning of the behavior; (3) establish behavioral patterns; (4) identify changes in behavior; and (5) evaluate the impact of the behavior on other clients, the staff, and the therapeutic milieu. When assessment occurs on an ongoing basis, the care plan can be modified in relation to changes in the cognitive, perceptual, affective, motor, and social spheres of experience.

Today, the majority of clients who have had schizophrenic episodes reside in the community. Many of the clients in this group have had repeated schizophrenic episodes that have required short- or long-term hospitalization. The community health nurse and other nurses who work in community agencies that serve this population assess the client's functioning in a community setting as well as the need for in- or outpatient treatment.

The following case study is the story of one client who might be assessed by the community health nurse on a periodic basis.

Bill S., age 40, had his first schizophrenic break at age 25. At that time he had become assaultive in a bar one night, convinced that the men at the bar were making homosexual overtures toward him. Bill spent 3 months in a short-term private psychiatric hospital and then was transferred to a state hospital when he did not improve and continued to be assaultive.

At the time of his first episode, Bill had completed college and was working as an electrical engineer in a research laboratory. He had always been a loner and liked the solitude of the laboratory. He had not seen his family since he graduated from college. His family was described as chaotic. His father, an alcoholic, had beaten Bill and his brothers on numerous occasions. Bill's mother was a tired woman, who had endured a lot of misery in her life and was frequently hospitalized for depression. His father finally abandoned the family when Bill was 13. Bill had to assume some of the responsibility for supporting the family. Bill went to college on scholarship, and once he graduated, vowed that he would not maintain contact with his family because his experiences had been so painful.

Over the past 15 years Bill has been hospitalized eight times for repeated schizophrenic episodes. At this point he would be considered chronically mentally ill (CMI). His level of integration has decreased with each episode. He is currently living in a single room in a state-approved boardinghouse. He works part time in a sheltered workshop assembling battery kits. His income is supplemented by disability checks. He goes to the medication clinic at the mental health center once a month. Bill refuses to participate in any of the social activities or therapy groups conducted at the center. He is suspicious of anyone who approaches him socially because he is convinced, although he rarely mentions it, that a group of FBI agents in Washington sends spies out to raid his mind and body for special secrets. Muriel W., a community health nurse, makes regular home visits to Bill's boardinghouse to assess his ongoing functioning in the community.

The following criteria are used by Muriel in evaluating Bill S.'s level of functioning and need for treatment.

1. Is the person able to meet basic human needs?
   a. Does the person have adequate living facilities?
   b. Does the person have enough money to pay for basic needs such as rent, food, clothes?
   c. Is the person able to buy food and prepare it so that basic nutritional requirements are met?
   d. Is the person appropriately dressed for the weather?
2. Is the person complying with the prescribed medication regimen?
3. Is the person involved in any kind of work or vocational rehabilitation program?
4. How does the person spend each day?
5. What is the person's level of involvement in a social or community network?
6. What are the person's support systems like (family, friends, community, agency contacts)?
7. Has the person experienced any internal or external stressors recently?
8. Is the person having any threatening thoughts or engaging in any bizarre or inappropriate behavior that is, either at this time or potentially, harmful to self or others?
9. Has the person moved or drifted from a room, apartment, group home, or other setting without notifying others?

The nurse will look for changes in the person's thoughts and behavior patterns that would indicate further ego disintegration that presents a threat to the safety of the client as well as others in the environment. The nurse will use the data for decision making about the need for hospitalization or other types of therapeutic interventions. (The reader is referred to Chapter 53, "The Chronic Mentally Ill in the Community," for an extensive discussion of such clients.)

Diagnosis

The nursing diagnosis is formulated from the data base that has been assembled during the assessment process. It includes identification of the client's strengths and problems. Table 37-7 illustrates the initial nursing diagnoses formulated for Cindy L. on the basis of the case study and assessment in Table 37-6. Table 37-8 identifies nursing diagnoses for Bill S. that reflect challenges for the community health nurse.

Nursing diagnosis occurs on an ongoing basis. As the nurse observes and interacts with the client and as the client's condition changes, patterns of additional problems and strengths emerge. Initial problems may be modified or resolved as the client's level of integration and wellness changes.

Outcome Criteria

Short- and long-term outcome criteria are developed for each nursing diagnosis. Short-term out-

Table 37-7 Nursing Diagnosis and Outcome Criteria for Cindy L.

Assessment	Nursing Diagnosis	Outcome Criteria
Huddles in a corner of her room; does not respond to or initiate communication; speaks in symbolic language; refuses to participate in unit activities.	Avoidance of interpersonal relatedness, stemming from feelings of mistrust	Client will tolerate an interpersonal relationship with one nurse, as evidenced by: 1. Allowing the nurse to remain with her for 15 minutes without leaving or telling the nurse to go away 2. Maintaining eye contact 3. Responding verbally to communication initiated by the nurse and by other clients 4. Initiating verbal communication with staff and other clients 5. Attending group therapy sessions 6. Participating in unit activities
Cindy: The devil is coming to get me. He says I'm a whore. I have to pray to keep him away.	Alteration in reality orientation manifested by auditory hallucinations and delusions of persecution related to unacceptable aggressive and sexual impulses	Client will maintain reality orientation as evidenced by: 1. Accepting the presence of a staff member 2. Verbalizing the content and occurrence of the hallucination or delusion 3. Verbalizing unacceptable feelings in a direct way 4. Identifying the relationship between anxious feelings and the hallucination or delusion 5. Utilizing distraction techniques 6. Interacting with others without becoming delusional or hallucinating
Cindy refuses to participate in unit activities; remains secluded in her room. Cindy has never dated, has few friends, and is unable to identify personal strengths	Social withdrawal related to feelings of low self-esteem and mistrust	Client will tolerate social relationships, as evidenced by: 1. Attending group therapy sessions 3 times per week without leaving 2. Attending art therapy and dance therapy 3. Interacting with her primary nurse 5 times a week for 30 minutes each day 4. Identifying feelings about social relatedness 5. Identifying the purpose behind her withdrawal 6. Participating in social activities on the unit
Cindy dropped out of school 6 months ago and has not been at work for 1 week. She says she is confused and cannot concentrate.	Inability to tolerate stress of college and work related to low self-esteem	Client will tolerate expectations of adult productivity, as evidenced by: 1. Assuming responsibility for the care of her room 2. Accepting responsibility for a unit job 3. Discussing feelings of low self-esteem as they relate to job and school 4. Identifying academic and career options 5. Returning to job, school, or vocational rehabilitation
Cindy: I don't want to eat. No, no; I won't drink, either. I can't trust it.	Inadequate nutritional intake; potential dehydration related to refusal to eat or drink	Client will maintain adequate nutrition and hydration, as evidenced by: 1. Increase in nutritional intake to 2500 calories per 24 hours 2. Increase in fluid intake to 2000 milliliters per 24 hours

(Continued.)

Table 37-7 Continued

Assessment	Nursing Diagnosis	Outcome Criteria
Cindy refuses to wash, shower, or change clothes.	Neglect of personal hygiene associated with low self-esteem and poor reality orientation	Progressive independence in self-care, as evidenced by: 1. Allowing the staff to meet her hygiene needs 2. Allowing the staff to assist her with hygiene needs 3. Assuming responsibility for self-care in hygiene activities
Cindy giggles when describing a knifelike sensation in her stomach. Her face is expressionless when she is saying that her stomach feels as if it doesn't belong to her and that she can't control it.	Flat or inappropriate affect related to fear of loss of control of behavior	Affect is appropriate for conversation.
Cindy: My mother tries to run my life. I've always been her baby. I can't do anything by myself.	Dependency-related fused and overclose mother-child relationship related to overfunctioning of mother and underfunctioning of daughter	Client will tolerate anxiety related to exploration of relationship, as evidenced by: 1. Acknowledgment by mother and daughter of the needs met by their relationship 2. Identification by client of dysfunctional aspects of the relationship 3. Client's beginning to identify personal likes and dislikes 4. Mother and daughter tolerate physical separation without becoming anxious 5. Client's beginning to make decisions independently without seeking help from mother 6. Withholding of advice by mother
Cindy: My mother tells me to grow up, but she treats me like such a baby. She also says we're a happy family, but we're not.	Double-bind communication associated with mixed message about dependence versus independence	Client will identify patterns of double-bind messages, as evidenced by: 1. Identifying different levels of messages 2. Verbalizing ways in which family members send mixed messages 3. Identifying ways of responding to mixed messages
Cindy: My mother and father hardly talk to each other.	Family projection process related to covert marital distance and conflict	Client will participate in restructuring family relationship boundaries, as evidenced by: 1. Identifying dysfunctional relationship patterns 2. Asking father to attend family sessions 3. Spending time with father to help establish closer relationship
Mrs. L.: My husband travels a lot for business. I don't know what I'd do if I didn't have Cindy.		
Mrs. L: I have no living family. My husband hasn't seen his family in years. We are not involved in the community.	Lack of extended family ties and isolation from local community related to emotional cutoff	Establishment by family of support systems, as evidenced by: 1. Identifying potential extended family and community resources 2. Initiating contact with a relative or community group 3. Participating in a community organization

Table 37-8 Nursing Diagnosis and Outcome Criteria for Bill S.

Assessment	Nursing Diagnosis	Outcome Criteria
Refuses to participate in therapy groups or social activities at the community mental health center. Has no friends, family, or community connections.	Social withdrawal related to mistrust and feelings of social inadequacy	Client will tolerate increased connectedness to others, as evidenced by: 1. Initiating verbal communication with the community health nurse on home visits 2. Attending a monthly social activity group for discharged clients 3. Attending a weekly current-events group at the community mental health center 4. Telephoning the community health nurse if problems arise 5. Permitting the minister of a local church to visit him after being notified of the visit
Spends time at home sitting and staring out the window.	Minimal leisure-time interests related to lack of social skills	Client will develop one leisure interest, as evidenced by: 1. Identifying potential recreational interests 2. Attending a recreational event at the center if picked up by a volunteer he knows 3. Joining a social skills training class
Bill: "I take my pills whenever I remember them. I don't know why I have to take them. I haven't been in the hospital for a year."	Potential problem of noncompliance with medication related to poor memory and inability to accept the need for ongoing medication	Client will comply with medication regimen, as evidenced by: 1. Taking medication regularly 2. Reporting any problems with medication to nurse at the clinic 3. Attending educational classes at the clinic 4. Verbalizing three reasons for continuing to take medication
Bill: "I can't let too many people know about the FBI. They might take it out on me, and then I would have to get back at them."	Potential destructive behavior directed toward self or others, associated with auditory hallucinations and with persecutory and grandiose delusions that are systematized, fixed, and periodically threatening	Client will decrease potential for disruptive behavior, as evidenced by: 1. Contacting nurse by telephone when hallucinations or delusions become threatening 2. Identifying ways in which he can keep anxiety at manageable levels 3. Following suggestions about how to distract attention from inner thoughts and perceptions
Bill is observed picking through garbage cans daily as he walks home from work. Neighborhood children shout, "There's that crazy guy again."	Potential increase in anxiety associated with negative labeling and stereotyping by neighborhood children because of bizarre behavior	Client will decrease bizarre behavior in public, as evidenced by: 1. Sharing negative experiences with the community health nurse 2. Accepting feedback from the nurse about his behavior 3. Considering modification of the behavior that is eliciting negative comments
Bill is informed that his landlord is selling the boardinghouse where he lives. He becomes very upset; his behavior becomes more disorganized; he stops going to work.	Behavioral disorganization related to anxiety precipitated by external stressors	Client will maintain reality orientation under stress, as evidenced by: 1. Verbalizing feelings in a reality-oriented manner 2. Identifying the external stressor 3. Accepting additional support to assist him in this crisis
Bill eats soup and cereal three times a day; no protein, vegetables, and fruit are included in his diet.	Inadequate nutritional intake related to unbalanced diet	Client will improve nutritional intake, as evidenced by: 1. Discussing menu planning with community health nurse 2. On shopping trips with community health nurse, selecting foods that have protein, carbohydrates, and fat 3. Preparing meals that are nutritionally balanced

come criteria consist of goals that the client will demonstrate in the process of working toward broader long-term goals. For example, a long-term goal might be that the client will initiate interpersonal relationships, as evidenced by:

1. Calling a person with whom he or she attends the day treatment center to ask about going to a movie
2. Making dinner plans with a former hospital roommate
3. Making a follow-up call to a college friend encountered at church

However, the first short-term goal might be that a mistrustful client will remain with the nurse for 15 minutes.

Goals should be realistic to avoid discouragement for both the nurse and the client. Both people need to be aware that these goals may take a long time to accomplish. For example, clients who utilize bizarre communication patterns such as neologisms and word salads are usually avoiding intimate relationships. They are reluctant to take the risk of communicating more directly. Accomplishing the goal of open, direct communication may take many months.

Goals need to be developed with the active participation of the client. They must be consistent with the client's ability to tolerate anxiety, since learning and change are anxiety-provoking experiences. Goals that are unrealistic and increase the client's anxiety level before he or she has the necessary coping skills and support systems may only reinforce the client's need for and use of dysfunctional coping behaviors. Goals must be revised on a regular basis. As goals are attained, new ones are formulated that reflect the client's current level of wellness and capacity for self-care. Tables 37-7 and 37-8 illustrate the goals identified for Cindy L. and Bill S. on the basis of the nursing diagnoses.

Intervention

The person's level of functioning will reflect the setting in which the nurse encounters the client. The goals of the setting as well as the nature of the client's problems will influence the formulation and implementation of nursing orders and interventions.

The acutely disturbed client is usually treated in a residential or inpatient setting. Nurses may encounter such clients in a short-term acute-care psychiatric unit whose goal is to assess the client's condition, intervene rapidly to restore the client to an optimum level of wellness, and return the client to the community as quickly as possible. In this setting, nursing interventions focus on alleviating the client's acute problems. Clients may also enter long-term residential treatment facilities which combine evaluative treatment and rehabilitative approaches. In this setting, nurses focus on both acute and ongoing problems.

The nurse will also encounter schizophrenic clients in outpatient settings. Many of these clients, discharged from inpatient facilities, are still unable to function independently and need further treatment and rehabilitation. Other clients receive treatment in outpatient settings as an alternative to hospitalization. Consequently, the nurse will encounter and work with schizophrenic clients in halfway houses, group homes, day care centers, community mental health centers, and medication clinics, as well as individual and group therapy. Programs offered in these outpatient settings give clients the chance to gradually adjust to life outside the institution or seek assistance in maintaining functional behavior in the community. They provide an opportunity for clients to continue working on problems that interfere with their ability to function independently. The focus of these programs is social rehabilitation.

The community health nurse also encounters clients who have been discharged from the hospital and require supervision, teaching, and support within the home setting. The home setting may be a family home to which the client returns, an apartment, or a single room in a boardinghouse. The same client may also be involved in one or more of the outpatient programs described above. The community health nurse often acts as a liaison between the client in the home setting and other outpatient facilities and services. (See Chapter 53.) The community health nurse may also intervene to initiate rehospitalization when the assessment data indicate that this is necessary. Nurses who work in the community also participate in primary prevention programs that address both healthy families and high-risk families.

Nursing intervention will vary according to the type of setting, the goals of the setting, and the role of the nurse in that setting. Individualization of care in both in- and outpatient settings will be a function of clients' problems and needs. This section will present interventions for dealing with clients' problems in both in- and outpatient settings.

Interventions with Clients

The client usually arrives at the treatment setting feeling confused, frightened, and isolated. The environment and people in it may be perceived as threatening. The client may respond with hostility and aggression or by withdrawal. The client and the family may be upset about separation.

The client requires skilled nursing intervention. The nurse must exercise judgment in assessing and responding to clients' needs. The nurse will need to meet their physical and safety needs and assist them with problems such as anxiety, mistrust, low self-esteem, dependency, social withdrawal, identity confusion, and difficulty evaluating reality. The nurse utilizes individual, group, environmental, and family interventions to address these problems.

CREATING A THERAPEUTIC ENVIRONMENT. When clients are admitted to the unit, they are often intensely anxious, confused, and frightened because of what are perceived as overwhelming internal and external stimuli. Their mistrust and inability to accurately test reality further inhibit their ability to make sense of what is happening. Each client should be assigned to a nurse who will work very closely with him or her. This will minimize the number of people to whom the clients must orient themselves at a time when they are having difficulty assimilating stimuli.[59] The nurse should orient clients to the unit. Because they may be having difficulty processing information, explanations may have to be repeated. Messages and instructions should be clear and direct. The nurse should provide directions that enable clients to follow the daily routine with a minimum of decision-making requirements. For example, instead of asking clients when they would like to take a bath, the nurse tells them that showers are taken at 8:30 every night. The same nurse should spend short periods of time with the client on a regular basis, whether or not the client responds, until he or she becomes less anxious on the unit. This will convey interest and respect and will contribute to the client's feelings of acceptance and comfort. The client, noting that attempts at understanding are being made, feels more secure and has more confidence in the nurse.

Immediate involvement in a variety of complex, stimulating activities such as community meetings, group therapy, or activity therapy may be contraindicated if clients are extremely anxious, confused, or frightened. These types of activities may be too stimulating or demanding at this time and may cause the clients' anxiety levels to escalate unnecessarily. Clients' involvement in such activities will be modified according to their capacity.

A therapeutic environment for schizophrenic clients needs to be orderly, consistent, and predictable. Different areas on the unit, such as the dining room, dayroom, activity rooms, and nurses' station, should be clearly labeled. Items such as clocks, calendars, schedules, and current magazines should be provided, to encourage clients to remain oriented to the environment. Environmental stimuli may need to be kept at a minimum during the initial phase of inpatient treatment, when clients are unable to effectively filter incoming stimuli. Sometimes the normal activity of the unit overloads clients, who may become increasingly agitated, confused, or out of control. A client may need to spend time in a quiet room alone or with a staff member.

During meetings or conferences in which clients are involved, all people should be introduced and the goals of the meeting stated. Clients should be spoken to in clear, understandable language. Clients' comprehension should be ascertained, and misunderstandings should be clarified insofar as possible.

MONITORING PHYSICAL AND SAFETY NEEDS. Clients in an acute schizophrenic episode are often too far out of touch with reality to be aware of grooming, nutrition, rest, medication, and safety. Even if they are aware of these needs, they may be too disorganized, apathetic, or negativistic to carry out the tasks required to meet them. For example, they might refuse to change clothes, shower, or get out of bed in the morning. Once they get up, they may refuse to go to bed at night. Clients who have chronic schizophrenia and reside in a hospital setting for longer periods of time may also have a poor reality orientation that interferes with their awareness of these needs. They may also, as a result of long-term hospitalization, become desocialized and either meet their physical needs in bizarre ways or depend on others to meet them. For example:

Annie loved to eat but insisted on using her knife to pick up her food. As a result, her vegetables, desserts, and soft meats spilled all over the place. She always had food on her clothes but did not appear to mind. When she was told to get her things together for a shower, she stood in the hall, not moving. When finally assisted into the shower and told to wash, she stood there with the soap in her hand, not washing, until the nurse came back and gave her step-by-step directions, which she was unable to follow. The nurse eventually finished washing her.

Nursing intervention involves assessing clients' ability to care for themselves. When a client is clearly unable to meet physiological needs at all, the nurse meets these needs in a way that preserves the client's dignity. The nursing staff may have to bathe, dress, and feed clients in order to prevent dehydration, malnutrition, and skin problems. For example, a client who is in a catatonic stupor may, if not helped to do otherwise, remain in the same position for hours without any seeming awareness of the need for food, drink, elimination, sleep, or any other basic requirements.

Clients who are partially able to care for themselves may work cooperatively with the nurse. The nurse may need to inform and remind them about the showering or mealtime schedule. The nurse may help clients identify necessary items for completing the task and may check that all items have been included. The nurse may need to supervise bathing, dressing, or eating to make sure that it is appropriately completed. A client who is having difficulty eating or dressing may need matter-of-fact, specific directions from the nurse in order to complete the task without additional assistance. In other situations a client, such as Annie in the example above, may perform self-care tasks such as feeding but do it in inappropriate ways. Such a client may be a candidate for behavior modification programs in which appropriate self-care behaviors such as daily showering and eating with a fork, knife, and spoon are systematically shaped and positively reinforced with praise or other tangible rewards such as cigarettes, coffee, and extra privileges.

A client who is partially independent in self-care activities needs to be encouraged to assume increasing responsibility for self-care. Having physiological needs met can provide positive nurturing experiences that have been absent in the client's life. However, this approach can foster dependency if it continues beyond the point when it is necessary. The client's ability to engage in self-care is periodically reevaluated so that this capacity is realistically identified and nurtured by the staff.

Nurses may also have to intervene with clients whose sleep patterns have been disrupted—for instance, those who have difficulty falling asleep or staying asleep. Data about at-home sleep patterns provide baseline information from which judgments about the client's current sleep patterns can be made. For example:

Sherry refused to go to sleep before 1:00 A.M. or get up before 10:00 A.M. without a battle. She would run up and down the hall yelling about how mean everyone was to her. She was more cooperative in the afternoon and evening. The nurse found out that Sherry did not work and had never had any limits imposed on her sleep hours. Her mother described her as a "night person." The staff negotiated with Sherry that she could stay up until midnight, if she stayed quietly in her room and got up by 9:00 A.M. each morning in order to get to group therapy by 10:00 A.M. Sherry cooperated in this program, because her needs were being respected. The staff felt good because the power struggle was eliminated and Sherry was ready to participate in unit activities when they began.

Other clients may show alterations in their sleep patterns because they are anxious or agitated. Assessment of the effectiveness of medication given at bedtime may be important. A warm drink, a massage, soft music, or relaxation exercises may be soothing to the client and promote rest. Sometimes just a chat for a few minutes with someone with whom the client can share nighttime fears or worries is sufficient to release anxiety, and the client is able to relax and sleep. Daytime naps should be avoided, as they often make clients wakeful at night.

Nursing intervention also includes monitoring the effectiveness of the psychotropic medication regimen; observing for side and toxic effects, such as photosensitivity, skin rash, parkinsonian symptoms, and tardive dyskinesia; coordinating initial and ongoing laboratory work; and implementing plans that educate clients about the medications they are taking, the potential side and toxic effects, and any precautions they can take. (See Chapter 26 for a complete discussion of the nurse's role in psychopharmacology.)

The inability to evaluate reality, the presence of command hallucinations, poor judgment, and impulsivity make it necessary to monitor clients' safety needs. Potentially harmful objects such as matches and cigarettes, razors, soda can tops, and even forks may have to be removed from clients' environment in order to protect them from their poor judgment and impulsivity. For instance:

> Sandy repeatedly burned herself with cigarettes in order to make sure she was still alive. Another client, Paul, would impulsively slash his arms and legs with soda can tops when he became angry.

A client who is standing at a window touching the glass should be removed from the area immediately. Command hallucinations, powerful voices telling the client to jump, may be so strong that the client would, if not removed, jump out the window without hesitation. Firm limits and controls must be set by the staff when clients' behavior is impulsive, destructive, or out of control. Such behavior is motivated by increased anxiety. Allowing it to continue only escalates the anxiety cycle. A client is often terrified but unable independently to provide the necessary controls and limits or to signal the occurrence of impending out-of-control behavior and request assistance from the staff. Therefore the staff must be alert to warning signals which indicate that anxiety is escalating and behavior is getting out of control. A frightened or agitated client may need to be removed to a quiet room or seclusion room until the anxiety level decreases and control has been restored.

Clients should not be restrained except as a last resort. When the nurse assesses a need for seclusion or restraint, sufficient physical assistance should be available in case the client loses control, but it should not be used unless the client actually does begin to lose control. The approach to the client should be firm but gentle, and the client should be constantly reassured about his or her safety. (See Chapter 32 for a complete discussion of out-of-control behavior.) For example:

> Willie F. has been pacing the dayroom all afternoon. He has been talking aloud to himself. The nurse, Nancy C., has approached him at regular intervals and walked with him around the dayroom. The nurse recognizes that Willie is frightened by voices and is also delusional. He believes that he is a victim of an FBI plot.

At 7 P.M., the nurse approaches Willie:

NANCY: Hi, Willie. You still look pretty upset.

WILLIE: What the hell do you think? You'd be upset if the FBI planted electrodes in your brain that had you programmed. I know that somehow you are all part of the plot. I'll find out! You wait and see; I'll get you all yet.

NANCY: That sounds very frightening, Willie.

WILLIE: No, I just have to be alert at all times. I can never relax. I have to protect myself. No one else cares, especially Joe (the nurse at the desk). He spies on me and feeds it into the FBI computer!

NANCY: Willie, you seem to be more upset. Let's sit down. We won't talk. Let's just sit.

WILLIE: No, I can't do that. I can't relax; I have to keep going.

NANCY: I'll be back in 15 minutes, Willie.

The nurse has recognized that the client, Willie, is becoming increasingly agitated and is losing control. She thinks that a quiet environment would be less stimulating and would make him feel safer. She requests the assistance of three staff members, and together they approach Willie:

NANCY: Willie, you are very upset. You are having difficulty with the voices and with your fears. You need to be quiet and rest until you feel calmer.

WILLIE: No, it's him; it's Joe. I just saw him talking to you. Now you're all part of the plot. Don't come near me.

NANCY: Willie, we won't hurt you. You must go to the quiet room now. You will feel safer and less frightened there.

WILLIE: No! I'm not going, I've got to get away from all of you. (Willie starts looking around the room.)

NANCY: Willie, walk with me to the quiet room. We understand that you're frightened. You need to be safe, and we won't hurt you.

WILLIE: Don't come near me!

NANCY: I'll stand away from you (backs away several feet), but you walk with us. You'll feel safer there.

WILLIE: Stay away from me! (But he walks down the hall toward the quiet room.)

NANCY: I have to pass in front of you to open the door.

WILLIE: All right. You can pass.

NANCY: Okay, Willie, you go in now. Put on your pajamas and lie down.

WILLIE: (Struggling and beginning to yell.) They're all out to get me. They can't do this to me. I'll get them all.

At this point, the client dashes for the door of the quiet room. The staff members recognize that he is losing control and may hurt himself or others. The four staff members approach him from either side in a quiet, calm manner. They walk with him as he struggles and walk him into the quiet room.

NANCY: Willie, we're going to help you get into pajamas. (Two staff members hold Willie while two others change his clothes.) Lie down in bed, Willie. We're going to wrap you in a blanket to keep you safe.

WILLIE: Don't let them get me.

NANCY: I won't, Willie. You'll feel safe in here. I'm going to be back to see you in 15 minutes.

This example highlights the importance of assessment, that is, recognition of early signs of impending loss of control and early intervention in meeting the client's safety needs.

THEMES IN THE NURSE-CLIENT RELATIONSHIP. *Anxiety.* Anxiety is one of the most crucial elements in the development of schizophrenia. Severe and panic-level anxiety contributes to many of the behaviors that clients exhibit. Nursing intervention is directed toward alleviating the anxiety.

To some extent the psychotropic medications alleviate anxiety and its accompanying symptoms such as delusions, hallucinations, agitation, aggression, and impulsivity. As clients become less anxious, they become more reality-oriented, their behavior becomes more appropriate, and they become more approachable and amenable to relatedness. Consequently, the nurse's role in monitoring the effectiveness of these medications is extremely important. The nurse observes clients for manifestations of anxiety and assesses the degree to which these behaviors are resolved as the medication takes effect. The nurse's observations are shared with the mental health team, so that appropriate adjustments in medications can be made. Medication is a valuable component of the treatment plan but should not be its only component.

Regression is often a manifestation of anxiety. The client returns to a less integrated level of functioning in order to protect the self from internal and external anxiety-provoking stimuli. Regression represents a dysfunctional attempt to reduce anxiety by returning to less mature behaviors which help the client tolerate the anxiety better. For example:

> Lillian was very frightened of relating to males. Whenever the unit had a party or dance, Lillian would refuse to dance with or talk to any of the male clients. She would become very agitated and then withdraw to a corner where she would sit and masturbate.

Lillian may have experienced an upsurge of unacceptable sexual feelings when approached by a male. She handled the anxiety that accompanied these unacceptable feelings regressively, by becoming agitated, withdrawing into a corner, and masturbating. This allowed her to retreat from an anxiety-provoking situation and to handle her sexual feelings in a less threatening way. The nurse needs to help the client identify what is frightening. The nurse describes the behavior that is occurring and encourages the client to talk about it in a reality-oriented way. The following dialogue illustrates one nursing approach that might be used with Lillian at this time:

NURSE: Hi, Lillian; you look upset. I'd like to sit with you awhile.

LILLIAN: (Silence, no eye contact.)

NURSE: Lillian, I noticed that you become agitated after Bob came up to you. Then I saw you come over here by yourself and begin masturbating. (Pause.) Can you tell me what upset you?

LILLIAN: Don't those men know enough to keep away? I hate them! When they're around, I feel terrible! (Looks angrily at the nurse.)

NURSE: I wonder if, when they approach you, you begin to have feelings that you're uncomfortable about and would rather avoid.

LILLIAN: Sex, sex—that's all that's on their mind. (Maintains eye contact.)

NURSE: Most people think about sex at certain times. Those thoughts or feelings can be upsetting, though, if they're unacceptable to you.

LILLIAN: They're scary feelings. (Pulls down her skirt and has direct eye contact with the nurse, but wrings hands agitatedly.)

NURSE: Lillian, why don't you and I get a cup of tea and talk some more about those scary feelings.

The nurse has described the behavior in a nonjudgmental way which demonstrates acceptance and encourages the client to describe and explore her anxious feelings on a less regressed level.

Regression may also be manifested by clients who have begun to progress or who are approaching discharge. They may suddenly, again, become delusional, withdrawn, or agitated, symbolic in their language, and inappropriate in their responses. The clients may be responding to inner or outer pressure to experience reality more completely. They may be communicating that the rate of progress is too fast or that discharge is approaching too rapidly. They may feel anxious about letting go of entrenched dysfunctional behavior patterns and taking a risk with new ones which, although more functional, are unfamiliar and perhaps more demanding. Clients often need to regress temporarily to a lower, but better-integrated, level of functioning to consider new feelings, thoughts, and behavior, before they feel comfortable enough to move forward again.[60]

When clients' anxiety occurs in relation to increasing independence and responsibility, they need assistance in identifying what is frightening them. It is important for nurses to convey understanding by sharing their perceptions about what is happening and providing opportunities to talk about it. Clients then feel safe and not abandoned. During such episodes, clients may need additional supportive measures such as medication, a low-stimulus environment, and extra one-to-one supervision.

Anxiety may also be manifested by resistance. *Resistance* is the behavioral mode the client uses consciously or unconsciously to avoid anxiety that is provoked when "security operations" are threatened.[61] Nurses' attempts to help clients clarify problems, explore feelings, or examine relationship patterns may be viewed by the clients as anxiety-provoking. Defensive maneuvers, such as resistance, will be utilized to ensure self-protection. Shame, guilt, embarrassment, low self-esteem, and hostility are but a few of the numerous feelings that may cause clients to develop resistance in the nurse-client relationship. The client may utilize resistive maneuvers such as superficiality, changing the subject, focusing on the nurse, becoming delusional, or hearing hallucinatory voices to avoid examination of painful areas of experience. For example:

Jim, a student nurse, had completed a nursing history with a client named Stanley. Stanley had been very cooperative and had supplied Jim with a lot of information. However, as Jim went back to explore significant problem areas, such as Stanley's inability to hold a job for more than 3 months, Stanley asked about Jim's work history, saying "I don't see that this is important, now that I'm in the hospital."

At such times the nurse needs to help the client notice the pattern of resistance and identify what it is that is anxiety-provoking. The nurse can also help the client explore whether the reluctance to share feelings is realistic in light of the nurse-client relationship. Sometimes transference is operating below the level of awareness. When the client feels that the climate for sharing both positive and negative experience is accepting, resistance often dissipates and the client becomes more willing to engage in self-disclosure.

After Jim had explored Stanley's work problem without being judgmental, Stanley said, "I can't believe you didn't put me down. I'm usually so ashamed of the fact that I get uptight on any job. I never want to talk about it because the responses I get from people are only a mirror of my own lousy feelings about myself."

Low self-esteem. The full extent of schizophrenic clients' low self-esteem may become apparent only after nurses have spent time interacting with them. Clients often do not have a coherent sense of identity. They may feel so worthless that they take on the identity of an important figure such as Napoleon or Christ in order to escape from their own identity, which they perceive as worthless. Clients often feel totally unlovable, inadequate, incompetent, and incapable of accomplishment. Such feelings may be derived from negative appraisals of others, rejecting relationships, and actual failures in relationships, school, work, or independent functioning. Poor self-concept pervades clients' experience and prevents them from incorporating positive feedback, expressing their feelings, and accurately assessing their personal strengths and weaknesses.

Guidelines for intervening with clients with low self-esteem include the following:

1. Spend a specified period of time with the client each day in an undemanding way. The nurse and the client may spend the time in comfortable silence. The nurse may provide broad openings for the client to initiate an interaction and may use active listening skills. Doing this indicates interest in and respect for what the client has to say and encourages the client to verbalize thoughts and feelings.
2. Respond to the client's communication in a nonjudgmental way. The nurse needs to convey that the client's thoughts and feelings are neither shocking to the nurse nor different from those of other people. The nurse should give the client permission to express both positive and negative feelings only if he or she is comfortable in hearing what the client has to say, has the time to listen, and is interested. The client may interpret the nurse's discomfort or lack of time or interest as a rejection, which reinforces low self-esteem.
3. Clarify communication that is not understood. When clients feel misunderstood, their self-esteem declines because they interpret misunderstanding as lack of caring. They often think that if people cared, they would try to find out what was really meant.
4. Provide opportunities for the client to experience success in interpersonal relationships. The nurse should gradually expand the client's relationship network. Initially, the client may be able to tolerate relating to the nurse on only a limited basis. The nurse may, over time, introduce the client to another client and act as a role model and facilitator for this relationship. As the client experiences success in this area, the nurse can initiate involvement of the client with other people.
5. Provide opportunities for mastering tasks. The nurse should involve clients in tasks that are structured in increasingly complex ways. Clients need to experience success, and tasks should be introduced in which they can experience success. Clients who experience success will be encouraged to attempt more complex tasks. Dance therapy is an activity which allows clients to experience the body in both positive and negative ways. It provides a vehicle for nonverbal expression of feelings in an accepting climate. Occupational therapy, recreational therapy, art therapy, and on-the-unit jobs and activities also present opportunities for individualized, graded mastery of tasks.
6. Provide opportunities for clients to be involved in hygiene and grooming activities. Personal hygiene is almost always neglected by people with low self-esteem. As stated in an earlier section, the nurse needs to assess clients' ability to complete such activities and supply the appropriate assistance.
7. Provide positive reinforcement for accomplishments in interpersonal relationships or at tasks. This should be given realistically. Too much praise may be regarded as insincere by clients or may be too incompatible with their self-concept to be incorporated as a real aspect of self. The nurse should avoid using words, such as *good, terrific,* or *bad,* that imply a value judgment about what the client has accomplished. Instead, describe the client's behavior. For example, "I think you look neatly dressed today," or "You did that puzzle by yourself."
8. Encourage the client to identify both strengths and weaknesses. This will help the client to modify a predominantly negative self-concept. If the nurse tells the client that a strength has to be identified for each weakness identified, the client may develop a more objective self-view.
9. Provide opportunities for decision making. Clients often feel inadequate about their ability to make decisions and implement them in an independent way. Many clients have been dependent on others for direction and feel unable to manage their lives without guidance. Initially, the nurse must assess the client's readiness in this area. For clients who are having difficulty processing information, choices should be kept to a minimum, because they will not be able to think of alternatives or establish priorities. As they improve, the nurse may engage them in a progressive process related to decision making.

These interventions will enable clients to incorporate positive experiences and feedback and in the process modify their self-concepts in a more positive direction.

Dependency. Dependency is a common problem among schizophrenic clients. It is closely related to low self-esteem in that clients lack confidence in their ability to be self-sufficient. If autonomy and independence have not been encouraged during childhood and patterns of dependency have been reinforced by care givers, clients will feel unable to be self-directing. If early dependency needs have not been met and abandonment is a dominant theme, clients will look to others, in current situations, to meet these unfulfilled needs. When these needs have been accompanied by ambivalence in the care givers, clients may remain confused or uncertain about the extent to which these needs are legitimate. Clients will then lack confidence in the reliability of others or in their willingness to be available to meet these needs.

Nurses strive to help clients become more independent, capable of both self-care and self-direction. Clients are helped to identify their thoughts and feelings. They are encouraged to express them and accept them as their own. For example, the nurse may ask clients, "What do you think about . . . ?" or "How do you feel about . . . ?" Such questions convey the expectation that the client does have ideas and opinions to share with others. The nurse can also focus on themes indirectly expressed by the client such as, "You seem uncertain about your ability to be in charge of your own life." This kind of statement focuses on the theme of dependency and opens it up for exploration in the nurse-client relationship. The nurse can also act as a role model who provides an example of how and when to be appropriately dependent and independent. The nurse may share his or her feelings about a dependence-independence issue. For example, the nurse might say, "I had been trying to make a decision about going back to school. It would have involved moving to another state. I was struggling with the idea of whether I was ready or willing to be totally on my own and separated from my family and friends." Selective use of personal disclosure may illustrate for clients the "normal" struggles most people have and the functional ways in which they resolve such conflicts. Many clients think that dependence and independence are all-or-none situations. Role modeling can help them learn that some of each is appropriate in different circumstances. It can also help them learn how to determine when each is appropriate.

Dependent clients try to cast nurses into a parental role. Rather than assuming this familiar role, nurses must be careful to relate to such clients as adults, conveying the idea that they are mature and capable of managing their own lives. However, clients may try to maintain their dependent position because it is familiar and secure. Becoming more independent carries with it the risk of change and increased self-responsibility which may be anxiety-provoking. They may become demanding and attention-seeking, trying to demonstrate their helplessness. Nurses must resist the urge to act like protective parents. Realistic requests should be consistently met. Limits should be set on inappropriate helplessness and demandingness, while at the same time appropriate behaviors should be identified. For example, "I will not prepare your bath or wash you, Nancy; you can do that yourself. However, I'll be glad to give you a neck massage, if you call me when you're ready." Appropriate behavior such as decision making and self-care should be positively reinforced by staff members with attention, praise, or privileges. Dependent or attention-seeking behavior is ignored, and inappropriate requests are matter-of-factly refused or ignored. Independent behaviors should increase if they are rewarded, and if dependent behavior does not result in gratification of needs.

Dependent clients often have difficulty with decision making. When clients are in the acute phase of a schizophrenic episode, their thoughts and feelings may be so confusing and disorganized that they are totally unable to make any choices or decisions. At times, nurses should minimize the need for decisions. The staff may initially structure clients' time and direct them to whichever activity is appropriate. Even filling out a menu may be too overwhelming for some clients; the array of choices for a whole day may be too much to deal with when clients are being bombarded by thoughts and feelings that they are unable to filter effectively. As clients' disorganization diminishes, the nurse may offer a few limited opportunities to engage in decision making. For example, a client may be asked to choose between two alternatives, "Do you want chicken or roast beef for dinner?" As the client's decision-making ability grows, the nurse helps to identify and evaluate alternatives. The client, reluctant to make decisions or to assume responsibility for their outcome, may try to involve the nurse. The nurse assists in evaluating the pros and cons of each decision and then supports the client's choice.

The client may demonstrate ambivalence in giving up a dependent position. The nurse must support the client's ability to move forward in this area even when the client temporarily regresses.

Social withdrawal. Withdrawn clients do not often respond quickly to nursing intervention. They usually need consistent, repeated approaches by nurses before they become convinced of the nurses' sincere concern. Such clients may be mute and immobile or reclusive. Intervention includes establishment of interpersonal contact, facilitation of communication, and facilitation of social participation.

Communication with withdrawn clients requires a great deal of patience on the part of the nurse. To sit in silence with a mute person can be uncomfortable if one is more accustomed to verbal clients. The nurse may be tempted to fill the silence with trivia or aimless chatter and may also communicate discomfort by fidgeting. The nurse facilitates communication with the client by:

1. Finding out about the client's concerns and using this information as a way of stimulating interest and participation by the client.
2. Avoiding filling up silences by talking about himself or herself, which conveys lack of interest in the client. Constant chatter by the nurse also conveys that the client is not expected to verbalize.
3. Utilizing open-ended questions followed by pauses that provide opportunities for the client to respond.
4. Avoiding direct questions which may be perceived as intimidating or not respectful of the client's privacy.
5. Attending to the client's nonverbal communication. A completely silent client may communicate a great deal through body movements, gestures, and posture. Withdrawn clients may indicate their nonverbal participation in an interaction through establishment of direct eye contact, particularly when it has previously been avoided. Relaxation or alertness in body posture may be a first sign of comfort with the nurse.
6. Using nonverbal methods of communicating with the client. Direct eye contact with the client conveys interest, concern, and caring. Leaning toward the client, but maintaining a comfortable distance, communicates that the nurse's attention is focused on the client. Touch should be used very judiciously with the schizophrenic, who is very mistrustful of any type of closeness. Providing physical care is an important way of conveying concern. Magazines and other objects, food, games, and walks are ways of promoting relatedness in a less demanding way because there is no requirement for verbalization. However, opportunities for talking may evolve out of experiences that both client and nurse have enjoyed.
7. Assisting the client in exploring negative relationships from the past that are influencing the way in which current relationships are perceived. This can help the client to remove distortions in current relationships that arise from transference and gain a more objective view of what is actually happening here and now. Transference can cloud clients' ability to evaluate people in their current life. This frequently occurs when the nurse is miscast by the client in a parental or authority role.

It is important to keep in mind that the client should play a key role in setting the pace for the development of closeness. The one-to-one nurse-client relationship provides the foundation for intervention with the withdrawn client. However, the nurse also strives to help the client to gradually develop social relationships with a variety of other people. As nurse and client become more comfortable with one another, the nurse may gradually include others in social situations with the client. Relatedness must proceed at a pace that meets the client's needs. A group walk, a movie, or an invitation to another client to join a card game allows for relatedness but does not demand communication. When such clients enter groups which have a verbal focus, they may initially need permission to participate on a nonverbal level. As their anxiety decreases, their verbal participation may increase and become more appropriate. At times a nurse may have to help a client withdraw from the group without losing face. Nurses also act as role models for appropriate communication and encourage clients to participate. Nurses must realize that clients need to be encouraged to establish their own standards for relatedness. Some clients may learn more appropriate ways of relating to others but may never feel comfortable in relationship situations; others may elect to lead lives that include few sustained relationships. Nurses should help clients learn to cope with their own choices of lifestyle; nurses should never impose their own values on clients' choices.

Mistrust. Nurses will find that schizophrenic clients display profound mistrust of self, others, and the world around them. When mistrust is most severe, the person experiences a loss of the meaning of life. This can lead to such strong feelings of despair, hopelessness, and withdrawal that the client feels disconnected and dead. An attitude of suspiciousness may be very noticeable in such clients. Mistrust has its origin in early interpersonal relationships which have been experienced as anxiety-laden, threatening, disappointing, and rejecting. Clients develop and utilize defensive strategies such as avoidance, ambivalence, testing, and manipulation to protect themselves from further assault in current relationships.[12]

With such clients, the goal of intervention is to help them establish trust in the nurse. The clients will then, it is hoped, also develop the ability to trust others and find renewed meaning in the surrounding world.[13] Trust can be described as a feeling that others are safe, dependable, and reliable. People demonstrate trust by making themselves accessible to others both physically and emotionally. Clients who do not avoid contact with the nurse and others and who are willing to reveal their thoughts and feelings are demonstrating trusting behavior. Trust develops gradually in any relationship. However, the process may be particularly slow when the client is mistrustful of other people in general.

Reliability and consistency are important factors to consider in trying to establish trust with clients. A sense of relatedness often helps to facilitate a feeling of connectedness and meaning with the client's world as well. When structuring the nurse-client relationship, nurses should be specific about the times and places of meetings. The duration of the relationship should also be outlined whenever possible. Nurses should follow through with the schedule as a way of demonstrating consistency and reliability. Many times clients appear indifferent to the nurse's presence. However, this indifference is often a facade. In fact, it often takes weeks to regain the client's trust when an unavoidable or unexplained absence occurs.

Mistrustful clients are often unable to tolerate prolonged interpersonal contact without becoming anxious. Their anxiety level rises because they anticipate threat or attack in each interpersonal encounter. Nurses may find it effective to schedule several short periods of relationship time spaced throughout the day. This will also reinforce the nurse's reliability in the client's eyes.

Clients interact with a variety of team members in the treatment setting. Assigning one or two staff members to work consistently with a client who has difficulty trusting others is helpful. However, other team members should also be aware of the care plan so that their approach to the client can be consistent with that of the major care givers, in order to promote development of trust in all the care givers.

Nurses must meet clients at their current level of behavior. They must be accepting as well as genuine with clients. Many clients have experienced conditional love, that is, caring attached to a demand or expectation. On the one hand, they are mistrustful of what others want or expect from them, and on the other hand, they have difficulty believing that others might like them for what they are as people. These clients may remain seclusive and unwilling to allow the nurse within their territorial boundaries. Nurses should nevertheless continue to spend time with them. Nurses may often work with clients for months without a smile, a greeting, a word of thanks, or even eye contact. If nurses expect such responses, clients' mistrust may escalate and the expectations of the nurse may seem unrealistic and not respectful of their needs.

Mistrustful clients are also very sensitive to the genuineness of others.[60] They are acutely aware of inauthentic behaviors of others. The nurse may, because a client's reality orientation is poor, think that the client is oblivious to what is occurring in interpersonal encounters. For example:

A student nurse was trying to utilize therapeutic communication skills with a delusional client. She could not understand why he laughed when she spoke to him and then walked away. The client finally told the student that she looked like a robot. She started to say, "No; I'm human like you." He interrupted her, saying, "Dead, mechanical, no life." It took the student some time to figure out that the client was referring to her robotlike, mechanical interpersonal style. When her responses became more natural and spontaneous, the client stopped laughing and walking away.

Honesty is also a component of genuineness. It demonstrates to the client that the nurse can be trusted. The client should be assured of confidentiality. Questions about care should be answered. Clients have a right to be informed about their treatment, to be involved in planning their care, and to know the rationale for any treatment.

The "need-fear dilemma" represents another barrier to trust in the nurse-client relationship. The client simultaneously needs and fears others. The need is derived from dependency requirements. The fear of others is derived from the anticipated threat of abandonment. Consequently, the nurse may observe the client engaging in approach-avoidance behavior. For example:

Dawn, a female client, would be waiting for her primary nurse each day at their appointed meeting time. However, each day for a week Dawn developed a stomachache within 10 minutes of the beginning of the session. She would excuse herself, go to the bathroom, and return 5 minutes before the end of the hour. At that point she would say, "I guess it's time for you to go now. I'll see you tomorrow." The client's feelings of ambivalence led her to look forward to the nurse's arrival each day but also caused her to dread her presence once she arrived.

Clients attempt to deal with the anxiety inherent in relationships by denying the need for relatedness and the accompanying fear of abandonment. For example:

Ray, a male client, had been very receptive when Barbara initially told him that she would be his primary nurse and would spend time working with him each day while he was in the hospital. Barbara thought that Ray was really beginning to trust her, when he suddenly began to miss appointments. His reasons were, "I forgot." "I was napping and forgot to set the alarm." "I was reading and I didn't notice the time. Don't worry, I'll be there tomorrow." He continued to miss appointments several times a week. Barbara brought this problem up at team conference. The staff decided that Ray was probably threatened by the closeness of the relationship. He wanted to relate to Barbara and wanted her help, yet at the same time he feared another disappointment.

Nurses need to realize that approach-avoidance behavior is motivated by conflicting feelings about closeness. Patience, reliability, and perseverance will usually demonstrate their sincerity and trustworthiness to clients. Nurses must also state their observations about the pattern of the approach-avoidance behavior to the client, so that the behavior can be discussed and dealt with in an open, direct way. They should comment on the theme underlying the content of the message. For example:

Barbara stated to Ray, "I noticed that you've missed quite a few sessions lately. I wonder if you have mixed feelings about your sessions with me. Could you describe how you feel when you have been with me for too long?"

Often a client will anticipate impending separations, such as vacations and job changes, and initiate termination before it is begun by others. For example:

One client refused to see his therapist at all before the nurse's scheduled vacation. When asked to explain his behavior, he responded, "I always take my vacations first; then at least I'm ahead of the game."

Consequently, changes in schedule and anticipated absences should be discussed in advance so that opportunities for fantasy about abandonment are minimized.

Testing is another aspect of mistrust. *Testing* refers to the client's attempt to determine the nurse's interest, caring, and sincerity. Clients may test the nurse by engaging in socially unacceptable behavior. For example:

Lillian would, in the initial stages of the nurse-client relationship, sit with her skirt up and masturbate. When that did not disturb the nurse, she would pick at scabs on her face. The nurse, recognizing the purpose of the behavior and its theme, intervened by identifying the behavior. She responded to Lillian by saying, "Are you wondering if you can drive me away with your behavior, or if I'm really being truthful when I say I want to work with you?"

Clients need to find out that nurses will not be put off by attempts to drive then away. As clients accept the nurse's sincerity, testing behavior diminishes.

Clients also test in order to find out if nurses will be scared away or destroyed by their hostility and aggressiveness. For example:

> Tony suddenly became very assaultive one evening, yelling, "Everybody's crowding me." He threw chairs and tables around the dayroom. He was removed by the staff to a quiet room where he was sedated. When his primary nurse, who was working evenings for the week, came into the quiet room where he was resting, Tony avoided eye contact but said, "I could have hurt you badly." His nurse replied, "Yes, Tony, I know that, but it takes a lot more than that to scare me. I wish you would tell me or the staff when you are feeling too closed in. We can help you cope with those feelings." Tony said, "I can't believe you're still talking to me." She said, "Yes, Tony, I am. I'm still counting on working with you."

The nurse can also help mistrustful clients learn how to expand the feeling of trust from the nurse to others. Nurses can help clients identify behaviors that are characteristic of trusting and trustworthy people, and differentiate between trustworthy and untrustworthy people. Clients then become more discriminating about whom to trust. The client who has a reliable set of criteria to follow regarding trustworthiness will feel more secure about initiating and partaking in relationships.

Identity confusion. Identity confusion includes both self-identity and sexual identity. Confusion about *self-identity* evolves from the loss of ego boundaries, that is, the inability to separate self from others or the environment. Anxiety, inconsistent feedback, and the loss of reality-testing skills inhibit the person's ability to formulate an integrated self-concept and define himself or herself as a separate person, a problem reflected in the difficulty the client has in differentiating "good me" from "bad me" and "not me." These factors also limit the degree to which the client is able to distinguish self from the environment and self from others. For example:

> Chris was observed walking around the unit with his arms stretched out in front of him. He looked as if he were unable to see; he seemed to be feeling his way around the dayroom and halls. As he approached a person or a wall, he touched it as if trying to make sure it was there. The nurse approached him to find out what was happening. The nurse said, "Chris, I'm Jay, the nurse. I see your arms stretched out. It looks as though you're trying to feel your way around. Can you tell me what's happening right now?" Chris responded, "It's so gray in here. It's all blended together; I don't know what's me and what's the room. I can't tell anything apart."

When clients demonstrate loss of ego boundaries, nurses can intervene in several ways. First, it is important to address clients by name and let them know who is approaching them. An example of that is the way in which Jay addressed Chris. Second, it is often helpful to orient clients to their surroundings. This defines the boundaries of the environment and provides an orientation about the client's position in that environment. For example, Jay might have said to Chris, "Chris, you are in the dayroom now, you are standing next to the windows, there is a couch next to you. I am Jay, the nurse, and I am standing on your right side. You are Chris C., and I hear you telling me that you are having trouble knowing where you are." Third, the nurse may focus the client on describing his or her perceptions as concretely as possible in order to provide feedback that confirms, in a reality-based way, the client's existence. For example, Jay might say to Chris, "Tell me what you see right now," and then provide feedback about what Jay, the nurse, sees. "I see you, Chris, a young man, dressed in jeans and a blue shirt, sitting on the chair in front of me." Fourth, the nurse should always use pronouns that convey a separation between people. For example, instead of saying, "It's time for our dinner," the nurse should say, "It's six o'clock, and it's time for *you* to go to dinner. *I* am going to walk to the dining room with *you*." This minimizes confusion for the client who does not know where his or her self ends and the nurse's begins. Fifth, some clients may touch other people in order to identify for themselves their separateness from others. The nurse may ask clients if they would like to touch the nurse in order to check out the separateness. Because many clients are frightened of physical closeness, this approach would be utilized following an assessment of the client's tolerance for touch. For other clients, touch only reinforces their sense of fusion with others. In this situation, touch should be avoided, as it would only reinforce identity confusion. When clients improve, nurses may be able to help them to begin sorting out the confusing aspects of their self-concept by encouraging them to describe their perceptions and ideas and to clarify their ideas, and then nurses can provide feedback for clients.

Clients who have never strongly identified with either parent may be confused about their *sexual identity* because of the perpetual rejection they have experienced in those relationships.[2] In addition, they may have had inadequate role models for male or female behavior. Role reversal in the parents may present confusing sex-role models for the child to identify with; that is, the child will have difficulty learning what behavior is normally expected of men and women. Parental expectations about gender-appropriate behavior may also contribute to this confusion.

Nurses can encourage clients to describe their perceptions of themselves as male or female. They can encourage clients to describe their ideas about gender-appropriate behavior and help them explore distortions and their origins. Nurses may need to provide sex education and information about role behavior that may modify clients' distortions and misinformation. Nurses can act as role models for gender-appropriate behavior.

Difficulty testing reality. People with healthy egos are able to differentiate between fantasy and reality most of the time. They utilize logical thinking processes, comparison with past experience, and consensual validation to accurately evaluate the contents of experience. When the ego is overwhelmed with anxiety, the ability to test reality is severely impaired. Behaviors in schizophrenic clients that illustrate loss of reality testing include magical thinking, hallucinations, and delusions.

Schizophrenic clients often indulge in *magical thinking*—that is, they have difficulty differentiating between thought, feeling, and action. They may consider having a thought or a feeling equivalent to acting on it. The nurse needs to help the client distinguish a thought or a feeling from an action. For example:

> A client with intensely hostile feelings toward her husband returned to the hospital from a 1-day pass in a frantic state. She believed that she had poisoned his food when she cooked dinner and was waiting for a telephone call telling her that he had died.

The following conversation took place between this client and the nurse:

NURSE: I know that you have been feeling very angry with your husband for some time now.

CLIENT: I poisoned him. I know he's dead.

NURSE: I hear you saying that you believe you poisoned him and that he is dead.

CLIENT: I know it. I'm waiting for the telephone to ring.

NURSE: Sometimes people feel so angry with others that they think about hurting them.

CLIENT: I know it! I just know it!

NURSE: Thinking of hurting someone doesn't mean you've actually done it.

CLIENT: You think . . . ? (Looks up at the nurse.)

NURSE: Feeling angry is not an unusual experience. It sounds as though your feeling was so strong that you seemed to be acting on it.

CLIENT: It was all so confusing. I couldn't think straight.

NURSE: Why don't I come with you while you call your house and check out what happened?

CLIENT: You think it's OK to do that?

NURSE: Yes. I'll come with you while you make the call.

The nurse acknowledged the client's feeling by verbalizing it aloud. She presented reality by indicating that having thoughts and feelings is not necessarily equivalent to acting them out. The nurse injected doubt about the reality of the client's perceptions, which gave the client the opportunity to consider a different perspective. The nurse acknowledged the healthy aspects of expressing anger; later she could go on to explore other options for expressing feelings. She also provided a way (the telephone call) for the client to consensually validate reality. This let the client know that feelings such as anger do not destroy others. The client's distorted sense of omnipotence was placed in a more realistic perspective as her magical thinking was clarified.

Hallucinations and delusions also represent disruptions in reality testing. They are very real and more vivid to the client than reality-based experiences. During the initial stages of the schizophrenic episode, such experiences may be very frightening and may be accompanied by intense anxiety.

They may be explained by the client as religious experiences. In an effort to defend against a hallucinatory or delusional experience, the client may begin to express interest in spiritual, religious, or philosophical questions, hoping to relieve the intense discomfort of the experience. Hallucinations and delusions tend to diminish or disappear as the client's overall anxiety level decreases. However, many chronic schizophrenic clients continue to have delusions and hallucinations and may learn to cope with them on a day-to-day basis.

In general, the nurse must try to understand the client's private world, what it means, and why the client has retreated into it. When clients sense that the nurse is trying to understand their conflicts, fright, and pain, they become more trusting and confident in the nurse and feel increasingly free to share their perceptions and feelings. The nurse can then become a bridge for the client in defining reality.

Hallucinations reflect a high level of anxiety and a projection of inner thoughts and feelings to objects outside the self. The attitude of the nurse who is interacting with a hallucinating client is very important. The nurse must be accepting and nonjudgmental. Attempts to reason with, argue about, or challenge the client's hallucinatory perceptions only serve to entrench them more firmly. However, the nurse should clearly indicate that the client's sensory perceptions are not shared by others. The nurse, while acknowledging the client's perception, indicates that he or she does not see or hear what the client is perceiving. The following example illustrates how the nurse might respond to a client who is having auditory hallucinations.

NURSE: Sherry, you say that you are hearing voices telling you that the devil is coming to take your baby. I understand that the voice is very real to you, but I don't hear that voice.

SHERRY: But he's saying it to me! I hear him saying he's coming to take my baby when it's born!

NURSE: It sounds as if the voices you say you hear are frightening to you.

SHERRY: I'm scared to death.

The nurse should be careful not to enter the client's hallucinatory world by agreeing with the hallucination. The nurse should cast doubt on the client's perceptions, while at the same time not denying the validity of the perceptions to the client.[8] For example:

> Gerald was standing at the window touching the glass. The nurse went over to him and asked, "How come you are standing there touching the glass?" Gerald replied, "The voices on the radio are telling me to jump. They say test the glass and then jump through." The nurse said, "You say you're hearing voices that make you feel like jumping through the window?"

The nurse would *not* want to say, "Wait a minute. I'll turn down the radio so you won't have to listen to those voices telling you to jump." Such a response would be nontherapeutic because it would serve to consensually validate and reinforce the client's idea that the voices on the radio were "talking" to him. The nurse can also cast doubt on the client's hallucinatory experience by presenting an alternative view of the situation. The client thus has two sets of data and can examine two views objectively, facilitating the possibility of choice. This provides a safe climate in which the client can validate the reality or unreality of the hallucinatory experience.[9]

The nurse tries to identify a pattern in the client's hallucinations. Behavior is rarely random. If it is observed over a period of time, an understanding of it usually emerges. The nurse may be able to gain such an understanding by observing the relationship between daily or special events and the occurrence of the hallucination. Relationship problems may also precipitate the experience. Often, nonverbal behavior such as moving lips or tilting the head to the side in a listening position provides clues that a hallucination is occurring. The nurse can use this behavior to elicit a description of the experience and the events preceding it. The nurse helps the client to make connections between anxiety-producing events or feelings and the hallucination.[9] The following example illustrates this process.

MICHAEL: I had asked this woman for a date, and I don't know what happened. She turned me down.

HELEN: How did you feel when that happened, Michael?

MICHAEL: I don't know.... (Stares wide-eyed at the wall and remains silent.)

HELEN: Michael, listen to me. What are you staring at?

MICHAEL: He's come. I told you he'd come. It's God; he's there on the wall.

HELEN: Michael, look at me. Michael, you and I were talking about the woman who refused to go out with you, and then suddenly you thought you were seeing God.

MICHAEL: (Turns to Helen.) God. I can always depend on him to make me feel better.

HELEN: Michael, is there a connection between being turned down by the woman and seeing God?

MICHAEL: It's funny; it always happens when I'm feeling awful about myself.

Michael's underlying low self-esteem and anxiety about being rejected called into play the hallucinatory image of God who came to confirm Michael's underlying goodness and acceptability. Helen tried to help Michael focus on feelings, situations, and people that evoked anxiety and triggered the hallucinatory experience by responding to the theme underlying his actual experience. Assisting the client to differentiate between long-standing religious beliefs and values, as contrasted with beliefs that have emerged as a result of dysfunctional reality testing, is an important aspect of clarifying the purpose served by the hallucination or delusion.

Encouraging clients to talk about reality-based issues is also helpful. Nurses may discuss current events or other subjects of interest to clients. They may involve clients in concrete activities such as games, exercise, art projects, and jobs which provide a reality-based focus. Clients often say that their auditory hallucinations are most bothersome when they are alone or not occupied. When a nurse sees a client actively hallucinating, it may be possible to distract the client's attention from the experience by saying, for example, "Listen to me; I'm here talking to you. I'm asking you to look at your menu with me right now." In using this technique, the nurse is essentially trying to set up a competing stimulus that is stronger than the hallucination. Another approach is to help clients to devise techniques for decreasing the intensity of their hallucinations. Teaching them to sing when hallucinations occur is one such strategy.[62] For example:

One client hallucinated a little man on his shoulder who talked to him. The client learned that the man would quiet down if he told him to shut up. Eventually, he became able to make the little man recede into the background by flicking his hand at him; the client would then be able to go about his business.

Sometimes clients who are hallucinating feel that they are losing control. At such times the nurse must supply external controls and set firm limits on the client's destructive tendencies. This approach was explained in detail earlier in this chapter, in the section on monitoring the client's safety needs.

Delusions are distorted thought patterns that are not based on a consensually validated view of reality. Nursing intervention with a delusional client requires great sensitivity. Delusional clients are convinced of the reality of their beliefs even though they are contradicted by logical thought and the perceptions of others.

The nurse needs to listen to the clients' descriptions of their thoughts in order to determine whether they are valid. Culturally determined thoughts and perceptions are sometimes interpreted by staff members as delusional or hallucinatory experiences. Such seemingly false beliefs should be validated with the family or others from that person's culture for accuracy.

The nurse's communication should avoid supporting and reinforcing the client's delusion. However, the nurse should not attempt to attack or challenge the delusion. This would strip the client of a necessary defense against overwhelming anxiety and might precipitate an outburst of uncontrolled assaultive behavior. Rational explanations will only make these clients adhere more firmly to their delusions. Instead, nurses may cast doubt on the validity of the clients' thoughts. For example, a client who expresses fear that someone is plotting to kill him may be able to listen to a nurse who responds by saying, "I sense that you are feeling frightened right now. You are safe on the hospital unit. I would like to spend time talking with you about the concerns you have that are frightening you right now." This shifts the focus from the imaginary killer to the client's real fears and concerns. As the client's anxiety level decreases, the delusion dissipates. The client needs to be helped to relinquish the delusion without losing face. The following example illustrates the client's growing awareness of the unreal quality of the delusion and the nurse's role in facilitating this process.

GERRY: I remember that when I first came here, I thought I was God. I heard voices, too. It feels like part of a different person.

NURSE: When you first came here, you felt very negative about yourself. Your identification with God was a way of eliminating those feelings. Now that you're understanding yourself better, you are able to look at yourself in different ways.

Some clients have well-entrenched delusional systems which never disappear. However, they may be able to function effectively in the community if the delusions remain nonthreatening and if they can learn not to talk about them except with people who are tolerant of their thoughts.

Delusions usually have a symbolic meaning for clients which may exist on an unconscious level. Unacceptable feelings relating to powerlessness, loss of self-esteem, inadequacy, sexuality, and anger are projected onto others or the environment, and thus the anxiety that accompanies these feelings is decreased. The nurse should respond to the theme that underlies the content of the message. For example, if a client talks about being God, the nurse may respond to the theme by saying, "It sounds as though it's important to you to feel powerful. I wonder how powerful you would feel as a regular person." This shifts the interaction to the real feelings that underlie the delusion and encourages the client to explore the purpose served by the delusion. In this example, the delusion increases the client's feelings of power and self-esteem.

Delusional clients are frequently suspicious. It is important to talk to them directly using clear, concrete terminology. This will minimize ambiguities and distortions in communication, which in turn will minimize opportunities for clients to think that they are being talked about. It will also encourage consensual validation.

The nurse should also focus the client on reality-oriented, unambiguous feelings that provide opportunities for success and positive appraisal which will realistically increase ego strength. When engaged in concrete tasks, the client will have less time to dwell on delusional thoughts. However, clients with delusions of grandeur may wish to participate in tasks or activities that may exceed their current capacity. Accomplishment of graded tasks may be more appropriate. Suspicious clients do better in activities which involve minimum levels of competition and which prevent them from dominating others. Such clients are forever trying to be "one up" on others and cannot tolerate losing. The nurse often has to help such clients gain satisfaction without losing face.

Interventions with the Family

Nurses have opportunities to intervene with clients and their families in different ways. Initially, family therapy sessions may not be appropriate. Severe disruption of cognitive, perceptual, and affective processes may make it difficult for a client to deal with the array of stimuli in a family session. Such a session might reinforce feelings of confusion and inadequacy. However, family therapy is viewed by many as crucial to the client's reintegration with the family and the community. It should be initiated as soon as the client's reality orientation improves, and it can be continued on an outpatient basis when the client returns to the community. Intervention includes providing support for family members, repatterning family communication patterns and role relationships, and expanding family and community support systems.[21,63,64]

Families experience a variety of feelings when a member has a schizophrenic episode. They may feel guilty about and take responsibility for the client's situation. The attitude of self-blame may be reinforced by what they have read or heard about parents "causing" psychosis in their children by faulty parenting. This perspective has little or no validity, because no parent intentionally "causes" a child to become psychotic. The nurse can intervene by remaining nonjudgmental and by redefining the problem as one for which nobody is individually responsible, but one in which each family member has participated in some way. This perspective distributes the responsibility more equally and alleviates the burden of responsibility on any one family member. It also equalizes the responsibility for changing things. When family members feel accepted by the nurse, they do not feel attacked or have to become defensive. They are thus receptive to change.

Family members may also exhaust their tolerance for one another and feel angry about the schizophrenic client's inability to cope. This is particularly true when the episode is not the client's first. The nurse needs to provide opportunities for families to express their feelings in an accepting climate. The nurse can also empathize with the upheaval created by the hospitalization of a member. This approach allows the intensity of these feelings to diminish so that when client and family encounter one another, they are not driven apart by a wall of hostility.

Family communication patterns may be characterized by indirect communication and lack of individuality. For example, a mother may approach the nurse who is providing family intervention and say, "I want to tell you about my son; but don't tell him I told you this, or he'll be angry." Becoming involved in the family's indirect communication patterns by agreeing to keep secrets can result in loss of the client's trust and does not provide a role model for open, direct communication. The nurse should encourage the mother to share the information in the presence of her son or not at all.

Another indirect communication pattern is the double-bind message. Family members will simultaneously communicate two messages which contradict one another. The person who receives the message will be confused about which message is intended and will not know how to respond. For example:

> David W., age 22, is being visited by his parents. When they enter the room, the mother smilingly says, "Aren't you delighted to see us, David?" As David says, "Yes, I am," and moves toward his mother to kiss her, she turns toward her husband with a frown and comments on the drab decoration of the unit. David withdraws and begins hallucinating.

The mother's initial message was, "Be glad to have a visit from your parents." However, when David tried to demonstrate his gladness, the second message, "I'm not glad to see you; don't come close," was communicated nonverbally as she turned away from David and spoke to her husband. This second message was reinforced by her remarks about the drabness of the unit, which could be interpreted as a way of scolding the son, whose illness was responsible for her being there.

The nurse, when dealing with family double-bind communication patterns, states observations about the communication process to highlight the lack of congruence and the difficulties inherent in responding to them. In the example above, the nurse might say, "I am hearing two messages at the same time. On one hand, you're saying, 'Aren't you glad to see us?' But on the other hand, when he responds in a positive way, you turn away from him." The nurse would then encourage each family member to clarify what he or she really means. The nurse would also point out how this communication leads to dysfunctional behavior. Describing David's withdrawal and hallucinatory behavior following that message would be a way of highlighting the situation for the family. The nurse also acts as a role model of clear, unambiguous communication.

Family communication may also reflect a lack of separateness or individuality that evolves from low levels of differentiation. People may speak for one another; one person may be the family switchboard or spokesperson, the one through whom all messages are funneled, the one who talks for the whole family. Communication may also have a "we" quality to it; that is, individual opinions are not expressed. One member may say, for instance, "We feel that Fred is not ready to move into a halfway house," without bothering to validate this thought with other family members. The nurse can deal with this by asking each family member to share his or her ideas or feelings and encouraging the use of the pronoun "I" saying, for example, "Fred, how do you feel about what your mother said?" If Fred's mother interrupts to answer for him, the nurse might say, "I've already heard what you think. Now I'd like to know what Fred and other people in the family are thinking, so please sit back and let each person speak. Then I'll be happy to listen to some more of your ideas." The nurse attempts to have the family focus on a topic until its meaning is shared by all family members.

Nurses help the families explore dysfunctional relationship patterns and identify ways in which they can be redefined. Nurses may intervene in structural ways to redistribute relationship patterns by redefining and clarifying boundaries. For example, seating may be restructured in order to separate an overclose parent and child and move a distant parent and child together. Relationship tasks such as having the distant parent take charge of the dysfunctional child would move the father, for example, closer so that he will be in a more active position, while moving the mother to a more distant, less involved position. A husband and wife might be instructed to spend a day together without their children in order to strengthen the marital boundary. Exploring protectiveness and devising ways to initiate growth and independence are difficult when dysfunctional patterns have been entrenched for long periods of time. However, nurses do have opportunities to offer help even under such circumstances. For example, they can encourage parents to support their child, the client, in a decision to move to a group home. Supporting the family as they "let go" of the client and helping them develop alternative sources of gratification are important; otherwise they will find ways to sabotage the client's progress in order to restore the family balance.

Intensity of relatedness characterizes many families with schizophrenic members. Such a family is frequently an overly close unit that has little or no connectedness with the extended family and also lacks a social or community network. This reinforces the family members' need for one another and contributes to an isolated, restricted lifestyle. The nurse can assist family members in establishing connections with community resources for help and socialization. Extended family cutoffs can be explored, and distances between family members can begin to be bridged. These support systems provide new relationships for the family at a time when they are trying to modify their interaction patterns to promote growth. (See Chapter 19.)

Interventions with the Community

A major form of community intervention focuses on lowering the incidence of schizophrenia in the general population, particularly high-risk groups. Outreach programs designed to identify such target populations in communities are very important. Once high-risk families are identified, they can be involved in a variety of programs that promote health. These programs are designed to increase people's capacity for caring for themselves, to improve their problem-solving skills, and to help them identify options for improving their lives. Following are examples of such programs:

1. Health maintenance programs provide periodic physical and mental health screenings that are designed to promote physical and mental health and provide early diagnosis of health problems. This is particularly important for high-risk groups. Both assessment of health needs and education about health are appropriate.
2. Parent education classes develop a knowledge base for parents who wish or need to enhance their parenting skills. These classes provide anticipatory guidance in relation to developmental patterns, appropriate stimulation and play modalities, setting limits, resolving conflicts, and parent-child interaction (see Chapter 47).
3. Community support programs help to strengthen support systems for both individuals and families. Among the groups that sponsor such programs are civic, social, educational, recreational, and religious organizations. Big Brother and Big Sister programs, newcomers' clubs, and the Boy Scouts and Girl Scouts are specific examples of programs that increase resources for family involvement in communities. Community agencies may also provide resources for individuals and families. Schools are another supportive community resource.
4. Community action programs can be effective in modifying the individual, family, or community environment. Inadequate housing, sanitation, nutrition, and employment are external stressors that contribute to problems in daily living and that should be priority items for social intervention. Additionally, some families need help in changing their home environment, to create order as opposed to chaos. Education about schedules, routines, and organization may help such families move toward more constructive self-direction.

Nurses may act as coordinators of primary prevention services or as liaisons between the family, the individual, and one or more community agencies. They may also play roles involving direct teaching, counseling, or technical activities in the delivery of primary-prevention health care.

Another important aspect of community intervention is planning for discharge from the hospital. When clients have acute schizophrenic episodes, the goal of treatment is to restore functioning at the clients' maximum level of health and to return them to the community. Planning for discharge begins when a client enters the treatment setting. Following an initial schizophrenic episode, it is likely that plans will focus on facilitating the client's return to family, work, or school. Modifications in work or school patterns are sometimes, but not always, necessary. For example, a client who has attended an out-of-town college may be encouraged to attend a local college for one semester and carry 9 credits instead of 15 in order to minimize external stressors. Alterations in family relationship patterns may be worked on in family therapy after discharge.

Plans for discharge may also include individual outpatient therapy so that the client can continue to work on individual problems. The first visits with the therapist, to get the client involved in that relationship, should ideally occur before discharge. Finally, referral to and initial contact with other community agencies, such as a medication clinic, a community support group, or Alcoholics Anonymous, is also part of the planning. Regardless of the specific needs of the client, nurses must remember that the transition from hospital to community is not easy. Efficient and comprehensive planning for adequate support systems will enhance the potential for success in reintegrating the client into the community.

People who have chronic schizophrenia and are considered chronically mentally ill may have a pattern of alternating hospitalization, treatment in outpatient community programs, and living with their families or alone without treatment. Community health nurses are often the professionals most intimately involved in the care of such clients. Chapter 53 provides extensive discussions of the chronic mentally ill in the community and the role of the nurse in working with such clients and their families.

Evaluation

Evaluation of the nursing care plan is important with schizophrenic clients who have experienced disintegration of so many aspects of themselves. Because they feel so overwhelmed by their alterations in thoughts, perceptions, affect, and behavior, documenting progress is valuable to the client. Nurses may also feel overwhelmed by the task of helping the client reintegrate the self. Since progress is often subtle and slow, evaluation that provides a realistic perspective on clients' accomplishments is valuable to nurses.

The following example shows how the evaluation process is used to appraise the effectiveness of nursing care for Richard N., a schizophrenic client exhibiting mistrust of himself and others (see Table 37-9, page 768):

> Richard N., a 25-year-old man, has been increasingly socially withdrawn. He states that people are not to be trusted; they want to "do him in." Recently he has been hearing voices which tell him that others are plotting against him and that he should not rely on or trust anybody. When Richard did not report to work for 3 days, his boss called him, and Richard said that he couldn't come to work because he couldn't trust anybody with whom he worked. His boss then called Richard's mother, who arranged for him to be admitted to the psychiatric unit of the general hospital. In the hospital, he has remained reclusive, sitting in his room muttering to himself about the evil that people are planning for him. The primary nurse assigned to Richard establishes a nursing goal of increasing his level of trust.

As new information about a schizophrenic client becomes available and as behavior changes, the assessment, diagnosis, and goals are refined. This process will be affected by the nurse's observations as well as by feedback from the client, the family, others in the client's support systems, and colleagues. The nursing care plan is modified as the nurse-client relationship grows and the client moves toward his or her optimal level of health.

SUMMARY

People who experience an overwhelming degree of anxiety and whose coping mechanisms fail to maintain their anxiety at a tolerable level may feel that they have lost control of their perceptions, thoughts, feelings, and behavior. A massive disintegration of ego functioning occurs, causing the person to be unable to deal effectively with self, others, and the environment. Patterns of dysfunctional reality orientation ensue. This chapter focuses on schizophrenia, one of the disintegrative patterns that occurs in psychosis.

Schizophrenia is characterized by perceptual, cognitive, affective, motor, and social changes. The person's patterns of interaction include biological and psychosocial theories that attempt to explain the development of schizophrenia. Family and environmental patterns of interaction also contribute to the development of schizophrenia. However, no single pattern has been identified as the underlying

Table 37-9 Evaluation for Richard N.

Assessment	Diagnosis	Outcomes	Intervention	Evaluation
Richard N. states that people are not to be trusted. He states that people want to "do him in." He reports that he has been hearing voices which tell him that others are plotting against him; they will get him and destroy him, and it's only a question of time. Richard remains in his room. He refuses to interact with staff or other clients on the unit. He states, "You are all dangerous."	Isolation of self from others related to mistrust	Richard will tolerate interaction with others, as evidenced by: 1. Consenting to allow the primary nurses to spend 10 minutes nonverbally sitting with him on each shift. 2. Verbally identifying times when relatedness is anxiety-provoking. 3. After 2 weeks, attending meals in the unit dining room. 4. Within 1 week, attending a group therapy session accompanied by the primary nurse and observing the meeting. 5. Within 2 weeks, attending group therapy sessions unaccompanied by the nurse and responding when spoken to. 6. Allowing another client on the unit to approach and talk to him without withdrawing.	1. Define the boundaries of the relationship for the client. 2. Be consistent and reliable about meeting with client at appointed time. 3. Use specific and concrete language. 4. Verbalize the implied contract and state observations about client's behavior. 5. Set limits on the client's attempts to reject the nurse. 6. Set up graduated contact with others on the unit. 7. Proceed at the client's pace. 8. Encourage evaluation of interpersonal experiences.	1. At the end of three sessions, Richard accepts the nurse's presence in his room without attempting to have her leave. 2. At the end of 8 days, the client begins eating in the unit dining room. 3. At the end of 1 week, the client begins attending group therapy but does not participate verbally. 4. At the end of 13 days, the client responds verbally when addressed by the therapist. 5. At the end of 3 weeks, Richard accompanies another client to music therapy when invited. 6. Richard verbally identifies sources of his mistrust.

significant factor in the development of this health problem.

In their encounters with schizophrenic clients, nurses assess the individual, the family, and the environment. Nursing diagnoses and outcome criteria reflect the clients' problems and strengths. Intervention is directed toward creating a therapeutic environment and monitoring clients' physical and safety needs. Problems related to anxiety, low self-esteem, dependency, social withdrawal, mistrust, identity confusion, and difficulty testing reality are addressed, as are family and community interventions. Evaluation provides a means of documenting and appraising clients' progress.

REFERENCES

1. Max Day and Elvin Semrad, "Schizophrenic Reactions," in A. M. Nichol, Jr., ed., *The Harvard Guide to Modern Psychiatry*, Belknap Press of Harvard University Press, Cambridge, Mass., 1978.
2. Silvano Arieti, *Interpretation of Schizophrenia*, 2d ed., Basic Books, New York, 1974.
3. M. Feffer, "Symptom Expression as a Factor in Decoding," *Psychological Review*, vol. 74, 1967, pp. 16–28.
4. L. J. Chapman and J. Chapman, *Thought in Schizophrenia*, Prentice-Hall, Englewood Cliffs, N.J., 1973.
5. R. W. Payne, "The Measurement and Significance of Overinclusive Thinking and Retardation in Schizo-

phrenic Patients," in H. Hach and I. Zubin, eds., *Psychopathology of Schizophrenia*, Grune and Stratton, New York, 1966.
6. A. H. Chapman, *Textbook of Clinical Psychiatry: An Interpersonal Approach*, 2d ed., Lippincott, Philadelphia, 1976.
7. B. Bloodstein, *Speech Pathology*, Houghton Mifflin, Boston, 1979.
8. K. H. Gavenkemper, "Hallucinations," in Shirley F. Burd and Margaret A. Marshall, eds., *Some Clinical Approaches to Psychiatric Nursing*, Macmillan, New York, 1963, pp. 184–188.
9. Sylvia Schwartzman, "The Hallucinating Patient and Nursing Intervention," *Journal of Psychiatric Nursing and Mental Health Services*, vol. 13, no. 6, 1975, pp. 23–36.
10. Janice Clark, "An Interpersonal Technique for Handling Hallucinations," in *Nursing Care of the Disoriented Patient*, Monograph 13, American Nurses Association, New York, pp. 16–26.
11. Mimi Dye, "Sexual Identity Confusion and Treatment of Schizophrenic Patients," unpublished paper, 1980.
12. W. M. Mendel, "Phenomenological Theory of Schizophrenia," in A. Byrton, J. J. Lopez-Iber, and W. M. Mendel, eds., *Schizophrenia as a Lifestyle*, Springer, New York, 1974.
13. A. E. Scheflin, *Levels of Schizophrenia*, Brunner/Mazel, New York, 1981.
14. G. Bateson et al., "Towards a Theory of Schizophrenia," *Behavioral Science*, vol. 1, 1956, pp. 251–264.
15. H. S. Sullivan, *The Interpersonal Theory of Psychiatry*, Norton, New York, 1953.
16. Norman Cameron, *Personality Development and Psychopathology*, Houghton Mifflin, Boston, 1963.
17. Frieda Fromm-Reichmann, "Loneliness," *Psychiatry*, vol. 22, 1959, pp. 1–13.
18. Hildegarde Peplau, "Loneliness," *American Journal of Nursing*, vol. 55, December 1955, pp. 1476–1481.
19. P. H. Lieberman, "Pathological Loneliness: A Psychodynamic Interpretation," in J. Hartog, J. R. Audy, and Y. A. Cohen, eds., *The Anatomy of Loneliness*, International Universities Press, New York, 1980, pp. 377–393.
20. D. Burnham, A. J. Gladstone, and R. W. Gibson, *Schizophrenia and the Need-Fear Dilemma*, International Universities Press, New York, 1969.
21. Murray Bowen, "A Family Concept of Schizophrenia," in M. Bowen, ed., *Family Therapy in Clinical Practice*, Aronson, New York, 1978, pp. 45–70.
22. American Psychiatric Association, *Diagnostic and Statistical Manual of Mental Disorders*, 3d ed., APA, Washington, D.C., 1980.
23. J. S. Strauss et al., "What Is Schizophrenia?" *Schizophrenia Bulletin*, vol. 9, no. 3, 1983, pp. 331–333.
24. P. O'Brien, *The Disordered Mind*, Prentice-Hall, Englewood Cliffs, N.J., 1978.
25. D. M. Turns, "The Epidemiology of Schizophrenia," in H. C. Denber, ed., *Schizophrenia: Theory, Diagnosis, and Treatment*, Dekker, New York, 1978.
26. J. E. Cooper et al., *Psychiatric Diagnosis in New York and London*, Oxford University Press, London, 1972.
27. E. Bleuler, *Textbook of Psychiatry*, Macmillan, New York, 1924.
28. H. E. Lehmann, "Schizophrenia: Clinical Features," in H. I. Kaplan and B. J. Sadock, eds., *Comprehensive Textbook of Psychiatry*, 4th ed., Williams and Wilkins, Baltimore, Md., 1985.
29. World Health Organization, *Report of the International Pilot Study of Schizophrenia. Vol. 1: Results of the Initial Evaluation Phase*, WHO, Geneva, Switzerland, 1973.
30. World Health Organization, *Schizophrenia: An International Follow-up Study*, Wiley, New York, 1979.
31. M. L. Kohn, "Social Class and Schizophrenia, A Critical Review and a Redefinition," *Schizophrenia Bulletin*, vol. 7, 1973, pp. 60–79.
32. H. W. Dunham, "Society, Culture and Mental Disorders," *Archives of General Psychiatry*, vol. 33, 1976, pp. 147–156.
33. M. Katz et al., "Ethnic Studies in Hawaii: On Psychopathology and Social Deviance," in L. C. Wynne, R. L. Cromwell, and S. Matthysse, eds., *The Nature of Schizophrenia*, Wiley, New York, 1978, pp. 572–585.
34. H. M. Babigian, "Schizophrenia: Epidemiology" in A. M. Freedman et al., eds., *Comprehensive Textbook of Psychiatry*, 3d ed., Williams and Wilkins, Baltimore, Md., 1980.
35. A. W. Loranger, "Sex Difference in Age at Onset of Schizophrenia," *Archives of General Psychiatry*, vol. 41, no. 2, 1984, pp. 157–161.
36. M. Foucault, *Madness and Civilization*, Vintage, New York, 1973.
37. K. S. Kendler and C. D. Robinette, "Schizophrenia in the National Academy of Sciences—National Research Council Twin Registry: A 16-Year Update," *American Journal of Psychiatry*, vol. 140, no. 12, 1983, pp. 1551–1563.
38. K. S. Kendler, "Overview: A Current Perspective on Twin Studies in Schizophrenia," *American Journal of Psychiatry*, vol. 140, no. 11, 1983, pp. 1413–1425.
39. R. Abrams and M. A. Taylor, "The Genetics of Schizophrenia: A Reassessment Using Modern Criteria," *American Journal of Psychiatry*, vol. 140, no. 2, 1983, pp. 171–175.
40. S. Kety et al., "The Biological and Adoptive Families of Adopted Individuals Who Become Schizophrenic: Prevalence of Mental Illness and Other Characteristics," in L. C. Wynne, R. L. Cromwell, and S. Matthysse,

eds., *The Nature of Schizophrenia,* Wiley, New York, 1978, pp. 25–37.

41. E. Kringlen, "Adult Offspring of Two Psychotic Parents with Special Reference to Schizophrenia," in L. C. Wynne, R. L. Cromwell, and S. Matthysse, eds., *The Nature of Schizophrenia,* Wiley, New York, 1978, pp. 9–24.
42. Robert Cancro, "The Genetic Studies of the Schizophrenia Syndrome: A Review of Their Clinical Implications," in L. Bellak, ed., *Disorders of the Schizophrenic Syndrome,* Basic Books, New York, 1979, pp. 136–151.
43. H. Y. Meltzer, "Biochemical Studies in Schizophrenia," in L. Bellak, ed., *Disorders of the Schizophrenic Syndrome,* Basic Books, New York, 1979.
44. H. Weiner, "Schizophrenia: Etiology," in H. I. Kaplan and B. J. Sadock, eds., *Comprehensive Textbook of Psychiatry,* 4th ed., Williams and Wilkins, Baltimore, Md., 1985.
45. S. H. Snyder, "Dopamine and Schizophrenia," in L. C. Wynne, R. L. Cromwell, and S. Matthysse, eds., *The Nature of Schizophrenia,* Wiley, New York, 1978, pp. 87–94.
46. R. Gruen et al., "Platelet MAO Activity and Schizophrenic Prognosis," *American Journal of Psychiatry,* vol. 139, 1980, pp. 240–246.
47. A. K. Pandurangi et al., "The Ventricular System in Chronic Schizophrenic Patients: A Controlled Computed Tomography Study," *British Journal of Psychiatry,* vol. 144, 1984, pp. 172–176.
48. N. Piran et al., "Motoric Laterality and Eye Dominance Suggest Unique Patterns of Cerebral Organization in Schizophrenia," *Archives of General Psychiatry,* vol. 39, 1982, pp. 1006–1009.
49. H. I. Kaplan and B. J. Sadock, eds., *Comprehensive Textbook of Psychiatry,* 4th ed, Williams and Wilkins, Baltimore, 1985.
50. L. George and R. W. J. Neufeld, "Cognition and Symptomatology in Schizophrenia," *Schizophrenia Bulletin,* vol. 11, no. 2, 1985, pp. 264–282.
51. M. A. Taylor and R. Abrams, "Cognitive Impairment in Schizophrenia," *American Journal of Psychiatry,* vol. 141, no. 2, 1984, pp. 196–201.
52. R. L. Cromwell, "Attention and Information Processing: A Foundation for Understanding Schizophrenia," in L. C. Wynne, R. L. Cromwell, and S. Matthysse, eds., *The Nature of Schizophrenia,* Wiley, New York, pp. 219–224.
53. A. McGhie and J. Chapman, "Disorder of Attention and Perception in Early Schizophrenia," *British Journal of Medical Psychiatry,* vol. 34, 1961, pp. 103–116.
54. L. S. Kubie, "Multiple Fallacies in the Concept of Schizophrenia," in P. Doncert and G. Lauren, eds., *Problems of Psychosis Excerpta Medica,* The Hague, Netherlands, 1971.
55. M. Foucault, *Madness and Civilization,* Vintage, New York, 1973.
56. T. Szasz, *The Myth of Mental Illness,* Harper and Row, New York, 1974.
57. R. D. Laing, *The Divided Self,* Penguin, Baltimore, 1965.
58. M. K. Opler, *Culture, Society, and Human Values,* Thomas, Springfield, Ill., 1956.
59. Helen Kreigh and Joanne Perko, *Psychiatric and Mental Health Nursing,* Reston, Va., 1979.
60. Frieda Fromm-Reichmann, *Principles of Intensive Psychotherapy,* University of Chicago Press, Chicago, 1950.
61. Alice Stueks, "Resistance," in Shirley F. Burd and Margaret A. Marshall, eds., *Some Clinical Approaches to Psychiatric Nursing,* Macmillan, New York, 1963, pp. 96–104.
62. W. E. Field and W. Ruelke, "Hallucinations and How to Deal with Them," *American Journal of Nursing,* vol. 73, 1973, p. 638.
63. L. P. Mosher and J. G. Gunderson, "Group, Family, Milieu and Community Support Systems for Schizophrenia," in L. Bellak, ed., *Disorders of the Schizophrenic Syndrome,* Basic Books, New York, 1979, pp. 399–452.
64. C. Christian Beels, "Family and Social Management of Schizophrenia," in Philip J. Guerin, Jr., ed., *Family Therapy: Theory and Practice,* Gardner, New York, 1976, pp. 249–283.

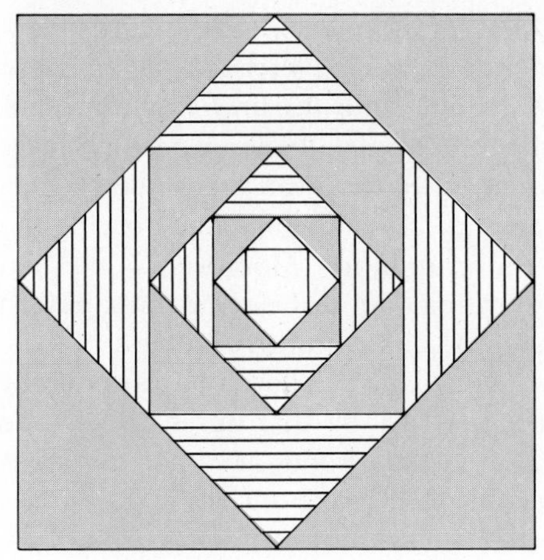

CHAPTER 38
Patterns of Sexual Dysfunction

Anita M. Leach

LEARNING OBJECTIVES

After studying this chapter, the student should be able to:

1. Discuss the individual, family, and environmental dynamics of dysfunctional sexual disorders.
2. Identify assessment factors for clients with sexual disorders.
3. Formulate nursing diagnoses and individualized goals for clients with sexual difficulties.
4. Discuss the techniques used in sex therapy.
5. Construct a nursing care plan for clients with sexual difficulties.

Problematic sexual behavior is behavior that precludes adult sexual relationships, is harmful to oneself or one's partner, or requires a victim. Since the three dimensions of the person—mind, body, and spirit—are involved in sexual expression, it cannot be seen merely as a way of meeting a physical or bodily need; the whole person is involved. The ability to differentiate lust from sexual intimacy evolves as one engages in meaningful relationships.

Sexual expression is not merely a genital act but is governed by thoughts, emotions, and the spiritual dimension. Using this framework, sexual deviation might be viewed as sexual expression that is out of balance—bodily or genital expression which excludes the emotional and spiritual dimensions. Deviations may also be seen as variations from heterosexual vaginal-penile intercourse.

The purpose of this chapter is to acquaint nursing students with sexual deviations. The nursing care of clients with gender identify disorders, paraphilias, and psychosexual dysfunctions will be discussed using the classifications of the *Diagnostic and Statistical Manual of Mental Disorders* (DSM III).

DYSYNCHRONOUS HEALTH PATTERNS

It is difficult to define normal sexual behavior. Any sexual act between adults that is consensual, does not involve force, and is performed in private, away from unwilling observers, should be considered normal. The key concepts here are *adult, privacy, consent,* and *absence of force.*[1] One might also view sexual behavior on a continuum, allowing for all the possible variations. Variations in sexual behavior are caused by biological factors; environment; and historical, social, spiritual, and cultural influences affecting each person's development. People who exhibit dysfunctional behavior are on a continuum from "not so sick" to "very sick," depending on their own experiences and those of the health care professionals with whom they come into contact.

The person to whom a specific *paraphilia* is ascribed has a personality structure which evolves from acts that are out of balance. For such people, sexual relationships involve only the sexual part of the self, rather than the whole person. Their sexual behavior is labeled *deviant* or "very sick." Generally, such clients indulge in unacceptable heterosexual acts in the hope of proving their sexual mastery and relieving anxiety, only to find that they are overwhelmed by the sexual object or partner: their anxiety is increased rather than alleviated. A perverse sexual act may also generate guilt, leaving the person even more unhappy. Moreover, a planned act of perversion may fail to be consummated on its own terms and thus result in shame and frustration. Clients who engage in deviant acts generally come to the attention of the nurse when the depersonalization that frequently accompanies perversion results in a psychotic episode, or the client develops a neurotic symptom such as hysterical paralysis or phobic aversion as a result of inhibition of the deviant behavior. Withdrawal is also used as a mode of dealing with paraphiliac acts, particularly when there are powerful family or environmental pressures.

The label *gender identity disorders* is used for clients who act out confusion about and incongruence between their subjective sexual feelings and their biological sexual identities. At one end of the continuum are clients who choose transsexual surgery; at the other end are those who experience developmental and fleeting confusion about sexual identity. The underlying dynamics of people who habitually cross-dress and people who choose transsexual surgery are believed to be early structuring of behavior by specific cross-sexual environmental influences, adoption of ritual acts to alleviate anxiety and escape the censure of the superego, and patterns of regressive, dysfunctional responses to stress.

Theoretically, *ego-dystonic homosexuality* also develops from underlying intrapsychic and interpersonal dynamics. A distinction is made between discomfort with a homosexual orientation and individual homosexual acts. People who become aware of, but are unhappy with, an orientation toward homosexuality either act out in ways that are incongruent with personal, family, or social values, or abstain from any sexual activity. For those who act out homosexual desires, discomfort generally takes the form of guilt, high levels of anxiety, and psychotic symptoms such as delusions or hallucinations. Those who choose to abstain from sexual activity and remain celibate may engage in meaningful relationships that stop short of sexual expression, or they may withdraw from any social contact. People who withdraw generally enter the health care system because of difficulties dealing with loneliness, depression, anxiety, or stress.

The term *sexual dysfunction* is used for clients whose subjective expectations about the sexual act and sexual enjoyment are incongruent with the reality they experience. Marital conflict is the most common underlying cause of sexual dysfunction, although physiological problems cause the greatest number of clients to seek out mental health care professionals. Sexual dysfunction may be transitory (as it is likely to be when marital discord exists) or permanent (for example, when it is caused by a spinal cord injury).

DSM III

The American Psychiatric Association's Task Force on Nomenclature and Statistics published DSM III in 1980. In DSM III, psychosexual disorders are divided into four groups: (1) *gender identity disorders,* (2) *paraphilias,* (3) *psychosexual dysfunctions,* and (4) *other psychosexual disorders,* which includes the classification *ego-dystonic homosexuality.*[2] (In this chapter, these will be taken up in the following order: gender identity disorders, ego-dystonic homosexuality, paraphilias, psychosexual dysfunctions.)

Gender identity disorders are characterized by incongruence between a person's biological sexual identity and subjective feelings about it. The gender identity disorder discussed in this chapter is transsexualism.[2]

DSM III categorizes ego-dystonic homosexuality with other psychosexual disorders. Ego-dystonic homosexuality is characterized by a sustained pattern of homosexual arousal which the client explicitly states is unwanted and which is a persistent source of distress.[2]

The paraphilias—sometimes referred to as *sexual deviations*—involve sexual arousal in response to sexual imagery or acts other than those generally considered normal in the society. DSM III categorizes fetishism, transvestism, zoophilia, pedophilia, exhibitionism, voyeurism, sexual masochism and sadism, and atypical acts as paraphilias.[2]

A sexual dysfunction is a psychosomatic disorder which makes it impossible to have or enjoy coitus. Both sexes may experience inhibited sexual desire or dyspareunia (pain associated with coitus).[2] DSM III classifies psychosexual disorders as inhibited sexual desire (ISD), inhibited sexual excitement (frigidity and impotence), inhibited female orgasm (orgasmic dysfunction), inhibited male orgasm (retarded ejaculation or ejaculatory incompetence), premature ejaculation, functional vaginismus, functional dyspareunia, and atypical psychosexual dysfunction.[2]

Epidemiology

The reported incidence of dysfunctional and deviant sexual behaviors does not accurately reflect the pervasiveness of the problems. Among factors that contribute to the difficulty of obtaining accurate statistics are the infrequency with which deviant sexual behavior and sexual dysfunction are the primary diagnoses and the intimate and private nature of sexual behavior.

A sexual dysfunction for example, may surface during marital counseling, or a newly admitted psychotic man may perform voyeuristic acts when he is feeling anxious. In the marital counseling situation, the sexual dysfunction is probably a symptom of marital discord, while the sexual deviation of the schizophrenic client is secondary to his major difficulty. In either case the sexual symptom is probably not reported statistically.

More than half the married couples in the United States have some sexual problem at one time or another. About 20 percent of clients seeking treatment for relief of sexual dysfunction are found to have a biological or physical cause for their difficulty, such as early diabetes, alcoholism, use of narcotics, local pathology of the genitals, sickle-cell anemia, neurological disease, or severe depression. Depression, stress, and fatigue can seriously damage sexual activity and are frequently the causes of dysfunction.[3]

PATTERNS OF INTERACTION: PERSON

Gender identity disorders generally involve disparity between clients' anatomical or biological sexual identity and their identification of themselves as masculine or feminine. *Ego-dystonic homosexuality* is the label used to describe clients who are emotionally uncomfortable with their sexual orientation. *Paraphilias* are characterized by a sexual response to objects or situations rather than reciprocal sexual activity with another person. *Psychosexual dysfunctions* are disturbances in the sexual response cycle. At one time or another, most couples will experience some degree of sexual dysfunction.

Gender Identity Disorders: Transsexualism

Gender identity disorders are characterized by incongruence between biological and subjective gender.[3] Gender identity is the sense of knowing the sex to which one belongs. It is awareness that "I am male" or "I am female." Gender identity disorders are rare; they occur when clients persist in behaving like members of the opposite sex. (This should not be confused with occasional feelings of inadequacy about masculinity or femininity.)

Transsexualism is the most commonly discussed gender identity disorder, although it is a relatively rare phenomenon. The term *transsexual* refers to a person who identifies psychologically with one sex but physically belongs to the other. The transsexual feels trapped in a body of the opposite sex. Some transsexuals seek sex-reassignment surgery out of a desire to make anatomy fit subjective gender identity. They generally seek surgery because they feel that their bodies are grotesque or inappropriate to their identities or because they hope that a changed role will improve their lives. Some transsexuals are sexually attracted to members of the same sex but maintain heterosexual drives and want to function in society as members of the sex with which they identify.[4]

Little is known about the developmental dynamics of the transsexual. Some literature suggests that there may be hormonal, genetic, and biochemical influences or that role modeling and socialization are major factors. Depression, isolation, and lack of self-acceptance are common problems of transsexual clients and can be worked on effectively. Becoming aware of and examining the total lifestyle of clients as well as their confusion over gender roles help nurses develop an attitude that conveys empathy and understanding.[4]

A person who chooses transsexual surgery generally becomes the subject of an intense evaluative process. Preparation for sex-reassignment surgery includes counseling and psychotherapy, hormonal therapy, lifestyle readjustment, cross-dressing and voice training, and (as appropriate) electrolysis for hair removal and plastic surgery in the form of breast augmentation, rhinoplasty, and reduction of thyroid cartilage. The preparation process may take up to 5 years. Legal documents are altered following the sex-reassignment surgery itself.

Ego-Dystonic Homosexuality

Ego-dystonic homosexuality refers to a dysfunctional behavioral pattern that features a desire to acquire a heterosexual relationship and heterosexual arousal and to deny the overt homosexual arousal and behavior that are present. This conflict is an unwanted and persistent source of distress. It is self-discomfort and stress about one's homosexual or lesbian behaviors or orientation. Loneliness, guilt, shame, anxiety, and depression are frequent experiences of clients experiencing ego-dystonic homosexuality.[2]

Paraphilias

A person with one of the paraphilias prefers nonhuman objects for sexual arousal, participates in repetitive sexual activity with another person that involves suffering or humiliation, or engages in repeated sexual activity with nonconsenting partners. The personality patterns of these clients are characterized by emotional immaturity and an inability to engage in lasting intimate relationships with members of the opposite sex. Table 38-1 defines the paraphilias and the characteristics common in each.

Psychosexual Dysfunctions

A psychosexual dysfunction, while primarily a physical impairment, also has emotional, intellectual, social, and spiritual dimensions.

It is generally believed that the immediate cause of sexual dysfunction is often an antierotic environment created by the couple which is destructive to the sexuality of one or both. Openness and trust, on the other hand, allow the partners to abandon themselves to the erotic experience. Among the specific causes of sexual dysfunction are failure or avoidance of sexual behavior that is exciting and effectively stimulating; fear of failure or an overanxiety to please or perform; perceptual and intellec-

Table 38-1 Paraphilias

Disorder	Definition	Distinguishing Characteristics
Fetishism	The act of deriving sexual pleasure from an inanimate object	Eroticizes certain nonsexual objects because of frequent associations with actual sexual parts and functions or because previous chance associations occurred under emotionally charged conditions. Prefers nonliving objects (fetishes) as the exclusive method of achieving sexual excitement.
Transvestism	Recurrent or persistent cross-dressing in the clothes of the opposite sex for release of tension or for sexual pleasure	Some transvestites are transsexuals. Some transvestites are homosexuals cross-dressing to attract other homosexuals. Transvestism is closely linked to fetishism. Intense frustration is experienced when cross-dressing is interfered with. Generally refers to males. Cross-dressing is generally used for the purpose of sexual excitement.
Zoophilia	The act of deriving sexual pleasure from animals	Sexual activity with animals is the exclusive method of achieving sexual pleasure; sometimes called *bestiality*.
Pedophilia	The act of obtaining sexual pleasure by molesting a child in the prepuberty stage of development	Pedophiles are often male and in the late thirties or early forties. These people lack feelings of emotional security and self-confidence and have often been recently rejected by an adult sex partner; a child represents a less threatening sex object. The offender is often familiar to the child and may be a relative, friend, or acquaintance. The child is generally at least 10 years younger than the client. Clients may be oriented toward children of the same or opposite sex. Legally referred to as *child molesting*.
Exhibitionism	The act of deriving erotic pleasure from briefly exposing the genitals to a surprised victim	Generally occurs in a public place. Pleasure stems from seeing the shocked reaction of the viewer. Masturbation sometimes accompanies the act of exposure. Occurs in males who have a weak sex-role identity and need to confirm their masculinity by showing their penises. Victims are generally female children or adults.
Voyeurism	The act of deriving sexual pleasure through viewing sex organs or sex acts of an unsuspecting victim	The voyeur's primary sex activity is viewing the sexual behavior of others. Family history usually involves an incident of viewing parents engaged in sexual intercourse. Behavior thought to be pursuit of parental behavior in the hope of coping with it. Generally occurs in early adulthood and is a chronic condition.
Sexual masochism	The act of deriving sexual pleasure and gratification by experiencing physical or mental pain and humiliation	The masochist desires to be dominated in the sexual relationship and is excited by the idea of being the recipient of pain; this is the person's repeated and preferred form of sexual activity. Involves being humiliated, bound, beaten, or otherwise made to suffer. The masochist engages in this activity intentionally. Activity sometimes involves self-mutilation.

(Continued.)

Table 38-1 Continued

Disorder	Definition	Distinguishing Characteristics
Sexual sadism	The act of receiving sexual pleasure and erotic gratification through infliction of physical or psychological pain on another	The sadist achieves orgasm from sadistic acts even when other sexual outlets are available. The desire to dominate is a primary dynamic. Generally involves a nonconsenting partner. Sometimes involves a consenting partner (masochist). Rape may be committed by persons with this disorder.
Atypical paraphilias	Includes the act of receiving sexual pleasure from various objects or actions:	Atypical paraphilias occur rarely. Victims of frotteurism are often oblivious to the action, because it occurs in crowded places.
Coprophilia	Feces	
Frotteurism	Rubbing	
Klismaphilia	Enema	
Mysophilia	Filth	
Necrophilia	Corpse	
Telephone scatologia	Lewdness on the telephone	
Urophilia	Urine	

tual defenses against erotic pleasure; and lack of communication about feelings, wishes, and responses. In contrast to clients who enjoy sex, dysfunctional clients suffer from inadequate sexual response and do not enjoy sexual intercourse.

The sexual response cycle is divided into four phases: *appetite,* or desire for sexual activity; *excitement,* or subjective sense of sexual pleasure with accompanying physiological changes; *orgasm,* or peak sexual pleasure with release of sexual tension; and *resolution,* or sense of general relaxation, well-being, and muscular relaxation. Sexual dysfunction may occur in any of the phases.

Masters and Johnson state that sociocultural deprivation and ignorance of sexual physiology constitute the cause of most sexual dysfunctions.[5] Freud believed that people who were in any way mentally "abnormal" would also be abnormal in their sexual life.[6] Other literature defines a positive but slight correlation between personality traits, psychopathology, and psychosexual dysfunction.

Sexual dysfunction may be lifelong or acquired, and generalized or the result of a specific situation. Dysfunction is not related to age, although occurrence is most frequent in early adulthood. There is an increased incidence of impotence, however, after age 55. Men with opportunities for satisfactory sexual activity enjoy intercourse well into their eighties. Lack of exercise of coital function, rather than the aging process, is thought to be the relevant factor in the cessation of sexual functioning in older men and women.[7]

Factors that may cause dysfunction include depression, alcoholism, diabetic or peripheral autonomic neuropathy, vascular disease, prescribed and abused drugs, pain, complications from surgery, trauma, and chronic illness. Dysfunctions may also be the result of congenital defects, infectious disease, or neurologic disorders. Specific psychosexual dysfunctions are defined in Table 38-2.

PATTERNS OF INTERACTION: FAMILY

People with dysfunctional psychosexual patterns of behavior, whether they suffer from gender identity disorders, paraphilias, ego-dystonic homosexuality, or a physiological sexual dysfunction, are frequently viewed by their families and spouses as deviant.

Gender Identity Disorders: Transsexualism

Because of the sensational nature of transsexualism, clients are often neglected by their families or completely cut off from family support. They are labeled *deviant* or *sick.* Family members mourn for

Table 38-2 Psychosexual Dysfunctions

Dysfunction	Definition
Inhibited sexual desire (ISD)	ISD is a disorder of the desire or appetitive phase of the sexual response cycle. Known also as *hypoactive sexual desire,* ISD is characterized by persistent and pervasive inhibition of sexual desire. Some persons with inhibited sexual desire have a lifelong history of lack of pleasure during sex, while others may acquire ISD following a physical or emotional trauma. Interpersonal conflicts, depression, and certain pharmacologic agents are seen as causative factors of ISD.
Impotence and frigidity	*Impotence* is the inability to achieve or maintain an erection. It is referred to as erectile dysfunction. It is analogous to *frigidity* or general sexual dysfunction in women. Both conditions are characterized by inhibition of the local vasocongestive phase of sexual response. In men the penis remains flaccid, while in women the vagina remains tight and dry. Fear of failure, or "performance anxiety," is the most common causative factor. Biological factors are also frequent causes of impotence and frigidity.
Orgasmic dysfunction	*Orgasmic dysfunction* is the specific inhibition of the orgasmic component of the female sexual response. A woman who suffers from primary orgasmic dysfunction is one who has never experienced orgasm.
Orgasmic dysfunction (continued)	A woman who has situational orgasmic dysfunction has previously experienced orgasm through masturbation or coitus but is currently nonorgasmic. If the disorder develops after a period of having been able to reach orgasm, it is considered secondary orgasmic dysfunction.
Retarded ejaculation	*Retarded ejaculation* is a condition in which men are able to respond to sexual stimuli with erotic feelings and a firm erection but, despite desire, are unable to ejaculate. It has also been labeled *ejaculatory incompetence.*
Premature ejaculation	*Premature ejaculation* is best defined as the inability of a man to exert voluntary control over his ejaculatory reflex. Once he is aroused, orgasm is reached very quickly.
Vaginismus	*Vaginismus* is defined as the irregular and involuntary contraction of the muscles surrounding the outer third of the vagina whenever there is an attempt at coitus. It results in the closing of the vaginal opening before penetration by the penis.
Functional dyspareunia	*Dyspareunia* is coitus associated with recurrent and persistent genital pain and may occur in males or females. Pain is not caused by another physical disorder (for example, cystitis or urethritis), lack of lubrication, or vaginismus but is rather a primary condition.

the "normal" sexuality of their loved one, usually have strong and persistent wishes for the transsexual to become "right" and often are apprehensive that what is happening may reflect negatively on them. Transsexuals generally are determined to have the sex reassignment surgery regardless of their family's reactions and often do not involve others until the actual surgical phase. Acceptance of the surgery by the family generally contributes to a favorable outcome. People who elect transsexual surgery may suffer loss of the family system or, of course, marriage. Clients and their families are known to become depressed after the surgery.

Ego-Dystonic Homosexuality

The family is a major factor in the development of ego-dystonic homosexuality. Lack of differentiation and too much concern with expectations of family members are often responsible for the emotional discomfort that characterizes homosexuals' discomfort with their sexuality. Family responses will vary with the religious, cultural, experiential, and educational background of the family. The key factor is family members' level of comfort with their own sexual concerns. The family's beliefs, values, and attitudes toward sexuality have a direct impact on whether family members deny, inhibit, or allow open discussion of homosexuality.

Classic explanations of the dynamics of homosexuality include theories about the early family life of homosexuals. Classic environmental explanations include the theory that the male homosexual's family life patterns include a mother who is unhappy with her marriage and turns to her son in a seductive, intimate way. Although this seductiveness stops short of physical contact, it is thought that the relationship engenders guilt in the son because of his desires toward his mother. This guilt causes him, eventually, to avoid all women. Generally, the father of a homosexual boy discourages masculine growth in a subtle way by favoring his daughters. The father resents his wife's attention to his son and may also be a weak, aloof, and ineffectual force in his son's life. Thus the boy comes to develop an excessive attachment to the mother, which he never outgrows.[8]

Some homosexuals have fathers who are harsh, overly aggressive, and too tough to allow their sons to enter into close relationships with them. In such a situation, a boy is unable to identify with his father and therefore does not learn a masculine role. The son becomes frightened of the masculine role epitomized by his father and is unable to accept it. Instead, he assumes a feminine role, with its implications of warmth and understanding. This is a defense against the unsatisfying relationship he has had with his father.[9] Converse dynamics can cause a young girl to choose a lesbian lifestyle. She may have been excluded by a rejecting mother and may seek from another older woman the maternal love that she was denied as a youngster.

The desire of parents to have a child of a specific sex may be another cause of homosexuality when they convey to their child that they reject his or her sex. Or a child's sex education may be faulty and laden with guilt. Finally, the relationship between parents is sometimes so bad that the child chooses homosexuality to escape from the feared and contemptible example of heterosexuality that is witnessed at home.

Paraphilias

A diagnosis of one of the paraphilias is often "public," particularly when the police or courts have been involved. However, the families and nurses of some clients may be unaware of these disorders. Even when they are aware, a client's attempts at dysfunctional closeness may result in tension or dishonesty in family relationships. Moreover, clients are entitled to privacy; and a client may request that his or her spouse and children not be included in treatment. Such situations can create feelings of anger and frustration in the nurse. On the other hand, when clients' families avoid sexually troubled clients, nurses may "triangle" with the client and express anger and annoyance at the family for their seeming neglect. The web of conflicting interactions contributes further to a client's already battered self-esteem.

Sexual Dysfunctions

Marital conflict is the most important of the dynamics underlying sexual dysfunction, and sexual dysfunction is a primary factor in marital conflict. Sexual functioning is only one strand in the bonding process of a marriage, but it is interwoven with other strands that keep couples together and reflect a married couple's total relationship. Sager described three categories for couples that reflect the extent to which discord precedes or results from sexual dysfunction:

1. Sexual dysfunction produces secondary marital discord.
2. Marital discord impairs sexual functioning because of interactions that generate anger, disappointment, or hostile feelings. There is an unsatisfactory environment in which to find sexual pleasure together.
3. Severe marital discord, usually with basic hostility, precludes the possibility of optimal sexual functioning.[10]

Couples who marry generally have defined their expectations of one another's ability to fulfill sexual desire. Sexual partners may fulfill expectations or create conflict around the issue of sexual functioning. Some people cannot allow themselves to choose a partner with whom they can enjoy sex. When partners have not clearly defined their expectations for themselves and each other, sexual dysfunction may result.[11]

There is limited evidence about the hereditary nature of sexual dysfunction. Bowen's theory about the multigenerational transmission process (see Chapter 19) suggests that a family history of a person with sexual dysfunction would reveal sexual dysfunction in other generations. Instability and disharmony in early family life and the lack during childhood of a person of the same sex with whom to identify have been shown to have had an impact on persons with primary orgasmic dysfunction. It is also known that sexual dysfunction between parents will affect the children, because anything that happens to one family member has an impact on the whole system.

People with sexual dysfunction may have grown up in a family in which sex was portrayed as dirty and sinful or in which parents punished children severely for sexual activity such as masturbation. People whose sexual responsiveness is inhibited were taught as children that no "nice" boy or girl is interested in sex or enjoys it.

PATTERNS OF INTERACTION: ENVIRONMENT

Attitudes toward sexuality are greatly influenced by the media and what society tolerates as "normal." Many forms of sexual conduct are not popular, for a variety of legal, historical, social, spiritual, moral, and psychological reasons. Generally, what is approved or disapproved by society at a particular time is a matter of social definition. Ideas of right and wrong, and whether or not an individual approves or disapproves of certain sexual activities, have to do with personal value systems. As a rule, private sexual activity between consenting adults is legally acceptable, but many forms may be considered immoral by some people.

The law does prohibit certain forms of public sexual activity; and (as noted earlier in this chapter) the American Psychiatric Association has labeled some activities *dysfunctional*. Many of the paraphilias, for example, are considered perversions or crimes against social order and are punishable by law. In general, community attitudes about transsexualism and the paraphilias are congruent with the legal system. Attitudes about ego-dystonic homosexuality are much more controversial. There is a considerable diversity of attitudes toward sexual dysfunction.[12] Some cultures view dysfunction as a normal occurrence; others condemn and ostracize people who are sexually dysfunctional.

The setting in which sexual acts occur (whether they are deviant or not) will influence or detract from enjoyment.[13] A lack of privacy (for example, because of in-laws or children in the household) may severely inhibit sexual activity and result in dysfunction; a secluded romantic setting may add to a couple's enjoyment of sexual activity.

Transsexuals usually come to the attention of nurses when they are hospitalized for the surgical phase of a change to the opposite sex. Paraphiliac behaviors are generally seen in the streets or as a secondary diagnosis in mental health settings where nurses practice. In both cases, censure by the community is likely. Ego-dystonic homosexuals, for the most part, are so integrated into the mainstream of their environment that they are not readily identifiable. Likewise, since most couples experience some degree of sexual dysfunction during the course of their marriage, and because of the intimate nature of the sexual act, people are not easily labeled *sexually dysfunctional* unless they have disclosed this fact about themselves.

Civil rights legislation prohibits discrimination because of sexual identity, but in reality known transsexuals, paraphiliacs, and those with an ego-dystonic homosexual orientation have difficulties finding housing and jobs when their sexual difficulties become known. A growing concern about AIDS and herpes has further encouraged discrimination.

NURSING PROCESS

Nurses, because of their holistic approach, consider clients' sexual functioning an important part of the total person and explore their sexual activity as a routine part of the nursing process. Many of the dysfunctions noted in this chapter may be discovered by basically prepared nurses during the assessment process; however, the main function of these nurses is limited to case finding and referral to appropriately prepared practitioners.

Assessment

Anatomical and physiological problems, pharmacological agents, and alterations of body image as a result of surgery or medicine contribute to sexual dysfunctions. Nurses are often the "frontline" diagnosticians of sexual dysfunction: their holistic approach to clients considers sexual functioning an important part of the total person, and nurses explore it as a part of assessment. It is not unusual for clients to confide sexual dysfunctions first to a nurse; but their statement of sexual problems may be veiled and vague: "I haven't felt much like sex lately"; "I haven't had sex since the surgery"; or "We thought we wouldn't be able to have sex any more"; or "I really don't enjoy sex." Very few clients will openly state, "I am unable to have an erection" or "I do not reach orgasm."

Nurses need to distinguish between what they themselves personally experience and consider appropriate and the preferences and experiences of their clients. Not all nurses are able to converse easily and comfortably about sexual concerns, dysfunctions, or orientations, but this ability is like most clinical skills and can be acquired.

A sexual history provides clients and nurses with a way to assess sexual concerns when sexual dysfunction is not the established diagnosis. When sexual dysfunction is a client's reason for seeking help, a sexual history provides the information necessary to distinguish causes and formulate interventions. A sexual history is an integral part of the physical, mental, and spiritual evaluation of clients and forms the basis of sexual counseling. It provides information about the needs, expectations, and behavior of the client's sexual role. A format for the sexual history is given in Chapter 23.

If clients are diagnosed as having one of the paraphilias, a gender identity disorder, or ego-dystonic homosexuality, nurses may ask the question listed below.

Assessment of Gender Identity Disorders

- Are you comfortable with your biological sexual determination?
- Do you wish you were a person of the opposite sex?
- Is your spouse or family aware of your desires?
- Are there social or cultural factors that influence your desires?
- Have you seen a therapist about your desires?
- What impact has your choice of transsexual surgery had on you, your family, your job, etc.?

Assessment of Ego-Dystonic Homosexuality

- When did your first homosexual encounter take place?
- Do you believe that you are homosexual?
- How often do you have homosexual experiences?
- Do you have a steady partner or do you prefer many partners?
- Are you emotionally comfortable with a homosexual orientation?
- Do your parents or siblings know about your sexual orientation?
- What is the response of your parents and siblings?
- Have you had difficulty at your job or where you live because of your homosexuality?
- Do you ever have sexual relations with someone of the opposite sex?
- Do you wish to change your sexual orientation?

Assessment of Paraphilias

- Do you prefer nonliving objects as a source of sexual arousal?
- Is dressing in the clothes of the opposite sex a source of sexual arousal for you?
- Do you experience sexual gratification as a result of physical or mental pain?
- Do you sexually enjoy inflicting pain on another?
- Is your spouse or family aware of your problem?
- Have you ever been arrested because of your sexual activity?

Diagnosis

A nursing diagnosis is a statement about health status that reflects the client's interaction with the environment. When a medical diagnosis includes one of the sexual dysfunctions, gender identity disorders, or paraphilias discussed in this chapter, or there is a determination that a person is experiencing ego-dystonic homosexuality, nursing diagnoses that call for intervention and referral to appropriate therapists need to be established. Table 38-3 lists several appropriate nursing diagnoses.

Outcome Criteria

Evaluation of nursing interventions is measured against the goals established for each client. Outcomes may be thought of as individualized, predictable goals or expectations that clients should achieve as a result of nursing intervention. Outcome criteria for clients with sexual dysfunctions, gender identity disorders, or paraphilias include the following examples. A client will be able to:

Verbalize an understanding of the interrelationship of sexual activity and physical, mental, and spiritual well-being

Decrease the number of instances of voyeuristic activity

Seek therapy to discuss discomfort with sexual orientation

Table 38-3 Nursing Diagnoses for Dysfunctional Sexual Patterns

Gender Identity Disorders
Depression associated with lack of family support for planned transsexual surgery
Gender identity conflict associated with psychotic behavior
Cross-dressing associated with sex change process
Ego-Dystonic Homosexuality
Anxiety related to confusion about personal identity
Inability to achieve desired sexual satisfaction with same-sex partner, associated with conflicts about sexual orientation
Social maladjustment associated with anxiety about sexual orientation
Paraphilias
Emotional insecurity and lack of self-confidence related to rejection by adult sex partner
Enjoyment of humiliation associated with sexually masochistic behavior
Orgasm related to sadistic sexual activity
Sexual Dysfunction
Limitation of sexual activity associated with spinal cord injury
Dysfunctional sexual activity related to lack of privacy
Altered sexual activity patterns related to altered body structure
Impotence associated with excessive alcohol intake
Inability to achieve desired sexual satisfaction associated with unresolved traumatic sexual experience in childhood
Sexual dysfunction related to misinformation and lack of knowledge

Verbalize feelings of loneliness, guilt, shame, and anxiety in a constructive manner

Respond positively to a referral for sex therapy for self and spouse

Intervention

Nurses have the responsibility to promote sexual health. The success of intervention with dysfunctional sexual patterns in clients will be dependent on the nurse's subjective experience and comfort with sexuality. A nurse's own strong emotions and personal religious ideation, a wide variety of attitudes and perceptions, and awareness of legal sanctions will influence responsiveness to clients with dysfunctional sexual patterns.

Self-Awareness

Self-awareness is a first step in the process of remaining nonjudgmental and therapeutic when interacting with these clients. Self-awareness may be facilitated by awareness groups and discussions with a clinical specialist or supervisor. Role-playing and responding to feedback about real situations are other means of increasing one's self-awareness.

Some nurses may deny sexuality either verbally or behaviorally. Avoiding the subject of sex and responding vaguely or unspecifically to clients' concerns are ways of expressing denial. Expressions such as "private parts" and "down below" in reference to the genitalia are indicative of avoidance by the nurse. In addition, some nurses are uncomfortable providing intimate physical care for clients of the opposite sex. Some hospitals have a rule that male professionals must care for male clients and female professionals for female clients; but where such rules are made, clients' comfort, not nurses' avoidance, should be the motivation.

Nurses are sexual beings who, as a group, experience the same sexual feelings and dysfunctions as their clients. They often experience insecurity and inhibition when confronted with clients' sexual concerns. Such responses interfere with therapeutic intervention, causing lack of objectivity and decreased sensitivity to the clients' needs. Fear of offending a client and embarrassment about sex also interfere with a therapeutic approach. In addition, the nurse's beliefs, attitudes, and values should not be imposed upon the client.

Nurses need to be aware of and secure enough about their own sexuality to encourage verbalization of clients' underlying sexual concerns. If they are comfortable with their own sexuality, they will respond to clients with empathy, reassurance, and respect for their feelings. A frank, warm, and objective approach will foster openness and encourage clients to discuss their difficulties. Nurses' effectiveness in this area will also depend on their educational background and expertise.

Levels of Intervention

Mims and Swenson have developed a model of sexual health that provides a framework for discussing nursing interventions with clients experiencing sexual difficulty (see Chapter 23).[14] Nurses may intervene at the "life experience" level; at the level of basic education and self-awareness; at an intermediate level; or at the level of expertise, with advanced training and education.

At the *life experience level* nurses respond with intuitive behaviors that may be helpful or destructive to clients. Taboos, myths, and stereotyped behaviors may be part of an intuitive response. To intervene effectively, nurses must examine their subjective values, concerns, and personal experiences and separate them from those of the client. Therapeutic responsiveness relies on empathy and genuineness.

Functioning and responding at the *basic level* involves awareness by nurses of their personal perceptions, attitudes, and beliefs about sexuality. The nursing process and basic communication skills are utilized. At the basic level nurses are expected to respond to clients objectively and to have basic objective knowledge about sexual dysfunction. They intervene directly by making referrals to skilled therapists. In inpatient settings, when dealing with clients whose sexual activity involves the paraphilias, nurses participate by setting appropriate limits to prevent sexual acting out. When such clients sense a nurse's sexual anxiety, they will distance from the nurse; they may make lewd remarks or behave seductively. Conveying a self-assured and comfortable attitude, as well as setting limits, is the appropriate intervention.

Nursing intervention at the *intermediate level* involves giving information and granting permission. Nurses assess clients and, by taking a sexual history, give them "permission" to discuss sexual concerns. Giving information involves imparting basic information about the client's problem—such as sexual dysfunction or ego-dystonic homosexuality—and its probable causes. Awareness of the training and credentials of local therapists is important information that nurses at the intermediate level acquire and give to their clients as part of the referral process.

Nurses at an *advanced level* of education in human sexuality intervene by offering suggestions, sex therapy, and sex education programs, and by participating in research projects. Self-awareness, accurate knowledge of human sexuality and sexual dysfunction, and acknowledgment of feelings, biases, prejudices, and attitudes about sexuality and sexual dysfunction in the self and others are essential to the nurse's therapeutic interventions. When a nurse is uncomfortable about intervening with clients with sexual concerns, the clients' care should be transferred to another professional.

Nurses encounter clients with gender identity problems and paraphilias in many settings. Nurses working in inpatient and outpatient mental health settings meet clients with defined problematic behaviors. Nurses in the community may be asked for help because of a client's or family member's problematic sexual behavior. The degree of intervention will depend to a great extent on the expertise, education, and comfort of the nurse.

There are several basic facts the nurse should keep in mind when intervening with clients who have sexual concerns or problems. Nurses need insight into clients' values and beliefs regarding sexuality. They must therefore be tolerant of values and behaviors that differ from their own, and they must avoid any judgment about the behavior or orientation of the client. They need to watch their nonverbal communication in order to avoid conveying personal values or a sense of discomfort to the client. When intervening with clients with rare or unusual psychosexual disorders, they must avoid the tendency to sensationalize and gossip.

Nurses must be aware of what they consider sexually normal and abnormal for themselves and others. They must think about and examine their values about persons whose sexual functioning has been labeled *unhealthy*. Except where legal or safety concerns are present, clients should be encouraged to arrive at their own answers when exploring sexual behavior. Clients need to discover for themselves what their personal values are regarding sexuality. Nurses need to assume a supportive, nonjudgmental attitude and avoid projecting their own concerns onto the client.

Sex Therapy

Nurses at an advanced level of practice intervene with sexually dysfunctional clients through sex therapy. Intensive interpersonal therapy, on the other hand, is the treatment of choice for clients with ego-dystonic homosexuality, one of the paraphilias, or gender identity disorders.

Sex therapy is the active treatment of sexual dysfunctions. Treatment is given to a *couple*, generally on an outpatient basis. It focuses on relief of the sexual problem and attainment of improved sexual functioning.

The generally accepted method of treatment for sexual dysfunctions involves the integrated use of systematically structured sexual experiences with conjoint therapeutic sessions. Once the assessment is complete and the diagnosis is determined, a behavioral program is planned with the couple. Techniques employed depend on the problem presented. Among the techniques used are self-stimulation (masturbation), sensate conditioning (bodily touching and exploration), "pause and squeeze" techniques (when ejaculatory control is the issue), cognitive and attentional imagery (to enhance fantasy activity in frigid women and impotent men), and dilators for the treatment of vaginismus. The mode of conjoint therapy sessions may be individual, group, co-therapy, or bibliotherapy.

Evaluation

Evaluation of nursing care related to sexual dysfunction, ego-dystonic homosexuality, and the paraphilias utilizes unique criteria based on a person's specific goals in therapy. Changes in the client's thoughts, feelings, and sexual functioning are identified. The replanning of the intervention process should be an ongoing process that involves both the nurse and the client.

Table 38-4 illustrates the proper use of evaluation in the form of a nursing care plan for the client described below:

> Jack L. is a 27-year-old married construction worker who is admitted to the medical unit of a local hospital with a diagnosis of acute gastritis. In addition to the obvious symptoms of alcoholism, Jack looks embarrassed as he tells the nurse that he has recently had difficulty in his marriage. His wife states that their sexual relationship has been troubled "since he started drinking."

The plan in Table 38-4 is an appropriate model for a nurse at the basic level of the Mims-Swenson model.[14]

Table 38-4 Nursing Care Plan for Jack L.

Assessment	Nursing Diagnosis	Outcome Criteria	Intervention	Evaluation
How much have you been drinking? Are you able to have an erection when you drink? Are there times when your sexual performance is OK? When? Have you been troubled by impotence in the past? Do you have trouble sustaining an erection at times when you are not drinking?	Dysfunctional sexual activity related to excessive alcohol intake	Jack L. and his wife will verbalize agreement to make and keep appointment at sex therapy clinic this week. Jack will verbalize agreement to attend Alcoholics Anonymous meetings twice weekly. Jack's wife will agree to attend Al-Anon meetings once weekly	Arrange for Jack to attend Alcoholics Anonymous. Arrange for Jack's wife to attend Al-Anon. Enroll client and family members in alcoholism education courses offered at hospital. Discuss relationship between excessive alcohol intake and impotence with client and his wife. Refer Jack and his wife to the sex therapy clinic.	Jack and his wife make an appointment with sex therapy clinic but fail to keep it. Follow-up telephone call will be made to assess reason for absence. Jack has been attending Alcoholics Anonymous meetings 3 times a week. Jack's wife has attended one Al-Anon meeting but is reluctant to attend others. Follow-up discussion will be held to assess her impression of Al-Anon and explore her resistance. Jack and his wife report that "things in the bedroom are OK again." Reinforce connection between alcohol intake and impotence.

SUMMARY

Normal sexual behavior is difficult to define but generally is characterized by the words *adult, privacy, consent,* and *lack of force.* Deviations are considered variations in sexual behavior. Psychosexual disorders are classified in four groups: (1) gender identity disorders, (2) paraphilias, (3) psychosexual dysfunctions, and (4) other psychosexual disorders, including ego-dystonic homosexuality.

The gender identity disorder discussed here is transsexualism.

Paraphilias involve sexual arousal in response to sexual imagery, objects, or acts that are not part of the normative arousal-activity patterns of society. The paraphilias include fetishism, transvestism, zoophilia, pedophilia, exhibitionism, voyeurism, and sexual masochism and sadism.

A sexual dysfunction is a psychomotor disorder that makes it impossible for a person to have or to enjoy coitus. The psychosexual dysfunctions include inhibited sexual desire, inhibited sexual excitement (frigidity and impotence), inhibited female orgasm (orgasmic dysfunction), inhibited male orgasm (retarded ejaculation or ejaculatory incompetence), premature ejaculation, functional vaginismus, and functional dyspareunia. Sociocultural deprivation and ignorance of sexual physiology are the causes of most sexual dysfunctions. Marital conflict is another leading cause. Social, cultural, religious, and family norms and mores figure largely as underlying dynamics in sexual dysfunction.

Ego-dystonic homosexuality is a behavioral pattern in which the person wants to acquire a heterosexual relationship and heterosexual arousal, but in which overt homosexual arousal and behavior are present and are an unwanted and persistent source of distress.

Nurses have feelings, beliefs, values, and attitudes about clients with sexual dysfunctions or ego-dystonic homosexuality. Nurses may respond with fear (feeling a threat to their own identity), anger, feelings of inadequacy, timidity, or shyness. Developing self-awareness is a first step when intervening with clients who exhibit sexual concerns. Taking a sexual history is an integral part of the psychological, social, and physical evaluation of clients; the sexual history forms the basis for sexual counseling. The nursing process is applied to clients and guides nurses in the formulation of nursing diagnoses, individualized goals for clients, and appropriate interventions. Nurses intervene according to their level of expertise; they should show respect and empathy for their clients' sexual concerns. Sex therapy, the active treatment of sexual dysfunction, is considered intervention at an advanced level of nursing practice. It involves the integrated use of systematically structured sexual experiences with conjoint therapeutic sessions.

REFERENCES

1. B. Goldstein, *Human Sexuality,* McGraw-Hill, New York, 1976.
2. American Psychiatric Association, *Diagnostic and Statistical Manual of Mental Disorders,* 3d ed., APA, Washington, D.C., 1980.
3. F. H. Mims and M. Swensen, *Sexuality: A Nursing Perspective,* McGraw-Hill, New York, 1980.
4. J. M. Atlee, "Dealing with the Emotional Needs of Persons Undergoing Transsexual Surgery," in Jeanette Lancaster, ed., *Community Mental Health Nursing: An Ecological Perspective,* Mosby, St. Louis, 1980.
5. W. Masters and V. Johnson, *Human Sexual Inadequacy,* Churchill, London, 1970.
6. S. Freud, *Three Contributions to the Theory of Sex,* Dutton, New York, 1962.
7. D. McIntosch, "Sexual Attitudes in a Group of Older Women," *Issues in Mental Health Nursing,* no. 3, 1981, p. 109.
8. J. J. Gill, "Homosexuality Today," *Human Development,* vol. 1, no. 4, Winter 1980, pp. 104–113.
9. A. E. Moses and R. O. Hawkins, *Counseling Lesbian Women and Gay Men: A Life Issue Approach,* Mosby, St. Louis, 1982.
10. C. J. Sager, *Marriage Contracts and Couple Therapy,* Brunner/Mazel, New York, 1976.
11. L. M. Hartman, "The Interface between Sexual Dysfunction and Marital Conflicts," *American Journal of Psychiatry,* vol. 137, no. 5, 1980, pp. 576–579.
12. J. S. Hyde, *Understanding Human Sexuality,* McGraw-Hill, New York, 1979.
13. E. R. Mahoney, *Human Sexuality,* New York, McGraw-Hill, 1983.
14. F. H. Mims, "Sexual Education and Counseling," *Nursing Clinics of North America,* vol. 10, no. 3, 1975, pp. 519–528.

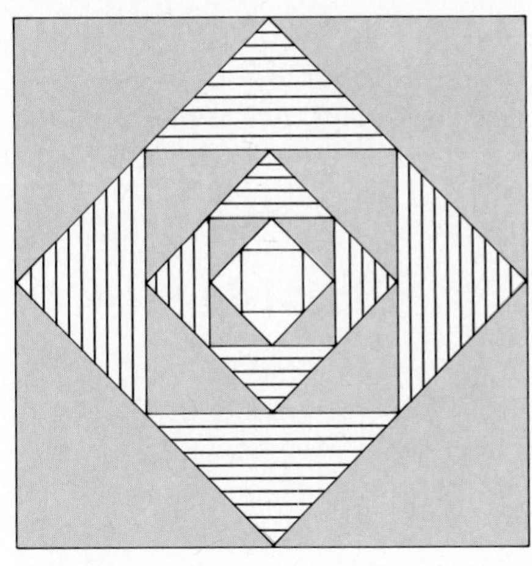

CHAPTER 39
Patterns of Dysfunction in Adolescence

Barbara Flynn Sideleau

LEARNING OBJECTIVES

Upon completion of this chapter, the student should be able to:

1. Describe the ways in which adolescents manifest dysynchronous physical, mental, and spiritual patterns of interaction.
2. Identify the DSM III diagnostic categories used with adolescents.
3. Discuss epidemiological factors associated with dysfunctional coping patterns in adolescence.
4. Describe dysynchronous patterns of interactions between adolescents and their families.
5. Describe environmental patterns of interaction associated with dysynchronous patterns of interactions between adolescents and their parents.
6. Assess adolescent, family, and environmental interactions to identify problems that can be addressed through nursing intervention.
7. Formulate nursing diagnoses related to dysynchronous patterns of interaction.
8. Collaborate with adolescents and their families in establishing outcome criteria that can be used to evaluate nursing interventions and provide feedback to clients on progress in resolving problems.
9. Select nursing interventions, derived from a holistic approach, that are appropriate to the diagnosed problems.
10. Evaluate the effectiveness of nursing interventions.

Patterns of dysfunction in adolescence emerge as a result of problems derived from the interaction of dramatic physical, social, mental, and spiritual changes with problematic separation dynamics. Adolescence is a transitional period between the end of childhood and the beginning of adulthood—roughly, from age 11 to the early twenties. It is a time of developmental change: physiologically, psychologically, socially, and spiritually. The changes in various areas interact with one another; but development in each area may proceed at a different rate, so that lags occur in one area but not another. Lags, or acceleration, in one or more developmental areas may be a source of problems for adolescents and for the parent-adolescent relationship.

Physical growth, emergence of secondary sex characteristics, and hormonal and neurochemical changes alter body awareness, self-image, and self-perception. The personality is reorganized. Cognitive processes evolve; logical and abstract thinking emerge. Moral development interacts with challenges from the peer group and society. Parent-child relationships are strained by the normative separation process and the adolescent's movement toward independence and the peer group.[1,2] Society and contemporary social issues interact with adolescents as they progress through this developmental stage.

The quantity, quality, and rapidity of these changes make them especially stressful. Moreover, preexisting childhood and family problems may interact and interfere with an adolescent's development. When this occurs, the adolescent may manifest serious dysfunctional patterns of interaction and consequently require psychiatric–mental health intervention.

The purpose of this chapter is to explore the dysfunctional patterns of interaction that occur in adolescence and are amenable to nursing intervention. Adolescent behavior patterns that are symptomatic of developmental and parent-adolescent problems are described. Disturbances in physical, mental, spiritual, and social development are addressed. Interactions among person, family, and environment that contribute to the development and maintenance of dysfunctional patterns are examined. The nursing process is applied to dysfunctional adolescent patterns of interaction from a holistic perspective. The dysfunctional patterns selected for discussion here may or may not result in hospitalization. They are preventable; or, if they are recognized early on, they may be altered by a holistic approach that helps the adolescent and family cope more effectively with developmental changes.

DYSYNCHRONOUS HEALTH PATTERNS

Depression and anxiety in adults are readily recognized and distinguished by the constellation of behaviors associated with each. Adolescents may present with adult symptoms of depression or anxiety; but more often, their depression and anxiety are masked[3] and manifested as acting out, self-destructiveness, problems with attendance and performance at school, running away, substance abuse, delinquency, problems with sexuality, cult membership, and somatic complaints. Dysfunctional family patterns of interaction that contribute to these dysfunctional patterns in adolescents involve centrifugal, centripetal, and delegating dynamics.

Socialization of a child is an interactive process. The quality of attachment, affective exchanges between parent and child, and the consistency or inconsistency of personal interactions influence the child's perceptions of and interactions with the world. An impaired or failed attachment, an affective climate that is characterized by depression or anxiety, and inconsistency in satisfaction of needs—any of these provides a foundation for depression or anxiety.[4]

Efforts to remedy deprivations, losses, or unpredictability are reflected in four coping styles that persist into adolescence:

- Prolonged, unresolved, chronic mourning characterized by unsuccessful attempts to recover what was lost
- A style of interacting, derived from rage generated by losses, which is characterized by anger directed toward self and others, and a sense of guilt for having created problems and caused losses
- Persistent attempts to care for others and to ignore self that eventually lead to feelings of emptiness, loneliness, and being overwhelmed by the needs of others
- Extensive use of denial—a fragile defense that inevitably fails, releasing a flood of feelings and creating a desperate need for relief

DSM III

Adolescents experience a wide variety of problems and manifest their anxiety and depression in many ways. In this chapter problems of adolescence associated with the following *Diagnostic and Statistical Manual of Mental Disorders* (DSM III)[5] categories of disorders are addressed: conduct, oppositional, anxiety, identity, adjustment, personality, and substance abuse disorders; and conditions not attributable to mental disorder (antisocial behavior, academic problems, phase-of-life problems, and parent-child problems).

Many diagnoses used with adolescents are also applied to children and adults. There is no one diagnosis that encompasses the various manifestations of masked or overt depression and anxiety in adolescence. Providers of health care are often reluctant to label adolescents with the DSM III categories of mental disorders; they may tend instead to use diagnoses categorized as "not attributable to mental disorder." Another problematic aspect of the labeling process with adolescents is that providers of health care may find it difficult to distinguish normal adolescent behavior from the degree of exaggeration that indicates psychopathology.

This chapter will not address disorders associated with impaired intellectual functioning with an organic basis, or attention deficit, schizophrenic, affective, and somatoform disorders. These diagnoses are, of course, used with adolescents; however, the nursing care of clients with these disorders is addressed in depth elsewhere in the text.[5]

Epidemiology

There are more than 30 million adolescents in the United States. Although as an age group they may appear to have more problems than other people, the incidence of mental illness is no higher among adolescents than among adults.

One out of every 600 adolescents dies each year, and 50 percent of these die violently. The suicide rate among adolescents in all racial and ethnic groups is reaching epidemic proportions in the United States.[6,7] Since 1970, it has risen 44 percent, while the overall rate has increased only 2.6 percent.[8] Statistics on adolescent suicide in this country do not reflect the extent of the problem, even though suicide is ranked as the second major cause of death in this age group. Accidents, the leading cause of death among adolescents between ages 15 and 19, include some "autocides" (one-car accidents) and motorcycle accidents that appear to be suicides but are not reported as such.[7,9] Statistics on accidental death among white adolescents reveal that two-thirds die as a result of vehicular accidents. This finding suggests that the actual extent of suicide among white adolescents may be much greater than statistics indicate. Local coroners and private physicians, either to protect families or because of social, religious, or legal taboos, may list vehicular suicides as accidental deaths.[7,10] Currently, nonwhite male adolescents are more likely to die as a result of homicide than in accidents. But in some of these incidents, adolescents may provoke their own murder rather than take their own lives.[8]

Most young people experiment with alcohol during their high school years.[11] Between 1965 and 1975, alcohol consumption by adolescents increased substantially; however, it has since stabilized.[12] According to a survey of high school seniors by the National Institute of Drug Abuse (NIDA), daily alcohol consumption has decreased 5.5 percent, but drinking at parties is still prevalent.[13] It is estimated that of all adolescents 14 to 17 years of age, 19 percent (3.3 million) are problem drinkers.[12] The NIDA survey also found a decrease in recreational drug abuse among adolescents.[14] Nevertheless, the United States reports the largest proportion in the world of young people involved with illicit drugs. By their senior year in high school, two out of three adolescents have used an illicit drug at some time. These figures may seem high, but statistics derived from surveys are conservative estimates of substance abuse. The samples include only those who were present in school the day the survey was administered and who were willing to complete the form; they do not account for chronic truants, dropouts, and possible abusers who refused to participate. The extent of substance abuse may be greater than is believed.[12]

One out of every four adolescents drops out of school. Dropping out leaves people ill-prepared for the work force in a highly technological society; for this and other reasons it is considered a problem.

One out of thirty adolescents runs away from home.[6] Over 1 million youngsters 10 to 17 years old run away each year.[15] Some of these young people gravitate to urban areas, where they become involved in prostitution, pornography, and criminal activities. Runaways, like dropouts, are a serious problem for our society.

Since there is no precise definition of *juvenile delinquency,* statistics about it are not readily available, and those that exist are incomplete. It is estimated that in 1 year more than 1 million young people (below age 18) appear in juvenile courts.[16]

One out of every two adolescents is sexually active.[6] These youngsters are at a high risk for sexually transmitted diseases, particularly since the number of partners has also risen in recent years. They are also at a high risk for unplanned pregnancy because they use ineffective methods, or no method, of contraception. Of all sexually active women, teenagers are more likely to have an abortion or unintended birth than any other age group. Of sexually active female adolescents, 34 percent become pregnant, and 65 percent of these use no method of contraception or an unreliable form.[17,18]

PATTERNS OF INTERACTION: PERSON

Acting Out

Definition and Description

Acting-out behavior in adolescents includes challenging the authority of parents and care givers, passively or aggressively resisting treatment, violating home or institutional rules, showing impaired ability to control impulses, threatening or inflicting physical violence and harm against people or property, and callously disregarding the rights and feelings of others. Mood fluctuations are inevitable during adolescence, as are dependency conflicts. In acting-out adolescents, these fluctuations and conflicts are exaggerated.

Such adolescents tend to be demanding, argumentative, irritable, and unpredictable. They see rules and limits as challenges; their response is to test them and then break them. Restrictions of any sort elicit temper tantrums. They will, initially, scream, yell at others, stamp their feet, and demand the removal of the restriction. If this behavior fails to produce a suspension of the restriction, they will resort to physical aggression, assault, and destruction. Their resistance to authority and to treatment is a declared war. They make it known that they will not conform, negotiate, or retreat, but will fight until death. They may impulsively destroy furniture, walls, and any objects at hand. As their rage builds, they seem unable to exert control, and vent it on people and property.

Dynamics

Underlying depression and anxiety, which are masked by aggressive and impulsive behavior, interact with developmental processes. The lifestyle and behavior of these adolescents are governed by mistrust, low self-esteem, a need for immediate gratification, and little tolerance for frustration.[4] Their needs are insatiable, and the failure to find satisfaction generates a defensive reaction. Rather than attempting to resolve their feelings, they externalize the solution and attack. Their behavior pattern is directed toward the avoidance of feelings of despair and helplessness. It is also used to coerce others into meeting their dependency needs. Their unrestrained, threatening, and sometimes reckless behavior and their lack of concern for others provoke anger in others, so that it becomes even more difficult for their needs to be satisfied.[4]

In their homes and in psychiatric institutions, these youngsters create chaos if they are allowed to control events through intimidation, threats, or actual violence. "They want what they want when they want it"—and they want to do whatever they please, whenever and wherever it suits them. This attitude inevitably brings them into conflict with authorities and with their peers.

Parent-child interactions which contribute to the development of an acting-out behavior pattern include impaired socialization; modeling by parents of explosive, hostile, and aggressive ventilation of feelings; losses, or impairment of the attachment process; and chronic failure to satisfy needs. Parental stress and interactions between the parents' temperaments and the child's temperament can also be influential. For instance, there will be a negative interaction between a difficult, colicky child who is easily distressed by change and an easily frustrated parent. The parent will be dissatisfied with his or her ability to provide care and will consequently feel inadequate and angry. The child has unmet needs and is developmentally unable to meet them, and the parent fails to "tune in." The pattern, once established, is reinforced by both. Adolescence, a time of turmoil at best, will escalate it. A chronically deprived adolescent, despite conflicts with the parents, has considerable difficulty separating and moving toward independence. The parents, however, may wish to be rid of the troublesome adolescent and may use hospitalization as a way of expelling the adolescent from the family.

Entry into Treatment

When a physical fight occurs between an adolescent and a parent, it may be so frightening that the family seeks counseling. An adolescent may experience acute anxiety or guilt or become a frequent visitor to the school nurse, complaining of minor health problems. In such an instance, and for other reasons, it may be the nurse who makes a referral for counseling. Sometimes acting-out behavior also appears at school. Verbal or physical attacks on peers or teachers may result in a recommendation by the school that the adolescent see a counselor or that the family seek counseling.

Not infrequently, admission to a psychiatric service follows a violent physical parent-child altercation: there may be damage to the home, parents and the adolescent may have been injured, and the police may have been called by a neighbor or a family member. Either because the police were involved or because the family senses that the situation is out of control, a decision is made to have the adolescent admitted for psychiatric treatment.

Self-Destructiveness

Self-destructive behavior patterns exhibited by adolescents fall into two categories: *self-harm* and *suicide*.

Self-Harm

DEFINITION AND DESCRIPTION. Self-harm occurs when adolescents consciously, willfully, and painfully injure themselves without intending to end their lives. These behaviors are sometimes labeled *self-multilation, parasuicide, focal suicide,* and *autoaggression.*

The behaviors characteristic of this syndrome include the examples listed in Table 39-1. Although these behaviors have been observed in elderly people with organic mental disorders, in children, and in schizophrenics, they occur more frequently among adolescents between the ages of 16 and 25 years.[19] Both males and females appear to be at risk. Also characteristic of the deliberate self-harm syndrome is the occurrence of multiple episodes suggesting a chronic behavior pattern, and the use of different (not lethal) methods in successive episodes.

Table 39-1 Deliberate Self-Harm Syndrome

Behaviors
Cutting or scratching wrists
Cutting or scratching forearms
Carving skin: forearm or abdomen
Self-biting: hands, wrists, arms
Self-burning: cigarette burns, application of lighter to skin, immersion of hand into scalding water
Eye enucleation
Self-amputation: tongue, finger joint, ear
Mutilation of genitals
Gouging skin with fingernails until ulceration occurs

SOURCE: E. M. Pattison and J. Kahan, "The Deliberate Self-Harm Syndrome," *American Journal of Psychiatry*, vol. 140, no. 7, 1983, pp. 869–872.

DYNAMICS. These youngsters experience depression, but do not verbally report feelings of helplessness, hopelessness, and worthlessness. An episode of deliberate self-harm is characterized by an overall depressed mood and an impulse to do something that will cause self-injury. These impulses are recurrent, and the adolescent feels unable to resist them. The impulses are associated with intolerable situations in which these youngsters feel trapped and from which they see no way of escaping. Anger, anxiety, depression, and agitation increase and reinforce the impulse to cause physical pain, which would decrease the mounting tension. The escalation of feelings constricts perception of alternative ways of coping. If not prevented by external influences, the adolescent inflicts a self-injury and immediately feels a sense of relief—sometimes even pleasure.[10,19]

Although deliberate self-harm may cause permanent physical damage, such as scarring or disability, it seldom causes death. Eventually, however, such behavior may become more dangerous, increasing the risk of suicide.[10,19]

Family patterns of interaction that contribute to this behavior pattern have not been delineated; research is needed to describe relevant early family situations and interactions.

ENTRY INTO TREATMENT. School nurses may recognize injuries or scars (for example, on forearms or legs) as evidence of self-harm, classmates may inform the nurse of self-harm behavior, or teachers may observe a student inflicting self-damage. In such instances the school system may refer the adolescent or family to counseling services. If episodes of self-harm cause serious disfigurement or physical disability, are occurring with increasing frequency, or are not resolved through outpatient treatment, then hospitalization may be recommended.

Suicidal Behavior

DEFINITION AND DESCRIPTION. Suicide attempts by adolescents vary in purpose and lethality. Adolescents who attempt suicide may be categorized as *intentional* and *unintentional.* Intentional attempters do want to kill themselves, recognize that they will die as a result, and choose a highly lethal method. Unintentional attempters do not intend to kill themselves, have not thought about the consequences of their actions or the finality of death, and choose a method that is not very likely to be lethal.

The processes leading to *intentional* suicide attempts include the following:[10]

- Perceiving problems remarkably accurately and maturely
- Experiencing an extended period of distress, usually dating back to early childhood
- Having a history of unsuccessful efforts to cope with problems
- Being driven to find solutions to problems when giving up and redirecting energy might be better
- Feeling isolated and lonely
- Thinking increasingly about problems caused by others, and feeling powerless
- Thinking obsessively about death and becoming involved in activities that seem to be directed toward an acceptance of death not as part of life, but as a way to escape it
- Overcoming moral and social constraints against suicide
- Arriving at a thoughtful decision to die, and planning suicide in a way that precludes rescue
- Choosing a lethal method, such as hanging or a firearm
- Implementing the plan thoughtfully rather than impulsively

Youngsters who intentionally attempt suicide experience despair, emotional pain, anger, and helplessness. When they are rescued (unlike those who deliberately harm themselves or make unintentional suicide attempts), they report no relief of tension and usually indicate increased distress because they survived.[19,20]

Adolescents who make *unintentional* suicide attempts have the following characteristics:

- They fail to consider the finality of death.
- They do not take time to plan a suicide attempt; the attempt is an impulsive gesture.
- They notify someone of the attempt immediately or make the attempt in the presence of people who will stop it and rescue them; they expect to be rescued.
- Their motivation may be to attract attention, to manipulate others, or to seek revenge.
- They may be attempting psychological blackmail or trying to control a relationship.
- They usually have a history of similar attempts; and they choose a method that is unlikely to be fatal.

DYNAMICS. Existing adolescent-family problems are compounded by normative problems generated by changes that occur during adolescence. Several risk factors are associated with adolescents' intentional suicide attempts.[7,9,10,19,21,22] See Table 39-2.

Motivation for an intentional suicide has two fundamental bases. First, these young people feel rejected and unwanted by their families; their need to be loved and their need to belong have been unfulfilled since childhood. Their feelings may have developed because their parents are physically absent or psychologically unavailable; or they may have been mistreated (physically abused, for example, or subjected to incest). Second, these youngsters experience an overwhelming sense of loss. The loss may be real or imagined, but in either case, from the adolescent's perspective it is permanent.[7] Loss of a parent before age 12 (from

Table 39-2 Intentional Suicide Attempts in Adolescence

Risk Factors
Academic problems coupled with unrealistic parental expectations
Family history of suicide attempts or completed suicides (parent, sibling, grandparent, relative)
Alcoholic parent
Chronically ill parent
History of and current child abuse (physical, sexual, hostile, or verbal)
Psychological unavailability of parents
Unstable or chaotic home environment
One or both parents absent from home
Living with a person other than a parent
Family history of high residential mobility
High number of school changes
Loss of significant relationship
Perception of self as unwanted or rejected by family
Perception of family conflict as extreme
Anniversary of a significant loss or crisis
Attempted or completed suicide by a close friend
Parental (or surrogate parental) denial or ignoring of signs of distress or previous suicide attempts

abandonment, separation, divorce, or death) is higher among suicide attempters than the general population.[23] These adolescents may be struggling with an unresolved mourning process. Some of these youngsters have been reared in intact families, but one parent has been chronically ill (particularly chronically depressed), or one or both parents were substance abusers and thus psychologically unavailable.[21]

In an attempt to compensate for emotional deprivation during childhood, these adolescents may become overinvested in an intense, emotionally charged relationship with a boyfriend or girlfriend. Their personal boundaries are not maintained. When the relationship ends, they may experience it as a loss of self and a further reason for killing themselves.[10]

At the other end of the continuum of parent-adolescent interaction are adolescents who experience parental "smothering." These youngsters have an ambivalent attitude toward the developmental struggle to separate from their parents: the transfer of love and desire from parents to peers is a source of conflict. The parents impede the separation process by failing to let go of the adolescent. Intense hatred of the parents occurs as a mechanism for separation, but this is countered by intense love and dependency. The "solution" is to turn hatred around toward the self, and thus suicide may become the only way to escape the symbiotic relationship with the parents.[24]

Among unintentional suicide attempters there is usually a history of parent-child problems, but not the extent of deprivation found among intentional attempters. Repeated impulsive gestures designed to manipulate and control the parents may have several outcomes. The family may live in constant fear that if they don't comply with the adolescent's wishes, he or she will become upset and make another attempt. In this situation the family becomes tyrannized by the adolescent. In contrast, some families ignore suicide attempts or deny their nature; these adolescents are at risk of "accidentally" committing suicide because no one comes to rescue them.[20]

ENTRY INTO TREATMENT. Adolescents who attempt suicide intentionally or unintentionally may be referred to treatment by the school system if the attempt was made on school property. If school nurses learn of attempts from an adolescent or from his or her peers, they may recommend that the family, including the adolescent, seek counseling. If the adolescent requires treatment in an emergency room, or hospitalization, for injuries sustained in the attempt, then psychiatric hospitalization is usually recommended.

Problems with School Attendance and Performance

Definition and Description

Problems with school attendance and performance that reflect underlying depression or anxiety include frequent absences, dropping out of school, a sudden and serious decline in academic performance, a history of underachievement, academic failure, and (sometimes) overachievement accompanied by isolation from the peer group. Some youngsters with school-related problems maintain a "tough," "know-it-all" facade as a cover for their low self-esteem and feelings of inadequacy. Others are shy and withdrawn, and have few if any friends.

Dynamics

The source of school problems is most often a dysfunctional parent-adolescent relationship that began in early childhood. For instance, four types of parent-adolescent interactions contribute to prolonged absences from school.

First, there is the chaotic family that places no value on education and makes no effort to promote attendance. Whether the adolescent remains in school, or even in the household, is of little concern. Inadequately socialized within the family, these adolescents are intolerant of the school structure that imposes limits on behavior and sets expectations for performance.

A second type of family has high expectations for performance and gives no positive feedback for accomplishments—only criticism. In these families adolescents perceive their value only in terms of achievement in schoolwork or sports that brings glory to the parents. There is little or no concern for the adolescent's wishes, preferences, and feelings. Parental approval is equated with public accomplishments rather than relationships within the family.

A third type of parent-child interaction is characterized by acute anxiety generated by the threat of separation. For the adolescent in such a family, problems with school attendance may peak with the transition from a neighborhood elementary school to a larger regional secondary school. The symbiotic parent-child relationship is intense; family equilibrium requires it. The parents' anxieties about separation and the adolescent's movement into a more peer-oriented milieu interact with those of the child. The threat to family equilibrium is reduced or eliminated if the adolescent develops a school phobia and remains at home, and the parents support this behavior.

The fourth type of parent-adolescent interaction occurs when chronic family anxiety escalates and reverberates. Anxiety may be generated by a parent's mental illness or a terminal illness, by the death of a parent or sibling, by divorce, by the alcoholism of a parent, by physical violence in the home, or by an incestuous relationship. The egocentrism of adolescence influences perceptions of such a family crisis and its consequences. An adolescent will be concerned for others in the family, but the focus of his or her anxieties is primarily the personal impact of the crisis, the threat to self. Thus the adolescent's ability to think clearly and logically and to concentrate is impaired; interest and participation in peer activities diminish; school performance declines; and attendance becomes sporadic. As withdrawal and self-absorption increase anxiety, the ability to cope deteriorates. The parents' own self-absorption may prevent them from recognizing the adolescent's distress.

Some adolescents whose achievements match their potential may be suffering from the equivalent of "success phobias" in adults. These youngsters are afraid of aggression and competition; their need is to have others like them. If their families urge them to compete aggressively and become successful, they have a conflict: success breeds envy and jealousy in others, which would interfere with their need to be liked. This conflict interferes with school performance.[10]

An overachiever may be able to win parental approval and love only through academic excellence. To maintain that excellence, the adolescent may be ignoring other areas of development. These youngsters have no time for peer relationships or recreation; they fail to develop social skills and are eventually alienated from and rejected by their peers.

Entry into Treatment

Many troubled youngsters do not receive treatment unless the school system has a counseling program for students who are chronically absent or whose grades show a sudden unexplained decline. Once an adolescent drops out of school, the school system may make little effort to follow through, to identify problems, or to make referrals for counseling, particularly if the adolescent is 16 or older. These teenagers come into treatment only if they are referred because of delinquency, running away, or substance abuse, or if their parents take the initiative. Those under age 16 who are chronically absent and may be school-phobic usually enter treatment because school authorities have insisted on it.

Running Away

Definition and Description

Running away (or *runaway behavior*) is defined as staying out of the home for at least 24 hours without parental consent or knowledge of the adolescent's whereabouts. Slightly more than one-half of runaways are males. There is little statistical difference between the percentages of white, black, and Hispanic runaways; and blue- and white-collar families are equally represented. One-half of all runaways travel less than 10 miles from home.[7] Some, following a heated argument with their parents, simply stay overnight at a friend's house. Others stay in cars, vans, or empty houses in the community. They may continue to attend school, work at a part-time job, and see their friends. With money from part-time jobs and with the help of friends, they manage to eat regularly. In time they return home; but most continue to run away periodically.

Seventy percent of runaways return home within a week.[15] Of those who stay away longer than a week, some eventually return home and others never return. One in twenty stays away a year or longer. Those who do not stay near their families and hometowns migrate to urban centers, where the struggle to survive inevitably creates problems. Since they are young, have no employable skills, have no place to live, and have no legal guardians, they cannot find jobs. Often they are ineligible for welfare or government training programs.[25] They may become "street people," living out of bags, foraging for food in garbage pails, and sleeping wherever they can find an unused doorway or hallway. They are hungry, dirty, tired, and scared. They become easy victims of pimps, pornographers, and drug dealers. To buy food and shelter they steal, shoplift, or panhandle or become muggers, pushers, or prostitutes.

The risk to health and life is high for these adolescents. They are vulnerable to physical abuse, rape, homicide, suicide, sexually transmitted diseases, unwanted pregnancies, and substance abuse. A chaotic lifestyle, inadequate nutrition, and poor hygiene—along with difficulties in getting sufficient restful sleep and the stress associated with continuous exposure to danger—increase the risk of a variety of health problems.

Typically, adolescent runaways are immature in many ways, despite the fact that they are on their own. Their attitude is sometimes sullen, hostile, and confronting. They have low self-esteem and feel rejected, inadequate, and lonely.[15]

Dynamics

Most adolescents who run away from home are doing so to escape an intolerable family situation. They hunger for affection and are seething with suppressed and repressed anger. They have had little opportunity in their families to express their anger directly. If they steal, it is usually only from the family to finance their running away. These adolescents may run away from home with the fantasy of punishing their families for real or imagined injustices and unkindnesses. They envision scenes and play out scenarios in which their parents are distraught and regretful.[25]

A variety of family-adolescent patterns of interaction contribute to runaway behavior. Some adolescents who are physically or sexually abused by a parent or surrogate parent may perceive running away as the only way to escape physical conflict, or an incestuous relationship. Living in poverty, in overcrowded conditions where the adolescent feels like an unwanted burden, may appear to offer little more than living on the streets. Living with a parent's alcoholism or criminal activity may become a chaotic or terrifying experience. An adolescent may seek relief by running away periodically or may decide to leave the family permanently.

Some families cannot tolerate the normative separation that occurs during adolescence. These families increase control and become more restrictive. The adolescent whose struggle to separate seems unsuccessful may run away to challenge parental control and to bring about a loosening of controls.

Oldest daughters are often given major household responsibilities and required to care for younger siblings while they themselves are still children. With the onset of adolescence and the need for independence and peer relationships, these burdens become intolerable. Running away becomes an escape from this "parentification," and a way of forcing the parents to assume their own responsibilities.

If an adolescent son or daughter has been used by a parent as a companion and as a way to maintain distance in the marital relationship, normative adolescent separation will threaten to upset family equilibrium, and the parent's efforts to obstruct this separation may precipitate runaway behavior. In such families, the absence from the household may be short-lived: the adolescent returns to restabilize the family and prevent the breakup of the parent's marriage, which is unable to stand the closeness that occurs when the adolescent is absent.

Parents who have always maintained a conforming, conservative lifestyle may fantasize a free-swinging, adventurous, risk-taking life even though they are too inhibited to experiment with nonconformity. These parents may unconsciously encourage adolescents to live their fantasy life. The adolescents actively participate by taking risks, running away, and participating in a variety of escapades, and by reporting these adventures to their parents. The parents, needing to escape from their conservatism, vicariously live out their fantasy life.

In divorced and separated families, adolescents may serve as go-betweens for the parents. Children in such families often have a "reunion fantasy" (mother and father back together again). If the children's problems force the parents to get together to talk, rather than using a child as a go-between, then an adolescent may use periodic running away as a mechanism for reuniting the parents.

In some families, an adolescent's running away precipitates a crisis. Parents' fears for the safety of the adolescent elicit efforts to find and return the youngster to the home. Frantic calls are made to friends, relatives, neighbors, and the police. In other families, little or no effort is made to locate the adolescent. No one is called; no search is initiated.

Entry into Treatment

Families may or may not seek treatment because of an adolescent's runaway behavior. If they do, they may initially seek outpatient counseling. If this treatment excludes the parents, however, focusing only on the adolescent, episodes of running away are likely to continue. Many parents do not seek inpatient treatment for the adolescent until the runaway pattern is well established. In some instances, school authorities make the referral.

If runaway teenagers are arrested as a result of criminal activity (such as pushing drugs, stealing, or prostitution), they may be sent back home or placed in a foster home or group home if they are under age 16. If older, they may be sentenced to a reformatory or jail. Individual counseling is often not available in these institutions. Recommendations for treatment are usually made but not always enforced if the adolescent returns home.

Substance Abuse

Definition and Description

Experimentation with drugs or alcohol does not indicate serious psychosocial dysfunctioning in the adolescent.[26] But prolonged regular and sometimes heavy use of mind-altering substances such as alcohol, cannabis, sedatives, opioids, cocaine, amphetamines, and hallucinogens is abuse. As a result of substance abuse, an adolescent's performance in school may be impaired, social relations may be disrupted by erratic and impulsive behavior, and automobile accidents or criminal behavior (such as stealing) may occur.

Adolescents may actually abuse only one substance, such as alcohol or cannabis, but they are likely to experiment with whatever capsules or pills they can acquire. They often mix these drugs with alcohol, even though they know it is dangerous. Sniffing glue, using PCP, tripping on LSD, skin popping, free-basing, and sniffing cocaine may all be tried for varying periods.

These young people will acknowledge the risk involved in taking "street" drugs, but they tend to shrug it off with a comment such as, "I've never gotten burned." Their risk taking and apparent lack of concern reflect their underlying depression and anxiety.

Dynamics

Research indicates that, rather than first emerging in adolescence, dysfunctional behavior patterns have been present throughout childhood. Five areas of social maladaptation in early childhood have been associated with increased risk of substance abuse in adolescence:[27]

1. *Shyness.* These youngsters are often timid and friendless.
2. *Aggressiveness.* They resist authority, lie, fight, and are disobedient.
3. *Immaturity.* They seek attention in disruptive ways, including tantrums.
4. *Underachievement.* Their performance in school falls short of their ability.

5. *Short attention span.* They are restless and easily distracted.

Adolescents' vulnerability to substance abuse is increased by long-standing underlying depressions, mismanagement of anxiety, and dysfunctional parent-child relationships.

When adolescents suffer from chronic emotional pain associated with depression and anxiety, they seek relief.[28] Use of drugs and alcohol to provide this relief is a function of sociodemographic, family, and individual interactions.[29] The choice of substance depends on availability. Initially these adolescents may tap their parents' liquor supply or steal their tranquilizers or sleeping pills. Once they experience release of tension from experimenting with what is available in the home, they seek out peers who either sell or can make contact with suppliers of drugs and marijuana, or they find someone older who can purchase alcohol.

Drug abuse is learned. Youngsters observe their parents' use of alcohol, tranquilizers, and marijuana to escape from anxiety and frustration. This behavior is reinforced by television, radio, magazines, and music. Commercials and advertisements "push" a variety of remedies to ease the tensions of daily living and to induce sleep. Adolescents see people in the adult world using drugs to escape from problems.

Substance abuse by adolescents closely parallels the patterns of their closest friends. Peer pressure, a need to conform to the peer group, and a substance-abusing peer group seem to be even greater influences than abuse of drugs or alcohol by parents or siblings.[30]

Interacting factors associated with substance abuse among adolescents are presented in Table 39-3. In addition, the effects of the substance used influence the behavior. Alcohol dependence, which is characterized by a need for daily use, an inability to cut down or stop drinking, and increased depression and anxiety when abstinence is attempted, reinforces continued abuse. Regular and heavy use of cannabis has been associated with memory problems (storage and retrieval), impaired motor coordination, bouts of acute anxiety, and generalized apathy.[31] These cognitive changes alter problem solving and decision making. The affective symptoms of anxiety increase the need for cannabis, and apathy interferes with motivation to stop using the drug.

Table 39-3 Substance Abuse in Adolescence

Interacting Factors
Peer pressure
Disrupted family structure (death, divorce)
Overrestrictive, overpermissive, or inconsistent parenting
Psychologically unavailable parents (lacking warmth, hostile, critical, not supportive)
History of behavior problems in childhood
Substance abuse by a parent or older sibling
Antisocial adolescent behavior pattern
Lack of religion
Poor performance at school—more failures than successes
Risk-taking behavior
Feelings of alienation

Entry into Treatment

Nurses interact with these youngsters in schools and in both inpatient and outpatient medical and psychiatric settings, and they may make referrals for treatment. Often psychiatric hospitalization is precipitated by an episode of running away, acting out, or delinquency. Sometimes, a substance-abuse treatment program is chosen to avoid imprisonment or is ordered after an adolescent has been arrested for possession or sale of controlled substances. Parents may have an adolescent committed because use of LSD led to a psychotic episode, or because they have recognized that the adolescent is having blackouts or anxiety attacks after drinking heavily. Adolescents who are simply avoiding imprisonment may be the most unwilling clients and may initially invest much time and energy devising ways to escape or to have drugs brought in to them. They flout hospital rules and policies and resist examining their feelings, exploring their behavior, and planning realistic changes in coping patterns and lifestyle.

Adolescent substance abusers tend to be manipulative. If there are any divisions among the staff, they find out and use their knowledge to cause disruption. Hospitalization does not mean the end of drug use for these clients. They will plot and plan to either smuggle in drugs or alcohol or have them brought in. Hence they, their activities, and their visitors require careful surveillance.

Delinquent Behavior

Definition and Description

The definition of *delinquent behavior* is to some degree socioculturally determined.

Juvenile delinquency is a legal and sociological term that has no precise psychiatric definition and is infused with value judgments. Whether a behavior is labeled *juvenile delinquency* or *youthful mischief* may be a function of who is attaching the label and what factors are influencing that person's perceptions. An adolescent from an affluent family that is powerful in the community will more than likely be treated very differently from an adolescent who is growing up in an urban ghetto. The latter is more apt to become a court case and spend time in an institution or on parole than the former. The label *delinquency* is appropriate when adolescents set fires, steal (in the form of shoplifting, burglary, or mugging), assault others, rape, murder, or engage in other criminal activities.

Delinquency is a continuum ranging from one or few minor illegal activities to many serious offenses. For example, stealing may range from pilfering of objects or money from family members or friends, to shoplifting, stealing a bicycle, stealing an automobile, and burglarizing an empty house without a weapon, and then to burglary and assault with a deadly weapon.

Dynamics

Delinquent young people are not constrained from committing deviant behavior by a moral code, a well-developed conscience, or consideration of possible consequences to themselves, their families, or society. They seem unaware of the moral implications of their behavior. They are totally self-focused and insensitive to the rights and feelings of others.

There is considerable difference among these offenders with relation to ego organization. Research findings also suggest that, for some, there are delays in cognitive development and deficiencies in other areas of neurologic development.[16,32] It may be that these developmental deficiencies contribute to academic problems, chronic inability to please adults, and persistent failure, with a consequent loss of self-esteem. These deficiencies may also impair the development of moral judgment. These youngsters' learning disabilities (which are related to developmental deficiencies) and anxious behavior when they recognized that they were lagging behind their peers may have been mislabeled in childhood as *lack of intelligence* or *misbehavior*.[33] Consequently, they may have been ridiculed or punished, with the result that their difficulties were exacerbated. These adolescents also tend to have language deficiencies which interfere with effective communication of their needs and problems.[16] Academic difficulties make them prone to drop out of school, and dropping out puts them at risk of antisocial behavior and substance abuse.

Overrestrictive or permissive parents, and parents who set limits inconsistently and illogically, have also been associated with development of delinquent behavior. Finally, some adolescents are following in their parents' footsteps when they begin a life of crime.[34]

Entry into Treatment

Delinquent adolescents admitted to psychiatric inpatient settings have often been remanded by a court (and are therefore involuntary clients), or they may enter treatment voluntarily while awaiting a court appearance for a serious offense. In either case, unmanageable, antisocial behavior or failure to participate in treatment can result in a transfer or sentencing to a correctional institution. This reality provides some leverage in engaging the adolescent in the treatment process.

Many adolescents admitted to an inpatient psychiatric setting for substance abuse, running away, or acting out also have a history of delinquent behavior that is not identified until treatment is under way.[35]

Dysfunctional Sexuality

Definition and Description

Problems of sexuality encountered by adolescents include ignorance about sexual matters (lack of accurate information about intercourse, fertility, masturbation, contraception, and so on), promiscuity, unintended pregnancy, sexually transmitted diseases, and sexual identity conflicts.[36,37] Biological development of secondary sex characteristics may precede psychological or social readiness to deal with sexuality, or biological development may lag behind psychological and social readiness. In either case, the adolescent may be distressed.

Dynamics

Conformity with peers is very important to adolescents. This need for conformity extends to sexual maturation and behavior: any perceived deviance is a cause for concern and may be a source of anxiety. Nonconformity entails a risk of rejection and exclusion.

Peer group pressure is associated with early sexual experimentation. Both males and females may succumb to this pressure in adolescence rather than risk "being different." These young people often lack basic information about anatomy and physiology, know little about contraceptives, and are emotionally unready for sexual experiences. Girls may be at a high risk of unintended pregnancy because they fail to use any form of contraception or use a form that provides inadequate protection.

If parents are uncomfortable about discussing sexual matters and reluctant to give fact-oriented sex education, they may fail to provide adolescents with opportunities to talk about relational aspects of sexual intercourse, premarital sex and abstinence, and feelings about sexuality. Discussions with adults, in an accepting, respectful atmosphere, are necessary if teenagers are to clarify values and moral issues, explore feelings, and make thoughtful personal decisions. Reluctance and embarrassment on the part of parents may convey to adolescents that sexual expression is not a normal part of human functioning and that there is something about it that is "not nice." When parents deny an adolescent's eroticism, punish it, or call it sinful or bad, they interfere with the adolescent's developing sense of identity, self-esteem, and sexual pleasure.[38]

Many adolescents engage in unprotected sexual intercourse, increasing the risk of unintended pregnancy. Some of these youngsters lack adequate information about or access to contraceptives. But many do have access to contraceptives, information, and services and simply choose not to use them; these adolescents may become pregnant intentionally.[39] Research has identified several factors that contribute to intentional teenage pregnancy; these are presented in Table 39-4. They encompass the adolescent's emotional need for pregnancy and dysfunctional parent-adolescent interactions.

Table 39-4 Intentional Pregnancy in Adolescence

Contributing Factors
Depression
Need to escape from personal problems
Poor school performance
Recent loss of a loved one
Acting-out behavior resulting from parent-adolescent conflict
Lack of love and approval in parent-adolescent relationship
Wanting someone to love them
Fear of abandonment by boyfriend
Wish to prove they are mature and independent
Need to affirm female identity
Repeated and cumulative experiences of failure
Parental complicity
Mother's need for another child but inability or unwillingness to become pregnant

Masturbation during adolescence is not in and of itself a problem unless an intervening situation or communication induces shame or guilt. It is normal for teenagers to explore their bodies and experience ejaculation or orgasm. Masturbation is usually accompanied by erotic imagery, and it is this aspect of the experience that makes the adolescent feel guilty, frightened, and troubled. Misinformation or ignorance about sexuality, and a poorly developed defensive structure, may cause masturbation to become a problem for the adolescent.[40]

Sexual promiscuity is a symptom of underlying depression and anxiety. Promiscuous adolescents are frantically seeking closeness and affirmation of their identity and sexuality in a series of sexual encounters which only leave them feeling lonelier and less accepting of themselves. The negative opinions of others concerning their promiscuous behavior reinforce their own poor self-concept. Even though they may find that their behavior fails to satisfy their needs for love and belonging and only aggravates their depression and anxiety, they seem unable to break the pattern. When sexual promiscuity occurs, the parent-adolescent relationship is and has been dysfunctional.

Intense same-sex friendships are a part of normal adolescent development. During this time, there may be experimental homosexual activity; evidence of same-sex affection is tolerated by society when it occurs between girls but is condemned between boys. This early adolescent stage usually evolves into a heterosexual orientation for love and desire.[41,42] Even during the stage of heterosexual orientation, adolescents may engage in homosexual activity when alternatives are not available (in a same-sex boarding school or a reformatory, for instance) but return to heterosexual interests and practices when circumstances change.[42] When adolescents experience warm, erotic feelings toward a friend of the same sex, they may interpret the experience as evidence of homosexuality and become anxious and depressed. Rarely will adolescents discuss their homosexual experiences. If an adolescent lacks a peer group and tends to be socially isolated, working through a fear of homosexuality may become difficult or impossible. Then, anxiety may escalate, and to reaffirm heterosexuality, the adolescent may become temporarily promiscuous.[43]

Homosexual characteristics appear to be established before adolescence. The self-conscious psychological orientation predates adolescence[42,44] but is not necessarily recognized as such until adolescence. Male homosexuals usually report that they became aware of their homosexual orientation during early adolescence; lesbians report this awareness in late adolescence.[42] Awareness of a homosexual orientation is not in and of itself problematic. Problems arise when adolescents experience acute internal conflicts, or when their orientation is known to heterosexual peers. The gender-role nonconformity of homosexually oriented adolescents often results in exclusion from the peer group, although this is more likely to happen with males than females. These youngsters are consequently more apt to be loners, feeling socially isolated and left out.[45,46]

Adolescents whose moral development is impaired or who act out to counter feelings of frustration, helplessness, deprivation, and anger may do so in a sexually aggressive fashion such as rape. In the community there is greater opportunity for heterosexual encounters and sexual mutuality. However, among institutionalized adolescents where only same-sex peers are present, these adolescents may participate in homosexual rape. Both the victims and the perpetrators may experience acute psychological distress after such an incident.

Entry into Treatment

Problematic sexual episodes that bring adolescents into treatment vary widely. Some adolescents are brought to a health care setting by parents who misinterpret normal sexual experimentation as evidence of deviant behavior. They may accuse the young person of being a "whore" or "gay." When youngsters are berated with these labels by significant others, the messages may become self-fulfilling prophecies. The adolescent's behavior begins to conform to the accusation, and these young people take the position that "if I am accused of it no matter what I say, I might as well do it."

Some adolescents are admitted to a psychiatric setting because of episodes of running away, poor school performance, or acting out. In the course of treatment, problematic sexual issues emerge. Adolescents in psychiatric treatment may try to use sex to manage feelings of depression and anxiety generated by the therapy. They may attempt sexual encounters with peers who are also in treatment, or they may act seductively toward staff members of the opposite sex.

Cult Membership

Definition and Description

Cults are, in contemporary usage, religious sects which (from the point of view of the society) promote deviant religions. They vary in size from small communes to international organizations. Regardless of size, they fall into two categories: "world savers" and narcissistic quasi-therapy groups. Both categories are led by charismatic authority figures who claim to be "messengers from God," and who dictate and regulate the behavior, thoughts, and interactions of their followers. Both categories have two primary functions: recruiting members and fund-raising. The cohesiveness of the membership is maintained through shared devotion and allegiance to the leader and the movement, and a system of beliefs and rituals.[47,48]

Some cults are dangerous to the emotional and physical well-being of members, their families, and society.[49] They tend to be first-generation entities with living leaders. Their goals include rapid expansion, aggressive conversion, and use of members to acquire large sums of money.[50] Table 39-5 lists characteristics of a destructive cult.

Adolescents who become involved in cults range in age between 18 and 25 years. Their induction into the cult usually occurs through a series of workshops, which are followed by a period of intense indoctrination. The characteristics of the

Table 39-5 Destructive Cults

Characteristics
Demand complete obedience to and subservience to one individual, who purports to be God, the Messiah, or some form of, or a messenger of, the deity.
Require separation from society. Association with non-members is discouraged except to gain money or proselytize.
Discourage any form of self-development. Education is scorned, and the self-image is totally destroyed.
Teach hatred of parents, organized religion, and sometimes the United States government.
Do not have concern for the material body; feel only the soul is important.
Take all material possessions (past, present, and future) for cult's use. Members are not permitted to own anything in their own names.
Make it almost impossible for a member to leave, either through the use of physical restraints or psychological fears.
Maintain the member in a "brainwashed" state through destructive behavior modification techniques.

Table 39-6 Indoctrination into a Cult

Indoctrination Process
Long, boring lectures on good and evil
Fatiguing rituals
Sleep deprivation
Rhythmic dancing and chanting
Disconfirmation of perceptions of self, beliefs, values
Isolation from society, family, friends, and familiar surroundings
Arousal of feelings of guilt, helplessness, and loneliness; belief that these feelings can be eased or eliminated by the leader
Warnings of inevitable physical death and loss of immortality if beliefs and rituals are not followed
Discouragement of questions, challenges, critical comments

indoctrination process are listed in Table 39-6; it has been described as a form of "brainwashing" or "mind control."[49]

Dynamics

Some investigators of cults have found no evidence of mind control or mental or physical harm and substantiate this finding by the high percentage of potential recruits who drop out early.[51] "Brainwashing" and "mind control" may be effective only with those people who are already susceptible. Many who join have recently experienced high levels of psychological distress—a broken romance, substance abuse (not necessarily drug addiction or alcoholism), interpersonal problems—or are at a turning point in their lives, such as beginning or ending college or starting a new job in a strange city. They find that the authoritarianism of the cult and its social and ideological cohesiveness provide structure in their lives. Membership helps them overcome loneliness and establish normative values, a sense of purpose, and freedom from decision making and individual responsibility. Cult members appear to be seeking standards and beliefs that provide them with a way of dispelling confusion and uncertainty. A cult is an escape from self-responsibility.[48,52]

Those who stay in a cult appear to have a pronounced need for dependency that is an exaggeration of the kind seen during childhood and early adolescence. The highly authoritarian structure characteristic of cults creates a milieu that fosters total dependency, a situation which is reinforced by idolization of the charismatic leader. All dependency needs are satisfied in the cult, and only in the cult.[48,52]

Some adolescents who join and remain in a cult have not engaged in antisocial behavior. They may be motivated by idealism or a search for a perfect life through austerity. Some are drawn into the cult and induced to stay through the initial stages by flattery, peer pressure, curiosity, and a need to "find themselves."

Those who drop out of cults have generally found the authoritarian structure and demands unacceptable; after they leave, they may continue to experiment with various groups and lifestyles.[52] An investigation of people who voluntarily left the Unification Church indicates that leaving a cult may reflect maturation. Initially, these young people need the cult's structure, authoritarianism, and values. As time passes, they experience conflicts between the norms of the cult and their own personal expectations and tend to become more psychologically stable. They become dissatisfied with certain aspects of the cult, such as lack of privacy and periodic geographical transfers. These findings suggest that formulation of self-concept and a movement toward independence have occurred.[47]

Vulnerability to cult membership reflects dysfunctional separation from the family. Parents and adolescents fear separation and independence from the family. These fears may precipitate adolescents' decision to join a cult: the cult represents a total break with the family they are unable to separate from in an orderly fashion and fear will never let them go. But this reactive step toward independence is in reality a transfer of dependency and enmeshment from the family to the cult.

Some parents believe that their children have been kidnapped and brainwashed, and therefore attempt to rescue them by means of kidnapping and deprogramming. Deprogramming is also a form of mind control or brainwashing. It is based on the premise that these young people do not voluntarily adhere to the beliefs and world views they have adopted as members of the cult but have been programmed by the cult.[37,48,49,53] The elements of deprogramming are shown in Table 39-7.

Entry into Treatment

While they are active members of a cult, young people do not seek mental health services; they see no need. Some who voluntarily leave a cult may seek outpatient counseling to help them adjust to living in a less structured society.

Those who have been deprogrammed often feel humiliated, ashamed at having been duped, and guilty about the emotional pain and worry experienced by their families. The involuntary separation from the cult, its structure, and its sense of purpose—and the recognition of responsibility for self following deprogramming—may be overwhelming.

Table 39-7 Deprogramming

Procedure
Interventions that elicit emotional excitement
Induction of intense anger, aggression, fear, and anxiety through confrontation and negation of cult beliefs
Confrontation on how the young person was duped or deceived into becoming a member
Imposing sleep deprivation and exhaustion
Moving the young people from place to place; forcibly retaining them in each location and during the moves
Interventions directed toward destruction of the use of repression, and induction of physical and emotional collapse

An acute anxiety reaction or a psychotic episode may occur, requiring hospitalization.[52]

Somatic Complaints

Definition and Description

When adolescents manifest their distress somatically, their complaints and problems range from minor psychosomatic symptoms to serious illnesses.[54,55,56] They may suffer from chronic headaches or stomachaches, rashes, episodes of dizziness, flare-ups of acne, ulcerative colitis, or eating disorders such as bulimia and anorexia nervosa (see Chapter 42).

Dynamics

These youngsters are experiencing chronic depression and anxiety, and they mismanage stressors in their lives. The biopsychosocial changes that are part of adolescent development may impair fragile coping mechanisms.

Somatic symptoms often reflect conflicts related to separating from the family and beginning an independent life, dealing with peer pressures, accepting sexuality, choosing a career, and dealing with concerns about body image. Their families tend to suppress feelings and enforce conformity. In addition, these families are usually experiencing difficulty "letting go" of the adolescent and recognizing the need for privacy.[54] Consequently, the adolescent's tension, created by suppressed feelings, is manifested somatically.

Entry into Treatment

Somatic problems are often brought to the attention of a school nurse. Teenagers may seek help from the school nurse for their symptoms, and only after a relationship has been established with the nurse will they reveal their anxiety, depression, fears, and family problems. The school nurse is then able to refer them for counseling. Those whose symptoms are treated by a physician may or may not be referred for psychiatric care. Physical symptoms and medical care are more socially accepted in this society than emotional symptoms and psychiatric care. Both medically oriented physicians and parents may resist seeing somatic symptoms as evidence of emotional turmoil.

PATTERNS OF INTERACTION: FAMILY

Adolescents whose behavior patterns are problematic have usually experienced a dysfunctional parent-child relationship since early childhood. The adolescent's developmental task of separation from the parents and becoming independent and the parents' developmental task of "letting go" and facilitating the adolescent's independence are interactive. The separation process influences the development of dysfunctional adolescent behavior patterns.

Separation Dynamics*

Steirlin[2] has categorized family separation dynamics which interfere with the adolescent's progress through this stage of development as centripetal, centrifugal, or delegating. His framework has to do with the issue of separation and the way transactional modes in the family system interfere with the process. Age-appropriate transactional modes are out of phase in these families. They are too intense, inappropriately mixed with other modes, or too distancing.

Centripetal Dynamics

Centripetal dynamics are forces within the family that interfere with the permeability of the family system's external boundary and influence the family's emotional system. These factors keep members within the family and prevent their individuation and separation. When centripetal dynamics are operating, the family employs a binding mode of transaction. Members operate under an unspoken assumption that needs can be satisfied *only* within the family system. The outside world is viewed as dangerous and unsatisfying. This sets up insurmountable barriers between the family and society and, in a collusive way, forces members to remain within the family. It fulfills some needs for security, support, and nurturing, but it does so at the expense of individual ideas, feelings, experiences, and behavior. Members are prevented from separating and differentiating, and that is destructive to the development of individual potential and freedom.[2]

* This section from Katharine J. Burns, "Adolescent Adjustment Reactions," in the second edition of this book.

The binding process corrals the members through the affective, cognitive, and superego levels. *Affective binding* is accomplished by offering the adolescent too much regressive gratification and thus infantilizing the youngster.[2] Awakening libidinal drives and the oedipal conflict are blocked from resolution in peer and societal relationships. The parents, particularly the opposite-sex parent, become the focus of reactivated symbiotic and incestuous feelings. Anxiety increases in youngsters who are blocked from moving away, and it must be defended against, yet running way or rebelling is not possible without feeling guilt and increasing anxiety. Even if these youngsters do manage to reach out to others, their ingrained, well-learned, excessive demands for regressive gratification are intolerable and unacceptable to peers or adults outside the family. These young people often use drugs or alcohol to quiet aggressive and sexual drives and to enable them to tolerate the smothering family life. Since substance abuse does not, at least initially, interfere with the mutual parent-child dependence, it is often covertly and unconsciously supported by the parents.[2]

Binding on the cognitive level occurs when the parents interfere with the adolescent's self-differentiated awareness and self-determination. The parents attribute to the adolescent feelings, needs, motives, and goals that disconfirm the child's position in these areas. Such an attribution process interferes with the ability of adolescents to perceive and differentiate what they are experiencing, want, and need by substituting or withholding meaning. An example of substituting meaning may occur when a daughter is angry because she cannot select her own clothes. Her parent tells her that she is just nervous, thus substituting anxiety for anger and disconfirming the daughter's own perception of the events and her feelings about them. Withholding of meaning is usually accomplished by parents who are silent or cryptic. Without reality-based feedback and shared perceptions, the adolescent is cognitively isolated and immobilized. The developing cognitive skills are blocked and distorted, leaving only fantasy, supposition, and untested hypotheses rather than logic and rationality.[2]

Binding on the superego level occurs when parents interfere with the process of loyalty transfer. These parents paint a picture of self-sacrifice, concern, and love. Any investment of feeling or interest in others is seen and interpreted as a rejection of them. The parental message to the adolescent is clearly, "How can you treat us like this and leave us? We live only for you." Consequently, if these adolescents attempt to initiate the normal separation process of this developmental stage, they feel guilty about abandoning their "loving" parents, who cannot exist without them. The conflict between parental requirements and developmental needs is intolerable, and they see self-destruction or incorporation back into the family system as the only alternatives.[2]

Centrifugal Dynamics

Centrifugal dynamics are forces within the family that diminish the integrity of the family system's boundaries and emotional system. These changes in family structure and function interfere with members' connectedness to the family and lead to premature separation. In centrifugal dynamics the parents are also coping with their own crises. The problems inherent in their adolescent's growth process are not the focus of their interest and are burdensome. Concerned primarily with their own needs, goals, and desires, they lack both the energy and the motivation to help the adolescent.

These parents do not want their children; instead, they want to pursue desired changes in their own lives.[2] They may not be ready or able to confront their own aging process. They may exhibit this expelling mode by becoming totally absorbed in their own recreation or work and simply ignoring their adolescents. They set no limits and provide no stability or support, and they may be unavailable physically and emotionally. If a youngster runs into problems at school or with the law, the parental attitude is, "What do you want me to do? I can't follow him (or her) around."

These youngsters may or may not be neglected or deprived materially; some live in the most luxurious of homes and are provided generously with food, clothes, money, and transportation. Others, however, lack even the bare necessities of life: warmth, food, adequate clothing, and a safe home. In either circumstance, they are seen by their parents as nuisances and also see themselves in that light.

In some instances adolescents are thrown out of the house; in others they run away because they are aware that they are unwanted. Sometimes the parent or parents go away—if not permanently, then for extended periods of time—leaving their children without financial support.

Youngsters caught in such a situation are left to spend their time as they wish. They collude in the lack of communication. They say little or nothing about their feelings, expectations, or activities; their parents ask no questions. The family may simply coexist under the same roof. All the relational aspects of family life are minimal or absent.

Some of these young people, left to their own devices, exhibit delinquent behavior, become drug abusers, or create violent turmoil in the home. When the school authorities or police confront the parents, they choose not to take active steps toward helping their children. Enraged that their lives are being disrupted, they expel the adolescent from the family system through a psychiatric commitment, surrender of guardianship, placement in a boarding school, or refusal to allow the youngster back into the home.

Delegating Dynamics

Delegating dynamics are forces within the family that influence adolescent members to act as emissaries or proxies for the parents; in doing so, they fulfill parental wishes, fantasies, or dreams at the expense of their own growth and development. Parental developmental crises contribute to the emergence of delegating dynamics. These ambivalent and conflicted parents select neither the centripetal nor the centrifugal solution to the problematic adolescent growth phase.[2] They are caught between their wish to consolidate existing relationships and positions and their desire to be rid of the adolescent. Consequently, they send conflicting messages to their adolescents: "Leave, but don't leave." They send the adolescent out on a mission as a proxy, while at the same time they hold on. The adolescent incorporates this ambivalence.

Steirlin[2] has identified four types of missions that adolescents may carry out to serve the ego needs of parents: (1) helping (work around the house, financial support of the household); (2) fighting (support of embattled parent); (3) scouting (serving as parents' experimenter); and (4) preserving (protecting fragile parents from conflict, activating emotions, and ambivalence).

A parent may vicariously enjoy and covertly support the acting out of dissocial impulses. An adolescent's dissocial behavior or successes in school may vicariously fulfill parental fantasies or experiences parents were deprived of in their own youth. The adolescent's behavior is directed not toward self-fulfillment but toward the affective and ego needs of the parents. Some parents may push their adolescent into the world to experiment with a single lifestyle before they themselves decide to get a divorce and pursue a similar lifestyle.

When parents have punitive and restrictive superegos, they may ascribe any one of three superego functions to the adolescent: (1) to serve as ego ideal, (2) to provide self-observation, or (3) to serve as a conscience.[2] If the first alternative is selected, the youngster's career choice will fit parental expectations and their own unfulfilled dreams regardless of the adolescent's personal preference. When given the self-observation mission, the adolescent must behave in ways that are contrary to the family's values and be "mad" or "bad." If the third alternative applies, the adolescent will be covertly encouraged to exhibit behavior that justifies punishment. The adolescent tends to exhibit antisocial behavior similar or comparable to that of the parent in the past. For example, the premarital pregnancy of a daughter and consequent maternal punishment resolve the mother's guilty feelings about her own out-of-wedlock pregnancy.[2]

Parents' Behavior Patterns*

Parents' perceptions of their role influence their behavior. Changes that occur with adolescence may threaten the parents, and the adolescent's behavior may interact with the parents' own residual adolescent fantasies and impulses. To protect and defend themselves and their status, they may act as omnipotent authority figures, become moralistic and self-righteous, or attempt to have a peer relationship with the adolescent. If the parents' ability to defend themselves is impaired, they may become overwhelmed and resort to suicide.

Omnipotent Authoritarianism

A parents' efforts may be directed toward supporting and preserving his or her self-concept as a strong, experienced, all-knowing adult with the privileges of seniority. To maintain this position, the adult must devalue the adolescent's accomplishments and activities. There is a need to keep the adolescent a dependent child; this frustrates the adolescent's developmental imperative for increasing independence. Frustration is generated in the adolescent by enforced regression, helplessness, and loss of opportunities to develop adult self-esteem and competence. Control over their own death or rebellious behavior may be seen by such adolescents as the only areas in which self-mastery is possible.[57]

Moralistic Self-Righteousness

In this pattern, interactions with adolescent offspring are characterized by moralizing and preaching directed toward eliciting demonstrations of respect and submission. To obey is paramount, to disobey catastrophic. This position, with its self-righteous, holier-than-thou proclamations, protects parents from acknowledging their revolt against their own parents and preserves their authority status with all its rights and privileges. At the same time it leaves the adolescent in a one-down position. To some adolescents this position becomes untenable. To rebel is to be bad. Truth, honesty, and morality appear to support the parental position. To confront and challenge it is unacceptable. Voluntary death or acceptance of the "bad" identity and role may be viewed as the only alternatives, since perfection is unattainable.

Peer Relationship

When parents define themselves as completely in tune with the adolescent and totally understanding of the adolescent's situation, they are suppressing their own terrified hostility in relation to adolescence. They identify with the ideal parents they would have liked and with the aggressivity of the adolescent. To protect themselves, they project a "nice-guy," "I am your friend" image. This position is designed to block the adolescent's hostile aggressive attacks and preserve self-images the parents find acceptable. In the process they obstruct the expression of developmentally necessary parent-child conflict. To attack "good" and "understanding" parents is perceived by the adolescent as unacceptable. But without parent-child conflict, maturation and hopes for becoming an adult seem

* This section from Katharine J. Burns, "Adolescent Adjustment Reactions," in the second edition of this book.

unattainable; self-identity is not possible, and loss of the remaining self is perceived as an inevitable outcome. Voluntary death by one's own hand blocks this fusion and disposes of the "bad, ungrateful" child.

These parents dress and behave more like than unlike their adolescents. They may attempt to socialize with their adolescents on a peer level. Rather than establishing the limits needed by their offspring, they tend to assume an overpermissive position and support it with a variety of rationalizations.

Another dimension of the "buddy" parent-child relationship is the need for the parent to remain young in order to dupe the adolescent and the self. The manipulation that occurs is designed to protect the parent from the danger of the adolescent's unmasking the "omnipotent" adult. The parent's regressive fixation and play-acting of the adolescent role deprive the offspring of an empathic parent and violate generational boundaries. In some instances the outcome is role reversal. The child consequently "parents" the parent. This dynamic interferes with the developmentally appropriate redefinition of the parent-child boundaries and relationship. The burden of parenting before maturation is complete may become too great for the adolescent to bear, and disturbed behavior develops.[57,58]

PATTERNS OF INTERACTION: ENVIRONMENT

Environmental patterns that influence the development of antisocial behavior are varied. In subcultures in urban areas, antisocial behavior conforms to the mores of the social system. Life in this subgroup operates on a survival basis for generations. Hopelessness and helplessness pervade, and morale is always at a low ebb. What is predictable in this environment is the continued subsistence level of living. Technological change is occurring rapidly in the rest of society, but people at this socioeconomic level do not benefit. Instead they continue to live with deprivation, which in one sense becomes greater as the disparity increases between their lives and those of people who reap the benefits of the changes.

Rapid, accelerated social change can have a disorganizing effect on the middle class as well. Adolescents need to participate in the life of the community to enhance their self-esteem and give meaning to their lives. When the society affords no meaningful opportunities for adolescents' involvement, the impact is experienced as a form of alienation and isolation. Cut off from society, the adolescent is ripe for participation in "us-and-them" dynamics which in turn can be perceived as a legitimate rationale for acting out toward society.

Adolescents in the upper socioeconomic strata of society may have ready access to material resources. However, if they fail to recognize their relationship to the total society and their responsibilities, they may feel as cut off and isolated as adolescents in other social classes. When this occurs, these adolescents are also vulnerable to a hedonistic and wholly self-oriented lifestyle. They view the environment as simply something to be manipulated for their own pleasure and excitement. The rights of others are ignored and negated. If the social environment is suppressed from censuring their behavior because of their parents' money and power, these adolescents fail to consider the rights and feelings of others and operate on a "what feels good" principle and from a "you wouldn't dare interfere" position in their interactions with society.

Environmental dynamics that may contribute to the popularity of questionable religious cults among some young people in our society may be related to today's secularism. Spiritual needs are not as clearly understood as physiological needs, but they are important. When religion is excluded from daily living and not assigned an important place in society, many people fail to develop skills in making religious choices. Without these skills, young people who are experiencing societal, family, and developmental pressures become vulnerable to proselytizers for cults.

Two major influences that disconnect adolescents from the family and from neighborhood social structures are (1) large suburban regional junior high schools and high schools, or busing of students from the inner city to other school districts or communities; (2) the accessibility of automobiles. Both can increase adolescents' alienation, susceptibility to peer pressure, and disengagement from childhood friends. They also lessen constraints against antisocial behavior. In a place far removed from home and neighborhood, there is anonymity and little risk that the family will find out about disapproved behavior—as compared with the neighborhood where one lives and is known. Consequently, adolescents who are geographically mobile may behave in ways they would not in their own neighborhood. The need to belong and to be accepted by peers may interact with feelings of anonymity and alienation, increasing vulnerability to peer pressures to act out, engage in delinquent activities or sexual promiscuity, abuse drugs or alcohol, or neglect school attendance or performance.

Cultural conflicts, economic trends, and working parents interact with adolescents' development. The threat of nuclear war also has an impact. Over half the adolescents in one survey named nuclear disaster or the threat of World War III as the most important problem facing the world. Adolescents in several studies seemed reluctant to talk about nuclear war in the presence of their parents; it appeared to the researchers that these young people were trying to protect their parents from their offspring's vulnerability and anguish.[59]

NURSING PROCESS

Assessment

A holistic approach to adolescents who exhibit dysfunctional behavior patterns and who have a dysfunctional parent-child relationship requires an assessment process that encompasses all interacting influences.

The Adolescent

In addition to identifying the elements of the dysfunctional behavior pattern, the nurse needs to identify the adolescent's perception of the situation, determine whether he or she sees a problem; and determine what the adolescent thinks should be changed, and how. Following is a guide for this aspect of the assessment process:

1. Does the adolescent think that he or she has a problem?
2. Does the adolescent think that the parents have a problem?
3. How does the adolescent feel about his or her situation?
4. What does the adolescent think will make the situation better?
5. Is there evidence of developmental lags or deficits?
6. How does the adolescent relate to peer and authority figures?
7. What is the adolescent's motivation for change?
8. What are the youngster's fears and fantasies about treatment?
9. How does the adolescent define and describe his or her relationship with the parents? Now? In the past?
10. Can the adolescent identify the situation which triggers anger, anxiety, or depression?
11. What problematic behaviors does the adolescent exhibit?
12. How does the youngster relate to care givers?
13. Was there a precipitating event for this emergency treatment or hospitalization? If so, what was it?
14. How does the adolescent distance people and reinforce a poor self-concept?
15. What needs are met by the maladaptive behavior?

SUICIDE ATTEMPTS. The school nurse is in a position to identify youngsters at risk of suicide. Attempted suicide is apparently a contagious form of behavior; therefore, after a suicide or an attempted suicide by a student, the school nurse—in collaboration with teachers and the school administration—needs to identify those who would be the most affected by the event and determine their risk. Warning signs of an increased risk of suicide are presented in Table 39-8. (The criteria presented in Chapter 36 are also applicable.)

Medical emergencies associated with suicide attempts and abuse of recreational drugs may cause the initial contact with a health care system. Many of these adolescents have been symptomatic for some time before this admission. They may have made several suicide attempts in the past or have a history of heavy substance abuse. Their symptomatic behavior may have been unrecognized or ignored by the family and the school personnel.

Table 39-8 Suicide Risk in Adolescents

Warning Signs
Decline in school performance or academic failure, particularly when coupled with high parental expectations for achievement
Sudden violent or rebellious behavior; increased irritability, temper tantrums
Frequent 1- or 2-day absences from school
Frequent visits to the nurse's office because of minor physical complaints
Accident-proneness; high-risk behavior
Withdrawal from peer activities; apathy, boredom; dropping out of clubs or sports activities
History of previous suicide attempts
Preoccupation with music, art, or literature with death themes
Writing of notes or poetry with death themes

Assessment of these youngsters needs to focus on their response to the rescue and their current suicidal feelings, and on identifying precipitating problems.

RUNNING AWAY. Once a pattern of running away becomes established and unrelated to external events, freedom becomes essential and confinement or restriction of any kind is seen as punitive, even if applied in a supportive way. If confined to an inpatient setting, runaway adolescents may suddenly decide to "elope" rather than confront members of a therapy group, participate in a family meeting, or follow through on discharge plans. These youngsters need to be assessed for their potential for elopement, particularly during periods of stress.

Adolescents who exhibit violent, aggressive, assaultive, or destructive behavior, or who have engaged in criminal activities such as burglaries, may enter mental health services through a court referral. School authorities tend to refer adolescents and their families for counseling when the symptomatic behavior is characterized by nonaggressiveness, exaggerated passivity, irrational inhibiting fears, or low school achievement. Newly admitted adolescents need to be assessed for potential acting out, aggressiveness, and assaultiveness.

The Family

Assessment of family parallels that of an adolescent. Following is a guide for this aspect of the assessment process:

1. Do family members think the adolescent has a problem?
2. Do they think they have a problem?
3. How do they feel about the situation?
4. What do they think will make the situation better?
5. What are their perceptions of the adolescent's development?
6. How do they describe past separation events in the adolescent's life?
7. Are they willing to participate in the treatment process?
8. What are their fears and fantasies about treatment?
9. What is the quality of the marital relationship?
10. How do the parents define and describe their relationship with the adolescent?
11. How do they relate to the staff?
12. What needs are met for the parents by having a dysfunctional adolescent?
13. What strategies are the parents using to avoid acknowledging themselves, or being seen, as bad parents?

The Environment

Throughout the period of treatment, from initial assessment to discharge, the environment is an important interacting influence. Whether treatment occurs in an inpatient or an outpatient setting, an assessment of the peer group is needed. Peer pressure is a significant influence on how an adolescent chooses to behave. Following is a guide for this aspect of the assessment process:

1. How well does the treatment team distinguish between behavior that is within the parameters of "normal" adolescence and that which is deviant?
2. Do physical and social environmental factors interfere with the development of the adolescent's responsible autonomy?
3. Does the physical environment provide opportunities for physical activities such as sports that would help channel the adolescent's energy?
4. When a number of adolescents are receiving care

on the same unit, how well are issues of power, authority, and control managed?

5. Do institutional policies facilitate or impede the therapeutic process with adolescent clients and their families?
6. What obstacles in the public school system interfere with nursing activities directed toward promotion of mental health and case finding among adolescent students?
7. What obstacles in the community health nursing system interfere with case finding, promotion of mental health, and effective treatment of adolescents and their families with chronic problems?

Diagnosis

Diagnosis of adolescents' problems may need to be both child-focused and family-focused. An adolescent's difficulties reflect dysfunctional interaction between the youngster and the parents; therefore, nursing diagnoses need to address this interaction. When an adolescent is hospitalized because of the severity of symptomatic behavior, nursing diagnoses will initially focus more on the adolescent's problematic behavior, but early in treatment there must also be a focus on family problems. Examples of nursing diagnoses are presented in Table 39-9.

Table 39-9 Nursing Assessment, Diagnoses, Outcome Criteria, and Interventions

Assessment	Nursing Diagnoses	Outcome Criteria	Interventions
Client 1 elopes from hospital following confrontation about violation of rule. Has history of runaway behavior.	Impulsive avoidance of reality associated with long-standing runaway pattern	Client will control impulse to flee from distressing situations; seek contact with others; talk about feelings.	Place client on close supervision when returned to unit. Enforce specified limits. Explore how feelings are managed. Assist client to examine consequences of his or her actions. Guide client in exploring alternative ways of dealing with feelings and problems. Encourage ventilation of feelings through physical activity and verbalization. Establish contract with client. When pressures seem unmanageable, client is to: Seek out nurse to talk about feelings. Write down a list of those things that seem to be causing the feeling of pressure. Write down how each of these sources of pressure can be lessened or eliminated. Encourage peers to share with client their feelings of anger, disappointment, and fear related to the elopement.

(Continued.)

Table 39-9 Continued

Assessment	Nursing Diagnoses	Outcome Criteria	Interventions
Client 2 makes aggressive, assaultive attack on peer. Yells and screams at staff and peers.	Impaired impulse control associated with inadequate socialization within the family	Client will develop adequate socialization and impulse control, as evidenced by: Arguing position in a modulated tone of voice Remaining quietly in room for specified period of time Accepting evening unit restriction without causing further turmoil among peer group Agreeing to participate in calisthenics Talking about feelings instead of behaving aggressively or assaultively	Use restraints to prevent assaultiveness and enforce limits. Facilitate verbalization of feelings. Enforce 30-minute "quiet time" alone in room. Suggest vigorous physical activity. Help client analyze situations to identify what provokes rage. Explore alternative ways of managing provocative situations. Enforce firm limits. Communicate behavioral expectations clearly. Help client to establish personal goals. Encourage other clients to confront the adolescent about their fears and concerns, and the impact on their ability to help.
Client 3 is preoccupied with religious beliefs and with perceived evil in the world. Sits alone in corner in a trancelike state. Talks obsessively about need for forgiveness for leaving the religious cult. Is underweight; shows evidence of muscle wasting. Gives stereotyped responses to questions. Reports terrifying nightmares; has difficulty falling asleep. Was admitted following a deprogramming attempt.	Religiosity associated with cult involvement	Client will exhibit decreased religiosity, as evidenced by: Interacting with other clients about various topics Participating in unit activities, initially with encouragement and later self-initiated Exhibiting varied facial expressions Defining needs met by joining the cult; exploring other ways of meeting them Talking about guilty feelings and their sources Questioning some of the tenets of the cult's belief system Showing decrease in good and bad dichotomies, and greater awareness of gray areas in situations	Encourage participation in unit activities. Talk with client for 15 minutes three times each shift about topics other than religion. Point out gray areas in situations dichotomized by the client. Encourage client to make decisions about daily living activities. Encourage client to talk about what was happening in his or her life before joining the cult.

(Continued.)

Table 39-9 Continued

Assessment	Nursing Diagnoses	Outcome Criteria	Interventions
Client 4 has anxiety reaction during first week away at college. Drops out of school and returns home. Stays in house with mother except for a movie one evening a week with girlfriend (3 months). Stays in bed most of day. Is frequently tearful. Parents are supportive, set no limits, make no demands.	Separation anxiety associated with entry into college	Client will initiate separation process with decreasing anxiety, as evidenced by: Talking about feelings related to staying versus leaving home Identifying one way parents interfere with independence, privacy, responsibility for self Making a decision to seek employment for the remaining semester and return to school in spring. Having discussions with parents; expressing feelings related to separation, independence, and self-responsibility	Point out strengths and areas of competence. Give positive feedback on efforts toward independence. Open communication between client and parents. Explore with client the role she plays in the family and how it affects her. Help parents examine their marital relationship. Explore with client her fears and fantasies about what will happen to her and her parents if she leaves home. Encourage other clients to share their perceptions of the client's predicament. Communicate societal expectations of people of the client's age. Require evidence of responsible behavior before full privileges are restored. Set up graduated, clearly specified responsibilities. Encourage peers to share with the client their perceptions and feelings about the episode.
Client 5 has disruptive and destructive temper tantrums at home and in school. Parents initiate increase in rules that confine adolescent to house and decrease contact with peers. Parents verbalize anxiety about peer group pressure and adolescent's increased involvement with peers.	Adolescent rebelliousness related to parents' authoritarian style of interaction	Client will decrease rebelliousness and parents will become more effective, as evidenced by: Parents' establishing and enforcing reasonable limits Parents' listening to adolescent's complaints empathically and providing logical responses calmly Adolescent's verbalizing feelings and arguing position calmly. Adolescent's not violating limits	Acknowledge parents' difficulty with managing the adolescent's temper tantrums. Encourage parents to listen to adolescent's complaints and verbal protests, and to respond only empathically, logically, and calmly. Help parents to clearly define a number of enforceable limits. Encourage parents to formulate reasons for the selected limits and communicate them to offspring. Encourage parents and adolescent to speak to each other in well-modulated tones.

(Continued.)

Table 39-9 Continued

Assessment	Nursing Diagnoses	Outcome Criteria	Interventions
(Client 5, continued)			Help adolescent selectively choose issues of disagreement with parents and verbally negotiate change. Help adolescent recognize benefits derived from talking about feelings. Suggest that adolescent repair or restore whatever he or she has destroyed.
Client 6 has conflict with parents during home visit. Violates hospital prohibition against drugs and alcohol on premises. Returns from pass with marijuana and bottle of alcohol hidden in clean laundry. Client and roommate become intoxicated after lights out.	Acting-out violation of hospital rules against drugs and alcohol, associated with limit testing and conflict with parents	Client will accept limit setting and cease substance abuse during or after home visits, as evidenced by: Verbalizing disappointment about interactions with parents during home visit Admitting having provoked fight with parents Making contract with parents to talk about feelings Returning from home visit and reporting no conflicts with parents Not using drugs or alcohol on home visit Not bringing drugs or alcohol back to hospital	Search client and belongings for drugs and alcohol. Confiscate drugs and alcohol. Restrict client to unit for 24 hours. Supervise client's activities and limit visitors to family only. Explore with client problems and feelings about home visit. Confront discrepancies between what client says and actual behavior. Help client to examine consequences of behavior. Provide opportunities for graduated assumption of responsibilities. Give positive feedback on effective management of frustrating situations and evidence of responsible behavior. Encourage other clients to verbalize their feelings of rejection and risk in reaction to client's behavior. Encourage client to discuss feelings and problems with parents.
Client 7 makes preadmission lethal suicide attempt. Communicates disappointment about rescue and survival to nurse. Isolates self from other clients. Is uncommunicative with nurse. Refuses to talk with or look at parents. Parents make two attempts to talk to client and decide to leave.	Suicidal depression associated with psychologically unavailable parents	Client will make commitment to living, as evidenced by: Talking about problems and feelings with other clients and staff Joining other clients watching television Agreeing to make no further suicide attempts while in therapy (signing contract) Participating in family therapy sessions	Place client on close continuous supervision. Encourage client to talk about feelings and problems. Encourage participation in unit activities. Initially select minimally demanding group activities. Provide opportunities for client to perform competently. Give positive feedback when tasks are handled well.

(Continued.)

Table 39-9 Continued

Assessment	Nursing Diagnoses	Outcome Criteria	Interventions
(Client 7, continued) Parents neither call nor visit for 3 days.			Require client to be escorted by others for all off-unit activities until client socializes voluntarily. Limit time client spends in room alone. Limit television watching by engaging client in conversation. Encourage other clients to involve client in unit activities.
Client 8 behaves seductively toward staff members and other clients of opposite sex. Client comes out of room onto unit partially disrobed. Client has history of sexual promiscuity and runaway behavior. Using loud voice, client tells obscene jokes to clients of opposite sex. During group therapy sessions, client talks about sexual escapades while a prostitute. Parents refuse to be involved in treatment. Client reports father-daughter incest relationship (when client was between 8 and 13 years old).	Dysfunctional sexuality associated with sexual abuse and abandonment by parents	Client will express sexuality appropriately, as evidenced by: Talking about sexual feelings and need for love Dressing appropriately in public Talking about feelings related to incest relationship Ceasing talking about sexual escapades Ceasing telling obscene jokes Talking about sadness and feelings of rejection and abandonment when parents refused to be involved in treatment	Confront client on use of seductive behavior as an attention-getting device. Positively reinforce authentic behavior and reactions toward others that are not laden with sexual overtones. Ignore sexually provocative behavior when used to gain attention. Explore client's thoughts, feelings, and attitudes about sexual feelings and behavior. Explore client's perceptions of the consequences of choosing sexual acting out. Set and enforce limits on socializing with other clients when seductive behavior occurs. Encourage other clients to share their feelings about client's behavior toward them. Encourage family to come in and discuss daughter's problems.

Outcome Criteria

Since adolescent problems reflect a dysfunctional parent-child relationship and the participation of all involved, outcome criteria should reflect expected changes in the client *and* significant family members. When a target child is the "symptom bearer" of the family's dysfunction, one nursing goal is to begin to move the focus of the family's projection process. Each family member is to be afforded space, time, and opportunities to grow and develop. No single member's ability to function effectively is to be impaired for an extended period of time.

Helping family members to increase their level of differentiation is a slow process. Increased self-awareness and efforts at self-definition require sustained motivation and work. The ability to see progress can be a source of positive reinforcement and motivation to continue with the process of change. Therefore, immediate outcome criteria that specify gradations of behavioral change are more useful than those that are stated in broad, general terms. For example, in the case of a violent, acting-out, unsocialized adolescent who is intolerant of frustration, the following specified sequential outcome criteria would be appropriate:

Stops struggling and yelling within 5 minutes after being placed in restraints because of violent assaultive behavior.

Goes into restraints voluntarily on direction from staff, when aggressive behavior begins.

Asks staff for restraints when feeling agitated and angry.

Talks to staff about angry and anxious feelings rather than acting on them.

Identifies elements in a potentially disturbing situation that he or she perceives as provocative of angry or anxious feelings.

Identifies relationship issues in the past that elicited similar feelings.

Additional short-term outcome criteria are presented in Table 39-9.

Desired behavioral outcomes for adolescent clients and their families also need to address accomplishment of developmental tasks. Developmental tasks for adolescents that can serve as long-term outcomes for nursing interventions are presented in Table 39-10. An adolescent's progress in accomplishing these tasks interacts with the parents' accomplishment of their developmental tasks, which are presented in Table 39-11.

Table 39-10 Developmental Tasks for Adolescents

Long-Term Outcomes
Progressively moving toward independence
Progressively separating from parents
Developing a value system
Developing abstract thinking and deductive logical reasoning
Exploring moral issues thoughtfully in interactions with others
Developing a positive self-concept (identity, body image, self-esteem)
Building relationships with peers of the same and the opposite sex
Developing control of impulses
Delaying gratification, in order to attain long-term goals
Managing sexual feelings effectively
Developing effectiveness in resolving conflicts
Preparing for gainful and satisfying employment in a highly technological society
Managing aggression effectively

Table 39-11 Developmental Tasks for Parents

Long-Term Outcomes
Progressively relinquishing control of areas of adolescent dependence
Progressively separating from the adolescent
Helping the adolescent clarify values
Encouraging and facilitating the adolescent's use of logical reasoning
Exploring moral and ethical issues with the adolescent, and facilitating opportunities for the adolescent to have similar discussions with other adults
Providing the adolescent with positive feedback, love, warmth, and acceptance
Allowing the adolescent time and space to establish peer relationships
Setting limits thoughtfully, realistically, and consistently
Helping the adolescent formulate long-term goals and encouraging him or her in working toward them
Recognizing the adolescent's developing sexuality; providing information and privacy
Modeling effective management of conflict
Facilitating the adolescent's acquisition of information about career choices, and analysis of needs and preferences
Recognizing aggression as inherent to adolescence and providing guidance in channeling it appropriately

Intervention

Symptoms and Treatment

When symptoms of dysfunctional adolescent behavior patterns occur, the turmoil and pain are distressing to all participants. Nurses working in school systems are in an ideal position to identify problems early and to develop prevention programs. However, educational systems contain many obstacles to an expanded role for nursing. School nursing is all too often considered by school boards and administrators as being confined to maintaining health records, screening for physical health problems, managing minor physical complaints, and collecting excuses for absences.

When dysfunctional emotional symptoms first appear and if they are mild, counseling on an outpatient basis may help family members enhance strengths and lessen weaknesses. In some instances, parents need to learn to understand adolescence as a developmental stage and a growth process. The nurse assesses the parents' knowledge of adolescence and provides the necessary information. Parents may have misinterpreted or mismanaged normal behavioral and emotional responses. With knowledge about the norm, the parents are better equipped to cope more appropriately. However, feelings are not always resolved by the provision of information alone. The nurse must also help parents and adolescents articulate their feelings and needs in a way that can be "heard." The nurse gives family members feedback on how their communications are received and encourages them to do the same. For example:

JOHN: (Yelling) Stop treating me like a baby. Keep your damn hands off me and quit the nagging.

NURSE: John, when you shout like that, I don't really "hear" what you say. I get angry when I'm yelled at, and I think that's how your parents react too. Is that true, Mr. and Mrs. B?

MR. B.: Sure, I get angry. And if he keeps it up, he'll be sorry.

NURSE: So you get angry too, and when this happens, it sounds as though you threaten John. How do you feel when that happens, John?

JOHN: I get madder.... He can't boss me around anymore.

NURSE: I'm wondering how each of you could tell the other how you feel, but in a way that the other could hear and understand, so that maybe you could work out the problem by finding another solution.

JOHN: I don't like being told so many times to take out the garbage or do my homework.

NURSE: What do you think are their reasons for telling you so many times?

JOHN: Because I forget.

MRS. B.: He needs to be reminded, but when we tell him, he blows up and there's a fight.

NURSE: Sounds as though John doesn't object to the chores but does have a problem remembering and being reminded.

JOHN: That's right.

MR. B.: That's about it.

NURSE: Well, then, if you could find a way of remembering or reminding other than by telling, the problem might be solved. Does anyone have some ideas about how this could be done?

By helping family members see how they participate in the conflict, the nurse refocuses the problem from being one person's burden and presents it as a shared difficulty. In this instance, the nurse focuses on the central issue and then attempts to help family members look at the conflict as a problem for which a solution can be sought.

Parents may learn to empathize with their children's difficulties if they are helped to get in touch with the struggles and distress that accompanied their own adolescence. In this process facilitating reminiscence and recall of how the parents felt and responded can be helpful. The parents also need to explore their feelings about their relationship and the changes they are experiencing. Interventions which help parents share needs, feelings, and concerns facilitate parental communication. Often the focus of their interactions has been their problematic adolescent. Refocusing onto their relationship defuses the parent-child conflict and provides an opportunity for them to explore their relationship as well as confront and resolve their conflicts. Both the parents and the adolescent may resist this type of intervention because the adolescent has been protecting the parents from this very activity.

Setting limits is a problematic issue for both the adolescent and the parents. Some parents may adopt an inconsistent and unstable permissive stance in order to protect themselves from the conflict which occurs when they attempt to enforce limits. Other parents are at the other end of the continuum, enforcing restrictive and inappropriate limits. The nurse models and facilitates the negotiation process as a way of defining and implementing limits. Parents and adolescents must be helped to listen to and analyze one another's positions. Sometimes each can be helped by role-playing the other's position or by alternating roles.

An adolescent needs to assume responsibility and to separate from the family gradually. The nurse helps each client explore how changes in various areas of life are experienced as well as the fears and fantasies that go with such changes.

An adolescent may need to be hospitalized if symptoms become so pronounced that the family can no longer tolerate the chaos, if the school system pressures the family, or if the law becomes involved because of delinquent behavior. When this happens, the dysfunctional family patterns may be well-established and the resistance to change strong. Both the parents and the adolescent may express a desire to change the situation, but underlying conflicts and the needs met by the maladaptive behavior may interfere with actualization of goals.

Often an adolescent is initially sullen, angry, and withdrawn. Flexibility and informality are necessary in the beginning of a relationship with the nurse. These young people need acceptance of *who they are* but *not* of their antisocial behavior. This distinction is difficult to communicate but necessary for the development of a trusting therapeutic relationship. No other group of clients can elicit a wider variety of feelings in care givers than mercurial adolescents. Their unpredictability is both a challenge and a burden.

These clients may initially feign meekness and, given their family histories of deprivation or abuse, may elicit sympathy in the care givers, who may entertain rescue fantasies. However, their compliant, meek behavior is usually short-lived. As the therapy proceeds and the need for conformity to hospital structure is made clear, these adolescents may become sullen, negativistic, hostile, or violent. Care givers become frustrated and angry when they must deal with impulsive acting out and monosyllabic responses to their interventions.

The adolescent's constant testing of people and limits seem endless. Attempts at exploring underlying conflicts may be met with intellectualizations or social criticisms which only serve to increase frustration and a feeling of futility in the nurse.

These youngsters attempt to put the nurse in various authority roles and to provoke exasperation and hostility, and they are often successful. They try to replay, with care givers, the patterns of interaction they participate in with their parents. Regardless of whether they display open opposition or negativistic silence, they manage to provoke anger in the nurse.[46]

The nursing staff, because of the acting out and resistence to treatment, may be reluctant to increase the adolescent's privileges, thereby prolonging dependency and impeding progress toward self-control and assumption of responsibility. In addition, nurses may assume a punitive parental role, which replicates the family dynamics and escalates the adolescent's anger.

Adolescents resist both in- and outpatient treatment. Such resistance frustrates the nurse and other care givers who seek to engage and maintain the adolescent in treatment.[58]

Treatment-Resistant Behavior Patterns

Adolescents employ a variety of strategies to defeat the structure of the treatment setting. If the social environmental dynamics support rather than resolve the use of the strategies, the context of care becomes antitherapeutic. Table 39-12 lists these behaviors, their purposes, and nursing interventions that facilitate their resolution.

Initially, adolescents who are brought to treatment by their families, or who are remanded by a court system, usually are unable to understand or admit their participation in the events that led to hospitalization. Because these youngsters are convinced that no adult could possibly understand them, they maintain a psychological barrier that at times feels impenetrable to the nurse. These adolescents, particularly those with long-standing problems, anticipate the recurrences of major traumas and participate in setting up a replay of these dynamics with their care givers.[58]

They expect that the care givers will retaliate punitively and hurt them. They therefore persistently provoke the staff, even to the point of threatening physical harm. The nurse and other care givers eventually react as the adolescent predicted. Frustrated by continual testing of limits, verbal barrages in response to the unit's policies, and threats of violence, staff members may impose limits in a punitive fashion. When nurses react with anger, after reflection they recognize the irrational emotionality of their behavior. They may then feel guilty. In response they may fail to consistently enforce limits or impulsively abolish them. Since adolescents are very concerned about justice, fairness, and rules, they react with further turmoil.

The nurses' emotionality supports the adolescents' ambivalent expectation that adults will prove that they are not perfect, blameless, omniscient, and omnipotent, and their expectation that adults will reject or abandon them. When adolescents' behavior is perceived as unmanageable by the nursing staff, there may be attempts by the treatment team to eject them from the setting. The nurses may recommend transfer to a more secure or "appropriate" institution or unit.

Table 39-12 Treatment-Resistant Behaviors

Adolescent's Behavior	Message	Dynamics	Nursing Intervention
Acts like "assistant nurse," "mother hen," "big brother."	"I act like you, so I'm not sick or crazy, and I don't need treatment."	Identification with the aggressor.	Give client feedback about how he or she uses this behavior to avoid dealing with own problems. Set limits that require focus on self and own problems.
Moves to develop a peer relationship with the nurse by asking personal questions, e.g., "Have you ever used pot?" "Do you have a boyfriend?"	"If I can prove that you are no better than me, then you have nothing to offer me."	Leveling.	Explore with client how this information would be useful to the treatment process. Point out that the purpose of therapy is for the client to use the time to talk about self and own problems.
Acts flirtatious or seductive.	"If I can seduce you, then you are not perfect or strong enough to help me."	Counterphobic way of dealing with sexual impulses that are frightening.	Encourage client to talk about beliefs, values, feelings, fears, and fantasies about sex.
Oversubmissiveness.	"I'm being good and you disapprove, so you want me to be bad. If you want me to be bad, you cannot help me."	Beat adults at their own game.	Express doubt and disbelief that anyone could be in specific situations and not feel angry or wish to rebel.
Persistent avoidance: daydreaming, refusal to participate in group therapy or group activities, pseudoseizures.	"I will provoke you to retaliate."	Prove that adults hate, hurt, and reject.	Persistent patience; firm limits consistently enforced without anger. Explore what it must feel like to stay out and just watch.
Manipulates a more disorganized peer to act out and calls nurse to help the "sick" peer.	"See how sick that person is; he or she needs you more than I."	"A scapegoat will divert the nurse's attention from me; no one understands and can help."	Continue to give attention to clients who seek help for other clients or provoke the latter to act out.
Tells peers rather than therapist about intimate details of problems.	"I can divide and conquer." "If I divide and conquer, then you can't be relied on to help."	Transference splitting.	Direct client to discuss problems with appropriate team members. Maintain clear, open communication with other team members.
Craziness and pseudo stupidity.	"I'm sick; don't trust me, but help me."	Ward off or protect staff from self-perceived dangerousness.	Acknowledge fears; encourage exploration of strengths.
Intellectual or artistic activities that exclude interactions with others.	"See how productive I am."	Avoid dealing with feelings.	Limit solitary activities. Talk about how difficult it is to interact. Acknowledge how difficult it is to talk about feelings, but how necessary to resolving problems.
Organizes or joins a disruptive peer group.	"We are more powerful than you."	"Us" against "them." "If our gang can disrupt your work, you can't help."	Firmly enforce preestablished limits. Exercise consistent patience. Confront client on avoidance of work in therapy. Deal with each adolescent as an individual.

SOURCE: D. B. Rinsley, *Treatment of the Severely Disturbed Adolescent*, Aronson, New York, 1980.

Nurses as well as other care givers working with adolescents often fail to recognize the normal behavior of adolescence. In these cases they may set unrealistic goals that reflect adult functioning. Failure to recognize normal adolescent emotional lability and unpredictability often leads nurses to label adolescents' fluctuant hostility, mood swings, and preoccupation with their bodies and sexual feelings as pathological even when this is not true.[58]

Nurses may have the same difficulties with adolescents as the clients' parents. If they themselves are well past the adolescent stage of development, they may have the same conflicts and defenses as the parents. When this occurs, it interferes with the therapeutic process. Nurses who are parents of adolescents or are the approximate age of the parents may be especially vulnerable to identification with the parents and to rejection of the adolescent. Students and younger nurses, on the other hand, are usually still resolving remnants of their own late-adolescent stage of development. Therefore, they may be more inclined to identify with the adolescent and cast the family in the "bad guy" role.

Because people tend to repress and deny adolescent experiences when they reach adulthood, their understanding of adolescents is impaired and their own self-awareness is blocked by their defenses. This compounds an already difficult situation. Consequently, according to Rinsley,[58] some adults who work with adolescents indicate a need to return to a kind of adolescence themselves. This is inevitably problematic. Such staff members may need to stimulate the adolescent clients to act out antisocially and thereby provide them with vicarious gratification of their own inhibited antisocial wishes.[58]

Adolescents need help in modifying and controlling their responses to irritating situations. By providing feedback and enforcing limits, the nurse initiates a socialization process directed toward helping the youngsters learn ways of interacting which are less abrasive, so that their expressed needs can be heard by significant others.

Adolescents living in residential treatment settings may experience increasing stress as they approach discharge. When the stress level is high, these adolescents may develop multiple minor physical complaints. These ailments reflect the way stress is being managed and may be used to gain attention. The physical complaints are often a physiological expression of their anxiety, manifested by nausea, headaches, diarrhea, or profuse perspiration.

Examples of nursing interventions are presented in Table 39-9.

Evaluation

Because of troubled adolescents' well-established, self-defeating patterns of coping, careful planning and intervention are necessary to help these youngsters follow through with the treatment program. They will impulsively and often unconsciously sabotage their own progress. Setbacks are inevitable and must be accepted as part of the natural course of events. Steps forward are often small. Staff members must recognize these small progressions and—more important—help adolescents see improvement not only in their behavior but in their overall situations as well.

If outcome criteria are clearly articulated and specified in terms of gradient change, they can be used to measure the effectiveness of nursing interventions. An example of an evaluation of the implementation of a nursing care plan is presented in Table 39-13.

SUMMARY

Dysfunctional patterns in adolescence emerge from interactions between problematic separation dynamics and the dramatic changes—physical, mental, spiritual, and social—that occur during this stage of life. Dysynchronous patterns include acting out, self-destructiveness (self-harm and suicide), problems having to do with attendance and performance at school, running away, substance abuse, membership in cults, and somatic complaints. Each of these patterns has distinctive dynamics and implications for entry into treatment.

The problems of adolescence addressed in this chapter are associated with the following categories in DSM III: conduct, oppositional, anxiety, identity, adjustment, personality, and substance abuse disorders; and conditions not attributable to mental disorder (antisocial behavior, academic problems, phase-of-life problems, and parent-child problems). Although as an age group adolescents do not have

Table 39-13 Evaluation of Nursing Care

Assessment Data	Nursing Diagnosis	Outcome Criteria	Intervention	Evaluation
On admission, client causes multiple self-inflicted cigarette burns on forearm. Day 1 after admission, carves initials on leg with piece of broken glass.	Deliberate self-harm associated with tension generated by psychiatric admission, fear of other clients, and rage toward parents	Client ceases self-harm behavior and manages feelings effectively, as evidenced by: Telling nurse when feelings of "tension" occur Identifying sources of increasing tension Signing contract with nurse to stop self-harm and talk about feelings instead Seeking out nurse to talk about feelings rather than initiating self-harm	Inform client that self-inflicted injuries will not be permitted. Provide continuous close supervision. Remove all items which could be used for self-harm or suicide.	
Verbalizes feeling better and exhibits elated mood after episode of self-mutilation. Day 2, pilfers thumbtacks from bulletin board and attempts to stick them into cheeks and nose. Day 3, verbalizes anger toward parents for bringing her to a psychiatric hospital and attempts to burn herself with cigarette lighter. Appears visibly anxious when other clients approach her. Refuses to acknowledge anxiety.			Explore feelings and events that precipitate self-harm or thoughts of suicide. Negotiate written contract with client to seek out nurse and talk about feelings when impulse to self-injure occurs. Be immediately available to client when she asks to talk.	Client begins to talk about situations that increase feelings of tension. Refuses to sign contract with nurse until day 4 but agrees to try to talk to nurse when feeling "tense." Day 1, attempts self-harm. Day 3, attempts self-harm. Day 4, seeks out nurse and asks for help in controlling impulse to injure herself.
Initiates and sustains interactions with nurse about problems and what "tense" feelings are like and when they occur.		Labeling "tension" as more specific feelings.	Encourage client to label feelings.	Labels feelings about particular clients as *fear*.
			Encourage client to identify situations associated with "tense" feelings.	Lebels feelings toward family as *anger*.
			Give positive feedback when there is appropriate management of feelings.	Day 5, no episodes of attempts to self-harm.
		Talks to parents during and after family and multifamily therapy groups, and during visiting hours.	Encourage client to discuss problems with family informally and in therapy groups.	Tentatively begins to disclose feelings and perceptions to each parent separately.

a disproportionate incidence of mental problems, problems of adolescence are widespread and have created serious concern.

Family patterns of interaction associated with dysynchronous health patterns in adolescence include "centripetal," "centrifugal," and "delegating" separation dynamics; and parents' behavior patterns—"omnipotent authoritianism," "moralistic self-righteousness," and "peer relationships" with their children. Environmental patterns of interaction are varied but affect adolescents in all social strata.

In the nursing process, assessment needs to encompass all interacting influences, and diagnosis may need to be both child-focused and family-focused. Outcome criteria should reflect expected changes in the adolescent and significant family members, and family members should be helped to increase their degree of differentiation; behavioral outcomes will address developmental tasks. Intervention may take the form of outpatient counseling, but hospitalization of an adolescent may be necessary if a family situation has become intolerably chaotic, if a school system is putting pressure on a family, or if the legal system has become involved. Adolescents resist both inpatient and outpatient treatment, and certain behavior patterns are particularly treatment-resistant. Evaluation must take into account the fact that setbacks are inevitable and must be accepted as natural; progress will occur in small steps which nurses must be alert to identify and share with clients.

REFERENCES

1. G. L. Valiant, "Adolescents, Parents and Peers: What Is One without the Other?" *Journal of Adolescence,* vol. 6, 1983, pp. 131–144.
2. H. Steirlin, *Separating Parents and Adolescents,* New York Times Book Company, New York, 1974.
3. K. Glaser, "Masked Depression in Children and Adolescents," *American Journal of Psychotherapy,* vol. 21, 1967, pp. 565–574.
4. C. P. Malmquist, "Depressions in Childhood and Adolescence," in S. I. Harrison and J. F. McDermott, eds., *New Directions in Childhood Psychopathology, Vol. 2: Deviations in Development,* International Universities Press, New York, 1982, pp. 827–859.
5. American Psychiatric Association, *Diagnostic and Statistical Manual of Mental Disorders,* 3d ed., APA, Washington, D.C., 1980.
6. B. N. Adams, "Adolescent Health Care: Needs, Priorities and Services," *Nursing Clinics of North America,* vol. 18, no. 2, 1983, pp. 237–247.
7. G. Keidel, "Adolescent Suicide," *Nursing Clinics of North America,* vol. 18, no. 2, 1983, pp. 323–332.
8. P. McCormack, "Watch for Warning Signs of Teen Suicide," *Bridgeport Post,* March 3, 1985, p. C-12.
9. W. T. Hamlin, "Adolescent Suicide," *Journal of the National Medical Association,* vol. 74, no. 1, 1982, pp. 25–28.
10. S. A. Husain and T. Vandiver, *Suicide in Children and Adolescents,* Spectrum, New York, 1984.
11. "The Risks of Teen Drug Use," *Science News,* August 4, 1984, p. 73.
12. L. Hennecke and S. E. Gitlow, "Alcohol Use and Alcoholism in Adolescence," *New York State Journal of Medicine,* vol. 83, no. 7, 1983, pp. 936–940.
13. "Going to Pot: Peer Group Connection," *Science News,* February 18, 1984, p. 107.
14. "Teen Drug Use Drops, but Problem Remains," *Science News,* February 18, 1984, p. 103.
15. A. Manov and L. Lowther, "A Health Care Approach for Hard-to-Reach Adolescent Runaways," *Nursing Clinics of North America,* vol. 18, no. 2, 1983, pp. 333–342.
16. W. M. Karniski, M. D. Levine, S. Clarke, et al., "A Study of Neurodevelopment Findings in Early Adolescent Delinquents," *Journal of Adolescent Health Care,* vol. 3, 1982, pp. 151–159.
17. J. F. Kantner and M. Zelnik, "Sexual and Contraceptive Experiences of Young Unmarried Women in the United States 1976 and 1971," *Family Planning Perspectives,* vol. 9, 1977, pp. 55–71.
18. J. G. Dryfoos, "Contraceptive Use, Pregnancy Intentions and Pregnancy Outcomes among U.S. Women," *Family Planning Perspectives,* vol. 14, no. 2, 1982, pp. 81–93.
19. E. M. Pattison and J. Kahan, "The Deliberate Self-Harm Syndrome," *American Journal of Psychiatry,* vol. 140, no. 7, 1983, pp. 869–872.
20. P. D. Stanford, R. L. Johnson, and K. Sprott, "An Analysis of Drug-Related Admissions on an Adolescent Service," *Journal of Adolescent Health Care,* vol. 3, 1982, pp. 114–119.
21. R. C. Friedman, R. Corn, S. Hurt, et al., "Family History of Illness in the Seriously Suicidal Adolescent: A Life Cycle Approach," *American Journal of Orthopsychiatry,* vol. 54, no. 3, 1984, pp. 390–397.
22. J. Herman, "Recognition and Treatment of Incestuous Families," *International Journal of Family Therapy,* vol. 5, no. 2, 1983, pp. 81–91.
23. E. Stanley and J. Barter, "Adolescent Suicidal Behavior," *American Journal of Orthopsychiatry,* vol. 40, no. 1, 1970, pp. 87–96.
24. L. J. Kaplan, *Adolescent: The Farewell to Childhood,* Simon and Schuster, New York, 1984.
25. M. P. Mirkin, P. A. Raskin, and F. C. Antognini, "Parenting, Protecting, Preserving: Mission of Adolescent Female Runaway," *Family Process,* vol. 23, 1984, pp. 63–74.
26. L. Pallikkathayil and S. Tweed, "Substance Abuse: Alcohol and Drugs during Adolescence," *Nursing Clinics of North America,* vol. 18, no. 2, 1983, pp. 313–321.
27. S. G. Kellam, D. L. Stevenson, and B. R. Rubin, "How Specific Are the Early Predictors of Teenage Drug Use?" *National Institute on Drug Abuse Research Monograph Series,* vol. 43, 1983, pp. 329–334.
28. R. S. Carman, B. J. Fitzgerald, and C. Holmgren,

"Alienation and Drinking Motivations among Adolescent Females," *Journal of Personality and Social Psychology*, vol. 44, no. 5, 1983, pp. 1021–1024.

29. H. B. Kaplan, S. S. Martin, and C. Robbins, "Pathways to Adolescent Drug Use: Self Derogation, Peer Influence, Weakening of Social Controls, and Early Substance Abuse," *Journal of Health and Social Behavior*, vol. 25, 1984, pp. 270–289.
30. M. Penning and G. E. Barnes, "Adolescent Marijuana Use: A Review," *International Journal of Addiction*, vol. 17, no. 5, 1982, pp. 749–791.
31. T. E. Smith, "Reviewing Adolescent Marijuana Abuse," *Social Work*, vol. 29, 1984, pp. 17–21.
32. I. Hurwitz, R. M. A. Bibace, et al., "Neuropsychological Function of Normal Boys, Delinquent Boys, and Boys with Learning Problems," *Perceptual and Motor Skills*, vol. 35, 1978, pp. 387–394.
33. C. Hodgman, "Current Issues in Adolescent Psychiatry," *Hospital and Community Psychiatry*, vol. 34, no. 6, 1983, pp. 514–521.
34. C. H. King, "The Ego and the Integration of Violence in Homicidal Youths," in S. I. Harrison and J. F. McDermott, eds., *New Directions in Childhood Psychopathology, Vol. 2: Deviations in Development*, International Universities Press, New York, 1982, pp. 913–916.
35. M. Lewis, "Adolescent Psychic Structure and Societal Influences," *Adolescent Psychiatry*, vol. 10, 1982, pp. 125–139.
36. T. J. Silber, "Adolescent Sexuality: A Developmental Viewpoint," *Pediatric Annals*, vol. 11, no. 10, 1982, pp. 793–796.
37. T. J. Silber, "Adolescent Morality—A Clinician's Viewpoint," *Postgraduate Medicine*, vol. 72, no. 5, 1982, pp. 223–224, 226.
38. M. S. Calderone, "On the Possible Prevention of Sexual Problems of Adolescence," *Hospital and Community Psychiatry*, vol. 34, no. 6, 1983, pp. 528–530.
39. S. J. Cohen, "Intentional Teenage Pregnancies," *Journal of School Health*, vol. 53, no. 3, 1983, pp. 210–211.
40. J. Noshpitz, "On Masturbation," *Pediatric Annals*, vol. 11, no. 9, 1982, pp. 748–749.
41. D. E. Greydanus, "Adolescent Sexuality: An Overview and Perspective for the 1980s," *Pediatric Annals*, vol. 11, no. 9, 1982, pp. 714–726.
42. R. Green, "Homosexual Behavior," in S. S. Gellis and B. M. Kagan, eds., *Current Pediatric Therapy*, Saunders, Philadelphia, 1982, pp. 719–720.
43. R. Jones and R. Shearin, "Communicating with Adolescents and Young Adults About Sexuality," *Pediatric Annals*, vol. 11, no. 9, 1982, pp. 733–736.
44. M. T. Saghir and E. Robins, *Male and Female Homosexuality: A Comprehensive Investigation*, Williams and Wilkins, Baltimore, 1973.
45. J. Harry, "Parasuicide, Gender and Gender Deviance," *Journal of Health and Social Behavior*, vol. 24, 1983, pp. 350–361.
46. A. Sondheimer, "Anticipation and Experimentation: The Sexual Concerns of Mid-adolescence," *Adolescent Psychiatry*, vol. 10, 1982, pp. 208–227.
47. M. Galanter, "Unification Church (Moonie) Dropouts: Psychological Readjustment after Leaving a Charismatic Religious Group," *American Journal of Psychiatry*, vol. 140, no. 8, 1983, pp. 984–989.
48. L. L. Schwartz, "Family Therapists and Families of Cult Members," *International Journal of Family Therapy*, vol. 5, no. 3, 1983, pp. 168–178.
49. E. Shapiro, "Destructive Cultism," *Family Physician*, vol. 15, no. 2, February 1977, pp. 80–83.
50. J. G. Clark, "Cults," *Journal of the American Medical Association*, vol. 242, no. 3, July 20, 1979, pp. 279–281.
51. L. Coleman, "New Religions and the Myth of Mind Control," *American Journal of Orthopsychiatry*, vol. 54, no. 2, 1984, pp. 322–325.
52. S. V. Levine, "Youth and Religious Cults: A Societal and Clinical Dilemma," *Adolescent Psychiatry*, vol. 6, 1978, pp. 75–89.
53. E. M. Levine, "Deprogramming without Tears," *Society*, vol. 17, no. 3, March–April 1980, pp. 34–38.
54. L. K. Zeltzer and S. LeBaron, "Psychosomatic Problems in Adolescents," *Postgraduate Medicine*, vol. 75, no. 1, 1984, pp. 153–164.
55. R. A. Oberfield, R. N. Reuben, and L. J. Burkes, "Interdisciplinary Approach to Conversion Disorders in Adolescent Girls," *Psychosomatics*, vol. 24, no. 11, 1983, pp. 983–989.
56. M. A. Wessel and W. B. McCullough, "Bereavement—an Etiologic Factor in Peptic Ulcer in Childhood and Adolescence?" *Journal of Adolescent Health Care*, vol. 2, no. 4, 1982, pp. 287–288.
57. A. Haim, *Adolescent Suicide*, International Universities Press, New York, 1974.
58. D. B. Rinsley, *Treatment of the Severely Disturbed Adolescent*, Aronson, New York, 1980.
59. B. Bower, "Kids and the Bomb: Apocalyptic Anxieties?" *Science News*, vol. 128, no. 7, 1985, pp. 106–107.

PART SIX

Health: Biopsychosocial Patterns

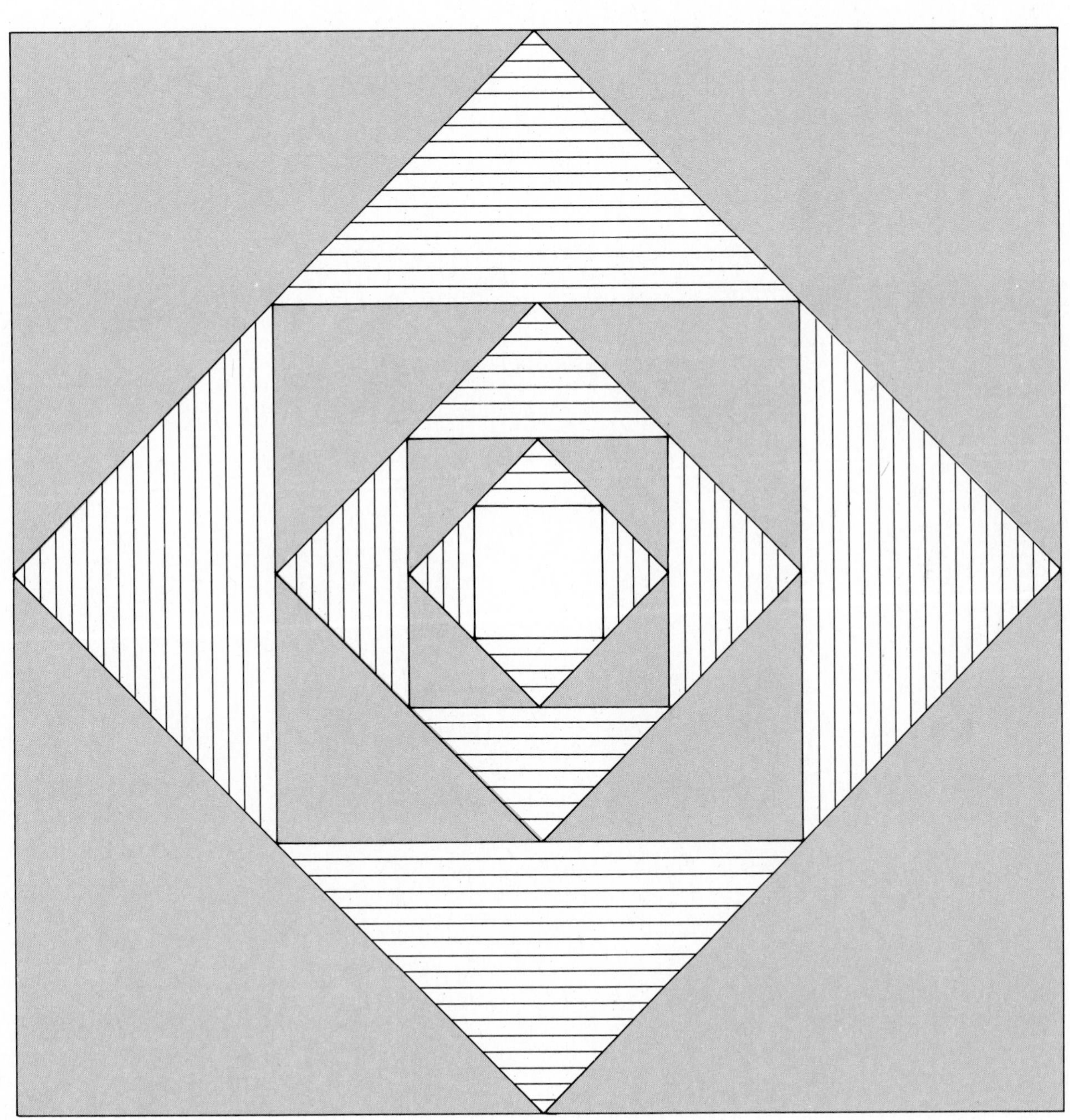

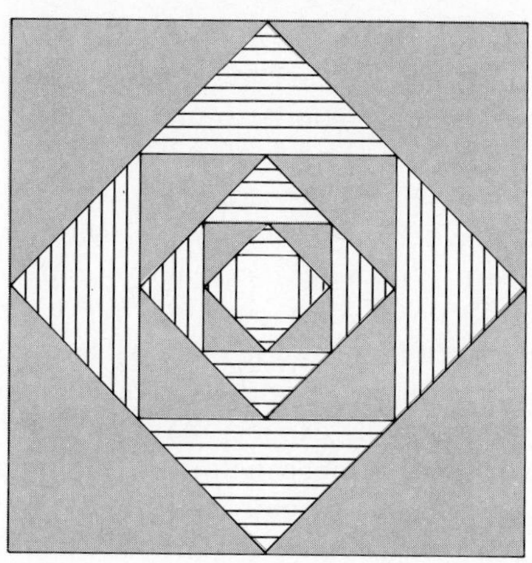

CHAPTER 40
Biopsychosocial Health

Judith Haber
Pamela Price Hoskins
Anita M. Leach
Barbara Flynn Sideleau

LEARNING OBJECTIVES

After studying this chapter, the student should be able to:

1. Elaborate on the definitions of *biopsychosocial health* and *biopsychosocial dysfunction.*
2. Relate the definitions of *biopsychosocial health* and *biopsychosocial dysfunction* to patterns of grappling with illness; the development, maintenance, and resolution of stress-related illness; disability and chronic illness; organic mental disorders; and the dying process.

The purposes of this chapter are to explore patterns of biopsychosocial health and dysfunction and their development and manifestation, and to provide an introduction and overview of Part Six. Dimensions of biopsychosocial health and dysfunction will be discussed from a holistic perspective. The problematic biopsychosocial patterns generated by illness and hospitalization, stress-related illness, disability and chronic illness, organic mental disorders, and the dying process will be discussed.

BIOPSYCHOSOCIAL HEALTH

Biopsychosocial health is a process in which a person's physical, mental, emotional, and spiritual patterns of functioning interact synchronously with each other and with the environment. Healthy biopsychosocial patterns of interaction foster effective and appropriate satisfaction of needs, physical well-being, and a productive and gratifying life. From a holistic perspective, synchronous patterns of interaction among person, family, and environment promote physical well-being.

Biopsychosocial patterns are a reflection of stress management. When these patterns are synchronous, exchanges with the environment are maintained at manageable levels and adequately meet physical, mental, emotional, and spiritual needs; bodily structure, function, and development are optimally maintained; and perceptions of events are realistic and generate appropriate interactive behavior. Thus emotions, feelings, and conflicts are recognized and managed effectively; thinking processes can operate independently of emotions; and behavior patterns reflect a thoughtful approach to life and its problems. Potentially problematic events are anticipated and efforts are made to prevent them or keep them manageable. Problem solving and effective decision making are used to maintain dynamic equilibrium among mind, body, and spirit and between self and environment.

Even in the presence of chronic illness, disability, and organic mental disorders—and during the dying process—optimal wellness and functioning may exist. Adherence to treatment regimens, rehabilitation, conservation of capacities when deterioration is inevitable, and a peaceful, dignified death represent biopsychosocial health within the limits of the situation.

Interacting family patterns that facilitate biopsychosocial health include effective management of emotions and feelings, efforts to maintain body systems at optimal levels of functioning, and human relationships that are mutually gratifying. Multigenerationally, the synchronous family is nurturing, respects members' uniqueness, is reality-oriented, can allow members to leave and reenter it as needed, supports self-identity and personal boundaries, tolerates disagreement, and seeks negotiated settlements. Such a family expects that only some human needs can be satisfied within the family's boundaries and that other needs require involvement in the larger environment.

An environment conducive to biopsychosocial health is one that generates manageable levels of stress. It provides needed resources and makes them accessible. There are opportunities for personal growth. Noxious physical, chemical, and interpersonal elements are controlled.

BIOPSYCHOSOCIAL DYSFUNCTION

Biopsychosocial dysfunction is a process in which physical, mental, emotional, and spiritual patterns of functioning interact dysynchronously with each other and the environment. Dysfunctional biopsychosocial patterns interfere with effective and appropriate satisfaction of needs, physical well-being, and the pursuit of a productive and gratifying life. From a holistic perspective, dysynchronous patterns of interaction among person, family, and environment contribute to physical illness.

RATIONALE FOR THE ORGANIZATION OF PART SIX

There are five chapters in Part Six, each of which contributes to an understanding of biopsychosocial dysfunction.

Chapter 41, "Grappling with Illness," provides an understanding of biopsychosocial dysfunction through a discussion of how personality, or personal style, interacts with the stress and anxiety of physical illness, hospitalization, the "sick role," and restoration of biopsychosocial health.

In Chapter 42, "Stress-Related Illness," person-family-environment interaction is explored in relation to mismanagement of stress and anxiety, change, conflict, and past and present factors that influence coping. These topics contribute to an understanding of the development and maintenance of physical illness and ways in which biopsychosocial health can be restored.

In Chapter 43, "Disability and Chronic Illness," understanding of biopsychosocial dysfunction is amplified through a discussion of the irreversible losses and changes that result from physical problems that permanently alter health patterns, maladaptive patterns that develop from mismanagement of stress, and ways in which optimal health can be achieved.

In Chapter 44, "Organic Mental Disorders," the irreversible and sometimes progressive deterioration of brain structures and function and mental capacities and the pervasive influence of these alterations on comprehension of the world, emotions, self-care, social interactions, and relationships illustrate biopsychosocial dysfunction as a holistic phenomenon.

In Chapter 45, "The Dying Process," death is examined as a personal interaction with family, society, and other relevant environmental systems. If death is considered a part of life, and if it comes peacefully and with dignity within a supportive context, it can illustrate how biopsychosocial health may extend to the end of biological existence. If it is considered a failure of life processes or is characterized by protest, avoidance, and loneliness in an unfamiliar context, without the comforting presence of significant others, it illustrates how biopsychosocial dysfunction can occur at the end of biological existence.

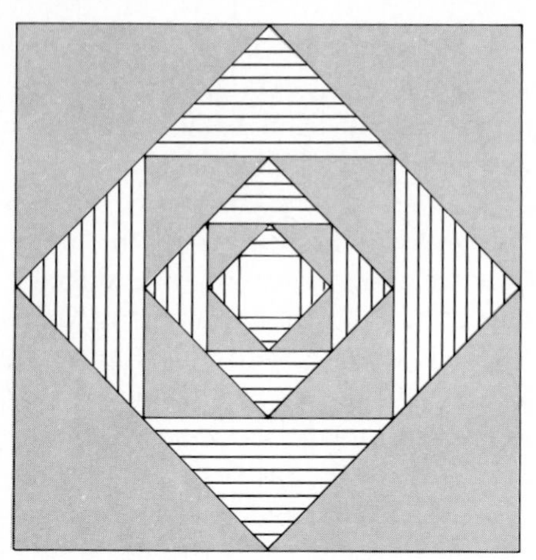

CHAPTER 41
Grappling with Illness during Hospitalization

Victoria Schoolcraft

LEARNING OBJECTIVES

After studying this chapter, the student should be able to:

1. Discuss the factors which affect the perception of illness.
2. Discuss the "sick role" and its interaction with illness.
3. Identify stressful factors in hospitalization.
4. Identify clients' behaviors which reflect healthy and unhealthy interactions with hospitalization.
5. Apply the nursing process to promote, maintain, and restore healthy patterns of interaction with hospitalization.

> Except for nurses, there would be no hospitals. They are personifications of a hospital's soul. Whatever a nurse is, a hospital is. (Anonymous, from recruiting materials, State of Oklahoma Teaching Hospitals.)

Hospitals were first established by nurses as places where the injured or ill who were homeless could find refuge and receive care that would otherwise be given at home by family members. Although hospitals have changed considerably, they still serve the function of providing care that families cannot give. And although modern hospitals have not been founded by nurses, nurses are the principal care givers within them.

Nurses are the people who consistently provide support and therapy to people who have been hospitalized. More than any other health care personnel, nurses observe and respond to all aspects of clients; regardless of the medical diagnosis, nurses must respond to each client's physical, mental, and spiritual dimensions and must be alert to indications of health or illness in any dimension. To provide optimal nursing care to a client who is physically ill, the nurse takes into consideration the interaction of the physical with the mental and the spiritual. If this is not done, mental and spiritual disturbances may impede attempts to deal with the physical illness.

The purpose of this chapter is to increase understanding of the psychosocial aspects of working with people who are ill and hospitalized, in order to promote effective use of the nursing process to help clients deal with hospitalization.

DYSYNCHRONOUS HEALTH PATTERNS

Illness is, in itself, a dysynchronous health pattern; but it also interacts with other factors to create other dysynchronous patterns. The factors which will be explored here are personality, culture and values, and perception of loss.

Illness

Illness has been defined as a dynamic pattern of interaction between stressors in the client and the environment—a dissonant, incongruous pattern manifested physically, mentally, and spiritually. This definition reflects the fact that illness is more than a physical problem. It is a state "characterized by feelings of helplessness, dependency, continuous discomfort, and narrowing of the focus of attention, with a corresponding increase in concern for somatic stimuli and constriction of goals."[1]

For centuries, people believed that illness and other afflictions were brought about by the intervention of evil spirits or disapproving gods. Today, even in the industrialized countries, some people still have mystical beliefs about the causes of illness; they believe that illnesses and afflictions are sent by God as a test or a punishment. But for many—perhaps most—people, beliefs about the causes of illness have changed as scientific experience and knowledge have increased. Initially, the scientific revolution led to identification of external agents or particular defects (genetic or organic) as causes of illness or disability; as a result, physical problems were found to be curable or preventable. In this century, scientific thought has been extended to influences of the environment—including other people—on health and illness and on psychological and spiritual factors in illness and disability.

Influence of Personality

Individual responses to the possibility of illness and the need for treatment range from being overly concerned, and seeking help for every minor ache or pain, to denying the significance of even major changes in physical or mental functioning. Within this range, there are, of course, many variations. Schontz[1] has identified factors which influence whether a person will seek or avoid professional help:

- Degree and extent of symptoms or distress
- Expectation of return to health if treatment is instituted
- Fear of diagnostic and treatment procedures
- Fear of discovery of serious illness
- Self-concept that one is always healthy

Some personality types seem to be more or less susceptible to certain types of physical problems. For example, Friedman and Rosenman[2] have considered how "type A" and "type B" personalities affect the development of coronary artery disease.

Portions of this chapter from Mary Jane Kennedy, "Impact of Illness and Hospitalization"; and June N. Brodie, "Critical Illness," in the second edition of this book.

Type A people are aggressive, driven, and time-conscious. Although more common among men than women, the type A pattern is seen in both sexes and all occupations and positions. Type A people tend to feel guilty if they relax and are likely to ignore or deny illness. Type B people are calm, confident, and able to live at a relaxed pace. They can relax without feeling guilty, and they can accept illness and seek proper treatment. Some people with type B personalities engage in behavior which is considered to increase the danger of heart disease, such as smoking and consuming a high-cholesterol diet, yet they seem nearly immune from coronary artery disease. People who have type A personalities are more likely to develop heart disease even if they avoid smoking and control their weight.

While there are serious criticisms of Friedman and Rosenman's findings, research is progressing on other personality types which may predispose people to particular illnesses. For example, the type C personality—characterized by a poor self-image, unresolved resentments, and difficulty in dealing with loss—may be prone to cancer. (See Chapter 42.)

People establish patterns or characteristic ways of dealing with life. These patterns of response influence how clients manage the stress of illness and hospitalization and interact with care givers; in fact, the stress and anxiety of illness and hospitalization may cause the patterns to become more pronounced. If they are not recognized by care givers, the client's uniqueness is denied, care is not individualized, and behavior is likely to be mislabeled as problematic. An approach to clients that ignores personal idiosyncrasies and personality styles may aggravate an already difficult situation. Personality styles may be considered as falling into the following categories: emotional, intellectual, fearful, suspicious, hostile, and avoiding. Each is discussed below.

Emotional Style

People whose primary response to life is emotional become disorganized, frightened, and overwhelmed by their feelings when they encounter problems. They have difficulty hearing or integrating information that might help them use a problem-solving approach or manage feelings more effectively. Information about their condition, its expected course, and procedures for treating it only increases their anxiety and depression. Their ability to use knowledge is overshadowed by emotionality. Discomfort may be perceived as life-threatening even when it is not. Discomfort, change of any sort, and pain are poorly tolerated and tend to be disorganizing. These people feel an acute need for family and care givers to be present at all times. Isolation from others, even for brief periods of time, seems to distort and exaggerate their perceptions of bodily sensations and of previous discussions about their health with family, friends, and care givers.

Intellectual Style

Clients who intellectualize use logic or reasoning in an attempt to avoid confrontation with the feelings evoked by illness, hospitalization, and threat to life. Feelings are denied, suppressed, and repressed to protect the self from acknowledging vulnerability. These people appear to have an exaggerated need for complete information about their condition, prognosis, and proposed treatments. Such knowledge is received calmly and followed by thoughtful questions; the response is characteristically detached and unemotional, even if the situation is very serious. But denial, suppression, and repression of feelings do not resolve them; and the unresolved emotions, because they affect physiological functions, aggravate the existing health problem.

Fearful Style

Fearful people approach life with the expectation that whatever happens will be inevitably catastrophic. Unfamiliar people, places, things, and situations evoke fear and dread. On some level these people may recognize that their fears are unfounded or exaggerated, but this awareness has little influence on the effective management of their fears and anxiety. When provided with information, they tend to hear selectively; they absorb more about what is threatening and less about what would help them understand and cope with the situation.

Suspicious Style

People whose personal style is characterized by suspiciousness have difficulty believing and understanding their situation. Regardless of what and how much they are told about their condition, they tend to suspect that some significant piece of information is being withheld. They are preoccupied with the motives of others and suspect that others do not act in their best interests. They may also believe that the care givers are not competent and for some unknown reason are deliberately placing them in jeopardy. They consider disclosure as threatening because it makes them more vulnerable, and therefore they may be reluctant to share their fears and fantasies about the situation. They may also distort and exaggerate the significance of treatments or bodily sensations and thus increase anxiety and unhealthy ego defenses.

Hostile Style

Some people approach problems with hostility. Change and stress make them irritable and angry. Their sarcasm, hostile interactions, and demanding behavior tend to push people away. The resulting isolation serves to increase their anxiety and anger. Their hypercritical assessment of care, the way it is provided, and the outcome is their way of dealing with a perceived loss of control over their lives and their bodies. These people may use information about their situation effectively, but they tend to be preoccupied with finding gaps, errors, or evidence that the data are incomplete.

Avoiding Style

Some people design and manage their lives so as to avoid confronting unpleasant thoughts, feelings, and situations. They seem to believe, "If I do not hear or see a problem, then it does not exist." They do not ask questions, because the answers might be unpleasant; anything disagreeable must be avoided. When information is provided, these people forget what they were told; sometimes they cannot remember anything at all about the interaction. Denial is their primary defense. They usually ignore illness or discomfort until it reaches crisis proportions, and then they express surprise that their situation could have become so serious in what they perceive as a short time.

Influence of Culture and Values

Hartog and Hartog[3] have identified value orientations which aid in understanding cultural and individual differences that influence responses to health and illness; the relevant components are presented in Table 41-1. Values are greatly influenced by culture, but there are vast individual differences within cultures. Therefore, although it is helpful to understand typical values of certain cultures, each client must be assessed individually. For example, it is characteristic of many Japanese people to value the ability to be dependent,[3] but a Japanese person raised, educated, and working in the United States may have adopted the western value of independence.

Table 41-1 Value Orientation

Components	Questions for Assessment
Relationship to nature	Is the person subjugated by, submissive to, in harmony with, or dominant over nature?
View of people as basically good or not	Does the person see people as responsible for bringing disease on themselves?
Dominant way of interpersonal relating	Does the person prefer to relate vertically (authoritarian structure), horizontally (communal structure), or in an egalitarian, sharing manner (individualistic)?
Time orientation	Is the person oriented toward the past (rejects new things), the present (follows medical regimes only when symptomatic), or the future (chooses prevention)?
Child or adult orientation	How does the age of an ill family member or self affect expected priorities, attention, and protection?
Independence or dependence orientation	Does the person accept the need for dependence and expect to be cared for; or does the person deny illness due to valuing independence?
Community or society orientation	Is the person oriented to small town, rural, family perspectives or to urban, large group, self-centered views?

SOURCE: Adapted from J. Hartog and E. A. Hartog, "Cultural Aspects of Health and Illness Behavior in Hospitals," *Western Journal of Medicine*, vol. 139, December 1983, p. 911.

Influence of Loss

The major impact of illness is usually loss. The person who is ill, of course, has the most intense experience of loss. However, the family, work group, and community also experience some impact, owing to the loss of a member or change in a member's role. For an acutely ill person, loss is temporary and limited to the time frame of the illness. For a chronically ill person, loss is continuous; this is further explored in Chapter 43.

Illness and hospitalization may cause people to experience a *loss of the sense of identity*. The degree of threat is influenced by the strength of the person's identity before hospitalization as well as by the actual effects of the illness. For example, someone who already has a poor self-concept and low self-esteem might be more distressed by a seemingly minor problem than someone who has a strong self-concept and high self-esteem and is facing a much more severe illness.

Another loss experienced by those who are ill and those who are hospitalized is *loss of control* over their own lives. Choices made almost unconsciously in everyday life may become major issues for someone who is in the hospital. Even simple decisions such as when to bathe, when and what to eat, and whether or not to watch television become complicated by the expectations and routines of hospital personnel as well as by the needs and rights of other clients.

Illness and hospitalization may also cause a *loss of sense of purpose*. People need to feel of value and to find meaning in life; hospitalization may threaten their capacity to make sense of life. Those who have a strong spiritual faith or a strong sense of higher values may tolerate illness and hospitalization better than those who do not. But some people's spiritual foundations are shaken by pain and suffering; and hospital routines and concomitant disruptions tend to interfere with clients' usual efforts to find spiritual peace.

The family must cope with the *loss of the hospitalized person*, whose usual roles and responsibilities may be interrupted. Other family members must make up for that loss and must also expend energy and time establishing their new roles in the hospital itself: they are now the "family of a hospitalized person."

Illness and hospitalization also constitute a *loss to the community*. First, the contributions of clients who work will obviously be affected. Moreover, these clients' employers must make decisions about how to respond to their absence. How much support clients receive from their employers and co-workers may be influenced by the value of their contribution and the amount of disruption their absence is causing. The second impact on the community is the loss of contributions to local concerns other than work. A hospitalized person may be unable to vote, participate in a public service group, or hold office in a professional or voluntary organization. A third loss of this kind has to do with resources used to help people interact with the environment in healthier ways. However, an extraordinary demand for resources need not have an entirely negative effect; it may unite a community. Many communities experience an increased sense of identity when people cooperate to raise funds for organ transplants or other extreme measures.

PATTERNS OF INTERACTION: PERSON

Hospitalization has an impact on one's individuality, and that in turn affects interaction with the environment. Individuality is reflected physically in rhythmic behavior, mentally in coping styles and autonomy, and spiritually through personal integrity; hospitalization influences each of these aspects.

Rhythms

All aspects of a person are rhythmic, as is most interaction between the person and the environment. (See Chapter 30.) When people are hospitalized, the hospital's expectations may be out of harmony with their own rhythms. For example, a person may be accustomed to going to bed after midnight and getting up no earlier than eight o'clock in the morning; in a hospital, it might be necessary to go to bed at nine in the evening, in order not to disturb a roommate, and get up at six in the morning, when a night nurse makes final rounds or delivers medication.

Disruptions to personal rhythms cause various changes, which might first be observed in measurements of blood pressure and secretions. In addition, there may be behavioral changes such as alterations in mood (depression or elation, irritability, impatience) and changes in communication style (becoming more or less talkative, for instance). Other effects of disrupted rhythms are increased fatigue and decreased energy, changes in food preferences and eating habits, changes in bowel and bladder function, changes in sleeping and waking patterns, and changes in self-perception.[4]

Although such disturbances have been observed and expressed by clients, their families, and health care professionals for years, little was done to alleviate them. Now, however, there is considerable interest in the role rhythms play in health and illness; recognition of their importance may lead to alterations in acute-care settings so that individual patterns can be supported if they are healthy and repatterned only if they are dysfunctional.

Coping Styles

One of the most important factors in people's reactions to illness and hospitalization is *what the illness means* to them. The "meaning" of an illness is partly conscious; the client recognizes that it is life-threatening or that it creates limitations. But some of the meaning is unconscious. For example, attitudes toward illness may have been acquired in childhood, and the client may be unaware of them. (As children, some people learn from their families or caretakers that illness implies being rejected, being rewarded, or simply being cared for.)

Another factor is *how the illness affects relationships with others.* Illness may disrupt or foster relationships, or it may have little effect on them. Illness can place such a strain on a relationship that the people involved become disassociated from one another. On the other hand, an illness may unite people or tie them together through guilt or pity. In many relationships, an illness is disconcerting but does not interfere with the usual pattern of interaction and involvement.

A third factor is *how the illness influences social or economic standing.* Illnesses that have social significance (such as venereal diseases and alcoholism) may cause social status to change. Awareness of stigmatization will obviously influence a person's response to having such an illness. An illness which interferes with a person's ability to earn a living will (other things being equal) be more of a threat than one which does not. The severity of the illness itself is not necessarily what determines whether it represents a threat to one's livelihood; a person who has inadequate finances or insurance, who will not be compensated for illness, or who cannot take sick leave may be devastated by even a relatively minor, short-lived illness.

How important any of these factors will be depends on personality, emotionally and socially learned responses, cultural differences, and past experiences with illness. They are also influenced by the nature and the psychodynamic and symbolic meaning of the symptoms.[5] Finally, the consequences of the illness—threat, loss, gain, relief—influence coping mechanisms[5] and patterns of interaction that develop.

As was noted earlier, illness represents *loss:* real, anticipated, and symbolic. Loss may generate anxiety and depression, lower self-esteem, and make it impossible to gratify needs. During an acute illness, the process of grief and mourning can lead to acceptance and thus to a healthy resolution of loss. Inability to grieve and subsequent denial of the importance of the loss are unhealthy responses. (The effect of loss is different in chronic illness; this is discussed in Chapter 43.)

Acute illness increases *anxiety* in two ways. First, there is a physiological arousal: the autonomic nervous system is activated in specific ways when the body is threatened. Second, this leads to affective symptoms of anxiety.

Perception of loss and increased anxiety during acute illness stimulate the person to seek relief through coping mechanisms. People tend to use coping mechanisms which they have used in the past. These mechanisms are influenced by personality style, described earlier in this chapter.

Autonomy

The first time people encounter the crisis of autonomy versus shame and doubt is at about 1 to 3 years of age. If this crisis is successfully negotiated, they incorporate a feeling that autonomy is valuable. Throughout life, they learn many things and grow increasingly competent at functioning autonomously. By the time they develop into healthy adults, their strivings for autonomy have usually been integrated with an ability to function cooperatively. Even though people are still expected to be willing and able to take care of themselves, they are also able to be trustingly interdependent in their personal relationships and at work.

The loss of autonomy associated with hospitalization is related to the extent of physiological distress as well as to the degree of autonomy allowed in the hospital. When clients are first admitted for care, they may experience relief. They are anticipating assistance and are therefore willing to endure a loss of autonomy. But as clients recover, they may want more autonomy than the hospital staff is ready to allow. The response to a loss or threatened loss of autonomy is like the response to any other loss: frustration and a lowering of self-esteem. This may be expressed by withdrawal, irritability, or hostility.

Integrity

Integrity is the functioning of the person as a whole being. It is the result of assimilating into the personality the knowledge and experience that enable people to function. Integrity is the harmonious interaction of a person's physical, mental, and spiritual dimensions. A person maintains integrity through the reinforcement of values and through acquisition of knowledge and experience related to each of these dimensions.

A threat to integrity is experienced as *abasement:* a state of feeling humiliated or degraded. Many of the experiences of a hospitalized client result in a sense of loss of integrity and an onset of abasement. People who must be hospitalized are in need of intrusions into their private daily activities. For example, assistance may be necessary for private functions such as elimination, and body parts which are ordinarily seen only by a person's most intimate associates are viewed by strangers. Procedures may be performed by nurses and others with little explanation, as if the client were an inanimate object. Procedures such as injections and enemas actually invade the bodily boundary. The client's need for spiritual or religious activities may be overlooked, interrupted, or viewed with disdain. In serious illnesses, clients may be dependent on technological devices for life itself, or at least for some supportive functions; and they may have periods of unconsciousness or disorientation because of physiological problems or the interventions performed to deal with them. Alterations in consciousness may threaten the client by increasing the sense of dependence on others or because alterations in behavior are brought about by disorientation and confusion.

The loss of integrity and the onset of a feeling of abasement may lead to behavioral manifestations which complicate clients' recovery. Clients may become *pseudo-independent,* or *noncompliant:* for example, a client may remove tubes, refuse medications, ambulate inappropriately, or leave the hospital against medical advice in an attempt to regain a sense of integrity. On the other hand, clients may become extremely dependent, expecting nurses, family members, and others to take even more responsibility than is indicated by their condition.

Table 41-2 Promoting Individuality

Nursing Interventions
1. Assess clients' patterns of waking, sleeping, and daily activity and adjust hospital routine to their rhythms as much as possible.
2. Observe clients for signs of disruptions in rhythms.
3. Assess what illness and hospitalization mean to clients, how their relationships with others are affected, and whether their social and economic standings are changed.
4. Encourage clients to be as autonomous as possible, given the extent and nature of the illness and considering what is age-appropriate.
5. Demonstrate concern for all aspects of the clients' individuality—physical, mental, and spiritual.
6. Call clients by name; include clients in making decisions; avoid doing things *to* clients which contribute to dehumanization.
7. Give complete explanations of procedures in terms clients can understand; encourage clients to discuss their feelings and their responses to hospitalization.
8. Introduce oneself and others to clients and explain the roles of personnel who are working with clients.
9. Remain kind, patient, and considerate even when clients are irritable, disoriented, or hostile.
10. Treat clients as normal, healthy people of the same age would be treated outside the hospital, making only those exceptions that are truly warranted by their illness.

Many of the considerations which will help nurses to preserve their clients' sense of individuality pertain to more than one of the facets described in this section. Table 41-2 lists important interventions.

PATTERNS OF INTERACTION: FAMILY

Illness and hospitalization for physical or emotional problems have an impact not only on clients but on their families as well. They constitute a crisis which can disorganize the individual and family unless they are dealt with constructively as an opportunity for growth and attainment of a higher level of wellness.

Families exhibit various behaviors when a member is hospitalized: they may become anxious, fearful, or angry. Some families rally around to support clients through the experience. They are nurturing, attentive, and *there*. This facilitates the client's acceptance of dependency and regression as part of the sick role. However, the family's support may interfere with the client's movement toward health, especially if family members fail to foster independence as the client improves physically.

Some families feel abandoned by the member who is sick, and burdened with the additional responsibilities incurred by the hospitalization. Their anger and frustration may be directed at the client and exhibited by infrequent visiting or minimal communication. The family may excuse this behavior by telling the client how burdened they are as a result of the hospitalization; then the client may feel guilty and anxious. Family members may also displace their anger onto the staff or the hospital itself and become critical or excessively demanding.

Differentiation (see Chapter 19) refers to the ability of family members to maintain their individuality and to balance intellectual and emotional processes so that they can be flexible and adaptable during an illness. When a family has a high level of differentiation, its members can function effectively and support each other during a crisis, despite the stress they are undergoing. If such a family becomes somewhat dysfunctional during the crisis, the disorganization is temporary, and more effective functioning is soon reestablished.[6]

When there is a low level of differentiation in a family system, the lack of flexibility and adaptability may have contributed to the illness; moreover, the family is less able to manage stress and is therefore likely to become dysfunctional during the crisis.[6]

Family members may not have the same level of differentiation; one member may seem to function at a higher level than others, and another member may seem to function at a much lower level and thus may become a recipient of a family projection process. A person's level of differentiation is usually stable; however, it may decrease if there are multiple, unforeseen problems and changes within a short period of time. Thus, ability to cope with an illness varies from one person to another and even within the same person from time to time.[6]

A critical illness casts a family into the context of a catastrophe. To some extent, however, the person who is ill may be shielded from the crisis. Clients in special-care units, for instance, are often not fully aware of the seriousness of their illnesses or its impact on their families. Also, during a physiological crisis, clients tend to use a variety of avoidance mechanisms. Such mechanisms help them conserve energy and keep them from becoming overwhelmed at a time when survival is at risk. Care givers will also make efforts to protect these clients from further stress and anxiety.

The burden of the catastrophic situation is, therefore, borne by the family. The family is usually the primary recipient of information about the nature of the client's critical illness and the degree of threat to the client's life. Consequently, family members may become confused and frightened about the outcome. Not only the client's predicament but also the special-care setting and the life-support technology generate acute stress in family members, which (as was noted earlier) can become a disorganizing force in the family system. Because a family is an emotional system, anxiety can be contagious; and a high level of stress and anxiety obviously increases emotionality. Family members feel a need to draw together, and this increases the risk of fusion. As a result, even families which usually have a relatively high level of differentiation may exhibit dysfunctional behavior.

When fusion occurs, the separateness and uniqueness of family members are negated. Individuals' needs, wishes, perceptions, and feelings are not recognized. Each member's sense of self is threatened because personal boundaries are no longer clearly defined. Thus, the anxiety experienced is exacerbated by a potential loss of self.

In every family there are members who hold a central, unifying position. They may be a primary organizing influence, may serve as the clearinghouse or mediator of information, or may be the focus of a projection process and thus have a significant influence on the equilibrium of the family system. When a central figure becomes critically ill, the impact may be greater because the illness is perceived as a threat to the existence of the family system.[6] The following case study provides an example:

> Sam was hospitalized in an intensive-care unit in critical condition after an automobile accident. The owner of a large construction company, in which he employed his four sons, he ran his business and his family with an "iron fist in a velvet glove." All decisions in the business required his stamp of approval, and

at home he controlled finances and social life. His hospitalization created a crisis in the business and the family. Since he had not groomed any of his sons to assume the leadership of the company, work schedules, supervision of the employees, and even the purchase of building materials were disrupted. Household crises were numerous. His wife could not sign checks to purchase food or pay bills. Sam had been the clearinghouse for the flow of information among family members. Consequently, there was a communication breakdown when he was hospitalized. The family members lacked accurate information about his condition and prognosis because no one else served as spokesperson for the family, nor had anyone established communication with the unit staff. Misperceptions and fantasies escalated the family's anxiety. Open conflict occurred among members. Sam's generous but controlling relationship had generated ambivalence: his family felt anger because of their dependence on him but at the same time loved him because of his warmth and generosity. This ambivalence influenced members' relationships with one another during his hospitalization. When family members gathered in the unit waiting room, they vacillated between tearful laments and loud, argumentative disagreements.

When the client is a recipient of a family projection process, the crisis precipitated by an illness may allow him or her to continue to serve as an organizing and stabilizing force. However, if the threat to life is great, the illness is prolonged and static, and the prognosis is poor, the family may need to find a new focus of projection. For example, if a client remains comatose but stable on life-support systems for several months, the crisis may diminish. Before the critical illness, the family balance may have depended on the client's symptomatic behavior. Now, the physical and psychological absence of the client may upset the balance, and in order to restabilize it, another family member may develop symptoms. The family then refocuses its attention. The critically ill client is abandoned emotionally if not physically. The family's interest and energy are reinvested in someone else. For example:

Mr. and Mrs. C.'s 17-year-old son Andy was hospitalized in a burn unit following a motorcycle accident in which the gasoline tank exploded. In addition to extensive third-degree burns, he had suffered a fractured skull and severe brain damage. Before the accident, Andy had been the "black sheep" of the family. His many arrests for drug-related offenses and vandalism had created turmoil in the household. The parents appeared to have endless patience, despite his repeated problems with the law and the costly legal fees. Just before this last incident the parents had verbalized anger and disgust at his behavior and said that they were giving up on him. But despite these statements, they had bought a new motorcycle for him, and they had continued to provide him with unlimited spending money. Immediately following his hospitalization, his parents visited frequently and appeared grief-stricken. At home, all communication among family members centered on Andy. When his condition did not improve and he continued to require life-support systems, the parents visited less frequently and stayed only a few minutes. Andy's 15-year-old brother Tim, who had maintained a low profile in the family, began to have problems at school. The use of marijuana became an issue between the parents and Tim. It was difficult to determine which came first, Tim's use of marijuana or the accusation that he would turn out like his brother. Regardless, the outcome was an increasing number of heated arguments between Tim and his parents, and Tim's increased use of marijuana and alcohol. Tim replaced Andy as the focus of the family projection process, and Andy was emotionally and to a great extent physically abandoned.

Over- and underfunctioning husbands and wives in families with a low level of differentiation are also significantly influenced by the critical illness of their spouse. Before the illness, overfunctioning spouses may have been able to regulate the extent of their responsibility. When an underfunctioning spouse becomes critically ill, all responsibility falls on the overfunctioning spouse. The ability to regulate assumption of responsibility is lost, and the burden created by additional responsibilities may be overwhelming. The overfunctioner may then become dysfunctional.[6]

When an overfunctioning spouse becomes critically ill, the underfunctioning spouse can either become completely disorganized and dysfunctional or move into the overfunctioning role. If overfunctioning is handled successfully, the spouse who has taken on this new role may not choose to abandon it when the ill spouse recovers. Then either a new functional arrangement develops between the spouses or there is so much conflict that the family disintegrates.

Both under- and overfunctioning spouses may, when the other spouse is critically ill, sustain their own original role by pulling a child into the opposing role. This is not necessarily problematic if the child is an adult. However, if the child is young or an adolescent, "parentification" occurs.

PATTERNS OF INTERACTION: ENVIRONMENT

The hospital environment may elicit behavior which is difficult to understand. As clients interact with it, however, recognizable patterns begin to emerge: territoriality, altered perception of time, uncertainty, depersonalization, reactivation of memories, regression, discontinuity and disassociation, the "sick role," and "clients' work." These are discussed below, along with specific stressful factors in hospitalization and the hospital environment.

Territoriality

Territoriality is "the state which is characterized by possessiveness, control, and authority over an area of physical space."[7] Territorial behavior helps to provide privacy, security, control, autonomy, and identity.[7] (See Chapter 3 for a discussion of this concept.)

It is important to emphasize the unconscious nature of personal space. Most people take their personal space for granted; they are not always aware that they are interpreting other people's behavior in terms of their own need for space. As a result, they may misinterpret the gestures and movements of others, and they may respond to a perceived "invasion" behaviorally rather than verbally. For example, if X is sitting alone on a couch and Y sits down immediately beside him or her (although other places to sit are available), X will tend to turn or edge away or may even get up and move somewhere else.[8] Personal space is space over which people want to exert control; but since the desire for control is not always expressed, an intrusion may cause physiological responses that in turn lead to withdrawal or flight—neither of which is entirely rational.

Allekian[8] found an interesting phenomenon in hospitalized clients. In most social situations, an intrusion into "intimate" space—bodily contact—is more discomforting than an intrusion into personal space. However, for hospitalized clients studied by Allekian the opposite was true: territorial invasions, such as going through a client's belongings or rearranging personal items, caused more uneasiness than intimate gestures, such as touching, or procedures which exposed the body. Allekian speculated that when people are hospitalized, they may be prepared for invasions of their intimate space but not for invasions of their wider personal territory.

Some researchers have estimated that people require 86 to 108 square feet of space in order to feel healthy and comfortable.[9] But Hayter[7] identified several factors which affect individuals' needs for territory: *age, gender, state of health,* and *culture.* Teenagers and the elderly may need more space than other people. With adolescents, the need for additional space appears to be connected with a struggle to establish identity. Older people, too, may need more space because they are threatened with loss of identity. Men seem to need more space than women, and they are more likely to invade other people's space than women are. People who are ill seem to feel a greater need to control their own territory; but although they are less tolerant of invasions, at the same time they are less able to defend their territory. Culture is a significant determinant of territorial needs. Westerners need more space than people from the far east or the middle east. People from Canada, Great Britain, and the United States need the most personal space; Latin Americans and Arabs need the least.[10] Within the United States, members of subcultures (such as Puerto Ricans, blacks, and Native Americans) may have attitudes toward space that differ from those of white people of British or European extraction.[7]

Privacy is the quality or state of being apart from company or observation. It is also freedom from intrusion of personal space. Most people respect others' right to privacy: they enter someone else's home only by invitation and leave family members alone who have asked to be left alone. However, it is a common practice in hospitals for nurses, physicians, and others to enter clients' rooms, draw back curtains from around beds, and uncover or undress clients with little or no explanation and without asking permission. Clients frequently complain about lack of privacy as part of the discomfort of hospitalization.

The need for personal territory may be expressed in a variety of ways by people who are hospitalized.

In a semiprivate room the clients may keep the curtain between their beds closed so that they cannot see each other. A client may place personal belongings on a piece of furniture or a windowsill to identify it as part of his or her personal space. Some clients keep special possessions such as letters, photographs, handkerchiefs, and mementos in bed with them. A client may create a "wall of noise" by wearing a headset connected to a radio or tape player.

Since, as was noted earlier, people are often unaware of the significance of their personal space, nurses should not assume that clients do not object to intrusions simply because they do not say anything about them. Clients seem to assume that health care personnel will invade their body; but they may nevertheless withdraw, fail to make eye contact, and speak as little as possible while nurses or others are performing invasive procedures. Silence should not be taken as consent; nurses should obtain permission for an intrusion and explain it. This acknowledges the client's need for control over intimate and personal space.

A list of considerations pertaining to territorial needs is given in Table 41-3.

Table 41-3 Meeting Territorial Needs

Nursing Interventions
1. Seek permission to enter clients' territory.
2. Allow clients to have control over personal space.
3. Leave time between intrusions so that clients have time to recover from one before being subjected to the next.
4. Organize work so that intrusions are minimal; enter clients' personal space only when warranted.
5. Include clients in the planning of care; design care to meet their preferences as much as possible.
6. Tell clients which things are part of their own territory in the hospital (e.g., bed, table, chair).
7. Expect clients to put their own belongings away; if this is not possible, have clients give directions and watch as the nurse stores their personal items.
8. Adjust lighting, temperature, furniture, door, curtains, and similar amenities to suit clients' expressed preferences as much as possible. Avoid making assumptions.
9. Seek clients' permission before examining or moving any personal belongings.
10. Stay within the limits of access granted by clients.
11. Use space in accordance with clients' individual needs, considering gender, age, culture, and illness.
12. Include territorial needs as part of the care plan.
13. Educate other personnel about the significance of territorial needs and how to meet them.
14. Provide adequate privacy for clients during procedures, treatments, or examinations; avoid exposing a client's body more than is necessary.
15. When interviewing a client, do so out of the hearing of other clients or staff members who do not need the information.
16. Provide times for clients to think, meditate, or pray; let clients know that this time will be uninterrupted and ensure that intrusions do not occur.

Perception of Time

Time is a conceptual experience, a way of perceiving the order of things. It is sensed both as motion (passing of time) and duration (length of time). (See Chapter 3.) Hospitalized people are generally more past- and present-oriented than future-oriented.[11] They tend to overestimate time intervals, and clock time seems to pass slowly for them. Factors that can affect clients' perception of time include *habits, metabolic rate, temperature, movement,* and *pain.*

Daily habits or patterns are an important influence on perception of time. For healthy people, the sense of clock time is based on the occurrence of expected, familiar activities and events: getting up, starting work, seeing other members of the household come and go. When these patterns are interrupted by hospitalization, clients may become disoriented with regard to time or sense it as passing more slowly.

People who have high metabolic rates perceive clock time as passing more slowly than other people do.[4] This implies that age can affect the sense of time. Since children have higher metabolic rates, they perceive time as passing more slowly than adults do. Conversely, as people age, their metabolic rate slows down, giving them the sense that time is passing more quickly.

Body temperature is also a factor in time perception. The higher the temperature, the slower clock time seems to pass.[4]

Studies have found that movement affects one's sense of the passage of time. The rhythm of people's movements is a physiological mechanism that helps preserve the integrity of the bodily system;[12] when it is altered, perception of time is altered too. Nearly all hospitalized people are restricted to some degree in their movement—even ambulatory clients are much more restricted than usual, and clients who are confined to bed or to a wheelchair or who must

Table 41-4 Promoting Time Orientation

Nursing Interventions
1. Provide clocks and calendars within sight of clients who have none—especially clients who are susceptible to disorientation (for example, those in special-care units).
2. Give clients specific information about time spans (such as duration of a treatment or time remaining until a medication may be given).
3. Allow clients to engage in as much normal activity as their physical condition warrants.
4. Provide some meaningful distraction when clients must endure unpleasant periods of waiting (for relief of pain or for some other anticipated event).
5. Give clients as much certainty as possible, by sharing adequate, clear information with them or helping other staff members to do so.
6. Orient clients to the environment.
7. Encourage clients to discuss memories which are reactivated by illness and hospitalization; encourage them to talk about feelings aroused by hospitalization to put memories in context.
8. Accept the amount of regression warranted by illness and hospitalization; nurture and support clients who have regressed and help them return to normal as they recover.
9. Call clients by name; treat them as individuals, not objects; acknowledge their cooperation in painful or uncomfortable procedures.
10. If clients' requests cannot be granted, acknowledge their needs and tell them how, when, and by whom their requests will be met.
11. Encourage clients to talk about their anxiety over illness and hospitalization.

use devices such as walkers and crutches are obviously severely limited.

Pain makes it difficult to think of anything else. The more severe it is, the more it interferes with awareness of other things. One significant effect is the sense that time is passing slowly. This is especially true for people who are waiting for some intervention that promises relief.

Table 41-4 lists important considerations for nursing care in regard to time.

Uncertainty

Uncertainty is the state of being doubtful, of being aware of things which are not clearly identified or defined. Mishel[13] has proposed a model of uncertainty in illness that helps to describe some behaviors seen in hospitalized clients. She identifies eight dimensions of uncertainty:

- Vagueness
- Lack of clarity
- Ambiguity
- Unpredictability
- Inconsistency
- Probability
- Multiple meanings
- Lack of information

When clients experience uncertainty, it is difficult for them to recognize or classify events: that is, they lack a cognitive structure within which situations can be defined. This limits their ability to evaluate an event as benign, challenging, or threatening. But they still make such evaluations and react accordingly: by direct action, for example, or by vigilance or avoidance.

When an event is marked by uncertainty, it is usually evaluated as a threat. Clients may initially respond with direct action; they seek information in order to establish certainty. If information is inadequate, uncertainty increases, and they resort to increased vigilance. Finally, if uncertainty persists, they may use avoidance, and withdraw in some way.

Depersonalization

Depersonalization is a disturbance in affect marked by feelings of unreality or strangeness with regard to the environment, the self, or both. People who have become depersonalized have a sense that they are no longer themselves; they may not even feel like human beings.

A person who is hospitalized must endure a myriad of unfamiliar experiences. Strangers come and go, demanding information, specimens, or compliance with treatments. The sense of self is severely threatened by an unfamiliar environment which is not at all like the everyday world. Personal space is invaded continually. Clothing and other belongings may have been taken away or may be under the control of hospital personnel. Decisions are made for clients, who may be treated as somehow inferior because they are ill. Nurses, physicians, and others may describe clients' behavior with labels that have strong emotional connotations: *crock, crybaby, uncooperative, noncompliant.*

Buffeted by unfamiliar experiences, clients may feel a substantial threat to their sense of self. Staff members may not address clients by name or may use the wrong names. Clients may feel "unreal" or "invisible" when they try unsuccessfully to get attention by calling out or making eye contact with staff members passing by their doors. Busy people bustle by without even acknowledging clients' distress. Clients must cooperate in procedures which may be uncomfortable or painful, without being consulted beforehand and without any acknowledgement of their cooperation. Such experiences make the client feel less than a person, even if the feeling is unexpressed at the time. Family members or nurses who hear the client describe such feelings later on may be surprised, since the client had seemed composed and unaffected.

Recognizing that depersonalization can happen, nurses can help to prevent or mitigate it by making efforts to preserve their clients' sense of self.

Reactivation of Memories

Hospitalization may remind clients of other occasions when they felt helpless, deprived, and unable to function independently. If these earlier experiences were never adequately resolved, manifestations of an emotional conflict may be observed. Memories of earlier losses or failures, and unresolved inadequacy or mistrust, can be reawakened; and enforced dependency in the past—particularly if needs were not met—may have generated anger or depression. The reactivated feelings may be as intense as those experienced originally. Moreover, present helplessness, dependency, and loss, especially loss of control, can themselves generate anger and frustration. If present feelings are aggravated by the reactivation of past feelings, clients may not be able to cooperate with care givers or conserve their own energy. Therefore, they may need help in expressing these feelings in order to prevent further stress that may disrupt the healing process.

Regression

Regression is reversion to an earlier level of functioning that was characterized by fewer demands, less responsibility, and less autonomy. For people who are hospitalized, it is likely to take the form of a return to a point in development when nurturing was needed and dependency was accepted.

If clients are to cooperate with care givers, they must accept some passivity and dependency; that is, some degree of regression must occur. Regression is also an effective way to conserve energy so that all available resources can be available for restoring and repairing the body. When considerable regression occurs, clients become egocentric. The world shrinks to include only needs and their satisfaction; survival may become the only goal; concerns about home, work, or significant others may be pushed out of awareness. The more severe the illness and the greater the physiological instability, the more the client is likely to regress. Regression can usually be measured by the client's willingness to accept dependency; as the client's health improves, regression usually diminishes and there is a movement toward more mature and independent functioning.

Regression is part of the "sick role" (which is discussed below), but it may not be accepted by all clients—it may conflict with their needs, expectations, and personalities. Nor is it invariably appropriate. For example, people who are hospitalized for diagnostic tests or minor elective surgery may feel quite well; and neither their physical status nor their personal needs may require nurturing and dependency. Expecting such clients to exhibit regression can create problems.

Discontinuity and Dissociation

Usually, people take their sense of continuity for granted and become conscious of it only when it is interrupted. Schontz[1] has described *discontinuity* as a process consisting of several stages. The initial effect is loss of continuity between past, present, and future. Next, operations used in the past no longer seem applicable. Finally, it becomes difficult to imagine oneself in the future; the future seems uncertain, bleak, or nonexistent. People who are in the acute stage of a serious illness may experience discontinuity as a result of changes in the sensorium accompanying delirium. Alterations in the state of consciousness may also be due to emotional or other physical factors.

Dissociation is a process by which aspects of an experience that are intensely anxiety-provoking are split off from conscious awareness. Clients who are gravely ill tend to dissociate from painful experiences and retreat from awareness of the seriousness of the situation. They sometimes describe this experience as being able to observe what is happening to their bodies without experiencing an emotional response to events or their meaning. This "emotional flight" allows them to conserve energy under extreme duress. (It can also occur in circumstances other than illness, such as overwhelming shame, debasement, fear, or anxiety.)

When a client is experiencing discontinuity and dissociation, what nurses will observe is unconcern or noninvolvement. Clients may be unable to recall instructions or information and may later forget interactions with nurses, physicians, and family members which took place during the period of dissociation. Some clients will try to figure out what happened by filling in the blanks with seemingly reasonable explanations, but their explanations may incorporate fantasies and distortions and thus can cause others to believe they are lying. Nurses can help clients fill in the blanks with accurate information, but they should not argue about notions the clients are unwilling to relinquish.

The Sick Role and Clients' Work

There are two ways of looking at people who are hospitalized. The classic way is in terms of what is called the *sick role*—a theoretical construct that Talcott Parsons[14] used within a broader analysis of western industrialized society. The sick role is characterized by passivity. In contrast, Strauss, Fagerhaugh, Suczek, and Weiner[15] have used another construct, *patients' work* (or *clients' work*), which recognizes clients' own efforts in getting well.

The sick role is characterized by four institutional expectations:[14]

- Sick people are exempted from normal social roles and responsibilities.
- Sick people cannot be expected to get well by "pulling themselves together," by an act of decision or will.
- But being ill is undesirable, and sick people therefore have an obligation to "want to get well."
- Sick people have an obligation, in proportion to the severity of their condition, to seek technically competent help, and to cooperate in the process of trying to get well.

The expectation of nurses, physicians, family members, and others that clients should assume the sick role accounts for many of the phenomena described earlier. Interruptions of autonomous functioning, invasions of territory, disturbances of time orientation, alterations in consciousness, and other experiences typical of hospitalization reflect the belief that people who are hospitalized should be dependent. Clients who take on the sick role are fulfilling these expectations and are seen as "good patients"; clients who do not fulfill expectations are seen as "noncompliant."

The concept of the sick role does not recognize clients as "workers" in the hospital. *Work* is the expenditure of physical or mental effort to achieve an objective. When nurses and other personnel do something like positioning a client, they consider that work; but when clients are expected to position themselves, that is not seen as work. This seems illogical. Clients in fact do a great deal of work—ranging from ordinary care of themselves (such as going to the toilet and keeping their hair neat) to monitoring intravenous administrations or managing machines at their bedsides.[15] Some activities that constitute clients' work are listed in Table 41-5. Although staff members do not usually define

Table 41-5 Clients' Work

Types of Work	Examples
Body work	Positioning self; ambulating as prescribed; coughing and deep breathing; participating in diagnostic tests (such as using a treadmill)
Monitoring work	Watching intravenous drips; notifying nurses of problems with machines; monitoring performance of staff members
Comfort work	Arranging self so as not to interfere with machines or personnel
Composure work	Maintaining control of emotions during painful procedures
Technical work	Setting up and maintaining complex equipment, such as dialysis machines
Resting work	Modifying activity as dictated by physical condition
Management work during chronic illness	Taking care of problems related to chronic illnesses not the focus of current hospitalization; helping staff modify care related to other illnesses
Decision work	Thinking and deciding about aspects of treatment
Biographical work	Deciding whether to live or die
Collaborative work	Consulting with other clients about a problem; monitoring for other clients

SOURCE: Adapted from A. L. Strauss, Shizuko Fagerhaugh, Barbara Suczek, and Carolyn Weiner, "Patients' Work in the Technologized Hospital," *Nursing Outlook*, vol. 29, July 1981, pp. 404–412. Used with permission.

these activities as work, each requires physical and emotional energy from clients, and clients are expected to comply with requests to do them. Clients who do not comply are likely to be considered recalcitrant or lazy and may be chided, scolded, or ignored (particularly if "composure work" is involved).

Clients may be asked to do some kind of work because their involvement is seen as a necessary aspect of recovery or improvement. Nurses may also involve clients in doing things for themselves because they see this as an aspect of clients' rights. However, much of the work clients are urged to do is not a matter of professional judgment or ideology; many tasks are turned over to clients for reasons having to do with nurses' personal needs. (For example, the nurse may need to leave; the nurse may be busy, and the task may have a low priority; the nurse may want to save personal energy; or the nurse may simply prefer not to do the task.)[15]

In order to coordinate the work of the care givers and the work of clients, Strauss and his associates advocate including clients in team conferences or having extended discussions with clients about the work they are doing in the hospital:

> It is our argument that the patient's relatively silent but genuine part in the ward's division of labor ought to be made explicit, generally recognized, and even perhaps built into the ward's accountability system.[15]

To help clients who are hospitalized, nurses must arrive at some integration of the sick role and clients' work. Clients do need to accept some degree of dependency, for example, but nurses must recognize that acceptance may require effort. If this effort is not acknowledged as work, clients may be perplexed or disturbed. For example, if a nurse simply orders a client to "let me do that for you" or chides the client for doing something without help, this threatens the client's identity. Instead, the nurse can make it clear that letting nurses do certain things is work for the client and thus is valued. With this approach, both nurse and client may develop more reasonable expectations and respond more appropriately.

Possible responses to illness can be thought of as forming a continuum (see Figure 41-1). At one extreme is rejection and denial of both the sick role and work the client must do to recover. This reaction is characterized by aggression toward care givers and family members who try to intervene, and by independence which is inappropriate under the circumstances.

The other extreme is characterized by secondary gain, hopelessness, helplessness, and overdependence. *Secondary gain* is acceptance of the sick role for the purpose of getting attention or special privileges. *Hopelessness* is the opposite of denial: the client acknowledges the illness and the circumstances of hospitalization and feels trapped. *Helplessness* is the opposite of aggression—it is a belief that everything that can be done has been done but will be of no avail. *Overdependence* can be seen as overacceptance of the sick role; the client behaves as if nurses and others should be completely responsible for all aspects of care, even if the illness or disability is not severe enough to warrant this.

A *healthy response* to the sick role lies between these extremes. The client must accept those aspects of the sick role which will conserve energy so that it can be applied toward getting better, and must also accept whatever work is appropriate. Instead of denying the illness or feeling trapped by it, the client should make efforts to perceive it accurately. The client should also make appropriate efforts to get better and to deal with frustration or

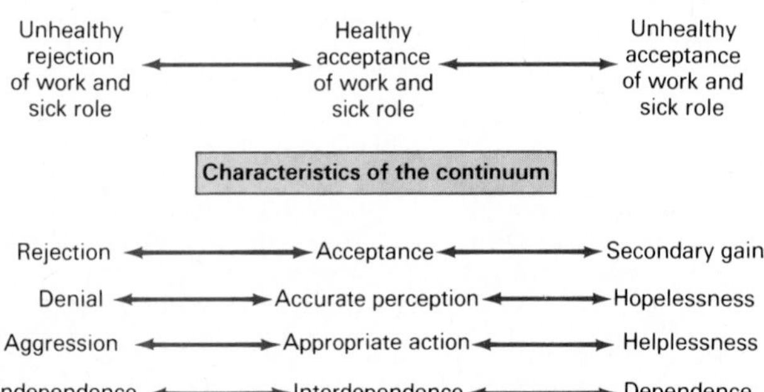

Figure 41-1 Continuum of responses to the sick role.

distress—and should not become aggressive or helpless. Finally, the client should have a flexible relationship with nurses and others; the client should be dependent or independent as appropriate and should determine what is appropriate in collaboration with the nurse. In short, the client should do the work necessary to achieve the best possible results; the nursing staff and family members should promote a healthy response and not reinforce unhealthy responses.

Stressful Factors in Hospitalization

The hospital is an unusual environment; its unfamiliar sights and sounds are a source of stress for clients and their families. Nevertheless, the client must interact effectively with this environment if the outcome of hospitalization is to be positive.

Hospital Environment

Hospitalization is inherently stressful, although the degree of stress will depend on the client's problem and the prognosis. In developing their Hospital Stress Rating Scale (HSRS), Volicer and others[16] identified 49 potentially stressful events, organized into 9 categories; these are listed in Table 41-6 (page 842). In a study of 535 medical and surgical clients in a community hospital, they found that surgical clients reported more stress than medical clients with regard to unfamiliarity of surroundings, loss of independence, and threat of severe illness. Medical clients reported more stress than surgical clients with regard to financial problems and lack of information. Although the medical clients had more serious illnesses than the surgical clients, it was the surgical clients who reported higher stress in relation to threat of severe illness; this finding suggests that preoperative surgical clients are more susceptible to this kind of stress than medical clients.[16]

The events noted in the HSRS are likely to be experienced by all hospitalized clients; but clients' personal experiences and perceptions determine which events are the most stressful.

Special-Care Units

The term *special-care unit* is used here to mean any unit in which clients receive intense nursing care for critical illnesses or traumas. This would include medical intensive-care units, coronary-care units, postsurgical intensive-care units, and neonatal intensive-care units. A special-care unit has a high ratio of nurses to clients.

Special-care units are stressful for clients for several reasons. First, of course, is the fact that the condition which has necessitated admission is itself a threat. Moreover, the condition—the illness or trauma—may have had a sudden and unexpected onset. Many clients are unconscious when they are admitted; when they regain consciousness, they must deal with pain or discomfort and with a life-threatening problem. The stresses of hospitalization are greatly intensified when special care is required.

A second source of stress is the environment of the special-care unit. Once they have become aware of their surroundings, clients begin to respond to the unit itself. Several elements of such an environment are stressors with which clients must somehow cope: immobilization, isolation from family and normal personal environment, sensory deprivation, sensory overload (particularly noise), lack of sleep, disorientation, and depersonalization. All this can lead to the "ICU syndrome."

IMMOBILIZATION. Ballard[17] studied clients in surgical intensive-care units and found that they were most distressed by immobilization and claustrophobia. These feelings were aroused because the clients were attached to monitoring equipment, had to wear oxygen masks, and had tubes in body orifices and intravenous and other lines in place.

ISOLATION. The next most common stressor noted by Ballard was clients' isolation from their families and their normal environment. This is intensified in most special-care units because of limitations on visiting.

SENSORY DEPRIVATION AND OVERLOAD. Sensory deprivation and sensory overload are also common problems in special-care units.[18] Sensory deprivation results from lack of meaningful—and familiar—stimuli. Clients in special-care units are constantly exposed to sights, sounds, smells, and touches of various kinds, but these sensations may be so unlike ordinary experience that they cannot help to establish and maintain contact with reality—that is, the stimuli may be highly intensified or may be unique to the special-care environment.

Table 41-6 Hospital Stress Factors

Category	Stress Scale Events	Category	Stress Scale Events
1. Unfamiliarity of surroundings	Having strangers sleep in the same room with you Having to sleep in a strange bed Having strange machines around Being awakened in the night by the nurse Being aware of unusual smells around you Being in a room that is too cold or too hot Having to eat cold or tasteless food Being cared for by an unfamiliar doctor	6. Lack of information	Thinking you might have pain because of surgery or test procedures Not knowing when to expect things will be done to you Having nurses or doctors talk too fast or use words you can't understand Not having your questions answered by the staff Not knowing the results or reasons for your treatments Not knowing for sure what illnesses you have Not being told what your diagnosis is
2. Loss of independence	Having to eat at other times than you usually do Having to wear a hospital gown Having to be assisted with bathing Not being able to get newspapers, radio, or TV when you want them Having a roommate who has too many visitors Having to stay in bed or in the same room all day Having to be assisted with a bedpan Not having your call light answered Being fed through tubes Thinking you may lose your sight	7. Threat of severe illness	Thinking your appearance might be changed after your hospitalization Being put in the hospital because of an accident Knowing you have to have an operation Having a sudden hospitalization you weren't planning to have Knowing you have a serious illness Thinking you might lose a kidney or some other organ Thinking you might have cancer
3. Separation from spouse	Worrying about your spouse being away from you Missing your spouse	8. Separation from family	Being in the hospital during holidays or special family occasions Not having family visit you Being hospitalized far away from home
4. Financial problems	Thinking about losing income because of your illness Not having enough insurance to pay for your hospitalization	9. Problems with medications	Having medications cause you discomfort Feeling you are getting dependent on medications Not getting relief from pain medications Not getting pain medication when you need it
5. Isolation from other people	Having a roommate who is seriously ill or cannot talk with you Having a roommate who is unfriendly Not having friends visit you Not being able to call family or friends on the phone Having the staff hurry too much Thinking you might lose your hearing		

SOURCE: B. J. Volicer, M. A. Isenberg, and M. W. Burns, "Medical-Surgical Differences in Hospital Stress Factors," *Journal of Human Stress,* vol. 3, June 1977, pp. 3–13. Used with permission.

People have a range of stimulation within which they can cope. When the limits are exceeded, they experience sensory overload, and their coping systems deteriorate.[18] Stimuli which can contribute to overload include continuous lighting, crowding, unpleasant odors, painful touches, unusual sights, uncomfortable environmental temperature, thirst, pain, discomfort from surgical wounds or other injuries, and noise.

Of all the stimuli, noise is most frequently identified as a cause of problems.[18] *Noise* is unwanted, undesirable sound. Whether a sound is noise is determined subjectively; it depends on individual perceptions of what is tolerable or intolerable, pleasant or unpleasant. Noise is created by machinery, monitors, and other kinds of equipment in special-care units as well as the usual buzzers, alarms, telephones, and paging systems; but the most disturbing noises seem to be those created by the activities of staff members, especially their communications with one another.[18] The response to noise—annoyance—is associated with measurable physiological changes such as constriction of peripheral blood vessels, increased cerebral blood flow, increased tension in skeletal muscles, and increased blood levels of cortisol and cholesterol. The degree of annoyance felt depends to some extent on perceived control over the source of the noise: the less the control, the greater the annoyance. In a special-care unit, clients are likely to feel that they have little or no control over noise. In addition to its physiological effects, noise has psychological effects. Many activities in special-care units create "moderately loud" noise—that is, sounds of 45 to 80 decibels (dB). These include administration of nasal oxygen (45 decibels), clattering bedpans (60 decibels), typical conversation in the nurses' station (65 to 70 decibels), and rattling side rails (80 decibels).[18] Noises like these cannot be controlled by clients and can lead to irritability, anxiety, and lack of sleep.

SLEEP DEPRIVATION. Lack of sleep, or sleep deprivation, is a serious problem for most clients in special-care units. Hilton[19] studied the sleeping patterns of clients in a respiratory intensive-care unit. Over a 24-hour period, the total amount of sleep for individual clients ranged from 6 minutes to 13.3 hours. Only about 50 to 60 percent of this occurred during the night, and not one client completed a normal sleep cycle. The most serious effect was that REM sleep (see Chapter 3) accounted for only 4.7 to 10 percent of sleep time—normally it is 30 to 35 percent of the sleep cycle. Regardless of time of day or night, the sleep of an average client was disturbed 20 minutes out of every hour.

DISORIENTATION. Many clients in special-care units report disorientation with regard to time, day, and place. Some units have clocks and calendars which help keep clients oriented, but many do not. If no windows are visible to clients, they often become confused about whether it is day or night. Events seem to be the same around the clock; clients therefore have difficulty in interpreting time of day.

DEPERSONALIZATION. Depersonalization (described earlier) is experienced by many hospitalized people, but it is especially common among clients in special-care units. Clients do not know what to expect in this unusual environment. Treatments and other procedures may be carried out with no warning and in no pattern that the client can discern. Clients in Ballard's study[17] complained of being unable to prepare themselves for painful events and of feeling that they were not in control of themselves. (These clients, however, were less concerned with lack of privacy and having to deal with unfamiliar physicians and nurses than clients who were not in special-care units.)

ICU SYNDROME. The unfortunate product of all the stressful elements in special-care units is inability to muster adequate coping mechanisms. Not surprisingly, some studies have found that as many as 70 percent of clients in such units experience high levels of psychological stress; what seems more surprising is that not all of them do.

ICU (intensive-care-unit) syndrome is an "altered emotional state occurring in a highly stressful environment, which may manifest itself in various forms such as delirium, psychosis, or neurosis."[20] It has four common manifestations, classified according to major symptoms.[20] (1) *Anxiety* or *fear* is the normal response to being in a special-care unit. Absence of fear or anxiety might indicate that a client has withdrawn and is becoming disturbed. (2) *Depression* is a more severe form of the syndrome. A depressed client has suffered a loss of self-esteem or some other significant loss because of the precipitating illness or confinement in the unit. (3) *Delirium* is impaired memory, disorientation, poor judgment, shallow affect, and disturbed intellectual functioning. (4) The most profound form of ICU syndrome is *psychosis*. The client is out of touch with reality, exhibits a high degree of anxiety (or even panic), is confused, and may have delusions and hallucinations which are usually paranoid in nature.

ICU syndrome usually appears 3 to 7 days after a client has been admitted to the special-care unit. The risk of a serious psychological reaction increases with length of stay in the unit.[20] It is also higher for people who have preexisting psychological problems (such as trait anxiety and schizophrenia) or are withdrawing from alcohol or other addicting substances. The syndrome usually disappears within 48 hours after a client leaves the special-care unit. Several studies cited by Ballard[17] have shown that the incidence of ICU syndrome can be decreased by providing clients with opportunities to discuss the experience. One significant factor was the development of supportive, positive relationships between clients and nurses.

Although most of these psychological manifestations can be attributed to the stress of being ill and hospitalized, similar conditions may have physiological causes. For example, delirium may be caused by toxicity or withdrawal from chemical substances. Dissociative reactions—accompanied by delirium, hallucinations, and bad dreams—often occur during recovery from dissociative anesthetics such as Ketamine. Clients with these reactions need a quiet environment, as little physical contact as possible, and reassurance that their experience is temporary.

NURSING PROCESS

Promotion of healthy interactions is the most significant nursing activity with regard to psychosocial aspects of illness and hospitalization. Acute illnesses and other life-threatening conditions demand immediate attention and take precedence over psychosocial and spiritual considerations, and the nature of physical illnesses and the circumstances of hospitalization often dictate priorities of nursing care. Nurses must therefore very deliberately provide for needs other than physical ones. This requires being alert for opportunities to promote psychological and spiritual well-being, and assessing clients regularly to identify potential and actual disturbances.

Assessment

Assessment of clients' reactions to illness and hospitalization is based on concepts explored in this chapter. Questions for assessment are found in Table 41-7.

Table 41-7 Questions to Assess the Impact of Hospitalization on Person, Family, and Environment

Person	Person
Personality: Do you tend to be aggressive, time-conscious, work-oriented? Or more calm and relaxed? Please describe your usual way of coping with very difficult circumstances.	**Integrity:** How "together" do you feel at this point? In what ways do you feel best about yourself? In what areas do you feel weak or vulnerable? Are you being treated with respect?
Culture and values: What is most important to you? Where would you prefer to live? How comfortable are you when you need something from somebody else? If you had a choice, what year would you like this to be? Why? In a work setting, with whom do you get along best? Do you think people are basically good or basically bad? How do you see the relationship of humanity to nature?	**Family**
	In what ways must the family change because you're in the hospital? How do you think family members feel about your illness and hospitalization? How understanding is your family of your needs? How worried are you about your family now that you're in the hospital? (See also Chapters 11 and 19.)
Loss: What is the hardest part of hospitalization for you? What do you miss the most?	
Rhythms: What adjustments have you made to go along with the hospital routine?	**Environment**
Coping style: How is this illness influencing the way you think about yourself? How is it influencing your relationship with family? Friends? How is it affecting your financial situation?	**Territoriality:** Do you have enough space? Privacy? How would you like the staff to address you? Are there particular habits that staff members have which bother you when they are in your room or helping you?
Autonomy: What is your impression of the degree of freedom you have to make choices about your treatment? Would you like more or less help from the staff at this point in your hospitalization? In what areas?	**Time:** Does time seem to pass slowly or quickly since you have been hospitalized? What are the most difficult times of the day for you? How could the staff help with your experience of time?

(Continued.)

Table 41-7 Continued

Environment

Uncertainty: Do some things seem confusing or uncertain to you? What are they? When you feel confused, what helps? When you feel confused or uncertain, how do you act?

Depersonalization: Do you sometimes feel like a stranger to yourself? Are you having unusual experiences? "Losing" yourself? How do you act when you feel this way? What helps when you're feeling this way?

Reactivation of memories: Does this experience remind you of other times in your life? What were those times? Who was involved? What happened? How much time are you spending remembering those times? How uncomfortable are you because of those memories?

Regression: Do you ordinarily do more for yourself than you are doing now? What's the best part about being sick? In the hospital?

Discontinuity and dissociation: (Observation.) What aspects of the current circumstance is the client not experiencing? What emotions would the client ordinarily be expressing? When the client talks, is the affect appropriate to the content?

Sick role: How comfortable are you with your illness? Hospitalization? How are you being treated (by family, friends, staff) because of your illness?

Clients' work: Are you comfortable with the amount of work you're expected to do for yourself? Do you think you should be doing more or less? How do you feel about being sick? About what's expected of you because you're sick?

Stressful factors: What do you find stressful about your illness? The hospitalization? What other stresses are occurring in your life right now? What stresses have you had to cope with in the past 6 months? What do you do to cope? What can the staff do to help you handle your stress?

Special-Care Units

Awareness: (Observation.) Did the client anticipate being in a special-care unit, or was the admission an emergency? Was the client oriented to what to expect in the unit?

Awareness (continued): How alert and aware is the client? How much of a threat does the client's condition pose to life? Does the client have an accurate awareness of the degree to which life is threatened? What information has been given to the client to promote understanding of what is happening in the unit?

Immobilization: How extensively is the client immobilized, and what is the client's response to immobilization?

Stimuli: What stimuli are within the client's awareness? Does the client understand them? Self-perceptions:

- Pain
- Touch
- Thirst
- Temperature
- Confusion
- Insertions of IVs, catheters, and other tubes
- Attachment to monitors or life support

Environmental perceptions:

- Sounds of monitors and life-support machinery
- Alarms and other signals
- Sounds and sights of other clients
- Presence and activity of personnel
- Noise
- Lighting

What is the client's response to stimuli?

Sleep: Is the client able to get an adequate amount of undisturbed deep sleep? What has been done to promote normal sleep cycles?

Orientation: Is the client oriented in terms of time, day, place, and person? What is being done to keep the client oriented?

ICU syndrome: Are there any manifestations of the ICU syndrome?

Interpersonal relations: How is the client able to summon staff members? Is the client aware of this method? What is the frequency and quality of visits with family members? What is the response of family members to the unit and the impact of these responses on the client? How much space does the client have around the bed? How able and willing is the client to talk about feelings, questions, and concerns?

Diagnosis

After making as extensive an assessment as possible, the nurse is prepared to formulate appropriate diagnoses for a client. The nursing diagnoses relate to the client's interaction with the hospital environment and focus on problems having to do with the illness and environmental stressors. Examples of nursing diagnoses are given in Table 41-8.

Client Outcomes

Client outcomes are statements of expected changes in the client's status as a result of properly implemented nursing interventions. These can be observed by the nurse or reported by the client. Examples of outcomes are also given in Table 41-8.

Table 41-8 Applications of the Nursing Process

Assessment	Nursing Diagnosis	Client Outcomes	Nursing Interventions
Client A. lives alone; becomes irritable if furniture in room is rearranged; cries when get-well cards are thrown away accidentally.	Threat to security and identity associated with loss of control over personal space.	Client will regain a sense of control over personal space.	Identify items in room under client's control. Avoid changing furniture without client's permission. Obtain permission before handling personal items. Assist the client in personalizing the room. Plan with client for uninterrupted times alone.
Client B. broke femur in automobile accident 2 days ago; bedfast in traction; suffering pain; complains, "It seems to take forever to get a shot."	Alteration in time perception associated with immobility and pain.	Client will regain more accurate perception of time.	Provide a clock or watch for client's use. Tell client how long the wait will be for pain medication. Return promptly with medication. Plan with client a regular schedule of isometric exercises.
Client C. objects to nurses' helping; denies severity of physical symptoms; becomes angry when encouraged to rely on staff to ambulate.	Inability to accept limitations imposed by illness associated with threat to autonomy and self-esteem.	Client will cooperate with nurses and accept the degree of dependence necessitated by illness.	Explain reasons for client's needing rest and assistance. Acknowledge client's rest and cooperation as work. Involve client in decisions about care whenever possible. Treat client with respect and positive regard. Help client to identify interesting activities which can be done without compromising medical or nursing goals.
Client D. is overly dependent; will not get up without help although needs to; asks nurse to make decisions client should make for self.	Secondary gain associated with accepting the sick role when no longer appropriate.	Client will give up sick role and function independently.	Help client to identify other, healthy ways of meeting needs for attention. Give client attention and time when functioning more independently. If family members are encouraging this behavior, help them to understand the importance of the client's becoming independent.
Client E. has lost a body part; spouse seldom visits; client is withdrawn and uninterested in participating in own care.	Alteration in body image related to loss of body part.	Client will grieve normally for the lost body part.	Encourage client to talk about loss and its meaning. Encourage ventilation of feelings.
	Alteration in marital relationship associated with spouse's inability to accept physical change in client.	Client will accept limitations imposed by loss of the body part and find ways to compensate for the loss.	Help client to identify ways to compensate for loss. Identify resource people who help clients with same loss. Help client identify things that client can do which are unaffected by loss.
	Dysfunctional grief related to loss of body part.	Spouse will accept client's body change, and marital relationship will be restored to precrisis level of functioning.	Talk with client and spouse together and individually about feelings and impact of loss on relationship.

(Continued.)

Table 41-8 Continued

Assessment	Nursing Diagnosis	Client Outcomes	Nursing Interventions
Client F. is in special-care unit; is irritable and flinches when nurse comes near or touches client; occasionally seems to be hallucinating; rarely sleeps more than 2 hours at a time.	ICU syndrome related to sensory overload and sleep disturbance.	Client will experience a healthy level of sensory stimulation. Client will have an adequate amount of undisturbed deep sleep.	Control unnecessary noise. Greet client by name and explain purpose of procedures and treatments. Explain noises and sounds. Warn client before touching or moving. Speak clearly, but no louder than required. Orient client to time, place, and person when necessary. Plan to talk to client at other times than during procedures. Provide comfort (such as back rubs) to promote rest. Provide a quiet period for undisturbed deep sleep. Identify any fears or other internal factors which may be disturbing client; discuss and help allay these.
Client G. is being transferred from a special-care unit; expresses fears about security.	Anxiety associated with move to unfamiliar and less technologically intense environment.	Client will experience less anxiety.	Encourage client to describe fears and anxiety. Provide information about new unit. Arrange visit by nurses on new unit. Involve family in planning for the transfer.
Client H. asks, "Why is God causing this suffering?" "Am I to blame for my own illness?" Feels alone and afraid.	Spiritual distress associated with self-blame. Fear and anxiety associated with feeling punished by God.	Client will find meaning in the experience of illness. Client will seek a restoration of former relationship with God. Client will recognize the reality of responsibility for illness.	Encourage client to talk about feelings. Plan with client for times to meditate and pray. Give client realistic information about illness. Encourage client to pray for understanding and help in dealing with illness. If client's feeling that the illness is a punishment is integral to religious belief system, encourage client to pray for forgiveness. Suggest a view of God as fair and loving.
Client I.'s family visits for long periods; client expresses mixed feelings and feels tired.	Ineffective family coping associated with client's illness.	Family will accept limits to visiting time.	Encourage family members to talk about their feelings about client's illness. Give family members complete information about the client. Explain client's need for rest. Involve family members in client's care when possible and appropriate.

Interventions

Nursing interventions are specific activities implemented by nurses to achieve desired client outcomes. Applicable interventions are included with nursing diagnoses and outcomes in Table 41-8. (Specific nursing interventions were also given in Tables 41-2, 41-3, and 41-4.)

Evaluation

The final step in the nursing process is *evaluation* of the earlier steps. Client outcomes should indicate the criteria for measurement of overall success of the care plan. In addition, the nurse should evaluate the success of specific interventions. Table 41-9 illustrates an appropriate evaluation for Ms. K., a client hospitalized for an acute illness:

Ms. K. was a 22-year-old secretary, single, and living alone. She was admitted from an emergency room to a general medical-surgical unit after suffering at home for 2 days with diarrhea, projectile vomiting, and abdominal pain. Her physician planned an emergency exploratory laparotomy. When she was brought to the ward on a carrier, she was rolling around, clutching her abdomen, crying, and moaning. When a practical

Table 41-9 Nursing Evaluation for a Hospitalized Client (Ms. K.)

Assessment	Nursing Diagnosis	Client Outcomes	Nursing Interventions	Evaluation
Ms. K. was experiencing extreme anxiety because of physical pain and uncertainty about what was happening to her. Her uncertainty had led her to perceive what was happening to her as a threat, and she responded by avoiding attempts to help her (which she interpreted as further threats to her integrity). Her personality style in response to the crisis of illness was emotional. She rejected the assumption of the sick role by denying that she could be helped, and by trying to be independent and aggressive.	Anxiety and uncertainty associated with an unfamiliar experience.	Client will: 1. Talk about feelings. 2. Express what she is uncertain about. 3. Cooperate in her care.	1. Explain what is happening and why procedures such as IV administration and insertion of a nasogastric tube are necessary. 2. Give information in clear, specific language. Reinforce explanations as needed. 3. Encourage client to ask questions and say what she is concerned about. 4. Be patient and assertive in persuading client to accept nursing procedures. 5. Be respectful and talk to her as an adult. 6. Stay with her or have another staff member remain with her while she is upset. 7. Acknowledge her efforts at cooperating as part of her work of getting better. 8. Ignore aggressive comments or clarify what is happening. (For instance, when she says that the nurse is *trying* to hurt her, acknowledge that she may feel that way, but point out that this is not true.)	**Outcomes** 1. Client expressed anger, fear, and dependency. 2. Client stated that she didn't understand her physical symptoms, her emotions, the purpose of the procedures, or why nurses like to make people suffer. 3. Client allowed nurse to start IV, insert NG tube, and give preoperative medication. **Processes** All nursing interventions were carried out. The same nurse worked with Ms. K. preoperatively.

nurse tried to take her temperature, Ms. K. became hysterical. When a registered nurse approached her to start an IV, she refused to cooperate and accused the nurse of hurting her intentionally. She responded similarly when the nurse said she needed to insert a nasogastric tube.

SUMMARY

Physical illness and hospitalization are stressful. Clients' responses to this stress are affected by individual styles of coping. Many of the problems which complicate hospitalizations are emotional or spiritual. To help clients, nurses must recognize symptoms of emotional or spiritual disturbances as well as physical symptoms.

The most significant nursing activities are those which promote healthy responses to illness and hospitalization and prevent unhealthy ones. Although prevention is not always possible where people are hospitalized for medical and surgical problems, nurses can learn to recognize unhealthy responses in their early stages. The principles discussed in this chapter can help nurses to intervene so that their clients will return to healthy patterns of functioning.

In the future, severely ill and injured people are likely to account for a greater proportion of hospitalized clients. Thus, critical physical problems will demand more attention, and nurses will see more emotional and spiritual disturbances. Nurses will need to be careful not to lose sight of the secondary effects of physical problems as those physical problems become more complex.

REFERENCES

1. F. C. Schontz, *The Psychological Aspects of Physical Illness and Disability*, Macmillan, New York, 1975.
2. M. Friedman and R. H. Rosenman, *Type A Behavior and Your Heart*, Fawcett, Greenwich, Conn., 1974.
3. J. Hartog and E. A. Hartog, "Cultural Aspects of Health and Illness Behavior in Hospitals," *Western Journal of Medicine*, vol. 139, December 1983, pp. 910–916.
4. M. B. Walsh, "Biologic Rhythms and Human Needs," in H. Yura and M. B. Walsh, eds., *Human Needs and the Nursing Process*, Appleton-Century-Crofts, New York, 1978, pp. 1–33.
5. A. J. Krakowski, "Hospital Encroachment on the Patient," *Public Health Reviews*, vol. 10, 1982, pp. 11–25.
6. M. Bowen, "Theory in the Practice of Psychotherapy," in P. Guerin, ed., *Family Therapy: Theory and Practice*, Gardner, New York, 1976, pp. 42–90.
7. J. Hayter, "Territoriality as a Universal Need," *Journal of Advanced Nursing*, vol. 6, 1981, pp. 79–85.
8. C. I. Allekian, "Intrusions of Territory and Personal Space," *Nursing Research*, vol. 22, May-June 1973, pp. 236–241.
9. A. J. Davis, "Don't Fence Me In," *American Journal of Nursing*, vol. 84, September 1984, pp. 1141–1142.
10. J. B. Meisenhelder, "Boundaries of Personal Space," *Image*, vol. 14, February-March 1982, pp. 16–19.
11. J. J. Fitzpatrick, "Patients' Perceptions of Time: Current Research," *International Nursing Review*, vol. 27, 1980, pp. 148–153 and 160.
12. E. S. Tompkins, "Effect of Restricted Mobility and Dominance on Perceived Duration," *Nursing Research*, vol. 29, November-December 1980, pp. 333–338.
13. M. H. Mishel, "The Measurement of Uncertainty in Illness," *Nursing Research*, vol. 30, September-October 1981, pp. 258–263.
14. Talcott Parsons, *The Social System*, Free Press, New York, 1951.
15. A. L. Strauss, Shizuko Fagerhaugh, Barbara Suczek, and Carolyn Wiener, "Patients' Work in the Technologized Hospital," *Nursing Outlook*, vol. 29, July 1981, pp. 404–412.
16. B. J. Volicer, M. A. Isenberg, and M. W. Burns, "Medical-Surgical Differences in Hospital Stress Factors," *Journal of Human Stress*, vol. 3, June 1977, pp. 3–13.
17. K. S. Ballard, "Identification of Environmental Stressors for Patients in a Surgical Intensive Care Unit," *Issues in Mental Health Nursing*, vol. 3, 1981, pp. 89–108.
18. C. F. Baker, "Sensory Overload and Noise in the ICU," *Critical Care Quarterly*, vol. 6, March 1984, pp. 66–80.
19. B. A. Hilton, "Quantity and Quality of Patients' Sleep and Sleep-Disturbing Factors in a Respiratory Intensive Care Unit," *Journal of Advanced Nursing*, vol. 1, 1976, pp. 453–468.
20. H. G. Kleck, "ICU Syndrome," *Critical Care Quarterly*, vol. 6, March 1984, pp. 21–28.

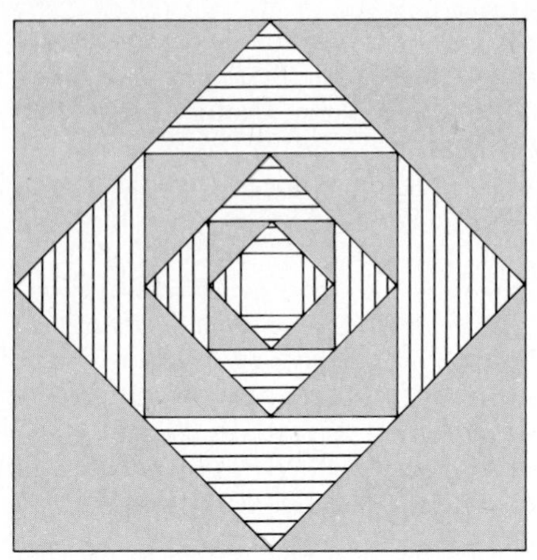

CHAPTER 42
Stress-Related Illness

Barbara Flynn Sideleau

LEARNING OBJECTIVES

After studying this chapter, the student should be able to:

1. Relate anxiety, conflict, and change to mismanagement of stress and the development of dysynchronous biopsychosocial patterns of interaction.
2. Discuss family patterns of interaction associated with stress-related illness.
3. Discuss environmental patterns of interaction associated with stress-related illness.
4. Discuss pain-, accident- and surgery-proneness in terms of past and present person-family patterns of interaction.
5. Discuss mismanagement of stress as it relates to dysynchronous patterns in body systems.
6. Discuss mismanagement of stress in relation to the eating disorders: anorexia nervosa, bulimia, pica, and obesity.
7. Apply the nursing process to clients with stress-related health problems.

The interaction between stress and physical illness has been studied from two major perspectives. According to the first perspective, illness develops because of personality characteristics which predispose people to certain emotional states, influence their appraisals of situations as either threatening or nonthreatening, and lead them to develop coping strategies characterized by behaviors or physiological responses that prolong stressful situations. According to the second perspective, the development of illness follows stressful life events that generate prolonged or exaggerated coping efforts; these efforts produce negative emotional states and alter effective functioning. The results of research using these perspectives, rather than supporting a relationship between a specific emotion and a particular disease or a particular stressful event and a disease, support a theory of multiple interacting factors in the development of illness. Person-environment patterns of interaction over time, stressful situations, the noxious quality of stressors, and even their neutralization interact and influence vulnerability to illness.

Recent research has been directed toward developing a greater understanding of the physiological processes involved in the development and continuance of health problems, the psychological processes which influence a person's interaction with the environment and generate or compound stress, and the interaction between self-regulatory or coping processes and bodily states that are precursors of disease.

Stress is inherent to life. Effective management of stress facilitates growth and development. Mismanagement of stress reflects disruption of the interaction of mind, body, and spirit. The holistic approach of nursing to the promotion and restoration of health and the prevention of illness addresses this interaction.

The purpose of this chapter is to examine dysynchronous patterns of interaction related to the mismanagment of stress and subsequent illness. Patterns of interaction in the person, family, and environment associated with stress-related illness are discussed. Selected health problems associated with the mismanagement of stress are examined. The application of the nursing process to clients with stress-related illnesses focuses on the promotion of effective coping and on ways to help people prevent, ameliorate, or resolve dysynchronous biopsychosocial patterns.

DYSYNCHRONOUS HEALTH PATTERNS

Stress is a primary factor in the development of health problems. Stress elicits physiological responses in the autonomic nervous system, endocrine system, hypothalamus, and cerebral cortex, which in turn influence other body systems and organs. There is no simple cause-and-effect relationship in the development of health problems; rather, it is the complex interrelationship of multiple factors which determines whether or not one will succumb to stress and become dysfunctional and how the body will manifest an inability to cope with stress.

Genetic, psychological, immunological, age-dependent, and environmental predisposing factors interact at a particular time in such a way that specific health problems develop. Because such a phenomenon is complex, research designed to explain it must overcome numerous methodological problems. However, each new research finding contributes to an understanding of the interactions between stress, pathophysiological changes, and health problems.

Stress and Anxiety

The model of the relationship between stress and anxiety in the development of biopsychosocial dysfunction encompasses the person-environment interaction. In this model, person-environment factors influence the processes of perception and interpretation. Perception and interpretation of threat are important aspects of stress-related dysynchronous patterns of interaction. Stressors (see Chapter 3) are linked to anxiety reactions by the perception of threat.

People's perceptions of events and the threats associated with the events differ. A person's appraisal of an event is a significant factor in relation to the judgment of whether the event is a threat, and the extent and intensity of the threat. A person's past experiences, present circumstances, aspirations, and appraisal of the degree of potential disruption influence if or how a threat is perceived.

The following are commonly perceived threats:

- Threat to life
- Threat to body integrity
- Threat to self-concept, identity, and future plans
- Threat to the fulfillment of customary social roles and activities
- Threat involving the need to adjust to a new physical or social environment

An event may be dangerous in fact, or it may be perceived and interpreted as dangerous because it symbolizes or implies a severe loss. How a person interprets an event is crucial. Once a person perceives a threat, physiological changes occur. The involuntary nervous system reacts specifically to the emotion generated.[1]

To understand the contribution of stress and anxiety to illness, one must differentiate between state and trait anxiety. The perception of a threat will increase state anxiety. Trait anxiety will increase the likelihood that an event will be perceived as threatening.[2]

Stress and Change

Change is inevitable in life. Some changes are minor or expected; they evolve and require minimal or gradual adaptation. Other changes are important, multiple in nature, and unexpected; they require radical adaptations in many spheres of life. Research has documented the relationship between change, stress, and loss and the development of psychological and physiological disorders.[3,4,5]

Stress and Conflict

Conflicts arise in all dimensions of a person's functioning. Stress-induced conflict is a biopsychosocial phenomenon. A person's internal milieu is maintained in equilibrium through the interaction of opposing physiological systems (for example, the sympathetic and parasympathetic systems).

Conflicts within the self that are stress-inducing include the following:

- Conflict among beliefs, values, and behaviors
- Conflict between perception of actual self and perception of ideal self
- Conflict between conscious and unconscious beliefs

Whatever the source, conflict generates stress that changes physiological processes, alters structures, and may thereby contribute to the development of health problems.[6]

PATTERNS OF INTERACTION: PERSON

Stress-related illness occurs when a person feels less able to cope. In such instances the person exhibits a withdrawal pattern, psychologically and physiologically, to conserve energy. Although specific personality types have not been positively correlated with the development of specific diseases, personality profiles and response patterns are evident in a variety of disease processes. Researchers have found a specific relationship between the way people feel and what they want to do about these feelings at the time they develop symptoms of disease. Their attitudes are seen not as being responsible for the development of the disease but as being part of the disease process.[7] For example, one does not have an *attitude* for hives; rather, the stress of conflict increases skin temperature, which increases the skin's susceptibility to this dermatological condition. The reasons for the increase in temperature and the skin's susceptibility are probably related to inherited predisposition, early conditioning, or both.

Past Experiences

In the maturation process, undifferentiated infantile patterns of hypersecretion, hypermotility, and hyperemia move from involuntary control in the oral stage, to combined involuntary-voluntary control in the anal stage, and finally to voluntary control in the genital stage. If people are confronted with stressors that tax them beyond their capacity to master events, regression may occur. The earlier undifferentiated physiological responses are decontrolled and their unregulated activity may become the basis for the development of psychosomatic health problems[7] or there may be lags in physiological development in some body systems.

Experiences in infancy influence the maturation of basic neuroendocrine processes, which in turn influence body organs and systems and the development of rhythms, such as the circadian rhythm in adrenal function. These experiences have lifelong effects on adrenocortical activity. Corticovisceral theorists postulate that psychophysiological disturbances may be caused in part by faulty signaling to internal organs that either inhibits or overstimulates organ functioning. The dysfunctions that result become an established pattern when stressful events occur repeatedly and are translated into altered psychophysiological states. These faulty regulatory mechanisms influence not only the development of health problems but their progression and severity as well.

These involuntary neuroendocrine reaction patterns which have been conditioned in the past may be elicited by social stimuli symbolic of previous experiences which influenced their development. Thus psychosocial stress mediated by these altered neuroendocrine reaction patterns can affect heart rate, blood pressure, the amounts of circulating free fatty acids (producing rapid changes), ovulation, renal water transport (causing changes that range from diuresis to suppression), insulin production and function, the growth rate of neoplasms, and the effectiveness of the autoimmune system.[8]

Past learning experiences also influence people to perceive a variety of situations as threatening and fearful. These fears distort perceptions of the here and now. Fear that is a product of the past interacts with and confuses the present. Memories of past fears and pain contribute to feelings of vulnerability in the present.

Fears from the past are evident in such statements as: "I can't," "It is impossible," and "I couldn't." Past fears block the person from recognizing freedom of choice. Symbolically, this blockage may be expressed by physical and physiological blockages. For example, the person who feels caught in a dilemma, blocked from acting, and fails to recognize the freedom to choose may express this blockage by exhibiting symptoms of obstructive vasoconstriction or bronchial constriction.[9]

An investment in holding on to old fears, angers, resentments, guilt, and pain heightens sensitivity to other people's behavior and leads to a tendency to interpret other people's behavior only as it relates to the self. Hurt feelings and perceived rejections programmed by old fears produce a continual state of upset and contribute to making the present miserable rather than pleasurable. Holding on to past fears, guilt, and resentments results in a perception that the future will be full of more of the same.[9] The chronic stress eventually impairs physiological processes, thus increasing susceptibility to illness.[10]

Present Experiences

Predisposing psychodynamic issues that have been associated with stress-related health problems are listed in Table 42-1. Also associated with stress-related health problems is the giving-up–given-up complex. This complex encompasses the relationship between the person's internal milieu and external milieu.[11] Characteristics of this complex are presented in Table 42-2 (page 854).

Coping

Coping is defined as action-oriented efforts directed at managing stressors in one's internal and external environment. It involves mastering, tolerating, reducing, or eliminating changes and conflicts that are stressful.[12] Coping involves an interaction between stress and functioning mediated by personal

Table 42-1 Predisposing Factors in Stress-Related Disorders

Psychodynamic Issues Associated with Psychosomatic Health Problems
Arrested and impaired social learning
A reliance on imitation and a loss of spontaneity
Childlike ways of thinking
Rigid and self-punishing moral standards and ideals
High and unrealistic expectations
Difficulties in assimilating and integrating life experiences
A reliance on securing love and affection and approval
An inability to master change or to learn new ways of dealing with frustration
Persistence of unconscious conflicts appropriate to earlier developmental stages (oral, anal, and aggressive conflicts)
Proneness to extreme emotional responses of fear, anxiety, and depression
Developmental lags
Stressful life events: births, deaths, marriages, divorces, retirement, economic success or failure, layoffs
Vacillation between active-seeking and passive-yielding behaviors
Unrealistic expectations related to need and wish fulfillment

SOURCE: H. Weiner, *Psychobiology and Human Disease,* American Elsevier, New York, 1977.

Table 42-2 Giving-Up–Given-Up Complex

Characteristics
Expressions of helplessness, hopelessness, and worthlessness
Disruption in the sense of continuity of the past, present, and future
Reactivation of memories of earlier situations that evoked similar feelings
Impaired interpersonal relationships
Resistance to seeking out and using new coping strategies
An inability to use environmental resources
An apparent surrender to the stress

SOURCE: G. Engel, "A Life Setting Conducive to Illness—The Giving-Up–Given-Up Complex," *Annals of Internal Medicine*, vol. 69, August 1968, pp. 293–300.

and environmental resources, cognitive appraisal, and coping processes.[13] *Coping resources* are a complex set of personality, attitudinal, and cognitive factors that provide the psychological context for coping.[13] A list of these coping strategies and explanations of how they function are presented in Table 42-3.

PATTERNS OF INTERACTION: FAMILY

When a family encounters a problem, the family members can perceive the situation as resolvable or unresolvable and they can act effectively or become disorganized. How they handle the problem is a function of the availability of resources and the family's capacity to use these resources. Resources within a family are those strengths and experiences a family uses to effectively manage situational and developmental crises. Family resources include integration and adaptability.

When families lack integration and adaptability, stress-inducing problems disorganize the family system. This disorganization leads to family dysfunction and individual dysfunction. The mismanagement of stress may become manifest in one member's physical or mental symptoms. The breakdown in the family's functioning compounds the problems of the symptom-bearing member because it often deprives that person of a needed supportive family system.

Personal resources of family members enhance the family's ability to cope. When these resources are sufficient, the family is better able to anticipate

Table 42-3 Coping Resources

Resource	Function
Logical analysis	Attempt to identify cause of a problem; careful scrutiny of each aspect of a problem using reality-based information, relevant past experiences, and rehearsal
Cognitive restructuring	Revising perception of a problem through the identification of positive as well as negative aspects; changing values and priorities in line with changing reality
Cognitive avoidance	Denying problem by trying to forget, refusing to believe, and engaging in wishful fantasies instead of thinking realistically about the problem
Information seeking	Asking or talking with someone, or using media to obtain information about problem and solutions that will guide action
Problem-solving action	Identifying options; making alternative plans; projecting possible outcomes; negotiating and compromising to find a solution to a problem
Developing alternative rewards	Changing from an activity that is problematic or not satisfying to one that is rewarding or satisfying; creating new avenues for satisfaction of needs or enjoyment
Affective regulation	Selection and use of strategies to moderate or control emotions generated by a problem
Emotional discharge	Verbal expressions or physical activity used to ventilate emotional tension
Requesting reassurance and emotional support	Seeking out professionals, family members, and friends and requesting help in solving problems, making decisions, or becoming less anxious or depressed
Social withdrawal	Avoidance of the problem and people that would initiate interactions about the problem
Intrapsychic processes	Use of defense mechanisms (denial, rationalization, repression, regression, reaction formation, undoing, displacement, projection, identification, substitution, conversion)

SOURCE: Constructed from R. H. Moos and A. G. Billings, "Conceptualizing and Measuring Coping Resources and Processes," in L. Goldberger and S. Breznitz, eds., *Handbook of Stress*, Collier-Macmillan, New York, 1982, pp. 212–230.

and prevent crises. These resources include economic well-being (adequate money to provide for goods and services needed by the family), education (knowledge and cognitive ability for problem solving), health (physical and emotional well-being), and integrated useful psychological patterns (self-esteem).[14] If personal resources are minimal, then vulnerability to stress and mismanagement of stress will contribute to members' health problems and to problems that interfere with restoration of health.

Families, when confronted with stress-inducing situations, even when family and personal resources are available, may need to strengthen these resources or acquire additional resources from outside the immediate family. The availability of social networks is important in these instances.[15]

PATTERNS OF INTERACTION: ENVIRONMENT

Crowding and population density have been considered potentially stressful factors contributing to the development of physical and emotional disturbance. Animal studies have revealed dramatic negative effects, particularly a breakdown in social behavior, when there was increased density of population in an enclosed area. However, crowding in human populations does not always seem to produce stress-related problems. What seems to make a difference is not the number of people living and working in a limited amount of space but other factors such as food supply, pollution, availability of needed resources, and the effects of having to interact with a large number of individuals. If people are protected from noxious environmental stressors, are able to meet their needs, and are not placed in situations where they are forced to interact with large numbers of others, then the density of the population does not seem to have an adverse effect on their coping capacity or health.

When a society is stable, has well-established and well-structured customs, traditions, and institutions, and has members who respond to a predictable sociocultural environment with integrated patterns of psychological adaptation, then blood pressure does not become elevated with age, and people are less vulnerable to stress-related health problems. People who live in a society experiencing accelerated change, uncertainty, and danger tend to develop health problems that reflect the stress generated through their interaction with the environment. Change and social chaos require psychological adaptations that may overwhelm people who are less flexible and less resilient. Weak links in a person's genetic makeup may predispose the person to particular health problems in such situations.

The physical environment in a technological society with a variety of heavy industries generates numerous noxious chemical, acoustical, and other stressors (see Chapter 3). Whether these physical stressors are disease-producing is a function of the degree of exposure and the coping capacities of those who are exposed.

The economic status of a society also influences vulnerability to stress-induced health problems. Economic contraction generates stress in the workplace, unemployment, and family stress. This increased stress increases vulnerability to illness.[16] On the basis of earlier research, it has been projected that the economic recession in 1981–1983 in the United States will have a negative impact on the health of the population.[17] An earlier study of the 1973–1974 recession revealed that death rates from cardiovascular disease peaked 3 years later. A recent study found that psychological distress was reported more often by those who had problems related to work and finances that developed as a result of economic contraction.[18]

Environments that lack resources and are under siege because of poverty, natural disasters, or war interact with families and individuals.[15] These interactions are stress-inducing and have potential for massive disruption of family functioning. Inevitably the more vulnerable families become disorganized, and their members are at risk of stress-related ailments. Those who have more personal and family resources mobilize, cope, and survive without major residual problems.

MISMANAGEMENT OF STRESS: DISORDERS OF PSYCHOGENIC ORIGIN

Acute and chronic stress have a deleterious impact on health and well-being. Stress has a disruptive influence on psychological and physiological processes. These disruptions result in a wide variety of health problems including sudden death.

Among the psychosomatic disorders there are four kinds that have physical symptoms with no organic basis: factitious disorders, hypochondriasis, panic disorders, and conversion disorders. People with these disorders are very likely to seek help from health care professionals—for them, seeking help is a way of coping with stress. (See Chapter 30.)

There are also general psychogenic disorders which do not present physical symptoms in quite the same sense but may be described as persistent or pervasive tendencies. Three of these—pain-proneness, accident-proneness, and surgery-proneness—will be discussed in this section.

Pain-Proneness

Pain is defined as a central perception (not just as a primary sensory modality) based on a complex system of psychological, neurochemical, and neurophysiological influences. These influences interact to activate or modulate the experience of pain. A part of the experience is the concept of suffering and the associated threat to the integrity of the self.[19] Pain is both a torment to the sufferer and a warning signal—a signal that something is amiss. Many theories have been postulated regarding the pain response mechanism. In addition to the physical stressors which elicit and sustain pain, there is also a psychological component.

To experience pain, a person must be conscious, attentive, and self-concerned. During the growth process, pain is perceived as a consequence of a variety of stimuli and is associated with feelings, ideas, actions, and people. Pain may become psychologically meaningful and influence adaptive behavior. Memories of painful experiences acquired in childhood may be reactivated, fantasized, or hallucinated later.[20] Symbolic stimuli are incorporated into the person's reward and punishment systems on the physiological level. Cognitive appraisal of a situation and the personal interpretation and meaning elicit a physiological and behavioral coping pattern.[21]

The term *psychogenic pain,* which is often used to describe pain not clearly related to a physical problem, is misleading. It tends to imply that the pain occurs as a result of mental or emotional problems. It also implies that since there is no evident physical problem which would cause the pain, the pain is not real and does not exist. However, studies consistently tend to support the idea that the reported pain is a real experience for the patient.[21]

Person-environment interaction is apparently influential in pain-proneness. People prone to pain tend to have a history of repeated chronic suffering from one or another painful complaint. For these people the pain has an adaptive function inasmuch as it serves as symbolic self-inflicted punishment for misdeeds.[22]

When children are punished, they experience both pain and anger toward the source of their distress. When anger and hostility are repressed, they often lead to depressive guilt feelings. The feelings of anxiety, anger, depression, and guilt and the fear of bodily harm or the loss of love become associated with situations that were punitive or characterized by loss.[22] Recent events elicit the emotional state associated with these past experiences, but the connection may go unrecognized. The more frequent or severe the punishment, the more intense and enduring may be the emotional states and the associated pain.[23]

When there are repeated punishing, guilt-provoking situations that are associated with relief of pain and reassurance or restoration of a nurturing relationship with the parents, then a pattern is established. This pattern leads to self-selected situations that "deserve" punishment. The punishment that follows is the pain. The reduction of guilt is expected and occurs. When this pattern is repeated across the life span, a pain-prone profile emerges.[24]

The punishment in childhood is associated with a way of controlling "bad" behavior and is exaggerated in retrospect. On the basis of childhood experiences, these people may as adults suffer pain as a symbol to evade guilt feelings generated by an impulse or action that is judged bad. This conditioning influences the development of "pain behavior" as a way of getting needed love and attention and relieving guilt.[22]

Pain occurs in many clinical syndromes through several mechanisms. It may be a secondary symptom of a psychophysiological disorder, or it may be a conversion symptom. *Conversion pain* originates in the mind but is experienced as if it were in the body. It is derived from reactivated memories of bodily functions that are used to represent unconscious conflicts in a symbolic manner. Conversion pain is a maladaptive process whereby an unacceptable idea, wish, or fantasy is expressed as a bodily pain.

Characteristically the pain-prone person denies conflicts; idealizes self and family relationships; and is a "work addict" before the chronic pain develops but becomes anergic, inactive, and fatigued afterwards. These people's emotions tend not to be differentiated and are not verbalized. They seem to lack self-awareness and to express emotions somatically, not verbally.[25]

Conversion pain may be considered an affect that is expressed somatically, and a way of seeking attention and communicating rejection, revenge, general dissatisfaction, helplessness, and anger. One who experiences chronic pain has an identity and a perception of self as an invalid and a suffering human being. The pain becomes a message to the environment.[26] The use of symptoms such as pain is an acceptable, legitimate excuse that frees the symptom bearer from the criticism and disapproval of others as well as self.[27] Chronic back pain and pelvic pain, with no identifiable organic pathology, are frequently encountered. In both instances the pain may represent displacement of conflicts. Unable to muster more effective coping, these people use conversion as an avoidance strategy. This defense achieves the primary gain of keeping the conflict out of awareness and the secondary gain of a supportive environment.[19] The secondary gains from the maintenance of the symptom are medical reasons for not working, for not being the breadwinner, for not having to be sexually active, or for postponing childbearing. These people remain unaware of the psychic pain related to conflicts, fears, and anxieties generated by unsatisfying interpersonal relationships and channel their emotions and invest them in their back or pelvic pain.[28,29]

Research findings indicate that family members of a client with chronic pain experience distress. Furthermore, families have been found to reinforce pain and worsen the prognosis. In these families the maintenance of the client's pain becomes psychologically important and provides a tertiary gain.[19,30,31,32] When the client and family agree on the severity of the pain experienced by the client, resistance to treatment may occur.[31] The client in pain and a family member taking care of the client may unconsciously collude in the maintenance of the chronic pain. This collusion is an unconscious agreement that provides for the satisfaction of needs for both parties. Roles are defined, and effort is expended in maintaining the status quo.[32]

Accident-Proneness

Accidents are the leading cause of death in the age range of 3 to 36 years, and even in later years accidents continue to be a significant cause of death.[33] The greatest number of these accidents occur in the home. Automobile, industrial, and sporting accidents account for the remaining bulk of accidents requiring hospital care and convalescence and sometimes resulting in physical, social, and economic loss.

Some people seem predisposed to accidents, suggesting an accident-prone personality type. The word *accident* implies an unplanned or unanticipated event occurring by chance or as a result of an unknown cause. Accidents elicit shock, surprise, and feelings of guilt and responsibility. However, when no direct cause is evident, chance explains their occurrence, and guilt and responsibility are resolved.[33]

Freud[34] described the relationship between severe psychoneurosis and self-inflicted injury. He suggested that many apparently accidental injuries are instances of self-inflicted injury. He proposed that mistakes have meaning, and when they occur repeatedly, they reveal a persistence that does not fit with the notion of chance. These mistakes are mental acts which have significance, intention, and tendency despite their apparent lack of motivation. He suggested that the impulse to self-punishment is present and unconscious. Circumstances arise which allow the person to act or fail to act so as to cause an accident that produces self-punishing injuries or losses.

Studies have found that among accident victims there seems to be a conflict. This conflict involves aggressive drives and a defensive sense of guilt, suggesting a link between aggression, guilt, suicide, and accidents. Reconstructions of events preceding accidents (particularly one-automobile accidents) appear to support Freud's theory that accidents satisfy the need for self-punishment and for dependency. In some instances people may also have an unconscious wish to escape or avoid a life situation. Humiliation and avoidance of new responsibilities are conveniently prevented by the accident.[34]

Several researchers have contributed to the development of a personality profile of accident-prone people—people with records of four or more accidents.[32] These people have a tendency to be impulsive rather than thoughtful. They have a low tolerance for frustration and impaired control over their hostility and aggressiveness. Generally they are more action-oriented than reflective.

Physical and environmental factors also appear to influence an accidental event. Whether these circumstances provide the accident-prone person with an opportunity for self-inflicted injury or whether the degree of exposure to dangerous situations increases the risk of accidental injuries has not been clearly delineated. However, the risk taking that leads to multiple accidents may reflect choices that have a self-destructive element.

Surgery-Proneness

Psychological factors influence surgical clients' preoperative and postoperative coping and may contribute to the tendency of some people to undergo numerous operations, sometimes for the same symptom, with unsatisfactory results.[35]

In some instances, symptoms treated with surgery have had no physical basis; nevertheless, the surgery effectively relieves the symptoms. However, among this group of clients, new physical symptoms develop; these new symptoms represent symptom substitution.[24] In these instances surgery-proneness may be explained as an unconsciously motivated masochistic need to suffer. These people may sacrifice a part of the body to avoid actual suicide. Among this group of surgical clients there is a pervasive unconscious guilt.[36] The surgery-prone tend to have a family history of repeated and multiple illnesses and surgical interventions which probably established a model for managing stress. These people also tend to have a personal history of pain-related operations dating back to early childhood. It would seem that past family and personal experiences have contributed to a dysynchronous pattern of conscious or unconscious use of illness to gain attention and as an excuse for giving up responsibility.[36]

People with psychogenic pain are at particular risk for unnecessary surgical procedures. It may be that the masochistic character structure associated with surgery-proneness is also an underlying characteristic of the pain-prone person.

The surgery-prone have repeated surgery which is either unnecesssary or needed to treat the scarring and complications of previous surgery. The unnecessary surgery continues to occur partly because of the persistent demands made by these people and partly because of the compliance of physicians who fail to recognize the underlying emotional problems.[24]

MISMANAGEMENT OF STRESS: DYSYNCHRONOUS BODY-SYSTEM PATTERNS

Mismanagement of stress can be influential in several body-system disorders. This section will discuss skin, respiratory, gastrointestinal, endocrine, and cardiovascular disorders; sudden death; and disorders of the immune system.

Skin Disorders

The skin interfaces with the environment and is a somatic sounding board for emotions. It is a major component in the body's homeostatic system. It plays a major role in heat and fluid regulation; its sense receptors for pain, touch, and temperature affect development and survival. States of fear, rage, and tension can induce increased sweat production, and excessive sweating under prolonged stress leads to secondary skin changes. This anxiety phenomenon is mediated by the autonomic nervous system. Tension, anxiety, and anger predispose the person to itching and scratching. Anxious and tense people may be more conscious than others of itchy sensations. Given this possibility and the skin changes which occur under stress, self-inflicted excoriations, urticaria, and aggravations of psoriasis can be better understood.[37]

Skin disorders may be classified as follows:

1. Exaggerations in skin color, such as blushing or pallor
2. Conditions caused when the person either consciously or unconsciously does something to the skin (self-inflicted scratching, picking, burning, carving)

3. Skin problems activated or aggravated by emotional states
4. Skin problems associated with disfigurement, pain, or itching that have profound psychological consequences

Problems with the skin involve both abnormal sensations and actual abnormal manifestations. One problematic sensation is generalized psychogenic pruritus (itching) for which there is no organic cause.

Patterns characteristic of the person may be important in skin disorders. Emotional conflicts have been found that account for psychogenic pruritus, for example. The emotions most frequently associated with this itching include repressed anger and repressed anxiety. An inordinate need for affection is a common characteristic among these people. Many of the skin ailments that develop in both childhood and adulthood are the consequence of deprivation of touching and caressing in early childhood.[37]

An anxious or angry person may self-inflict scratches, often violently. This rubbing or scratching of the skin is derived from reflexive movements. Scratching is an activity also found among animals, particularly when they are caught between conflicting drives. The same may hold true for people who scratch to express frustration. Rubbing the skin may also provide a substitute gratification of the need for affection; violent scratching, particularly when it produces excoriations, may represent aggression turned against the self.[37]

Research indicates that people who develop dermatological disorders exhibit a muted responsiveness to the environment. As a group they tend to accept things as they are and to minimize the negative rather than to maximize the positive. They are not motivated to seek resources outside themselves or to change the environment. They are self-sufficient to a fault and maintain distance in relationships. If they are distressed by the environment, they choose withdrawal rather than confrontation.[38] They organize their lives according to self-imposed rules.

Several physiological phenomena seem to be of greatest importance with respect to their emotional associations to skin sensations, cutaneous vascular changes, and sweating.[39] These are presented in Table 42-4.

Table 42-4 Skin Disorders and Associated Psychodynamics

Condition	Psychodynamics
Delusions of skin parasites	A way of protecting the self from unbearable anxiety or guilt.
Pruritus; self-inflicted irritations, inflammation and excoriation	Fixations or aggressions lead to conflicts and intolerable impulses. Involved body part is often symbolic of the conflict, e.g., pruritus of the genital area when there is a sexual conflict.
Acne	Anger results in hypersecretion of sebum that is followed by guilt and depression, which produces hyposecretion and plug formation; a recurrence of anger and hypersecretion leads to inflammatory processes.
Blushing; heightened vascular responsiveness	Sensitivity to heat, hot drinks, spiced foods, and emotions. Abnormally high self-esteem in a continuous state of threat from everyday situations. Strong, unreasonable feelings of inferiority, guilt, and shame. Compulsive wish to please others. Element of confession and self-punishment suggested by visible manifestation of blushing.

Respiratory Disorders

Psychological, cultural, social, and occupational factors interact to produce and aggravate many pulmonary diseases. The effects of psychosocial stress are easier to recognize in respiratory ailments than in other system disorders because of the rapidity with which symptoms are manifested. Changes in the rate, depth, and regularity of breathing may be brought about voluntarily or may correlate with many different emotional and behavioral states, with physical illness, and with changes in the ambient temperature and the stage of sleep.

Breathlessness and Hyperventilation Syndrome

Breathing is regulated by the autonomic nervous system and can also be voluntarily controlled.[40] Changes in the rate, depth, and rhythm of breathing may have a somatic or psychogenic basis.[41] *Breathlessness* (dyspnea) is the unpleasant feeling of difficulty in breathing or inability to breathe based on the perception of real, threatened, or fantasized impairment of ventilation.

Breathlessness accompanies fear, anxiety, anger, and depression. The psychological responses to chronic obstruction pulmonary disease may also generate fear which produces dyspnea and hyperventilation. Everyday stress and exceptional stressful situations have been associated with episodes of breathlessness. During the fight-flight response, when the sympathetic nervous system is activated, the breathing pattern is altered. This change from relaxed, deep, diaphragmatic breathing to chest breathing is designed to meet the expected increased oxygen demand of the fight-flight response. If there is no physical fight or flight behavior and the change in breathing pattern persists, then hyperventilation occurs. Thus, emotional arousal appears to be a major consideration in the hyperventilation syndrome and in precipitating asthmatic attacks in predisposed populations. It has been proposed that chronic chest breathing can perpetuate or recreate the sympathetic response to produce a state of constant or chronic anxiety.[40] Psychogenic factors appear to contribute significantly to the person's condition regardless of the presence or absence of underlying pathophysiology.[41]

Some people who exhibit the hyperventilation syndrome have repeated attacks of loss of consciousness not related to epilepsy, narcolepsy, or other forms of syncope. If these people breathe rapidly and deeply for 2 to 3 minutes, they experience the feelings and sensations of derealization, fear, and buzzing in the ears. Anxiety is a significant precipitating factor in the development of these attacks. The profile of people vulnerable to attacks of hyperventilation includes evidence of hysteria, hypochondria, anxiety, or depression and exaggerated or bizarre descriptions of beathing problems.

Hay Fever

Hay fever is an allergic disease of the mucous passages of the nose and upper air passages. Hay fever sufferers react differently to the offending substances depending on their psychological state. When these people experience stress to the point where they feel helpless, nasal secretions are increased, hypervascularity occurs, and the membrane edema and obstruction follow. If they are feeling secure and have a sense of well-being, exposure to the offending substance does not elicit symptoms.[42]

Asthma

Asthma is a recurrent, obstructive disease of the airways which tends to respond to a variety of stimuli by bronchoconstriction, edema, excessive secretion of mucus, and formation of mucous plugs.[43]

Physiological mechanisms related to the hypothalamic, limbic system; autonomic nervous system, immunological system, and peripheral tissue functioning interact with genetic and environmental factors to produce this condition. Genetic factors play a role in the predisposition to bronchial asthma. However, twin studies suggest that environmental factors (such as social, familial, psychological, infectious, allergic, occupational, or industrial factors) interact with the genetic factor (which is probably an inherited defect in pulmonary functioning and in the formation of specific antibodies). Immigration to a new environment appears to play a significant role in the onset of bronchial asthma. The exposure to new substances and the inherent losses and stressful changes imposed by the move may interact to produce the condition.[43]

Several researchers point to conditioned visceral learning, mediated by the autonomic nervous system, as significant in the development and aggravation of asthma. However, the importance of psychosocial stressors lies in their influence in triggering diffuse pulmonic obstruction, hypersecretion, mucosal edema, and the consequent acute respiratory status. This physiological response resembles the regressive undifferentiated reaction of infancy. It is notable that such attacks often occur when the environment has generated feelings of helplessness and exclusion which have potential for reactivating memories of similar events in the past, thus escalating the impact of the stress.[42] Potential or actual separations, fear of rejection, immature ways of coping with the environment, and a tendency to become depressed and helpless are significant in the development of a bronchial asthmatic episode.

Some asthmatics also respond to the power of suggestion, which raises the question whether or not these people respond to a self-fulfilling prophecy generated in interpersonal relationships with significant others. Studies have revealed a high level of nonspecific characterological anxiety with a disregard for symptoms among those who have more frequent hospitalizations and more intensive steroid therapy.[42,44,45]

During a period of emotional conflict, asthma-prone people use regression as a major defense; they move from activity and problem solving to fantasy which cannot be fulfilled. When fantasies and other defenses fail to protect the self, the asthmatic attack occurs. When defenses preclude the resolution of anger, fear, anxiety, or guilt, the person is vulnerable to an asthmatic attack. The prevention of the expression of feelings produces mounting tension. This tension is discharged either partially or completely through the attack.

Emphysema

The emphysemic resembles the asthmatic during a severe attack. Both types of episodes are precipitated by activating emotions such as anger, anxiety, or elation which require increased ventilation. A hyperventilation syndrome develops. Thus psychosocial stressors are significant in the development of the disability once the disease is present.

These people tend to avoid any emotionally charged life experiences; nevertheless they experience disabling depression and anxiety, and fear of dyspnea.[44,46] They employ repression, denial, regression, and isolation to ensure their comfort and survival. Despite their efforts, they are preoccupied with their bodies. Episodes of dyspnea have been associated with increased depression and expressions of helplessness and hopelessness.[42,44,45] Moreover, others in their environment also tend to avoid conflict to prevent precipitating an attack. As a result of this avoidance of authentic conflict and emotional release, their frustration may be further increased.[47]

Gastrointestinal Disorders

Organic bowel disorders such as regional enteritis, irritable bowel syndrome (colitis, spastic colon, diarrhea), and malabsorption syndromes are stress-related problems characterized by riddance and retention. *Regional enteritis* (Crohn's disease) is an inflammatory disease of the small bowel and sometimes the colon. It is distinguished by pathological lesions called *granulomata* in the bowel as well as in other parts of the body such as the mouth and skeletal muscles. The psychological issues associated with this condition are similar to those found among clients with ulcerative colitis. The conflict between physiological functioning and the socializing demands for bowel control and cleanliness influences the role of the bowel in psychogenic disorders.[48]

Research suggests that gastric erosion and ulceration depend on factors which decrease the competence of the gastric mucosa. The normal hypersecretion and hypermotility patterns of infancy—which may be in part genetically determined and in part learned in the mother-child relationship—are significant factors in the development of gastrointestinal disturbances. Psychic tension ebbs and flows in the *hunger-crying-feeding-satiation-sleep* sequence of infancy. Reduction of tension is regulated by the relationship with the nurturer and oral satisfaction. Incongruence in the mother-child relationship may interrupt the sequence, so that satiation and sleep are delayed or blocked. If this occurs, it may intensify and ingrain in the child strong oral-dependent wishes. Current psychosocial stressors may trigger these physiological changes and produce disease.[48]

People with gastrointestinal illnesses, particularly ulcers, exhibit oral character traits and conflict around dependence and independence. Some present as dependent, passive people, while others deny their needs and appear highly independent, self-reliant, aggressive, and continually overactive.

People vulnerable to gastrointestinal disorders manifest high responsivity to and much interaction with the environment. As a group they are impulsive, easily excited, and spontaneous. They are pursuers by nature, and at risk of loneliness if relationships are unavailable. Nevertheless, close relationships are difficult for them to manage.[48] As a group, these people are controlling and unconsciously have their needs met by this behavior. Some may mask this control by being outwardly compliant, ingratiating, compulsive, overconscientious, and demanding in a passive-aggressive way, obtaining satisfaction of needs from the secondary gains of manifest illness. The sequence of events which culminates in illness has been described as follows:

1. Intensification of psychological and social devices usually used in satisfaction of needs

2. Failure of these devices, with increasing anger, which is suppressed or denied if it threatens satisfaction of needs
3. Internalization of aggressive impulses
4. Perceived inability to cope, accompanied by feelings of helplessness and hopelessness

Irritable Bowel Syndrome

Irritable bowel syndrome (IBS) is a common motility disorder that is modified by psychosocial factors.[48] The abnormal motility patterns affect both the large bowel and the small bowel. These people may have "nervous diarrhea," abdominal cramps, or alternating constipation and diarrhea. The constipation may present as reduction in frequency of stools, passage of hard pellets, or pencil stools. The diarrhea may be accompanied by the passage of large amounts of mucus. Motility patterns include hypermotility, hypomotility, and postprandial motility patterns. *Hypermotility* of the sigmoid colon is associated with cramping, smooth muscle contraction in the bowel walls, increased intestinal wall tone, and reduced propulsion of contents. *Hypomotility* of the sigmoid colon produces a painless diarrhea that is probably due to a pressure gradient from the proximal colon to the distal colon causing a drop in intraluminal pressure and rapid transport of colonic contents. *Postprandial motility* pattern is characterized by an increased contraction rate of the bowel.[48,49]

Peptic Ulcers

Peptic ulcers are circumscribed erosion of the mucosa in the lower end of the esophagus, in the stomach, in the duodenum, or on the jejunal wall. Certain families have an increased incidence for peptic ulcers. However, there have been reliability problems in establishing a diagnosis for this condition. If genetic factors do play a part, it is probably related to the stomach's greater secretory capacity, which is a precursor of peptic ulcers. Some researchers have attempted to identify genetic markers that either characterize persons who are predisposed to the disease or correlate significantly with the disease itself. An ectomorphic body build (thin, frail) is frequently correlated with peptic ulcer. Blood type O, which may be related to high serum pepsinogen levels which are associated with the formation of ulcers, has also been correlated. Genes may not play a direct role in causation; rather, they may help to determine the severity of the ulcer indirectly, through the control of blood group O.

Conflicting research findings regarding personality traits among people with peptic ulcers are explainable as variations in the ways people express dependency and oral passivity. It appears that these infantile needs are exaggerated in the person prone to peptic ulcers. Problems do not arise unless and until the significant person or persons that are depended upon become unavailable as a source of gratification. Situations which trigger or exacerbate the ulcer include losses, the birth of a grandchild, gynecological surgery, and the pregnancy of a younger female relative.[50] A common finding among these people is the history of rejection by or loss of a parent and a strong need to be taken care of with defense against recognition of this need. Also common to both men and women is the apparent role of vacillation between active-seeking and passive-yielding behavior in triggering the onset or recurrence of the ulcer. Conflict related to the suppression of resentment, anger, guilt, fear, and fear of helplessness also plays a significant role in exacerbation of ulcers. Preulcer conflicts may be long-standing but appear to become acute approximately 3 months before the appearance of symptoms.[50]

Surgical treatment of peptic ulcers that have not responded to medical intervention often results in symptom substitution, which supports the hypothesis that psychological factors influence the development of ulcers. Following a gastrectomy, many of these people complain of a variety of psychosomatic symptoms.[49,50]

Endocrine Disorders

The endocrine system plays an important role in a person's management of stress. The hypothalamus directs much of the pituitary activity, which, in turn, influences the other endocrine glands either directly or indirectly. The neurohumoral link between the hypothalamus and the pituitary appears to be important to the function of neuroendocrine mediating mechanisms. This system, acting either directly or through a variety of complex interactions with the nervous system, may have a pervasive influence upon the enzyme system, metabolic processes, and membrane permeability at the molecular and intracellular levels. These, in turn, influence processes such as cell division, growth, maturation, energy metabolism, fluid and electrolyte metabolism, the inflammatory process, the immune system (specifically antibody production), and ovulation or spermatogenesis.

The endocrine glands are interdependent to varying degrees. Their relationships provide an important feedback mechanism. The endocrine mechanisms appear to be a signaling system between cells, and the system itself constitutes a physiological mechanism of adaptation.

Gonadal Dysfunction

Menstrual dysfunction, particularly amenorrhea, has been associated with psychogenic causes such as depression and postpsychic trauma after rape or abortion.[51] Fertility and infertility have psychogenic bases resulting from psychologically based impotence or frigidity, premature ejaculation, and aberrant sexual behavior. Hypothalamic dysfunction, psychogenically or physically based, leads to infertility. In women, it can cause anovulation, an inhospitable viscous cervical mucus, or an improperly prepared uterus. In men, hypothalamic dysfunction may cause oligospermia or inadequate motility of sperm.[52]

Psychogenic influence on testicular function is not well understood; however, stress appears to decrease the urinary excretion of testosterone.

Hormonal changes associated with menopause produce discomforts. However, women who have negative psychological sequelae have had previous emotional difficulties such as low life satisfaction and low self-esteem. Premenstrual tension syndrome appears to be related to the interaction of psychological, social, and biological factors.[52]

Thyroid Dysfunction

THYROTOXICOSIS. The personality pattern of people with *thyrotoxicosis,* hyperactive thyroid function, described by several researchers is characterized by premature assumption of responsibility with suppression of dependency needs. These people express an exaggerated fear of death and injury. They appear to be particularly vulnerable to the loss of significant people and situations that are severely frightening. The meaning of these findings in relation to predisposition or cause of thyrotoxicosis is not clear. The premorbid personality traits, genetically vulnerable autoimmune system and thyroid tissue, and acute emotional stress may interact to produce the biochemical and physiological changes and excess thyroid hormone.[52–55]

HASHIMOTO'S DISEASE. Research has not yet validated the role of stress; however, when the thyroid-stimulating hormone (THS) and vasoconstrictor substances associated with increased tension are secreted, both act together to traumatize the thyroid and expose cell walls to the body's immune system. The immune system, in turn, may respond by causing long-acting stimulation of the thyroid and eventual exhaustion as seen in *Hashimoto's disease.*[54]

Adrenal Dysfunction

Addison's disease is characterized by diminished function of the adrenal glands leading to decreased levels of circulating corticosteroids. Research suggests that Addison's disease may be an autoimmune disease. *Cushing's syndrome,* which is characterized by a chronic excess of circulating cortisol, has been associated with stress; however, the findings are not conclusive.[56]

Diabetes Mellitus

Diabetes mellitus is a hereditary disease; however, why it becomes manifest at a particular time is not understood. There is some evidence that major life events, particularly family losses, increase the demands for insulin and accelerate the burnout of beta cells, of the islets of Langerhans, or of other mechanisms, precipitating the diabetes.[57] Psychological stress may influence the course of the disease. Acute and chronic complications of diabetes mellitus may be precipitated or aggravated by the person's emotional status. These complications in and of themselves generate feelings which may create further stress. This additional stress may interfere with physiological processes and insulin utilization, increasing the risk of shock and coma.

Cardiovascular Disorders

Cardiovascular disorders are a leading cause of death in the United States. They develop through the interaction among biological, environmental, sociocultural, genetic, and psychological factors. The neuroendocrine mechanisms play an important role in their development. Emotions not only increase blood pressure, heart rate, and oxygen consumption but also cause sudden and marked increases in serum cholesterol and decreases in clotting time and hemoconcentration. These responses predispose a person to migraine headaches, hypertension, stroke, and coronary heart disease.

Headaches

Headaches are common complaints that can produce mild, transitory discomfort or can become disabling. They are sometimes vague and at other times rhythmically or arrhythmically throbbing, and they may or may not be accompanied by other somatic complaints.[58] Somewhere between 10 and 25 million people experience the debilitating pain of migraine headaches.[59]

The National Institute of Neurological Diseases and Blindness identified four major types of head pain in which psychological factors are implicated: muscle-contraction; migraine; combined migraine and muscle-contraction; and conversion, or hypochondriacal. The most common types of migraine or vascular headaches include classic, common, and cluster headaches.

Blood flow, nerve receptors, and enkephalins (pain-relieving chemicals in the brain) play a role in migraines and may also be involved in a different fashion in cluster and tension headaches. Stressful stimuli which affect these mechanisms can be triggers for these headaches.[59]

Person-environment interaction affects headaches. The combined migraine and muscle-contraction headache presents a clinical picture that includes characteristic features of both types. Since the headache is a subjective symptom, delusional, conversion, and hypochondriacal states are difficult to identify. However, the delusional and hypochondriacal people usually exhibit excessive preoccupation with their headaches as well as the malfunctioning of other body organs. These people also frequently report inability to concentrate and poor sleep patterns, and they express irritability. They characteristically and primarily focus on these symptoms and describe them compulsively and repeatedly. An in-depth interview usually reveals a serious internal body-image disturbance and frequently reveals delusional beliefs as well.[58]

Migraine and tension headaches tend to occur in a life setting that engenders frustration, resentment, anxiety, emotional tension, and fatigue. Anxiety has been found to be the predominant predisposing factor. No one specific personality type is associated with chronic recurring headaches; however, personality disorders such as passive aggressiveness, obsessive compulsiveness, perfectionism, orderliness, moralistic rigidity, hypochondriasis, and hysteria and their underlying conflicts seem to predispose people to such headaches.[60]

Repressed and suppressed hostile impulses seem to be the chief source of the neurotic conflicts that precipitate an attack. In some instances the headache may be caused partly by this rage and partly by hysteria. Positive or negative identification with a parental figure and introjection of that figure also play a role when symptoms arise from the person's wish to gain affection or attention. The headache may reflect a need to be dependent.

Headache pain, particularly among married people, is a transaction that provides the symptom bearer with a self-perception and identity of a suffering human being and affects the spousal relationship in the following ways: it regulates sexual activity; provides a substitute for intimacy; elicits caretaking; serves as a power strategy to control the spouse; legitimately extricates the person from situations he or she needs to avoid; and serves as a strategy for avoiding open hostility and divorce.[61,62]

Hypertension

Hypertension is sustained elevation by multiple causes of systolic or diastolic blood pressure or both above an arbitrarily established level. It is a symptom of internal disequilibrium. Hypertensive disease is a major health problem in our society. It is a significant contributing factor in the development of coronary heart disease and cerebrovascular accidents. Genetics (genes for the precursors of atrial natriuretic factors) and hormones are believed to play a part in hypertension.[63] Elevation of the blood pressure is a component of the fight-flight response. Research findings indicate that a familial tendency toward heightened cardiovascular reaction to psychological stressors exists. The physiological mechanism that appears to be influenced by psychological stress is sodium retention in persons who have a family history of hypertension and who have a high sympathetic nervous system response to stressors.[64,65,66] A wide range of environmental stimuli generate the fear, anger, and frustration that elevate the arterial blood pressure. The stress of combat, technological change, and natural disasters as well as high noise levels have resulted in prolonged elevations of blood pressure.

The physiological mediating mechanisms for hypertensive responses to events perceived as stressful include activity in the cerebral cortex, limbic system, reticular formation, and hypothalamus. Involvement of these structures leads to activation of the sympathoadrenal system and in some instances increases plasma renin activity.

Person-environment interaction can influence hypertension. Hypertensives may learn—through conditioning and as an adaptive response—to screen out of awareness potentially noxious stimuli, but they continue to respond to these stimuli physiologically with their conditioned or inherited hyperreactive pressor systems.[65,66]

These people often suffer from chronic rage or guilt over their aggressive tendencies. However, they may present the "nice person" image, repressing or suppressing angry and aggressive feelings. They often appear outwardly calm, easygoing, restrained, and not overtly assertive; they suffer the consequences of this tension physiologically, through sustained diastolic elevation.[67]

When chronically elevated blood pressure results in a stroke, the person has usually experienced a period of sustained and relatively severe emotional disturbance which was intensified before the onset of illness. As a group, these people assume an unusual degree of personal responsibility for their situations. They tend to perceive others as dangerous and untrustworthy. Consequently, they maintain distant relationships with others while at the same time behaving provocatively and generating in others the very anger they fearfully expect. Before the stroke, they felt pressured to meet goals which they had set for themselves; but they often felt that they were not in control of either their lives or the environment and were failing to meet their own expectations. They appear to lack the psychological capacity to integrate, manage, and resolve conflicts related to aggression.[68]

Coronary Heart Disease

Coronary heart disease is myocardial damage due to insufficient blood supply that is caused by pathological changes in the coronary arteries. Coronary heart disease is the leading cause of death in the United States in spite of an overall trend that reflects a decline among young and middle-aged adults. Major postulated risk factors for the premature development of coronary heart disease include not only diet, smoking, and physical inactivity, but the influences of a specific behavior pattern, job or marital dissatisfaction, work overload, exposure to loud noise over an extended period of time, disturbing emotions of anxiety and depression, and a family history of premature death from cardiac problems.[69,70]

There is ample evidence that coronary heart disease is genetically based, and this predisposition interacts with daily living habits, environmental stressors, and personality factors. Life stress has been identified in studies of twins as the primary environmental factor contributing to coronary heart disease. The hectic life appears to trigger heart attacks.[69]

THE PERSON: MYOCARDIAL INFARCTION, ANGINA, AND CORONARY BYPASS SURGERY. The heart has symbolic meaning and may be used to communicate psychological conflicts and distress. Psychological stress is known to produce certain physiological conditions that increase the impact of known risk factors for heart attack.[69,70]

There is some correlation between personality type and manifestation of heart disease. People susceptible to heart attacks have been described as type A personalities.[71] Characteristic behaviors of type A personalities which appear to be associated with a predisposition to coronary heart disease reflect inner tension. The personality profile of these people is presented in Table 42-5. As a group, these people are outwardly controlled and apt to be successful in repressing and denying anxiety, anger, and depression.

Other psychological variables which also seem to play an important role are upward mobility, significant loss, multiple life changes, overwork, and job dissatisfaction. An unfamiliar social or work environment, increased responsibilities, and discrepancies between the expectations of the culture

Table 42-5 Type A Personality

Profile
Aggressive, ambitious, unable to delegate authority
Possesses intense physical and emotional drives
Concentrates on career and has no hobbies
Experiences a chronic sense of time urgency
Preoccupied with deadlines
Exhibits excessive competitive drive
Exhibits easily aroused hostility under very diverse conditions
Meets challenges by expending extra effort
Takes little satisfaction from accomplishments
Obsessed with numbers
Obsessed with money
Presents as self-assured and self-confident
Measures self by number of achievements
Insecure about status
Restless during leisure time and guilty about relaxing
Thinks of or is doing two things at once
Schedules more and more activities into less and less time
Hurries the speech of others
Becomes unduly irritated when forced to wait in line or when behind a slowly moving car
Believes that if you want something done right, you have to do it yourself
Gesticulates when talking
Frequent knee jiggling or rapid finger tapping
Makes a fetish of always being on time
Plays every game to win
Rapid eye-blinking or ticlike eyebrow lifting
Explosive speech

of origin and the current cultural situation place demands on the individual's capacity for psychosocial coping. Bereavement is a significant factor, particularly with regard to losses in relationships, roles, and status. Surviving spouses during the first year after the death of a husband or wife are particularly vulnerable.[72]

Recent research designed to identify and describe a stress-resistant personality style has distinguished this style and conceptualized it as *hardiness.*[73,74] The characteristics associated with hardiness include commitment, positive response to challenge, internal locus of control, perception of life events as positive and under one's control, and a tendency to perceive situations and events in ways that are less stressful.[73,74] Hardiness appears to alter perception and thus mitigates the influence of stress on health. Type A personality style and hardiness operate independently.[74] Type A personality and a low level of hardiness appear to interact and contribute to the greatest risk of psychological distress and physical illness following events perceived as undesirable or less than totally controllable.[74,75] People with these characteristics have a tendency to perceive in these negative ways and to respond with type A coping behaviors. It is the combination of type A personality and a low level of hardiness that increases vulnerability to stress-induced illness. A high level of hardiness helps protect a person from stress-induced psychological problems and physical illness,[74,76] even if the person has a type A personality.

Myocardial infarction and angina. Survivors of myocardial infarctions and those who succumbed to sudden coronary death were found to have had statistically significant elevations in reported life changes over a period of 6 months immediately preceding the episodes.[69] Adverse life events producing anxiety, anger, or depression have been associated with sudden life-threatening cardiac problems. Likewise, an increase in business, social, or domestic problems preceding myocardial infarction has also been noted.

The stressful circumstances preceding a heart attack are often characterized by failures to achieve, actual or threatened losses, or a combination of these. The following stressful situations are often related to a breakdown in health: actual or threatened loss of a job, transfer to a new place of work, conflict between work and family demands, bereavement, adultery, divorce, and confrontation with rebellious offspring.

Symptoms before a heart attack that reflect the stress associated with life change, loss, and various problems include fatigue, reduction in customary activities, excessive sleeping, irritability, and a marked decrease in sex drive. People who have myocardial infarctions have been found to be more compulsive, to repress emotions, and to have a poor fantasy life.[69]

A large percentage of people who complain of chest pain and seek medical help for this symptom have no coronary artery obstruction; instead, they suffer from angina pectoris. People with angina pectoris differ psychologically from those who develop myocardial infarctions. These people manifest stress-induced somatic symptoms of anxiety and hyperventilation.[77] Overt anxiety, emotional lability, somatic concerns in response to stress, and a lower pain threshold are characteristic of people who exhibit angina.

Unstable angina patients fare better if they use denial of their illness and its life-threatening nature.[78] Precipitants of anginal attacks are similar in nature to precipitants of myocardial infarctions: heightened autonomic arousal characterized by anger, fear, anxiety, elation, and excitement.[69] If the person is unable to master the stress of these situations, the fight-flight response, which was designed for short-term emergency situations, is prolonged and becomes detrimental. The homeostatic mechanisms remain chronically mobilized, and this leads eventually to exhaustion. Often the illness strikes not at the peak of the stressful experience but rather shortly after the pressures of the situation have diminished, when exhaustion begins to occur. It is during this *letdown* period that the viscosity of the blood increases, clotting time decreases, and there is a sudden drop in cardiac output and oxygen consumption, creating a period of maximal vulnerability consequent to the lowering of coronary blood flow.[79,80]

Physiological and biochemical correlates of type A behavior have been linked to acute cardiac episodes and the genesis of the atherosclerotic process. These changes, which are influenced by emotions and probably by a low level of hardiness, include:[69]

Extensive narrowing of coronary arteries

Accelerated deposition of thromboembolic components of the blood on the plaque

Intensification of the initial growth of coronary artery atheroma

Accelerated rupture of the plaque

Predisposition to potentially lethal arrhythmias

Following a myocardial infarction, anxiety and fear are inevitable. How a person defends against this anxiety and copes influences survival, convalescence, and rehabilitation. Acute, conscious fear and anxiety in the immediate postinfarction time period increase the blood pressure and heart rate, heighten the risk of lethal arrhythmias, activate the sympathetic nervous system (causing the release of epinephrine), and cause electrical instability of the heart.[81,82,83]

Coping styles used by clients to defend against anxiety may or may not be helpful.[82] Some of these coping styles, behavioral examples of coping, and the advantages and disadvantages of these styles are presented in Table 42-6 (page 868).

Research findings indicate that even discrete social interactions can cause enough anxiety to affect the heart activity of clients in a cardiac-care unit (CCU). Changes in heart rate, rhythm, and frequency of ectopic beats can occur. A significant increase in the number of deaths following medical ward rounds in the CCU has been documented.[84,85] These findings suggest that even interactions with nurses and doctors can influence cardiac functioning. If nursing interventions are dysynchronous with the client's coping style, then there is a risk that acute anxiety may be generated and cardiac functioning consequently compromised.

Clients in CCUs may be reassured by the speed, efficiency, and expertise of the staff in responding to emergencies. Nevertheless, they harbor a strong fear of dying. Exposure to others in the unit with the same diagnosis who are suffering cardiac arrest or who have died is anxiety-producing. To defend against these realities and identification with the victims, clients tend to perceive themselves or their condition as different from that of the others.[82,83]

When clients suffer cardiac arrest, they often exhibit symptoms of organic mental disorders, which may be either transient or permanent. Most of these people do not confront or explore the implications of their arrest, but they do report violent dreams with sudden-death scenarios. They also suffer from insomnia and exhibit cognitive impairment. They feel that their experience has made them unique, and they may have unspoken fears and fantasies about their "death" experience.

Cardiac rehabilitation following discharge from the hospital may be obstructed by denial, fantasized fears, or family interference. For these reasons, invalidism after a myocardial infarction is often prolonged. Secondary gains may interfere with the recovery process and foster noncompliance with the rehabilitation program. However, fear is probably the most influential factor in resisting participation in the program. Fear that physical exertion could be fatal is a powerful deterrent.[86]

Coronary bypass surgery. Coronary bypass surgery has become an increasingly popular treatment for coronary artery obstruction. Those who undergo this surgery are at risk of postoperative arrhythmias. No association has been found between these arrhythmias and health-risk factors such as obesity,

Table 42-6 Defensive Coping Styles of Cardiac Clients

Coping Style	Behavior	Advantage	Disadvantage
Avoidance	Uses denial and repression Negates stress of the experience Negates implications of illness Avoids acquisition of information Forgets information provided Rationalizes symptoms as "indigestion" or "bursitis" Euphoria	Immediate survival value Lessens risk of increased blood pressure and pulse Lessens risk of arrhythmias	Hyperindependent behavior can lead to failure to comply with treatment regimen and to conserve energy. Tendency toward global, intense, diffuse overreaction if confronted with reality. Risk of noncompliance during convalescence.
Regression	Adopts sick role Becomes compliant Surrenders control	Conserves energy during acute phase of illness Protects against conscious anxiety and consequent risk to lethal arrhythmias and extension of infarction First stage of acceptance of health problem	If there is resistance to regression required of sick role, it can cause (1) hostility toward care givers and significant others, resulting in isolation or (2) anxiety, resulting in increased cardiac dysfunction. Excessive dependence impairs appropriate assumption of self-care activities.
Obsessive-compulsive	Attempts to structure the environment Attempts to structure events Seeks information Raises questions Develops tendency to intellectualize	Emotions kept in check if able to structure events and environment and to acquire information	Imposition of hospital routine or failure to provide required information is disorganizing and increases anxiety.
Depression	Withdraws socially Shows sad facial expression Cries Expresses hopelessness Talks about losses incurred by illness		Associated with mortality.
Transient psychosis	Becomes delirious Experiences perceptual distortion Experiences visual or auditory hallucinations Becomes disoriented Experiences paranoid delusions and suspiciousness Becomes fearful	Warning signs of physiological derangement in some instances	Increased risk to lethal arrhythmias and extension of infarction if physiological functioning is accelerated.

heavy use of tobacco, or even the number of bypasses performed. High preoperative anxiety is associated with a low frequency of atrial arrhythmias. People with type A behavior have increased risk of ventricular arrhythmias. Those who have high levels of depression and anxiety have fewer atrial arrhythmias; however, when these people use denial, they tend to have an increased risk of atrial arrhythmias. These findings indicate that after surgery, denied emotions are more problematic than those that are overt and recognized.[87]

THE FAMILY. At the time of an infarction, family members experience feelings of loss, depression, and guilt. As the client's physiological status stabilizes, the fear of death lessens but insomnia and appetite disturbances continue. Many family members, particularly spouses, complain of stress-response symptoms such as headaches, chest pains, and shortness of breath. These symptoms may persist through the acute and convalescent periods. Some spouses tend to be overprotective, which often leads to marital discord and sexual problems. Spouses and children often avoid conflict, and the client, too, tends to avoid arousing activating emotions. Suppression of feelings and the failure to recognize and resolve conflict increase and escalate tension within the family.

Research findings reveal that a year after the heart attack, spouses felt marital relations to be different from what they were during the premorbid period. When relations were markedly changed, the wife had assumed a managing role and tended to be overprotective, while the husband with coronary problems remained irritable and less independent.[88]

Families experience financial strains as a result of the costs of the hospitalization, which are compounded after discharge by layoffs, job changes which mean lower pay, forced retirement, dependence on disability pensions, or difficulty in finding employment. Socioeconomic problems often interfere with the resumption of the earlier lifestyle. Often these clients are unable to get automobile or life insurance, keep their homes repaired or as clean as they had been, or maintain their premorbid standard of living. Role reversals in the marital dyad and a shift in parenting responsibilities further strain the family's ability to cope. When this stress is experienced as intense or prolonged and solutions seem unavailable, the family may become disorganized and family members may become predisposed to stress-related disorders.

THE ENVIRONMENT. The development of cardiovascular disorders, particularly stroke and coronary artery disease, is related to societal patterns of interaction. Fast foods, a sedentary lifestyle, fast-paced work environments, rapid technological change, and turnovers in company ownership and goals contribute to the development of stress and its mismanagement.

The American diet has been high in salt, fat, and sugar, all of which have been linked to heart disease. The time pressures of daily life and the two-career family influence not only what is eaten but also how it is eaten. Fast foods and prepared quick-cooking foods tend to be high in salt, fat, sugar, and calories, increasing the tendency for obesity, and they tend to be eaten "on the run." This society has only recently become nutrition-conscious. Food companies are beginning to market low-salt, low-fat, low-calorie foods, but tastes and eating patterns are slow to change. A preference for a healthy diet develops slowly if at all for some people. The foods people eat and the way they eat them interact with other aspects of daily life. Entrenched use of fast foods and use of food to cope with stress or to socialize will be resistant to modification.

Daily exercise has also only recently been recognized as important to health, and particularly to effective cardiovascular functioning. For those who continue to live a sedentary life, the risk of cardiovascular disorders is high.

As technology grows and provides faster ways to perform work, time pressures increase. Acceleration of the pace of living increases and compounds the demands on coping capacities. The perception of time pressure is in itself a source of stress. The mismanagement of stress is a common occurence in the face of rapid change and the perceived need to continually increase the work pace. Rapid technological change places a demand on employees to learn and adapt new skills or new ways of performing old tasks.

The interactions between employer and employee are also undergoing rapid change. Job security and satisfaction and a sense of job competence have been derived, in part, from stable company identity and integrity. Company reorganizations and changes in ownership as a result of takeovers threaten job security and company loyalty and generate stress.

Sudden Death

The relationship between sudden death and emotional trauma has a long and persistent history. Examples of people dying while exhibiting extreme fear, rage, grief, humiliation, or joy can be found in the Bible and in historical texts. Clinicians have described people with heart disease who died suddenly after coming to an "impasse" in their lives.[89]

Engel[89] found that events preceding sudden death correspond to the circumstances that he found preceding illness in general. An analysis of the life circumstances surrounding 275 sudden deaths revealed four major categories:

1. An exceptionally traumatic disruption of a close human relationship or the anniversary of the loss of a loved one (135 deaths; 57 of these deaths were immediately preceded by the death of a loved one)
2. Situations of danger, struggle, or attack (103 deaths)
3. Loss of status, self-esteem, or valued possessions, as well as disappointment, failure, defeat, or humiliation (21 deaths)
4. Moments of triumph, public recognition, reunion (16 deaths)

Disorders of the Immune System

The immune system significantly influences the development of a range of health problems. The immune response maintains bodily integrity in relation to foreign substances such as bacteria, viruses, tissue grafts, organ transplants, and neoplasms. Immune mechanisms may also fail to recognize body cells and respond as if they were foreign substances and destroy them.

Studies suggest that stressful psychosocial situations may affect the immune system and that the immune response is subject to learned and conditioned effects. A number of studies report changes in immunoglobulin levels in relation to psychological conditions.[90,91] Substantially lower T-lymphocyte proliferation and less effective action of "killer" cell lymphocytes has been observed in studies of animals in "learned helplessness" situations.[90] Lymphocytes, the main immunocompetent cells, proliferate significantly less in people who are depressed.[92] In a study of medical students, "natural killer" (NK) cell activity declined among those with high scores on scales of stressful life events and loneliness. Research findings support the theory that a relationship exists between psychological stress and immunosuppression.[93,94]

In a study of psychiatric inpatients, high levels of loneliness were associated with lower levels of NK cell activity, poorer T-lymphocyte activity, and higher urinary cortisol levels.[93] A study of middle-aged and elderly people under acute stress found that the elderly, particularly those with severe symptoms of depression, excrete larger amounts of urinary cortisol.[94] If responsivity to stress is exaggerated in the elderly, as indicated by the increased urinary cortisol and severe depressive symptoms, then their vulnerability to immune incompetence is increased. This might explain the increased risk of cancer and vulnerability to overwhelming flu and other infections in the elderly.[94]

Neuroendocrine pathways may mediate psychosocial influences on the immune system. Changes in corticosteroid levels have been noted in relation to separation, mourning, and clinical depression. Corticosteroids, which also are increased with emotional changes, usually suppress various immune system functions, but in some instances they enhance functioning. The increase in epinephrine and norepinephrine that occurs during stress decreases immune responses.[95]

Infection

Multicausation is generally accepted in relation to infection. Host-microorganism interaction influences the development of infections. Psychosocial factors have been found to influence susceptibility to pathogens. It is postulated that these psychosocial factors alter immune system function, which in turn increases or decreases vulnerability to infections.

Relationships between psychosocial factors and infections which have been substantiated through clinical research include the following examples.[96–100]

Recurrent herpes simplex lesions and depression

Stressful life events and decreased resistance to tuberculosis

Anger-inducing life experiences and changes in the bacterial composition of the intestines

Maladaptive aggression and upper respiratory infections

Acute and chronic family stress and streptococcus infections

Recovery rate from infectious mononucleosis and psychological variables

Susceptibility to the common cold and psychological variables

Cancer

Cancer is not just one disease. It is a number of related diseases that affect different parts of the human body in various ways. The link between malignancies and emotions was recognized at least 1800 years ago. In the eighteenth and nineteenth centuries the relationship between a person's life history or personality and cancer was widely accepted. Depression and despair before the diagnosis of cancer, particularly in response to loss, were noted by Paget in 1870. Until recently there was little interest or effort in researching or treating cancer from this vantage point. In recent years, however, research findings and clinical observations have suggested that psychological stress and emotions are linked to the development of cancer, its response to treatment, and its prognosis.

Studies indicate that psychological disturbance affects endocrine and immune system functions and appears to have a role in the development and course of certain kinds of cancer. The NK cells have been implicated in both fighting tumor growth and aiding the body's surveillance of new tumors. Recent findings indicate that the activity of these cells is compromised among younger cancer clients who report "fatigue." This fatigue may represent passivity, a perception of helplessness, and a decreased willingness to fight, diminishing the body's resistance to tumor growth. A study of a group of women with recurring breast cancer revealed that those who manifested the most psychiatric and psychological symptoms had the best chance of surviving longest. These findings indicate that psychological distress may elicit a "fight" response that influences the progression of disease.[101,102] It has also been demonstrated that remissions of cancer occur when underlying depression is relieved. It appears that brain mechanisms can influence immunological competence. Thus, the person's mood can influence the course of malignant disease.[103] The holistic model supports the possibility that psychological as well as physical and environmental factors interact and contribute to the development of cancer.

Person-environment interaction can be significant in cancer. Over a 21-year period LeShan[103] used a short, personal, structured interview and the Worthington personal-history questionnaire to collect from 455 people with cancer information about major unconscious stresses, ego defenses, functioning, and ways of relating to others. In addition, over a 14-year period 250 people with cancer were interviewed from 2 to 8 hours each. Another 200 people with cancer were interviewed in relation to adjustment problems that either they or their physician saw as needing intervention. The close relatives of 50 people with cancer were interviewed for between 1 and 3 hours each, and 40 close relatives were seen for between 20 and 50 hours in total.

LeShan found that 95 percent of the people with cancer and only 10 percent of the people without cancer in the control group exhibited a basic emotional pattern. A cancer-prone profile that includes LeShan's, the Simontons', and other researchers' data is presented in Table 42-7. This profile predates the development of cancer and is associated with both rapid tumor growth and a poor prognosis. (A profile of family patterns of cancer-prone people is presented in Table 42-8.) In contrast, people who experience spontaneous remissions and who live longer and more fully exhibit a different profile.[104] The characteristics of these cancer "superstars" are presented in Table 42-9.

Table 42-7 The Cancer-Prone Person

Profile
Establishes a single role or relationship with spouse or child that gives meaning to life
Disruption of this meaningful relationship increases susceptibility
Impaired ability to establish another meaningful relationship
Losses both recent and past generate despair and lead to invalidation of their existence
Impaired ability to develop and maintain meaningful long-term relationships
Poor self-image: self-dislike, self-alienation, self-distrust
Sees self as a victim; tendency toward self-pity
Presents self as "martyr" or "saint"
"Nice person" type—easy to get along with; avoidance of conflict
Values conformity; denies genuine feelings
Lacks flexibility and resiliency
Maintains unrealistic standards based on "shoulds"
Tendency to hold resentments and a marked inability to forgive or forget
Feelings of helplessness and hopelessness; depression
A characteristic inability to express emotions, particularly anger, resentment, or aggressiveness

Table 42-8 Families of Origin of Cancer-Prone Individuals

Family Profile
Lack of warmth in parent-child relationship
Lack of closeness in parent-child relationship
Physical or emotional neglect of the child
Child feels neglected by one or both parents
High incidence of parental loss through death with consequent residual guilt and feelings of responsibility that extend into adulthood
Child learns to expect pain, desertion, loneliness, and despair
Child learns to believe that the situation is the result of own faults and failures
Child learns and continues into adulthood to view life as predetermined and joyless, and opportunities for satisfaction are limited
Child learns to believe that love and approval are out of reach

Table 42-9 People with Above-Average Remissions of Cancer

Profile
Tend to be generally successful people
Tend to be intelligent and highly creative
Feelings of personal adequacy and vitality
Tend to be receptive to new ideas
Absence of rigidity
Have a freedom from overconventional behavior
Rebellious spirit; refuse to give up
Lack of ethnic prejudice
Permissive morality
Hostile, compulsive, demanding
Are highly verbal, confrontive, and sometimes scrappy
Psychological insight
Psychologically aggressive (have more-aggressive immune systems)
Strong sense of reality
Open to examining their lives to identify factors that serve as psychological stressors
Have an internal locus of control; recognize and take personal responsibility
Continue to grow intellectually and emotionally
Continue to seek out new worlds to conquer
Seek out the "best" medical treatment
Seek out both traditional and less well substantiated cures

INVOLVEMENT IN TREATMENT. According to the Simontons,[104,105] beliefs about cancer and its treatment significantly influence the course of the disease and the efficacy of treatment. Most people with a diagnosis of cancer see it as synonymous with death. They tend to feel that their situation is hopeless. They also have negative feelings about their treatment. They see themselves as victims and do not see how they participated in the development of the disease or what they personally can do to help themselves get well.

This negative belief system is reflected in the way these people tend to visualize their cancer, their treatment, and their personal resources and capacities. They see the cancer as big and powerful, and their own immune systems as either weak or nonexistent. In contrast, people who experience spontaneous remissions tend to visualize themselves as effectively combating the cancer and see themselves as getting well.[104,106]

The cancer may be (1) a means of inflicting self-punishment to relieve perceived guilt, (2) a way of proving that others are incompetent to be of help in dealing with loneliness, depression, or guilt, or (3) a way of attacking those who have failed to meet needs or making them feel guilty for failing to be available or supportive. Because cancer is meeting these needs or other needs, it serves a purpose for these people. They may seem surprisingly passive about their care. Some seem accepting of their situation and appear resigned to a "fate" that need not occur. They may accept postsurgical recommendations for or against follow-up chemotherapy or radiation without question. Some turn down treatment altogether.[103]

In spite of media coverage about the importance of a second opinion when a significant decision must be made regarding one's health, many people with cancer are satisfied with one physician's opinion. The importance of one's frame of mind in relation to effective coping and recovery from cancer has been an issue discussed on many television talk shows. Despite exposure to such information, many people with cancer are not motivated to increase their understanding of themselves, and they may reject psychological help. It appears that they would rather die than increase their understanding of self or the situation, or actively participate in getting well.

Refusal to take or benefit from treatment may be a way of repeating earlier experiences that were characterized by illness and childlike helplessness that elicited nurturing and the satisfaction of dependency needs. Invalidism and pain may be perceived as mere inconveniences that are endurable because they lead to the attention and care these people so desperately need, or they may serve as mechanisms for self-punishment for past misdeeds. These people may feel that they "deserve" the punishment, or that through their "selfless" giving they have "earned" the right to be cared for by others.[103]

Among those who refuse traditional medical-surgical care and accept *only* nontraditional, controversial treatments, there may be a self-destructive dimension. The search for and acceptance of treatments that have been shown to be ineffective or are unsubstantiated are substituted for a genuine attempt to find a cure.

When the cancer is an unconscious defense against anxiety generated by an otherwise unavoidable situation, it serves an important function for the person. A cure would mean the loss of an important source of protection against the reemergence of the dreaded anxiety.

Research suggests that people with schizophrenia (except for paranoid schizophrenics) develop cancer less frequently than the general population. Alteration in lymphocyte activity in people with schizophrenia may alter the immune system's response to neoplastic cells. However, the findings are not conclusive; the influence of phenothiazines on lymphocyte activity needs further study. Some suggest that schizophrenia is an autoimmune disorder which provides protection from the proliferation of cancer cells.[101,107,108] Others theorize that malignant diseases and the regressive psychosis associated with schizophrenia could be alternative expressions of proneness to illness.[109,110]

INTERACTION WITH TREATMENT MODALITIES. The person with cancer usually undergoes a wide variety of treatments that cause physical discomfort, changes in body image, and derangements in physical structures and physiological functioning in ways that generate symptoms. Some psychological symptoms develop consequent to the discomfort; others, however, are side effects of the treatment or pathophysiology. Metabolic encephalopathy, tumor and metastases, and side effects of treatment have all been implicated in the manifestation of psychological symptoms, but the organic bases for these symptoms are often not recognized.[110,111]

Table 42-10 Cancer: Physical Disorders and Treatments and Psychological Symptoms

Disorder or treatment	Symptoms
Hypercalcemia, with bronchogenic carcinoma and multiple myeloma	Depression, anxiety, paranoid psychosis
Hyponatremia	Fluctuating confusion, restlessness, emotional lability
Hypomagnesemia	Personality change, nervousness, irritability, restlessness, depression
Hypoxia	Sudden change in mood, thought, and behavior
Hypothyroidism, with disturbance in cortisol metabolism	Depression, mania, psychosis
Carcinoid tumors	Depression, anxiety, confusion
CNS tumor or metastasis	Change in personality, intense depression, euphoria, paranoia, extreme anxiety, sense of impending doom
Radiotherapy	Changes in mood and attitude (secondary to physical side effects)
Chemotherapy	
Cimetidine	Confusion, depression, agitation, delirium
Vincristine	Depression
Mustargen	Confusion
Methotrexate	Dementia
Narcotics	Clouded consciousness, lassitude, confusion
Pentazocine	Dysphoria
Steroids	Depression, irritability, euphoria, psychosis

SOURCE: R. J. Goldberg, "Psychiatric Symptoms in Cancer Patients," *Postgraduate Medicine*, vol. 74, no. 1, 1983, pp. 263–273.

Examples of these physical and treatment factors and the psychological problems they generate are presented in Table 42-10.

Autoimmune Disorders

The optimally functional immune system recognizes and distinguishes between foreign substances and the body's own cells. Cell-mediated and humoral responses may become dysfunctional in relation to recognition of and response to the body's cells. Psychosocial stress has been associated with the onset and course of diseases of the autoimmune system. Dysfunction and hypofunction are mediated by neuroendocrine mechanisms. Immune dysfunctions may be induced by unmanageable psychosocial stress. Research suggests that the onset of dysfunction follows closely on emotional decompensation in predisposed individuals.[112,113] An autoimmune factor has been associated with ulcerative colitis, arthritis, Hashimoto's disease, systemic lupus erythematosus, psoriasis, myasthenia gravis, and pernicious anemia.[112]

ULCERATIVE COLITIS. *Ulcerative colitis* is an inflammatory disease of the mucosa of the colon, primarily affecting the rectum and the sigmoid colon. It may be mild, moderate, severe, or lethal. Toxic megacolon involving perforation and massive hemorrhage is a major life-threatening disease. Genetic, immunological, and personality traits have been implicated in its occurrence. Experiences and attitudes related to stressful life events have also been related to the onset and course of ulcerative colitis.[48]

Ulcerative colitis has frequently been associated with anticolon antibodies. Confronted with unmanageable stress, the neuroendocrine mechanisms create disequilibrium in the immune system, thus allowing these destructive antibodies to proliferate. People with a predisposition for ulcerative colitis respond to activating emotions with a marked increase in bowel motility, hyperemia, increased fragility of the bowel wall, and a marked increase in lysozyme levels, producing effects similar to those caused by strong cholinergic stimulation. It is possible to observe the development of small ulcerations and petechial hemorrhages when these people are experiencing rage, resentment, and anger. Strong activating emotions appear to decrease bowel-wall defenses and increase the levels of proteolytic enzymes.[114]

Person-environment interaction seems to have significance in ulcerative colitis. People with ulcerative colitis have been portrayed in the literature as passive, conforming, oversensitive, egocentric, dependent, conscientious, indecisive, and obstinate. However, when they have schizoid or paranoid tendencies, messiness and disorderliness predominate. People with ulcerative colitis tend to exhibit guarding of affectivity, overintellectualization, rigid attitudes toward morality, a defective sense of humor, and extreme sensitivity to rejection and hostility from others. They are also likely to expend considerable energy warding off potential rejections. Their outward manner, which is often energetic, ambitious, and efficient, may mask feelings of inferiority. They possess an acute sense of obligation and a close bond with one or two parent figures on whom they depend for guidance. They tend to act on the conscious or unconscious wishes of these figures and then to experience hostility, which cannot be discharged because of fear of rejection.

ARTHRITIS. *Rheumatoid arthritis* is a systemic disorder of unknown cause and crippling effects. It is characterized by inflammatory changes found in articular and associated structures. Stress plays an important part in the causation and exacerbation of arthritis. The psychophysiological mechanisms are complex and unclear. Hormones involved in the regulation of connective-tissue synthesis (the growth hormone, thyroxine, androgens, estrogens, and adrenal corticosteroids) interfere with the immune mechanisms and with the production of collagens. The neuroendocrine mechanisms also affect the network of capillaries and nerve fibers surrounding the synovium.

Alterations of antibodies occur in arthritis. The altered antibodies fail to recognize the body's tissue; this leads to tissue damage and inflammation. Stress and emotional distress may influence the immunological system through the CNS and endocrine mediation.

People who develop juvenile rheumatoid arthritis have been found to have experienced more life changes in the previous year than control subjects. Life changes, particularly those involving loss, are of major importance in generating the activating emotions and the level of stress capable of altering neuroendocrine mechanisms.

MISMANAGEMENT OF STRESS: DYSYNCHRONOUS EATING PATTERNS

Extreme weight loss or gain reflects dramatic changes in a person's eating patterns. Stress is a significant influential factor in the development of problematic eating patterns. Psychogenic malnutrition may occur in clients exhibiting agitated behavior or disordered thinking. Extreme overactivity, apathy, or delusions which lead people to believe that their food is poisoned and therefore not edible may lead to psychogenic malnutrition. Depressed people may also experience excessive weight loss. Their retarded motor activity and mood interfere with appetite and the motivation to feed themselves.[115]

Some people who are experiencing either acute or chronic stress may eat excessive amounts of food and choose high-calorie foods. This eating pattern may become stable and persistent and thus a way of life, or it may be episodic in nature and characterized by alternating periods of strict dieting and severe weight loss followed by binge eating and excessive weight gain. Malnutrition and overnutrition, without evidence of underlying pathology such as cancer or brain damage, are psychogenic in nature. Anorexia, obesity, and the consumption of nonedibles reflect maladaptive ways of coping with stress.

The eating disorders discussed in this section of the chapter are anorexia nervosa, bulimia, pica, and obesity. In the past, anorexia nervosa and bulimia were considered separate clinical entities, and in this section each is presented separately. Recently, however, research has indicated that anorexia nervosa and bulimia represent a spectrum of eating disorders. It appears that a considerable number of people with these disorders do not completely recover after one episode. Those who have a 10- to 20-year history have experienced several transitions between food-restricting anorectic episodes, binge-and-purge episodes during periods of low weight, and intervals of relatively normal weight with frequent binges and purges.[115]

Anorexia Nervosa

Anorexia nervosa is characterized by drastic weight loss, a refusal to maintain a minimal normal body weight, disturbance of body image, a cachectic appearance, slow pulse, amenorrhea, and a morbid and irrational fear of being fat.[116] People who develop anorexia nervosa are usually female (90 to 95 percent), white, and 12 to 25 years old. Onset after age 30 is rare. These young people tend to come from upper- and middle-class families. Anorexia nervosa appears to be increasing rapidly to epidemic proportions in most affluent countries with a significant number of well-educated people. Approximately 40 percent of anorectics recover spontaneously; 20 percent respond to treatment; and probably 40 percent become chronic.[116,117,118] The risk increases for sisters of anorectics. In many instances the anorectic's parents have an explicit history of significantly low adolescent weight or weight phobia. Research findings indicate that the average age of these parents at the time of the birth of the child with anorexia was higher than the average for the population as a whole.

Patterns of Interaction in Anorexia Nervosa

THE PERSON. In some people the onset of anorexia nervosa is associated with a stressful life situation. About one-third are mildly overweight at this time.[119] Before the appearance of overt symptomatology, the anorectic person often becomes increasingly irritable, develops eczema and other skin disorders, complains of abdominal discomfort, reports headaches, exhibits hyperactivity and heightened energy output with no apparent fatigue, and develops amenorrhea. Depresssion and anxiety may occur, and the person may react to menstruation with horror and rejection. The overactivity and the beginning of social withdrawal from friends and family may be masked by the choice of activities. The high level of investment in schoolwork, running, or in perfecting performance in a sport may be overlooked as a symptom and meet with parental approval. Many of these people are described as overly perfectionist, "model" children.[120]

The onset of self-starvation may occur some time after this prodromal period. Once self-starvation has begun, these young women exhibit an obsessional preoccupation with the desire to be thin and a compulsive avoidance of food. As a group they exhibit a remarkably high level of activity in spite of their frail appearance. Often these young women are shy, timid, neat, and controlled adolescents. Frequently they have a history of excess weight before the development of the symptoms of anorexia. They diet to lose this weight, but fail to recognize the attainment of their optimal weight. During the weight-reduction process, they become counterphobic to avoid obesity. The failure to recognize their emaciation reaches delusional proportions. They have a morbid fascination with collecting recipes, with eating, and with cooking. It is not uncommon for them to prepare gourmet meals or fancy, rich desserts for others and then refuse to even sample what they have prepared. They deny their hunger.[115,120]

The dieting usually is done secretively although they have a sense of pride in their eating behavior. At mealtime, when it cannot be avoided, they take a small portion and spend time rearranging it on their plates and frequently take pains to cut everything into small pieces. If there is family pressure to eat, they may secretively hide the food in their pockets or in a napkin and dispose of it when they leave the dinner table.[116–120]

The loss of appetite does not occur early in the disease process. Voluntary restricted consumption of food may be difficult. Consequently, the anorectic person may engage in binge eating. If a quantity of food is consumed during such a binge or because of parental pressure, the person may stick a finger down the throat in order to induce vomiting. With time anorectics learn to disgorge the contents of their stomachs at will. They may also take large doses of cathartics or use self-administered enemas to rid their bodies of the unwanted food.[115,116]

They narcissistically admire their emaciated bodies in the mirror. The degree of body-image distortion, which is reflected in persistent overestimation of the size of the body and its parts, appears to be related to the severity of the disease process. Those who manifest the greatest body-image distortion have the greatest denial of their problem and have the poorest progress when in treatment. Their perceptions of their bodies are delusional, and their fear of being fat is phobic.[121,122]

Sexual adjustment problems are common among these young people. They tend to lack accurate information about sexual matters. They have little or no sexual activity. As the malnutrition increases, interest in sex decreases. Generally these young women have delayed psychosocial sexual development. A small group have a history of sexual promiscuity, drug abuse, or both.[116]

These young people are highly motivated for academic achievement. They work hard and attain above-average grades.

During the acute phase of the disease process, obsessive-compulsive behavior, sleep disturbances, crying spells, acute anxiety, suicide attempts, somatic complaints (particularly epigastric discomfort), and compulsive stealing are more likely to occur.

Weight loss of these clients exceeds 25 percent of original body weight. If the client is under 18 years of age, the degree of weight loss must also include both the amount of the loss from the original body weight and the projected weight gain expected on the basis of pediatric growth charts.[116]

When the weight loss is profound and malnutrition is severe, hospitalization is required. A strict behavior modification program is usually employed when the physical condition becomes life-threatening.

After nutrition has been restored and the threat to life removed, the symptoms and dynamics often continue, although with less severity, even after discharge from the hospital. Both the family and the anorectic may resist individual, family, or group follow-up therapy in spite of evidence of "picky" eating habits, anxiety about sexuality, and perfectionist attitudes.[116]

As the disease progresses, anorectics develop hypotension, cyanosis of the extremities, brownish pigmentation and blotchiness and a yellow-orange hue of the skin, and increased lanugo. The breasts atrophy; axillary and pubic hair are reduced. Leukopenia, lymphocytosis, anemias, hypoglycemia, hypocholesteremia, and hypoproteinemia develop. Generally there are no notable changes in hormone levels with the exception of the gonadotropins and ovarian hormones. Amenorrhea, which is characteristic of the disorder, occurs in 50 percent of these women before weight loss; the menstrual cycle may not return to normal for some time even when the nutritional status has returned to and been maintained at a normal level. These facts suggest psychogenic causation.[123,124]

As the disease progresses and the physiological status deteriorates, these clients experience psychiatric and medical emergencies. Somewhere between 5 to 21 percent die of malnutrition, some unknown derangement of metabolic or cardiac function, or intercurrent infections.[123]

Amenorrhea preceding weight loss is usually the first notable physical symptom. No disturbance in the central control of appetite has been identified. Secretion of the luteinizing hormone and estrogen is depressed. These endocrine alterations may not return to normal for some time after the restoration of normal weight. The changes that occur in relation to pituitary, thyroid, and adrenal hormones are thought to be related to malnourishment.[123,124,125]

The metabolic changes that occur (hypothalamic alkalosis, dysfunctional diuresis, electrocardiographic changes, fall in body temperature, decreased blood pressure, decreased cardiac output) appear to be related to the self-induced vomiting, malnutrition, and abuse of purgatives and diuretics. Pericardial effusion has been found when an anorectic dies as a result of starvation.[126] The decrease in gastrointestinal tract activity and constipation that occur are also a result of the state of starvation and reflect a conservation-survival adaptation.[115] Various hematologic and immunological abnormalities such as bone marrow changes, abnormal red blood cells, leukopenia, and defective bactericidal activity of granulocytes have been found. Dietary and psychogenic factors are thought to play a role, since these abnormalities are reversible with increased nutritional status.[127] These people also manifest severe acid-base derangements. The hypokalemic metabolic alkalosis, intravascular volume depletion, and hypotension that occur probably contribute to death.[128,129]

A genetic predisposition has been postulated for anorexia nervosa on the basis of family histories and the association with other inherited diseases. Hypothalamic dysfunction has also been proposed on the basis of the independent development of amenorrhea before the emaciation. Increased catecholamine activity has also been implicated.

Psychological theories have focused on phobic avoidance of food resulting from sexual and social tensions generated by the physical changes associated with puberty.

Anorexia nervosa is usually precipitated by traumatic events centering on actual or potential separation, the bodily changes of puberty, and sexual experiences and failures. Food comes to symbolize evil and self-indulgence, and severe dieting is used to control the body, its impulses, and sexuality. These clients may starve themselves to dangerous levels but do not seem aware of the lethal implications of their behavior. In the clients' hatred of food, their internal signals of hunger are disrupted and signs of satiation are misinterpreted or lost. The cachexia is seen as a way of becoming inconspicuous, while the disease process enables the victim to avoid both responsibility and the need to deal with the emerging secondary sex characteristics and their implication. If there has been sexual activity, even masturbation, these women may feel guilty and use the strict dietary regimen for self-punishment. Misconceptions causing fear of pregnancy are not uncommon.[116] Some fear a fantasized pregnancy. The starvation is aimed at preventing any abdominal protrusion. They seem to hold a deep-seated wish to remain tiny and immature and to retain an intrauterine type of passive dependency on parental figures. Their behavior reflects a maturational conflict.[116]

PERSON-ENVIRONMENT. Cultural pressures for thinness may also initially influence the development of behavior resulting in anorexia. Pressure to conform to the ideal body configuration promoted by the media and exemplified by emaciated high-fashion models interacts with the anorectic's mother's heightened concern about weight control and may be supported by the anorectic's perfectionist and obsessive-compulsive personality traits. Another possible influence may be the changing value that society gives to motherhood. The fear of being fat may mask a basic conflict between the biological drive toward motherhood and its diminished societal value.[124,125]

PERSON-FAMILY. Food and its consumption become a control issue in anorectics' families. Overprotectiveness, overconcern with dieting, overconscientious perfectionism, repression of emotion, infantilized decision making for the anorectic, and intrusiveness are characteristics of these families.[124]

A dependent, seductive relationship with a warm but passive father and guilt over aggression toward the mother have been cited as contributing factors. Other findings reveal an overly dependent relationship with the mother, who is dominant, solicitous, and chronically depressed. These findings suggest that a family projection process may be operating.[120]

These families appear to function well; however, fusion is pervasive. Boundaries are not respected and thus become blurred. "Mind reading" is prevalent; thus there is a general failure to discriminate between who owns which thoughts and feelings. The anorectic cannot even claim ownership of her body. The adolescent's developing sense of independence is sabotaged. Politeness, apparent genuine parental concern for the welfare of the children, and superficial pleasantness mask the covert interference with separation and differentiation. The recognition and expression of anger, anxiety, aggressiveness, and depression are blocked.[120] Differences of opinion and arguments are not allowed. Unitary perceptions and feelings are enforced. Togetherness is prized, and efforts toward independence and separation are viewed as traitorous. The need for loyalty is exaggerated. The family, which is usually intact, caring, and overinvolved, uses avoidance of conflict as determinedly as the anorectic uses avoidance of food and avoidance of maturation as a style of coping.[125] The treatment dropout rate is very high for anorectics; often the anorectic leaves treatment as a consequence of family resistance to treatment and sabotage. This high dropout rate probably reflects the tendency to use avoidance coping strategies.[130] Perfectionism and excellence in school, hobbies, and sports are highly valued. Excellence is the standard. Since perfection in all spheres of life is unattainable, parental criticism is inevitable. Rather than rebel against these standards, anorectics seek love, approval, and recognition by trying harder and by becoming more obsessive and perfectionistic. Family transactional patterns foster somatization; therefore, the anorectic expresses feelings of anxiety and depression through physical complaints.[120]

In spite of the superficial politeness characteristic of these families, tension at mealtimes is common. Both parents appear to be continually defensive against their own low self-esteem and unacceptable feelings and impulses. They invest considerable energy in pretending that all is well. The investment of energy in maintaining this facade contributes to their rigidity.[125] When the family recognizes the anorexia and initiates or is referred for treatment, that is perceived as an indictment of the parents. The parents usually exhibit hopelessness, anger, and guilt.[130]

The family becomes focused on the adolescent. Overt and covert domination and negation of individuality threatens the adolescent's identity formation. The only apparent avenue for control lies in what the anorectic allows herself to eat. Control of her own sensual desires, maturing body, and her parent's intrusiveness and dominance is symbolized and acted out through her control over her eating patterns.

Many families of anorectics have no male children. Consequently, the girls are expected to make up for this family deficiency by becoming outstanding, particularly in fields traditionally occupied by men. The mothers of these girls have often given up careers for marriage and taken on the role of submissive housewives. These women defer to their husbands but do not respect them. When the anorectic is no longer the symptom bearer for the family, the polite facade crumbles and marital discord develops.

Males with Anorexia Nervosa

Anorexia nervosa in males is rare. Males with anorexia nervosa tend to have been obese before the onset of symptoms. In early adolescence they begin a self-starvation pattern in pursuit of thinness which is similar to that of female anorectics. They also develop a distorted perception of their body size, avoid becoming what they perceive as fat, and engage in self-induced vomiting that is often followed by binge eating. There often exist significant psychosexual conflicts, including unconscious homosexual conflict, before the onset of the disorder.[131,132] The male anorectic also exhibits hyperactivity and an exaggerated drive for achievement. The development of symptomatic behavior is usually preceded by a change that threatens the anorectic's position as a superior achiever. It appears that despite a history of excellent performance, particularly in relation to academic pursuits, the male anorectic doubts his competence and experiences insecurity in relation to his ability to sustain his outstanding performance. Bruch noted that despite the "stubborn, aggressive and violently negative behavior following the development of symptoms, this sense of personal ineffectiveness is pervasive."[131]

The family dynamics associated with the development of this condition among males are characterized by a controlling mother, who imposes her concept of the son's needs and wishes. This mother-child transactional pattern is symptom-free, since the child complies. However, the developmental imperative during adolescence for independence and separation threatens this fusion. The son gains autonomy and self-control through regulation of the eating pattern.[131]

Bulimia

Bulimia is episodic, uncontrolled, rapid ingestion of very large quantities of food over a short period of time (binge eating), followed by attempts to avoid weight gain through self-induced vomiting and the use of laxatives. It usually occurs in females. No causes for the development of bulimia have been supported by research. The episodic nature of the condition suggests an epileptic-type problem; however, the problem has not responded to antiseizure treatment approaches.[116]

The Person

A person with bulimia tends to eat high-calorie, easily digested foods in an inconspicuous fashion. Physical discomfort is the reason given for terminating the binge. Feelings of guilt, depression, and self-disgust follow a binge.[116]

These people become so frightened of weight gain that vomiting becomes a necessity.[116] The vomiting symbolically expresses an outpouring of rage. These people, unlike anorectics, are aware that their eating pattern is abnormal, and their fear is that they won't be able to stop eating voluntarily.[116] A pattern of gorging and self-induced vomiting develops. They may engage in this cycle of gorging and vomiting for years without anxiety. During this time they may thrust fingers down their throats to induce vomiting so aggressively that they traumatize the tissue. Generally this self-induced vomiting is done secretively, or with a friend who is also bulimic.[116,117]

Evidence of a pattern of self-induced vomiting is often discovered by a dentist or doctor when the oral cavity is inspected during a physical examination. Inspection of the oral cavity reveals chemical erosion of the tooth structure due to the high acidity of the vomitus. These people may also complain of dental sensitivity due to the loss of tooth enamel and inflammation of the salivary glands.[129]

It is not until these people attempt to stop the self-induced vomiting that they recognize they cannot.[132] Then they become afraid of gorging. These people tend to exhibit wide fluctuations in their weight patterns, ranging from being markedly overweight to being underweight. Their weight loss is not severe enough to classify them as anorectic, and amenorrhea may or may not occur.[115,116] The bulimic, unlike the anorectic, acknowledges an enjoyment of eating, a voracious appetite, and a fear of not being able to stop eating; like the anorectic, the bulimic has a fear of being fat.[131]

As a group bulimics are slightly older than anorectics and tend to come from a lower social class. The underlying personality of bulimics is predominantly histrionic. They tend to be impulsive. They are unable to accurately identify and deal with emotions. They channel their emotions into their abnormal gorging and vomiting, a fear of being fat, and dissocial behavior.[115,116] They tend to be drug or alcohol abusers, to engage in stealing, and to engage in aggressive and sexual acting out. They become sexually promiscuous or delinquent. Many exhibit depression, pathological guilt, worrying, poor concentration, obsessional ideas and rumination, nervous tension, tiredness, self-depreciation, and irritability.[115,116] Their perceptual distortion is an overestimation of their size and an underestimation of their nutritional needs.

Bulimics are also at risk of premature death. They may die because of hypokalemic cardiac arrhythmias, renal damage, or suicide, or because of metabolic derangements that have yet to be identified.[115,133]

The Family

The patterns of interaction in the bulimic's family have not been documented in as great detail as those in the anorectic's family. Similarities in family histories of anorectics and bulimics reveal an excessive interest in food and dieting. Parental weight problems and controlling parent-child interactions have been identified. Families of bulimics also tend to use avoidance patterns in coping with life stresses.

Pica

Pica is the persistent ingestion of nonnutritive substances such as dirt, clay, starch, and paper. The medical problems that result from this behavior are extensive and sometimes serious.

Women, particularly while pregnant, and children appear to exhibit this behavior more frequently than men. The factors that contribute to indiscriminate ingestion of nonnutritive substances are thought to be (1) nutritional deficiencies or (2) unmet oral needs. Among children this eating pattern may be a symptom of a pervasive developmental disorder. Among pregnant women the eating pattern usually disappears after delivery. Cultural beliefs have been cited as a factor when pregnant women adopt this eating pattern. In spite of the cultural influences and traditional family practices, there is thought to be a psychological factor that contributes to this behavior.

Obesity

Obesity is a condition marked by excessive, generalized deposition of fat. It is a complex health problem associated with the development of many chronic diseases and with premature death. Age, sex, height, and relative fat content must be considered in judging whether overnutrition and obesity are a problem. The most commonly used criterion of caloric overnutrition is found in tables of desirable weights for men and women based on age, height, and body frame. Skinfold measurements, which are more scientific, are also useful in determining body fatness.[134,135] There is no universal agreement on the degree of overweight that defines obesity. A deviation of from 10 to 20 percent over desirable weight presumes obesity.

Being overweight predisposes people to cholelithiasis, hypertension, diabetes mellitus, cardiovascular disease, surgical complications, and accidents.[135]

The following factors have been identified as contributing to the development of obesity: sociocultural factors; genetic predisposition; an increase in size of fat cells (hypertrophic obesity); an increase in number of fat cells (hyperplastic obesity); an increase in both size and number of fat cells; energy expenditure; caloric intake; and interaction between the person and the family.

Person-Environment Interaction

There are approximately 30 million overweight and 15 million obese Americans. In some societies, because of the limited availability of food, only the wealthy have access to enough food substances to become overweight. In such societies obesity is restricted to the privileged class. When famine and starvation occur in a society, people will eat anything that relieves the acute symptoms of hunger, regardless of whether it is digestible or nutritious. When food is plentiful, people are more selective and are more apt to choose foods for their emotional value. When one can choose freely what, when, where, and how much one eats, then there is opportunity to satisfy hunger without problems. Appetite based on desire rather than need consequently influences eating and nutritional patterns. Obesity in our society is more prevalent among women and children of low socioeconomic status than among those from higher-status groups. At age 50 this prevalence drops significantly, presumably because of the high mortality of the obese from cardiovascular disease. Since food is generally available in our society, appetite based on desire rather than the satisfaction of hunger may influence the choice and quantity of foods eaten.[135]

During periods of emotional stress, some people in affluent societies will use food to meet security needs. One study cited an increased consumption of milk products during situations in which a sense of security is threatened. The study also noted that people seeking gratification of needs or approval or an antidote for self-pity consumed chocolate, hot dogs, candy, or nuts. "Fetish foods" dominate the diet when there is a need for strength to compete on a social, intellectual, physical, or job-related activity; a need to overcome an adversity; or a need to stay healthy. Whatever the society defines as "energy foods" become fetish foods. This thematic use of food is illustrated by Popeye's need for spinach when he wishes to be strong. Children in our society are influenced by the media. Advertisements that promote certain foods for "quick energy" influence the choice of fetish foods.[135] In most instances the foods used to meet emotional needs are high in calories and are consumed in excessive amounts.

Families assign meanings to food and eating and thus influence the development of eating patterns. Maternal emotions during feeding and attitudes toward feeding influence infants' and children's eating patterns. When the mother's anxiety, anger, tenseness, resentment, and lack of nurturing qualities are associated with eating and satiation, the infant or child is more likely to develop dysfunctional eating patterns that lead to obesity.

Maternal overfeeding, which is based on unconscious grief, and underfeeding, which is rooted in resentment, also help to establish dysfunctional eating patterns that in many cases continue into adulthood. Dysfunctional eating patterns, particularly obesity, reflect disturbances at the oral stage of development. Selecting and eating food acquire an anxiety-reducing function that persists into adulthood.[135]

Social learning within the family is a significant dimension in the choices one makes related to when, where, why, and how much one eats. Recognition, love, and approval may be communicated through the use of food. Food may become a symbol of family togetherness and security. Holiday celebrations usually center on meals and traditional foods. For families that have had stress experiences related to immigration or to natural or technological catastrophies, food, family mealtimes, and holiday feasts often symbolize security. Consequently, overeating and the consumption of fatty and high-calorie foods are equated with togetherness and security.

When parents have emotional problems or are experiencing marital conflict, they may exhibit these disturbances in their own excessive caloric intake or through their relationship with their children, particularly as that relationship centers on food and its consumption. Overfeeding becomes a pattern. The overprotective, oversolicitous parent needs the cooperation of the child for the development of an eating pattern. The child's cooperation may be based in the following dynamics: imitation of the parent's eating habits; the assumption of a passive, accepting position when food is provided and eating is encouraged; the management of aggressive and hostile feelings by excessive ingestion of food; or an identification with a person whom the family, particularly the mother, has idealized, and who is a heavy eater.[135]

The psychological factors that may contribute to the development and maintenance of eating patterns which lead to overnutrition and obesity are presented in Table 42-11.

Food can be used as a substitute for unobtainable love; as an expression of rage, hatred, or a wish to become pregnant; or as a source of power. Foods having a texture, temperature, and taste that symbolically recapture past pleasurable experiences are included in the diet when the person is lonely or sad. When people need to reinforce their concept of themselves as adults, they tend to overindulge in such foods as coffee, tea, and beer. These foods are chosen because they tend to be associated with being "grown up."[136]

Table 42-11 Obesity

Psychological Factors
Faulty responses to emotional tensions such as loneliness, anxiety, and boredom
Use of food as a substitute gratification for states of tension and frustration resulting from unpleasant or intolerable life situations
Symptomatology of an underlying emotional disturbance such as depression
Feeling that one is not leading one's own life but is simply reacting to outside influences
Impaired ability to recognize physical hunger
Compulsive eating in the form of an addiction to food
Chronic hostility
Profound feelings of isolation
Difficulty adjusting to change
Obsessive preoccupation with food

Most obese people suffer psychologically from their excessive size. Psychological stress arises from difficulty with sexual identity and role and with overall self-concept. Unhappiness perpetuates fatness. Obesity perpetuates obesity. Depression, anxiety, hostility, alienation, and low self-esteem may trigger overeating and the consequent fatness. Being overweight in a society that views thinness as attractive may aggravate these moods and feelings and lead to further overeating, thus causing a vicious circle.

People of normal weight seem to regulate their body weight without special efforts. Lifetime weight histories of obese people usually show that they have never sustained their weight within the defined range of body weight for their sex, age, and build. Many obese people respond to external cues to eat rather than to internal cues that nutrients are needed—that is, they respond to external factors rather than to hunger. With respect to food preferences and rate of consumption, eating responses of obese people differ from those of people who maintain optimal weight. Obese people tend to choose high-calorie foods and to consume them quickly.[130]

Physical inactivity contributes to obesity. Recent studies suggest that inactivity may contribute to an increased food intake, and increased physical activity may decrease the food intake. A complex and powerful central regulatory system influences the balance between energy intake and expenditure. The interaction of the limbic system with the neuroendocrine and enzymatic systems is undoubtedly a dimension of this regulatory system.

Intestinal-Bypass Surgery and Jaw Wiring

Intestinal-bypass surgery and jaw wiring have been used to treat obesity.[126,136] A survey of one group of women following bypass surgery revealed that "striking" changes occurred in their marital relationships following the surgery; these ranged from brief episodes of conflict to upheavals that led to divorce.[137] Many marriages do not survive the multiple postsurgical stresses.[138] The disturbances appear to be related to the spouse's feelings of insecurity and sense of threat. After the surgery, increased sexual demands by the spouse who has undergone surgery lead to marked sexual problems.[139] Conflicts also occur in response to the spouse's resistance to the client's desire for increased independence. A wife's obesity appears to have a stabilizing influence in a marriage. The weight loss following the surgery disturbs the dynamic equilibrium in the family.

In a study of obese women who elected to have their jaws wired, all participants lost weight initially and were enthusiastic about the effectiveness of the intervention. However, over time most became discouraged, apathetic, and irritable. Weight loss gradually decreased and most regained the weight they had lost.[126]

Bypass surgery and jaw wiring may be generally ineffective if the needs that had been satisfied through eating remain unsatisfied. Unless alternative means of satisfaction are found, the continued state of deprivation becomes acute. Old eating patterns reemerge to satisfy these needs.

NURSING PROCESS

Assessment

Clients who have psychophysiological disorders exhibit a wide variety of disease processes and symptoms. The one thing they have in common is that all exhibit dysynchronous patterns of coping with stress; their health problems are manifestations of this failure. For their bodies to do the work of health maintenance or repair, energy must be diverted to this task. Thus, nursing is primarily concerned with helping these people learn how to cope more effectively, to manage their environments, to modify the number and intensity of existing stressors, and to modify stimuli which would generate further stress. The assessment process is conducted within a holistic framework that encompasses the person-environment interaction and focuses on identifying stressors and determining their impact on the client; identifying problematic perceptions, attitudes, feelings, and behavior; examining real or imagined threats; and assessing self-esteem, conflict management, recent changes, and coping styles. When a holistic approach is used in the care of a client, a systematic assessment of the client, family, environment, and interactions that occur among them is needed to formulate an appropriate plan of care.

Assessment of the Person

LOW SELF-ESTEEM. Low self-esteem has been associated with dysfunctional coping and feelings of helplessness and hopelessness. When people feel incompetent and unable to cope with life, they experience chronic stress and are vulnerable to becoming overwhelmed, even by usual life events. An assessment guide for the identification of low self-esteem is presented in Table 42-12.

LONELINESS. *Loneliness* is a subjective, sometimes unpleasant experience of feeling separate and alienated that results from deficiencies in a person's social relationships.[140] It has been linked to the development of disease, accident-proneness, surgery-proneness, and premature death. When self-esteem is impaired, vulnerability to loneliness increases. People who lack self-worth have difficulty initiating and maintaining reciprocal relationships.

People who experience chronic loneliness erect barriers between themselves and others. Their self-protective distancing, which supports a self-fulfill-

Table 42-12 Self-Esteem

Assessment Guide
When you are faced with a new or challenging situation, how do you feel?
How successful do you expect to be in such a situation?
In your family, how appreciated or unappreciated do you feel?
In your work or in a social setting, how appreciated or unappreciated do you feel?
In new situations and when meeting new people, how do you feel?
How powerful, influential, or in control do you feel in family, social, and work situations?
What do you view as your accomplishments?
How do you feel about your accomplishments?
How do you prefer to handle disagreements with others?
How do you feel when you encounter conflict or opposition?
How do you feel about yourself in general?

ing prophecy, sustains their position and can become an obstacle in developing a therapeutic nurse-client relationship. In addition, during a period of acute loneliness, a person is often unable to talk about it without risking acute anxiety. Consequently, the assessment of loneliness can be difficult.

Evidence of loneliness emerges through the nurse's use of therapeutic communication skills. The assessment questions that are listed in Table 42-13 can be used by nurses in identifying a client's loneliness.

Table 42-13 Loneliness

Assessment Guide
Does the client describe self as separate and alienated from others?
Does the client report the loss of a significant relationship through death, divorce, or geographical move?
Does the client believe that when people are acting friendly "they want to use you"?
Does the client express feelings of helplessness?
Does the client describe dissatisfaction with various aspects of life: work, colleagues, family, and social relationships?
Does the client talk about having friends but avoid describing these relationships?
Does the client respond to the question, "Who can you count on if . . . "? with a reply that supports the notion that "One stands on one's own feet—you can't count on others"?
Does the nurse experience the client as remote?
Is there a history of drug and alcohol abuse?
Is there a history of pursuing relationships with others frantically and with little success or satisfaction: multiple, casual sexual encounters? Does the client describe days as endless?
Does the client do a lot of talking but focus on things that are superficial?
Does the client talk about always waiting for something but not engage in an activity that would help it to occur?
Does the client seem to look for other people's weaknesses?
Does the client vacillate, and is the client indecisive?
Does the client attempt to reverse roles with the nurse?
Does the client blame others for dissatisfactions and problems?
Does the client describe self as different from others?
Does the client describe self as inferior or inadequate?
Does the client describe difficulty in acting assertively or sociably?
How does the client communicate needs and feelings?

IMPAIRED COPING. Assessment of coping must address the person's cognitive appraisal of the situation: is it or is it not objectively threatening or perceived as threatening? Some degree of threat is present in any health problem; therefore, the person's perception of threat or failure to perceive it is important information. If no serious threat is objectively present, but the client perceives a serious threat, then revision of perception needs to be addressed.

The assessment also needs to include identification of current coping strategies. It is important to remember that whatever the coping style—approach, avoidance, or any combination of the two—it is the *best* that the person can do at that time. Awareness of or knowledge about other ways to cope in the situation may be lacking. In formulating judgments about the usefulness of a coping style, nurses must consider this evaluation from the client's perspective and from a professional, health-promotive perspective; the nurse must consider the hierarchy of unmet needs that must be addressed and help establish priorities and a time framework for meeting these needs. The assessment of the effectiveness of a person's coping is not as straightforward as one might think. The assessment one makes regarding the effectiveness of another's behavior is always a value judgment. The time, the circumstances, and the particular needs being met by the behavior must be considered. For example, when physiological needs are paramount because the person is in a life-threatening situation, interpersonal conflicts may be denied or avoided. In this situation the denial is useful because it conserves energy and attention. Once the physiological crisis is resolved, a continued use of denial may increase the risk of another physiological hazard. In this situation, the denial is dysfunctional. Coping mechanisms can be judged functional or dysfunctional in reference to a particular situation at a particular time.[141] A guide for assessing coping styles is presented in Table 42-14 (page 884).

MISMANAGEMENT OF CHANGE. Change is inherent to life. When it occurs, it places a demand on coping capacities. Anticipated gradual change is usually more easily and effectively managed than unexpected abrupt change, unless there are symbolic losses that threaten self-integrity. When situations arise that impose radical change, then coping ca-

Table 42-14 Coping

Assessment Guide
What is the client's perception of the cause of his or her health problem?
What is the client's perception of the implications of the disease process?
How is the client coping with current stressors?
Which coping mechanisms is the client employing?
Are these coping mechanisms helping the client cope effectively and conserve energy or are they generating additional stress?
What are the client's expectations of the care giver?
What are the client's self-expectations?
What is the client's support system?
How does the client perceive this support system?
Is the client able to explore alternatives in lifestyle?
Is the client exhibiting behavior that interferes with conservation of energy and effective coping?
How does the client solve problems and make decisions?
Does the client have financial burdens?
What changes in lifestyle has the health problem imposed?
What will the client lose if he or she changes lifestyle or behavior?

pacities may be overwhelmed. One's perception of the impact of the change and one's ability to adapt influence coping. Assessment of stress generated by change needs to address the person's expectation of change, the person's perception of what the change means, the objective stressors inherent in the change, and the person's resources. A guide for this assessment is presented in Table 42-15.

Table 42-15 Change and Stress

Assessment Guide
What changes have occurred in your life in the recent past?
What do you think caused these changes?
Which changes do you view as positive in your life?
Which changes do you view as negative in your life?
What did you need to do because of the change?
Describe how you felt when the change occurred.
Who or what has been helpful in coping with these changes?
What else would have helped you at that time?
How do you feel about these changes now?
What do you think would help you cope with these changes right now?

MISMANAGEMENT OF CONFLICT. Many people who suffer from health problems that result from stress have difficulties with conflict management and resolution. These people may attempt to avoid confronting the conflict, and in doing so, suppress and repress emotions which continue to elicit a physiological stress response. Others tend to fight rather than collaborate. The anger associated with this behavior elicits a physiological response that may also lead to or aggravate illness. Assessment questions designed to identify conflict-avoidance patterns are presented in Table 42-16.

Assessment of the Family

Person-family interactions influence vulnerability to stress-related health problems and the effective resolution of these problems. An assessment guide for the identification of problematic family interactions is presented in Table 42-17.

Table 42-16 Avoidance of Conflict

Assessment Guide
Does the client . . .
Forget to say or do something that might generate disagreement or conflict with another?
Delay doing or saying something that might be rejected or be a source of disagreement with another?
Tell an uninvolved person about perceived problems or "hurt" feelings related to another person?
Change the subject when an issue comes up that would generate overt disagreement?
Fantasize, daydream, or concoct unrealistic ways of escaping a situation that cannot be or are never realized?
Tease and kid ("I was only fooling . . .") rather than own up to and support a statement with potential for conflict?
Take whatever comes his or her way willingly and smile even when there is obvious rejection, hostility, or imposed inconvenience because client is unwilling to "rock the boat"?
Agree to do something but never act?
Present self as fragile and easily intimidated?
Use tears or somatic complaints to respond to another's statements or demands or to avoid acting?
Respond to another's demands or requests with statements that cast self as a martyr or "good person" and the other as a "bad person" who is inconsiderate and ungrateful (intending to generate guilt in the other person)?
Say "we" to avoid taking a position that might elicit disagreement?

Table 42-17 Family Patterns

Assessment Guide
What behaviors does the family foster in the client?
Is the family relationship supportive or destructive of the client's effective efforts at coping?
How does the family handle conflict?
How does the family handle change?
How does the family handle feelings?
How are needs being met within the family?
How does the family relate to the staff?
Does the family need information or support?
What is the family's perception of the health problem and its implications?
How does the family make decisions?
Does the client's health problem reflect a family pattern?

Table 42-18 Environmental Patterns

Assessment Guide
What stressful factors are present in the physical environment (light, temperature, noise, odors, technology)?
What is the level of sensory input?
What is the response of care givers to the client?
What is the degree of environmental flexibility?
Are care givers sensitive to client's "need to know" and to participate in his or her own care?
How do care givers deal with feelings and their behavioral manifestations?
What are the care givers' perceptions of the causes for the client's illness and distress?
Is the client's source of emotional, social, and economic support threatened by this health problem?
How predictable or unpredictable is the environment?

Assessment of the Environment

Patterns of person-environment interaction influence the development, maintenance, and resolution of stress-related problems. A guide for the assessment of these patterns of interaction is presented in Table 42-18.

Diagnosis

Once a holistic data base is assembled, it must be analyzed and conceptualized. The result of these processes is the formulation of nursing diagnoses. These diagnoses reflect the client's unmet needs and problematic interactions that influence the development and maintenance of stress-related health problems. The following are nursing diagnoses appropriate to clients with stress-related health problems:

- Anxiety associated with inability to use problem-solving skills as a means of coping with stress
- Depression associated with the failure to mobilize effective cognitive coping skills
- Respiratory distress associated with conflictual relationship with parents
- Unrealistic "workaholic" schedule related to a need to avoid dealing with feelings
- Obesity related to the use of overeating to relieve depression
- Persistent purge-and-binge eating pattern related to inflexibility and inability to use cognitive restructuring
- Hypertensive episode associated with conflict avoidance
- Generalized pruritus associated with recent multiple changes
- Loneliness related to inadequate social skills
- Chronic psychogenic pain associated with low self-esteem
- Unrealistic expectations of self and others related to impaired ability to engage in cognitive restructuring
- Life-threatening, food-restricting diet associated with impaired ability to develop alternative ways of coping with developmental changes

Outcome Criteria

The number of potential or actual stressors and their intensity are examined to determine which can be prevented, modified, or eliminated to lessen the demands on the client and promote effective coping. The person's previous and present coping patterns provide data on how stress is managed and suggest areas that need modification. The roots of dysfunctional neuroendocrine responses go deep into the client's past, and behavior patterns tend to be entrenched. Therefore, changes may be small, slow, and almost imperceptible. Goals that are realistic and useful in evaluating care must reflect this very gradual, step-by-step process of change.

In many instances the nurse helps the client to initiate the process of change. It is the client who must, over time, work on modifying lifestyle, perceptions, and the environment. Motivation to change is an important, complicated, and problematic issue. A first step toward resolving the issue of motivation is to determine the client's needs, the ways in which they are satisfied, and what alternative, functional ways of meeting them may be available. All behavior, functional and dysfunctional, satisfies needs. The nurse's perception of the client's problems and priorities for the fulfillment of needs may not agree with the client's perception. From the nurse's viewpoint, the emaciated anorectic adolescent has a primary need for adequate nutrition, but to the adolescent, the need to manage the fear of obesity or to be dependent has priority. Therefore, the nurse must also determine which needs take priority for the client. If primary needs are satisfied, then the needs that the nurse sees as important for the restoration of health will emerge.

Examples of nursing outcomes include the following:

1. Client will exhibit flexibility. Evidence:
   a. Exploring new ways to meet needs
   b. Changing from activity that is problematic to one that is rewarding
2. Client will use effective problem-solving and coping mechanisms. Evidence:
   a. Identifying options
   b. Making alternative plans
   c. Projecting possible outcomes
   d. Negotiating with others to get what is needed or wanted
   e. Compromising to get some aspect of what is needed or wanted
3. Client will exhibit effective coping with anxiety (generated by mismanagement of stress). Evidence:
   a. Labeling feelings as *anxiety*
   b. Making connection between anxiety and physical tension
   c. Making connection between physical tension and increased arthritic pain
   d. Exploring alternative perceptions of stress-inducing situation as partially related to own expectations
   e. Identifying positive and negative aspects of a stressful situation
4. Client will exhibit effective management of stress after myocardial infarction. Evidence:
   a. Developing interest outside workplace
   b. Using relaxation technique daily
   c. Pacing work schedule within realistic limitations
   d. Limiting assumption of responsibility

Interventions

People encounter stress from many sources throughout their lives. The inevitability of stress is unquestioned. However, stress may be growth-promoting rather than destructive if a person is able to cope effectively. Stress becomes destructive when coping is not directed at effectively managing, lessening, or eliminating the stressors. Mismanagement leads to biopsychosocial dysfunction. Mismanagement may be caused in part by deficient or nonexistent social supports and by an impaired ability to acquire and maintain a social support system. Nursing interventions related to altering patterns of mismanaging stress are directed toward promotion, maintenance, restoration, and rehabilitation of health.

Levels of Intervention

PROMOTION OF HEALTH (PREVENTION). Prevention has great importance in the area of psychobiological dysfunction. This level of intervention is directed primarily at the family, the growth and development of the individual, and the prevention of dysfunctional neuroendocrine responses. Therefore, the more functional the family, the better able it will be to provide a milieu that is conducive to the effective management of stress.

Prenatal care which maximizes maternal health and adaptation influences the child's neuroendocrine development and later functioning. Maternal stress level during pregnancy influences circulating hormones in the fetus. These hormones, particularly norepinephrine, may help to organize and accelerate fetal neuroendocrine processes, increasing responsivity to stress-inducing stimuli. The process of birth may also have a profound impact on how the person interacts with the environment throughout life. A serene birth process may influence the neuroendocrine system in ways that enhance physiological coping with external stressors.

The process of forming attachments and the ongoing relationship of the child to family members are basic to helping the child mediate the stresses that will be encountered throughout life. A healthy family system helps the child develop a positive self-concept, self-esteem, effective coping patterns, the ability to perceive and interact realistically with the environment, and the ability to engage in effective problem solving and decision making.

Nursing interventions include teaching, counseling, role modeling, and supporting activities directed toward helping the family develop healthy patterns of interaction. There are several significant factors in the development of effective relational patterns supportive of an emotionally healthy family system.[142] Nurses intervene with families to facilitate the development of the following healthy characteristics:

1. A climate which encourages members to reach out and to expect caring, support, and empathy
2. A climate in which it is safe and acceptable to talk about feelings
3. The acceptance of conflict, disagreement, and differing views as a part of family life
4. Assumption of responsibility by each member for his or her own feelings, thoughts, and actions
5. Firmly established and maintained gender and generation boundaries; parental coalition and complementarity that support these boundaries and defend against emotionally charged alliances with children, particularly those of the opposite sex
6. The capacity to tolerate personal autonomy of members, differentiation, and the separation of the children from the family in a gradual way that is appropriate to each child's developmental age
7. The judicious use of parental power, and use of logical limit setting and negotiation rather than authoritarianism
8. Effective problem solving and decision making
9. Recognition, acknowledgement, and acceptance of complex motivations for behavior
10. Respect for family and individual initiative as reflected in the ability of members to reach out to the community constructively and become involved, and to have many interests and relationships outside the family.

Health-promotive interventions directed toward the adult population need to address the increasing awareness that multiple life changes predispose people to illness and need to help people explore options for stabilizing their lives through ongoing, effective management of stress. Anticipation of inevitable life changes allows for preparation. Interventions need to help people identify projected changes such as the physical signs of aging, separation of children, and the impact of societal trends on the workplace. Clients need to learn strategies that will help them control their environment and the number of stressors they must cope with at any given time.

Emotional coping strategies have biopsychosocial consequences. People who do not express emotions verbally and whose emotions intensify with time are at risk of expressing these emotions through stress-related illnesses.[12] Some theorists encourage open expression of emotions as a path to psychological well-being.[143,144] Such a recommendation is not appropriate for all people, since each person is unique. For some people, the expression of some emotions, particularly strongly negative emotions such as anger, may in and of itself be highly stressful. Person-environment interaction in the expression of emotions must be considered. Expression of feelings must be considered in terms of relevance, appropriateness, and the ability of the object of the feelings to tolerate their expression at a particular time. Otherwise, the expression may aggravate an already problematic situation. Is the expression appropriate to the relationship with the person who will receive it? Is the feeling expressed appropriate to the time, place, and person? Is the receiver, at that time, able to cope with the expression of feelings, or is the receiver too vulnerable? Will the ventilation of the feelings or emotions result in a desired change? Will the expression of feelings and emotions be a useful catharsis, or will it escalate emotions and generate a more painful feeling such as guilt?

Avenues for emotional release are needed by those who suppress and channel the discharge of emotions through physical symptoms. The approach to helping clients with this emotional release must be individualized and must take environmental interactions into consideration. The effective expression of feelings requires a thoughtful appraisal of the situation, the people involved, the appropriateness, and the consequences.

MAINTENANCE OF HEALTH. Nursing interventions directed toward health maintenance include those taken to weaken the impact of an inevitable situation which is potentially or actually stressful. A person's perception of an event is a significant mediating factor in the impact of the stressor.

Research indicates that when people are warned of and prepared for stressful events such as pain, change, or conflict and given sufficient realistic reassurance, fear may be controlled and will be less likely to generate an acute emotional disturbance.[145,146,147] Nursing interventions that effectively prepare people for potentially stressful events include these:

- Interfere with the person's spontaneous efforts to ward off total awareness of the impending threat; this will help the person use cognitive strategies for anticipating and coping with the event.
- Provide information that gives a realistic but not fear-inducing picture of the impending situation.
- Provide information in "titrated doses"; the gradual presentation of information allows the person to contain anxiety and use a cognitive problem-solving approach.

When the person's knowledge base is inadequate and perceptions concerning an inevitable impending stressful event are absent or distorted, anxiety and tension increase. By maximizing realistic communications, the nurse can assess the person's perception of the event, provide the requisite information that helps the person structure (or give meaning to) the event and understand its ramifications, and help the person identify the most effective way of coping with the event. For example clients who must undergo surgery or a painful procedure are better able to handle their anxiety if they are given just enough information about what the procedure will be like and how it will affect them but are not overwhelmed by graphic descriptions which would elicit fear.

The nurse can also manage the environment so as to minimize external stressful stimuli such as noise, light, and interpersonal contacts. Reduction of environmental stressors conserves the person's energy and facilitates the coping process.

Prevention of potential disability is a primary nursing concern when a health problem exists. Threats can become challenges that can be mastered. The circumstances that facilitate people's perceptions of their health problems as challenges and nursing interventions that promote these circumstances are presented in Table 42-19.

Early identification of emerging dysfunctional patterns provides opportunities for preventive intervention. For example, anorexia nervosa is on the increase. Early recognition and intervention may stop the development of chronic eating disorders.

RESTORATION AND REHABILITATION OF HEALTH. Restorative and rehabilitative nursing interventions are directed toward relief of acute or chronic stress. People in stressful situations may feel that no solution is available. They may blame themselves and thus not be motivated to act on their own behalf, believing that the distress they are experiencing is a punishment for past misdeeds. In some instances the only solutions they are able to envision seem more threatening and devastating than the stress they are experiencing. In such instances the nurse can help these people examine the situation, identify alternative solutions, explore the consequences of these alternatives, and accept feelings without guilt or fear. A coronary client who has followed a fast-paced work schedule with no time out for rest or relaxation or a client with cancer who has lost a loved person may see the situation as one that cannot be changed. Exploration of alternatives may help such a client learn how to identify and examine new ways of coping.

When people have difficulty expressing their feelings and perceptions, nurses use a variety of communication techniques and actively listen to what is related in an accepting and empathic manner.

Personal Change

People suffering from psychophysiological disorders often need to alter their lifestyles and ways of relating to others. In order to change basic values, attitudes, and behavior, one must go through a change process which is demanding and time-consuming. These people often resist recognizing the need to change and to engage in a process of change.

Mastery of destructive stress requires more than a repertoire of patchwork activities. It is an active process which is responsive over time to ever-changing environmental demands. These demands are often ambiguous and intangible, since they arise out of the social fabric and climate.

Effective stress management may require some people to make a commitment to an exercise

Table 42-19 Translating Threats into Challenges

Issue	Nursing Intervention
Noxious environmental influences	Neutralize these influences: Direct manipulation of circumstances in behalf of the client. Help the client to recognize these influences and explore ways of altering them.
Negative events and realities	Facilitate (depending on the point in time) avoidance, denial, toleration, replacement, or acceptance: Support denial when the person is in physiological crisis. Explore the ramifications of the disruption gradually. Help the person identify and use strengths and resources. Help the person identify and explore alternatives. Help the person formulate a realistic perception of the situation. Help the person gain ego strength and satisfaction from the use of existing potentials.
Impaired self-image	Facilitate the development of a positive self-image: Help the person focus on strengths and accomplishments rather than on losses and disabilities. Help the person clarify the values associated with the self-image. Help the person formulate values which enhance a revised self-image.
Emotional disequilibrium	Facilitate the recognition of emotions (depression, fear, anxiety, and anger) and develop ways of managing them effectively: Reinforce the notion that such feelings are normal responses to situations of threat, loss, change, and conflict.
Emotional disequilibrium (continued)	Encourage ventilation of feelings. Help the person relate feelings to particular situations and symptoms. Help the person become hopeful in relation to the management of feelings. Help the person explore ways of discharging emotional states. Help the person begin to define boundaries of and responsibility for self in order to prevent or lessen the influence of another's emotionality. Help the person verbalize own perceptions, thoughts, and feelings and accept them as valid. Help the person make a distinction between his or her needs and wishes and those of another.
Perceived lack of a social support system	Facilitate the client's recognition of and effective utilization of a support system: Use genogram as a tool for identifying potential sources of support. Encourage the person to connect with family members and friends. Encourage the person to ask clearly and directly for what is needed. Identify resources and alternative people that can provide support. Help the person use initiative in contacting potential resources and assessing how they can be useful. Help the person recognize that by being the recipient of help, he or she is also giving.

program, a diet, or modified work habits. Others may need to learn and practice social skills or to develop a social support system. Expectations for oneself and others may need to be revised or given up. Whatever the change, it will not be easy. There will be a need for support and motivation. Nurses need to work collaboratively and supportively with the client and significant others throughout the change process.

Change is a complex phenomenon. It is difficult to accomplish because multiple interacting influential forces are involved. The past and present interact in ways that are often unrecognized and therefore unchallenged. Important needs may be satisfied by perceptions and behaviors that disrupt self-regulatory patterns and cause dysfunction.

Change is a process that evolves across space and time. Progression through a change process is

Table 42-20 Change Process

Client's Task	Nursing Intervention
Step 1	
Recognize that the problem is serious enough to require a change.	Challenge the client's position that the problem is not serious.
Recognize that there are undesirable consequences in the present coping pattern that should be avoided.	Provide reality-based information on the severity of the consequences if no change is effected.
Consider the possibility that there are other, alternative ways of living, relating, and behaving.	Explore other alternatives and their consequences.
Step 2	
Experience doubt about the present coping pattern.	Point out the deleterious effects of present coping pattern.
Seek information about alternatives.	Provide data regarding alternatives.
Appraise alternatives from the standpoint of averting negative consequences.	Support examination of alternatives.
Discard alternatives which appear to be unsafe or too costly.	Assist client to examine consequences of alternatives—the risks and benefits.
Identify feasible alternatives.	
Step 3	
Examine pros and cons of feasible alternatives.	Assist client to identify the advantages and disadvantages.
Identify the alternative that meets realistic personal criteria.	Assist client to clarify how realistic his or her personal criteria are and the relevance and appropriateness of the selected alternative.
Step 3 (continued)	
Examine utilitarian gains or losses to the self and to significant others.	
Examine the possibility of approval or disapproval of significant others.	Help client explore impact of change on the self and significant others.
Examine whether there will be self-approval or disapproval.	
Step 4	
Decide to adopt change.	Support decision to change.
Tell others that client is going to adopt the selected alternative way of living, relating, or behaving.	Reassure client that change is possible. Support telling others to maximize commitment.
Implement the alternative.	Give positive feedback when change is implemented. Empathize regarding the difficulties expressed by client.
Step 5	
Confront whether persistence in change will be possible in face of problems encountered.	Assist client to employ a problem-solving approach when difficulties occur.
Examine negative social feedback, both covert and overt disapproval.	Explore perceptions that the change is not supported by significant others.
Examine expectations when they are not met.	Help client clarify the importance of negative social feedback. Help client to examine expectations.

not linear. It reflects a series of gains and setbacks and plateaus. The model presented in Table 42-20 provides guidelines for nursing involvement in helping people to change and criteria for assessing a client's progress using behaviors which reflect the various tasks in effecting change.

Nurses must keep in mind that they are only facilitators of the change process in the care-giving situation. Their role is to work *with* clients. The clients have the rights and responsibilities in relation to change. More important, nurses cannot be sensitive facilitators of change if they themselves are not personally involved in an ongoing change process directed toward personal growth and self-understanding.

SCHEMATA AND STRESS MANAGEMENT. A *schema* (plural, *schemata*) is a cognitive structure used to organize experience. It is an abstract representation of regularly occurring experiences that includes imagined plans for dealing with them. Schemata are constructed through interactions with the environment and are automatically activated by particular situations.[148] When the schema is one of hopelessness or passivity in stress-inducing situations, it must be changed, or effective coping will not occur. For example, in a stressful interpersonal situation a person may perceive himself or herself as a victim and see the predicament as hopeless. The perception of having no control over events or their impact on the self may increase the stress experienced. If the person tends to perceive many situations as beyond personal control, then a negative schema is operating and chronic stress characterized by hopelessness is likely to be present. The nurse-client relationship is a vehicle for helping people to revise their negative schemata through the following interventions:

- Facilitating an increased awareness of a schema and how it is influencing perception and behavior
- Helping the person identify and describe situations in which the schema is evoked and coping is impaired
- Exploring alternative views of provocative situations
- Encouraging the person to experiment with alternative ways of interacting with the environment
- Teaching the person assertiveness skills
- Helping the person analyze the use of modified or new schemata

FACILITATING SELF-MANAGEMENT. Self-management approaches to stress responses are derived from the "participant model" for health care. The argument in favor of this approach is based on the following points:[149]

Most behavior patterns are not easily accessible for modification except by the client.

Many problematic behavior patterns have associated thoughts, fantasies, and feelings that are inaccessible to all but the client.

Many people verbalize the desire to change problematic behavior patterns but are motivated only to alleviate present discomfort.

People need to develop self-managed assessment and coping skills to deal with future situations effectively.

Acceptance of responsibility and motivation to actively seek change are critical elements in self-management. A contract is a useful strategy for helping clients evolve self-management approaches. It helps both the client and the nurse to clarify a problem, a direction for resolution, and criteria for evaluating progress.

The initial work of the nurse with clients is directed toward helping the client recognize the necessity for change and develop clear personal objectives in relation to the change. The client needs to begin to clearly identify and delineate areas for cognitive and interpersonal action that will promote the behavioral change. Rewards reinforce the repetition of behaviors. In a self-management approach, the incentives and rewards used to reinforce new behaviors must be defined, assigned, and applied by the client and not by the nurse.

The nurse uses a negotiation model in helping clients through this process. The nurse serves as a sounding board for ideas, and asks thought-provoking questions. The role is one of consultant to the client in relation to the "how" of implementing change rather than prescribing the change and its implementation. Helping the client identify options and choices is a significant nursing role. This aspect of nursing intervention is important because people tend to become more highly motivated and more successful when:

They believe that they have responsibility for some action.

A successful outcome occurs because of personal competence.

Their behavior is voluntary and not controlled by external threats or rewards.

They have chosen among alternative courses of action.

The "how" of implementing change is not geared toward suggesting specifics; rather, it is directed toward helping the client use self-monitoring of behavior. Self-observations are measured against self-developed performance criteria. The nurse encourages the client to examine when and where these criteria have been met and uses the previously identified rewards. When criteria have not been met, the focus of interactions with the client is on using a problem-solving approach to identify obstacles and to seek ways to remove these obstacles.

A person who changes behavior patterns must contend with external environmental influences. Because of the continual presence of various obstructive environmental factors, the nurse needs to help clients establish favorable conditions for implementing the behavior change and developing self-control. A continuing series of decisions must be made to maintain the original commitment to the change. The nurse can help the client identify potential pitfalls and rehearse how to best deal with each so as to stick with the change. The nurse may initially need to provide extensive guidance and support in relation to the client's tasks of selecting and using strong reinforcing consequences, rearranging powerful contingencies that influence behavior, and tolerating temporary discomforts, dissatisfactions, and deprivations.

Self-management implies self-responsibility. The idea of personal responsibility for one's health problems is a difficult one for both care givers and clients to accept. As long as people see the source of the health problem as outside of the self, they will believe that they have no control over the problem. People tend to equate personal responsibility for their health problems with blame. Thus, accepting responsibility is seen as taking the blame for a situation—as having done something wrong. If one causes one's own disease, then one is guilty. Responsibility, however, is not blame; it is recognizing that one has control over one's life and body. Responsibility for one's health problem means first recognizing that the mind and body are mutually influential. It is difficult for both nurses and clients to ask themselves: "Why did I need to become ill at this time?" Health problems meet a need. Feelings and perceptions of one's life or present situations that predate the onset of a health problem reflect problematic conflicts, losses, and changes. The health problem is a solution to another problem. The mind, influencing the body, produces the "solution." Once this is understood, then the client can begin to see the possibility of using the mind to heal the self, and seek other solutions.

ATTAINING AND MAINTAINING PEACE OF MIND. Jampolsky[9] proposes that the development of love fosters internal peace and harmony. Healing, the maintenance of health, and sensitive nursing are functions of letting go of fear and other destructive emotions and allowing love to flourish. He proposes that people have been given everything that is needed to be happy. To be able to fully experience the moment for what it is without the overlay of past fears and anxieties is to be at peace. Personal fulfillment, which is a part of inner peace, lies within the person. However, people tend to think that personal worth and satisfaction are dependent on external symbols and people. Jampolsky proposes that to achieve peace of mind, people need to let go of past belief systems and associated fears and resentment and to practice living within the reality of the present moment.

To begin to live in the present and exert freedom of choice over one's life one needs to believe that:[24]

> Forgiveness is the way to achieve peace of mind.
>
> One can *choose* to live in the present and let go of old fears by putting a halt to being critical and judgmental, and by not projecting the past into the future.
>
> One can *choose* to learn to accept direction from the inner self and give up listening to fear-based directions that come from the past.
>
> A commitment can be made to a personal goal even when there is no readily apparent way of achieving it.
>
> One can *choose* how an event is perceived and how one will feel about the event.
>
> One can *choose* to see someone who is attacking or critical as being afraid and thus not a threat to the self.

Forgiveness is an integral part of learning how to love oneself and others and of achieving peace of mind. It is letting go of the past and the misperceptions of the present that reflect past fears. It means using selective forgetting to let go of beliefs about what we think we have done in the past that generated guilt feelings and what we believe others have done to us that generates fear and resentments.[9] People tend to believe that what one gives away one loses. What often goes unrecognized is that one must give in order to receive. Forgiving and giving do not mean that one stands above and dispenses forgiveness and love to others below, nor do they represent a martyrlike toleration of another. They are part of "generosity of the moment."[9]

The nurse needs to help clients find ways to let go of obstructive belief systems, the need to control and predict, and the old guilts and fears that are being continually recycled. Clients need encouragement to experiment with giving and forgiving.

To help clients let go of the past, nurses must help clients explore their perceptions, thoughts, and values. The client may need help to look at past decisions not as bad decisions but as the best decisions that could be made at that time.[150]

The nurse and the client must also stop and examine statements such as: "He makes me angry";

"I feel unhappy when you . . ."; "She hurt my feelings when . . ." Each of these statements reflects the perception that another *makes* one happy, unhappy, angry, or sad. One experiences these feelings in a situation because one chooses to perceive and to feel that the other person is a cause. People need to think about the fact that they *choose* the way they define situations and the way they will feel about them. Once there is recognition of the fact that a choice is made, people can explore alternative choices that lead to other perceptions and feelings. People become immobilized by believing that a situation cannot be changed. The first step toward becoming unstuck is to fantasize about what would happen if the situation changed, and if one acted differently.

RESISTANCE TO CHANGE. People who have become dysfunctional because of excessive stress in their lives, their mismanagement of stress, their inability to cope effectively, or any combination of these factors need to recognize the need to change and to cooperate with a therapeutic regimen. Resistant behavior may take many forms. Clients may openly reject a treatment program or covertly sabotage its implementation. Some clients terminate treatment prematurely, while others cooperate only partially. Forgetting, making up complex alibis and excuses, or proposing alternatives that are less demanding and effective may be used to avoid involvement in activities that promote health.

Nursing interventions that reduce or remove resistance include:

- Increasing the person's awareness that an actual or potential health problem exists
- Helping the person believe that the diagnosis of the problem is accurate
- Helping the person believe that the health problem is a threat and that harm will come if it is not treated or if personal changes do not occur
- Helping the person believe that the prescribed treatment or suggested changes will help
- Helping the person believe that the benefits of the prescribed treatment or suggested changes outweigh the risk, discomfort, or inconvenience
- Identifying and recruiting resources to support the person through the process of change and cooperation with the treatment regimen

Further nursing interventions and the theories from which they are derived are presented in Table 42-21 (page 894).

MANAGING EMOTIONS DURING A CHANGE. When a person becomes aware of a health problem and is told of the changes needed, he or she often experiences feelings of anxiety, depression, and anger. If these feelings are not recognized by the care givers and worked with, then they may obstruct the client's ability to develop health-promotive behavior. Care givers often immediately focus on the desired changes and the education related to what must be done and how and why the changes in lifestyle must be implemented. Clients need this information; however, knowing or having insight does not automatically alter behavior. Required changes generate feelings and inevitably result in losses that must be worked through.

Feelings are an important dimension of behavioral change. They may obstruct compliance if clients are unaware of them or suppress them. Many people believe that one must not talk about or express negative emotions. When such a situation occurs, nurses need to facilitate the ventilation of these feelings. Modeling is a useful facilitating mechanism. The nurse, may say to the client, "If I were in your shoes, I would be feeling angry about . . . , sad about . . . , or confused about what I should do first." Such a statement acknowledges that feelings do occur in relation to life events, and—more important—that it is acceptable to talk about feelings with another person.

Some clients deny, rationalize, or distort reality in an attempt to defend against awareness of risks or symptoms. They may fail to hear what has been explained to them by care givers or to follow through on suggestions. When this happens, the nurse assesses whether these defenses are useful to the client at that particular time. If they are useful defenses, efforts to alter them are postponed. If the defenses are obstructive, then interventions which help the person feel secure, hopeful, and able to cope may lessen the need for their use.

Sundberg[151] points out that obese people in a weight-reduction program grieved for the loss of foods which were of great psychological and emotional value to them. Initially these people persistently discussed foods and eating and tended to be depressed. Food and eating had become so highly

Table 42-21 Nursing Interventions and Theories: Resistance to Change

Theory	Nursing Intervention
Cognitive dissonance: Proposes that people are motivated to act in ways consistent with their beliefs, values, and perceptions. When there is inconsistency between behavior and beliefs, values, and perceptions, people experience cognitive dissonance and are motivated to change.	1. Provide information about the nature of the health problem. 2. Provide information about proposed treatment: the rationale for choosing it and a detailed description of the treatment process. 3. Provide information about the desired outcome, side effects, and benefits. 4. Point out to the client problems associated with current coping. 5. Point out how current coping compounds problems. 6. Encourage the client to compare consequences of current coping and more effective coping. 7. Generate doubt about effectiveness of current coping through discussion of past and present problems. 8. Explore with the client alternative ways of coping. 9. Encourage the client to experiment with more effective coping.
Attribution: Proposes that a person formulates an idea about the causation of events. Logical devices are used to explain why a phenomenon occurs.	1. Help the client estimate the nature of the threat to life inherent to noncompliance. 2. Help the client recognize the probability that a health problem will be compounded unless there is compliance with treatment regimen. 3. Help the client recognize the severity of the situation. 4. Help the client identify ways of preventing, lessening, or resolving a health problem. 5. Explore with the client gains and losses associated with compliance and noncompliance.
Social reinforcement: Proposes that behavior is modified by its consequences. Consequences either increase or decrease the probability that a particular behavior will occur again.	1. Give the client positive feedback when compliance occurs. 2. Help client identify self-administered rewards for compliance. 3. Establish reward system for compliance that enhances self-esteem and personal control. 4. Prompt client to identify and use desired behavior. 5. Help client recognize gain derived from desired behavior. 6. Deliver reinforcements immediately, contingently, and consistently when desired behavior is exhibited. 7. Gradually decrease external prompting and reinforcement.
Interoceptive conditioning: Proposes that reinforcers arise from within the person (nausea, decreased libido, tachycardia) and cause conditioning. The conditioned learning influences behavior.	1. Help client recognize the relationship between noncompliance and side effects from treatments (chemotherapy, radiation, antihypertensives). 2. Teach client to use a relaxation exercise or meditation to cope with unpleasant side effects. 3. Help client anticipate changes related to side effects of treatment and take steps to lessen the impact of the changes.

SOURCE: I. Barofsky, "Sociological and Psychological Aspects of Medication Compliance," in I. Barofsky, ed., *Medication Compliance: A Behavioral Management Approach*, Slack, Thorofare, N.J., 1977, pp. 29–44.

valued that they might actually be considered a love object with special symbolic meaning. The deprivation incurred by dieting represented the loss of a significant source of need gratification.

One cannot alter lifestyle or change behavior without incurring losses. Recognizing a grieving process provides direction for nursing interventions. The client is encouraged to talk about the losses that have resulted from the behavior change. The nurse acknowledges the "normality" of feeling anxious, depressed, and angry and helps the client to see these feelings as part of the process of letting go of old ways and learning new ways of behaving. If clients are helped to understand the reasons for these feelings and to ventilate their feelings and thus tolerate them, compliance will be facilitated.

When people are kept waiting for appointments for extended periods of time or when they see different care givers at each appointment, they are less likely to keep appointments and less likely to understand their situation and comply with recommendations. Therefore, health care settings need to establish a schedule for appointments that minimizes the time a client must spend in either the waiting room or the examining room. Time must be allowed for each client to talk about concerns privately. When nurses appear rushed and the focus of their interactions with clients is on the physical aspects of care, significant psychological determinants of compliance may be overlooked.

The family may support either compliant or noncompliant behavior. Family members need accurate information about how they can be helpful to the client. In some instances, dysfunctional family dynamics may interfere with the client's compliance. If the family needs a member in a sick role to maintain intrafamily dynamic equilibrium, multilateral forces may be unconsciously exerted to maintain the client in this role. Unconscious sabotage may be used to sustain the client in the sick role.

Increasing family members' awareness about how the family operates is a first step toward resolving family interference. Fears as well as underdeveloped capacities to manage conflict and change must also be addressed. Helping the family to talk about the way it operates and providing feedback will help the family increase its awareness. As with the individual, however, significant needs are satisfied through the existing operations. Unless equally satisfying alternatives are tested, change will not occur.

Helping the lonely can be a frustratingly slow process. The nurse needs to help these people recognize their participation in the development of loneliness, and encourage them to experiment with relationship behaviors. Successful supported experiments with these relationship behaviors may positively reinforce their continued use.

Individual therapy and group therapy are useful therapeutic modalities for these people. Each provides human contact and opportunities to share feelings, practice new behaviors, and recognize that fears, fantasies, and feelings are not unique.

The nurse helps clients with this work by providing information and feedback that emphasize the need to practice interest, patience, and concern for others. By questioning and doubting the usefulness of having expectations of others, the client is encouraged to experiment with operating without these expectations. These efforts combined with efforts to attain and maintain peace of mind help these people move out of a chronic state of loneliness that contributes to the development and maintenance of health problems.

To learn to love is never easy, because it involves constant change. The person must be helped to invest time and energy in accepting and appreciating the self—to love the self. The nurse can help people accept these activities as growth-promotive rather than as selfish. Appreciating and valuing self-discovery and one's own uniqueness are prerequisites to appreciating others and giving love. Since neither can occur within superficial, temporary relationships, the nurse needs to encourage these clients to reconnect with people with whom they have had a viable relationship, and, more important, to work on existing relationships so that they become stable and long-lasting. These people need help to become sensitive to other people's needs, and develop the ability to give to others to help them meet their needs. Most important, they need to learn how to ask for help and take risks connected with being dependent on others.[150]

A long-term nurse-client relationship is a useful vehicle for helping these clients begin to experience trust in a relationship. Within the context of the nurse-client relationship the client practices relationship behavior. The nurse provides feedback that helps and encourages the client to transfer to social relationships the ability to participate in the therapeutic relationship.

CONFLICT RESOLUTION. The nurse can help clients develop more effective ways of managing interpersonal conflicts with family members and with people in work and social contexts. People who attempt to avoid problematic conflicts through denial and a variety of avoidance behaviors need to:

1. Recognize the existence of the conflict
2. Recognize the impact on health of the avoided conflict
3. Explore fears and fantasies about what would happen if the conflict were confronted
4. Identify the sources of these fears and fantasies and the basis of each in reality
5. Take self-responsibility in situations rather than blame or avoid

The nurse helps the client through this initial phase by providing realistic feedback about conflict avoidance as a chronic stressor and the problems created by residual resentments when one loses a conflict by default. Each of the client's fears and fantasies also needs to be addressed in relation to its basis in reality. These clients need to verbalize the worst thing and best thing that could happen if they did face up to the conflict. Throughout the process, these people need support, empathy, genuine concern, respect, and realistic reassurance. The nurse needs to recognize and accept the fact that those clients have learned to avoid conflict. The learning may have taken place throughout their early lives within the family, or it may be the consequence of aversive conditioning. The avoidance of conflict may be deeply ingrained, and changing this style of operating may be a slow and difficult process. It may mean much more besides altering manifest behavior if, in changing, the person violates basic family and cultural norms and rules.

Once one recognizes and accepts the need to change the style of dealing with conflict, skills in acting in one's own behalf must be learned. Assertiveness training can provide useful skills that can be valuable to the client in other interpersonal situations as well.

The target behaviors the nurse encourages and supports include those which reflect taking an "I" position and a problem-solving approach to conflict. The development and application of these behaviors in various family, social, and work situations can be facilitated in the nurse-client relationship. Role playing and rehearsing can be used by the nurse with the client to help the latter practice these new behaviors. It may be useful if the client practices using assertive statements in imaginary situations and also practices using these statements while playing the role of the other person. The nurse can also model the desired behavior for the client to imitate in the nurse-client relationship as well as in other situations.

PROMOTING RELAXATION. People who wish to prevent or more effectively manage stress-related health problems benefit from relaxation exercises. Nurses can teach these exercises and encourage clients to use them on a regular basis.

The nurse needs to advise clients to prepare for these exercises by assuming a comfortable position in a quiet environment. The client is told to select some neutral, peaceful, or pleasant thought or object and to focus full attention upon it while at the same time maintaining a passive attitude. The client is told to ignore environmental distractions by shifting attention back to the preselected thought or object.[152]

Recognizing the opposing feelings of tension and relaxation is important to being able to relax. Alternate tensing and relaxing of large muscle groups is a way of developing this recognition.[152] Initially the nurse coaches the client to begin by taking several deep abdominal respirations and to exclude unpleasant thoughts. The client is then told to tighten in sequence the following muscle groups: dominant hand and arm, nondominant hand and arm, facial muscles, shoulders and upper torso, abdominal, and legs and feet. The client is instructed to tense the muscles from 5 to 7 seconds and relax them for 20 to 30 seconds.[152] Following completion of the muscle tensing and relaxing, the person is told to sit quietly and to focus attention on the preselected thought or object.

Disorder-Specific Interventions

CORONARY HEART DISEASE. People with coronary heart disease need to alter their perceptions and style of operating and learn more effective ways of dealing with the stress in their lives. Participation in cardiac rehabilitation programs is a function of the ability and motivation to comply with recommendations. To enhance compliance with these programs, diets, and exercises, the nurse may encourage these clients and their families to participate in group psychotherapy, self-help groups, individual counseling, and behavior-modification programs.[153]

Early involvement with "resource people" related to work analysis, preparing for return to work, and retraining have been found to be related to both successful rehabilitation and a positive emotional state. People not provided with assistance frequently return to work too soon and experience physical and psychological problems. They also are more vulnerable to lack of confidence, financial worries, and depression. The nurse may need to take the initiative in helping clients gain access to resources by recommending and making referrals to occupational-vocational counselors and social workers.[153]

These people also benefit from group interventions. The support derived from the group experiences appears to be ego-strengthening. Ventilation of feelings and sharing help in realistic future planning. When significant family members are included, they are also provided with opportunities for support and for evolving a more realistic perception of the client's status. They are helped to recognize and respect personal boundaries, which allow the client and themselves to become self-responsible. This helps stabilize interpersonal relationships and facilitates health-promotive personal growth and health-promotive relationships. Behavior-modification programs have been used successfully to change type A behavior patterns. These programs help people learn to identify physical and psychological stress, to rehearse alternative ways of coping using visual imagery, to experiment with these alternatives, and to examine related difficulties. Behavior-modification techniques using relaxation responses have also been used to treat arrhythmias that are a threat to life.[154,155]

ANOREXIA NERVOSA. Resolution of anorexia nervosa may need to occur in two phases if a threat to life exists. Phase 1 addresses severe life-threatening malnutrition and is directed toward reestablishing a nutritionally adequate eating pattern. This phase of treatment usually occurs in the general hospital setting. Nursing measures are directed toward the client's undernutrition, dehydration, electrolyte imbalance, sleep disturbances, fatigue, difficulty in concentrating, obsessive ruminations about food, and resistance to the program as evidenced by surreptitious and manipulative behavior.[156]

A strict behavior-modification program (Tables 42-22 and 42-23) is used.[156] Examples of the restrictions imposed during phase 1 of the program are presented in Table 42-22. The program imposes social isolation and the deprivation of pleasurable activities. Progressive weight gain is rewarded by a stepwise granting of visitors, access to television, radio, stereo, and so on. Nurses restrict their interventions to those of a technical nature. Communication with the client is utilitarian, and not facilitative or supportive. Only when these clients show a weight gain may the nurse interact on a facilitative level. Relationship time with the nurse is used as a reward for weight gain.

Phase 2 begins following the resolution of the

Table 42-22 Anorexia Nervosa: A Behavior-Modification Program (Phase 1)

Restrictions
Until target weight is attained, client . . .
Is not allowed out of bed
Has no bathroom privileges
Is segregated from other clients
Must submit to daily weighings
May eat only food provided during allotted time
Must clean up own vomitus
May have no visits from friends
May have only limited visits from family members
May have only limited interactions with staff members

Table 42-23 Anorexia Nervosa: A Behavior-Modification Program (Phase 2)

Recognizing and Respecting Personal Boundaries
Encourage client and family members to verbalize thoughts, perceptions, and feelings.
Point out areas where the client and a family member disagree.
Emphasize the uniqueness of each person's viewpoint and the right of each to maintain his or her position.
Check out each person's perception of what another has said to reinforce listening skills.
Emphasize with client and family members the importance of using "I" and taking responsibility for self.
Facilitate the definition of areas for client self-responsibility and self-regulation.
Facilitate the client's self-control of these areas.
Support the client's attempts at self-determination.
Provide the parents with information concerning developmental needs of their adolescent daughter's or son's gradual separation, self-responsibility, and self-determination.
Provide parents with opportunity to ventilate fears and anxieties about their child's well-being and provide realistic reassurance.
Provide sex education to client when evidence of fantasized fears and misinformation is present.
Redirect conflicts related to the issue of control between client and parents away from food onto developmental issues related to curfews, school activities, etc.

acute threat to life. Improving nutrition continues to be a concern. Realistic feedback and education enhance the behavior-modification program. However, engagement of both the anorectic and the family in therapy is a primary interest during this phase. Dysfunctional intrafamily communication and relationship patterns and controversial issues are addressed. This phase begins during hospitalization and continues after discharge either to an inpatient psychiatric facility or to the client's home. Nursing interventions which facilitate change are presented in Table 42-23.

Alternative Approaches to Stress Management

Stress management is becoming a societal concern. Many people are seeking ways to better manage their lives, their internal milieu, and the external environment with which they interact. Scientists are studying a wide variety of untraditional approaches to promoting health, as well as preventing and remedying health problems. A holistic approach to health problems encompasses the interaction between the person as a unified whole and the environment. The emphasis of this approach is on harmony within the self and with both the physical and the human environment. Increasing awareness of self and of one's physiological processes are important aspects of a holistic approach to health care (see Chapter 25).

The nurse's role in relation to various alternatives such as the use of visual imagery, meditation, hypnosis, biofeedback, and autogenic training includes the following activities:

1. Inform clients and their families that these alternatives exist.
2. Describe the alternatives.
3. Provide information about the advantages and disadvantages of each.
4. Provide information about where these interventions can be obtained.
5. Help clients and their families analyze the usefulness of each alternative and clarify their feelings about each.

Evaluation

Evaluation is a necessary component of the nursing process. The effectiveness of nursing interventions must be determined to make sure that goals have been met. Purposeful assessment of effectiveness includes not only observations made by the care giver but also assessment of documentation by others involved in the care and, most important, subjective validation by the client and family. Long- and short-term outcome criteria are examined in light of assessment data on the client's present status. Evidence that outcome criteria are not adequately met indicates that the situation must be reassessed, further planning initiated, and alternative interventions identified. The client and family are included in this process to increase the possibility that outcome criteria will be successfully met by the revised plan and identified interventions.

An example of the full application of the nursing process in a case of stress mismanagement (anorexia nervosa) is presented in Table 42-24.

SUMMARY

The mismanagement of stress is a pandemic health problem related to anxiety, conflict, and change. It is associated with the development of a wide variety of illnesses, sudden death, and proneness to pain, accidents, and surgery. The patterns of interaction of the person's mind, body, and spirit, within the context of past and present experiences, and the person's family and environment are important factors in the management of stress. Various coping resources are available to people and used by them.

Stress-induced respiratory, skin, gastrointestinal, endocrine, cardiovascular, immune, and autoimmune disorders are related to the mismanagement of stress and the existence of dysynchronous family and environmental patterns of interaction. Dysynchronous eating patterns associated with anorexia nervosa, bulimia, pica, and obesity are also related to these.

The application of the nursing process to clients experiencing stress-related health problems focuses on low self-esteem, loneliness, impaired coping, and the mismanagement of change and conflict. Nurses assess these characteristics of the person as well as family and environmental patterns of interaction. They form diagnoses and establish outcome criteria for clients. Nursing interventions for the promotion, restoration, and rehabilitation

Table 42-24 Full Application of the Nursing Process (during Hospitalization and after Discharge): Anorexia Nervosa

Assessment	Nursing Diagnosis	Outcome Criteria	Nursing Intervention	Evaluation
Stage 1				
Cachectic appearance. Profound weight loss. Food-intake restriction. Dehydration. Fluid and electrolyte imbalance. Secret self-induced vomiting. Excessive laxative use. Hoards rather than consumes food. Excessive secretive exercising. Perceives self as fat.	Life-threatening weight loss associated with self-starvation and delusions about body size	Adequate nutritional status. Evidence: a. No dehydration b. Rebalanced electrolytes c. Cessation of self-induced vomiting d. Cessation of laxative abuse e. Consumption of food at mealtime. f. Cessation of food hoarding g. Progressive weight gain h. Accurate perception of body size	Monitor during and after mealtime. Until required pounds are gained, the following restrictions are enforced: a. Remain in bed b. No bathroom privileges c. No peer or extended-family visitors d. Parental visiting on Sundays, 2–4 p.m. only e. No radio, TV, cassette player f. No socializing with other clients or staff members g. No phone calls Weigh daily.	Fluid and electrolyte balance restored. Complies with daily weigh-ins. Ceases self-induced vomiting. Ceases laxative abuse because of unavailability. Hoards food day after parental visiting. Uses bedpan but complains. Still sees self as fat. Family violates visiting restrictions. Monitoring required to keep client from socializing. Periodic plateaus in weight gain. Violates bed restriction to exercise vigorously. Eats only part of each meal.
Stage 2*				
Violates bed restriction to exercise vigorously. Periodic plateaus in weight gain. Monitoring still required to keep client from socializing. Still sees self as fat. Hoards food.	Treatment resistance related to misperception of body size and nutritional status	Restoration of nutritional status and body weight. Evidence: a. Limiting physical exercise voluntarily b. Finishing all meals c. Progressive weight gain d. Cessation of food hoarding e. Recognition of drastic underweight status f. Following restrictions	Continuous observation. Maintenance of restrictions. Give feedback on thinness during daily weigh-ins. Reinforce target weight for age and height. Enforce no exercising.	Requests permission to walk around room, visit with other clients, and have stereo brought in from home. Fails to recognize cachectic appearance. Ceases exercising. Ceases food hoarding. Progressive weight gain.
Stage 3*				
Adheres to restrictions. Substantial progressive weight gain. Still fails to see self as thin.	Adherence to treatment program restrictions related to wish for restriction reduction	Continued progressive weight gain as restrictions are lifted	Lift restrictions one at a time as long as there is a weight gain.	Continues to gain weight. Approaching desirable target weight. Perception of body size unchanged.

(Continued.)

Table 42-24 Continued

Assessment	Nursing Diagnosis	Outcome Criteria	Nursing Intervention	Evaluation
Stage 4* Client and family express fear and reluctance to participate in scheduled family therapy. Client reports difficulty setting limits on parent's intrusiveness. Client reports difficulty in being able to make and implement decisions without parental interference.	Resistance to family therapy related to fear of unknown and impaired boundary maintenance	Engagement of family members in therapy. Evidence: a. Attendance at all sessions b. Active participation in sessions c. Discussion of potential postdischarge problems outside sessions d. Confrontation of parents by client on interference with decision making	Answer family questions about what will happen in therapy sessions. Encourage family and client to participate in therapy. Encourage client to take "I" position. Encourage client to discuss conflicts with parents.	Family participation in therapy. Client takes steps to limit parental intrusiveness. Client initiates family discussion about potential postdischarge problems.
Stage 5* Family violates visiting restriction: comes in twice in evenings during the week; arrives at 10 A.M. on Sunday. Family advises client to increase food intake *very* gradually and not to worry if there is no weight gain in a week. Family sneaks in reading material and cassette player.	Family efforts to sabotage treatment regimen related to need to maintain client in role of "identified patient"	Compliance by family with treatment regimen. Evidence: a. Visiting only when permitted b. Not discussing food or weight gain with the client c. Bringing nothing to client unless permitted by staff members	Enforce family visiting hours. Instruct family to refrain from discussing food or weight gain with client. Encourage client to remind family of visiting restrictions.	Family becomes angry when told to leave because they are violating visiting restrictions. Family conforms to visiting schedule when requested to do so by client.

(Continued.)

of health and for the prevention of illness play an important role. Nursing interventions can facilitate personal change, the revision of problematic schemata, self-management, the achievement and maintenance of peace of mind, the resolution of conflicts which cause resistance to health-promotive change, effective management of emotions, and relaxation. In intervening, nurses can use both traditional and nontraditional approaches. The alternative approaches include the use of visual imagery, hypnosis, meditation, autogenic training, and biofeedback. The effectiveness of any nursing intervention is determined through the evaluation process.

REFERENCES

1. F. Cohen and R. S. Lazarus, "Coping with the Stresses of Illness," in G. C. Stone et al., *Health Psychology: A Handbook*, Jossey-Bass, San Francisco, 1979, pp. 217–254.
2. C. D. Spielberger, "Anxiety as an Emotional State," in C. D. Spielberger, ed., *Anxiety: Current Trends in Theory and Research*, vol. 1, Academic, New York, 1972.
3. L. E. Hinkle, "The Concept of Stress in the Biological and Social Sciences," *International Journal of Psychiatry in Medicine*, vol. 5, no. 4, 1974, pp. 335–357.
4. R. Ader, "Role of Developmental Factors in Suscep-

Table 42-24 Continued

Assessment	Nursing Diagnosis	Outcome Criteria	Nursing Intervention	Evaluation
Stage 5* (continued)				
Family bombards client with questions about interactions with staff members. Client engages in self-induced vomiting after parents' visit.				
After discharge†				
Reports fear of being fat. Reports difficulty eating with family. Increasing exercise. Indicates lack of peer relationships. Stays in room alone after school. Reports feeling left out but is reluctant to join peer groups.	Anxiety related to distorted body image Parents-adolescent conflict related to dysfunctional separation dynamics Social and emotional loneliness related to ambivalence about being an adolescent	Continued adequate nutritional concerns about weight Continued engagement therapy with family Establishment of realistic exercise program Initiation of relationship with peers Participation in one after-school activity	Provide reality-based feedback on weight and appearance. Encourage client and family to continue in therapy. Nutritional teaching. Explore factors contributing to lack of social relationships. Encourage client to participate in an after-school activity. Encourage experimentation with assertive and social behaviors. Help client to inventory reality-based strengths and weakness and desired changes.	Continues to struggle with accurate perception of body. Continues in therapy. Attempts to select foods and maintain a well-balanced diet. Verbalizes awareness of own participation in loneliness. Socializes after school and weekends with male and female friends and initiates some activities with friends.

*Assessments in this stage developed on the basis of evaluations in previous stage.
†Assessments developed by school nurse.

tibility to Disease," *International Journal of Psychiatry in Medicine,* vol. 5, no. 4, 1974, pp. 367–376.

5. C. M. Parkes, "Broken Heart: A Statistical Study of Increased Mortality among Widowers," *British Medical Journal,* March 1969, pp. 740–743.
6. S. Epstein, "Conflict and Stress," in L. Goldberger and S. Breznitz, eds., *Handbook of Stress,* Collier-Macmillan, New York, 1982, pp. 49–68.
7. R. S. Lazarus, "Psychological Stress and Coping in Adaptation and Illness," *International Journal of Psychiatry in Medicine,* vol. 5, no. 4, 1974, pp. 321–333.
8. H. Wolff, *Stress and Disease,* Thomas, Springfield, Ill., 1953.
9. G. G. Jampolsky, *Love Is Letting Go of Fear,* Bantam, New York, 1979, p. 22.
10. F. Henker III, "Psychosomatic Illness: Biochemical and Physiologic Foundations," *Psychosomatics,* vol. 25, no. 1, 1984, pp. 19–24.
11. G. Engel, "A Life Setting Conducive to Illness—The Giving Up–Given Up Complex," *Annals of Internal Medicine,* vol. 69, August 1968, pp. 293–300.
12. J. A. Ogden, G. Von Strumer, "Emotional Strategies and Their Relationship to Complaints of Psychosomatic and Neurotic Symptoms," *Journal of Clinical Psychology,* vol. 40, no. 3, 1984, pp. 772–779.
13. R. H. Moos and A. G. Billings, "Conceptualizing and Measuring Coping Resources and Processes," in L.

Goldberger and S. Breznitz, eds., *Handbook of Stress*, Collier-Macmillan, New York, 1982.

14. C. Figley, "Catastrophes: An Overview of Family Reactions," in C. R. Figley and H. I. McCubbin, eds., *Stress and the Family*, vol. 11, Brunner/Mazel, New York, 1983, pp. 3–20.
15. C. R. Figley and H. I. McCubbin, eds., *Stress and the Family*, vol. 11, Brunner/Mazel, New York, 1983.
16. R. Catalano and D. Dooley, "Health Effects of Economic Instability: A Test of Economic Stress Hypothesis," *Journal of Health and Social Behavior*, vol. 24, 1983, pp. 46–60.
17. D. E. Rosenbaum, "Deep Recession Is Expected to Harm American Health," *New York Times*, June 28, 1984, p. A16.
18. D. Dooley and R. Catalano, "Why the Economy Predicts Help-Seeking: A Test of Competing Explanations," *Journal of Health and Social Behavior*, vol. 25, 1984, pp. 160–176.
19. W. L. Webb, "Chronic Pain," *Psychosomatics*, vol. 24, no. 12, 1983, pp. 1053–1063.
20. J. C. Nemiah, "Somatoform Disorders," in A. M. Freedman, H. I. Kaplan, and B. J. Sadock, eds., *Comprehensive Textbook of Psychiatry*, 3d ed., Williams and Wilkins, Baltimore, 1980, pp. 1525–1544.
21. W. Kiely, "From the Symbolic Stimulus to the Pathophysiological Response: Neurophysiological Mechanism," *International Journal of Psychiatry in Medicine*, vol. 5, no. 4, 1974, pp. 517–529.
22. R. A. Ramsay, "Psychiatric Considerations in Chronic Pain States," in E. D. Wittkower and H. Warnes, eds., *Psychosomatic Medicine*, Harper and Row, New York, 1977, p. 60.
23. W. E. Fordyce, *Behavioral Methods for Chronic Pain and Illness*, Mosby, St. Louis, 1976, p. 29.
24. R. A. Devaul and L. A. Faillace, "Surgery-Proneness: A Review and Clinical Assessment," *Psychosomatics*, vol. 21, April 1980, pp. 295–299.
25. D. C. Turk and P. Saloney, "Chronic Pain as a Variant of Depressive Disease: A Critical Appraisal," *Journal of Nervous and Mental Diseases*, vol. 172, no. 7, 1984, pp. 398–404.
26. R. A. Sternbach, *Pain Patients: Traits and Treatment*, Academic, New York, 1974.
27. P. Watzlawick, J. Bevin, and D. Jackson, *Pragmatics of Human Communication*, Norton, New York, 1967.
28. C. C. Nadelson, M. T. Notman, and E. A. Ellis, "Psychosomatic Aspects of Obstetrics and Gynecology," *Psychosomatics*, vol. 24, no. 10, 1983, pp. 871–883.
29. K. R. R. Krishnan, R. D. France, and J. L. Houpt, "Chronic Low Back Pain and Depression," *Psychosomatics*, vol. 26, no. 4, 1985, pp. 299–302.
30. S. B. Shanfield, "Pain and the Marital Relationship: Psychiatric Distress," *Pain*, vol. 7, 1979, pp. 343-351.
31. D. Swanson and T. Maruta, "The Family's Viewpoint of Chronic Pain," *Pain*, vol. 8, 1980, pp. 163–166.
32. J. Delvey and L. Hopkins, "Pain Patients and Their Partners: The Role of Collusion in Chronic Pain," *Journal of Marital and Family Therapy*, January 1982, pp. 135–142.
33. E. D. Joseph and A. H. Schwartz, "Accident Proneness," in A. M. Freedman, H. I. Kaplan, and B. J. Sadock, eds., *Comprehensive Textbook of Psychiatry*, 3d ed., Williams and Wilkins, Baltimore, 1980, pp. 1953–1956.
34. Sigmund Freud, "The Psychopathology of Everyday Life," in *Standard Edition of the Complete Psychological Works of Sigmund Freud*, vol. 6, Hogarth, London, 1960.
35. J. G. Modell and F. Guerra, "Psychological Problems in the Surgical Patient," in F. Guerra and J. A. Antonio, eds., *Emotional and Psychological Responses to Anesthesia and Surgery*, Grune and Stratton, New York, 1980, pp. 155–176.
36. C. W. Wahl and J. S. Golden, "The Psychodynamics of the Polysurgical Patient: Report of Sixteen Patients," *Psychosomatics*, vol. 8, 1966, pp. 65–72.
37. W. D. Engels and E. D. Wittkower, "Skin Disorders," in A. M. Freedman, H. I. Kaplan, and B. J. Sadock, eds., *Comprehensive Textbook of Psychiatry*, 3d ed., Williams and Wilkins, Baltimore, 1980, pp. 1930–1940.
38. D. F. Greenwald, "Responsivity/Nonresponsivity in Psychosomatic Disorders," *Journal of Clinical Psychology*, vol. 40, no. 1, 1984, pp. 40–51.
39. R. S. Medansky, "Dermopsychosomatics: An Overview," *Psychosomatics*, vol. 21, no. 3, 1980, pp. 195–200.
40. S. R. Langner and C. Innes, "Breathing, Holism, and Health," *Topics in Clinical Nursing*, vol. 2, no. 3, 1980, pp. 1–10.
41. M. N. Starkman and N. H. Applelblatt, "Functional Upper Airway Obstruction: A Possible Somatization Disorder," *Psychosomatics*, vol. 25, no. 4, 1984, pp. 327–333.
42. G. K. Fritz, "Childhood Asthma," *Psychosomatics*, vol. 24, no. 11, 1983, pp. 959–967.
43. P. H. Knapp, "Psychotherapeutic Management of Bronchial Asthma," in E. D. Wittkower and H. Warnes, eds., *Psychosomatic Medicine*, Harper and Row, New York, 1977, pp. 210–219.
44. J. F. Dirks, A. Paley, and K. H. Fross, "Panic-fear Research in Asthma and the Nuclear Conflict Theory of Asthma: Similarities, Differences and Clinical Implications," *British Journal of Medical Psychology*, vol. 52, 1979, pp. 71–76.

45. J. F. Dirks and R. A. Kinsman, "Clinical Prediction of Medical Rehospitalization: Psychological Assessment with the Battery of Illness Behavior," *Journal of Personality Assessment,* vol. 45, 1981, pp. 608–613.
46. R. A. Kinsman, R. A. Yaroush, E. Fernandez, et al., "Symptoms and Experience in Chronic Bronchitis and Emphysema," *Chest,* vol. 83, 1983, pp. 755–761.
47. G. D. Greenberg, J. J. Ryan, and P. F. Bourlier, "Psychological and Neuropsychological Aspects of COPD," *Psychosomatics,* vol. 26, no. 1, 1985, pp. 29–33.
48. S. Cheren and P. H. Knapp, "Gastrointestinal Disorders," in A. M. Freedman, H. I. Kaplan, and B. J. Sadock, eds., *Comprehensive Textbook of Psychiatry,* 3d ed., Williams and Wilkins, Baltimore, 1980.
49. S. Bonfils and M. Dem Uzan, "Irritable Bowel Syndrome vs. Ulcerative Colitis: Psychofunctional Disturbance vs. Psychosomatic Disease?" *Journal of Psychosomatic Research,* vol. 18, 1974, pp. 291–296.
50. L. Levi and A. Kagan, "Adaptation of the Psychosocial Environment to Man's Abilities and Needs," in L. Levi, ed., *Society, Stress and Disease,* vol. 1, Oxford University Press, London, 1971, pp. 399–404.
51. G. A. Fava, G. Trombini, G. Grandi, et al., "Depression and Anxiety with Secondary Amenorrhea," *Psychosomatics,* vol. 25, no. 12, 1984, pp. 905–908.
52. L. Koran and D. Hamburg, "Psychophysiological Endocrine Disorders," in A. M. Freedman, H. I. Kaplan, and B. J. Sadock, eds., *Comprehensive Textbook of Psychiatry,* 2d ed., Williams and Wilkins, Baltimore, 1975.
53. C. G. Lindemann, C. Zitrin, and D. F. Klein, "Thyroid Dysfunction in Phobic Patients," *Psychosomatics,* vol. 25, no. 8, 1984, pp. 603–606.
54. L. D. Young, "Organic Affective Disorder Associated with Thyrotoxicosis," *Psychosomatics,* vol. 25, no. 6, 1984, pp. 490–492.
55. M. S. Gold and H. Rowland Rearsall, "Hypothyroidism—Or Is It Depression?" *Psychosomatics,* vol. 24, no. 7, 1983, pp. 646–656.
56. M. F. Reiser and L. Whisnant, "Endocrine Disorders," in A. M. Freedman, H. I. Kaplan and B. J. Sadock, eds., *Comprehensive Textbook of Psychiatry,* 3d ed., Williams and Wilkins, Baltimore, 1980.
57. A. M. Jacobson and J. B. Leibovich, "Psychological Issues in Diabetes Mellitus," *Psychosomatics,* vol. 25, no. 1, 1984, pp. 7–15.
58. S. H. Frazier, "Headaches," in A. M. Freedman, H. I. Kaplan, and B. J. Sadock, eds., *Comprehensive Textbook of Psychiatry,* 3d ed., Williams and Wilkins, Baltimore, 1980.
59. J. Arehart-Treichel, "Migraines: Unmasking the Cause," *Science News,* vol. 118, October 11, 1980, pp. 237–238.
60. H. J. Featherstone and B. D. Beitman, "Marital Migraine: A Refractory Daily Headache," *Psychosomatics,* vol. 25, no. 1, 1984, pp. 30–38.
61. E. M. Waring, "Conjoint Marital and Family Therapy," in R. Roy and E. Tunks, eds., *Chronic Pain: Psychosocial Factors in Rehabilitation,* Williams and Wilkins, Baltimore, 1982.
62. L. C. Kolb, "Attachment Behaviors and Pain Complaints," *Psychosomatics,* vol. 23, 1982, pp. 413–475.
63. "At the Heart of Blood Pressure," *Science News,* vol. 126, 1984, p. 40.
64. "How Stress Causes High Blood Pressure," *Science News,* vol. 123, 1983, p. 261.
65. A. Steptoe, D. Melville, and A. Ross, "Behavioral Response Demands, Cardiovascular Reactivity, and Essential Hypertension," *Psychosomatic Medicine,* vol. 46, no. 1, 1984, pp. 33–37.
66. S. B. Manuck, J. Proiette, S. J. Rader, and J. M. Polefrone, "Parental Hypertension, Affect and Cardiovascular Response to Cognitive Change," *Psychosomatic Medicine,* vol. 47, no. 2, 1985, pp. 189–194.
67. P. E. Baer et al., "Assessing Personality Factors in Essential Hypertension with a Brief Self-Report Instrument," *Psychosomatic Medicine,* vol. 41, no. 4, 1979, pp. 321–330.
68. R. Adler et al., "Psychological Process and Ischemic Stroke," *Psychosomatic Medicine,* vol. 33, 1971, pp. 1–29.
69. Z. J. Lipowski, "Cardiovascular Disorders," in A. M. Freedman, H. I. Kaplan, and B. J. Sadock, eds., *Comprehensive Textbook of Psychiatry,* 3d ed., Williams and Wilkins, Baltimore, 1980.
70. "Airport Noise Linked with Heart Disease,"*Science News,* vol. 123, 1983, pp. 294.
71. M. Friedman and R. Rosenman, *Type A Behavior and Your Heart,* Fawcett, Greenwich, Conn., 1974.
72. A. M. Razin, "Psychosocial Intervention in Coronary Heart Disease: A Review," *Psychosomatic Medicine,* vol. 44, no. 4, 1982, pp. 363–387.
73. S. C. Kobasa, "Stressful Life Events, Personality and Health: An Inquiry into Hardiness," *Journal of Personality and Social Psychology,* vol. 37, 1979, pp. 1–11.
74. S. C. Kobasa, S. R. Maddi and S. Kahn, "Hardiness and Health: A Prospective Study," *Journal of Personality and Social Psychology,* vol. 42, 1982, pp. 168–177.
75. F. Rhodewalt and S. Agustsdottr, "On the Relationship of Hardiness to the Type A Behavior Pattern: Perception of Life Events Versus Coping with Life Events," *Journal of Research in Personality,* vol. 18, 1984, pp. 212–223.
76. S. C. Kobasa, S. R. Maddi, and M. Zola, "Type A and

Hardiness," *Journal of Behavioral Medicine*, vol. 42, 1983, pp. 168–177.

77. C. Bass and C. Wade, "Chest Pain with Normal Coronary Arteries: A Comparative Study of Psychiatric and Social Morbidity," *Psychological Medicine*, vol. 14, 1984, pp. 51–61.
78. J. L. Levenson, R. Kay, J. Monteferrante, and M. V. Herman, "Denial Predicts Favorable Outcome in Unstable Angina Pectoris," *Psychosomatic Medicine*, vol. 46, no. 1, 1984, pp. 25–29.
79. C. M. Parkes, *Bereavement*, International Universities Press, New York, 1972.
80. H. Russek and L. Russek, "Is Emotional Stress an Etiologic Factor in Coronary Heart Disease?" *Psychosomatics*, vol. 17, no. 2, 1976, pp. 63–67.
81. J. L. Levenson and R. O. Friedel, "Major Depression in Patients with Cardiac Disease: Diagnosis and Somatic Treatment," *Psychosomatics*, vol. 26, no. 2, 1985, pp. 91–101.
82. Alma Wooley, "Excellence in Nursing in the Coronary Care Unit," *Heart and Lung*, vol. 1, no. 6, 1972, pp. 785–792.
83. H. Cassem et al., "Reactions of Coronary Patients to the Coronary Care Unit Nurse," *American Journal of Nursing*, vol. 70, no. 2, 1970, p. 319.
84. J. Lynch et al., "The Effects of Human Contact on Cardiac Arrhythmia in Coronary Care Patients," *Journal of Nervous and Mental Disease*, vol. 158, no. 2, 1974, pp. 88–99.
85. K. A. J. Jarvinen, "Can Ward Rounds Be a Danger to Patients with Myocardial Infarction?" *British Medical Journal*, vol. 1, 1955, pp. 318–320.
86. P. H. Soloff, "Effects of Denial on Mood, Compliance, and Quality of Functioning After Cardiovascular Rehabilitation," *General Hospital Psychiatry*, vol. 2, 1980, pp. 134–140.
87. A. M. Freeman, L. Fleece, D. G. Folks et al., "Psychiatric Symptoms, Type A Behavior and Arrhythmia Following Coronary Bypass," *Psychosomatics*, vol. 25, no. 8, 1984, pp. 586–589.
88. M. S. Dominian, "Psychological Stress in Wives of Patients with Myocardial Infarction," *British Medical Journal*, vol. 2, April 14, 1973, pp. 101–103.
89. G. Engel, "Emotional Stress and Sudden Death," *Psychology Today*, November 1977, p. 114.
90. "Depression and the Lymphocyte Link," *Science News*, vol. 125, 1984, p. 341.
91. "Study Shows Decrease in Immunity," *Science News*, vol. 124, 1983, p. 7.
92. J. K. Kiecolt-Glaser, D. Ricker, J. George, et al., "Urinary Cortisol Levels, Cellular Immunocompetency, and Loneliness in Psychiatric Inpatients," *Psychosomatic Medicine*, vol. 46, no. 1, 1984, pp. 15–23.
93. J. K. Kiecolt-Glaser, W. Garner, C. Speicher, et al., "Psychosocial Modifiers of Immunocompetence in Medical Students," *Psychosomatic Medicine*, vol. 46, no. 1, 1984, pp. 7–13.
94. S. Jacobs, J. Mason, T. Koster, et al., "Urinary Free Cortisol Excretion in Relation to Age in Acutely Stressed Persons with Depressive Symptoms," *Psychosomatic Medicine*, vol. 46, no. 3, 1984, pp. 213–221.
95. M. Stein, S. Schleifer, and S. Keller, "Immune Disorders," in A. M. Freedman, H. I. Kaplan, and B. J. Sadock, eds., *Comprehensive Textbook of Psychiatry*, 3d ed., Williams and Wilkins, Baltimore, 1980.
96. R. Rimon and P. Halonen, "Herpes Simplex Virus Infection and Depressive Illness," *Diseases of the Nervous System*, vol. 30, 1969, p. 338.
97. N. G. Hawkins, R. Davies, and T. H. Holmes, "Evidence of Psychosocial Factors in the Development of Pulmonary Tuberculosis," *American Review of Tuberculosis and Pulmonary Diseases*, vol. 75, 1957, p. 768.
98. M. A. Jacobs, A. Spilken, and M. Norman, "Relationship of Life Change, Maladaptive Aggression and Upper Respiratory Infection in Male College Students," *Psychosomatic Medicine*, vol. 31, 1969, p. 31.
99. L. Luborsky et al., "A Herpes Simplex Virus and Moods: A Longitudinal Study," *Journal of Psychosomatic Research*, vol. 20, 1976, p. 543.
100. R. Totman, S. E. Reed, and W. J. Craig, "Cognitive Dissonance, Stress and Virus Induced Common Colds," *Journal of Psychosomatic Research*, vol. 21, 1977, p. 550.
101. S. Greer and P. M. Silberfarb, "Psychological Concomitants of Cancer: Current State of Research," *Psychological Medicine*, vol. 12, 1982, pp. 563–573.
102. "Giving It Up—At the Cellular Level," *Science News*, vol. 124, 1983, p. 148.
103. L. LeShan, *You Can Fight for Your Life*, Evans, New York, 1977.
104. O. C. Simonton and S. S. Simonton, "New Dimensions of Habilitation for the Handicapped," unpublished paper presented at the University of Florida, Gainesville, June 14, 1974.
105. O. C. Simonton, S. Matthew-Simonton, and T. F. Sparks, "The Psychological Causes and the Psychological Treatment of Cancer," unpublished paper.
106. C. Holden, "Cancer and the Mind: How Are They Connected?" *Science*, vol. 200, June 23, 1978, pp. 1363–1368.
107. J. Acterberg, I. Collerain, and P. Craig, "A Possible Relationship Between Cancer, Mental Retardation and Mental Disorders," *Social Science and Medicine*, vol. 12, 1978, pp. 135–139.
108. N. C. Rassidakis, M. Kelepouris, K. Goulis, and K. Karriaossefidis, "Malignant Neoplasms as Cause of

Death among Psychiatric Patients," *International Mental Health Newsletter*, vol. 14, 1972, pp. 1–3.
109. C. B. Bahnson, "Psychophysical Complementarity in Malignancies: Past Work and Vistas," *Annals of the New York Academy of Sciences*, vol. 164, 1969, pp. 319–333.
110. G. Bennett, "Psychic and Cellular Aspects of Isolation and Identity Impairment in Cancer: A Dialectic of Alienations," *Annals of the New York Academy of Sciences*, vol. 164, 1969, pp. 352–363.
111. R. J. Goldberg, "Psychiatric Symptoms in Cancer Patients," *Postgraduate Medicine*, vol. 74, no. 1, 1983, pp. 263–273.
112. W. Meissner, "Family Process and Psychosomatic Disease," *International Journal of Psychiatry in Medicine*, vol. 5, no. 4, 1974, pp. 411–430.
113. A. Amkraut and G. Solomon, "From the Symbolic Stimulus to the Pathophysiologic Response: Immune Mechanisms," *International Journal of Psychiatry in Medicine*, vol. 5, no. 1, 1974, pp. 541–563.
114. F. Backus and D. Dudley, "Observations of Psychosocial Factors and Their Relationships to Organic Disease," *International Journal of Psychiatry in Medicine*, vol. 5, no.4, 1974, pp. 499–515.
115. A. E. Andersen, "Anorexia Nervosa and Bulimia: A Spectrum of Eating Disorders," *Journal of Adolescent Health Care*, vol. 4, 1983, pp.15–21.
116. K. A. Halmi, "Pragmatic Information on Eating Disorders," *Psychiatric Clinics of North America*, vol. 5, no. 2, 1982, pp. 371–377.
117. A. J. Plumariega, P. Edwards, and C. B. Mitchell, "Anorexia in Black Adolescents," *Journal of the American Academy of Child Psychiatry*, vol. 23, no. 1, 1984, pp. 111–114.
118. A. Hall, "Deciding to Stay an Anorectic," *Postgraduate Medical Journal*, vol. 58, 1982, pp. 641–647.
119. A. W. Root and P. S. Powers, "Anorexia Nervosa Presenting as Growth Retardation in Adolescents," *Journal of Adolescent Health Care*, vol. 4, no. 2, 1983, pp. 25–30.
120. J. A. Sour, *Starving to Death in a Sea of Objects*, Aronson, New York, 1980.
121. R. C. Casper et al., "Disturbances in Body Image Estimation as Related to Other Characteristics and Outcome in Anorexia Nervosa," *British Journal of Psychiatry*, vol. 134, 1979, p. 71.
122. I. Story, "Anorexia Nervosa and the Psychotherapeutic Hospital," *International Journal of Psychoanalytic Psychotherapy*, vol. 9, 1982–1983, pp. 267–303.
123. B. M. Lippe, "The Physiologic Aspects of Eating Disorders," *Journal of the American Academy of Child Psychiatry*, vol. 22, no. 2, 1983, pp. 108–113.
124. C. P. Wilson, "The Fear of Being Fat and Anorexia Nervosa," *International Journal of Psychoanalytic Psychotherapy*, vol. 9, 1982–1983, pp. 233–255.
125. A. H. Crisp, "The Psychopathology of Anorexia Nervosa: Getting the 'Heat' Out of the System," *Research Publications Association for Research in Nervous and Mental Disease*, vol. 62, 1984, pp. 209–234.
126. P. Castelnuovo-Tedesco, D. C. Buchanan, and H. D. Hall, "Jaw-Wiring for Obesity," *General Hospital Psychiatry*, vol. 2, 1980, pp. 156–159.
127. J. Kay and R. B. Stricker, "Hematologic and Immunologic Abnormalities in Anorexia Nervosa," *Southern Medical Journal*, vol. 76, no. 8, 1983, pp. 1008–1010.
128. D. R. Mars, N. Anderson, and F. Rigall, "Anorexia Nervosa: A Disorder with Severe Acid-Base Derangements," *Southern Medical Journal*, vol. 75, no. 9, 1982, pp. 1038–1042.
129. D. Peterson, "Oral Signs of Frequent Vomiting in Anorexia," *American Family Physician*, vol. 27, no. 4, 1983, pp. 199–200.
130. W. Vandereycken and R. Pierloot, "Drop-out During In-Patient Treatment of Anorexia Nervosa: A Clinical Study of 133 Patients," *British Journal of Medical Psychology*, vol. 56, 1983, pp. 145–156.
131. I. L. Mintz, "Anorexia Nervosa and Bulimia in Males," in C. P. Wilson, ed., *Fear of Being Fat*, Aronson, New York, 1983, pp. 263–303.
132. I. L. Mintz, "Psychoanalytic Description: The Clinical Picture of Anorexia Nervosa and Bulimia," in C. P. Wilson, ed., *Fear of Being Fat*, Aronson, New York, 1983, pp. 83–113.
133. C. G. Fairburn, "Cognitive-Behavioral Treatment for Bulimia," in D. M. Garner and P. E. Garfinkel, eds., *Handbook of Psychotherapy for Anorexia Nervosa and Bulimia*, Guilford, New York, 1985.
134. J. P. Foreyt, ed., *Behavioral Treatments of Obesity*, Pergamon, New York, 1977.
135. A. J. Stunkard, "Obesity," in A. M. Freedman, H. I. Kaplan, and B. J. Sadock, eds., *Comprehensive Textbook of Psychiatry*, 3d ed., Williams and Wilkins, Baltimore, 1980.
136. R. McLain and F. W. Widlak, "Patient's Self-Concept and Weight Reduction: Use of Covert Sensitization," *Issues in Mental Health Nursing*, vol. 2, no. 2, 1979, pp. 1–19.
137. "Bypass: Surgery on Marriage," *Science News*, August 12, 1978.
138. C. S. W. Rand, K. Kowalske, and J. M. Kuldau, "Characteristics of Marital Improvement Following Obesity Surgery," *Psychosomatics*, vol. 25, no. 3, 1984, pp. 221–226.
139. J. R. Neill, J. R. Marshall, and C. E. Yale, "Marital Changes after Intestinal Bypass Surgery." *JAMA*, vol. 240, 1978, pp. 447–450.

140. L. A. Peplau and D. Perlman, "Perspectives on Loneliness," in L. A. Peplau and D. Perlman, eds., *Loneliness,* Wiley, New York, 1982, p. 3.
141. F. Cohen and R. S. Lazarus, "Coping with the Stresses of Illness," in G. C. Stone et al., eds., *Health Psychology,* Jossey-Bass, San Francisco, 1979, pp. 227–228.
142. J. Lewis et al., *No Single Thread,* Brunner/Mazel, New York, 1976.
143. F. S. Perls, *Gestalt Therapy Verbation,* Real People, Lafayette, Calif., 1969.
144. W. C. Schutz, *Here Comes Everybody,* Harper and Row, New York, 1971.
145. R. Dumas and R. Leonard, "The Effect of Nursing on the Incidence of Postoperative Vomiting," *Nursing Research,* vol. 12, no. 1, 1963, pp. 12–15.
146. M. Meyers, "The Effect of Types of Communication on Patients' Reaction to Stress," *Nursing Research,* vol. 13, no. 2, 1964, pp. 126–132.
147. Irving Janis, "Vigilance and Decision Making in a Personal Crisis," in G. Coehlo, D. Hamburg, J. Adams, eds., *Coping and Adaptation,* Basic Books, New York, 1974.
148. G. Mandler, *Mind and Body,* Norton, New York, 1984.
149. F. H. Kanfer, "Self-Management Methods," in R. H. Kanfer and A. P. Goldstein, eds., *Helping People to Change,* 2d ed., Pergamon, New York, 1980, pp. 334–389.
150. L. Buscaglia, *Love,* Slack, Thorofare, N. J., 1972.
151. M. C. Sundberg, "Framework for Nursing Intervention in the Treatment of Obesity," *Issues in Mental Nursing,* vol. 1, Fall 1978, pp. 26–44.
152. G. Rosen, *The Relaxation Book,* Prentice-Hall, Englewood Cliffs, N. J., 1977.
153. K. A. Frank et al., "Psychological Intervention in Coronary Heart Disease," *General Hospital Psychiatry,* vol. 1, no. 1, 1979, pp. 18–23.
154. R. M. Suinn et al., "Behavior Therapy for Type A Patients," *American Journal of Cardiology,* vol. 36, 1965, pp. 269–270.
155. B. Lowen et al., "Decreased Ventricular Contractions Through the Use of Relaxation in Patients with Stable Ischemic Heart Disease," *Lancet,* vol. 11, 1973, pp. 380–382.
156. K. A. Halmi, "Anorexia Nervosa: Treatment in the General Hospital," *Current Psychiatric Therapies,* vol. 24, 1983, pp. 181–185.

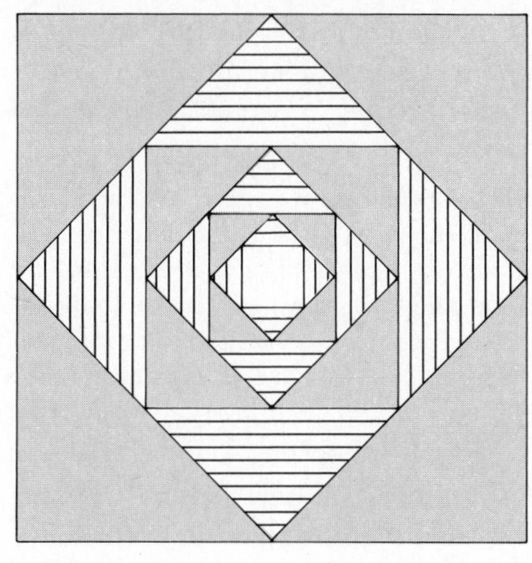

CHAPTER 43
Disability and Chronic Illness

Judith Gregorie D'Afflitti

LEARNING OBJECTIVES

After studying this chapter, the student should be able to:

1. Identify the stages of adjustment to chronic illness and disability.
2. List the changes imposed by chronic illness and disability.
3. Discuss patterns of interaction in person, family, and environment that influence chronically ill and disabled clients and their families.
4. Describe behaviors of clients and families that reflect a disturbed response to chronic illness and disability.
5. Discuss the significance of environment in rehabilitation of chronically ill and disabled clients.
6. Apply the nursing process to the care of chronically ill and disabled clients and their families.
7. Construct a plan of care for clients who are chronically ill or disabled.

Health, defined by nurses as a synchronous pattern of interaction in the person-environment system, is often defined more rigidly by clients as the absence of illness or disease. When clients become ill, they think of becoming "better"—that is, they believe and hope that an episode of acute illness is temporary and that physical, mental, and spiritual immobilization are transitory. They expect their sense of well-being and their usual lifestyle to be restored.

However, when illness or injury leaves residual impairment and return to a previous level of wellness is highly improbable, clients and families must confront the imposed changes and evolve altered ways of living. They experience at a deep level the impact of altered self-image, self-concept, self-esteem, body image, and personal identity. Clients' bodies, as well as their abilities to think and feel, are changed. Hopes and ambitions are reconsidered and revised, and questions about personal goodness and one's relationship with God are raised. Frequently, nurses hear clients despair that they can no longer achieve their goals. They also hear clients express anger at God, as once familiar patterns change or become stagnant. Many clients with chronic health problems no longer feel that they have a right to choose a life purpose. They become less visionary and more disillusioned.

Achievement of an optimal level of functioning becomes a lifelong struggle for those who are developmentally challenged. The purpose of this chapter is to discuss supportive and educational interventions, which are an ongoing challenge to nurses who believe that wholeness is more than body integrity. It looks at ways in which clients who are despondent because of chronic illness, and the losses inherent in it, can be helped to transcend their physical problems and achieve a greater sense of mental and spiritual well-being.

DYSYNCHRONOUS HEALTH PATTERNS

Chronically ill, disabled, or developmentally challenged clients vary greatly in the severity, pervasiveness, and prognosis of their problems. Initially, a chronic condition may interfere with their lifestyle very little or not at all. In time, however, chronic illnesses are likely to produce moderate to severe impairments and in many instances to shorten life.

Some definitions will help clarify the meaning of several commonly used labels. The Commission on Chronic Illness defines *chronic diseases* as follows:

> All impairments or deviations from normal which have one or more of the following characteristics: are permanent, leave residual disability, are caused by nonreversible pathological alteration, require special training of the patient for rehabilitation, may be expected to require a long period of supervision, observation, or care.[1]

Disability is a legal definition: a lack of legal qualification to do something. A person who has an observable and measurable physical or mental impairment, whatever the cause, is called *disabled. Impairment* is the actual disturbance in structure or function that results from anatomical, physiological, mental, or spiritual abnormalities. The term *handicap* implies that total readjustment is necessary as a result of an impairment. The term *handicapped* is gradually being replaced by the term *developmentally challenged.* All these terms refer to physical, mental, or spiritual disadvantages that make achievement in some area of functioning unusually difficult. A handicap, impairment, or developmental challenge occurs when there is a decrease in the quality or quantity of a person's functioning as a result of the impact of disease or injury and a negative self-image or negative social attitudes toward the disabled person.

A person's response to chronic illness or disability is an interacting and complex process involving many variables. The factors in the person, family, and environment that influence responsiveness to chronic illnesses and disabilities are shown in Figure 43-1. Of concern to nurses are the dysynchronous behavioral patterns that result from these influences. Common behaviors exhibited during a client's adjustment phase are protest and denial, depression, anxiety, anger, detachment, and reinvestment. Common dysfunctional health patterns include generalization of the disability, rebelliousness, and independence-dependence conflict. A chronically ill or developmentally challenged person also experiences alterations in self-concept. The extent of these alterations is affected by changes in functional status, changes in physical attractiveness, the visibility of the problem, the feasibility and availability of rehabilitation, and the time factor in the development of the disability or illness.

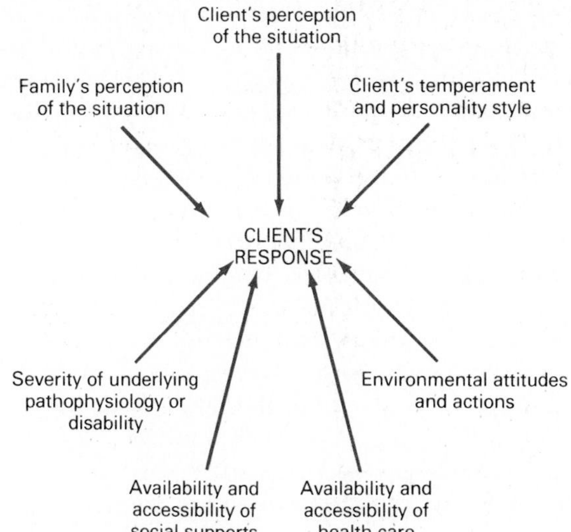

Figure 43-1 Responses to chronic conditions. How person, family, and environment influence clients' responses to chronic illness and disability.

Stages of Adjustment to Chronic Illness and Disability

When clients are confronted with the fact of permanent and chronic illness or with the knowledge that severe limits have been imposed on their physical, mental, or spiritual functioning, their responses will vary. People's responses to loss are dependent on a variety of factors: constitutional factors that help determine cognitive capacities, temperament, and personality development; perception of loss and change; personal resources available at the time of the loss; established patterns of coping; ability to transcend the past; and acceptance of a loss as part of life's purpose.

Twelve stages of adjustment to a disabling condition have been noted: (1) shock, (2) anxiety, (3) bargaining, (4) denial, (5) mourning, (6) depression, (7) withdrawal, (8) anger, (9) hostility and aggression, (10) acknowledgment, (11) acceptance, and (12) adjustment.[2] People respond in unique ways; their responses range from "normal" grieving to overt dysfunctional behavior such as massive denial or severe depression. Some persons progress through the stages in a short period of time, while others may never complete the grieving process. Moreover, although there is evidence from research to substantiate the universality of the dynamics of grieving, not all clients will overtly experience all the stages of adjustment. Dysfunctional adjustment to chronic illness is indicated by some degree of protest and denial as well as depression, anxiety, and anger.

Protest and Denial

Initially people attempt to protect themselves from becoming overwhelmed by the growing awareness of the extent of disability and threat to life. They protest the facts of the situation ("It couldn't be"), the extent of the imposed changes ("I can't have lost . . ."), and the fact that it has happened to them ("This is a nightmare—this isn't happening to me"). Denial intervenes when the threat to life and self-concept becomes intolerable. The denial that predominates during this period is a combination of existential, psychological, and nonaccepting denial.

When the physical impairment is sudden and massive, the physiological shock that follows elicits psychological defenses. There is a need for conservation of energy and protection from further stress. Consequently, as a defense against psychosocial stressors, the capacity to acknowledge what has occurred is limited. When the person becomes physiologically stable, the need to defend ego integrity lessens and reality is allowed to intrude. Protest and denial give way to growing awareness. People no longer say, "It can't be true," "You people are getting unnecessarily upset; this problem will be all over in a day or two," and "This is just a nightmare. I am going to wake up, and this nonsense will be forgotten." Instead, they ask questions directed toward collecting and integrating information that enhances their understanding of what has happened.

Temporary and periodic use of denial allows for the gradual acknowledgment and working through of the changed lifestyle imposed by the chronic illness or disability. On the other hand, when a client extensively screens out of awareness all significant realistic information regarding the extent, permanence, or degenerative nature of the chronic illness or disability, *massive denial* has occurred. It involves exaggerated use of psychological and nonaccepting denial that results in the following dysfunctional behavior:

Noncompliance with treatment regimens. Client with Parkinson's disease: "I won't take those pills any more—they make me shake and keep me from walking right."

Nonparticipation in planning treatment. Client with hemiplegia: "No, I don't want to hear about any rehabilitation program—I just bruised the nerves when I fell. When the bruising heals, I'll be okay."

Unwillingness to modify living arrangements. Client with advanced multiple sclerosis: "What is this nonsense about moving my bedroom downstairs? Once I go home and get some decent food, my strength will come back and those stairs will be no problem."

Refusal to participate in vocational counseling. Client with extensive permanent cardiac damage: "Being a garbage man isn't hard work. Once I get back in shape, this shortness of breath will be gone and I'll be able to lift anything. I just need to work out with some weight lifting. I don't need to get stuck in some desk job, so I don't want any retraining."

Chronically ill people protest, plan, and behave as though they were invulnerable, their deficits were temporary rather than permanent or progressive, and their return to a previous level of wellness and activity were expected. They resist efforts directed toward developing accommodations in activities of daily living and adapting living arrangements. They may adamantly refuse vocational rehabilitation on the assumption that the previous employment will be resumed. They may spend excessive time fantasizing about being in their preillness state of health. They cannot achieve their maximum potential, because they continue to refuse to collaborate in treatment planning and to participate in rehabilitation activities.

Depression

Depression occurs when chronically ill or disabled people stop putting energy into futile attempts to recover what has been lost and allow themselves to feel the empty spaces created by the loss. People experience painful disorganization, restlessness, and depression. The person thinks and says, "How am I going to manage now?" The realization is emotionally painful. Hope is threatened, as the more pessimistic view of the situation creeps into awareness. Cognitive ways of dealing with the losses are temporarily unavailable and emotionality dominates. Tears are common. Memories about "how things were" generate deep sadness, and the person cries openly for that which has been lost. The organized, automatic behavior seen during the period of shock and disbelief is replaced by anxiety that is characterized by a degree of disorganization and confusion. There is a greater dependency on others for structure and a reluctance to make decisions. Explanations and instructions must often be repeated, and even then the person may fail to clearly understand what is expected or the full implications of what has been said. Complaints of pain and discomfort may increase as the anxiety and depression increase. Expressions of frustration and anger in response to the limitations imposed by the deficits and impairments can be expected.

Some degree of depression is expected when clients face the reality of a disabling, chronic illness. However, severe depression, characterized by total apathy and massive social withdrawal from family, friends, care givers, and other clients, is pathological. People experiencing such depression verbalize expressions of helplessness ("I can't ..."), hopelessness ("There is no point ..."), and worthlessness ("I'm no good to ..."). Most important, the depression extends to all aspects of the self, including identity, roles, and relationships. Interest and participation in self-care deteriorate. Eating and sleeping patterns are severely disturbed. These people may become totally involved in their symptoms and thereby exaggerate the extent and seriousness of minor aches and discomforts, or they may develop an overlay of hypochondriacal symptoms. For example:

> Mrs. L., confined to a wheelchair with multiple sclerosis, stayed in her room with the door closed in spite of the fact that her ranch-style home permitted free access to all rooms. She refused to see family or friends when they visited and spent her waking hours staring out the window. The only subjects she would talk about to her immediate family or the visiting nurse were problems related to her bowels and the advantages and disadvantages of various laxatives and bowel softeners. Efforts to involve her in self-care were met with "I can't" and even greater apathy.

Anxiety

The losses incurred, predicted, and expected by people with chronic illness and disabilities generate anxiety. Depending in part on the individual's personality and style of responding to stress, the anxiety is converted into anger or depression. Some people find angry feelings and their expression frightening, in which case they tend toward a depressive reaction, while others automatically respond defensively with anger.

When people still see help in terms of regaining what has been lost, they are anxious (they complain of nervousness, loss of appetite, and insomnia). They feel depressed and hopeless ("Nothing—no one—can help me!"). Such a client often lashes out at family members and the hospital staff because they are unable to do the impossible—bring back what has been lost. People are feeling and expressing the agonies of loss. The displacement of the anger is a manifestation of the underlying anxiety.

A degree of anxiety is expected. On the other hand, severe anxiety indicates that the client is experiencing a state of defenselessness. Severe *free-floating anxiety* consists of a feeling of dread that the client cannot assign to a specific cause. The person is irritable and hypersensitive to ordinary light and sound. Cardiac palpitations, breathlessness, giddiness, nausea, dryness of mouth, diarrhea, compulsive eating, frequent urination, blurred vision, and a feeling of confusion are experienced. Coping mechanisms used to defend ego integrity from overwhelming threats to self fail or are severely weakened. When anxiety escalates to severe or panic proportions, the experience is extremely uncomfortable, and the energy expended may aggravate the disease process. The drive for activity to relieve the tension may result in behaviors and decisions that interfere with effective management of the disease process. If the disability limits physical activity, there may be a regression to primitive defenses such as hallucinations and delusions. Demanding behavior may be excessive, hysterical, and clinging in nature.

The chronically disabled may become totally self-absorbed and preoccupied with their symptoms and bodily functions. Feelings of insecurity are great; to ease them, these people may overvalue authority figures and unrealistically invest care givers with the power to meet their infantile dependency needs completely. Since care givers are fallible and needs are insatiable, disappointment and rebound anxiety are inevitable. For example:

Mr. A., whose father had died at a young age as a result of a stroke, reacted to the diagnosis of his own hypertension with free-floating anxiety several weeks after treatment had been instituted. He experienced an acute episode of panic, characterized by cardiac palpitations and shortness of breath, and reported a feeling of dread and terror. He was admitted to the emergency room on the basis of his expressed fear that he was having a heart attack. When cardiac problems were ruled out and the assessment of his status was completed, a diagnosis of acute anxiety attack was made. Further discussion with the nurse revealed that he could not identify the source of his anxiety and that he was resistant to exploratory attempts to make the connection between his father's death and his concern about his own health.

Anger

Commonly, people initially convert the anxiety generated by losses and their implications to anger. Blame may be placed on the self or projected or displaced onto family members or care givers. When anger occurs, it tends to remain in force until the person gives up what has been lost. Depression sets in when this "giving up" develops. Grieving for what has been lost is initiated. The mourning process becomes the mechanism for working through and letting go of past capacities, self-images, dreams, and expectations. This grieving process is necessary before an accurate reintegrated perception of self and of one's capacities can begin to evolve.

While anger is a feeling commonly experienced by chronically ill and disabled people, they have difficulty expressing it directly because of the degree to which they depend on their families and professionals not only for basic needs but for survival itself. Their fantasy is that the expression of anger will lead to abandonment and rejection. Knowing that their lives depend on those around them, they choose not to risk expression of anger, since the stakes are too high. However, unexpressed anger may be acted out in ways that sabotage treatment or create sufficient stress to cause other physical problems or psychopathology.

Anger becomes pervasive and exaggerated when it is sustained for extended periods of time. Behavior may at times include explosive, irrational expressions of anger or aggressiveness; diffuse and indiscriminately displaced anger; and acting out toward objects and people. There may be physical or verbal abuse of family members and care givers. Communications are bitter, overtly hostile, sarcastic, and highly critical. Medications, treatments, and exercise programs may be angrily refused or abruptly terminated. An example will help illustrate the expression of dysfunctional anger:

> Mr. B., age 23, was convalescing at home following spinal injuries and the amputation of both legs as a result of a work-related accident. During a home visit the community health nurse was the recipient of verbal abuse and observed Mr. B. exhibit an irrational tirade because the ice cubes in his orange juice had melted. Further discussion with his parents revealed that on several occasions he had become combative when they were attempting to help him move from his bed to a chair.

Detachment and Reinvestment

Detachment, the letting go of the past, and *reinvestment,* the making of new commitments, are slow processes involving a working through of losses. Clients require open awareness and acknowledgment of changes and losses that have occurred and their present and future implications. Such awareness is often acutely painful emotionally; letting go of "what was" is difficult and must be experienced time and time again until the emotional investment and associated feelings fade to a more tolerable level. The ongoing nature of this process can be emotionally deenergizing. Thus, people must have periods of respite. To deal with this painful process, people use temporary psychological, nonaccepting, and nonattention denial because constant confrontation is too stressful. Periodic use of denial supports progress toward the resolution of the loss.

Realization and acknowledgment may be suddenly replaced by denial of the prognosis, particularly in relation to specific consequences that impose permanent limitations on mobility and lifestyle. Some people who employ nonaccepting denial may for periods of time seem to ignore certain aspects of their limitations that had previously been a focus of concern. Nonattention denial is evident when people redirect preoccupation with their disease or rehabilitation to an area in their lives not related to their disease. This refocusing serves as a distraction and may provide a way of restoring ego integrity. For example:

> Mr. C., despite increasing disability as a consequence of multiple sclerosis, channeled his energies into devising more sophisticated computer games and developing creative ways to teach children how to use computers in daily life. This work became totally absorbing. It helped him feel alive and useful; more important, it distracted him from many of the discomforts imposed by immobility.

When the disease process is progressive (as with Mr. C.), there is no end to the losses until life itself is lost. Thus, the phases of denial, anger, depression, detachment, and reinvestment are cyclical. Each new loss or extension of an old loss reactivates the cycle. Total reinvestment in life is an ideal. In reality, the challenges of each new day may confront the existing level of accommodation and reinvestment.

When detachment and reinvestment are being negotiated, people are able to detach themselves sufficiently from the lost objects to have the energy for new investments and relationships. They begin to accept what they have and to work with that. They may have, and act on, thoughts such as: "I won't be able to travel the way I used to, but with good planning we could have an occasional trip." "I couldn't manage my old job, but my sister needs some help in her office, and I could handle that work now." There is growth in new directions with personal rewards. Rather than seeing life as a glass half empty, these people begin to see it as a glass half full.

The time it takes a person to deal successfully with a loss is highly variable and dependent on the nature of the loss, the individual's personality, and many environmental and interpersonal factors. Those who are not involved in the grieving often expect the person to resolve the loss quickly. A year is not a long time in dealing with loss; it is a logical time frame for mourning. It provides opportunities to experience the seasons and the significant holidays and anniversaries, and the altered self throughout. The feelings that are generated by each significant day or season, if worked through, facilitate the resolution of the losses and reinvestment.

Problems of Adjustment

Generalizing a Disability

When clients generalize a disability, they extend impairment and consequent limitations to many activities that would be possible if attempted. For example, some paraplegics or hemiplegics who could participate in their care and take responsibility for some activities of daily living adopt a passive position. They request or demand that care givers assume full responsibility for their physical care. After discharge they use their disability as an excuse for not participating in family activities, socializing with friends, or attending social or recreational events. These people define themselves as bystanders and as more dependent than their condition warrants. They experience an escalation of dependency needs and are extremely sensitive to deprivation of these needs. Invalidism becomes a way of deriving secondary gains. For example:

> Mrs. W. had symptoms of Parkinson's disease but was still able to ambulate and participate in her own care. Nevertheless, she refused to dress, feed, or wash herself, or to leave a recliner chair in the living room except to return to bed. Suggestions to continue socializing with friends, to take vacations, and to continue her involvement in social activities outside the home fell on deaf ears. In spite of the physical capacity to remain active with assistance, she chose to adopt the role of an invalid.

Rebelliousness

Some clients experience dependence as totally intolerable. The reactivated feelings associated with the loss of control and dependence on others for satisfaction of needs are so frightening and unpleasant that regardless of the consequences these clients act to eliminate the feelings. Rebelliousness and acting out result. Refusal to accept medications, to participate in planning care, and to permit care to be given is not born out of denial or anger and frustration regarding the losses; rather, the hyper-independent stance is a function of the need to defend against dependence. The "I don't care" protests are an expression of a priority that places independence over and above even survival. For example:

> Miss V., a 20-year-old newly diagnosed diabetic, seemed interested and capable while receiving instruction about her disease and its management. She appeared to be managing well throughout the summer. When it was time to return to college in the fall, the family expressed concern about her leaving home, living in a dormitory, and eating in the school cafeteria. As a result of these family pressures, she decided to remain at home and attend a local college. During her first semester her school performance dropped markedly, and the management of her diabetes also suffered. She was admitted to the hospital in diabetic coma as a result of dietary indiscretions. During the Thanksgiving holidays she "forgot" her insulin and was admitted to the hospital in serious condition. Reminders and efforts by the community health nurse to help her understand the importance of compliance had been rebuffed with, "I don't care—so leave me alone." The decision to remain at home escalated the dependence-independence conflict that she had managed well while she was able to live away at college. This conflict was escalated by the expressed concern of her family about her diabetes and her perception of increased dependence. She reacted with rebelliousness, using the diabetes as the issue of control.

Dependence on Technology

The relationships of chronically ill and disabled people with those around them are easily interfered with by the amount of emotional energy that is expended in dealing with the stresses presented by the illness or disability. Family, friends, and business colleagues are viewing the client differently and feeling stress because of increased responsibilities and perhaps role changes imposed by the illness or disability. But there is also a unique relationship that must be considered in an attempt to fully understand the situation of the client whose life depends intimately and directly on technology: the relationship between the person and a machine or mechanical device.

Today, everyone is dependent to a large degree on technology. There would be no way to feed the population of the United States, for example, without a mechanized farming and transportation system. When they are ill, most people depend on technology for diagnosis and treatment, but they are not directly, intimately, and regularly dependent on a machine for life itself. This, however, is the situation of clients on dialysis and those who have implanted pacemakers.

Some clients who have been dialyzed say that they feel dehumanized by their dependence on a machine for what should be a normal function of their own bodies. These people do not feel entirely human. Some liken themselves to "zombies," people risen from the dead, or "androids," robots who appear human. On the other hand, they may project human feelings onto the machine, at times even having delusions that the machine is performing well or poorly with some direct intent to benefit or destroy them.

Clients understandably feel a great deal of ambivalence about dependence on a machine or other device and focus considerable frustration and anger upon others. One client spoke of this relationship by saying, "I find it impossible to make friends with the monster." Because clients to some extent incorporate the artificial or mechanical device as a part of themselves, they also project their own feelings onto it. It should also be remembered that people who are seriously enough ill to need mechanical assistance to maintain life are often experiencing some organic brain syndrome. Resulting confusion could increase the distortion in their minds concerning their relationship to a machine or other device.

Conflict between Independence and Dependence

The conflict between independence and dependence is one of the most troublesome for the person with chronic illness. Although this is an important conflict for any chronically ill person, it is perhaps more salient for clients who are involved with frequent, direct dependence on a machine, injections, or physical therapy and the person who is assisting with the use of that machine, administering the life-sustaining drug, or helping with the exercise program. It is most difficult to be dependent in the area of treatment of an illness and then to function independently in the rest of life. There are some people who are able to accomplish this well, but many clients exhibit either excessive dependence in all areas of their lives or a rebellious, adolescent type of counterdependence which does not allow effective medical management of the illness. The client's behaviors can include resistance to treatment, sabotage of treatment, or demands for assistance in activities which could be managed unaided.

DSM III

While there are no specific medical diagnoses which apply uniquely to the mental health problems of the chronically ill and disabled populations, several subcategories of *adjustment disorder* and the diagnosis of *psychological factors affecting physical condition* may serve as appropriate labels. The subcategories of *adjustment disorder* include codes for clients with depressed and anxious mood; clients with mixed emotional features, with disturbance of conduct, and with mixed emotions and conduct; clients with work (or academic) inhibition, with withdrawal problems, and with atypical features. When a client's emotional difficulties interfere with maximizing physical function, the label *psychological factors affecting physical condition* may be appropriate.[3]

Epidemiology

Chronically ill and disabled clients constitute a major health care population. However, it is believed that although more than 10 percent of the world's population have physical disabilities, only about 3 percent receive any health care.[3] Even fewer clients receive any mental health intervention. The community health issues created by this population are numerous. To cite statistics here is beyond the scope of the chapter; students are referred to community health nursing texts for specific data. It is sufficient to remind the reader that chronically ill and disabled clients have an impact on every area of the health care system. It is also remarkable that only recently has legislation been adopted to prevent discrimination against this population. A multitude of mental health, rehabilitative, and vocational services are necessary to help restore clients to optimal psychosocial wellness.[4]

PATTERNS OF INTERACTION: PERSON

Losses and changes are inherent in chronic illness and disability. Losses and changes vary in extent, severity, and timing. In some cases massive accommodations are required and the level of optimal functioning is severely limited, while in other instances the level of functioning is only minimally affected. The number and severity of the losses influence the person's ability to accommodate, attain an optimal level of functioning, and continue to enjoy life.

Physical losses include loss of independence, comfort, physical functions, and familiar surroundings. Loss of mental functions and alterations in self-concept constitute the major mental losses. Spiritual losses include loss of well-being and of one's role in society.

Loss of Independence

From the moment of birth people struggle for an appropriate amount of personal independence in their environment and human relationships. Events throughout their lives help form patterns of dependence and independence. If all goes well, as they reach adulthood, a balanced personality structure that allows for maximum creativity and integrity emerges. When people become ill, however, they are forced back into patterns of dependence they had long since abandoned.

Loss of Comfort

It is both distracting and frightening to be physically uncomfortable. The discomfort is an ever-present reminder of vulnerability and does not allow a person to focus well on other aspects of life. The more severe the discomfort, the more severe the disruption of activities, ranging from care of one's own body to interpersonal relationships. Different conditions cause different types and levels of discomfort. The person with chronic kidney disease suffers pain, itching, weakness, and some periodic mental slowness and confusion. The paraplegic must learn to live with frequent muscle spasms. Some medication regimens involve intramuscular or subcutaneous injections; each injection is a source of discomfort. Additionally, the injection sites may become scarred, making penetration of the needle difficult, impairing absorption, or both. Catheters and ostomy appliances may be a constant source of physical discomfort and embarrassment. Procedures for changing and cleaning these appliances usually produce some degree of physical and psychological discomfort. Skin irritations are not uncommon, and unpleasant odors are distressing.

People who are ill must often depend on others for assistance with bodily needs and functions, from help with personal hygiene and mobility to help with using the toilet. Other adults, from family members to professionals who are strangers, often take over decision making for a person who is ill. It is at best frightening and conflicting for adults when they are suddenly forced to revert to patterns of dependence they have not experienced since childhood.

People who are suffering from acute temporary health problems can look forward to regaining independence. However, chronically ill and disabled people must confront either sudden or eventual, and inevitable, loss of independence. Rehabilitation and health supervision may be able to help restore or conserve independence in some areas of functioning. However, the end result is more often than not some degree of dependence on a hospital and its personnel, a machine, a diet, appliances, prosthesis, medications, possibly a shunt for dialysis, perhaps society for financial assistance, and many other things which together make up a "program" to maintain life.

People with some disabilities may in reality be able with appliances to regain physical function, but initially this is not easily accepted because the implication is a loss of independence. Clients with pacemakers and brittle diabetics are also dependent on the health care system for periodic care and emergency treatment. Not since infancy have such people been so dependent for survival on people and things outside themselves. At the same time that they have lost adult independence in so many areas, they are expected to maintain independent adult behavior in areas of work, finances, family relationships, and other social relationships. This is a difficult task at best, requiring the development of new self-concepts and patterns of dependence and independence. The degree to which people are successful in working with the human condition of dependence and independence before illness will directly affect the degree to which they can adjust creatively to the demands of chronic disease.

Loss of Physical Functions

Many people with chronic illnesses experience intermittent or permanent loss of various physical functions. People with kidney failure are no longer handling fluids and urination as they once did. They often complain of an overall weakness and malaise which prevents them from performing usual and desired activities. With many chronic illnesses, active participation in sports or jobs requiring physical strength or stamina must be abandoned. Neurological deficits may be so great that not only is mobility impaired but, as in the case of multiple sclerosis and amyotrophic lateral sclerosis, the ability to chew and swallow food may be severely altered. Some motor diseases of the nervous system interfere with coordinated purposeful movement, speech production, and facial expression. These changes interfere with initiating and maintaining interpersonal relationships and with a myriad of job-related and recreational activities.[5]

Physical attractiveness is culturally determined but universally desirable. Alterations in bodily structure and function may detract from a person's appearance or be invisible but negatively influence the person's self-perception. A negative self-image, and particularly a negative body image, can result in unilateral or mutual social withdrawal. The person who perceives the self as unattractive may also see the self as undesirable as a companion and a sex partner. Alterations in physical attractiveness that are highly visible may include scars from extensive surgery, skin discolorations, a flaccid limb, or bizarre movements of the face or extremities. Such changes may be distressing to the person and significant others. Ostomies may not be visible under clothing, but the fear that they are odoriferous may put them in the same category as more visible disfigurements.

Another important physical loss is the loss of sexual function. Sexual problems arise as a result of the physical effects and psychological stress of the illness or disability. Sexual functioning of clients is altered when they experience vascular disease, psychogenic stress, physical illness, and diseases affecting the nervous system. Certain medications that affect the central nervous system and vascular system also alter sexual performance. Lack of muscular coordination, joint pain and impairment, and the presence of catheters can all interfere with sexual interest and performance, and with the perception of oneself or another as a desirable sexual partner. Malaise, chronic pain, ongoing grief, and negative responsiveness of a sexual partner can affect sexual functioning. Multilating surgery has an impact on sexual functioning, either temporarily or permanently. Those who have suffered injuries to the spinal cord usually have neurological impairments that permanently affect sexual performance. They also face body-image changes, probable decrease in self-esteem, and difficulty with gender identity because of forced changes in role functioning. Decisions about marriage and parenthood and finding new ways to express and experience sexuality are also dimensions of changed sexual functioning. The view that sexual function is a private concern, cultural attitudes that make people uncomfortable about sexuality, abounding misinformation, and myths about the sexual needs and concerns of disabled and chronically ill people contribute to the difficulty people have in acquiring accurate and helpful information, thus compounding their loss.

Loss of Familiar Surroundings

If the onset of a chronic illness is sudden, the illness is inherently catastrophic. At a time when clients could most use the reassurances of the place and people they know best, they are forced to move to a hospital, which is a strange environment, and to relate in a dependent manner to many strangers who purport to help them. When the illness is chronic, the person faces repeated hospitalizations. In the case of chronic kidney failure, for example, the treatment of hemodialysis is often done in the hospital setting. No matter how familiar a setting the hospital becomes, it is never a place where the person controls the environment.

Extensive loss of the ability to move purposefully interferes with self-care. Following the acute phase of a disease, a person may be transferred to another unit or hospital for rehabilitation. The length of residential stay in such a program varies according to the extent of the need for rehabilitative intervention and the person's capacity and ability to participate in the program. If the rehabilitation program is extensive, the person may be confined to this setting for months. With time, the unfamiliar becomes familiar, predictable, and comfortable. When residential rehabilitation is temporary, clients must eventually again endure a change of environment.

If after rehabilitation the person is still unable to manage self-care and needs some level of skilled nursing care, the decision for long-term hospitalization may be made. Relocation to another treatment center again exposes the person to the loss of familiar surroundings and the need to accommodate to a new setting.

Discharge to one's own home may not necessarily be a return to familiar, comfortable, or predictable surroundings. If the person still has major limitations in relation to mobility and self-care, the home environment may need to undergo major changes. The client may not be able to return to his or her bedroom, to a favorite family room, or to certain other parts of the home because of the inability to climb stairs or the need to have bathroom facilities accessible. Clients may find themselves relocated to a converted dining room, for example, that has been turned into a combined bedroom and sitting room. To simplify the caregiving process, the family may have outfitted the room with hospital furnishings, further depriving the person of what is familiar. In some instances the financial burden imposed by the illness and the loss of income may have resulted in a relocation to more affordable quarters.

Loss of Mental Functions

The emotional stress of trying to cope with the many losses of chronic disease results in states of anxiety and depression. People are often less able to concentrate and organize thoughts efficiently, so that they cannot think as clearly as they did before the illness. In addition, many illnesses result in organic changes which affect mental functioning. Fluid and electrolyte imbalances and the buildup of toxins or waste products caused by kidney or liver dysfunction can result in organic brain problems such as language or memory impairment. Medications such as diuretics and antihypertensives can also cause mental confusion. Brain-tissue damage caused by trauma or cerebrovascular accidents also influences cognitive and affective functioning. People suffering from Huntington's chorea eventually exhibit severe psychiatric disturbances, and symptoms during the latter stages of multiple sclerosis include confusion, disorientation, and memory deficits.[6]

Loss of Well-Being

Health and illness are incorporated into self-concept. Before they become ill, people usually perceive themselves as healthy, perhaps even vigorous and enthusiastic about life. Chronic illness and disability alter this dimension of the self-concept. Healthy thinking about self is lost. Assuming the sick role and the "client" identity reinforces this revision and clarifies the associated losses and changes.

A person may experience a physical crisis and respond realistically with great fear and anxiety for life itself. People around the ill person offer reassurance about what realistically can be done. If treatment does indeed help the person's physical functioning, fear of extinction moves into the background. If there are residual impairments, attempts must be made to deal with many changes. However, the fear of death is a backdrop for all the less catastrophic fears to follow.

A sense of well-being, the capacity to learn self-care tasks, and the ability to participate in pleasurable preillness activities may be lost. The dependence on care givers, families, and machines may cause emotional distress, and the disease process may produce physical distress. Discomforts, impediments, and, at times, episodes of pain emphasize the loss of health and reinforce the status of being ill.

Loss of Self-Concept

As noted above, before the onset of a chronic illness or the development of a disability, a person has the concept of self as healthy. After an initial episode of illness, if recovery is not complete, the concept of self is altered and the person views the self as impaired, disabled, or handicapped. The degree of response to alterations in self-concept is a function of:

- Functional significance of the body part, identity, or role involved
- Importance of physical appearance, identity, status, or role to the person
- Visibility of the part, identity, or role
- Feasibility and availability of rehabilitation
- Speed with which the change occurred
- Previous coping patterns and their effectiveness[7]

The significance to the person of the particular body part affected by the chronic illness or disability will influence the degree of dysynchrony experienced by the person. Some body parts are more highly invested and endowed with emotional significance. For example, the heart is commonly viewed as the symbol of life; the seat of love, hate, pain, joy, and sorrow; and even the location of the soul. The brain, genitals, and breasts are also perceived as highly significant. Some people also place a high emotional value on other body parts not commonly conceived of as highly significant. Involvement of these specially invested body parts elicits a greater psychobiological response than may be expected.

The functional significance of certain identities and roles is in part due to societal influences, as in the case of the male's role as breadwinner. For some people their professional identity is a significant and perhaps overdetermining dimension of their self-concept. Loss of significant identities and roles can be perceived as catastrophic.

The visibility not only of the body part or parts involved but also of the person's identity or role is another significant factor affecting the self-concept.

The alterations in body structure and function that occur with chronic illness and disability may be viewed as overwhelming losses. If rehabilitation is feasible and available, the prospect of recovering and reversing some or all of the losses offers hope, and self-esteem is less likely to be severely affected.

Whether a chronic illness or disability develops slowly or suddenly is another factor that influences the person's ability to work through the changes and losses and maintain self-esteem. Sudden, traumatic, and massive alterations in body structure and function may prolong the period of shock, disbelief, and denial, particularly if the person's physiological status is unstable. A slower onset allows a person time to acknowledge what is occurring and work through the losses gradually. Being able to anticipate provides opportunities to plan future accommodations. When the progressive changes are known to be evidence of complete loss of function and control, leading to death, they may be dreaded. Such changes generate a greater response, even if they impose only minimal limitations, than changes that produce severe limitations but do not shorten life. Regardless of whether the changes and losses are sudden or gradual, there is usually some degree of lag between occurrences of the alterations and the person's awareness of the extent of these alterations and revision of self-concept.

Whether the person is willing and able to maximize available rehabilitative resources is in part a function of past experiences with problems and the degree of hope he or she can muster when confronted with a crisis. A self-perception of being a strong, competent survivor enhances participation and persistence in the rehabilitation process.

When the conception of self is disturbed and distorted by chronic illness or disability, feelings of insecurity and fear develop. When the innermost level of bodily experience is affected, as in the case of Cushing's syndrome, kidney failure, or cirrhosis, it is a profoundly frightening feeling. Changes and associated sensations at this physiological level are experienced as life-threatening.[8] Some bodily changes have observable results such as muscle flaccidity, bizarre movements, or severe mood swings. These changes may be accompanied by feelings of shame. When a hereditary component exists, as in the case of Huntington's chorea, there may be feelings of guilt and fear about passing on the defective genes to children. Some bodily changes disturb the ability to relate to the environment. The stroke client whose hemiplegia affects the facial muscles has distorted facial expressions which interfere with nonverbal communication. If aphasia is also present, interactions with others are either unsatisfactory or almost impossible.

It has also been pointed out that the ability to function with control—relative to the time and place of activities—is held in personal, social, and cultural esteem. To achieve what is desired precisely at the right time and in the right way gives people a sense of accomplishment and self-esteem. A stroke victim with emotional lability is deprived of the ability to use emotions as an expression of what is experienced, to communicate feelings coherently, and to do so when and where it is appropriate. Self-respect is measured by these as well as more sophisticated accomplishments. Interference with the ability to derive satisfaction and respect from accomplishments leads to frustration, anxiety, and fear. To lose complex, coordinated, and controlled functional abilities which have been achieved and integrated into the personal system is to lose or be threatened with the loss of self.[8]

Loss of One's Role in Society

People develop lifestyles which include participation in travel, theater, church, community, work, sports, school, and social groups. Such activities may be disrupted temporarily or permanently by chronic illness or disability. Our society stresses independence as a virtue, and the dependence forced on people by illness results in a loss of cultural as well as personal esteem.

PATTERNS OF INTERACTION: FAMILY

The families of people with chronic illness or disability suffer fear and loss in much the same way as clients. They experience fear about the permanent loss of the loved one through death as well as the constant losses and changes in role and functioning that are responses to the changes in the client. The family goes through a process of denial, grief, and mourning, and it is subject to many situational stressors, some of them related to special problems created by home care. Family dynamics can evolve in effective or ineffective ways. The "spectator–care giver" pattern is an example of ineffective family dynamics; the pattern of "mutual participation" is an example of effective family dynamics.[9]

Denial

Family members use denial to cushion the feelings brought about by loss and to avoid confronting the inevitable changes in their own lives that will occur as a result of the illness and disability. When the initial shock begins to dissipate, reality overcomes the denial; fear, anxiety, and depression are experienced. Sometimes the timing of the development of these feelings varies among family members, or between family members and the client. When this occurs, the member who realizes the full implications of the situation feels unsupported and isolated if the rest of the family persists in denial. If the aware member attempts to confront the other members' denial, he or she may become the recipient of the family's anger.

Some families have an intolerance for the expression of feelings. There is an unspoken expectation that regardless of the situation one must keep the proverbial "stiff upper lip." Encounters between the client and family members are superficial and directed toward "cheering up" the client. Painful feelings and anxiety-provoking subjects are avoided. Family members expect the client to "cheer up," minimize his or her losses, and make no complaints or demands. These family expectations are often derived from the need to have the sick member be more comfortable and to be themselves less pained and burdened by what they see their loved one experiencing.

Anger, Anxiety, and Depression

When the family members are depressed and anxious, they may become so preoccupied with their own distress that they are unavailable as a support system to the client.

Whether there is full realization or continued denial, the family has a need to survive. The day-to-day adjustments and accommodations may become a burden because of the added responsibilities. The client has the support of the treatment or rehabilitation team, but the family members may perceive themselves as struggling alone and unsupported. Overburdened and inconvenienced because of the chronic illness or disability, and the deprivations it entails, they become angry. However, anger toward a loved one who is chronically ill and suffering, and whose life is threatened, is intolerable, and guilt is experienced.

Family members also experience a sense of helplessness because they are not able to alleviate the ill person's suffering or bring back life as it used to be. There is great frustration and mourning for all the dreams for the future that must be abandoned.

Situational Stresses

There are multiple situational changes for families over and above the changes in the client's status. Finances are usually a problem as work gets interrupted and the expense of treatment has to be met. Daily schedules and routines are altered. The family's dietary habits may not be compatible with the client's needs, and there may be requirements necessitating the preparation of special meals in special ways. Relationships with friends change, sometimes gradually, usually in the direction of deterioration, resulting in a loss of support. Often social contacts are narrowed to the nuclear family. People find it difficult to deal with chronic illness, and the client may have limited energy, so that there is mutual withdrawal.

Chronic illness and disability often jeopardize roles and relationships in a family. Once the initial crisis of accommodation has passed, the family settles into new roles and divisions of labor and responsibilities. If the family and client sustain the latter's sick role and the former's care-giver role, there is a tendency to use these roles as excuses to allow dependence, to avoid responsibility, and to ignore demands for involvement and participation in the family and the community. The stresses on the family are very great, and hostile feelings toward the client are sometimes acted out by the family in life-threatening ways: medical appointments are missed and dietary restrictions are not supported or perhaps even directly violated. With home care there is sometimes large, ominous equipment which serves as a constant reminder of the client's problem, its severity, and the responsibility it imposes on the family member or members who must assist the client. For example, home care with hemodialysis or home care of people who are totally disabled poses increased problems for the relationship between the client and the person assisting with the dialysis or the physical care, usually a spouse. The person manipulating the machinery is constantly fearful that the loved one will die as a result of some mechanical malfunction; this is, of course a real possibility.

Anger is often repressed but constantly fed by a situation in which the person giving the care feels that there is a great deal of "giving" and little "getting" in return. Denial is the usual defense used to cope with the difficulties, and this, of course, interferes with the quality of the relationship.

Home care of people who are totally disabled is known to be stressful, perhaps to the point of being contraindicated in some cases. Clients such as those who are confined to beds and wheelchairs and those who have progressive weakening and wasting of muscles have problems maintaining authentic relationships because of their unavoidable dependence. The client's dependence and the family's care-giving burden are known sources of stress. Loyalty bonds and a family ethic, "We take care of our own," sustain the relationship but not without cost.

A family's socioeconomic status can influence the way in which the family members manage imposed losses and changes. Problem solving and access to resources are enhanced by a higher socioeconomic status. When there is a sound financial basis, the family is better able to make the physical alterations in the home that facilitate care and to afford help with the household chores and the care of the disabled member.

Losses Experienced by Children

Not enough is known about the reaction of children to a parent who is chronically ill or disabled. Children are, however, exposed to vast changes in family life, particularly frequent parental absences, losses in family life, and frightening scenes such as hemorrhages.

When a parent is chronically ill, the stress within the family is often characterized by inconsistency and instability in setting limits, giving affection, demonstrating love, letting go appropriately, separating, and balancing dependence and independence. Discipline is often a problem as children act out their angry and depressed feelings around the loss and deprivation in their lives. School performance may decline, and aggressive or withdrawal behavior may develop.

If the parent is absent or bedridden at home, children may be expected to assume household responsibilities beyond their developmental capacities. This "parentification" of the child disturbs the child's growth and development and initiates a multigenerational loyalty imbalance. The child feels more loyal and more "parentlike" toward the sick parent than the parent feels toward the child. Without intervention and change, this imbalance will affect the child's own offspring.

Subtle learning occurs regarding the way one's dependency needs are met in a family. The children in a household that revolves around the needs of a disabled parent learn that the sick role is a way to be nurtured and to control others. The multigenerational transmission process will operate. Even if these children later become overnurturing parents initially, in time the burden of the parent role will become too stressful, a sick role will be assumed, and a child in the next generation will also be parentified.

If the disabled parent is demanding and irritable and seeks satisfaction of dependency needs in the parent-child relationship, the child may feel angry, resentful, and deprived. However, children learn at an early age that the sick, be they animals or people, are fragile and need nurturing. Consequently, they will feel guilty about their angry feelings. This guilt may create a need for self-punishment. Such children become vulnerable to unconscious self-destructive behavior or high-risk behavior.

Adolescence is a time of turmoil and identity formation. Parents continue to be a source of introjections. If the parent is disabled or disfigured, the introjections may include these impairments and contribute to an adolescent's poor self-image. Adolescents are sensitive to impairments in body image. Their anxieties related to "being different" may be so great that they avoid the disabled parent or respond with hostility. The latter is both anxiety-producing and guilt-producing. Adolescents who experience such stresses may act out with substance abuse or antisocial behavior.

Family Dynamics

"Spectator–Care Giver" Dynamics: Ineffective Functioning

When a client is an inactive bystander and the family members become overresponsible and take over his or her care, the resulting interactions can be described as "spectator–care giver dynamics." These dynamics are maintained only with the implied consent of everyone involved. The spectator could not sustain his or her role unless the family supported it, and the family could not be overresponsible unless the client passively or actively "gave up" some aspect of personal responsibility.[9]

The spectator role is characterized by refraining from family activities; constantly watching television; loss of future orientation; exemption from all productive or constructive activities; and abandonment of socialization with extended family and friends. The spectator is preoccupied with physical status or discomfort. These people seem immobilized in their position and overwhelmed by fears of abandonment, confusion, depression, and anxiety. Deprived of their original roles, they seem unable to compromise and renegotiate modified versions, evolve new roles, or even become interested in avocations. They generalize their impairments and remain inactive. The dependency of the spectator becomes a manipulative device that is recognized on some level by the family members, who suppress and repress their anger because they perceive the spectator as "sick."[9]

Family members support the "spectator role." They may feel guilty for leaving the spectator alone and for continuing their lives outside the family. They participate in the process by making no demands, acting in an overprotective fashion, and denying evidence that the spectator is indeed capable of acting productively and constructively in areas not affected by his or her disability.

"Mutual Participation" Dynamics: Effective Functioning

When a disabled member actively participates in family life and activities within the limitations imposed by the disease process or the disability, and the family members "do for" or "act for" the person *only* when and where the disability totally impairs the person's capacity to act in his or her own behalf, the resulting pattern can be described as "mutual participation." Parties, picnics, and other social events, as well as household management and support, become family projects. If the disabled member cannot perform physical chores, he or she may become the planner, delegator, or coordinator.[9]

The disabled family member is encouraged and supported in efforts to work. The illness is redefined as a handicap. If work outside the home is or becomes physically impossible, the family supports the person in finding and developing a new avocation. Social relationships are maintained. If the client becomes discouraged, the family is supportive and encouraging. Likewise, the client recognizes family members' needs for help and support and "gives" in ways that are possible despite physical limitations. Traditional roles may be modified, but the client's preillness status as a worthwhile person and authority figure is sustained.

PATTERNS OF INTERACTION: ENVIRONMENT

All societies, to varying degrees, respond negatively to those members who are disfigured, different, or deviant. The presence of these imperfections in society confronts the well members' vulnerability. This confrontation is anxiety-provoking and leads to self-protective distancing maneuvers. Societal attitudes vary from pity and protectiveness to hatred and cruelty, from prejudice to humor. Job discrimination and physical and emotional barriers isolate and alienate chronically ill and disabled people.[7]

Personal worth is a function of both personal self-definition and societal definition. A stigma is attached to an attribute, either physical or psychological, that is deeply discrediting—one that makes an individual different from others and less desirable. Social stigma is associated with deformities, disfigurements, chronic illnesses, and disabilities. Disabled people are used by society as a reference group for gauging the dimensions of normality and for maintaining a sense of identity and personal integrity for the rest of society.[10]

In our society there are four barriers that prevent those who are developmentally challenged from leading "normal" lives: (1) confused value system, (2) problems of mobility, (3) obstacles to entry into the world of work, and (4) lags in implementing technology.[11]

Confused Value System

Our society has espoused "rugged individualism" as a basic philosophical tenet since its foundation. Therefore, the concept of interdependence of individuals in a society, which has greater relevance for a highly technological urbanized society, is less acceptable. Lack of support for the principle of interdependence is best illustrated by the government's and the citizenry's meager support of handicapped people.

The ability to make money and attain affluence, based on rugged individualism, is highly valued in our society. Consequently, a primary thrust of rehabilitation is achievement as measured by acquiring job skills, and a primary thrust of societal responsibility is the promotion of hiring handicapped people.

Still another societal value, the traditional supportive family, is in reality more myth than fact. The high divorce rates and the prevalence of blended families and geographically scattered family members negate the traditional conception of a family as mother, father, child or children, and an extended family nearby. All too often handicapped and chronically ill people do not have intact families, and among those who do have traditional families, many find that these families are either unable or unwilling to fulfill a supportive role.

Problems of Mobility

In spite of the recent governmental efforts to remove obstacles to transportation and mobility, there are still many barriers. Newer architecture tends to accommodate the special needs of handicapped people; however, proportionally there are far more older buildings which have barriers such as narrow bathroom doors that prevent entry of a wheelchair, telephones placed out of the reach of someone in a wheelchair, and access to upper floors only by stairs because there are neither elevators nor ramps. Special buses exist, but in most instances their availability and accessibility are limited. Resorts for handicapped and chronically ill adult vacationers are becoming more common. Many more affluent places have accommodated their facilities on a limited basis. However, the larger poor and middle-class population does not have access to this type of facility. The societal message again is that only those who are financially productive can have access to leisure activities and vacation resorts.

Obstacles to Entry into the World of Work

The previously cited lack of availability and accessibility of transportation is a significant barrier to finding and maintaining employment. The sheltered workshop has been promoted as a source of employment for handicapped people. However, in such a setting the work tends to be characterized by simple repetitive tasks that do not challenge the intellect or creative abilities. Workers are usually paid the minimum hourly wage, and promotions that would provide greater responsibility, prestige, and more money are nonexistent. Meaningful employment, integration into the job market, and a living wage are not always readily available to chronically ill and disabled people.

Participation in the working world for many who are able is also discouraged by disability compensation. Rather than accommodating the workplace or providing meaningful job retraining, some companies prefer to support and encourage premature retirement from the system and not to define significant roles for disabled people.[11]

Lags in Implementing Technology

Accelerated development of technology characterizes our society. Massive amounts of money have been invested in space programs, and great technological advances have been accomplished. However, there has been a considerable lag in applying these technological advances to helping disabled people. Spin-offs that are profitable and widely marketable have developed quickly because money from the private sector has been invested in their development. The same investments of time and money have not been made by either private industry or government in applying this technology to helping chronically ill and disabled people overcome or compensate for their impairments. If the same energy, time, and money were invested in developing technology for handicapped people, those who are blind might be helped to "see," those who are deaf to "hear," and those who have uncontrolled muscle coordination to function purposefully.

Breakthroughs have occurred, but funding and public interest do not support refining these discoveries or promoting rapid dissemination among those who could benefit. Because such technology is not highly profitable and because of the devalued position of people who are socially stigmatized, a lag exists.

NURSING PROCESS

Applying the nursing process to people who are disabled or chronically ill involves careful assessment of the person, the family, and the environment. Nursing diagnoses will be varied in nature and will need periodic review and revision as the client moves through the various stages of adjustment. Intervention should be consistent and will vary in degree from complete wholly compensatory care of the client to self-care. Evaluation, scheduled at periodic intervals, is necessary to keep goals and plans current.

Assessment

Clients with chronic illness and disability experience biopsychosocial response to the imposed losses and changes and their perception of the situation. The assessment of these clients is directed toward finding out how they are managing changes and losses. Since the grieving process is a significant dimension of this management, it is vital that distortions of the grieving process be identified as early as possible. Monitoring "grief work" is, therefore, a significant nursing activity.

The Person

A client's responses to the following assessment questions will provide health care professionals with the data needed to determine the client's reactions to the chronic nature of the disability.

- What was the client's emotional response to information about the diagnosis and its long-term implications?
- Has the client verbalized sad and angry feelings about his or her situation?
- Has the client shed tears in response to talking about the losses and changes imposed by the disease process or disability?
- Has the client been able to talk about what the implications of the situation mean to him or her?
- How does the client deal with the depression, anxiety, and inevitable frustrations and angry feelings related to the losses?
- Has the client been able to talk about what his or her life was like before the present situation, particularly those aspects that will be drastically altered by the chronic disease or disability?
- Does the client have an accurate perception of the situation and still retain either expectations or hope?
- What efforts does the client make to remain maximally functional and active?
- How is the client making decisions regarding choice and timing of treatment approaches?

The assessment process focuses on determining whether the person is expressing anger, depression, anxiety, or denial; how these are being expressed; and whether the expression is being accepted by care givers and significant others as a normal and necessary part of the process of dealing with the imposed losses. If the expression of feeling is producing interpersonal problems for the client, steps can be taken to help all concerned to understand and accept the situation. The assessment of feelings in chronically ill and disabled clients focuses primarily on the inhibition of direct expression and the consequences of that inhibition which impair accommodation to the imposed changes and losses. The following questions are useful:

- What is the client's ability to verbalize feelings of frustration?
- What effect does the displacement of anger have on the client, family, and care givers?
- Is there evidence of noncompliance and subtle sabotage of the plan of care?
- Is the client able to follow directions concerning medications and their side effects?
- Does the client have the capacity to attend and relate to others or the environment?
- What is the client's perception of his or her dependency?
- To what degree does the person initiate self-care and self-responsibility, given the extent of im-

pairment imposed by the disease process or disability?

- Does the client verbalize feelings about dependency and the losses and changes that have been experienced?
- What is the client's emotional tone while receiving care; what changes occur when the care is initiated and terminated?
- What is the degree of change imposed by disease or disability?
- Does the client participate in planning care and selecting and implementing the treatment regimen?
- What defenses does the client use to cope with the disability?
- Is denial used to screen out the frightening aspects of the situation?
- Is fantasy used to gratify frustrated desires through imaginary accomplishments that enhance ego integrity?
- Is rationalization used to justify self-worth?
- Is projection used to fix blame outside the self and protect ego integrity?
- Is repression of emotionally painful thoughts and feelings being used?
- Is reaction formation used to prevent the expression of threatening wishes?
- Is regression used to increase the client's tolerance of depression?
- Is identification used in the process of redefining identity?
- Is introjection used in incorporating values consonant with the altered self?
- Is compensation used to mask weaknesses and emphasize strengths?
- Is displacement used to rid the self of feelings that militate against reintegration and preservation of ego identity by venting them on an external object or person?
- Is emotional isolation used to protect the self from emotional pain?
- Is intellectualization used to dampen emotional pain and compartmentalize incompatible attitudes?
- Is acting-out behavior used to discharge the tensions produced by the losses?
- Is sublimation used to gratify unsatisfied needs?

The Family

The nurse should interview each family as a unit as soon as possible after admission of the client so that communication and the flow of accurate information will be facilitated right from the start. The nurse needs to know how each member perceives and is affected by the illness and what areas of strength and weakness need support and intervention as the family tries to cope. There should be periodic family meetings to facilitate accurate monitoring of the family's adjustment and, when necessary, intervention. In this way, crises can be prevented.

Assessment of the family must focus on the interaction that occurs within the family and its effect on the management of stress associated with chronic illness and disability. As more and more clients are cared for by their families or health care professionals at home, an important component of the family assessment becomes the family's readiness to care for the client for an indefinite period of time. The following factors need to be considered when assessing family needs:

- What is the nature of the family's way of responding to the client?
- What is the family's tolerance of the expression of emotionally painful feelings?
- Does the family have the ability to foster the client's self-determination?
- What is the family's capacity and willingness to be available and accessible as a support system?
- Does the family recognize and attempt to meet members' individual needs?
- Is the client or the client's sexual partner able to discuss and work through the changes in sexual functioning imposed by the illness or disability?
- Are the family's personal resources supportive of home care?
- What is the family's process for making decisions regarding the client's care when the latter's capacity for self-determination is impaired by the disease process?
- Does the family have the ability to grieve over the loss of the member when his or her identity is severely altered by the disease process?
- What was the client's previous level of sexual functioning?
- What meaning does sexual activity have for the client?
- What is the client's cultural environment?
- What significance does physical wholeness have for the client?

- Has the client accepted or rejected the current illness or surgical alteration?
- What is the client's sense of body image and self-esteem?
- What is the client's outlook for the future?
- What is the client's sensory status?
- What are the alterations in the client's perception and sensitivity to touch?
- What is the client's capacity for mobility?
- What degree of assistance does the client need to fulfill sexual needs?
- What is the family's understanding of the client's future sexual functioning?
- Is the client's sexual partner open to and willing to explore alternative means of sexual enjoyment?
- Does the client have a supportive sexual partner?
- Does the client have other family members who can offer support?
- Is the client isolated or cut off from family members?
- Is the spouse or another family member capable of and willing to learn the care necessary for meeting the client's needs?
- Is the client able to assume independent functioning?

The Community

The use of a systems framework for conceptualizing the problems of chronic illness and disability emphasizes the importance of environmental influences. Questions useful in assessing the environment include:

- Are necessary resources, such as home care support, transportation, physical therapy, and financial aid, available and accessible?
- To what degree does social stigma interfere with the normalization process?
- How sensitive are care givers to the special needs of the client?
- What is the capacity of the treatment team to facilitate the client's and family's participation in the care-giving process?
- What physical aspects of the environment enhance self-care?
- Is technology to lessen or remove the impact of the disability available and accessible?
- What meaningful employment opportunities exist for the client?

Diagnosis

Analysis of the assessment data provides the basis for conceptualizing the client's problems and formulating nursing diagnosis. The following are examples of nursing diagnoses representative of some of the major problems and needs confronted by these clients:

- Noncompliance with treatment regimen related to excessive use of denial
- Inability to comprehend content of teaching plan associated with high levels of anxiety
- Pattern of withdrawal from relationships related to depression
- Inappropriate expression of anger related to family disorganization
- Inconsistent work habits related to abandonment by the family
- Sexual dysfunction associated with chronic pain
- Rejection of physical limitations related to denial of disability

Outcome Criteria

When the data base regarding the client's and family's responses to the chronic nature of the disease and its ramifications has been assembled and diagnoses have been formulated, outcome criteria are determined. Outcome criteria are set by the nurse to provide direction in the formulation and planning of intervention. They also provide a way of evaluating care. The following represent selected outcome criteria established for clients with chronic illnesses:

- Client will verbalize insight into use of excessive denial after six therapy sessions with clinical specialist.
- Client will exhibit independence in the organization and completion of activities of daily living after three instruction sessions with nurse.
- Client will report decreased levels of anxiety following instruction in stress-alleviation techniques.
- Client will attend vocational rehabilitation workshops for six meetings.
- Family will visit client twice weekly after supportive intervention by nurse.
- Spouse will verbalize improved sexual function following sex therapy sessions.
- Client and family will attend family therapy sessions once a week.

- Client and family will effectively express sad, anxious, and angry feelings.
- Client will experience periods of appropriate depression, indicating that the loss of functions is being faced and ramifications are being felt.
- Client will resume some old and begin some new relationships and activities, with recognition and integration of the loss as part of life.

Intervention

Intervention with the Person

GRIEVING PROCESS. Clients coping with loss are dealing with feelings of disbelief, anxiety, anger, depression, and fear. They are using many defenses to soften the impact of the loss so that feelings can be faced and worked through. The nurse's first responsibility is to understand the human feelings of grief and the process of mourning so that the client's emotional responses can be understood.

Acceptance of clients' feelings about the changes in their lives is the way in which nurses can best help these people to endure the painful period of grief and continue to some resolution of their loss. This can be a difficult task, because everyone prefers to avoid feelings such as fear, despair, and anger. Genuine acceptance of whatever a person needs to feel supports that person's self-concept and prevents isolation. This support allows the person to work through the necessary painful feelings and resolve the losses.

> One young man with diabetes suddenly developed irreversible renal failure. His brow was always knit, his eyes were open wide, and his gaze darted from object to object in the room. He was sweating and sighing a great deal, but his only comments were that he was sure his kidneys would be fine, and that any hour now the doctors would discover this, too. This man was very appropriately in the initial phase of grieving for his lost kidneys. Part of him did not believe that this loss had occurred, but somewhere there was a beginning realization of the loss as he exhibited anxiety and depression.

In the case of the young man with diabetes and renal failure, the nurse need not confront his verbal denial. Instead, comments such as, "It must be very hard for you to believe this has happened to you," are most helpful, because they recognize, acknowledge, and accept what is happening to this person. Such an approach should eventually encourage this client to talk about anxieties.

When clients use denial to the degree that it interferes with treatment, the nursing intervention is aimed at helping them accept themselves as worthwhile. Illness does not diminish one's value as a person or one's dignity. The nursing task is to help the person confront, *a little at a time,* the losses imposed by the disease and to mourn these losses effectively.

Clients will at times fail to cooperate with the treatment program. Uncooperativeness must be recognized as meeting a need for the client and not interpreted as a rejection of the nurse, the team, or the program. Reassessment of the client's physical, social, and psychological status may reveal the need to use denial at that time. Management of other impinging stressors may lessen the need for denial.

When the client displays anxiety, depression, or both, the appropriate nursing intervention is acceptance of these feelings and constant reassurance about what is positive in the situation, so that these clients do not add isolation to their list of discomforts and have some help in keeping their feelings in line with reality.

The client should be encouraged to express all feelings, especially the difficult ones like anger and depression. Without expression the feelings become buried; however, they may continue to influence behavior in destructive ways. Buried feelings may also reemerge later, at a time when they seem inappropriate. When this happens, support may not be readily available, and the feelings may seem confusing to the client and significant others.

Nurses need to let clients know that anger is a normal part of dealing with loss and that they can allow themselves to feel and express anger without fear of abandonment. If anger is repressed, expressed only indirectly through sabotage of treatment, or turned into sarcasm, the clients will become more depressed as they turn the anger inward and focus it on themselves. The sad reality is that staff members often do withdraw from the angry client.

Nurses must expect some anger to be directed at treatment and at them as a part of that treatment. Becoming angry or defensive in return is not an objective response. Instead, the nurses need to just acknowledge the anger and let the client express feelings. This kind of acceptance gives people permission to express themselves and work with their anger. Once again, it is helpful to remember that chronic illness and the effort to adjust to many traumatic life changes—in addition to being constantly fearful for one's very life—make any human being feel frustrated, anxious, and depressed. Anger will be expressed in some manner in such an uncomfortable situation, and it is most constructively expressed openly and directly.

The "working through" dimension of the grieving process involves helping clients look back and talk about the areas of their lives that have been altered. Reviewing the memories and experiencing the related feelings are a process of gradually "letting go" of what has been lost. This can, initially, be painful for the client, and the wish to avoid it is experienced by both the client and the nurse. However, if these losses are not dealt with, the ability to get on with life as it is will be impaired.

The nurse, as the professional who spends the most time with the ill or disabled person, is responsible for understanding and treating the client's response to disease and treatment. This makes the nurse uniquely able to facilitate the expression of feelings, to explore alternative solutions to problems, and to clarify situations for the client. Ill persons will continually and often repetitively ask questions about their situations as they work to understand and accept the changes in their lives.

The nurse needs to support positive movement through the process of mourning and to support and advise about constructive change as it occurs in the person's life. Through knowledge of human responses and the process of a chronic illnesses, the nurse facilitates adjustment. Figure 43-2 illustrates this process.

Figure 43-2 Cycle of nursing intervention during mourning.

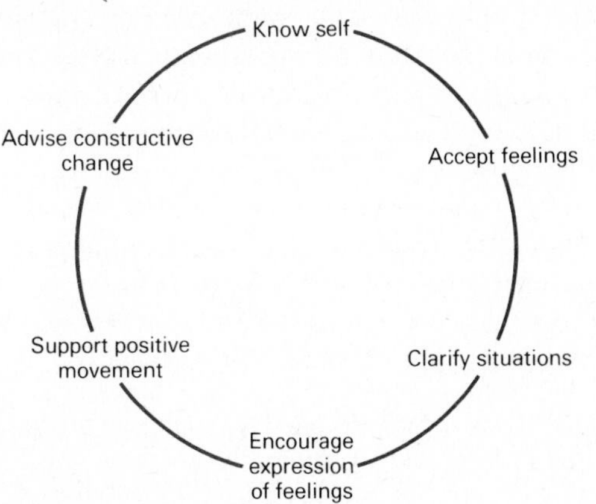

NEUTRALIZING ENVIRONMENTAL OBSTRUCTIONS. Nursing interventions must also be directed toward neutralizing obstructive environmental influences that diminish the client's self-worth and contribute to noncompliance. Clients who are struggling to repattern behavior and redefine lifestyle need realistic positive feedback. Since discouragement and frustration are inherent in this process, nurses can help clients identify criteria for an evaluation of their progress that is sensitive to minuscule changes. Making progress or maintaining the status quo becomes very important to people who are in a rehabilitation program or who are dealing with progressive deterioration. Realistic reassurance is best accomplished by providing objective data that are also accessible to the client. For example, a client with amyotrophic lateral sclerosis who expresses concern about the status of his impairment and the rate of change can be told, "You were able to use the card shuffler today just as well as you did last week."

EXPECTATIONS. Many clients with chronic disease or disability entertain unrealistic expectations regarding themselves, their families, and their care givers. Such expectations tend to produce continual disappointments and frustrations. Preoccupation with these perceived "failures" detracts from the areas of strength and competence and negates the support that is available.

Nurses can help clients revise these unrealistic expectations by facilitating the client's perception of life without them or with lowered expectations. They can ask the client, "What would it be like for you if . . . ?" The explorative discussion that would follow can help the client address his or her fears and fantasies, as well as limitations, and apply a problem-solving process to life with revised expectations.

SEXUAL FUNCTIONING. Because many chronically ill and disabled clients must deal with impairment of sexual functioning, nurses must provide clients with help in this area. Sex education, clarification of attitudes and values, and counseling regarding sexuality as a disabled or chronically ill person must be available to these clients. Given the high incidence of sexual problems among the general population, the incidence of sexual problems among chronically ill and disabled people is probably much higher. Most disabled and chronically ill clients either overcompensate or withdraw and experience sexual dysfunction.[12]

When disabled clients are confronted initially with the impact of their disability on their sexuality, their anxiety is intensified by existing attitudes, misapprehensions, and misunderstandings. Thus, opportunities must be provided for more than ventilation of feelings. Facts regarding the extent of the impairment must be communicated using vocabulary, drawings, and printed materials that best help the client and partner accommodate to changes and losses. If the assessment reveals a lack of knowledge about sexual function, the needed information must be provided before the impact of the impairment is presented.

Usually this information is presented by either the primary physician or a consultant to the treatment team whose expertise includes sexual therapy or counseling. Since sexuality and its impairment are emotionally charged topics, clients and their spouses may have difficulty "hearing" what has been said. Thus, the nurse's role is to help the couple thereafter further clarify and discuss what was said to them and to express feelings.

Nurses and other members of the health team may not have the solutions to the problems, but they can provide options, particularly alternative ways available for sexual satisfaction. Clients and their spouses need to examine these options and alternatives in light of their values, religious beliefs, and personal needs. Nurses can help such couples by facilitating this examination process, particularly by helping the couple communicate with each other about needs and feelings.[13]

PERSONAL WORTH. The self-definition of chronically ill and disabled people is based to a large extent on their values related to being a "doing" person. Our achievement-oriented society, which places a high value on "rugged individualism," influences these clients' values and self-definition. To be a worthwhile person in this society, one must be a "doing" person. Therefore, illnesses and disabilities that impair "doing" also redefine one as a worthless member of society. The feeling of worthlessness is a function of the value placed on productivity.

When people feel worthless, they also distort past and future time. They are unable to fully conceive of themselves having been productive and worthwhile or to value past accomplishments and derive satisfaction from them. They perceive the changes and losses that have occurred as precluding future accomplishments and consequently perceive themselves as forever worthless.

The interventions needed to alter these values and perceptions must be directed toward changing self-defeating attitudes to self-benefiting attitudes. This requires changing from a "doing" orientation to a "being" or "being in becoming" orientation. A "being" orientation is the valuing of behavior for its own sake. Satisfaction can be derived from such activities as exploring, manipulating, being curious, choosing, organizing, simplifying, playing, and just being unique. A "being in becoming" orientation values spontaneous activities that are not intrinsically purposeful but are nevertheless enjoyable. Activities which enhance self-development and self-actualization flow from this orientation.

All too often rehabilitation programs reflect the societal "doing" value. The client is acutely aware of the goals of rehabilitation and experiences interpersonal pressures exerted by care givers and family members to accomplish these goals. Maximization of self-responsibility and self-care is useful to the client, particularly when it will enhance self-esteem. However, when the client is severely limited or subjected to degradation because of the progressive deteriorative nature of the disease process, it is not a sound basis for self-worth.

Helping clients move from a "doing" orientation and the need to accomplish something in order to be worthwhile is a slow process along yet uncharted byways. Nurses who attempt to work with clients on developing a "being" orientation must first challenge the "doing" orientation of their profession. Nurses must evolve a sense of comfort in just "being there" with their clients, not performing tasks or procedures or engaging in goal-directed interactions such as teaching or exploring feelings. One must be able to experience sights, sounds, smells, and all the various aspects of daily living and derive pleasure and satisfaction from doing so before helping a client to explore these experiences. Deemphasizing achievement and productivity requires a continual positive reinforcement of activities that do not reflect these values.

Interactions with clients which focus on the following enhance clients' "being" orientation:

Tuning in and enjoying sights, sounds, and smells that were previously ignored

Deriving pleasure from comfort

Choosing from the menu or the shows available on television, or the time schedule for the exercise program, and enjoying the good feelings related to regulating and controlling certain aspects of one's own life

Pursuing information regarding a subject that aroused curiosity

Noticing many facets of a common object that has been taken for granted but on closer inspection offers new features

As clients begin to experience the pleasures of "being," they also begin to find the search for the meaning of their lives absorbing, satisfying, and less anxiety-provoking and steeped in regrets.

Intervention with the Family

NEEDS. The families of chronically ill and disabled people need to learn when, how, and where to seek help for themselves. Too often the needs and care of the client become paramount. Family members not only become burdened by their responsibilities but may use them as a way of avoiding the confrontation of their own unmet needs and the related feelings of deprivation.

Nursing interventions need to be directed toward helping families recognize that their needs and feelings of deprivation are legitimate and deserving of attention. Families need to know that taking care of oneself is not "selfish;" they need help to work through their guilt feelings. When nurses find time to explore concerns with family members and to listen to their fears and feelings empathically, they are legitimizing the family's needs. Likewise, when nurses emphasize the importance of family members' acting to meet their own needs, they are "giving permission" from a position of authority.

Family members may need to be encouraged to use the nurse and other members of the treatment team as resources for themselves when they feel overburdened, anxious, and depressed and when problems of daily living seem insurmountable. Ventilation of feelings and help with problem solving can be used to relieve intra- and interpersonal tensions. When family members experience relief, if only temporarily, as a result of encounters with the health team, they will be more apt to seek help when they encounter difficulties in the future. Because of the chronicity of the client's situation, tension within the family will ebb and flow. It may be aggravated by other stressors such as maturational problems or situations external to the family system.

When there are children in the home, the well parent may need help in recognizing a child's need for dependency and nurturing. Otherwise, "parentification" of the children may occur, and the family may be unaware of its implications. The well parent may need help in finding and using extended family, friends, and community resources. The use of support systems can make time, energy, and emotional resources available for more effective parenting.

EXPECTATIONS. The expectations of both the family and the client may be a source of problems for all. If family members experience the client's situation as acutely frightening and anxiety-provoking, there may be a need to deny the extent, permanence, and seriousness of the disability. Some families may pressure clients to subject themselves to extensive tests and assessments in search of a "cure."

Nursing interventions need to be directed toward helping family members begin to explore their fears and fantasies about what life will be like with the disabled member and how their lives will change. Such discussions help family members confront reality and can lead to the identification of prospective problems and their solutions. Exploration of the members' fears and fantasies and realistic feedback help to desensitize them and free energy for problem-solving activities.

When family members persist in maintaining the chronically ill member in the sick role, they may need realistic feedback on the extent and seriousness of the disability. This information can help the family develop a more realistic way of managing roles, relationships, and responsibilities.

In spite of having been given accurate information, some family members continue to participate in maintaining the client in the sick role. When this happens, there is a need to explore the members' feelings and perceptions about the client and the cause of the disability. If members believe that their negligence or the burdens they placed on the client contributed to the development of the chronic illness or disability, they may experience guilt feelings. To relieve these feelings, they may attempt to "make up" to the client for their real or fantasized negligence.

Intervention with the Community

Chronically ill and disabled people, once discharged from an acute-care setting or rehabilitation facility, must begin the arduous task of readjustment to their home and community. The period of time immediately following discharge is crucial to the recovery of a client's optimal level of functioning. It is frequently the time, however, when clients are most neglected by providers of health care. Resolution of the many crises that occur in this time of reentry need the attention of nurses.

Multifamily group meetings or smaller group meetings of specific family members have been found to be very useful ways of increasing communication; decreasing isolation, guilt, depression, and anxiety; and promoting constructive adjustment to the illness and its treatment during the adjustment phase.

Regular home visits by the nurse can be indispensable in the promotion of constructive family adjustment. Difficulties for a family—both physical and emotional—are often much more easily recognized when the nurse can evaluate them in the home setting. Also, clients and families live with their problems at home; it is often more effective to deal with the problem in that environment.

Families may need facilitation of their problem-solving and decision-making activities. Issues which need examination and areas for counseling often include allocation of resources (money, space, and time); rearrangements around division of labor; giving and receiving affection and esteem; setting limits and establishing consistency in child rearing; understanding feelings generated by the disruption in family life, that is, how various members express these feelings and how each may be supported in their resolution; and resolving conflicts effectively.

In particular, children need to be supported, helped to understand, and enabled to feel some control over the changes in their lives. They need to explore their fears and fantasies and express their concerns and needs verbally so that intellectual and emotional growth will not be impaired.

Disabled people are affected by the social stigma imposed on them by society. Nurses have a professional role in helping to reduce and eliminate prejudice toward those who are physically disabled. Following are approaches that would facilitate the alteration of the social stigma attached to physical disability.

Increase the amount of meaningful contact between disabled and nondisabled people.

Provide disabled people with the facts about stigma and improve their behavioral skills in dealing with nondisabled people.

Influence the media to present more realistic views of disability and disabled people.

Include the disabled person's family and significant others in the treatment program.

Help to politically organize disabled people.

Pressure elected officials to review and repeal legislation that restricts the lifestyle of disabled people.

Promote the removal of social barriers (institutional abuse in housing, education, and employment).

Advocate the removal of physical barriers that deny access to the disabled.

Promote the availability and accessibility of rehabilitation services and residential treatment.

Promote a humanistic philosophy of care.

Evaluation

Outcome criteria provide a means for the evaluation of care. However, the care of chronically ill and disabled clients does not usually proceed in an uninterrupted pattern toward the resolution of problems. Interventions may eliminate or lessen the severity of problems; however, when there is progressive deterioration, these problems reemerge periodically. Thus, there are periods of apparent accommodation accompanied by little or no distress and periods of upheaval when new or reactivated feelings and problems create stress. Table 43-1 illustrates an evaluation of the nursing process as it is applied to the care of a chronically ill, disabled client, "Bill T.":

> Bill T. is a 41-year-old married man who was recently diagnosed with amyotrophic lateral sclerosis, a progressive weakening and wasting of muscles. He has experienced explosive and uncontrolled outbursts of laughing and crying; his speech is slurred. He has been fired from his job because of these symptoms. His wife and three teenage children are supportive, but Bill is frequently depressed and noncompliant with physical therapy and his medication regimen.

Table 43-1 Nursing Care Plan Illustrating Evaluation (Bill T.)

Assessment
What is Bill's level of anxiety about his illness?
Are there any realistic hopes for improvement that can be offered to Bill?
Has he accepted his illness?
Has Bill's family been involved in his therapy?
Will Bill consent to see a counselor?
How depressed is Bill?
Can he verbalize the reasons for his depression?
Has Bill's family allowed him the opportunity to grieve?
Is the family able to cope with the degenerative nature of his illness?
What financial and environmental supports are available to Bill?
Diagnosis
Noncompliance with medication regimen related to denial of illness.
Depression associated with unresolved grieving process.
Overinvolvement of family related to anxiety about illness.
Financial difficulty in family related to Bill's unemployment.
Outcome Criteria
Family will agree to ongoing participation in multifamily support group after two educational sessions with the public health nurse.
Bill will verbalize acceptance of the limitations imposed by his disease.
Bill will exhibit overt signs of grieving after five sessions with counselor.
Spouse will contact social welfare agencies for financial support.
Bill and his wife will consent to attend marital counseling sessions after 1 month of intervention by the nurse.
Intervention
Educate family about the disease and its consequent limitations.
Arrange weekly visits from the public health nurse.
Arrange referrals for family members to multifamily support group, social welfare agency, and marital therapist.
Refer Bill for counseling.
Allow Bill to mourn the loss of his health.
Evaluation
After 1 month of intervention, Bill and his family continue to deny his progressive deterioration and the seriousness of his illness. The team members working with Bill agree to continue their plan for another month, but they also arrange for the family to consult with a mental health nurse clinician on a regular basis. The team will evaluate the clinician's interventions in 1 month.

SUMMARY

Loss and change are inevitable when people develop chronic illness or disability. Feelings generated by the losses are experienced by clients and their families. The patterns of interaction in the person, family, and environment influence the ways in which a person maximizes strengths, works through the losses and changes, and attains and maintains an optimal level of wellness. Individuals respond in unique ways; their responses range from "normal" grieving to overt dysfunctional behavior such as massive denial or severe depression. Clients experience loss of physical function, independence, comfort, mental function, well-being, self-concept, and roles in family and society. Changes in family roles can occur in concrete functions and interpersonal relationships. Chronic illness can force changes in these functions and relationships. Anger or impatience toward the sick member may evoke feelings of guilt in family members. The conflicts generated by the normal frictions of living together may not be openly and authentically resolved, causing increased tension. This tension, if unresolved, may be acted out in ways which interfere with the treatment plan, isolate the client within the family, or cause behavioral or physical problems in other members. The nursing process is used to help chronically ill or disabled people, their families, and their communities adjust to loss and change by developing healthy patterns of interaction.

REFERENCES

1. A. L. Strauss, *Chronic Illness and the Quality of Life,* Mosby, St. Louis, 1975.
2. H. Levneh, "The Process of Adjustment to Disability: Feelings, Behaviors, and Counseling Strategies," *Psychosocial Rehabilitation Journal,* vol. 4, 1980, pp. 26–35.
3. American Psychiatric Association, *Diagnostic and Statistical Manual of Mental Disorders,* APA, 3d ed., Washington, D.C., 1980.
4. National Center for Health Statistics, U.S. Public Health Service, *Current Estimates from the Health Interview Survey,* U.S. Department of Health, Education, and Welfare Publication 1980 82-1061, May 1982.
5. L. K. Hart, J. L. Reese, and M. O. Fearing, *Concepts Common to Acute Illness,* Mosby, St. Louis, 1981.

6. J. Luckmann and K. C. Sorenson, *Medical-Surgical Nursing*, Saunders, Philadelphia, 1980.
7. M. S. Brown, *Distortions in Body Image in Illness and Disability*, Wiley, New York, 1977.
8. R. Rubin, "Body Image and Self-Esteem," in V. A. Christopherson et al., eds., *Rehabilitation Nursing: Perspectives and Applications*, McGraw-Hill, New York, 1974.
9. P. W. Power, "The Chronically Ill Husband and Father: His Role in the Family," *The Family Coordinator*, vol. 28, October 1979, pp. 616–621.
10. D. C. Turk and R. D. Kerns, *Health, Illness, and Families*, Wiley, New York, 1985.
11. L. D. Park, "Barriers to Normality for the Handicapped Adult in the United States," in R. P. Marinelli and A. E. Dell Orto, eds., *The Psychological Impact of Physical Disability*, Springer, New York, 1977, pp. 25–33.
12. A. B. Ford and A. P. Orfirer, "Sexual Behavior and the Chronically Ill Patient," *Medical Aspects of Human Sexuality*, vol. 1, no. 2, October 1967., p. 51.
13. K. Burkhalter and L. Donley, *Dynamics of Oncology Nursing*, McGraw-Hill, New York, 1980.

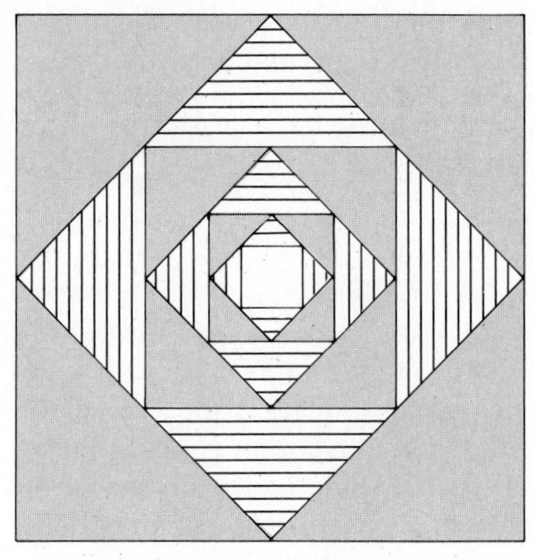

CHAPTER 44
Organic Mental Disorders

Barbara Flynn Sideleau

LEARNING OBJECTIVES

After studying this chapter, the student should be able to:

1. Describe the clinical picture associated with organic mental disorders.
2. Distinguish between behavior symptomatic of dementia and behavior symptomatic of pseudodementia (depression).
3. Provide an epidemiological description of organic mental disorders.
4. Provide an overview of known causes and theories related to the development of organic mental disorders.
5. Discuss dysynchronous patterns of interaction in the person that are associated with dementia, delirium, paroxysmal disorders, and attention deficit disorders.
6. Discuss dysynchronous family patterns of interaction associated with organic mental disorders.
7. Discuss dysynchronous environmental patterns of interaction associated with organic mental disorders.
8. Apply the nursing process to the care of clients with organic mental disorders, their families, and the environment.

The biopsychosocial disorders discussed in this chapter involve organically based impairment of personality, mood, and language patterns; loss of intellectual functioning related to memory, abstract thinking, and judgment; disturbances of the sensorium; and social and occupational dysfunction. These impairments are associated with transient or permanent brain dysfunction. The changes that occur have a devastating impact on mind, body, and spirit, and on patterns of interaction with others and with the environment.

Organic mental disorder (OMD) can be categorized as either acute or chronic. The onset of an acute brain disorder is often sudden, with rapid impairment of orientation, memory, intellectual function, judgment, and affect. The client may be delirious or in a coma, and in some instances psychopathology may be present. The cause of acute OMD is usually a temporary, reversible, diffuse disturbance of brain function. With time and treatment, organic symptoms are resolved. The onset of chronic OMD is often but not always insidious. In some instances, acute OMD may deteriorate and become chronic. Consciousness is not usually impaired, at least in the early stages, but there are varying degrees of disorientation in relation to time, place, and person; failing memory (remote and recent); intellectual impairment; impaired judgment; and disturbance in affect. The alterations in the brain tissue are irreversible; in some instances, the pathology progresses over time, intensifying and extending the symptoms.[1]

The purpose of this chapter is to examine the impact of organic mental disorder on patterns of interaction in the person, family, and environment. An epidemiological profile of these disorders is presented. Factors associated with the development of organic brain-tissue dysfunction are identified. A holistic application of the nursing process to the care of people with OMD and their families is presented.

DYSYNCHRONOUS HEALTH PATTERNS

The dysynchronous health patterns associated with an organic mental disorder reflect a drastic alteration in the person's self-concept and ability to interact meaningfully with the environment. The sudden loss or deterioration in mental functioning diminishes or destroys the ability to perform even basic activities of daily living. Loss of memory interferes with the recall of personal experiences as well as world events, robbing the person of his or her past. The present is experienced as alien. Familiar people and places may not be recognized. The essence of the person is lost, as are hope and anticipation of the future.

With chronic OMD, person-family interactions are irrevocably altered. Changes in the ill person's personality and capacity to share past and present experiences diminish for the family the satisfaction and pleasure of a relationship with the afflicted member. The burden of either caring for the family member or placing the person in a residential care facility further disorganizes the family.

Attention Deficit Disorders

Some adults suffer from impaired brain function that has persisted since childhood. Intellectual capacities may be relatively intact, but distractibility and impulsivity interfere with the acquisition of information and a thoughtful approach to problems.

The persistence of attention deficit disorders (ADD) into adulthood has been overlooked generally. Its existence has been concealed by the application of a variety of diagnostic labels. The connection between ADD and psychopathology has been inferred from data obtained in longitudinal, retrospective, and family studies. Research has revealed that a subgroup of adults diagnosed as *schizophrenic* respond well to psychostimulants which are effective in managing the behavioral symptoms of children with ADD. These findings suggest that this group of adults may have ADD rather than schizophrenia. It has also been found that some adults with hysterical, explosive, and antisocial personalities and some alcoholics have responded similarly to stimulant drugs, suggesting that their behavioral problems may be the result of the persistence of ADD into adulthood. Thus, some adults who have been diagnosed as having major psychiatric disorders, who are chronic alcoholics, or who become involved in criminal activities may have unrecognized ADD.[2–6]

People who have suffered accidental head trauma may develop symptoms of ADD. These clients are often young people who have been involved in automobile or motorcycle accidents. Their situation is further complicated if they recognize the losses and consequently experience a sense of helplessness and hopelessness.

Seizure Disorders

A seizure is caused by uncontrolled excessive activity of either a part of the central nervous system or all of it. A seizure occurs when the level of excitement of the nervous system rises above a certain critical threshold in a predisposed or vulnerable person. The abnormal electric discharges in the brain tissue interfere with the sensorium. A seizure is not a disease; it is a symptom of a problem in the central nervous system which is causing it to produce abnormal discharges. A seizure signals that neural, humoral, metabolic, and vascular regulatory systems of the brain are imbalanced.

Paroxysmal disorders of cerebral function occur as a consequence of hyperpyrexia, infections of the central nervous system, metabolic disturbances, cerebral hypoxia, brain lesions (tumors or hemorrhages), brain defects, cerebral edema, cerebral trauma (accidental or surgical), anaphylaxis, the presence of toxic substances (poisons ingested or inhaled), and withdrawal from addictive drugs such as alcohol, hypnotics, and tranquilizers.

Epilepsy is a term used to describe a state of impaired brain function characterized by paroxysmal seizure activity that disturbs mental functioning and behavior. The two basic types of epilepsy are *generalized epilepsy,* which involves essentially all parts of the brain at once, and *focal epilepsy,* which involves a limited portion of the brain.[7]

People who suffer from seizures, particularly when they are not adequately controlled by medication, may be limited in their vocational choices and may not even be able to operate a vehicle. The alterations in brain function may alter their perceptions of self and environment. Superstition and fear have influenced societal perceptions of and interactions with these people. The suddenness and bizarre quality of behavior during seizures often sets these people apart from others.

Dementia and Pseudodementia

Senility is not a medical diagnosis. It is a term frequently used with older people when there is evidence of increasing difficulty thinking, remembering, communicating, relating to others, and self-care.[8] The use of the term *senility* is problematic because it is a poorly defined label that may be applied to older people experiencing benign senescence, pseudodementia (depression), primary degenerative dementia, or multi-infarct dementia.[9] Assignment of the label may preclude a holistic assessment, an accurate diagnosis, and the implementation of appropriate interventions.

"Forgetting" is a universal phenomenon. Recall begins to decline sometime around age 40, but people tend not to complain about forgetting until they are in their sixties or seventies.[10,11,12] *Benign senescence,* or aging, is accompanied by changes in intellectual functioning.[9] Alterations in attention, naming ability, and abstraction have been noted.[11] The changes that may be most disturbing to the person and that may be mistaken as evidence of senility are related to memory. Elderly people who are well do not lose either recent or remote memory, but their reaction time to the initiation of information retrieval is slowed as a normal aspect of aging. In addition, they need more information before acting than young people do.[9] With time, minimal prompting, and sufficient information regarding the need to act, elderly people are able to retrieve and recall both recent and remote stored memories.

The term *pseudodementia* is used to describe a syndrome of cognitive and memory impairment that appears in the course of functional psychiatric disorders such as depression, and leads the diagnostician to believe that the impairments are related to a neurological disease.[13] Usually, multi-infarct dementia can be distinguished from pseudodementia and primary degenerative dementia because it develops after a series of abrupt episodes in which widespread neurological deficits occur. Significant overlap exists between elderly people who meet the criteria for primary degenerative dementia and those who meet the criteria for pseudodementia (depression), both of which may develop over time and progressively worsen. Many people with Alzheimer's disease and other progressive dementias may present with depressive symptoms in the early stages of their diseases. However, there are behavioral patterns that distinguish dementia from pseudodementia.[9,14–18] Examples of these differences are presented in Table 44-1.

There are also differences between normal forgetting, the memory loss associated with the de-

Table 44-1 Pseudodementia (Depression) and Dementia

Pseudodementia (Depression)	Dementia of Alzheimer's Disease
Family history of affective illness.	Family history of Alzheimer's disease (sibling or parent).
Posture stooped.	Stands erect.
Refuses to undertake normal social activities; loss of interest.	Gradually gives up shopping or attending social gatherings alone because of difficulty remembering how to get there and how to return home.
Slow to answer questions.	Answers spontaneously.
Answers questions with one or few words.	Answers with many words but not fluently. ("Dysfluent.")
Answers to questions are vague.	Answers are not relevant to questions. ("Confabulation.")
Gives "I don't know" answers.	Makes up answer rather than admit not knowing.
Understands what is asked; able to select appropriate words to convey relevant response.	Does not comprehend questions; pathological, repetitious use of spoken words and phrases (palilalia) or misuse of words or word combinations (paraphasia).
Oriented to time and place.	Disoriented to time and place; becomes lost in a familiar environment.
Is able to perform tasks that require the incorporation of new information.	Is unable to perform tasks that require the incorporation of new information and repeatedly asks questions about what to do.
Is able to follow a conversation between two people.	Has difficulty following a conversation between two people and may interject irrelevancies or comments on a subject discussed previously.
Is able to recall recent events.	Has difficulty recalling both personal and nonpersonal recent events.
When asked to recall distant past, person talks about memories of losses and disappointments.	As disease progresses over time, forgetting increases and past memories are erased.
Exaggerates extent of mental impairment; is aware of some cognitive impairment and complains about poor memory and concentration.	Denies or underestimates mental impairment.
Discrepancy between person's complaints and observable impairment of memory and attention.	Absence of complaints is discrepant with observable impairment of memory and attention.
History of depressive episodes.	No history of depressive episodes.
Presence of persistent, bizarre structured delusions.	Delusions are sporadic, poorly structured, and tend to be paranoid in nature.
Hallucinations may occur.	Hallucinations are rare.
Able to concentrate on ruminations about past, helplessness, hopelessness, worthlessness, and regrets.	Diminished concentration.
Sleep problems: early-morning awakening (EMA).	Nocturnal confusion: awakens in middle of night, is confused, and behaves as if it were daytime.
Loss of appetite.	Appetite unchanged.
Observably depressed affect.	Affect shallow and labile.
Insecure with others.	Demanding of others.
Relatively rapid onset and rapid progression.	Insidious onset, gradual progression.
Depression precedes dementia.	Dementia present before depression, and depression transitory.
May be best at night.	Apt to be worst at night.
Temporary impairment of intellect that is restored when depression decreases.	Deterioration of general intellect.
Affective distress unchanged by location.	Distress or anxiety less apt to occur in home surroundings.
Spatial orientation intact.	Impaired ability to recognize cues and clues to negotiate a familiar or new area.
Knows how to dress and undress.	Does not remember how to put clothes on or take them off.
Recognizes persons, places, and objects and their meanings.	Fails to recognize persons, places, and objects and their meanings.
No disoriented wandering.	Wanders away from home or hospital because nothing seems familiar and is searching for the familiar.
Retains social inhibitions unless psychotic.	Reduced social inhibition and modesty in interactions.
If delusions are present, they are persistent and structured.	If delusions are present, they are sporadic, poorly structured, and tend to be paranoid in nature.

mentias, and amnesia. With few exceptions amnesia results from structural brain pathology. It is characterized by normal *immediate* recall unless delirium or aphasia is present. The ability to learn new material is compromised. There are deficits in long-term memory, but the ability to retrieve *very old* information, learned before the amnesia, may be relatively normal. Both cognition and personality are intact. The memory loss associated with the dementias involves both recent and remote memory, and personality changes are evident.

Causes of Organic Mental Disorders

Brain-tissue dysfunction can stem from a variety of causes.[10,19,20,21] Examples of these causes are presented in Table 44-2. People of all ages are vulnerable to OMD. It can be found among children with lead poisoning, adolescents injured in motorcycle accidents, adults with head injuries related to automobile and other accidents, fire fighters who suffer smoke inhalation, alcoholics, drug abusers, and elderly people who suffer from Alzheimer's disease.[22] In addition there are people with OMD who are the survivors of attempted suicides or homicides that destroyed brain tissue.

With increasing societal attention to environmental pollution and the efforts to enforce the Occupational Safety and Health Act, there is an increasing awareness of the damage to brain tissue caused by industrial chemicals. Occupational exposure to toxic substances may produce symptoms of OMD ranging from the mild and transient to those which cause severe destruction and dysfunction. People exposed to repeated courses of electroconvulsive therapy are also subject to permanent residual brain damage. Given so many possible causes and variations in symptoms, diagnosis requires an extensive assessment of the client.

The interacting pathophysiological factors related to the development of progressive dementia and multi-infarct dementia include genetic predisposition, impaired neurochemistry, circulatory deficiencies, cellular degeneration, disorders of the immune system, and slow-acting viruses.[10,12] Recent findings suggest a genetic influence on the early and late development of Alzheimer's-type dementia. The disease tends to cluster in certain families, and there is a 60 percent risk among identical twins and a 40 percent risk among fraternal twins. Findings also suggest a link between dementia and

Table 44-2 Causation of Organic Mental Disorders

Cause	Examples
Volatile agents	Gasoline, aerosols, glues, paint removers, solvents, lacquers, varnishes, dry-cleaning agents, home-cleaning products (alone or when mixed)
Heavy metals	Lead (paints, ceramic glazes, moonshine whiskey), mercury, arsenic, manganese
Insecticides	DDT, parathion, malathion, diazine
Brain trauma	Concussion, contusion, hemorrhage, thrombosis, penetrating wounds, blast effects, electrical trauma
Drugs	Alcohol, barbiturates, opioids, cocaine, amphetamines
Infections	Meningitis, encephalitis, neurosyphilis (*tabes dorsalis*), tuberculosis, viral diseases, Creutzfeld-Jakob disease
Neoplasms, tumors	Astrocytoma, medulloblastoma, meningioma
Metabolic and endocrine disorders	Hepatic disease, uremic encephalopathy, prophyria, thyroid dysfunction, parathyroid dysfunction, adrenal dysfunction, Wernicke-Korsakoff syndrome
Nutritional deficiencies	Lack of protein, deficiences in vitamin C and the B vitamins (folic acid, niacin, pyridoxine, riboflavin, thiamine, B_{12}), fluid and electrolyte imbalance
Seizures	Petit mal, grand mal, focal seizures, psychic seizures
Hypoxia-ischemia	Anoxia related to delayed or prolonged cardiopulmonary resuscitation
Multiple small or large cerebral infarcts with occlusion of small terminal arteries	Atherosclerosis; vascular, circulatory, or valvular disease; emboli; vasculitis
Brain changes related to loss of neurons, senile plaques, neurofibrillary degeneration and tangles, loss of dentritic tree, choline acetyl transferase (CAT), inherited genetic influence, or interactions among these factors	Alzheimer's disease
Possible genetic influence	Parkinson's disease, Huntington's chorea

leukemia that involves proteins coded on chromosome 16, and between Alzheimer's disease and Down's syndrome involving chromosome 21.[16,23,24,25]

Nerve cells (cholinergic neurons) that use acetylcholine as neurotransmitters are also impaired in OMD. These neurons play a significant role in memory. The hippocampus, an important structure related to memory function, is rich in cholinergic neurons.

Additional studies also suggest that protein material which should be incorporated into antibodies may become plaques in the senile brain. These antibodies may act against the brain neurons, destroying functional tissue and producing a scar tissue that interferes with normal function. The development of senility may depend on an accumulative disability to fight off an inherited toxin. Further studies are attempting to correlate the level of such antibodies in the senile brain with the degree of mental impairment.[23,24]

Autopsies comparing the brains of people who have been diagnosed as senile with those who are normal reveal no overall differences in size, weight, number of neurons, or size of the ventricles. The only visible pathology found in the senile brain is the presence of numerous plaques and tangles. On analysis the plaques have been found to contain an abnormal protein called *amyloid* that is surrounded by paired helical filaments, and the neurons have been found to contain twisted fibers in the cytoplasm. These cellular abnormalities have been found primarily in the frontal and temporal lobes of the cerebral cortex.[23,24] The plaques that have been found in senile brains have also been found in the brains of people who have slow-virus diseases. This finding raises the question whether a slow virus might also be involved in producing the tangles and plaques in the senile brain.

Premature death has been associated with senility.[24] However, the pathophysiological factors associated with senility are such that they would neither contribute to death nor explain the fact that death comes sooner than in the case of benign senescence.[24] Furthermore, in spite of the previously cited physical and physiological changes associated with senility, many people remain alert and intellectually active into advanced old age.[22] When these losses do occur in the older person, environmental factors, underlying pathophysiological conditions, and other factors yet to be determined suggest multicausation.

DSM III

DSM III makes a distinction between organic brain syndrome (OBS) and organic mental disorder (OMD) based on whether the etiology is known or presumed. OBSs are constellations of symptoms of organic brain dysfunction. They include the following six categories: (1) delirium and dementia, (2) amnestic syndrome and organic hallucinosis, (3) organic delusional syndrome and organic affective syndrome, (4) organic personality syndrome, (5) intoxication and withdrawal, and (6) atypical or mixed organic brain syndrome. OMD is a broad category of organic brain dysfunction that encompasses the symptoms of OBS and a known or presumed etiological factor that is determined through a history, physical examination, or laboratory tests. Organic mental disorders are heterogeneous. Differences among these disorders are related to the clinical picture, which includes the nature of the onset, progression and duration of symptoms, and the pathophysiological process. The dementias of OMD may occur before (presenile) or after age 65 (senile). These dementias include two major categories: primary degenerative dementia and multi-infarct dementia. Diseases encompassed by the diagnosis of dementia include Alzheimer's disease, Pick's diseases, and Huntington's chorea, as well as a rarer condition, Creutzfeld-Jacob disease.

Attention deficit disorder (ADD) is described in DSM III as a behavioral disorder, usually associated with children. It is a neurological condition that produces "soft" neurological signs, motor-perceptual dysfunction, and problematic behavior related to distractibility, impaired ability to concentrate, and impulsivity.[1]

ADD is commonly recognized by 3 years of age but often is not fully evident or diagnosed until the child enters school. In some instances the condition may be self-limiting and resolved by the time the person is an adolescent or adult. In other instances residual impairments continue into adulthood.[1]

Epidemiology

The increased number of elderly people in this society reflects a decreased death rate in youth and middle age, and a recent dramatic reduction in the death rates of elderly people. The "very old" (over 75 years of age) are an increasing portion of the elderly. It is estimated that during the 1980s the number of those over 85 years of age will increase by 52.4 percent.[26] The incidence of psychopathology increases with age; however, 80 percent of elderly people who need psychiatric care are not being served.[26] From 5 to 7 percent of the population over 65 years of age show symptoms of dementia, and 20 percent of those over 80 years of age have symptoms of severe cognitive dysfunction.[27] Five out of every 100 persons over age 65, and 20 out of every 100 persons over age 80, experience cognitive impairment.[8]

Between 60 and 70 percent of the population with irreversible dementia suffer from Alzheimer's disease, between 15 and 25 percent from multi-infarct dementia, and between 10 and 20 percent from a combination of both conditions.[28] These figures do not include those in the early stages of Alzheimer's disease or those who are cared for at home. The declared cases (some 4 million) represent only the tip of the iceberg.[16] As the population in the United States ages, the number of cases will increase. Nursing home costs for these people were estimated at $10 billion in 1980.[29] The cost of home care by family members and privately employed caretakers and companions probably far exceeds what is spent in nursing home care. According to demographic projections, the number of those affected by dementia will increase 50 percent in the next generation.[30] Between 5 and 10 percent of those who are in medical hospitals and 40 percent of those who are in geriatric institutions exhibit delirium at some time.[31]

The numbers of younger people with organic mental disorders related to brain trauma, chemical toxicity, substance abuse, and other causes and the cost of their care are unknown. In most instances these people are not institutionalized and are dependent on their families for their care.

PATTERNS OF INTERACTION: PERSON

The wide variety of behavioral symptomatology associated with OMD reflects the complexity of the central nervous system. OMD is characterized by behavioral manifestations of the underlying tissue dysfunction or metabolic derangements. These clients may and often do exhibit psychopathological behavior along with the manifestations of their deficits. It is no simple matter to determine which abnormal behaviors are based solely on physiological deficits and which are maladaptive responses to the deficits—responses caused by previously impaired coping abilities. This difficult distinction requires extensive assessment by a team of specialists representing several different professions.

Behaviors characteristic of OMD with which psychopathology may coexist may be classified as dementia, delirium, paroxysmal disorders, and attention deficit disorders.[32]

Dementia

Dementia is a loss of intellectual abilities of sufficient severity to interfere with social or occupational functioning. In this group of clients OMD is characterized by amnesia (dysmenesia); impaired intellectual functioning; disorientation; affective dysfunction; motor, sensory, perceptual, and language impairments; and personality changes. Some of these symptoms may also occur in delirium, but in delirium, inattention and a fluctuating level of awareness predominate. Decreased adaptability to changing circumstances and to external stimuli, loss of control over reactions, and loss of problem-solving and decision-making abilities affect the person and the family.

Deficits Associated with Dementia

DYSMENESIA. *Dysmenesia,* which is an impairment in the ability to retain and recall information, is the most prominent symptom of dementia.[32] Initially the person may be forgetful and absentminded. For example:

> Ms. A., an elderly woman, puts a kettle of water on the stove to make a cup of tea. While waiting for it to boil, she forgets why she is waiting and decides to do a household chore. In the meantime the water boils away and the kettle handle or spout burns. If her sense of smell is poor (as is often the case with older people), a fire may start and spread before she becomes aware of its existence.

In Alzheimer's disease, dysmenesia develops gradually.[33] In the early stages as dysmenesia progresses, the client remains, at least initially, able to recall events that occurred before the memory failure began. Such a client may reminisce in great detail about life as a child or youth, the adventures of that time, marriage, and the birth of sons and daughters. Dates are easily remembered, rooms described in detail, and social events recalled with attention to minor incidents. However, events of the recent past are either less easily recalled—with descriptions that are less precise—or not remembered at all.

People past the age of 65 may have minor increased forgetfulness. In contrast people who develop dementia exhibit severe, pervasive memory loss which may include failure to recognize significant others, familiar names, and how to use common household objects. These people are unable to find familiar places, and they get lost if they leave their homes.[33] As their perception of the physical and social environment becomes distorted, suspiciousness becomes pronounced and may be accompanied by restless behavior, tactlessness, and even aggressiveness.[34] There may be misperception of a spouse's sociability toward friends, and acute jealousy may occur. The spouse and friend may be accused of flirting. If disordered thought processes also include delusions that their friends and families intend to poison or otherwise harm them, these people may withdraw from social interaction with others. When this happens, they are further deprived of both realistic feedback and the social stimulation all people need.

Memory loss may be very mild and almost undetectable, but with progression of the underlying destructive process, the memory loss gradually extends to the remote past, so that not only recent events but past ones as well are no longer recalled.[35,36] In the final stages of Alzheimer's disease, even the memory needed to perform self-care activities is impaired, and the person requires wholly compensatory physical care.[33] In addition to the impairment of the retention of established memory, these people's abilities to register and store memories and to learn and integrate new experiences also deteriorate.[37]

IMPAIRED INTELLECTUAL FUNCTIONING. Impaired intellectual functioning includes disturbances in the following activities: calculating, comprehending, recalling and using a general fund of information, and learning new tasks. When abstract reasoning is impaired, the initial deficit may be mild and uneven. The affected person may be able to continue working for a considerable time if the job does not require decision making or the ability to deal with sensitive interpersonal situations. As the impairment progresses, it becomes more evident to coworkers and family because judgment becomes unreliable and decisions and behavior become inappropriate. For example:

> Mr. B., an investment broker, was noted for his conservative stance in managing investors' portfolios. He first manifested his impaired judgment by selecting speculative stocks more frequently; but this went unnoticed initially. However, he began progressively to counsel investors away from blue-chip stocks until one day he advised a long-standing customer to close out his portfolio and invest all the cash in a risky company that produced avant-garde movies.

Many such people are highly defended against awareness and discovery of their growing impairment. Consequently they will provide long and involved rationales for their actions. In many instances, family, friends, and coworkers tend to deny the character changes until the behaviors become blatant or the social indiscretions become embarrassing.

DISORIENTATION. *Disorientation* is a loss of one's bearings or position with respect to time, place, identity, or some combination of these. Disorientation is closely related to dysmenesia. When disoriented clients do not know who they are, the time of day, the date, or to whom they are speaking, they have dysmenesia or memory impairment as well. In its earliest stages, disorientation is characterized by an impaired sense of time. The abilities to assimilate, retain, and use cues are impaired.[36] For example:

> Mr. C. was able to recall what work he had done the day before but not what tasks he had done in the morning as opposed to the afternoon or evening. In Mrs. D.'s case, time confusion took the form of arising in the middle of the night or very early in the morning and preparing to leave her home to go shopping or to go to church.

Time orientation involves recognition of the following: (1) public time markers (year, month, date), (2) cued time (time of day, season of year), and (3) personal time (subjective experience of the passage of time). People with dementia have impaired recognition of public time markers and cued time. In the last stages of Alzheimer's disease, recognition of personal time is also impaired.[34]

As time disorientation increases, clients cannot recall the day, month, week, or year. They also have increasing difficulty orienting themselves to place and even to familiar surroundings. As Alzheimer's disease progresses, so does disorientation; those who have multi-infarct dementia maintain better contact with the environment.[38]

Disorientation becomes more pronounced in twilight and as the night progresses. A strange environment, such as a hospital or convalescent home, can also aggravate this condition, as can abnormal levels of sensory input. Overstimulation can be confusing, and sensory deprivation may have an equally disturbing effect.[39]

When confusion occurs, the person is experiencing temporal-spatial disorientation and has a tendency to mistake the unfamiliar for the familiar. The hospital room may be mistaken for a bedroom at home; a close relative is not recognized and is believed to be an imposter.[34]

A loss of one's personal orientation is experienced as not knowing oneself. When the dementia is progressive, as in the case of Alzheimer's disease, the person's identity eventually becomes totally obliterated.[34]

The following example illustrates severe disorientation:

> Mr. E., suffering from increasing disorientation and dysmenesia, walked away from his daughter's home. When he was picked up by the police at 3 A.M., wandering in the downtown district, he was unable to give either his name or his address and did not know the time, day, or year. When his daughter arrived at the police station to retrieve him, he refused to go with the "strange woman."

AFFECTIVE DYSFUNCTION. *Emotional lability,* which is an affective disturbance characterized by excessive emotional responses, is sometimes a consequence of OMD, particularly multi-infarct dementia.[38] The person experiences strong emotion in the absence of either intrapsychic or environmental stimuli. The feeling tone may shift suddenly and excessively, without warning, from sadness and crying to euphoria and laughter, or the felt emotion may be inappropriate to the situation. When this occurs, it is disturbing to both the client and the family, particularly when they do not understand that it is a consequence of brain-tissue dysfunction.[19]

Other people with OMD manifest affective disturbance by exhibiting a blunting and shallowness of emotion or a lack of responsiveness.

MOTOR IMPAIRMENT. Motor performance is also often impaired with dementia. The exaggeration of gait that occurs with aging—decreased stability, narrow-based step, and shuffling—may develop. Alterations in muscle tone, decreased gait balance, and increased unsteadiness appear as Alzheimer's disease progresses.[10] Because of changes in gait, the use of a walker or the assistance of another person may be needed. These people are vulnerable to falling and to associated traumas such as fractured hips, wrists, and arms. Admission to the hospital for the treatment of these injuries further disorganizes thinking and feeling processes and produces severe disorientation.

SENSORY AND PERCEPTUAL IMPAIRMENT. Organic alterations in brain tissue may cause delusions and hallucinations. When hallucinations occur, they involve any of the sensory modalities (olfactory, gustatory, visual, or auditory).[19] When these clients also suffer from visual impairment, hearing loss, or other complicating physical problems, social isolation may be greater. Sensory deprivation may contribute to the development of confusion. A monotonous environment, impaired vision and hearing, and social isolation may interfere with the sensory stimuli needed to maintain the arousal mechanism in the reticular formation of the brain. When this arousal system is depressed, the person experiences thought disorganization and sleep and psychomotor disturbances and expresses somatic complaints and inappropriate affect. It is not uncommon to find that disability is exaggerated when either somatization or hypochondriasis occurs. There is a preoccupation with symptoms such as heaviness in the chest, dry mouth, and gastric upsets.[40] There is physical deterioration as well as decreasing self-esteem and self-acceptance. Psychotic symptoms such as illusions, delusions, and visual hallucinations may emerge; or there may be neurotic symptoms such as depression, anxiety, obsessions, compulsions, or phobias.[10,18]

Compulsive, ritualistic behavior is a common means whereby these people attempt to compensate for their disabilities. For others, alcohol abuse, promiscuity, and impulsivity develop as maladaptive responses to the impact of loss.[18]

The client's disturbed perception of the inner and outer environments creates a climate for the development of delusions. Paranoid ideation is reflected in expressed beliefs about being mistreated or threatened. Clients talk about being rejected, neglected, and spied upon. They express fears that their family or care givers are poisoning them in order to steal their money or jewels. Sometimes the delusions involve their own bodies. They may believe that their insides have rotted away and consequently refuse to eat or swallow food. The more cohesive delusions reflect the person's real-life situation and everyday irritations, particularly feelings of loss, helplessness, loneliness, and abandonment.[32] For example:

> Mrs. F. had been living with her son and daughter-in-law ever since her increasing forgetfulness had begun to worry her children. Before her husband's death, Mrs. F. was active in senior citizen groups. In spite of neighborhood deterioration, an increased crime rate, and the loss of old friends, the couple were socially active. After her husband's death, Mrs. F. withdrew from friends and dropped out of club activities. The sudden social isolation and grief over the loss of her husband contributed to feelings of loneliness, helplessness, and a distorted sense of time. She became preoccupied with the fear that burglars would break in and take her money, leaving her nothing; she squirreled away her money here and there around the house. She hid dollars in books, vases, pillows, and couch cushions and then promptly forgot where she had put them. After searching vainly one day for a particular envelope of money, she accused her daughter-in-law of taking her money and belongings.
>
> The loss of her home and familiar surroundings and the resettlement in her son's home required adaptation beyond Mrs. F.'s coping capacity. Her impaired thinking processes, the stress generated by the move, and the need to defend against recognition of her deficits created the need to link her daughter-in-law with her losses and to develop the delusion that her daughter-in-law was taking her possessions from her. What was particularly painful for the daughter-in-law was the element of truth that she had urged her husband to bring his mother into their home, fearing that her forgetfulness would result in an accidental injury or that she would set fire to her home while preparing meals.

The environment influences the way in which people with OMD experience their deficits. If the environment makes demands on the person which are beyond his or her ability to cope, disorganization will be accelerated and maladaptive behavior is more likely to emerge. When support is inadequate—when the family or care-giving structure is rigid, demanding, confronting, or rejecting—it causes the person to feel isolated, abandoned, and anxious. If situational supports are adequate, flexible, accommodating, and focused on conservation of capacities and enhancement of strengths, they protect the person from unnecessary stress, anxiety-producing confrontations, and awareness of deficits.

To protect themselves from full awareness of their disabilities, these people will deny their deficits. When a request is made—such as "Clean your room" or "Make your bed"—they may refuse to comply, not because they are truly negativistic but because they may not remember where their room is or how a bed is made. If pressured, they may not do what is requested but rather perform a substitute task with which they can cope, such as straightening the room in which they happen to be at the time.[32]

These people may convey disorderliness in their dress or hygiene but be compulsively orderly in other areas of their lives. They may arrange holy statues on their dressers in a set pattern; if the pattern is disturbed for any reason, they experience considerable distress. Some carefully wrap or sew into bags odds and ends such as holy medals, buttons, broken jewelry, or other small items which they store carefully in specific places. Some tend to simplify their environment so that they will be able to negotiate it with a minimum of distress. Others hoard or save almost everything that comes into their possession, fearing that they will not be able to tell the difference between what is worth keeping and what is not.

LANGUAGE IMPAIRMENT. Dementia has been associated with language impairment that interferes with the ability to interact with others. If the dementia progresses, as in Alzheimer's disease, or if multi-infarct dementia is present, there is a loss in use, understanding, and comprehension of language.[41] These people lose the ability to name objects and actions.[42] The *aphasia* (inability to express oneself) that develops may extend to all areas of communication, as does *apraxia* (inability to understand the meanings of things and inability to perform certain movements in the absence of impaired motor power or coordination).[9] Comprehension of verbal messages is impaired. For example, a person may be told that the television is broken and cannot be used until it is repaired. When comprehension is impaired, the person may continue to try to turn on or tune the television or to wait expectantly for a show to come on. Those who do not remain fluent may exhibit pathological repetition of words or phrases (*palilalia*) or misuse spoken words or word combinations (*paraphasia*).

Communication is an area these people can and often do control. During the early stages these people may refuse to speak or to converse unless they themselves have chosen the subject; they attempt to manage the environment so as to avoid a confrontation with their deficits. A question may be met with stony silence, a rationalization about why they cannot answer, a fabrication of events rather than actual facts, confabulation, or a tangential monologue that is not a true response but an attempt to bind anxiety.[31] For example:

> One client, Mr. G., confronted a nurse, who was reminding him that it was dinnertime, by replying, "Stop hassling me! You don't want to help me; you only want to make me upset so that I'll have to stay here."

PERSONALITY CHANGES. The personality changes that accompany dementia involve one or more of the following: emotional lability; impaired impulse control; suspiciousness; lack of judgment, social tact, grace, reliability, or foresight; apathy or euphoria; and lack of inhibition.[31,43] People with Alzheimer's disease experience progressive deterioration in personality, with disturbance in the abilities to make choices, indicate preferences, and be self-determined. In time these people deteriorate to a vegetative state.[41]

Emotional Responses to Dementia

Many factors influence the way a person responds to dementia. When confronted with these losses, a person has an emotional reaction and makes efforts to adapt. The premorbid personality, the rate of deterioration, environmental demands and support, stresses, and the state of overall health all affect the person's response to the deficits.

Initially, depression and anxiety occur. The person may exhibit classical signs of depression such as sadness, anergia, and declining interest in personal appearance and the environment, or become overtly anxious.[37] Fear may become so great that regression occurs. When this happens, dependency is greater than brain function warrants. Incontinence, falling, and failure to attempt self-help may occur. Some people mobilize a manic defense and exhibit euphoria in the face of failing capacities. Others use denial to avoid awareness of their diminishing capacities. Frustration may become evident in others as the losses increase. As deterioration progresses, the person may respond to daily demands with irritability and hostility and may become aggressive and assaultive.[37]

The person's difficulty in perceiving the outside world extends to the internal milieu as well and thus interferes with self-awareness. Because of this impaired sensitivity to the self, the range of emotional responsivity and the congruity between affective state and ideation may be disturbed. Since this disturbance is manifested by excessive or inappropriate emotional responses, lability, and blunting or shallowness of affect,[19] it becomes difficult to discriminate between a maladaptive emotional response and alterations of affect caused by disturbance in brain tissue.

People who are experiencing mental deterioration may be aware of these changes. Feelings of helplessness, hopelessness, and worthlessness may become pervasive and contribute to a wish to die. Self-esteem and self-confidence are diminished, and a sense of failure, humiliation, and shame develops. Because of their progressive deterioration, these people lose physical, mental, social, and economic resources as well as a sense of purpose. They grieve over these losses and to varying degrees recognize their permanence. Initially, affected persons may be apathetic. They become listless and lose interest in others, their appearance, and the physical environment. Initiative is also lost. Token compliance and a slowing of speech and movement are evident. Attempts to facilitate involvement in activities with others are not infrequently countered with anger and even assaultive behavior.

Maladaptive behavioral responses are exaggerations of the ways in which the person coped in the past. Gregarious, outgoing people become more so, and their behavior often becomes socially obnoxious, while solitary and suspicious people become more withdrawn and paranoid. Often the personality that emerges because of the deficits and the emotional response to them is a caricature of the previous personality. Previous life events, past and present stresses, interpersonal factors, and the current environment influence the adaptive process.

Initially such coping mechanisms as sublimation, denial, and repression serve to protect the person from confronting the deficits. However, with increasing impairment, these mechanisms become ineffective and inefficient and are replaced by more primitive defenses.[32] Rigid, negativistic behavior then predominates. Unable to defend against awareness of the deficits or to interact effectively with the environment to fulfill needs—a difficulty which is compounded by a constant misinterpretation and distortion of reality—the person is vulnerable to catastrophic anxiety reaction, profound depression, or sudden assaultive aggressiveness. Also, as anxiety increases, sleeping and eating problems develop, with consequent weight loss and susceptibility to other physical problems.

Delirium

Delirium is a clouding of consciousness, a decrease in attention, and a decreased level of awareness. The term *delirium* refers to a number of illnesses of organic origin that are usually reversible and characterized by dysmenesia, disorientation, and disturbances in the regulation of sleep and wakefullness such as insomnia, somnolence, fluctuating awareness, and dysattention.[32] It is a syndrome which is a transient disturbance of brain function characterized by a global impairment of cognitive processes. Symptoms usually develop rapidly and fluctuate widely, and usually last only a few days. The level of consciousness is altered, but the person may not be out of touch with the environment. He or she may exhibit only a slight reduction in alertness or be comatose.

Since thinking, memory, perception, and attention are disturbed, the ability to understand and interpret the internal and external environment in accordance with past experience is reduced.[17] These changes in the sensorium interfere with the person's ability to gratify needs. The disruption in the metabolic processes of the brain produces the behavioral symptoms; however, psychological factors strongly influence the content of the delirium.[17]

Manifestations of delirium vary widely. The person may be quiet and experience only brief periods of inattentiveness which are not easily detected. However, as the level of awareness decreases, responsivity to external stimuli slows and the impaired thinking becomes more evident. In extreme cases, the person becomes delusional, enters a hallucinatory state, and is likely to be moribund.[17]

Factors associated with the development of delirium include sensory deprivation, sleep and dream deprivation, severe anxiety, immobilization, and psychological stress. Delusional thinking is not uncommon; it is persecutory in nature but poorly organized, and the content of thought changes rapidly. Consequently, the person may call out for help despite reassurances and the presence of a supportive person. If hallucinations occur, they are usually visual in nature, but they may be auditory as well.[31] The person tends to misidentify objects, people, or voices in the environment and then to generate hallucinatory experience. This misidentification also occurs in the form of illusive pseudorecognition. Clients suffering from sensory disturbances may, in a poorly illuminated room, mistake the nurse or other care givers for people they have known in the past.[32] For example:

> Mr. H., a client in serious metabolic disequilibrium, greeted the nurse one evening with the words, "Margie, how did you know I was here? I haven't seen you in years." Even when the nurse (whose name was not Margie) approached his bed and identified herself, he continued to relate to her as Margie, a friend from the past.

Four stages of delirium which delineate changes in the sensorium have been identified.

In the *first stage* the person is restless and talkative, experiences distortions of time and space, has difficulty remembering what is said or taught, is mildly suspicious, has increased sensitivity to stimuli (particularly visual and auditory stimuli), and exhibits moods which range from elation to irritability or bewilderment. Insomnia and day-night reversal may occur, and sleep is accompanied by vivid dreams or nightmares.[31]

In the *second stage* speech becomes incoherent and slurred, the ability to concentrate is even more impaired, and the disorientation to time, place, and person increases as misinterpretation of the environment becomes more marked. There may be overactivity which seems purposive, and emotional tone is labile.[7]

If the underlying problem is not resolved, the person enters the *third stage*. Hyperactivity continues but becomes purposeless, speech is disorganized, there is global disorientation, dysmenesia and easy distractibility predominate, hallucinations and delusions develop, and feelings of depression and fearfulness are pervasive.

If the person enters the *fourth stage*, the extreme of delirium may be manifested by either excitation or stupor or progress from the former to the latter. In either case, there is no meaningful relationship with the environment.[32]

Delirium is a medical emergency. The underlying cause must be treated promptly if permanent damage to brain tissue is to be prevented.

Paroxysmal Disorders

Generalized seizure activity, which includes grand mal epilepsy, is characterized by extreme neuronal discharges originating in the brain stem of the reticular activating system that spread throughout the entire central nervous system, to the cortex, to the deeper parts of the brain, and into the spinal cord.[7]

The clinical picture associated with this type of seizure activity includes: an aura* followed by an outcry; loss of consciousness; falling; extreme tonic spasm followed by clonic alternating flexion and extension of the body muscles. Cyanosis is marked until the seizure terminates. There is also deep, noisy breathing; profuse sweating; excessive salivation; and urinary and fecal incontinence. In the male there may be an erection and ejaculation of semen. The attack usually lasts from 2 to 5 minutes, after which the person is often in a confused state ("postictal twilight state").[7]

Some people are immediately alert after regaining consciousness. Frequently people lapse into a normal sleep that lasts from several minutes to 1 or 2 hours. There are often complaints of muscular aches and pains and a ravenous appetite following recovery. If recovery is rapid, the person is likely to complain of feeling depressed. Many people report feeling less tense, less depressed, and more alert during the days after a seizure than they did before it.[7]

Petit mal seizure activity also originates in the brain stem reticular activating system. These seizures, which last only 5 to 30 seconds, are characterized by clouding of consciousness, with several twitchlike contractions of the muscles, usually in the head region (for example, eye blinking), followed by a return to consciousness and resumption of previous activities.[7]

Focal seizures can involve any part of the brain, either localized regions of the cerebral cortex or deeper structures of both the cerebrum and the brain stem. This type of seizure activity usually arises from a localized lesion of the brain such as a tumor or scar. When rapid discharge occurs in the neurons in the specific area affected by the lesion, it gradually involves adjacent areas. In the case of the psychomotor seizure the person may experience any of the following: a short period of amnesia, an attack of abnormal rage, sudden anxiety or fear, a moment of incoherent speech or the repetition of a particular phrase, a "motor attack," such as smacking the lips or rubbing a body part.[7] Awareness of the seizure varies with attacks.

If localized discharge spreads over the motor cortex, it produces a progressive "march" of muscular contraction throughout the opposite side of the body. The Jacksonian seizure, which usually begins at the corner of the mouth or the thumb with a twitching muscle and extends downward to the legs, is an example of this process. As long as the seizure is unilateral, the person remains conscious.

In some seizure clients, particularly those whose conditions have been poorly controlled, there is an insidious dementia with narrowing interest, slowed mentation, and apathy. These people may also be vulnerable to a variety of emotional disturbances which are complicated by family and societal attitudes toward seizures.

Focal, sensory, psychomotor, and autonomic seizures have psychiatric implications. The organically based apathy characteristic of these people reflects an empty indifference that differs markedly

* *Aura:* A warning sensation that an epileptic usually experiences before a seizure.

from the apathy of depressed clients, which is accompanied by a preoccupation with worrisome thoughts.[44] These people are subject not only to alterations in consciousness but to changes in cognitive and affective processes as well. They may become suddenly irritable and impulsive and exhibit angry outbursts or periodic interictal violence. These people differ from those with character disorders inasmuch as they accept responsibility for their anger and are less likely to claim amnesia or irresistible impulse as the reason for their outbursts.[45] Some also become suddenly paranoid and engage in bizarre behavior. Seizures may also be accompanied by déjà vu phenomena; dreamy states; changes in self-awareness; a sensation of growing larger or smaller; forced thought in which a phrase, melody, or scene occupies the mind; hyposexuality or sexual arousal in the absence of stimuli.[31] Temporal lobe seizures and central nervous system tumors, particularly those in the occipital lobe, are associated with visual hallucinations that may include brightly colored, diffuse forms; colored patterns; or well-formed images.[31] Paroxysmal attacks of anxiety and the impression that objects in the environment are growing larger or smaller also occur. These people exhibit circumstantial behavior (behavior irrelevant to the situation), bizarre humor, and philosophical interests.[45] There is evidence of profound deepening of emotional responses, particularly an intensification of moral, ethical, cosmological, and religious feelings and concerns. These people often are unable to distinguish between trivial details and important matters in everyday life, and are often preoccupied with unimportant details.[31] They tend to scrutinize the right and wrong of every situation in a way similar to the religiosity seen among schizophrenics. Such phenomena are similar to those experienced by the schizophrenic or the person labeled *emotionally disturbed*, and this fact has implications for adaptation. Many people with seizure problems suffer from the psychotoxic effects of their anticonvulsant therapy; these include drowsiness, depersonalization, and dysmenesia. If these side effects are not remedied by alteration of dosage or drug, the person may develop disturbance of impulse control or judgment, depression, conversion symptoms, dissociative states, or delirium. Since time labeling is located in the dominant temporal lobe, people who have temporal lobe epilepsy experience subjective time disturbances.[32,37]

Anticonvulsant toxicity and a history of repeated seizures have an impact on lifestyle and self-perception. They interfere with the attainment of personal goals and elicit fear and avoidance on the part of others in social situations. In addition, the symptoms contribute to the client's low self-esteem, low self-acceptance, fear of insanity, and difficulty in obtaining gainful employment.

Body image is often disturbed by the side effects of the medications. Self-consciousness in relation to the gingival hypertrophy caused by the anticonvulsant therapy may cause the person to avoid smiling or to speak with minimal lip movement to prevent displaying the puffy gums. Hirsutism, acne, eczema, and loss of hair cause further embarrassment and alteration of self-concept.

People who suffer from seizure disorders are misunderstood and discriminated against. They are restricted in driving; they are excluded from many jobs, including military service; and they experience difficulty in obtaining life, automobile, and health insurance. This ostracism is damaging to the person's self-esteem and may contribute to the development of antisocial behavior such as alcoholism, drug abuse, and criminal activity. Recent studies that surveyed prisoners in several correctional institutions in various states revealed that the percentage of prisoners suffering from seizure disorders requiring anticonvulsant medications is more than 3 times the percentage in the general population. The findings from these studies suggest that onset of seizure disorders in childhood or adolescense predisposes these young people to poor social adjustment in adulthood. Impaired self-esteem and social adjustment may contribute to unemployability and social rejection. Alienated from society and lacking economic stability, they are prone to antisocial or criminal behavior.[46]

Attention Deficit Disorders

Behaviors that reflect the persistence of attention deficit disorders into adulthood include the following: impairment of attention, restlessness, emotional lability, impulsivity, rage reactions, aggressiveness, and impaired ability to form meaningful relationships with others. The intense rage reactions exhibited by these people are characterized by verbal or physical agressiveness which is both unpredictable and strikingly different from their usual behavior. They are often regretful and repentant after such outbursts. Between the outbursts they are generally easily excited and overresponsive to environmental pressures.[5]

Some people who have symptoms of hyperactivity, particularly those with antisocial behavior, do not outgrow their problems. As adults many continue to be distractible, emotionally immature, unable to maintain goals, and lacking in self-esteem. A significant number of these people are substance abusers. They are also at risk of involvement with the court system with respect to disturbance of the peace, theft, aggression, drug abuse, and traffic offenses.[47]

PATTERNS OF INTERACTION: FAMILY

Families are disrupted when a member suffers from OMD, regardless of the age of the person with the dementia.

A family with a young adult who suffers from OMD may be disorganized by grief and lack of support within the community. Financial and caretaking burdens may deprive the parents and siblings of family resources. Conflicts may emerge when continual supervision is needed. One parent may need to become the caretaker, usually depriving the family of either a second income or a portion of this income if a companion must be employed during the work day.

Most elderly people who develop OMD are living with a spouse who is not always physically well. Dementia in the older person disrupts the final developmental stage as well as the couple's plans and fantasies related to retirement.[48] The elderly couple are often isolated, less aware of community resources, and less able to seek out these resources. Even if they live near their children, there is no guarantee of support. Middle-aged sons and daughters may experience conflicting loyalties. The needs of their spouses and children may compete with the needs of the demented parent and the caretaking parent.[49] The geographical mobility of the younger generation and the dual-career marriage are phenomena that increase the difficulties encountered by adult children when they wish to be supportive of their parents. Spouses and unmarried adult children who are left alone to provide the caretaking are vulnerable to the stresses inherent in caring for a demented family member.

When a family member has OMD, the other members may experience a wide range of feelings that are in and of themselves disturbing. Acceptance of the diagnosis is preceded by anxiety and depression or denial. When denial occurs, family members experience a misplaced sense of shame.[37] The deterioration of the family member and the increased burden on the caretaker are not recognized. Open communication, which would facilitate support, problem solving, and decision making, does not occur, because all are involved in keeping the situation out of awareness and a secret. In such instances the family may fail to mobilize personal resources or seek community resources. Consequently the energy within the family may be rapidly depleted. Failure to use rehabilitation services that would maximize the client's strengths, self-responsibility, and self-determination may lead to premature institutionalization.

When OMD develops in adulthood and among the elderly, the manifest problems of the disorder can mask and exacerbate serious relationship problems within the family.[50] The client may become the focus of irrational feelings. The changes in the person's moods, personality, and self-sufficiency are difficult for family members to accept.[34]

In some families hostility and rejection occur, indicating that the relationships with the affected family member or with both the demented parent and the caretaking parent have a history of difficulties. Rejection and hostility may lead to the physical abuse of the family member with dementia. In other instances, these feelings generate guilt which is followed by expiation and overcompensation.[37] Overprotectiveness and restrictiveness, whether based on anxiety or guilt, may interfere with the dimensions of self-determination and self-responsibility that could be preserved and maximized. Imbalance of the family system may result in excessive attention and devotion to the client at the expense of other family members.[37]

Efforts that are directed toward minimizing family anxiety may not be constructive. For example, family members may deal with the client's disorientation and dysmenesia by failing to correct the client's misperceptions and confusions; thus they fail to provide realistic feedback. The family may operate on the false assumption that to correct errors would be either upsetting or a waste of time. Consequently the family further contributes to perpetuating the disorientation and dysmenesia.[51] When deterioration involves mental and emotional processes, it is more difficult for the person to retain any degree of self-responsibility and more difficult for the family to recognize the person's intact dimensions, foster maximization of these dimensions, and not take over. In the name of love and protection, families may deprive these older people of all self-determination and every shred of self-respect.[51]

In the family's eyes the person with dementia dies a little at a time as the personality, intellectual capacities, and self-care deteriorate. To the family, psychological death is occurring, and all are involved in an ongoing funeral, but lack the comfort of formalized religious rituals. Mourning may extend across years and remain incomplete until physical death occurs.[48]

The problems associated with the dementia that are the most difficult for family members include the following: incontinence, anger and aggressiveness, difficulty lifting and moving the person while giving physical care, lack of communication, risks of accidents such as burns and falls, and wandering.[52]

Families that are able to manage effectively during the early stages of the person's progressive mental and physical deterioration may encounter difficulties during the latter stages. A spouse may, however, become socially isolated. These people may live in social limbo, feeling neither married nor single. The way love is given and received is altered. Sexual interactions are impaired. Lack of sexual interest; insensitivity toward the unimpaired spouse; or incessant, inappropriate demands may occur.[48] If during the night the person wanders about the house, leaves and roams the streets, becomes more disoriented and shouts out, or develops urinary and fecal incontinence, family members' sleep will be disrupted. Over time, sleep deprivation and worry about the person's safety will become chronically stressful. When this occurs, family members may become impatient and easily frustrated with each other and with the person.

When placement in residential care becomes a necessity, it is a difficult decision and one that inevitably produces a crisis in the family. Families may be split on how to handle the problem. If there are members who are denying the situation or caught up in the anger related to their grief, their anger may be displaced onto the caretaking member or the member who recognizes the increasing burden and is urging the decision for placement. The caretaking member or other members who have accepted the situation may be accused of neglect or cruelty. Deciding on placement and implementing that decision have major implications for the complex network of family relationships. The family which decides impulsively or procrastinates by agonizing over the decision may aggravate an already difficult situation. Old family conflicts and rivalries may surface, preventing careful exploration and evaluation of alternatives. The turmoil that occurs may result in the total exclusion of the client, even when it is inappropriate. The person designated as the one responsible for the decision may be the recipient of blame and hostility regardless of the outcome. The person may experience the decision-making role as burdensome, and after the decision he or she may feel depressed and guilty.

Separation from the loved one precipitates or aggravates grieving and influences the way other family members separate from the family in the future. If, for example, the placement of an aged grandparent proceeds in a deliberate, orderly, and empathic fashion that preserves emotional connectedness, then the separation and departure of the young adult grandchildren will be more likely to proceed in the same way.

If the client's relationship with the family is severely disturbed and characterized by an emotional cutoff, the emotional ties may be too weak or negative to support even the sense of social obligation. In these instances the person is abandoned, and social agencies assume responsibility for physical safety and care.

Seizure-prone people, including people who simulate seizures, are members of family systems; consequently, when maladaptive behavior occurs, it is a symptom of the family's problems in coping with the disease process. Thus, interventions are directed toward helping the family to manage the interpersonal difficulties consequent to the paroxysmal disorder.

Family and adoption studies indicate that psychopathology is a common occurrence in the families of clients with ADD. Studies reveal that alcoholism and antisocial and hysterical personality disorders are common among family members. The occurrence of similar symptoms from generation to generation may be a function of genetic factors. However, learning during childhood in a symptomatic family may also contribute to the transfer of problematic behavior from one generation to another. From a holistic perspective this transgenerational phenomenon is probably a product of the interaction of inherited predisposition, environmental factors, and the multigenerational transmission process.[2,6]

PATTERNS OF INTERACTION: ENVIRONMENT

Young and middle-aged adults with OMD wish to retain and maximize their autonomy.[50] The deficits imposed by their condition may seriously affect their participation in the working world and their ability to be totally self-responsible. Our society systematically undermines the position of elderly people and deprives them of major functions.[53] Furthermore, in a materialistic culture, decreased income and social status are viewed as catastrophic. The youth orientation in our society also aggravates the elderly person's response to the changes that are occurring as a result of the disease process. Behavior and dress that would be accepted or ignored in the young may be considered evidence of mental incompetence in the elderly and become grounds for incarceration in a nursing home.[53]

Placement of the elderly person with OMD is usually in a nursing home. These facilities vary greatly in relation to the philosophy that guides the care-giving process and the delivery of services. They generally tend to provide for basic nutritional, hygiene, and safety needs in a monotonous, routinized fashion. Sensory stimuli are minimal, aggravating the disorientation and dysmenesia. The staff members tend to relate to the clients as if they were children, fostering further regression. Cut off from friends and family in strange surroundings, deprived of meaningful sensory stimuli, these clients deteriorate and die more rapidly than they otherwise would.[54]

Nursing homes are not organized to provide care to people with dementia. For example, the wandering behavior which is meaningful exploration for these people is problematic in these settings. Nursing homes do not routinely lock the unit doors, but if doors are not secured, the demented person may wander out of the institution and not know how to return. All too often clients are restrained in chairs or beds to prevent this behavior. This restrictiveness interferes with maximizing their potential.[55] Total institutional care all too often interferes with even limited self-determination and self-responsibility. Institutional policies, pressures for conformity, and the lack of meaningful activities promote a loss of social competence and a vegetative, dehumanized existence.

All too frequently there are no residential services for the young adult in or near the community. A state psychiatric facility may be the only option if the young person becomes unmanageable. Since these agencies are not designed to meet the particular needs of people with organically based psychosocial deficits, the placement becomes mere "warehousing."

Home care has the potential to provide the greatest opportunity for meaningful relationships and adequate sensory stimuli. However, as the deterioration progresses, the required physical care and continued monitoring may become a physical and emotional burden for the family. Sensitivity is lost and care giving becomes ritualized and emotionally distant.

Family members who have access to extensive personal and community resources may be able to fulfill their role functions in their relationships with each other and particularly in the relationship with the family member they are caring for at home. A stressful home environment and the overburdening of family members who are emotionally drained lead to self-protective distancing of the disabled family member. Likewise, generalizing or extending the effects of the person's organic deficits leads to negation of his or her humanity. Communication during care giving may be nonexistent, depriving the person of reassurance of worth and the opportunity to share concerns. The care-giving process and isolation within the home context may accentuate loneliness and further disorganize the person.[56]

Many families wish to keep the person with dementia at home and to provide humanistic, loving, and sensitive care. These families need relief from the 24-hour-a-day care and the inherent burdens.[55] Supportive services can often maintain elderly people in their homes longer. Lack of these resources may precipitate premature and inappropriate placement in an institution that prevents these people from maximizing their strengths and instead focuses on their pathology. Adult day care, if available, can help meet these needs. When this service is unavailable, inappropriate commitment to an institution may occur. Wandering and self-neglect are not necessarily indications of dangerousness to self. Only 42 percent of elderly people with dementia are committed because of unmanageable aggressiveness and assaultiveness. Even this population would need not be committed if stress within the family or care setting was managed effectively and medication was prescribed to decrease behavioral symptoms.[53]

Single-room-occupancy hotels (SROs) in cities are populated by residents who have multiple health problems including varying degrees of OMD. These are alienated people who live a marginal existence in substandard housing. They are in desperate need of outreach health care services. However, health and welfare services are either totally lacking or grossly inadequate because of budgetary limitations. People with OMD may not have the capacity to provide for their basic nutritional, hygiene, and safety needs. They suffer from malnutrition and often sustain injuries that remain untreated.[57] Their accommodations are often infested with vermin. Because their thinking is disordered, they are unable to seek help when their quarters are without heat in the winter or their water supply is cut off. During a heat wave they may become dehydrated and die in their unventilated apartments, wearing layers of winter clothes.

Funding of services for people with OMD is inappropriate and inadequate. As the number of people with these disorders increases, as projected, the problems associated with their care will mount. The cost of providing care is staggering and will become even more of a burden if action is not taken to fund services that are appropriate to the needs of these people and their families. Medicare provides continued care for the elderly poor; however, in most states Medicaid budgets are underfunded. Mental health services have been underfunded historically. Indigent people who are institutionalized are often kept in state hospitals beyond therapeutic need because of the difficulty of placing these people in more appropriate and less costly settings. Per diem costs in state hospitals are almost 2 times those in nursing homes and 4 times the cost of psychiatric day care. In addition, nursing homes are inappropriate settings for these people.[53] Since family members, particularly unimpaired spouses, may deplete their financial base in providing home care, funding of supportive services for home care and appropriate day care and institutional care is needed.

NURSING PROCESS

Many of the behaviors exhibited by clients with OMD distance care givers. Impulsivity, irritability, slowness to respond, and negativistic behavior generate feelings of impatience which, with time, grow into anger. Poor personal hygiene and inappropriate behavior may elicit feelings of disgust and the wish to avoid the client. These negative feelings may cause care givers to succumb to pressured time schedules and sacrifice individual needs of the client; care givers may sometimes even coerce clients to conform when it is not necessary.

Responsibility, appropriateness, self-control, responsivity to others, social awareness, and rationality are attributes we assign to adulthood. These qualities are components of what we consider to be human dignity. When nurses must care for clients over time and watch irreversible, progressive deterioration of these human qualities, they experience feelings of impotence and helplessness. It can be depressing for nurses to work with perseverance and caring, only to find their clients becoming more vegetative, aggressive, or disorganized. The nurse's distress is, of course, compounded by the fact that there are no interventions available to arrest the progressive deterioration. As a defense against such distress, nurses may appear to withdraw physically and emotionally from clients. This response is often exhibited by the mechanical, technical, and impersonal way in which care is delivered.

Nurses respond to symptoms of delirium differently depending on the setting. In the hospital and when there has been a diagnosis, the symptoms are interpreted as a medical emergency and treated as such. If the symptoms begin when the client is not in a medical setting, they can be misinterpreted. If the lack of attention, hallucinatory behavior, suspiciousness, talkativeness, elation, depression, and incidents of illusive pseudorecognition are not recognized as signs of acute and severe brain dysfunction, the nurse may respond with bewilderment and frustration or as if the problems were psychogenically rather than physiologically based.

Seizure disorders can also be misinterpreted. If the care givers share the perception that there is an emotional component, the assessment process may be skewed toward interpreting data in a way that fails to attend to the client's needs. The nurse may become impatient and nonsupportive, and the client may be baffled and anxious about the symptoms and lack of empathy from care givers.

Elderly clients who have been able to compensate for their mental deterioration while in the familiar surroundings of their own homes may become severely disorganized by a sudden medical or surgical hospitalization. Not infrequently these older people are admitted for the treatment of a fractured hip on an emergency basis. The underlying OMD that may have contributed to their accident becomes blatantly evident after hospitalization. They become noisy, shouting and rattling the side rails incessantly, particularly at night. In spite of their injuries, they may attempt to climb over the side rails on their beds. Basic care such as bathing and feeding often precipitates yelling and combative behavior. Medications are often spit out. When these patients are turned, they may dig their fingernails into the nurse's arm or pinch the nurse angrily. These clients generate frustration in their care givers. In response, nurses tend to avoid them. When they provide care, their anger may be expressed by a lack of empathy, rough handling, and the issuing of orders in a loud, angry voice ("Stop your yelling, Mazie. Be quiet! You're acting like a pest!").

As other clients on the unit increase their complaints during the night and, unable to sleep, become more demanding of the nurse's time and attention, the nurse becomes increasingly angry at the disruptive elderly client.

Some elderly people with OMD respond to their confusion by becoming overcompliant and apathetic. Because they present no nursing management problem, they may be treated with benign neglect or be infantalized by the staff members. Interactions with these clients may resemble those with a toddler. Respect and efforts to preserve the client's dignity may be totally lacking. Because this type of client is neither disruptive nor demanding, he or she has a low priority in the delivery of care. In spite of the client's urinary or fecal incontinence and need for frequent nutritional supplements and fluids, the nurse may enter the client's room infrequently and leave the client unattended for long periods of time.

The responses that clients with OMD generate in the nurses who provide care for them are not preventable. They are real and unavoidable and require ventilation. However, these feelings need not interfere with the delivery of comprehensive, individualized, and sensitive care. Awareness that such feelings are developing is the initial step in their resolution. When nurses begin to get in touch with these feelings, clients' behavior can be examined in light of what is known about the effects of organic damage on functioning; this process will redefine the situation to some extent. Behavior which may have been perceived as purposely frustrating, inappropriate, and destructive may be redefined as the client's only available way of defending against deficits and the awareness of a changing self-concept.

Being able to "put oneself in another's shoes" is an important approach to understanding the client's problem and desperate need to protect and conserve the self. From this vantage point, the nurse's perception is altered. Empathy can emerge, and this expands and sensitizes the nurse's perceptions of the client's needs and environmental factors which influence coping.

Clients' impulsivity is yet another problem. Knowing that the condition is organically based is not always sufficient. The behavior may be provocative, disruptive, an obstacle to providing needed attention to other clients, and continuously frustrating. However, such situations need not be hopeless. Nurses can cope more cognitively than affectively if they are supported by a cohesive multidisciplined team which maximizes communication, plans knowledgeably and collaboratively, and evaluates plans nonjudgmentally, thus sharing the burden of helping clients learn some dimension of control.

The nurse who cares for a client with OMD will often respond to the situation on the basis of his or her own identification with the client or family. If the nurse is struggling with the burden of caring for a family member with OMD and values maintaining the person at home, a family which decides in favor of institutionalization will be viewed negatively. Regardless of the objective reality of the family's situation, the nurse may condemn the decision and express impatience and hostility toward the family. If the decision for placement has been difficult for the family and infused with ambivalence, the nurse's behavior will escalate their feelings of guilt and anxiety.

Many nurses who work for extended periods of time with mentally disabled elderly people in nursing homes develop self-protective emotional distance from the clients and their situation. Care giving becomes routinized and ritualistic. Getting the "job" done is paramount and the recipients of the care become nonpersons. When this happens, families who visit frequently and make numerous requests of the staff members are viewed and treated as nuisances. Little or no information about the client is shared with the family. If the family expresses concern about a problem, the nurses respond in a matter-of-fact fashion and often covertly communicate that such concern is ridiculous.

In these situations when the client becomes moribund and death is imminent, the nurse may not notify the family members. The presence of the family at this time is not perceived as important, since the client is confused or comatose. There is a total lack of recognition of family members' need to be present.

If nurses perceive the family's direct or indirect involvement in the client's predicament, they may blame the family. For example, if the client is a young person whose OMD is the result of a motorcycle or automobile accident, the nurse may believe that the family is to blame and may overtly and covertly exclude the family from the care-giving process. Rescue fantasies in relation to clients are not uncommon in these situations.

The management of a person with OMD in the home is often a difficult burden for the family. If the nurse who is making home visits identifies with the family's burden and can see himself or herself trapped in a similar situation, that nurse may campaign for institutional placement. Instead of supporting family members, helping them use a problem-solving approach to difficulties, and involving community resources, the nurse may focus the work with the family on the decision for placement.

Nursing care plans for clients with problems related to OMD are presented in Table 44-3. The assessment, diagnosis, outcome criteria, and intervention components of the nursing process are illustrated.

Table 44-3 Nursing Care Plans

Client 1		Client 1	
Assessment	Disoriented to time, place, and person. Expresses acute distress when family member is not recognized. Wanders continuously around unit in an agitated state, looking for bedroom at home. Demands to be fed at odd hours, forgetting when meals are eaten. Agitated at change of shift or when visitors or physicians enter unit.	**Diagnosis**	Disorientation related to dementia and loss of familiar surroundings.
		Outcome criteria	Client will check time by looking at clock and will tell nurse correct time of day. Client will wait for family members to identify who they are. Client will wander but in an explorative way, and without visible agitation. Client will ask to eat at appropriate times.

(Continued.)

Table 44-3 Continued

Client 1	
Nursing interventions	1. Frequently orient to time, place, and person, using clocks, calendars, and visual aids. 2. Establish a set, well-known routine for the client to follow. 3. Address the client by name and title ("Good morning, Mr. Tate") to reinforce a sense of identity. 4. Repeat basic information frequently during the day. 5. Orient the client when he or she wakes up during the night. 6. Do not agree with the confused client's incorrect statements, argue, or insist on your viewpoint. 7. Correct the client gently but not insistently. 8. Do not allow the client to ramble incoherently. 9. Respond to the client openly and honestly. 10. Create a calm, quiet, and unhurried atmosphere. 11. Speak slowly and distinctly. 12. Moderate or avoid stressful situations to decrease stimuli which would distort perceptions or cause sensory overload. 13. Convey warmth and concern. 14. Respond patiently and consistently. 15. Patiently explain procedures, reasons for equipment, and changes in routines or personnel. 16. Instruct family members and visitors to introduce themselves whenever they come on unit or are face to face with client. 17. Orient client to unit daily for 1 week by taking a tour and explaining each room and its use. 18. Allow client to wander without restriction on unit except for entering other client's rooms.
Client 2	
Assessment	Distractible when nurse is talking to client. Abruptly walks away when being given an explanation. Fiddles with clothes or possessions when someone is attempting to talk with client.
Diagnosis	Dysattention associated with deficits of memory and language comprehension caused by dementia.
Outcome criteria	Client will maintain eye contact with nurse during an interaction. Client will admit to not knowing the answer to a question; will say, "I don't know." Client will attempt to respond appropriately to verbal messages. Client will ask nurse, "May I leave, please," rather than leave abruptly.
Nursing interventions	1. Look directly at the client when communicating. 2. Position self in client's line of vision when communicating. 3. Give clear, distinct, simple directions in a step-by-step fashion. 4. Direct conversation toward concrete, familiar subjects. 5. Provide simple activities that will encourage purposeful motion. 6. Repeat messages slowly, calmly, and patiently until the client shows some signs of comprehension. 7. Vary media and words to fit the client's ability to comprehend the message. 8. Modify environmental stimuli which affect attention.
Client 3	
Assessment	Makes no attempt to interact with other clients or staff members. Wanders alone or isolates self in room. Does not join other clients watching television. Takes seat at empty table at mealtimes. Becomes agitated when other clients attempt to interact. No visits from family or friends. No phone calls from family or friends. Becomes agitated when asked questions about family visiting.
Diagnosis	Social isolation related to 1. Impaired communication capacities 2. Attempts to avoid anxiety 3. Abandonment by family and friends.
Outcome criteria	Client will join other clients watching television. Client will join other clients at mealtimes.

(Continued.)

Table 44-3 Continued

Client 3	
Outcome criteria	Client will stay out of room during day. Client will appear comfortable when staff members or other clients accompany client during wanderings.
Nursing interventions	1. Support statements in which the client describes significant others as caring, concerned, and helpful. 2. Help the client seek and accept reasons why the behavior of significant others is not meeting the client's expectation. 3. Encourage the display of mementos. 4. Actively listen to the client's viewpoints and perception of the past and present. 5. Modify environmental factors affecting feelings about significant others. 6. Help the client maintain communication with significant others.

Client 4	
Assessment	Becomes visibly agitated when unable to remember facts or when possessions are misplaced. Feigns deafness when asked questions or directed to do something. Becomes irritable and hostile when reminded to go to meals or get ready for bed.
Diagnosis	Dysmenesia related to organic brain impairment.
Outcome criteria	Client will seek help in finding misplaced possessions. Client will accept reminders to go to meals or get ready for bed. Client will follow nurse's assistance and lead in accomplishing tasks.
Nursing interventions	1. Give simple, clear, step-by-step directions even for routine, uncomplicated activities. 2. Interpret feigned deafness or refusal to perform certain tasks as a defense against memory loss. 3. Repeat policies, routines, and other information regarding daily living activities when the client's behavior suggests that he or she cannot remember this information. 4. Initiate assistance in the performance of a task if the client shows hesitancy or refuses to do it, giving verbal reminders for each step the client is expected to perform. 5. Avoid confrontation or exposure of fabricated stories or untruths, and interpret these behaviors as defenses against memory impairment. 6. Interpret anger and irritability as possible defenses against the client's realization that he or she cannot cope with the demands of the situation. 7. Interpret difficulty with abstract reasoning and inability to conceptualize as possible symptoms of organic dysfunction, and avoid making unnecessary and inappropriate demands. 8. Recognize negativistic behavior and substitute activities as defenses against dysmenesia; avoid confrontation.

Client 5	
Assessment	Becomes aggressive and assaultive when unable to perform a task, when reminded of unit schedule, or when client sees two other clients or staff members talking privately. Wanders constantly. Becomes more aggressive and assaultive in late afternoon. Acknowledges fatigue at dinnertime.
Diagnosis	Catastrophic fear reaction and suspiciousness related to awareness of deteriorating intellectual functioning.
Outcome criteria	Client will ignore or deny deficits. Client will ignore clients and staff members who are conversing. Client will not exhibit assaultive behavior. Client will take afternoon nap without objection. Client will express interest in people and events "here and now."
Nursing interventions	1. Support client's efforts to ignore or deny intellectual impairments. 2. Avoid confrontation of inappropriate behavior and probing for feelings.

(Continued.)

Table 44-3 Continued

Client 5	
Nursing interventions	3. Communicate in a way that does not increase the client's awareness of deficits or need for defensive coping mechanisms. 4. Accompany the client during wanderings, gently providing guidance back to the specified area. 5. Avoid use of restraints or incarceration, which will cause greater feelings of inadequacy and helplessness. 6. Interpret suspiciousness as a possible regression to a lower level. 7. Do not make false promises. 8. Include client in conversations when possible. 9. Encourage client to take short afternoon nap. 10. Encourage client's interest in and discussion about unit activities.

Client 6	
Assessment	Newly admitted client who makes no attempt at self-care. No motor or coordination deficits. Follows verbal directions. Resists self-care activities; complains about physical ailments and cites them as reasons for not acting in own behalf.
Diagnosis	Dependence fostered by family's failure to maintain independence and unrelated to physical capacity.
Outcome criteria	Client will function with minimal assistance in performing daily living activities: feeding, bathing, dressing.
Nursing interventions	1. Support maintenance of personal hygiene through verbal step-by-step directions, and avoid "doing for" the client. 2. Provide maximum personal freedom within the bounds of safety. 3. Foster the maintenance of established daily living activities. 4. Actively listen to somatic complaints and help the client remain physically active within medically defined limits. 5. Modify the environment to facilitate independent functioning. 6. Help the client perform a task only when there are data indicating sensory and motor impairments which would prevent the client from functioning without help.

Client 7	
Assessment	80-year old man hospitalized for fractured hip. Calls out loudly for help and rattles side rails during evening and throughout night. Calls evening nurse his granddaughter. Tells nurse he sees people sitting in chair placed in corner of room.
Diagnosis	Misinterpretation of reality related to delirium and sudden placement in unfamiliar setting.
Outcome criteria	Client will not exhibit illusive pseudo-recognition. Client will cease calling for help and rattling side rails. Client will cease reporting people present in his room at night.
Nursing interventions	1. Give reality-oriented feedback. 2. Avoid use of physical restraints; instead, use "othereness" and calming verbal reassurance. 3. Support medical treatment for underlying medical problem. 4. Give reassurance that the client is safe. 5. Protect the client from excessive noise level and restricting the number of people in the environment. 6. Provide a modulated level of stimulation that prevents both excitement and sensory deprivation. 7. Provide sufficient light in the client's room at night so that the client will be able to identify surroundings correctly and thus avoid developing illusions. 8. Have people who come in contact with client identify themselves each time they enter the client's room.

Assessment

Clients exhibiting behavioral symptoms of OMD are encountered by nurses in a wide variety of settings: emergency rooms; clinics; medical and surgical units in a general hospital; special-care units such as the intensive-care unit (ICU) or cardiac-care unit (CCU); convalescent and continuing care settings; psychiatric hospitals; mental health centers; and their own homes. These settings may alleviate or aggravate the display of symptoms. Nurses must be knowledgeable about the symptoms characteristic of OMD and their causation so that they can be alert to finding cases of OMD and can be sensitive to the needs of their clients and their clients' families.

Nurses have a major advantage in the care of clients who are potential victims of OMD. In inpatient settings, nurses are provided with an opportunity to observe and document clients' behavior in many situations and with various people 24 hours a day. These data become a valuable base for the physician's and nurse's diagnoses as well as the planning, implementation, and evaluation of care.

Nursing is primarily concerned with clients' responses to illness. Thus the assessment of clients suspected of or diagnosed as having OMD focuses on their behavior and their response to existing or progressing deficits. Table 44-4 presents a general framework for assessing clients in a variety of settings to determine whether there is a possibility that OMD may be interfering with their ability to function optimally. The mental status questionnaire and scoring system presented in Table 44-5 are a way of making a rapid assessment of the extent of a client's disability. The questions may be asked sequentially or integrated into the admission interview. Table 44-6 presents a series of questions that are designed to elicit data which can be analyzed to determine how the person diagnosed as having OMD is coping with the organic dysfunction.

Language impairment associated with OMD often interferes with the client's ability to express needs and feelings. Nurses need to recognize the use of codelike language.[58] For example, when feeling afraid, a client may talk about monsters lurking in dark corners. If feeling a loss of identity, the client

Table 44-4 Case Finding

Assessment
1. Are there personality changes which can be observed over time or described in behavioral terms by significant others?
2. Is the person oriented to time, place, and person?
3. Is there evidence of absentmindedness which is creating problems or indicating potential problems of a serious nature?
4. Is remote memory more accessible than recent memory, and is there evidence of extensive use of confabulation to mask memory gaps?
5. Is the person's judgment becoming unreliable or dangerous to self or others?
6. Is speech more impoverished than it has been in the past?
7. Is self-care deteriorating?
8. Is there evidence of emotional lability or inappropriate affect, blunting, shallowness, or unresponsiveness in interpersonal relationships?
9. Is the sensorium disturbed?
10. Does the person exhibit behavior suggestive of a paroxysmal disorder?
11. Are there changes in the person's behavior which violate social conventions and have potential for causing embarrassment or being labeled *deviant?*

Table 44-5 Mental Status Questionnaire (MSQ)

Questionnaire
1. Where are we now?
2. Where is this place located?
3. What is today's day, day of month?
4. What month is it?
5. What year is it?
6. How old are you?
7. What is your birthday?
8. What year were you born?
9. Who is president of the United States?
10. Who was president before him?

Scoring

Number of errors	Mental status
0–2	OMD absent or mild
3–5	OMD mild to moderate
6–8	OMD moderate to severe
9–10	OMD severe
Nontestable	OMD severe

SOURCE: Modified version, A. I. Goldfarb, *Aging and Organic Brain Syndrome*, Health Learning Systems, Bloomfield, N.J., 1974, p. 12.

Table 44-6 Client's Response to OMD

Asessment
1. What coping mechanisms is the client using to defend against awareness of the deficits?
2. Is the client becoming isolated and withdrawing from social contact with others?
3. Does the client exhibit affective dysfunction or increasing disorganization at certain times or in specific social situations?
4. Is inappropriate behavior elicited by specific situations or communications?
5. Does the client avoid situations which would expose the loss of intellectual functioning?
6. Do the client's deficits require protection from self-injury and the environment and interventions to preserve human dignity?
7. Are the client's family or care givers flexible, supportive, and sensitive to the client's needs?
8. Are sleeping and eating problems developing or worsening?
9. Are the client's judgment and decision making becoming less reliable?
10. Is there behavioral evidence that delirium is worsening?
11. Is there evidence suggesting a toxic reaction to anticonvulsant therapy?
12. Is there evidence that the client with a seizure disorder is receiving secondary gains from the illness that interfere with effective functioning?
13. Is the client using substitute or negativistic behavior when requested to perform a designated task?

may talk about getting to work on time—to a place where he or she was known and respected and had an identity. When this codelike language is recognized and interpreted, statements that seem out of touch with the reality of the client's situation are seen not as inappropriate comments but rather as the best possible effort at communicating feelings.

Wandering is a common behavior associated with dementia. If there is no accompanying agitation, then this behavior is meaningful to the person and a means of exploring and becoming oriented to an unfamiliar environment.

To determine how rapidly the client is deteriorating and to be able to project when home care may become a burden to the family, the nurse needs to establish a baseline of functioning and to compare this baseline periodically with the client's current status. A framework for this kind of baseline assessment is presented in Table 44-7 (see page 958).

Since the impact of a family member's OMD on the family is significant, the nurse needs to assess family coping. The framework presented in Table 44-8 (page 959) is designed to serve as a guide for this assessment. The interacting institutional environment also influences the coping of people with organically impaired mental functioning. The assessment of this environment for factors that interfere with optimal functioning of both the person and the family is presented in Table 44-9.

Diagnosis

The planning phase of the nursing process begins with the formulation of nursing diagnoses. During this phase of the nursing process, priorities are set regarding which problems require immediate intervention and which require long-range planning or attention at a later time. The problems that are identified—for example, "Excessive drowsiness interfering with participation in unit activities"—may not be under nursing's purview; if that is the case, a report or referral is made to professionals with the requisite expertise.

The data collected during the assessment process are analyzed, categorized, compared, and synthesized to determine the existence of problems and strengths. Once this work is completed, decisions are reached as to whether problems do in fact exist and whether there are areas where intervention would enhance existing strengths and help the client to achieve the highest possible level of wellness given the existing organic damage. The nurse then formulates the nursing diagnoses, which will guide planning and implementation.

The following are examples of nursing diagnoses related to OMD:

Severely limited self-care activities related to organically based memory impairment

Wandering related to temporal-spatial disorientation

Emotional lability related to brain tissue dysfunction

Impaired language comprehension related to brain tissue dysfunction

Table 44-7 Framework for Monitoring Functioning

	Unaided	Minimally Compensatory	Extensively Compensatory	Wholly Compensatory
Self-care:				
Eating				
Bathing				
Toileting				
Dressing				
Preparing food				
Moving about				
Shopping				
	Intact	**Minimal Impairment**	**Extensive Impairment**	**Totally Obliterated**
Mental functioning:				
Time orientation				
Place orientation				
Person orientation				
Recent memory				
Distant memory				
Concentration				
Attention				
Judgment				
Comprehension of questions				
Comprehension of directions				
Use of words (language)				
Ability to follow a conversation				
Sleep-wake cycle				
Affect				
Interest				
Ability to participate in a conversation				
Capacity to adapt to change				
	None	**Occasional**	**Pervasive**	**Unresponsive to Envrionment**
Problematic behaviors:				
Hallucinations				
Delusions				
Disinhibition				
Confusion				
Wandering				
Restlessness				
Aggressiveness				
Agitation				
Pathological repetition of words or phrases				

Table 44-8 Family Functioning

Assessment
1. Is the family involved in the care of the client, or is there rejection and hostility?
2. Have all family members accepted the diagnosis?
3. If some members are denying the diagnosis, how is this influencing interactions with the client? Other family members?
4. Is one family member responsible for the client's care, or is the responsibility shared?
5. Does the caretaker member feel burdened and unable to gain relief?
6. Does the client require supervision 24 hours a day?
7. How is the client's condition affecting the family financially?
8. Are family members who are not directly involved in the client's care supportive of those who are caring for the client?
9. Are family members able to talk about their feelings, fears, and fantasies?
10. Does the behavior of family members aggravate or minimize the client's coping?
11. How do the family members feel about eventual institutionalization?
12. Has the family openly discussed institutionalization?
13. Who will make the decision for institutionalization?
14. Will the decision maker be supported by other family members?
15. Do family members perceive the psychological death of the client?
16. How are members managing the grieving process?
17. Is the care giver able to have periods of time free from the supervision of the client?
18. Is there potential or actual abuse of the client related to care giver burnout?

Table 44-9 Environment

Assessment
1. Is there safe, adequate space for the client to wander without interference?
2. Is there an adequate number of staff members or family members to permit unhurried, patient assistance with daily living activities?
3. Are there clocks and calendars visible to help the client maintain a time orientation?
4. Do various rooms, such as the dining and television rooms, and the client's own room have designating signs to help the client maintain space orientation?
5. Are staff members and family members knowledgeable about how the brain dysfunction influences the client's behavior, and do they structure daily schedules that reflect this understanding?
6. Are opportunities provided to help the client, when possible, be informed of community and societal events?

Substitute activity related to memory impairment

Unpredictable rage reaction related to interictal period

Impulsiveness related to impaired judgment

Hoarding related to recognition of increasing memory loss

The following are examples of diagnoses for clients with OMD who are having problems coping with their deficits and environments:

Persecutory delusions related to changes in daily routine

Aggressiveness and assaultiveness related to confrontation of deficits

Apathetic withdrawal from others related to being restrained in a chair and not allowed to wander

Combative behavior associated with hurried assistance with daily living activities

Pilfering of other clients' possessions related to loss of personal possessions when institutionalized

The following are examples of diagnoses of family problems related to coping with a member with OMD:

Deepening depression related to increasing caregiving burden and lack of relief from responsibilities

Adult child's spousal conflict related to financial stress

Conflict among adult siblings related to the issue of institutionalization

Acute anxiety related to client's wandering

Abuse of client related to family members' unresolved childhood conflicts with demented parent

Anxiety of spouse related to depletion of financial security

Acute grief related to client's psychological death

Secondary gains from seizures related to family overprotectiveness

Incontinence and lack of self-care effort related to family's failure to recognize client's abilities and their own fostering of dependency

Outcome Criteria

The outcome criteria for clients with OMD must often accommodate progressive deterioration and at the same time provide criteria that reflect concern with attaining maximum health potential. When OMD is a major contributing factor to the problem behavior, it must be remembered that total resolution of the client's difficulties may not be possible. Thus, the outcome criteria need to reflect the client's best efforts, given the circumstances. Examples of these outcome criteria are:

Client will cease being combative.

Client will abandon persecutory delusions.

Client will make effort to bathe with supervision.

Client will exhibit orientation to time of day.

Client will participate nonaggressively in group art project.

Client will participate in relaxation exercise when agitated.

Examples of outcomes for family problems are:

Family will achieve decrease in depression. Evidence:

1. Absence of insomnia
2. Increased appetite
3. Decreased tearfulness
4. Decreased complaints of fatigue

Spouse will resolve marital conflict related to finances and care giving. Evidence:

1. Seeking and receiving financial assistance from other family members
2. Seeking and receiving assistance for part-time home health aide

Adult siblings will resolve conflict. Evidence:

1. Ability of siblings to discuss parent's impairment realistically
2. Ability of siblings to discuss parent's prognosis
3. Ability of siblings to collaborate in setting criteria for when institutionalization of parent will be necessary

Intervention

Intervention with the Client

There is a difference between reversible and irreversible OMD. When OMD is reversible, nursing goals and interventions are directed toward (1) supporting medical treatment of underlying pathophysiology, (2) helping the client to respond adaptively to the temporary deficits, and (3) reassuring the client that a return to health is a realistic expectation. When OMD is irreversible, nursing interventions focus on helping the client to function optimally given existing and progressive deterioration. If abilities are impaired because they have not been conserved and supported, then retraining takes top priority. Efforts are made to keep these clients mentally active, but always within the parameters of their limitations. Independent functioning, self-responsibility, and self-determination are also fostered. These clients are never encouraged to explore feelings and must be protected against developing insights into their problems. It is very important to help them avoid awareness of their deficits and deterioration. This approach contradicts the nurse's usual way of helping clients with mental illness. Confrontation and recognition of deficits only heighten these clients' anxiety and encourage maladaptive behavior. Insight only serves to damage the self-concept and interfere with a dignified decline.[32]

HELPING CLIENTS TO FUNCTION. Clients may be resocialized through the use of discussion groups.[59] Clients with OMD, given support, may be able to participate in these groups. Topics that help these people become more aware of the environment, holidays, time markers, and their own past are usually manageable.[58]

Many maladaptive behaviors stem, in part, from disturbances in sensory perception and interpretation.[39] Impaired cognitive functioning interferes with the ability to regulate and interpret sensory input; consequently, sensory deprivation or overload occurs. People with OMD need sensory stimulation that is appropriate and regulated, and they need help in comprehending what the stimuli mean.

Behavior-modification strategies are useful with clients who have OMD when they are designed to reinforce and reward appropriate behavior. Nurses have the opportunity to monitor behavior and implement a behavior-modification plan of care in the institutional setting, and to teach an family to use such a program in the home setting.[39]

Day care for people with OMD is helpful to the client and family and often maintains the client in the home longer by helping to relieve the family from the burdens of care. Day care can help provide opportunities for socialization and reinforcement and maintenance of functioning. It can provide stability, meaningful relationships and activities, and opportunities to increase and maintain self-esteem.

Clients with irreversible and progressively deteriorating OMD are a challenge to nursing regardless of the setting. Hospitalization or institutionalization often aggravates their symptoms, and increased disorientation often leads to noisy and disruptive behavior. The application of restraints to prevent a client from climbing over side rails will ensure safety but also usually increases the disruptive behavior unless a concerted effort is made to implement a program of reality orientation. Table 44-10 shows a format for a reality-orientation program. Nurses working in convalescent homes may provide less direct care to these clients, but they are responsible for planning the care and helping

Table 44-10 Reality-Orientation Program

Format
1. Place large, easily readable clocks and calendars in the client's room and in community rooms.
2. Introduce yourself whenever you enter the client's room or engage client in an interaction.
3. Tell client the day of the week, time of day, date, and season at least once each shift.
4. Tell client the name of the institution, or that he or she is at home, and the name of the room whenever you initiate an interaction.
5. Name utensils and foods when feeding or assisting the client to eat.
6. Ask client which food is preferred for each forkful or spoonful.
7. Look directly at client and stand or sit in the line of vision.
8. Hold the client's hand if that helps to reduce distractibility.
9. Give clear, concise, one-step-at-a-time directions.
10. Repeat information about activities frequently.
11. Talk about concrete, here-and-now subjects.
12. Use guiding assistance in performing daily living activities.
13. Name articles of clothing while assisting dressing and undressing.
14. Name objects such as television, chairs, sofas when settling client in a room.
15. Guide client to bathroom, dining room, activity room.
16. Help client clarify a confused message.
17. Suggest use of bathroom or bedpan at specified intervals.

the nonprofessional care givers to understand the clients' predicament and the importance of following nursing orders.

Recognition of a possible underlying neurological deficit is important to identification of an appropriate care plan. Since many of these people have been misdiagnosed, case finding includes the assessment of people with various diagnostic labels who are not responding to treatment. Symptomatic behavior is not always a clear indicator. Psychological and physical testing is more likely to be done with children, particularly when they encounter problems in school. Adults with ADD may have been overlooked in the past because educators and health care personnel were less aware of this condition. Thus if ADD is suspected, it is important to refer the client for testing and to communicate clearly and concisely to other health professionals the data base which suggests an organic cause for the problem. Community health nurses may encounter such people in the homes of families they visit for other reasons. Extending care to them may be a significant factor in increasing the community's awareness of the problem and the development of relevant services for the client and the family.

SOMATIC TREATMENT. Once a diagnosis of OMD has been confirmed, a variety of therapeutic modalities are employed to reverse, arrest, or ameliorate the tissue destruction. When OMD has been caused by toxic substances, the cellular damage cannot always by reversed. However, prevention of further exposure to the substance arrests cellular toxicity and destruction.[60] In the case of poisoning from heavy metals such as lead, the chelating agent EDTA may be prescribed. However, this is useful only in the treatment of acute poisoning and lead encephalopathy; it is not effective in chronic cases except in the presence of plumbemia (toxic levels of lead in the blood). Unless it is treated immediately, mercury poisoning will cause irreversible damage.

With metabolic and endocrine problems, treatment of the underlying disorders prevents irreversible neuronal damage. Hypoglycemic encephalopathies require interventions which focus on helping clients understand, accept, and manage their diabetes and life stress more effectively.

Circulatory disorders which contribute to the development of OMD require treatment of the underlying pathophysiology. Anticoagulants, vasodilators, and lipotropic enzymes are used to alleviate the problems of atherosclerosis; however, no controlled studies have been conducted which clearly prove their value.[17,61] Other encephalopathies can usually be controlled or reversed by treatment of the underlying pathophysiology.[17]

Anticoagulants, vasodilators, and neuropeptides have been used to treat blood "sludging" and red blood cell aggregation with a modicum of success in reversing and halting the symptoms of multi-infarct dementia. Where the symptoms have appeared to be related to impaired acetylcholine activity, physostigmine and lecithin have been administered. These drugs inhibit the action of the enzyme that normally destroys acetylcholine. The increase in acetylcholine that then occurs appears to enchance the learning and memory functions of the brain.[12,62,63]

When OMD is related to inherited or acquired progressively degenerative diseases such as Alzheimer's disease, there is no specific treatment; care is directed toward helping clients to cope effectively and comfortably within the limitations imposed by their deficits.

Antipsychotics and psychostimulants are sometimes used with dementia clients for the management of functional symptoms. On the basis of the hypotheses that adrenergic receptors in the aged are supersensitive because of the reduction of cerebral catecholamines and that neurotransmitter and related enzymes are reduced in the brain's cholinergic system, several cholinergic agents as well as tyrosine and 5-hydroxytryptophan have been used experimentally. There has also been recent experimentation with replacement or metabolic regulatory therapy involving vitamins, hormones, and enzymes.[62,63]

Psychotropics can be valuable in relieving symptoms of anxiety, impulsivity, hyperkinesis, depression, and paranoid ideation in clients with OMD. Antidepressants are also useful in the management of psychomotor retardation and may improve intellectual functioning and social performance.[32] However, drugs with anticholinergic properties must be given with caution to avoid prostatic obstruction, constipation, glaucoma, and hypotension in older clients.[32] The nurse's documentation of changes in mood, behavior, and performance of activities of daily living provides valuable data which will guide the physician's choice of drug and titration of dosage. If the client is living with his or her family while on medication, the nurse teaches the family how to assess the client's response to the regimen, the side effects, and signs of toxicity.

Brain traumas present a different picture. The reduction of increased intracranial pressure and removal of foreign objects or bone fragments may be all that is necessary to alleviate symptoms of acute OMD. However, where damage cannot be relieved or completely repaired, rehabilitation and retraining are employed to maximize functioning.[17]

When adults with ADD have been diagnosed and medications for the management of symptoms have been prescribed, the nurse can help the client and family understand the importance of adhering to the prescribed regimen and devise ways to remember when to take the medications. The community health nurse, who has opportunities to assess and intervene with the family system, can play a significant role in helping these clients work through obstacles to following the prescribed treatment.

Intervention with the Family

When clients living alone show a degree of dysmenesia that threatens their safety, they need help in relocating to an environment which better meets their safety needs. In these cases, the nurse works with the client, the family, and in some instances social services in providing for safer living arrangements. The community health nurse can serve as a resource for and coordinator of the services needed and used by the client and family. These services may include medical treatment, day care or home assistance, legal and financial counseling, individual or family therapy, and support groups for families with OMD. If the person has been abandoned by his or her family and placement in a residential care setting is necessary and desirable, then consistent care givers sensitive to the client's needs may in some measure replace the lost family.

Families may need facts about the OMD, how it affects functioning, and the prognosis. This information is helpful in dispelling myths and in developing an accurate understanding of the problem. Family recognition of the impairments allows the nurse to help the family provide a safe environment and an approach to care giving that maximizes the client's strengths and capacities.[64]

Joining a support group may enhance family members' personal coping and help them feel that they are not alone with their burdens. These groups provide opportunities to share feelings with empathic people who understand the problems and the painful feelings because they are confronted with similar situations. Group members are also able to help one another find solutions and strategies for managing problems encountered in providing care to a family member with OMD in the home.[48]

When clients with progressive OMD are living with their families, the first task the community health nurse may need to accomplish is to help the families stop denying the deficits. In the case of the older client, it saddens and distresses adult children when they must make decisions for their parents because the OMD has impaired intellectual capacities and judgment. Whether clients with OMD are young or old, their behavior may be frustrating and demanding, requiring continual supervision. Under such circumstances even a relatively healthy family will experience stress. As a result, symptoms of distress may appear in any one family member (manifested, for example, in marital discord) or lead to family disorganization. The nurse may be able to help the family identify changes in lifestyle, ventilate feelings, analyze responsibilities, clarify values, and examine both division of labor and allocation of resources. Once communication in these areas has been facilitated and issues have been examined, the family may be ready to effectively engage in problem-solving activities relevant to the difficulties engendered by living with a member having OMD. This helping process also includes helping the family understand that some of the client's behavior is a consequence of the organic pathology and of the need to defend against confronting these deficits.

Families may need to be taught strategies for providing assistance without "taking over" and "doing for" the client and for providing the client with opportunities to retain as much independence as possible. Some dysfunctional behavior may stem from a maladaptive response to illness. Working with family members, the nurse helps them understand the manifestations of the disorder and analyze the circumstances of daily living to identify situations which may tend to generate maladaptive behavior. Family members also need help in seeing how they are interfering with or failing to maximize the client's independence and participating in the development of maladaptive behavior. Family members may also need assistance in looking at these data, developing awareness of their own and the client's needs, and planning ways to modify responses and relationships to extinguish maladaptive behavior and develop more effective functioning in all members. By engaging family members in this problem-solving activity, the nurse can help them resolve present difficulties and strengthen their ability to deal with problems in the future.

In some instances, the family is unable to care for the client at home, and members must confront the decision to place the client in a residential care setting. If the nurse has been working with the family for some time and deterioration was inevitable, then long-range planning regarding placement will have been initiated and feelings will have been dealt with during the early phases of care.

Periodic assessment of the client's ability to cope with activities of daily life provides the nurse and family with objective data that can be used as a guide to measure the rate of deterioration, identify the need for increasing supportive services, and provide information to assist in deciding when institutionalization may be appropriate. It is most helpful to the family if they can use this guide when symptoms first appear to formulate criteria for eventual institutionalization. If these criteria are established before home care becomes burdensome, the family may be able to approach the decision more rationally; the feelings generated by the placement will be in response to the separation and loss. The nurse intervenes to help the family become aware of and work through the grieving process. Placement that is sudden and poorly thought out or poorly worked out is likely to occur when the family feels desperate. In these instances the family tends more often to feel guilty and anxious and to perceive the placement as abandonment. The anxiety generated around the placement will be more likely to be expressed through intrafamily conflict or by making a scapegoat of the person who made the decision.

If the community health nurse enters the picture when family members are recognizing the fact that they can no longer manage the client in the home, then nursing interventions focus on helping them with their decision-making process, the selection of a care setting, and the feelings generated by the placement. The placement and the preceding period of decision making are always a time of crisis for the family. Guilt feelings usually predominate. In some families blaming of one member or a care giver may occur. When this happens, there is usually denial of the client's status and an unwillingness to assume responsibility for the decision. The community health nurse intervenes by helping members ventilate feelings and develop an understanding of each other's burdens and position. Helping family members recognize the client's deterioration and their increasing inability to cope can sometimes be accomplished by either identifying or helping them identify significant incidents which illustrate the problem and the need for placement. The community health nurse who works with the client and family over an extended period of time is in a position to facilitate this work.

People with ADD, brain injuries, and seizures who exhibit rage reactions can be frightening to family members. The unpredictability and violence characteristic of such outbursts can disorganize the functioning of the family as a whole and individual members. If the client's behavior cannot be adequately modified through the use of pharmacotherapy, the family may need to address the placement of the client in a long-term residential institution to protect the life and well-being of its members. But even if the client has a history of multiple outbursts that have resulted in the destruction of property and injury to members, the family may be reluctant to decide on placement. Nurses can play a significant role in helping family members ventilate their feelings, examine the impact of the behavior on various members, and explore options for resolving the problem.

When symptoms appear in the client and other family members, the family may be disorganized or chaotic. A long-term helping relationship with the nurse may be used to help family members anticipate problems and evolve solutions that prevent the occurrence of crises. The family may need ongoing support. Such support would more than likely include interventions that both stabilize the family's emotional system and provide access to resources such as financial aid, counseling services, or job training.

Intervention with the Community

The drastic alterations in personality and intellectual functioning, the wandering, the impaired social inhibition, and in some instances the unpredictable aggressiveness and combativeness associated with OMD often generate shame in the family and fear among outsiders. Friends and strangers may be embarrassed for the client or family or be terrified by the client's unpredictable violence or bizarre ramblings.

When family and society do not understand dementia and are frightened or embarrassed, the client is often hidden away in the home or an institution and the dementia becomes a shameful secret. When a community operates on an "out of sight–out of mind" principle, then it fails to provide support to either the family or the client. Those affected by the disease remain isolated and burdened. Community awareness is needed before an appreciation of the problems can develop and resources can be allocated to help those who must cope with the disorders.

Community interventions which may help to alleviate the family's and the client's isolation, and also help the community to understand OMD, are ones that are directed toward educating people about the causes of OMD and how organic brain dysfunction alters behavior. Nurses assume a leadership role when they initiate public education forums in the community, speak to community groups about the needs and problems of people with OMD, participate as guests on radio talk shows that accept call-in questions while on the air, and collaborate with other health care professionals in educating the public.

Since a great many people with OMD are cared for at home, the families of these people need a supportive community to ease their caretaking burden. Community health nurses may initiate and organize regularly scheduled self-help groups for family members. These groups need to be designed to help members through the process of sharing feelings that may be perceived as unacceptable and feelings that cannot be disclosed either within the extended family or to friends. These feelings are received empathically and are accepted by the members of such a group because they are shared and their source is understood. Group members can also help one another cope with pragmatic issues by searching for solutions or sharing solutions they have used successfully. The nurse is a facilitating member and resource in these groups and a recruiter of new members.

The daily burden of caring for people with OMD in the home may become overwhelming or impossible because of the caretaker's need to work. Families need either periodic relief or daily relief, and the community needs to provide supportive resources. People with OMD usually require continuous supervision, as well as appropriate stimulation and assistance in maximizing their capacities. If finances are not a constraint, then families may employ companions. If families have limited or no financial resources, they may have a problem caring for a demented member. Day care centers for people with OMD are practical and economic solutions. Nurses can assume a leadership role in introducing this model of care to a community, serve as liaison in helping families locate such services, or provide professional nursing care in the day care setting.

Nurses have a responsibility in helping communities establish day care services for this population. These settings provide a safe, predictable, and appropriately stimulating milieu that conserves and maximizes the person's capacities. In some instances they are able to help people regain abilities that were lost through overdependency on their part and overprotectiveness on the part of the family. In addition, the client has opportunities to socialize with peers and staff members and to be helped to maintain social skills.

Evaluation

Determination of the effectiveness of interventions is an important step in the nursing process. Validation of the effectiveness of the interventions includes not only objective data but subjective information as well, if this is at all possible. The following case study and the nursing care plan presented in Table 44-11 (page 966) are provided to illustrate the evaluation component of the nursing process:

> Carla F., 18 years old, received severe head injuries in a car accident which left her with residual brain damage. Her impulsivity became intolerable for her family, and a psychiatric admission resulted. Her first week on the unit was stormy. Temper tantrums—including the throwing of food and objects, the slamming of doors, and the destruction of furniture—characterized her impulsivity.

SUMMARY

Many factors influence the development of organic mental disorders. Hazardous environmental pollutants, trauma, genetic factors, brain lesions, and progressively degenerative diseases have been implicated in the development of these disorders.

Dementia, particularly the dementia associated with Alzheimer's disease, is an increasing problem given the expanding population of elderly in our society. Nurses must also be alert to the need to distinguish between dementia and pseudodementia, since the latter can be remedied. Attention deficit disorders are often unrecognized, and other psychiatric diagnostic categories are assigned. Accurate diagnosis can lead to appropriate treatment and amelioration of symptoms. Nurses' observation and documentation of symptomatic behavior contribute to the formulation of accurate diagnoses. People with seizure disorders must cope with their symptoms, alterations in consciousness, the side effects of their medications, and a social stigma that influences various dimensions of their lives.

The manifestations of organic mental disorders include disturbances in thought, affect, perception, self-determination, and self-care. Many clients with OMD suffer from dementia. The problems presented by these clients include the following: dysmenesia, impaired intellectual functioning, disorientation, affective dysfunction, motor impairment, sensory and perceptual impairments, language impairment, personality changes, and emotional responses to deficits. Clients also exhibit problems related to delirium, ADD, and paroxysmal disorders.

Interaction among the client, family, and environment influences the client's, family's, and care giver's management of the presenting problems. Nurses also need to recognize their own responses to the behavior of clients and their families in order to continue to act therapeutically.

The application of the nursing process is a systematic way of case finding; determining deficits; establishing realistic goals; and identifying interventions that maximize the client's potential, preserve dignity, and help the family cope effectively with the person in the home and engage in rational decision making related to appropriate institutionalization.

Table 44-11 Evaluation (Carla F.)

Assessment	Diagnosis	Outcome Criteria	Intervention	Evaluation
History of head trauma. Organically based recent memory impairment. Misuses spoken words. Aggressive, assaultive, and destructive behavior when unable to find words to communicate needs or to perform self-care activities.	Temper tantrums related to emotional response to neurological deficits and environmental provocation.	Client will refrain from assaultive behavior. Client will refrain from destructive behavior. Client will be able to say, "I can't remember," when unable to recall how to perform a task. Client will attempt to express and label feelings in an appropriate fashion.	Immediate restriction to room for 1 hour following an assaultive or destructive outburst. Use restraints if client physically resists quiet time in room. Provide explanation that assaultive and destructive behavior will not be tolerated. Listen patiently and attentively when client speaks. Help client find and use appropriate words in an unhurried fashion. Encourage client to ask for and accept help in relearning activities. Explore ways for client to communicate and label feelings (written notes, art).	Needs to be put into restraints on 2 consecutive days. Accepts quiet time on third day with only loud verbal complaints. Accepts quiet time on fifth day with no complaints. No outbursts on seventh day. Makes attempts to relearn appropriate use of words. Is able to ask nurse to help her relearn how to tie shoelaces. Uses acrylic paintings to communicate emotions: (red pictures = anger; blue pictures = sadness; yellow pictures = happiness; purple pictures = anxiety).
Object of ridicule by adolescent clients on unit.		Client will be able to walk away from adolescents.	Educate adolescents on unit about relationship between head injury and client's behavior.	2 of 7 adolescents continue to be provocative.
Becomes assaultive toward provocative adolescents.		Unit adolescents will refrain from being provocative.		Becomes verbally abusive, frustrated, and depressed when taunted by two adolescents. Joins other adolescents in volleyball.

REFERENCES

1. American Psychiatric Association, *Diagnostic and Statistical Manual of Mental Disorders,* 3d ed., APA, Washington, D.C., 1980.
2. D. R. Wood, "Diagnosis and Treatment of Minimal Brain Dysfunction in Adults," *Archives of General Psychiatry,* vol. 33, December 1976, pp. 1453–1460.
3. L. Y. Huey et al., "Adult Minimal Brain Dysfunction and Schizophrenia: A Case Report," *American Journal of Psychiatry,* vol. 135, no. 12, 1980, pp. 1563–1565.
4. H. A. Hanford, "Brain Hypoxia, Minimal Brain Dysfunction and Schizophrenia," *American Journal of Psychiatry,* vol. 132, 1975, pp. 192–194.
5. J. R. Morrison and K. Minkoff, "Explosive Personality as a Sequel to the Hyperactive-Child Syndrome," *Comprehensive Psychiatry,* vol. 16, 1975, pp. 343–348.
6. J. Morrison, "Adult Psychiatric Disorders in Parents of Hyperactive Children," *American Journal of Psychiatry,* vol. 137, no. 7, 1980, pp. 825–826.
7. F. Ervin, "Organic Brain Syndromes Associated with Epilepsy," in A. Freedman, H. Kaplan, and B. Sadock, eds., *Comprehensive Textbook of Psychiatry,* 3d ed., Williams and Wilkins, Baltimore, 1982, vol. 1, pp. 1138–1157.
8. R. N. Butler, "Charting the Conquest of Senility," *Bulletin of the New York Academy of Medicine,* vol. 58, no. 4, 1982, pp. 362–381.

9. B. Gurland and J. Toner, "Differentiating Dementia from Nondementing Conditions," in R. Mayeux and W. G. Rosen, eds., *The Dementias: Advances in Neurology,* vol. 38, Raven, New York, 1983, pp. 1–17.
10. R. W. Hamill and S. J. Buell, "Dementia: Clinical and Basic Science Aspects," *Journal of the American Geriatric Society,* vol. 30, no. 12, 1983, pp. 781–787.
11. M. Albert, "Assessment of Cognitive Function in the Elderly," *Psychosomatics,* vol. 25, no. 4, 1984, pp. 310–317.
12. Benson, "Neuropathology of Memory Disorders," *Psychosomatics,* vol. 25, no. 12, 1984, pp. 12–15.
13. G. L. Klerman and J. M. Davidson, "Memory Loss and Affective Disorders," *Psychosomatics,* vol. 25, no. 12, 1984, pp. 29–32.
14. V. A. Kral, "The Relationship between Senile Dementia (Alzheimer Type) and Depression," *Canadian Journal of Psychiatry,* vol. 28, no. 4, 1983, pp. 304–306.
15. A. F. Schatzberg, B. Liptzin, et al., "Diagnosis of Affective Disorders in the Elderly," *Psychosomatics,* vol. 25, no. 2, 1984, pp. 126–131.
16. M. K. Hasan, N. L. Slack, and R. P. Mooney, "Diagnosis and Treatment of Alzheimer's Disease," *West Virginia Medical Journal,* vol. 79, no. 5, 1983, pp. 98–102.
17. J. L. Cummings, "Treatable Dementias," in R. Mayeux and W. G. Rosen, eds., *The Dementias: Advances in Neurology,* vol. 38, Raven, New York, 1983, pp. 165–175.
18. W. G. Rosen, "Clinical and Neuropsychological Assessment of Alzheimer Disease," in R. Mayeux and W. G. Rosen, eds., *The Dementias: Advances in Neurology,* vol. 38, Raven, New York, 1983, pp. 51–64.
19. J. Nelson and L. Gutman, "Dementia: An Overview," *West Virginia Medical Journal,* vol. 78, no. 9, 1982, pp. 219–225.
20. "Senile Dementia Linked to Immunity Genes," *Science News,* vol. 124, 1983, p. 5.
21. D. S. Dahl, "Diagnosis of Alzheimer's Disease," *Postgraduate Medicine,* vol. 73, no. 4, 1983, pp. 217–221.
22. M. Storandt, "Understanding Senile Dementia: A Challenge for the Future," *International Journal of Aging and Human Development,* vol. 16, no. 1, 1983, pp. 1–6.
23. G. Schmidt, "Mechanisms and Possible Causes of Alzheimer's Disease," *Postgraduate Medicine,* vol. 73, no. 4, 1983, pp. 206–213.
24. A. H. Ropper and W. S. Williams, "Relationship between Plaques, Tangles and Dementia in Down's Syndrome," *Neurology,* vol. 30, 1980, pp. 639.
25. L. L. Heston, "Alzheimer's Dementia and Down's Syndrome: Genetic Evidence Suggesting an Association," *Annals of New York Academy of Science,* vol. 396, 1982, pp. 29–37.
26. J. W. Rowe, "Physiologic Changes of Aging and Their Clinical Impact," *Psychosomatics,* vol. 25, no. 12, 1984, pp. 4–10.
27. M. Albert, "Assessment of Memory Loss," *Pychosomatics,* vol. 25, no. 12, 1984, pp. 18–20.
28. M. L. Freedman, "Organic Brain Syndromes in the Elderly," *Postgraduate Medicine,* vol. 74, no. 4, 1983, pp. 165–176.
29. A. A. Fisk, "Management of Alzheimer's Disease," *Postgraduate Medicine,* vol. 73, no. 4, 1983, pp. 237–241.
30. B. Cooper and H. Bickel, "Population Screening and the Early Detection of Dementing Disorders in Old Age: A Review," *Psychological Medicine,* vol. 14, 1984, pp. 81–95.
31. M. A. Fauman, "The Emergency Psychiatric Evaluation of Organic Mental Disorders," *Psychiatric Clinics of North America,* vol. 6, no. 2, 1983, pp. 233–257.
32. T. Detre and H. Jarecki, *Modern Psychiatric Treatment,* Lippincott, Philadelphia, 1971.
33. L. Gwyther, "Alzheimer's Disease," *North Carolina Medical Journal,* vol. 44, no. 7, 1983, pp. 435–436.
34. G. E. Berrios, "Disorientation States and Psychiatry," *Comprehensive Psychiatry,* vol. 23, no. 5, 1982, pp. 479–491.
35. K. Hamsher, "Mental Status Examination in Alzheimer's Disease," *Postgraduate Medicine,* vol. 73, no. 4, 1983, pp. 225–228.
36. H. Omer, J. Foldes, et al., "Screening for Cognitive Deficits in a Sample of Hospitalized Geriatric Patients," *Journal of the American Geriatric Society,* vol. 31, no. 5, 1983, pp. 266–268.
37. L. Hemsi, "Living with Dementia," *Postgraduate Medical Journal,* vol. 58, 1982, pp. 610–617.
38. G. Bucht and R. Adolfsson, "The Comprehensive Psychopathological Rating Scale in Patients with Dementia of Alzheimer Type and Multi-infarct Dementia," *Acta Psychiatrica,* vol. 68, 1983, pp. 263–270.
39. N. Leng, "Behavioral Treatment of the Elderly," *Age and Aging,* vol. 11, 1982, pp. 235–243.
40. L. Gimbel, "The Pathology of Boredom and Sensory Deprivation," *Psychiatric Nursing,* vol. 16, no. 5, September–October, 1975, pp. 12–13.
41. J. C. S. Breitner and M. F. Folstein, "Familial Alzheimer Dementia: A Prevalent Disorder with Specific Clinical Features," *Postgraduate Medicine,* vol. 14, 1984, pp. 63–80.
42. W. G. Rosen, "Neuropsychological Investigation of Memory, Visuoconstructional, Visuoperceptual, and Language Abilities in Senile Dementia of the Alzheimer Type," in R. Mayeux and W. G. Rosen, eds., *The Dementias: Advances in Neurology,* vol. 38, Raven, New York, 1983, pp. 65–73.
43. E. W. Massey and C. E. Coffey, "Frontal Lobe Personality Syndromes," *Postgraduate Medicine,* vol. 73, no. 5, 1983, pp. 99–106.

44. D. Blume and D. F. Benson, "Personality Change with Frontal and Temporal Lobe Lesions," in D. Blume and D. F. Benson, eds., *Psychiatric Aspects of Neurologic Disease,* Grune and Stratton, New York, 1975, pp. 151–170.
45. D. Bear, K. Levin, D. Blume, et al., "Interictal Behavior in Hospitalized Temporal Lobe Epileptics: Relationship to Idiopathic Psychiatric Syndromes," *Journal of Neurology, Neurosurgery and Psychiatry,* vol. 45, 1982, pp. 481–488.
46. "The Crime of Epilepsy," *Science News,* August, 1978, p. 101.
47. L. Hechtman, G. Weiss, and T. Perlman, "Hyperactives as Young Adults: Past and Current Substance Abuse and Antisocial Behavior," *American Journal of Orthopsychiatry,* vol. 54, no. 3, 1984, pp. 415–425.
48. L. Kapust, "Living with Dementia: The Ongoing Funeral," *Social Work in Health Care,* vol. 7, no. 4, 1982, pp. 79–91.
49. F. Sheldon, "Supporting the Supporters: Working with the Relatives of Patients with Dementia," *Age and Aging,* vol. 11, no. 3, 1983, pp. 184–188.
50. E. M. Brody and G. M. Spark, "Institutionalization of the Aged: A Family Crisis," *Family Process,* vol. 19, no. 1, 1980, pp. 76–90.
51. P. H. Meyer, "The Choice in Aging," *The Family,* vol. 5, no. 2, 1980, pp. 48–50.
52. N. B. Levine, D. P. Dastoor, and C. E. Gendron, "Coping with Dementia: A Pilot Study," *Journal of the American Geriatric Association,* vol. 31, no. 1, 1983, pp. 12–18.
53. L. R. Jones, R. R. Parlour, and L. W. Badger, "The Inappropriate Commitment of the Aged," *Bulletin of the American Academy of Psychiatry and the Law,* vol. 10, no. 1 1982, pp. 29–38.
54. J. Meyers and C. S. Drayer, "Support Systems and Mental Illness in the Elderly," *Community Mental Health Journal,* vol. 15, no. 4, 1979, pp. 277–286.
55. D. Sands and T. Suzuki, "Adult Day Care for Alzheimer's Patients and their Families," *Gerontologist,* vol. 23, no. 1, 1983, pp. 21–23.
56. V. Wood and J. F. Robertson, "Friendship and Kinship Interaction: Differential Effect on the Morale of the Eldery," *Journal of Marriage and the Family,* vol. 40, no. 2, May 1978, pp. 367–375.
57. C. I. Cohen and J. Sokolovsky, "Clinical Use of Network Analysis for Psychiatric and Aged Populations," *Community Mental Health Journal,* vol. 15, no. 3, 1979, pp. 203–213.
58. L. J. Novick, "Senile Patients Need Diverse Programming," *Dimensions in Health Service,* vol. 59, no. 9, 1982, pp. 25–26.
59. R. G. Bennett, "Care of the Demented: Long-Term Care, Institution, Home and Family Care, and Hospice," in R. Mayeux and W. G. Rosen, eds., *The Dementias: Advances in Neurology,* vol. 38, Raven, New York, 1983, pp. 253–263.
60. G. Peterson, "Organic Brain Syndrome Associated with Drug or Poison Intoxication," in A. Freedman, H. Kaplan, and B. Sadock, eds., *Comprehensive Textbook of Psychiatry,* 3d ed., Williams and Wilkins, Baltimore, 1982, pp. 1108–1121.
61. T. Ban, "Psychopathology, Psychopharmacology and the Organic Brain Syndromes," *Psychosomatics,* vol. 17, no. 3, 1980, pp. 131–135.
62. H. E. Lehmann, "Psychopharmacological Approaches to the Organic Brain Syndrome," *Comprehensive Psychiatry,* vol. 24, no. 5, 1983, pp. 412–430.
63. L. J. Thal, A. Fuld, M. Masur, and N. S. Sharpless, "Oral Physostigmine and Lecithin Improve Memory in Alzheimer Disease," *Annals of Neurology,* vol. 13, no. 5, 1983, pp. 491–496.
64. C. Steele, M. J. Lucas, and L. E. Tune, "An Approach to the Management of Dementia Syndromes," *John Hopkins Medical Journal,* vol. 151, no. 6, 1982, pp. 362–368.

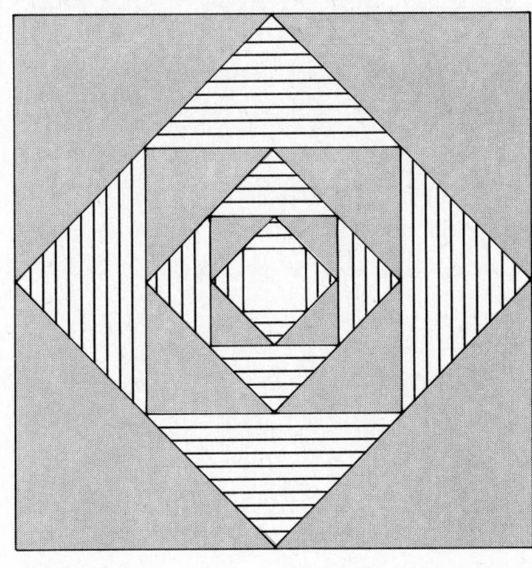

CHAPTER 45
The Dying Process

Elise L. Lev

Thomas Francis Nolan

LEARNING OBJECTIVES

After studying this chapter, the student should be able to:

1. Discuss the system of death in this society.
2. Discuss the interactions of person, family, and care giver and the setting in which a person dies.
3. Discuss nursing care in relation to the dying process.
4. Discuss the dying process in relation to the physical, mental, and spiritual dimensions of the person.
5. Discuss family patterns of interaction during the dying process and after the death of a loved one.
6. Discuss patterns of interaction related to grieving over the losses implicit in dying.
7. Identify dysynchronous patterns of interaction in the person associated with the dying process.
8. Discuss contexts of awareness of dying in relation to interactions of person, family, and care giver.
9. Apply the nursing process to the care of people who are dying and their families.

The process of living and dying is integrated into a universal rhythm.[1] One cannot speak about dying without also speaking about living. Indeed, a human being begins the process of dying from the very first moment of existence. Dying is as much a part of the life process as living. Dying and death are events that happen to all. People can postpone death or gain reprieves, but ultimately all must die. Many people react to this with the feeling that there is something morbid in paying attention to death. They comment that they are more interested in life than in death. La Rochefoucauld epitomized this viewpoint in his remark, "One can no more look steadily at death than at the sun."

When death is imminent, the physical, mental, and spiritual dimensions of the person are confronted. Change in the physical dimension alters self-concept. Thoughts about the meaning and purpose of life and death are intertwined with the person's spiritual dimension. Beliefs about life after death or continued existence as a part of the universe are reviewed and sometimes challenged. For some there is a return to the spiritual beliefs held during youth, while for others there is a repudiation of and anger toward these beliefs and a sense of injustice about facing death. Grieving over the losses implicit with death and facing the unknown aspect of death inevitably generate feelings that are painful.

In the course of life, all people relate in their own way to the knowledge that death is certain. Throughout human history, the idea of death has posed the eternal mystery which is at the core of religious and philosophical systems of thought. And it is quite possible that this idea is the basis of human anxiety. Insecurity may well be a symbol of death. Any loss may represent total loss of the self. One of the distinguishing characteristics of human beings is the capacity to grasp the concept of a future, including the inevitability of death. And it is in this anticipation of death that people discover the hunger for immortality.

In the twentieth century, thinking about the problem of death entails profound contradictions. Tradition assumes that a person is both terminated by death and capable of continuing is some other sense beyond death. Death is viewed by some as a wall, the ultimate personal disaster, and suicide as the act of a sick mind; by others death is seen as a doorway, a point in time on the way to eternity.[2]

The purpose of this chapter is to explore the dying process and what it means to the one who is dying, the family, and the nurse. It is written to help nurses understand the thoughts, feelings, perceptions, and interactions that occur, and how all involved can experience personal growth through their interaction with the dying process.

PATTERNS OF INTERACTION: ENVIRONMENT

Death is a personal event, but it is a social one as well. Reactions of the person and the family to death and dying are greatly influenced by the social context. Therefore, the environmental interactions of the dying process will be examined first in this chapter.

The contexts of death and dying in this society include the sociocultural milieu, contexts of awareness, and the settings in which people die. Each of these contexts is discussed below.

Sociocultural Milieu of Death

The prospect or fact of death has been interpreted in many ways in this culture. Most of these interpretations are derived either from one's family heritage (from previous generations) or from earlier cultures that have influenced contemporary culture. Some of these interpretations are more easily accepted than others, and the current cultural milieu may be generating significant new variations on ancient themes and also developing new approaches to death and dying.

This society tends to foster the idea that it is futile to contemplate death; at the same time, it communicates that the only proper way to conduct one's life is through the daily contemplation of that inevitable moment toward which one is moving. It is believed by some that fear of death is instinctive, deeply rooted in human nature, and some contend that no one can truly understand or even accept mortality.

Healthy people who contemplate death do so with nervous laughter, composure, denial, resignation, intensity, indifference, doubt, or certainty. Critically ill people and others who face imminent death maintain silence, sometimes an agitated silence and sometimes a stoical, tranquil, or enigmatic one. Or they face death with desperate maneuvers, eager anticipation, dread, apathy, or mixed feelings.

Death as a Background of Life

Four conditions from the past contributed significantly to the general background against which interpretations of death emerged. The *first* and most obvious condition was the rather short life expectancy that confronted people throughout most of history. Relatively few people survived beyond the years of early maturity. A *second* and related condition was exposure to death, to the sight of dying and dead persons and animals. The average person had relatively little insulation from witnessing death. A *third* condition was the sense of possessing relatively little control over the forces of nature. The world was an untrustworthy abode, sometimes comfortable and dependable, but sometimes crushing and devastating to its inhabitants. For many centuries, people had rather limited resources for altering the unfavorable circumstances in which they frequently found themselves. The *fourth* factor is that the psychosocial concept of individualism was poorly developed in the ancient world. The person was primarily a social component, a unit that fulfilled an expected role within the dictates of custom. The extended family and the clan, tribe, or city provided the needed strength and continuity. Most persons in most societies were not expected to make individual decisions about basic issues or ultimate matters, nor was the emotional satisfaction or fate of the individual as an individual considered to be of primary significance. The well-being of the individual was important chiefly as it related to the carrying out of obligations for the group.

Thus, in earlier cultures, the individual's hold on life was quite precarious, with death occurring within what is now regarded as the first half of the life span. Dying and death were visible, and one generally did not expect to exercise control over the environment.

The "Death System"

Words and actions concerning death may be considered as jointly constituting a system. All societies have developed one or more death systems through which they have tried to come to terms with death in both its personal and its social aspects.[2]

For example, the Egyptians of antiquity developed a death system that was quite explicit and detailed. Their *Book of the Dead* provided an outline of a comprehensive death system cast largely in the form of prescriptions for funerary practice.[3,4] This system was intended to transmit a relatively integrated approach that would enable people to think, feel, and behave with respect to death in ways that they might consider to be effective and appropriate. It offered an explicit world view which was sponsored by the governing authorities, shared by the community, and linked to individual behavior in specific terms.

Within the death system, the individual's belief was the community's belief. The individual was not alone. People had important actions to perform with regard to death, ranging from the dying process through the care of the dead. The most important function of this system seemed to be that of giving people something to do in situations which otherwise might have exposed them to feelings of utter helplessness. Belief in magical control over the powerful forces of death and the afterlife further encouraged the Egyptians to think of death as an event that was well within their province of action.[3]

The American System Of Death

Every culture has myths, rituals, and taboos related to death and dying that help people cope with the fragility of life. Before the nineteenth century, dying was an integrated part of the life cycle, shared by the immediate and extended family. Since World War II, advances in technology have escalated health care costs and encouraged the depersonalization of the care of people who are dying. The idea that every technological advance is synonymous with progress was the impetus for newer, more expensive technologies. This trend was reinforced by commercial exploitation and by public and professional interests. The results were fragmentation and dehumanization of care; a person was reduced to the composite of various systems, independently analyzed and treated. Aggressive, impersonal approaches to the cure of diseases were encouraged by health care institutions as the control of a person's fate shifted from the individual and the family to the institution and its staff. Institutions rarely addressed a dying person's social pain (the consequence of social isolation), emotional pain (the consequence of the perception of inability to control fate), or spiritual pain (the consequence of an inability to conceptualize the meaning of life within the person's belief system). A care giver who helped a person to verbalize pain was frequently accused of creating pain.

American society today differs from most earlier cultures in that we no longer have to contend with a short life expectancy, constant exposure to death, a feeling of helplessness against the powers of nature, and a lack of individualism. What is the "death system" like in this society?

The American medical system emphasizes the impersonal, mechanical aspects of disease and is interested primarily in disease itself rather than the reaction of people to disease. In contrast, the British health care system has a different emphasis. The *British Medical Dictionary* defines *disease* in terms of the person, as experiencing "a departure from the normal state of health."[5]

The current American society denies the need for acceptance of pain, sickness, and death. The goals of modern society are to kill pain, eliminate sickness, and control death; these goals are different from those of previous cultures. By transforming pain, illness, and death from personal challenges into technological problems, modern society has changed the expectation that people will deal with their human condition as a part of life to the expectation that modern technology will conquer death. Life expectancy in the United States today is more than twice as long as it was for most of our ancestors on this planet. Today, people are less likely to regard death as a knife at their throats, or a scourge at their children's bedside. Death stands at a more reassuring or *proper* distance from the young and the middle-aged. It is old people who die! This line of reasoning is, of course, highly biased in the direction of youth. This is a youth-oriented society. The power and glory belong to the young. Increasingly, then, death is becoming detached from the valued core of society: the young. In a sense, natural death is becoming obsolete. Death is an event that happens only to those people who have already become obsolete. In today's society death is rarely viewed as an appropriate part of the life cycle. Even the deaths of elderly people are commonly viewed as sad, and the deaths of young people are viewed as tragic.

Illness and death, like illness and recovery, is a sequence that is becoming removed from household management. Americans "pull through" or die on the crisp white sheets of an institutional bed. There is now a choice regarding how children will be informed of death. Not so many years ago there was no choice: children saw what was happening because death occurred in the home and was part of the family experience.

As a society, we are insulated from the perception of death. The insulation is not perfect, yet it protects people from the sights of dying and death to an extent that could not have been imagined in most previous cultures. The sequence of dying and death in this culture is increasingly handled by teams of specialists. Providers of health care and funeral directors perform their functions in special settings, inviting families to participate only at certain approved stages of the process. Participation is peripheral, and people can, in fact, completely avoid experiencing the dying and deaths of others if they so wish.

The very nature of modern health procedures hides from both care givers and clients the contradiction between death as a natural process and the reality of clinical death.[6] Within hospital walls there are implicit rules and choices. Hospitalized clients are not supposed to die in just any place at any time. It is deemed important that they not expose other clients, staff members, or visitors to the phenomenon of death except under carefully specified circumstances. The obliging terminal client will first provide clear evidence, either through clinical symptoms or laboratory findings, that his or her condition is worsening. This enables the hospital administrative personnel to add the person's name to the "danger list." Clear signs of further deterioration or jeopardy require either that special treatments begin in a private room on the present unit or, preferably, that the client be transferred to an intensive-treatment unit or one specializing in the care of dying people. Death is expected. The approved sequence is approaching its finale. The chaplain and other nonhospital personnel can enact their roles in the customary manner. This reflects a technological ritual of death. Standardization of procedures related to those who are dying in institutions meets the system's needs—not the clients' needs—for effective utilization of time, energy, and resources.[6]

Those involved feel a sense of discomfort and sometimes even express rage when a client dies in the wrong place at the wrong time. People have become accustomed to cultural insulation from the impact of death, and they accept it. Even the "death specialists," who are delegated the responsibilities that formerly belonged to the family, demand a certain insulation.

This general situation is also related to an attitude toward the physical environment. The growth in scientific knowledge and its visible technological applications has greatly increased the ability to reshape the world. This has led to expectations of being able to control and master events. There is an implicit assumption that with the help of science and money, problems ought to be solved when there is a sufficient investment of time and resources, but the reality is that society cannot sweep death back from daily life. Present difficulties in the care of clients during the sequence of dying and death stem mainly from the expectation that technological answers can be found for all problems, and from the idea that people can remove or remake whatever stands in the path of their desires, including death.

Finally, our society is no longer dominated by tradition, lineage, or accepted dogma. The older systems of social control and stability have lost much of their ability to shape behavior and support people in times of crisis. These systems have never been adequately replaced. This situation generates anxiety. The individual is the primary unit now, and people are free to pursue their own self-actualization. But they also face more doubt and anxiety than did their ancestors, who grew up in a milieu which had firmly entrenched ideas and practices regarding life-and-death matters. Increasingly, individuals are held responsible for their own ideas and actions. Decisions that once were almost automatic must now be made without guidance from tradition.

These decisions are particularly evident in the realm of death. The orientation of healthy people toward their own deaths, the orientation of the dying person, and people's attitudes toward funerary practices are no longer predictable or constant; therefore, they call for decisions by the individual. Death, in this sense, has lost a stable context. There is not the reliable, heavily reinforced social fabric that enabled the ancient Egyptians to know that the right thing was being done in the right way. The need to make individual decisions arises more often for those who encounter death repeatedly in their professional lives. It also weighs upon people in various walks of life who occasionally find themselves in life-and-death situations. Decisions and responsibilities, then, are salient characteristics of a relationship with death in the present cultural milieu, but people do not always accept the responsibility for making and abiding by their decisions.

Awareness of Dying

Glaser and Strauss[7] studied the situations of people who are dying in relation to their recurrent interactions with the people in their environment during hospitalization. On the basis of their observations, they developed a schema for describing the contexts of awareness of dying people as *closed, suspected, mutual pretense,* and *open.* Contexts of awareness include the following dimensions:

1. What each significant person (care givers, family members, client) believes ("knows") about the client's diagnosis and prognosis
2. What each significant person believes every other significant person "knows" about the client's diagnosis and prognosis
3. What each significant person believes about others' awareness of his or her perceptions of the client's diagnosis and prognosis
4. The influence of these perceptions on interactions among these significant people

The schema is presented in Table 45-1 (page 974). The interactions that occur in each context have a significant impact on the participants, and influence whether the client is able to use denial effectively and maintain self-determination.[7]

Settings for the Sequence of Dying and Death

Emergency Room and Trauma Center

Threats to life are occurring continually in an emergency room or trauma center. As the word *emergency* implies, this setting is a context of unforeseen circumstances that call for immediate action. In this setting the unexpected catastrophe becomes the expected. The orientation of care tends to focus on physiological crises and rescue of the

Table 45-1 Contexts of Awareness of Dying People

Awareness	Characteristics
Closed	Absence of disclosure about the impending death to the client and sometimes also to the family.
Suspected	The version about health status that is given is not fully accepted by the client, or by the family in some instances. Assessment of the situation, interventions, and evidence of deterioration provide the client and family with data that lead to suspicions about the explanations that have been provided.
Mutual pretense	Staff, client, and family know about the impending death, but no one openly discusses the situation. Questions that would uncover the situation are avoided.
Open	Staff, client, and family have full and accurate information about the client's diagnosis and prognosis, and discuss the situation with one another in an open manner.

client. Death is not uncommon. However, the continual demands and needs of the living overshadow the accelerated dying process that occurs in this setting. Because of the critical nature of the care being delivered, family members are often relegated to the waiting room. They may also be excluded from the moment of death and acquire information about their loved one after the fact. This situation deprives both the family and in some instances the dying person of the support needed to face death.

General Hospital Unit

Death is a frequent visitor in a general hospital unit, but care giving in this setting is less dramatic because dying is a slow process here. Often clients are in and out of hospitals several times before the final admission, that is, before the hospital becomes a permanent abode because care at home is no longer possible. On some of these units, there are increasing numbers of clients who are socially dead because they have suffered partial or complete loss of brain activity yet who are biologically alive and sometimes kept among the "living dead" with the assistance of life-prolonging machinery.

Hospital policies and the tendency to adhere to schedules and routines often interfere with the client-family relationship. Because the hospital has become oriented primarily to acute physical and physiological problems, there is often a lack of sensitivity to the needs of people who require only comfort measures and basic care giving such as feeding, bathing, and positioning. Management of pain in these settings tends to be organized to provide relief from acute, temporary pain. But the chronic pain associated with many terminal diseases needs a different approach and a different guiding philosophy. Addiction to pain-relief drugs is not an issue; therefore, rigid adherence to prescribed time schedules and dosages is inappropriate and interferes with adequate management of pain for dying people.

Special-Care Unit

A hospital is organized primarily to promote the saving of lives, and this activity assumes critical importance on the special-care unit, where rapid action can make the difference between life and death. Here top priority is given to recovery-oriented, medically delegated nursing tasks, and "comfort care" is essentially relegated to a secondary position.

In this setting families of people who are dying encounter many barriers to being with and comforting the family member whose death may be imminent. Visiting is usually severely limited. When the family is allowed at the bedside, the various machines, monitors, and tubes have an intimidating effect and interfere with interactions.

Home Care

Care of people who are dying by families at home traditionally has been supported by community health nursing agencies. In the past this support focused primarily on helping the family meet the physical needs of the dying person. The mental and spiritual needs of the client and family were considered the responsibility of others, were ignored, or were addressed only if they interfered with the delivery of physical care to the client. A family was left to seek out other support systems or to manage without them.

Caring for a dying person at home is a challenge to the family and to health professionals. Success or failure depends in part on the availability of the family's personal support system and the extent of accessible community resources.

This context allows the client to remain in familiar surroundings. Institutional barriers to interactions with loved ones are nonexistent. Family participation in the care often helps members work through the feelings associated with grieving. Accessibility to medical personnel and coordination of care may be problematic and require greater effort on the part of the family's and the community-based nurse. Consequently, management of pain and relief of symptoms may not run a smooth course, but the security of being with the family and at home may in some instances more than outweigh these disadvantages.

The SHANTI project, a community-based volunteer counseling program for clients and families facing life-threatening illness, was organized as an alternative model for meeting the psychosocial needs of these people. It is designed to alleviate the social distancing and emotional alienation that plague the dying process. Volunteers provide peer counseling, companionship, emotional support, and information about resources to the client, family, and care givers. Their help also extends beyond the dying process and includes supportive services for the survivors.[8] This type of resource is particularly useful when home care is the setting chosen by the dying person and the family.

Providing physical care, meeting clients' psychosocial needs, and educating those involved are objectives included in home care. Time, knowledge, and skill are needed by nurses who explore the thoughts, feelings, and perceptions of the dying person and family members, and intervene supportively. The education of client and family may need to address the dying process and how to provide care and comfort throughout; it may also involve people in the environment who are not related to the family. For example:

> While making home visits to Mr. G, a client dying of lung cancer, the nurse identified the need to educate his neighbors. They had been avoiding the client and decontaminating the washing machine whenever the client or his family members used the common laundry room. The neighbors needed information on the causes of lung cancer and the fact that it is not a contagious disease. Once provided with this information, the neighbors resumed socializing with the client and discontinued the decontamination process.[9]

Nursing or Convalescent Home

Sometimas a family may attempt to care for the dying member at home, then become overwhelmed as the person deteriorates significantly. Sometimes this occurs after a hospitalization, when the person becomes significantly less self-sufficient and requires around-the-clock nursing care. In these instances the decision may be made to place the dying person in a nursing home. This is particularly true for an elderly person whose aged spouse or adult working children are unable to manage the care needed. Death in a nursing home is expected, and in some instances the setting is oriented toward providing a dignified and peaceful death.

Convalescent homes tend to set up barriers between the dying person and the family. There is a tendency to focus primarily on the physical care of the client rather than to take a holistic approach. Services such as bereavement counseling are not available to family members. There is often a tendency to discourage their presence except during prescribed times. Sometimes families welcome instititutional policies that limit visiting, because these rules are a desired protection against confrontation of the dying process. Relief of pain is provided but may not be managed in ways that promote alertness and involvement in living.

Hospice

The hospice concept was developed by Dr. Cicely Saunders and implemented by her with the founding of St. Christopher's Hospice in London. This institution provided the terminally ill with a more humanistic treatment setting and model for care.[10]

The hospice system of care is designed to provide highly specialized care to people who are dying. The goal of hospice care is to maintain the dying person fully alert, comfortable, and pain-free during the final phases of living. Control of pain is a major aspect. It includes relief from physical, psychological, social, and spiritual pain.[10]

The components which follow form the basic philosophical and organizational framework for this concept of care. Each of these components is necessary, and none of them can be omitted without violating the concept.

Care is provided by an interdisciplinary team. Home care is available 24 hours a day, 7 days a week. While the person is being maintained at home, there is collaboration between those providing home care and the professionals in the residential facility. When home management is no longer desirable or appropriate, the person is admitted to the residential facility. The dying person and the family are defined as the unit of care. The organizational structure and delivery of care are designed to eliminate the institutional barriers that interfere with communication among the care givers, families, and dying clients. Support and giving between the family and the dying person are enhanced. Efforts are directed toward protecting the client from dying alone and from feelings of abandonment. The family members are helped to feel that they have done all that was possible for their loved one and to accept the death without feelings of guilt. Bereavement counseling for the family is made available after the death of the client.[6]

Within the hospice framework people are helped to live through the dying process, experiencing it with strength, confidence, and alertness; to find meaning in their lives through the experience of dying; and to die with dignity and respect.[10]

The hospice is a relatively new concept in the United States for the care of people who are dying. Those hospices that have been developed are modeled after St. Christopher's in England. Nurses, particularly Florence Wald, provided leadership in bringing the hospice concept to the United States.[11] The time was right for the introduction of this approach. People were beginning to demand participation in decisions relative to their own care.[12]

In the United States, the word *hospice* is used to denote a place, but more important, to describe a specialized health care program that emphasizes the needs of dying people and their families. The hospice philosophy recognizes disease as a process which calls for active treatment, but views dying as an eventuality in the life cycle.[13] The goal of hospice care is to provide a context of care and interventions that are appropriate and relevant to individual client's needs. Care is available 24 hours a day, 7 days a week. Bereavement counseling for the family is provided during and after the dying process. An interdisciplinary team of care givers, including doctors, nurses, social workers, clergy, and volunteers, assists the client and family with the physical care and provides a support system to help people live while facing death. The settings in which hospice care may be given vary from one community to another. Home health agencies, hospital-based services, palliative-care units, and independent institutions provide care to dying people and their families from a hospice perspective.[13]

The standards of care for hospices are developed by the National Hospice Organization. This agency also acts in an advisory capacity to those who accredit or certify hospice programs.[14]

Nurses in hospice programs function as a vital part of the interdisciplinary team, which develops the plan of care for each client. Nurses in a home health agency may or may not provide for more than physical care and include psychosocial support and bereavement and nutritional counseling in their services. Nurses in a hospice program provide care that encompasses the physical, mental, and spiritual needs of client and family and do so through collaboration with a team of professionals. For example, a hospice client whose care plan focuses on the management of pain may have a social worker to help the family defray the cost of medication; a physical therapist to address relief of pain by heat or cold therapy; a nurse and a pharmacist collaborating to establish medication doses; nurses teaching relaxation exercises; and family members acting as informed, active participants in planning and implementation. Family members are also clients and may use the services of a social worker or participate in bereavement counseling. The hospice nurse continues to visit the client and family if and when there is a need for an admission to a general hospital.

Support for the nurses and other care givers is a dimension of the hospice program and usually involves members of the team meeting on a regular basis with a support person not affiliated with the hospice staff.[14] During these meetings clients, families, and self are discussed.

PATTERNS OF INTERACTION: NURSE

Before 1960, the scientific study of issues associated with death and dying was limited. Twenty years after Feifel's[15] book *The Meaning of Death* was published in 1959, the professional literature on death and dying expanded from a few hundred to thousands of citations.[11] During this period of time, a theme mentioned in numerous studies was the degree to which dying clients were avoided.[16,17] One study of nurses' responses to dying clients revealed that nurse took longer to answer calls from clients with terminal prognoses than from those who were less seriously ill. They also lacked awareness of this "undemocratic" behavior.[18]

Patterns of Avoidance

One of the factors contributing to nurses' avoidance of dying clients is the perception of the *social loss* of clients.[19] Factors such as age, education, personality, social class, and skin color influence whether the nurse perceives the client's death as a great loss to family or society, a premature death before life has been fully experienced, or an appropriate time for life to end. For example, a dying child or a young mother, on the basis of perception of social loss, may receive considerable nursing concern and attention, while an old person, representing low social loss, may receive minimal care.

Professionals share the public's attitudes in the United States, as in all societies. Avoidance of interaction with dying people is characteristic of this society.[17] In the 1960s, nurses were concerned about whether or not the care they gave to dying people was adequate and appropriate. Frequently, nurses expressed guilt over their perceptions of inadequate physical care as well as inadequate emotional support of clients.

Verbal behavior reflects the professional's discomfort with the topics of dying and death. For example, a study by Kastenbaum[20] of nurses' responses to clients who spoke of their deaths ("I think I am going to die soon"; "I wish I could just end it all") revealed five categories of responses that reflected discomfort:

1. *Reassurance.* "You're doing so well now. You don't have to feel this way." "You're going to be feeling better soon; then you won't be thinking this way. You'll be feeling more like your old self again."
2. *Denial.* "You don't really mean that." "You are not going to die. You're going to live to be a hundred."
3. *Change of subject.* "Let's talk about something more cheerful." "You shouldn't say things like that; there are better things to talk about."
4. *Fatalism.* "We are all going to die sometime, and it's a good thing we don't know when." "When God wants you, He will take you. It's a sin to say that you want to die."
5. *Discussion.* "What makes you feel that way today? Is it something that happened, something somebody said?" "Tell me why. I'd like to know."

Nurses who were inclined to "turn off" clients often explained that they did not like to see their clients looking so glum. Mention of death was equated with a state of fear or surrender that was unacceptable to the nursing personnel. The nurses felt that clients should want to live and should expect to live. Therefore, they considered it appropriate to try to get the client's mind off death. Some of the respondents were direct enough to say, "Talking about death upsets me." In general, silencing a client who speaks about death seemed to derive from both humanistic ("I like to see them happy") and self-protective ("It shakes me up to talk about death") viewpoints. When the facts of the situation were too obvious to permit an easy denial, then fatalistic response was deemed appropriate. This response came naturally to those attending staff members who held it as a personal belief.

Fatalism, denial, and change of subject occur most often when nurses are uncomfortable in the dying context. Few nurses are at ease exploring clients' thoughts and feelings about death and dying. It would seem that unless nurses become sensitized to the needs of dying clients and helped to develop communication skills and to clarify their own feelings about death, these clients are unlikely to find a nurse who is able and willing to help them verbalize and deal with the dying process.

Nurses experience many feelings about their dying clients but often try not to let them show, even when the clients' deterioration increases these feelings.[20] Nurses are not always able to insulate themselves from the emotional implications of their work. Nurses care about what their clients are experiencing but often believe that they should not "give in" to their feelings, even to the extent of letting them show. In such instances nurses may be trapped by their role image. If the prevailing professional ethic disapproves of the expression of feelings or the nurses believe this to be true, fear of censure serves to suppress and repress emotional responses to clients.

Sociocultural Patterns

In Kastenbaum's study, typical nurses considered themselves to be devout people with a strong belief in some form of life after death. This included the conviction that they would be personally accountable to God after death. Very few nurses agreed that we are each entitled to do as we like with our lives as long as no one else is hurt or that suicide is nobody else's business. Few reported that they had ever wished someone else to die, and few were in favor of "mercy killing" under any circumstances. Most of the nurses agreed that "the length of people's lives is pretty much decided when they are born, and that no matter what you do, when it's your time to go, you go."[20] This cluster of attitudes and beliefs was discernibly different from that of staff members at the same hospital who had different educational and occupational backgrounds.

It seems fair to suggest that the ethnic, religious, and socioeconomic backgrounds that people bring with them to a situation affect the way they think and behave when they become care givers. The degree of influence that background and the professionalization process have on practice has yet to be studied adequately. However, it is probable that personal background and professionalization come together at certain points to emphasize a particular behavior. For example, the nurse may, because of a particular ethnic heritage, have a fatalistic outlook on death. If this is reinforced by an ethic not to show emotion on the job, then for that person it may be easier to control the outward expression of feelings than it is to live with the feelings that continue to percolate inside.[20]

Patterns of Professionalization

A nurse's "bedside manner" is a learned behavior.[21] Students may reinforce or learn to deny their real feelings about their dying clients, and to replace these feelings with what they believe they "should" feel. These "should" feelings are learned through watching the seemingly unemotional reactions to dying clients of more experienced nurses and nursing faculty members. If students' perceptions are not altered, they contribute to the development of an avoidance pattern in providing care to dying clients.[22] The coping mechanisms that develop, to manage the "should" feelings, restrict personal involvement with dying clients. Nurses become too busy with tasks to spend time talking to clients. Although experienced nurses tend to avoid dying clients, those over age 40 have more positive attitudes toward dying than younger nurses.[23] It may be that once an avoidance pattern is learned, it is not easily replaced, even when the fear of death lessens with age. Lack of knowledge and skill related to therapeutic communication may inhibit these older nurses from engaging in an exploration of dying clients' thoughts and feelings.

A focus of recent nursing research has been on how nursing education can generate more positive attitudes about death and dying clients and assist care givers in providing more humane care to dying people. Both classroom and clinical experiences can reduce student nurses' fears of death and dying.[24] Interactions with dying people during nursing education is an important factor in reducing students' fears that would otherwise lead to an avoidance pattern.[25] Research findings indicate that the more education about death student nurses receive, the better able they are to focus on dying clients' psychological and spiritual as well as physical distress.[26]

Attitudes and Values

When nurses have difficulty coping with the emotional needs of dying clients and their families, the sources of these problems are multidimensional. The less these nurses are aware of their feelings, the less able they are to work sensitively and supportively with those who are dying. They will be more apt to fall back upon whatever guidelines are available from other sources: the life-and-death orientations that have been learned as part of a particular ethnic and socioeconomic background, the pressure of colleagues to conform to their definition of what constitutes a good nurse, personal experiences, and unchallenged beliefs. The influence of these orientations will be lessened if the nurse has had guidance, supervision, and sensitization to clients' needs; if communication skills have been developed; and if the nurse has a broad knowledge base as well as a theoretical framework to guide practice.

When nurses sense inadequacy in themselves in caring for dying clients—if they have not developed an awareness of how they perceive death or worked through the concomitant feelings—they tend to become invested in routines and rituals of a technical nature that help them defend against anxiety. This approach denies the clients' emotional and social needs and may serve to alienate and isolate clients. Moral, ethical, and legal considerations, including the client's "right to know," may be overlooked.

Enormous attention may be given to life-prolonging techniques and to the most tenuous hopes of recovery, while little effort is made to provide comfort to dying clients. It is difficult to strive to keep clients alive at all costs and simultaneously to help them die in a dignified and comforted manner. These conflicting goals become more difficult to resolve if the nurse fails to attend to the nurse-client relationship, exploration of the thoughts and feelings of both the nurse and the client, and the primacy of the client's needs and rights.

One of the most significant influences on the lifelong development of a nurse's attitudes and feelings about dying is the nurse's own family of origin. The family of origin provides a person with an intense learning experience from the first moment of life, in which thoughts, feelings, and perceptions about the important issues in life are born and shaped. If a nurse's own family is characterized by open and supportive emotional relationships, whereby family members have been allowed to express their feelings with one another about the deaths of significant family members, it is likely that the nurse will be more at ease, and hence more professionally competent with the dying client. Conversely, if a nurse's own family experience with death has been characterized by inability or unwillingness to express feelings associated with loss and grief, chances are that the nurse will transfer to professional practice this mode of relating to people who are dying.

It is important for the nurse to recognize that some, even many, of one's own feelings and perceptions of a currently stressful, intensely emotional situation are related to the way similar situations have been experienced in one's family of origin. Consequently, nurses are directed to work through the unresolved emotional aspects of these situations with members of their own family as well as with people they encounter in the present.

Authority and Control

While it is always important not to get involved in power struggles with clients, this is especially true in the case of dying clients. Sometimes nurses become very withholding when it comes to providing information or administering pain medication. Or, conversely, they become pushy in an effort to see that clients take their medications. The issue is one of who is in charge rather than of doing what is best for clients and allowing clients to retain control over their lives.

Perhaps the reason why nurses are so controlling around a dying patient is that, since the client is losing control over everything, their own anxiety is high. The loss of the client's control reminds nurses of their own potential loss of control; because of this reaction, nurses work overtime at being "in charge" on the unit.

Identification

Some nurses develop a strong identification with their dying clients. The projective identification and the transference and countertransference phenomena are potentially disruptive to the quality of a relationship which would otherwise be facilitative, therapeutic, and supportive.

Transference is a distortion of the client's perception of the nurse. The dependency and regression that occur in illness, along with the need for personal physical care and comfort by the nurse, distort the relationship. Feelings generated in the client have their roots in past childhood relationships of a similar nature. These feelings of dying clients and the resulting behavior are normal; they are not directed at the nurse personally but are distortions of the present based on remembrances of the past.

By the same token, it is natural for the nurse to have distorted feelings about the client. This distorted perception of the client is *countertransference*. Countertransference feelings are heightened when the dying client reminds the nurse of a relative or friend who has died.

Countertransference and transference can be both positive and negative. The feelings generated may be warm, supportive, and nurturing or hostile and rejecting. These feelings and their consequent expression may interfere with sensitive and accurate assessment of needs and delivery of care.

When the nursing staff has invested considerable time, energy, effort, and feeling in the care of a dying client, the death of the client causes acute feelings of loss. Consequently, nurses may react with anger which is not recognized. Since they are unaware of the roots of this feeling, the anger gets projected onto others. This is often evidenced by the staff's irritability toward ancillary helpers or toward the housekeeping department or another department with which they interface.

Nurses who care for dying clients may develop rescue fantasies. Clients of "high social value" have a greater potential for generating these fantasies in their care givers. Such fantasies prompt nurses to try to help the client whether or not the "help" they wish to give is appropriate or desired. When this happens, the nurse's needs are not congruent with the client's needs.

> Mr. A., a client dying of cancer, worked persistently and with great effort at self-care and maximum independence. Mr. C., his nurse, motivated by a rescue fantasy, intervened in ways that fostered dependence and regression. These interventions met Mr. C.'s need to be helpful and needed, but they generated anxiety and helplessness in Mr. A.

"Chronic helpers" do things for others constantly and without being asked. They operate under the assumption that what they do is helpful, never checking to see whether their interventions actually help others cope more effectively. Their behavior is indicative of their own underlying dependency needs. Their helpfulness engenders inappropriate dependency in the client which blocks the client from assuming responsibility and maintaining mastery. This dependency generates feelings of helplessness and anger in the client. Care givers are puzzled and hurt when their "help" is rejected or sabotaged by the client. The helper's dependency need is not being met, and the client's compensatory independence is not being effected. Thus, feelings of rejection, failure, and anxiety surface. Such helpers may say, "What a fool I am for letting myself be used" or "This is what being kind and helpful gets you." The theme becomes, "I'm not approved of; therefore, I must be bad." The development of self-awareness is the most effective way of preventing and managing rescue fantasies and chronic helpfulness.[27]

Helplessness and Hopelessness

People in the health professions, including nurses, tend to have a "cure" orientation which interferes with the care of dying clients and their families. When dying clients fail to improve, and even worsen despite the efforts expended, discouragement is inevitable if a cure orientation is present.

The personal investment and the intensity of working with dying people and their families can be emotionally exhausting. The psychic exhaustion that occurs after prolonged exposure to these clients is a product of "death saturation."[28] The feelings of helplessness and hopelessness related to this phenomenon are inherently stressful. These feelings may become acute if the nurse develops "exaggerated compassion." This identification with the dying person is an attempt to undo past guilt, relieve past shame, restore personal self-esteem, and rework personal experiences of death.[29] The overinvolvement that develops is emotionally draining. The nurse's vulnerability to physical and psychosocial problems increases. Depending on the nurse's personal physical and psychological vulnerability, symptoms of burnout may include any of the following: increased absenteeism; conflict at home or work; depression; increased susceptibility to infections, accidents, or serious mistakes.

Some nurses who wish to address dying clients' psychosocial needs may be frustrated by restrictions imposed by the health care setting.[30] Nurses who carry a heavy caseload of dying clients may eventually withdraw physically or psychologically to protect themselves. Some leave the setting or the profession. Those who remain and do not evolve constructive ways of resolving problematic feelings use self-protective distancing maneuvers that dehumanize the care-giving process. They may interact minimally or superficially, avoid gathering data about the client's premorbid lifestyle, or avoid developing a relationship with the family. Preoccupied with the very necessary physical ministration and technical procedures, they defend against experiencing the client's predicament and humanness.

They may relegate a dying client to the room farthest from the nurse's station, rationalizing the decision by saying, "It's quieter, and the client will be more comfortable." They may also avoid the client's predicament by failing to initiate communication about the client's perception of the prognosis or its impact on his or her lifestyle and future. This game of avoidance occurs when staff, family, and client know the seriousness of the illness but there is a mutual unwillingness to talk about it. This "conspiracy of silence" is further reinforced by visitors who also deny the facts. When the client, in spite of obvious deterioration, asks, "Don't I look better today?" the nurse will hastily reply, "Yes, you *do* look much better."

Angry clients are often exasperating and generate hostility in their care givers. Staff members are tempted to retaliate in kind, but if they do so, they will, of course, further isolate and alienate clients who are already overwhelmed by the dying process.

When nurses fail to recognize their anxiety and depression in relation to the care of dying people, these feelings evoke defensive behaviors that are detrimental to the families' and the clients' ability to cope. If nurses are consciously or unconsciously uncomfortable with the questions family members ask about the dying person, their tears, the way members relate to the dying person, or members' critical appraisals of the nursing care, they may avoid the family and any meaningful interactions with members.

Effectiveness with dying clients and their families increases when collegial support enables nurses and other care givers to better handle their own feelings and uncertainties.

"Care-Cure" Conflict

One of the tenets of nursing is that *care*, which is characterized by nurturing, supportive behavior, is always possible, even though *cure* may not be. This tenet is especially important for nurses who work with dying clients.

Society rewards life-saving activities and technical achievement rather than achievement of job satisfaction derived from working with clients whose main needs involve human, care-oriented concerns.[31] The development of nursing was significantly influenced by historical associations with "women's work" and more recently has been affected by the "productivity" model of business, which devalues a care orientation. Nurses need to transcend the traditionally dependent role and the emphasis on productivity in order to provide the kind of care required by dying clients.

PATTERNS OF INTERACTION: THE DYING PERSON

Dying is a process that leads to death. It occurs in space and time and interacts with the physical, mental, and spiritual dimensions of the dying person and significant others in the environment.

Clinical Phases of Dying

Three clinical phases of dying have been identified: the acute crisis, the chronic living-dying phase, and the terminal phase. This section focuses on the chronic living-dying phase and the terminal phase.[29]

The *chronic living-dying phase*[29] is that period of time when a person has the knowledge that the expected life span has been foreshortened. It is the period of time between the crisis during which knowledge of death is absorbed and the point of death itself.

This phase is characterized by a constellation of fears that include fear of (1) loneliness, (2) sorrow, (3) the unknown, (4) loss of self-concept and alteration in body image, (5) loss of self-control, (6) suffering and pain, and (7) regression and dependency.[32] The intensity of each of these fears and the degree to which each becomes problematic vary. These fears and their sources are presented in Table 45-2 (page 982).

The *terminal phase* is that period of time when the dying person knows that death is imminent and certain and significant others also have this knowledge. The person's physical status is such that there are no ambiguities about the time frame or the certainty. The precise onset of this phase is difficult to determine. According to Saunders,[33] people enter this phase when all active treatment

Table 45-2 Fears of Dying People

Fear	Source of Fear
Loneliness	Distancing by family, friends, and care givers
	Client's debilitation, pain, and incapacitation
	Inherent loneliness of hospitalization
	Fear of dying alone
Sorrow	Awareness of personal mortality
	Anticipatory grief
The unknown	Confrontation of the unknown dimensions of death
	Concerns about what will happen to the self after death
	Concerns about what will happen to loved ones
Loss of self-concept and alteration in body image	Impact of mutilating surgery, chemotherapy, and debilitating changes imposed by the disease process
	Partial or total loss of role and status
Regression and dependency	The instinctive regression that threatens ego integrity
	Perceived inevitable physical deterioration
Loss of self-control	Loss of control of bodily functions, daily living activities, decisions, thought process, and emotions
Suffering and pain	Physical, social, psychological, and spiritual pain
	Organic changes caused by the disease process
	Alterations in relationships with significant others
	Multiple losses incurred and impending
	Anxieties related to the disease process and treatments

of the disease becomes ineffective and irrelevant to their real needs. However, some people remain active for extended periods of time after treatment has been terminated, and in some instances treatment is continued regardless of its relevance until death occurs.

Characteristic of this phase, which may and should be brief, is physical and psychological withdrawal. There is usually a marked decrease in anxiety, and what has been described as a turning away from the outside world and a turning into the self.[32] While anxiety diminishes, depression may tend to increase during the terminal phase. Debilitation decreases the client's available energy, and withdrawal is in part an energy-conserving maneuver. *Expectational hope,* which is a composite of beliefs and a set of expectations that have some possibility of fulfillment and is characteristic of the chronic living-dying phase, is replaced by *desirable hope*—it would be nice to live, but that is not expected. Periods of remission, relief of symptoms, and active interventions are no longer occurring and reinforcing expectational hope. Replacement of expectation with desire is the beginning of movement toward acceptance of death. Acceptance is in part the movement from expectational hope to desirable hope. It is also a regression into the self as the physical capacities are markedly deteriorating and psychological energies are diminished. This phenomenon is characteristic of psychic death and precedes biological and physiological death.[8,32]

Patterns of Dying Clients

Fears about death and dying, revisions in hope, and physiological changes related to the disease process interact with the dying person's physical, mental, and spiritual dimensions of self.

Kübler-Ross's[34] work with dying people and with medical students learning how to care for them contributed to the health profession's and the public's awareness of people's responses to dying. She identified the following specific patterns of response to the dying process: initial shock and disbelief, denial, anger, bargaining, a sense of loss and depression, and acceptance.

There has been a tendency among providers of health care to view these reactions as occurring in stages and to believe that if people are successful in negotiating the initial stages, they will attain the state of acceptance. Clinical observations do not support this; research findings suggest, rather, that each person tends to adopt a pattern of behavior that characterizes his or her dying process.[7,35] The reactions described by Kübler-Ross[34] do occur. However, there is no solid evidence that the reactions occur in a uniform and predictable sequence, or that failure to experience a particular stage interferes with acceptance, the ability to continue to live with hope until death, and a peaceful death.[29]

The uniqueness of each person, family, and environment, and the interactions that occur produce an individualized way of working through the dying process. The responses described by Kübler-Ross[34] are ways that people cope with dying. Knowledge about these responses contributes to an understanding of the dying process.

Shock and Disbelief

Shock and disbelief occur when a person receives information that he or she will die in the very near future. These reactions may occur immediately upon pronouncement of the diagnosis of disease or after the person is told definitely that there is no cure or remedy, the disease is progressing, and life will be cut short. Confrontation of the mortality of the self generates feelings that influence interactions with others and self-perceptions.

Denial

When reality is perceived as threatening to biological survival, competent behavior, and responsible conduct, denial is a useful way of excluding the most frightening aspects of this reality from awareness.[36] Denial is not an all-or-nothing response. It can be used selectively and in a limited way. When it excludes only the most threatening dimensions of reality and protects people from feelings of acute anxiety and dread, it helps them participate more actively in other areas of living.[34] Denial helps people protect themselves by allowing time for gradual management of the crisis and mobilization of more effective defenses.

Denying is a process composed of four successive steps:[36]

1. Acceptance of an environmental perception of the situation
2. Rejection of a portion of the situation
3. Replacement of the painful, rejected portion of the situation with a more agreeable interpretation of the situation
4. Revision of reality that excludes the intolerable, and restoration of conditions as they were before the crisis

For a person to be able to deny a diagnosis, a prognosis, and the physical and psychosocial alterations caused by the disease process, the social environment must participate in this denial. For whatever reason, there must exist either a conscious or unconscious collusion to avoid some aspects of the reality of the situation. Sensitive issues such as a radical change in the person's appearance or evidence that the disease has progressed rapidly and is not responding to treatment may be excluded from all conversations. For example, symptoms of metastasis may be redefined with the help of significant others and even physicians who suggest that they are due to a bursitis or to food that might have been improperly prepared.

Closed awareness, suspected awareness, and mutual pretense support denial to varying degrees.[7] Ambiguities may also exist even when there is an open awareness that allows some denial. The time and manner of death are often unknown by the client, and information about these aspects of the dying process may be withheld even when there is open awareness.[7]

When reality is rejected by negation or a blocked perception, a psychological gap develops. People fill in this gap by replacing the anxiety-producing reality with a revised perception and redefinition that is more comfortable and therefore more acceptable. This revised perception allows people to exclude the threatening and anxiety-producing aspects of reality and to restore the precrisis psychological stability and comfort. Symptoms of progression of a disease can be more easily ignored or explained away. For example, "As soon as the vitamins start working, I won't feel so fatigued," or, "I think this pain in my back is arthritis."

Four levels of denial have been identified: existenial, psychological, nonacceptance, and nonattention. *Existential denial* is a fundamental approach to mortality that allows people to proceed with living free of the threatening awareness that life is temporary. *Psychological denial* is an unconscious defense mechanism that protects the person from conscious awareness of the implications of terminal illness and the dying process. It allows the person to remain hopeful and actively engaged in living within the limits imposed by the disease.[29] *Nonacceptance denial* is the active suppression of recognized facts about the terminal prognosis and the dying process. *Nonattention denial* is a strategy by which people focus their interest and energy on activities that distract them from being aware of their discomforts and from thinking about illness and impending death.

Anger

Feelings of anger, rage, envy, and resentment may occur during the dying process in response to limitations placed on life and well-being by the disease process and by the health care system. The anger may be diffuse and displaced in all directions. It may be projected onto the environment at random, or focused on specific people, situations, or the self. Concern for personal safety and fears of abandonment usually mediate the choice of people and circumstances on which the anger is vented.[36] Anger at this point is normal. Death causes separation from loved ones and a loss of self. The dying person is frustrated by the inability to change the situation.

The anger experienced during the dying process can also be generated by the dehumanizing therapies and care-giving process, and the loss of control over lifestyle and bodily functions.[34] The expenditures for treatments and care may deplete financial resources that are viewed as a source of security, the means needed to pursue enjoyable hobbies or travel, or a legacy for survivors.[7]

Some people become angry as a defense against the painful procedures and treatments, the discomfort in performing daily living activities, the losses they are incurring, their increasing dependency on others, and their helplessness and hopelessness.

Bargaining

Bargaining, which is an attempt to postpone pain or death by offering good behavior, is helpful to the client for brief periods of time. It sets a self-imposed deadline and includes an implicit promise that the client will not ask for more if this postponement is granted.

Most of these bargains are made with God and are usually kept secret or mentioned only implicitly. It is not uncommon to hear, "I promised God that if He would let me live, I'd go to church every day for the rest of my life." The husband of a dying wife said, "If she gets better, we'll go on the vacation she has always wanted." One mother whose deterioration was becoming more evident said, "I only want to see my children graduate from college and start their own lives." Psychologically, promises like these may be associated with guilt for not attending church more regularly; for feeling as though one has not done enough for one's family or has treated them badly; or, in the case of family members, for not having done enough for the dying person.

Sense of Loss and Depression

The dying person is no longer able to deny the illness when certain symptoms appear. Then the numbness, stoicism, anger, and rage that may have been experienced initially are replaced with a sense of great loss and a feeling of deep depression which may be reactive, preparatory, or both.

Reactive depression may be the response to change of body image, financial burdens, inability to function, or loss of job. *Preparatory depression* occurs in anticipation of impending loss and is necessary to facilitate acceptance. The client is in the process of losing everything and everybody: the spouse or other survivors, on the other hand, are losing only one person, the client. This preparatory depression is more silent than reactive depression, in which the client has much to share and requires many verbal interactions. This silence is difficult for the client's family and other visitors to accept because they instinctively want to cheer up the client. But nothing could be more hollow than the sometimes banal efforts that well-wishers make to humor those who are on the verge of losing their entire world. Such efforts are thin disguises for the anxiety that stalks beneath. The dying grieve for their anticipated loss of life. When some family members are unsure of how to respond to the client's grief and depression, they may pretend that everything will be all right, thus causing the dying person to feel that efforts to communicate with others are useless.[37]

Unhappiness and depression influence perceptions of bodily sensations, particularly painful experiences. Thus, tolerance of bodily pain decreases. The increased discomfort reinforces the sense of loss and depression.

Acceptance

Acceptance is a psychological state almost devoid of feelings. It is not a capitulation, nor is it happy. Survival is no longer necessary. Hope exists but transcends its conditional dependency on survival.[7,35] There is a sense of closure. Unfinished business that was a source of concern either no longer matters or has been resolved. The separation from significant others is no longer acutely painful.

Kübler-Ross[34] noted that people are often fatigued and physically weakened by the disease process when acceptance occurs; they have a need to extend the hours of sleep. She observed that the sleep pattern is very similar to that of a newborn child but in reverse order, and it is not an avoidance strategy.

Acceptance is not necessarily an absolute and stable state. It may fluctuate with changes in the person's psychological or physical status. When it exists, a person is able to derive a sense of purpose and meaning from his or her life and death.[36]

When there is acceptance, the person does not mind being alone and is not disturbed by feelings of loneliness. The person is no longer in a talkative mood. Communication becomes more nonverbal than verbal. Occassionally the dying person can actually articulate what is happening and can do so casually, and this startles those present. One young man, the day before his death, said in a matter-of-fact voice to the nurse who came to give morning care, "You know, I'm dying."

PATTERNS OF INTERACTION: FAMILY

The family's interactions with the dying client and care givers significantly influence the context of dying. Family members experience a process that parallels the client's responses to dying. However, the family's response pattern may or may not be in synchrony with the client's. Furthermore, the dying client's problems have an end in view, while the family sees its problems as continuing.

A family may participate in or be excluded from awareness of the dying person's situation. The unaware family can remain so only if the care givers collude to forestall their awareness. As the client's situation deteriorates, suspicions develop. Family members may hide these suspicions from one another and attempt to mutually sustain their belief in the client's recovery.[7] In some instances selected family members are aware of the situation and communicate with one another about it but exclude other family members. When this occurs, it is often perceived as a way of "protecting" those excluded from awareness. Such a secret in a family is divisive. When mutual pretense exists, the family colludes with staff members to keep the client in the dark about the situation.[7]

When a context of open awareness is lacking, the family system is closed, and it operates with an automatic emotional reflex that protects against anxiety. Most people will say that they avoid taboo subjects so that they will not upset others. Because death is a taboo subject, there are at least two emotional processes operative when someone's dying is an issue. One is the process that protects all of us all the time: the existential denial of death. The other is the closed relationship system in which people cannot communicate the thoughts they do have lest they upset the family or others.

Most terminally ill people know they have a disease with a poor prognosis. Even children are aware of their impending death, even when it is accompanied by the denial of the diagnosis on the part of both parents and the hospital staff.[6,36,38] They also know when death is imminent. When the family system is closed, there is often an attempt to deny the dying person's knowledge of the facts and to prevent the care givers from discussing the predicted death with the client. The conspiracy of silence, born of the wish to be protective, condemns both the client and the family to an inauthentic relationship. This loss of openness deprives them of the support and the interactions which would facilitate dealing with feelings. For example:

> One young woman dying of cancer said to the nurse, "Please don't tell my mom and dad how sick I am; I don't want them to be upset." Later that day, the parents instructed the same nurse, "We don't ever want our daughter to know what she has, or that she is dying."

Lack of communication denies both the client and family the right to an orderly separation, and the right to share a part of the living-dying experience.

Acceptance is facilitated by an open relationship in which people are free to communicate most of their inner thoughts, feelings, and fantasies to others who can reciprocate. No one ever has a completely open relationship with another, but it is a healthy state when a person can have a significant relationship in which a reasonable degree of openness is possible. An open system of family communication is also valuable in restabilizing a family after the death of a member.[39]

An open relationship provides opportunities for both the family members and the client to separate in an orderly and mutually supportive way. Meaningful interaction allows both the dying person and the family members to give to each other, receive from each other, and grow as persons in the process.

Death or threatened death is one of many events that can disrupt a family. A family unit is in functional equilibrium when it is calm and each member is functioning at reasonable efficiency for that period. The equilibrium of the unit is disrupted by the loss or impending loss of a member. The intensity of the emotional reaction is governed by the functioning level of emotional integration in the family at the time and by the functional importance of the one who is lost to the family.

Just as the dying person may experience anger, so too may family members. They may be bewildered by feeling openly angry or by finding themselves feeling resentful. Sometimes they are angry at the dying relative because they feel that the person did not take care of himself or herself, and they feel confused by their anger. Some turn their separation anger toward other family members, while others focus it on one or more care givers. Some family members proceed through the grieving process more quickly than the client; their feelings and behaviors may be incongruent with those of the dying person, who may feel abandoned. On the other hand, a client may experience acceptance and be at peace before the family reaches this point; in this case, the family will feel closed out of the client's world.

When death occurs suddenly, with little or no warning, members of the family of the deceased are generally told about the death after the fact. In such instances, the family members are the clients. They need help in working through their shock, anger, and guilt. Their feelings of helplessness are heightened by the fact that they have not been able to "do anything" for the deceased. They may be overwhelmed by guilt feelings rooted in earlier conflicts with the deceased or aroused by their failure to recognize the seriousness of the illness.

The Emotional Shock Wave

Emotional shock wave is a term coined by Bowen[40] to describe the network of "underground aftershocks" that can occur anywhere in an extended family system in the months or years following a serious emotional event in a family. It occurs most often after the death or the threatened death of a significant family member. It is not directly related to the usual grief or mourning reactions of people close to the one who died. It operates on an underground level of emotional dependence of family members on one another. The emotional dependence is denied, the serious life events appear to be unrelated, the family attempts to camouflage any connection between the events, and there is vigorous emotional denial when anyone attempts to relate the events to each other.

The symptoms of a shock wave can be any human problems. They can include the entire spectrum of physical illness, from an increased incidence of colds and respiratory infections to the first appearance of chronic conditions, such as diabetes or allergies, to acute medical and surgical illnesses. It is as if the shock wave is a stimulus that can trigger physical processes. The symptoms can also include the full range of emotional symptoms, from mild depression, to phobias, to psychotic episodes. The social dysfunctions can include drinking, failures in school or business, abortions, illegitimate births, an increase in accidents, and the full range of behavior disorders. In one study focusing on the families of leukemic clients, 50 percent of the families needed psychiatric intervention.[41] In another study of an inpatient pediatric psychiatric sample, 50 percent of the children had suffered from the death of a family member before admission.[42]

Another subtle but not always recognized shock-wave effect that occurs after the death of a significant family member is the naming of a child after the deceased person. In effect this creates a living memory of the lost person, and sometimes it is an attempt to recreate or replace the person.

Not all deaths have the same importance to a family. Some deaths are very likely to be followed by a shock wave. On the other hand, some deaths are a relief to the family and are usually followed by a period of better functioning. If the nurse can know ahead of time about the possibility of an emotional shock wave, steps can be taken to prevent it or to make the family aware of how it may influence functioning.

Anniversary Reactions

Anniversary reactions are time-specific psychological or physiological events that occur or recur in response to a traumatic event in one's own past or in the past of a person with whom one closely identifies.[43] A person who experiences an anniversary reaction attempts to relive or reexperience the traumatic event again in order to master it.[43]

Many clinicians have noted an anniversary reaction among surviving family members. As the anniversary date of the loss of the significant family member approaches, surviving members feel anxious or depressed, develop symptoms that had been experienced by the dead person, become ill, or have an accident. Family members are often unaware of the connection between what is happening to them and the fact that it is the anniversary of the death.

The reason for the occurrence of this phenomenon is not clearly understood. It seems to be related to the emotional shock wave; and it tends to affect family members' feelings, behaviors, and well-being while often remaining at the unconscious level. Because of anniversary reactions, people are more vulnerable to physical, psychological, and social ills during the time just before, during, and just after the anniversary of the death of a significant family member.

DYSYNCHRONOUS PATTERNS OF INTERACTION: THE DYING PERSON

Many of the behaviors exhibited by a dying client that contribute to a stressful dying process are exaggerations of the client's coping style and psychological and behavioral responses to the dying process. Whether behaviors become dysynchronous patterns or are perceived as problematic by the care givers is dependent in part on the expectations that influence perceptions and judgments about the behavior, and whether the context of care facilitates or obstructs people's ability to recognize and meet the dying person's needs.

Denial, anger, depression, and pain are common among the dying. They become problematic for clients when they cause distress and interfere with the ability to derive daily satisfaction of needs and eventual peaceful acceptance of death. When exaggerated, they aggravate an already difficult situation. Pervasive, inappropriate use of denial; overt problematic expression of anger; pervasive depression; giving up on life without acceptance; and intractable pain are core problems for dying people that must be resolved if they are to maximally participate in self-determination and die peacefully.

Dysynchronous Patterns of Denial

Some degree of denial is useful because it gives the client breathing space after the initial reception of devastating news. However, denial becomes dysfunctional when it keeps the client from deriving satisfaction from living, interferes with meaningful family interactions, blocks the use of resources, prevents coming to terms with the impending death, and interferes with self-determination.

In some instances, despite the prognosis the person can live a satisfactory and productive life for an extended period of time, and sometimes until shortly before death. Massive denial can lead to the use of even more primitive defenses such as delusions, perceptual hallucinations, and depersonalization.[32] Denial may interfere with a client's safety and well-being and even precipitate premature death.[1]

When people deny the facts about a disease, deny the implications of the changes that occur, fail to make plausible inferences about tests or treatments, or fail to seek explanations, they may not follow through on recommended treatments that might make life more comfortable. These people fail to "hear" or "remember" what they have been told, or they redefine the situation so that it negates reality.

Denial can been seen in a variety of behaviors. There may be an unwillingness to look at or examine the site of an operation, for instance, or to look in a mirror. For example:

> Miss A., a client who had undergone a midthigh amputation, refused to watch or participate in dressing changes. She pulled the sheets over her head so that she could not see the procedure.

> Mr. B., a client with a large, disfiguring facial tumor, was asked by the admitting nurse why he had not sought health care before. He replied that he had not been bothered by it and had learned to live with it.

In some instances because of denial the client may engage in life-threatening activities:

> A client in a coronary care unit who massively denied

the reality of his condition and the possibility of precipitating his death was found doing chin-ups despite warnings to limit his physical activity.

Thus, extensive, nonuseful denial prevents clients from recognizing the inappropriateness or the dangerous aspects of their behavior:

A high school football player who was diagnosed with stage 4 Hodgkin's disease could describe in detail the process of the disease, but he skillfully avoided discussions about alterations in his physical activity. In fact, he continued to talk about making plans for doing heavy labor as a construction worker.

People need to confront dying in "manageable doses."[44] No one is strong enough to look at this alarming reality without some relief. However, indiscriminate and continuous use of tranquilizers to "get through" or prevent coming to grips with the situation only distorts the grieving process and displaces it in time. Without realistic feedback, dying clients may make inappropriate plans and attempt to implement them. Pervasive denial also interferes with meaningful interaction with family members. Conversations tend to be social in nature and suggestions regarding the need for a will fall on deaf ears.

Dysynchronous Patterns of Anger

Some clients who are having difficulty coping with the dying process displace and project intense anger in ways that are upsetting to them and the people in their environment. The expression of this anger may be painful and bewildering to dying people and those around them.[28]

The dependent client who expresses anger often feels guilty and fears retaliation. It is frightening for clients to express anger to the care givers or family members upon whom they feel dependent for survival. To control or hide anger, clients may withdraw from all self-assertive behavior and become emotionally inaccessible. Or such a client may become the classic "difficult patient," the one who is uncooperative with the staff, complains about everything, and never seems satisfied. Some clients may show intense, overt anger.

When anger builds, these clients scan their environment for someone to blame. The target selected is usually perceived as the safest focus for the anger and blame, but this is not always the case. Unrestrained expression of anger toward care givers and family members may result in further isolation and feelings of helplessness if the recipients of the anger withdraw. Angry clients may berate the chosen target for perceived failures or incompetence. They may explode into temper tantrums because the coffee is cold or the wrong lotion was purchased. Others may respond sarcastically or critically to whatever the targeted person says or does. The client is apt to perceive the targeted person's behavior globally as "always" wrong or unsatisfactory.

Some clients enraged at their incurable status focus their blame and anger on the physician who made the original diagnosis. This compartmentalizes the anger and keeps it out of relationships the client perceives as a vital support system.

When an exaggerated fight pattern occurs, the dying client confronts and challenges the social environment. This confrontation may be characterized by insistent questioning, demanding behavior, or a search for a magic cure. Care givers do not view anger, aggressiveness, or even assertiveness as compatible with the sick role; such behavior may be labeled as problematic regardless of its intensity.

Usually, however, the anger is more subtly expressed:

Mrs. Q., a superficially sweet elderly woman, frustrated the nursing staff during her dying process because she would neither swallow her pills nor spit them out. She would just let the pills sit in the back of her throat. This was her way of controlling the last manipulable piece of her life.

The client may feel guilt in relation to hostile thoughts and feelings and overtly angry behavior. Clients may view their illnesses as punishments visited upon them for past sins, though they usually cannot tell what they have done that is so bad. Clients are often distressed over their anger and do not always understand its derivation or how to resolve it. For example:

Mr. J. prayed out loud on the day before he died that God would forgive him for trying to bite the nurse who routinely gave him his injection. This prayer was his way of expressing guilt for his angry feelings and an attempt to resolve the hurt he felt he had caused.

Dysynchronous Patterns of Depression

When the periodic sadness and unhappiness associated with the dying process become intense and pervasive, they are pathological and increase the client's suffering. There is a decreased tolerance of bodily pain.[45] Sleeping, eating, and elimination are disturbed. Insomnia increases feelings of fatigue. Loss of appetite may accelerate weight loss and further decrease energy. Some clients may be tearful at first, but as the depression deepens, they may become vegetative and exhibit a flat affect and a lack of spontaneity.

Self-esteem may be drastically diminished if extensive bodily mutilation and distortion result in a rejection of the altered self. If the self is unacceptable, the ability to relate to others is impaired.

There is a withdrawal from physical and social activity. The social isolation and alienation that develop intensify the self-focus, magnify distressing emotional and physical sensations, and contribute to forgetfulness and mental dullness.[36] The alienation and accompanying loneliness erect barriers that reinforce their existence. The sense of powerlessness and meaninglessness that is experienced is immobilizing. The grieving process is at a standstill. Movement toward acceptance is blocked. There is a capitulation, and if significant others are emotionally unavailable, the "giving up–given up" complex develops.

The Giving-Up–Given-Up Complex

Engel[46] has identified a complex of behaviors that seem to contribute to the emergence of life-threatening disease and persist throughout the downhill course of illness. This set of behaviors is referred to as the *giving-up–given-up complex*.

In clinical and phenomenological terms, Engel delineates the characteristics of the complex as follows.

1. It has an unpleasant affective quality, expressed in such terms as, "Too much," "It's no use," "I can't take it anymore," "I give up." It encompasses two different affective qualities: *helplessness,* where these feelings are ascribed more to failures on the part of the environment; and *hopelessness,* where feelings are ascribed more to one's own failures and include a sense of being beyond help from others.
2. The self is perceived as less intact, less competent, less in control, less gratified, and less capable of functioning in a relatively autonomous fashion.
3. Relationships with significant others are felt to be less secure and gratifying; the client may feel given up by these or may give up the self.
4. The external environment may be perceived as differing significantly from expectations based on past experience, which no longer seems as useful a guide for current or future behavior.
5. There is felt to be a loss of continuity between past and future and an inability to project oneself into the future with hope or confidence. Hence the future may appear relatively bleak or unrewarding.
6. There is a tendency to revive feelings, memories, and behavior connected with occasions in the past which had a similar quality.

This description represents a composite of overlapping phenomena, not all of which are represented to an equal degree in every client. Hence it is called a *complex,* having configurational, temporal, and quantitative aspects. It may exist very briefly or for an extended period of time, may begin or end abruptly or gradually, may wax and wane over a period of time, and may be of greater or lesser intensity.

Helplessness and hopelessness have been identified as characteristics of two distinct types of the giving-up–given-up complex. These affects reflect ego awareness of an inability to defend against a loss of two different types of autonomy. *Helplessness* reflects a loss of ego autonomy combined with a feeling of deprivation; it results from the loss of gratification from objects other than the self. *Hopelessness,* on the other hand, reflects a loss of autonomy accompanied by a feeling of despair; it comes from an awareness of the self's inability to provide the desired gratification. Not all life situations which engender true hopelessness or helplessness evoke giving-up–given-up responses. Central to the complex is the psychic perception of failure or unavailability of resources: hence real, threatened, or symbolic psychic object losses constitute the most common provocative situations.

The giving-up–given-up complex is only one of innumerable possible responses to loss and is not employed by everyone in the same situation. Hence, the response is not present in all who are dying: when it is present, however, it seems to hasten death. It appears that there is a direct connection between the giving-up–given-up complex and the various biological processes that occur at the same time.[46]

Dysynchronous Patterns of Pain

Pain—the anxiety it produces and the fear of it—is a major concern of people who are dying. Chronic pain is very different from acute pain, not only in duration but also in quality. Saunders[47] defines *chronic pain* as a reaction between the stimulus and the whole person. Chronic pain may no longer be functional; when that happens, it must be seen as an illness in its own right.

When clients experience intense anger, depression, or anxiety, the pain associated with the dying process is aggravated. People who experience severe, prolonged pain without relief become chronically anxious and fearful that they will never again be free of pain. Consequently, there is a decreased tolerance of both the chronic pain and the acute discomfort associated with diagnostic procedures and treatments.[45] These clients may seem to overreact to injections, intravenous therapy, and even care-giving activities such as a bed bath. They may cry out, clutch the bed, or cling to the care giver. Whimpering, crying, moaning, gasping, or screaming may occur in anticipation of a painful experience. The words selected to describe pain tend to reflect the client's perception of its severity. The physiological response to pain may also be severe. Acute nausea, weakness, and muscle tension may occur both during and in anticipation of a painful experience.[45,48]

Clients may lie very still with their eyes closed in an attempt to control pain, avoid stimuli that might increase pain, and conserve energy. There is a massive withdrawal from the environment and an increased focus on the self and bodily sensations. This response often escalates the distress.

When clients have minimal or no control over their pain, medications become a primary concern. The lack of control and the dread associated with pain increase the perception of pain and diminish the effects of pain-relief medications. Requests for these medications may become insistent demands for more frequent administration and larger doses. When this happens, the management of the pain may result in an unnecessary, extensive use of drugs that decreases alertness and prevents social interaction prematurely.

NURSING PROCESS

Application of the nursing process to dying clients and their families provides a systematic way of delivering nursing care. It provides a framework for identifying problems, planning to remedy the identified difficulties in collaboration with the client and family, and selecting interventions that facilitate living until death and death with dignity.

Assessment

The first step in the process requires the collection of a data base needed to provide comprehensive care to dying clients and their families. The interactions of person, family, and environment that occur are influential and must therefore be addressed. Consequently, the assessment process must be directed toward the client, the family, and the context of care.

The Client

The assessment of the client needs to address the physical, mental, and spiritual dimensions in interaction with the family and the environment.

The following questions are a guide for the assessment of the client:

1. How is the client behaving?
2. Is the client's behavior helping or hindering the dying process?
3. What is the client's emotional response pattern?
4. How is the client managing these feelings?
5. Has the client been told the diagnosis and prognosis? If so, what was the response?
6. Does the client feel supported by significant others?
7. Is the client able to "ask" and "take" to satisfy needs?
8. Is the client able to grieve over the impending losses?

9. Is the client able to begin to say good-bye to significant others?
10. Is the client able to settle business affairs—for example, make a will?
11. How is the client dealing with pain?
12. If drugs are being used, do they relieve the pain and allow the client to be alert and able to relate to others?
13. What does the client fear most about dying?
14. Is the client where he or she wishes to be, that is, at home or in the hospital? If not, then why not?
15. Does the client have realistic expectations in relation to the dying process?
16. Are there resources available for meeting these expectations?
17. At what stage of growth and development is the client? How is this influencing the client's and the family's response to the impending death?
18. What is the client's relationship with care givers?
19. Has the client been able to talk with anyone about the meaning of life and death?

The Family

The total family configuration, the position of the dying person in the family, and the overall level of adaptation to life are important for the nurse to assess in attempting to help a family before, during, or after a death. It is also important for the nurse to assess the developmental level of each member of the family, and in light of that level to weigh the impact of the impending death on each member. It is one thing for a 65-year-old person to lose a parent, and quite another for an adolescent. Nevertheless, no matter how young or old a daughter or son is, the death of a parent always raises issues associated with one's "child relationship" to the parent. It is helpful for survivors if these issues can be brought into the open and discussed before and after the parent dies.

The following questions are a guide for the assessment of the family:

1. What role does the client play in the family system?
2. Does the family recognize and acknowledge that the client is dying?
3. How does the family manage angry feelings?
4. How does the family respond to the expected loss of the client?
5. Who in the family will be most affected by the loss of the client?
6. What plans are family members making to cope with the loss?
7. What is the family's perception of the diagnosis and prognosis?
8. What feelings are being experienced by family members?
9. What influence do these feelings have on the dying person?
10. How do family members communicate?
11. What influence does this style of communication have on the dying person?
12. What are the family's needs?
13. What resources does the family have for gratification of these needs?
14. How does the family relate to the care givers?
15. How does the family communicate with the dying person?
16. Is the family able to use the care givers as a resource?
17. What other stresses is the family experiencing at this time?
18. How do these stresses interact with the stress of having a dying family member?
19. How is the family coping with these stresses?

The Environment

The assessment of the environment is essential. The context of care is a major interacting influence in the dying process. These clients are often confined to the context, physically unable to escape it, and sometimes lacking the energy to initiate changes that would make it more satisfying.

The following questions are a guide for the assessment of the environment:

1. What is the context of the dying process?
2. Is the environment designed to help the client to cope effectively with dying?
3. Is the client's room set off from others?
4. Is relief from pain and discomfort readily available and under the client's control?
5. Does the client participate in planning his or her care?
6. Are people available to facilitate communication with the client and family?

7. Is there a staffing pattern that facilitates communication with the client?
8. Do staff members have adequate time to spend with the client?
9. Do staff members have ample opportunity to develop an ongoing relationship with the client and family?
10. Is community support available to the client and family?

Diagnosis

Nursing diagnoses are formulations of what the nurse sees as the client's problematic patterns of interaction that require nursing intervention. They are so stated as to identify the problem and define it conceptually and thus provide a basis for the further development of the nursing-care plan.

The problems of clients vary a good deal and are dependent upon a combination of circumstances, including (1) the phase of the illness (chronic living-dying or terminal), (2) the type of assistance that is needed (lifesaving care, direct physical care, teaching-socialization, emotional support), (3) the amount of time that is involved (short-term, long-term, or permanent contact), and (4) the social context in which care is provided (ambulatory care, home care, institutional care).

The following are examples of nursing diagnoses:

- Pervasive depression associated with massive physical deterioration and infrequent family visiting
- Global overt anger related to loss of control over bodily functions and previous lifestyle of "being in charge"
- Acute loneliness related to admission to nursing home and separation from family
- Family confused and bewildered in relation to client's decreased communication
- Family imposing closed awareness related to history of dysfunctional communication patterns

Outcome Criteria

The purposes of nursing in the care of a dying person and his or her family are: (1) helping the client to live more fully and comfortably until death, (2) helping the family to give support to the client, and (3) helping both the client and the family to move toward acceptance of the death. There is a time to live and a time to die. Death asks for one's identity, and meaningfulness is crucial. Being a part of life is often difficult, but to experience it is to truly live.[49]

In the latter stages of many terminal illnesses, pain is a constant companion. Pain itself is the strongest antagonist to analgesia.[45] Pain can exclude all other aspects of life, requiring only endurance until relief comes. Relief from pain need not mean loss of conscious awareness and alertness.

Most dying people know the truth, whether they are told or not. But their hope is taken away when they try to talk about reality and find family members engaging in avoidance. Hope is frequently confused with magical solutions. People sometimes say that they do not want to tell clients they are dying for fear of taking away their hope. Hope involves more reality than magic, though. Hope can be maintained right up to the moment of death; it does not mean taking death away but rather supporting the dying person to the end. With hope, clients can *live* until they die.[49] Humans cannot bear very much reality and often need a "day off";[49] thus intermittent periods of denial occur.

Aside from pain, loneliness, and abandonment, one of the things clients fear most about dying is the unknown. Death itself is *the* great unknown. Even though some clients have a strong religious belief in the life hereafter, the experience of making the transition from this life to the next is still unknown and frightening. Such fear of the unknown can extend and be generalized to the hospital and nursing procedures.

Mourning is not forgetting. It is untying each knot that holds persons, things, and memories to the self. Grief is a personal experience and a part of the matrix of humanity. Grieving has psychological, sociological, and somatic components. People need relatedness to one another to survive, to experience life, and to die. The dying person needs to be able to gradually withdraw his or her emotional investments in others.

Although each person's and family's experiences throughout the dying process are unique and vary in time and context, there are commonalities among all who face imminent personal death or the death of a loved one. The outcome criteria that follow reflect these shared experiences and their effective management.

1. Effective coping, by client and family, with the unknowns that accompany death. Evidence:
   a. Conversations between client and family about what the final days and hours will be like
   b. Conversations between client and family about spiritual beliefs and about existence beyond death
   c. Interactions between client and nurse related to the meaning of life and fears related to dying
2. A separation process that is beneficial for client and family. Evidence:
   a. Client's giving special mementos to individual family members
   b. Client's saying good-bye to family members individually
   c. Exchanges of verbal expressions of love between client and family
   d. Client's making out a will
   e. Discussion between client and spouse about how to tell the children about the death and how the children can participate in the funeral services
3. An alert, active, comfortable life for the client until death occurs. Evidence:
   a. No expressions of distress related to pain
   b. Communication with visitors (although client will increasingly become a listener—paying attention but making fewer comments)
   c. Watching television or reading alone
4. Grieving by client and family over their impending losses, and mutual consolation. Evidence:
   a. Talking with each other about their feelings
   b. Crying together
   c. Physically comforting each other (as by hugging)
   d. Being able to sit quietly and maintain physical contact for periods of time as the client's physical status deteriorates

Intervention

Intervention with the Client

The delivery of nursing care to dying people requires an attitude of attention and an atmosphere of security and caring. Clients experiencing the dying process have explained that they fear being abandoned while at the same time they feel distressed about being a burden to their families. As they confront the inevitability of death and physical deterioration, much of the effectiveness of nursing care is contingent upon the quality of the nurse-client relationship.

The focus of nursing during the dying process is not on "cure." It is on helping the client achieve and maintain the maximum quality of life possible. This includes encouraging clients to make decisions that effect their lives. It means providing dying people with a context within which it is safe and helpful to express feelings, describe what is happening to them, and articulate their needs. These people need opportunities to express their feelings, sort out the realistic outcomes from the unrealistic fears, understand and accept themselves and their families and friends, and accept the validity of their own feelings rather than judge themselves. The quality of the nurse-client relationship influences the development of a context within which these opportunities can occur. The core dimensions of the nurse-client relationship, the use of facilitative communication skills, and the nurse's acceptance of death as a part of life and the dying process as a stage of growth contribute to a sensitive and supportive context.

When loss of energy and physical deterioration are occurring, previously gratifying activities cannot be sustained. It is at this point that dying people may need help in structuring time in ways that they find satisfying. This may also be a time when they try to explore the meaning of their life and their death. The nurse's contribution is to listen to clients as they review their lives—their achievements, their successes and failures, their joys and sorrows—and to "be there" with them throughout this disclosure.

"RIGHT TO KNOW." Withholding of knowledge from one who is dying isolates the person from meaningful relationships with self, family, and others. Unless the truth is shared, much energy is consumed in "keeping the secret." The intention may be protection of the client from confronting imminent death. The outcome deprives the client of experiencing the dying process fully and precludes growth in the last stage of life. It also keeps the person in a form of "solitary confinement," deprived of authentic human relationships.

Nursing interventions are directed toward helping clients acquire information, process this information, and work through the feelings generated by the information.

When the diagnosis is made initially and when complications arise during the illness, the client has the right and the need to be told. This does not mean that the client will necessarily show evidence of *hearing*. Even if there has been direct and truthful communication, the client may act and speak in ways that deny the reality. However, the facts have been given, and the brain has recorded the message. When the client is able to cope with the message and its implications, it will be recalled in part, and then the client will seek confirmation of what is feared but known to be a possibility.

When the diagnosis is made initially, the medical treatment tends to generate optimism. The client is usually eager to talk, and there is a minimal need for defenses.[50] A client at this point is able to articulate his or her need to know; the client asks questions about what he or she is able to deal with. Open and honest answers to these questions lay the foundation for functional communication throughout the dying process. However, the client may not be able to handle all the implications of the condition; therefore, it is important to respond to what is asked and to find out how the client perceives and experiences this information before offering further elaboration.

Once a dying client has accepted the fact of dying, the issue of control over his or her remaining time can be faced. Clients have a basic human right to have a major voice in the decisions that are made regarding further treatment protocols, management of pain, and place of care. Clients must know what is happening to their physical being and what is projected to happen in the near future if they are to make informed decisions about how they will spend their final days on earth. The nurse can be useful as a facilitator for clients and families in their decision-making process.

If there have been open channels of communication and support, the client will continue to ask questions when the disease process has advanced. However, the questions are now different. The client may complain to friends or ancillary staff members but never ask the nurse or physician, who could give the correct information. Areas of communication that still exist focus on symptoms and remedies. Clients who were formerly open and direct exhibit a "loss of memory" for previously discussed facts and implications. Such clients are often compliant and seem to project a "nice person" image, which is a defense against fears of rejection and abandonment.[50] During this phase the nurse supports the denial and provides the desired information regarding the client's complaints. Patience, acceptance, and realistic reassurance may help the client to be less fearful of abandonment.

No single event, with the exception of death itself, has greater impact on the life of a family than being told that a member has a fatal illness. Honesty, frankness, and a kind, warm, supportive attitude may be more important than exactly what is said. Initially, much of what is told to a client and family is not remembered: it is too emotionally charged. The client's and family's education about what is occurring is a slow process of receiving information that is asked for; exploring thoughts, feelings, and perceptions; and clarifying misconceptions. Periodically the client and family may experience a "loss of memory" with regard to what they have been told. In some instances this is ignored by the nurse, particularly if it is not hindering the dying process or the mutual supportiveness of the family. But sometimes there is a need to facilitate recall. Periodically, clients and families need denial ("temporary memory loss") to escape from the emotional intensity of the grieving process.

When the disease process is irreversible, deterioration is evident, and as the time of death draws closer, fear, depression, a sense of loss, and loneliness predominate. These feelings are replaced by positive withdrawal and acceptance if an orderly, progressive separation from life and significant relationships has been occurring. These clients tend to become uncommunicative verbally but retain a need for continual support. They do not want to talk about death or dying but will explore the possibility that their death may have a meaningful purpose. Even though these clients do not express their anxieties or fears easily and tend to withdraw, it is essential that the nurse continue to communicate, sometimes with words and at other times with touch and presence.[50]

MANAGEMENT OF PAIN. Pain often occurs during the terminal stage of the disease process. The client experiences pain associated with obstruction, inflammation, bone destruction with infarction, infiltration or compression of nerves, infiltration or distension of body tissues, and tissue necrosis. This bodily pain may be compounded by social, emotional, and spiritual pain. Approaches used during the earlier stages may continue to be effective; however, the extent of the disease process and the acute psychic pain related to the loss of self may be too great to be managed using traditional approaches.[1]

The pain during the latter part of the dying process is often intolerable and unrelenting. The pain heightens anxiety, which in turn intensifies the pain. Thus, control of pain is essential if the client is to cope effectively and feel some degree of comfort.

At St. Christopher's Hospice, selective use of antidepressants, psychotropics, and nonbarbiturate sedatives has been found to be useful in alleviating the feelings that create psychological pain. The efficacy of these drugs, according to care givers, lies not in their pharmacological properties alone but in appropriate combinations and dosages offered in an atmosphere of genuine caring and concern for the client's comfort and well-being.[5] If alertness without pain can be provided for the client, the client will have a greater opportunity to participate in life and its remaining pleasures.[49]

Saunders[49] recommends anticipating pain for the client and stresses the importance of this. These clients must be monitored very closely for the early prodromal signs of pain; their patterns of relief and distress must be defined. If the nurse administers pain-relieving medications and institutes comfort measures before the pain has reached the client's conscious awareness, the client is provided with maximum relief continuously. In this way, the clients are not reminded of their dependence on the care giver, since they do not have to watch the clock or ask for pain relief. Addiction is not an important issue or concern in the care of the terminally ill. When pain relief is consistent and accompanied by sensitive care, tolerance and ever-increasing dosages do not seem to be a problem. Dosages are usually maintained at levels which permit the client periods of drowsiness and periods of alertness until the disease itself clouds the consciousness.

For some, bodily discomfort is overshadowed by emotional and spiritual pain related to depression, anxiety, grief, and the sense that life and death are meaningless and that one's life has been without purpose or benefit to self or others. Combined interpersonal, psychotherapeutic, and chemotherapeutic interventions can be successful in alleviating symptoms and promoting peace and calmness. Interpersonal interventions require the availability and accessibility of the staff and family. Empathic, active listening facilitates the expression of grief. "Thereness" sometimes involves implementing a comfort measure, and at other times sitting with the person in silence. Loneliness is painful, and providing times for extended, uninterrupted opportunities to talk decreases the sense of isolation and loneliness.

Care givers' beliefs can shape their assumptions about others; these assumptions must be validated before they are used in planning care. For example, care givers may assume that clients who do not complain of pain do not experience pain. Unvalidated, this assumption leads the nurse to conclude that a client who stoically does not complain of pain does not need to be assessed or treated for pain.

FEELINGS. The dying person experiences the broad spectrum of human emotion; this can be both rewarding and painful. The feelings which present the greatest problem to the client and care giver are fear, anger, anxiety, and depression. However, when the client is dying, these feelings on the part of the client and others are normal and to be expected. The anxiety and depression accompany a real and catastrophic situation and are not necessarily related to an underlying neurotic component. Therefore, the usual approach to working through these feelings—which is helpful when there is a neurotic basis—is not applicable. Moreover, the reality of the client's death and the absence of remedies generate feelings of inadequacy, helplessness, and insecurity in the nurse. However, the emotions the client experiences need not be overwhelming and can be resolved. Identification of the factors which are contributing to an intensification of the feelings associated with the normal stages of resolution and grieving is the first step toward intervention. Once these factors have been identified and labeled in the nurse-client relationship, joint problem solving offers the client an opportunity to master what has previously caused helplessness and hopelessness. The more the client is able to control and modify the environment, even indirectly, the more likely feelings of anxiety, depression, and anger will decrease.

Following are two examples of how dying clients' feelings can affect both themselves and their care givers:

> Ms. N., a hospitalized woman dying of cancer, has difficulty falling asleep at night. She watches television until the early morning hours and sleeps only a few hours, since the hospital routine requires her to be awake for early-morning care and breakfast. Fatigued and anxious about her condition, she feels depressed and helpless. If care givers help her find ways to control her environment—to eat, sleep, and participate in her care in a way that meets her individual needs—her anxiety and feelings of helplessness can be greatly reduced.

> Ms. P., a woman in the same predicament, lashes out at the staff angrily and has been labeled a "difficult patient." The staff avoids and isolates her. In response, she has withdrawn, and her feelings of anxiety, guilt, and abandonment have thus been intensified. This cycle of mutual withdrawal can be ended if her behavior is assessed within the environmental context and is seen as an expression of unmet needs.

Dependency on others may generate conflict and anger. The anger felt and expressed by the dying person activates fear of abandonment and guilt, which in turn fosters depression. Minimizing the client's perception of dependency and need to be dependent, while also maximizing the client's power to control what is happening, lessens the client's need for defenses and feelings of distress.

ALTERED BODY IMAGE. A client who has suffered an alteration of body image as a result of radical surgery or the ravages of disease experiences a crisis and must engage in the grieving process. Initially, when confronted with the reality of the alteration, the client will experience a period of denial, including a retreat from reality, and may have fantasies about his or her body and its functions in its earlier, healthy state. Some people may experience a temporary euphoria or may rationalize what has happened to them. With a healthy course of events, the client will eventually acknowledge the reality of the new image and redefine the self. This means cooperating with the goals that are set, the treatment plan, and the care given. The client's personal goals will be realistic. The crisis is successfully resolved if the client tries new coping mechanisms and sets out with a renewed sense of worth. It is unsuccessfully resolved if the client permanently tries to avoid reality, regresses in behavior, and withdraws from social contacts.

During the actual crisis of physical alteration, the client should be encouraged to mourn. The process includes facilitating acknowledgment and expressions of anger, rage, depression, and phantom pain.

The client should be encouraged to look at the dressing if surgery has been involved and to feel the stump if there was an amputation. This will help the client actualize the loss. The client will watch others' reactions closely; the nature of these reactions will influence the client's own perception and acceptance of the loss.

If the client exhibits denial, reinforcement and argumentation are neither useful nor therapeutic. When denial is present, it is a defense against more anxiety than the client feels able to cope with; it must not be shattered by another. Interventions which reassure the client, increasing self-esteem and self-acceptance, will in time diminish the need for such a defense. The client will then slowly and carefully begin to confront well-defined bits and pieces of reality. The client who copes successfully with these bits and pieces will be encouraged and motivated to venture further in acknowledging the loss.

SEXUALITY. Chemotherapy, the debilitating effects of radiation, the illness itself, and the emotional response to the illness and impending death interact to adversely affect sexuality. There is little in the literature on sexuality during the dying process, and the need for research is evident.

Some people with cancer lose sexual function early in the disease process as a consequence of surgical intervention or the disease itself. This physical and physiological impairment need not eliminate all sexual activity. The psychological impact of surgery and the quality and satisfaction of the person's preoperative sex life seem to have a major impact on sexual interest and activity. If the person chooses to live life to its fullest and maintain his or her lifestyle as much and as long as possible, then enjoyment and satisfaction can be derived from masturbation, petting, and exchange of affection.[51–53]

The dying client is a human being, with all the feelings that go with being human. Sexuality is a part of one's total identity, and the fact that clients may be dying does not reduce them to asexual beings. Consequently, it should be expected that dying clients may sometimes want to express themselves sexually. This expression may take the form of genital behavior, speech, or touch; it may be overt or covert. Its occurrence need not disturb nurses unless they are already uncomfortable with their own sexuality or sexual feelings.

Discussion of sexual issues should not be taboo when caring for dying people. These people need factual information about their capacity for sexual activity. Alternatives to the expression of sexuality must also be identified and explored. Inappropriate sexual behavior is minimized or eliminated if sex education and counseling are initiated early in the disease process and continued until satisfactory and comfortable adjustments and adaptations have been made.

HOPE. Although people differ in their need to find meaning in their lives and deaths, Frankl[54] noted that people who lost hope were doomed to premature death. Hope is a very personal experience and a mediating process which influences perception. Failure and success tend to be cumulative. These outcomes contribute to a schema which is a perceptual set, telling the person that he or she will succeed or fail in an endeavor. The nurse who cares for the client expressing hopelessness must direct activities toward building and evoking a hopeful schema. This includes emphasizing the client's strengths and intervening to desensitize the client to that which is feared and provokes anxiety. To accomplish this, the nurse must build a relationship in which the client has confidence that the nurse will consistently facilitate the satisfaction of needs. When the client has confidence in the nurse, the resulting feeling of security encourages risk-taking behavior. If goals are simple, attainable, and graduated, the client will build and strengthen the schema of hope as success is experienced. Success begets success. Clients' participation in defining and reaching goals in itself increases their sense of mastery, thus reducing anxiety and supporting movement toward goals. This reduction of anxiety, the activity, and the mastery all serve to diminish feelings of hopelessness.

Intervention with the Family

Sometimes, the family may wish to prevent the dying client from discovering the diagnosis and prognosis. In such a case, the family must be helped to understand why it is important for authentic, open communication to occur between the client and family members, and among family members. They need to see that if secrecy about the diagnosis and prognosis is allowed to prevail, it will interfere with the mutual support that can be derived from the sharing of feelings and experiences. Families must also be helped to recognize that people coping with the dying process at some point recognize their progressive deterioration and know they are dying. Mutually protective dynamics supported by family secrecy prevent opportunities for saying good-bye, resolving old misunderstandings, and forgiving past transgressions. These families need realistic reassurance that an open and honest relationship is important to all.

It is especially important for the family members to deal openly with unfinished business with their dying member. A useful way for people to focus on the issues that need resolution is to project ahead to the person's death, and to imagine attending the funeral services. It helps if one can think about all the things that should have been said or done while the dead person was still alive. These issues are the ones that family members should be encouraged to express with one another and the dying person now, while there is still time. Sometimes the most difficult thing for sons and daughters to do is tell dying parents directly that they love them, and even to embrace their dying parents, especially if this is not a usual way for them to express themselves. It seems that male family members especially need encouragement and support to express verbally and physically their tender feelings for one another. For example:

> One young father, who was very reticent about expressing his feelings, witnessed the death of his cancer-ridden son. It was only when the boy breathed his last that the father was able to take him in his arms and say, "I love you, son."

Initially, family members need support when talking to the dying person about issues that provoke their fears and generate anxiety. A nurse who listens empathically and explores fears, fantasies, and feelings will help family members understand what the dying person is experiencing, deal with their own problems, and support the client through the dying process.

Nurses caring for a dying person need to establish a relationship with the family. The grieving experienced by family members generates painful emotions. Family members are often at different points in the grieving process, and this may be a source of conflict among members. For example:

> In one family the youngest adult child, who had been the mother's "favorite," was the family member who brought gossip, humor, and fun to her visits with her dying mother. Both looked forward to the visits. The mother was alert, at times animated, and seemed to enjoy the visits. The spouse and three older offspring, who were more directly involved in the home care before hospitalization, were experiencing depression and a sense of loss. Their emotional pattern was dysynchronous with that of the youngest daughter. The mother vacillated between periods of depression and denial of her imminent death. The visits by the youngest provided temporary relief from her depression and were not experienced as dysynchronous. Conflict developed between the older depressed siblings and the youngest, who shared in her mother's temporary periods of denial.
>
> Nursing intervention was needed to help the family understand the basis for the conflict, and to accept each other and what each contributed to helping their loved one through her dying process. They also needed to recognize that the youngest had not shared their anticipatory grieving and would, when the mother died, need support when the full impact of the loss hit her.

Family members who mourn prematurely or who are overwhelmed by their feelings of inadequacy, helplessness, and hopelessness may withdraw from the dying person, leaving him or her isolated and abandoned. Some family members will visit less frequently, offering transparent excuses, while others will continue to visit faithfully but will tend to talk among themselves, excluding and even discussing the dying client as though he or she were not present. The nurse, who may initially feel anger toward the family in such instances, must work at understanding why the members are behaving in such a manner and must reach out to them to help them deal with the feelings generated by the situation. The members may need to learn how they can still communicate with and support the dying person by their presence. If the client's acceptance and consequent withdrawal are contributing to these dynamics, the family needs help in understanding this phenomenon and in finding ways to continue communicating care and support to the dying person.

Families need to know that anger, depression, guilt, and a sense of loss are normal and a part of grieving. Nurses need to be available to members throughout the dying process and to help them ventilate feelings appropriately.[55] In supporting the family, the nurse must intervene to help family members adapt to changes that have occurred and will occur with the client's death. These interventions need to assist members in redefining their roles and responsibilities, engaging in collaborative problem solving with other members, and accepting the death.

If the dying person was central to the family's pattern of communication in terms of disseminating information and bringing members together, the death may disorganize interactions and relationships among family members. Interventions that help family members begin to reorganize their communication patterns before the death, and to recognize the need for this reorganization, are necessary.

The client's physical deterioration and helplessness may generate helplessness, anxiety, and a need to be useful in family members. In such instances the nurse may enlist the help of family members rather than exclude them when giving physical care to the dying person. The family can help the nurse provide such care and comfort measures as bathing, turning, massaging, and feeding. This participation in the nursing care may help family members deal more effectively with their feelings. It gives them a sense of having done something for the person, which will help them in their own grieving after the client's death.

Evaluation

The effectiveness of nursing interventions is assessed using outcome criteria. Evidence that the outcomes have not been attained requires reassessment of needs and reexamination of the interventions and rationales. If outcome criteria have been satisfactorily attained and related needs met, then higher-order needs will emerge. These will call for assessment and subsequent reinitiation of the nursing process.

Ethical standards of behavior require that nurses allow clients to live in their own ways during the dying process rather than coerce them into a standard way of dying. Although some clients achieve an acceptance of death, people should not be forced to adopt any particular mode of behavior.

The nursing care plan presented in Table 45-3 illustrates how the components of the nursing process interact and how the evaluation process is accomplished using outcome criteria.

Table 45-3 Evaluation of Nursing Care

Assessment	Diagnosis	Outcome Criterion	Intervention	Evaluation
Client is uncommunicative with family members when they visit. Client feigns sleep when family visits. Client asks family members to leave because they interrupt her sleep. Client is sociable, talkative, and alert with nurses. Client is confined to bed and unable to perform self-care without considerable assistance because of physical limitations.	Discrepancy between interactions with family and with nurses related to impaired family communication.	Client will verbalize reason for discrepancy in behavior.	Explore the discrepancy in socializing and interacting with family and with nurses.	Client verbalizes anger toward family for putting her in a nursing home.
	Covert problematic anger toward family related to admission to nursing home.	Client will discuss how the decision was made.	Facilitate client's examination of how the decision was made.	Client talks about family discussions, in which she was included, that focused on (1) her need for nursing care 24 hours a day, (2) the fact that adult children are all working full-time and have several offspring each to support, (3) the financial constraints of each, and (4) lack of any other option.
		Client will discuss the reasons given by adult children and list objections to nursing home.	Encourage client to think about and talk about the reasons and her objections.	Client acknowledges that she did not object during the discussions. Client acknowledges the validity of the family's reasons, but feels abandoned. Client refuses to talk about nursing home.

(Continued.)

Table 45-3 Continued

Assessment	Diagnosis	Outcome Criterion	Intervention	Evaluation
	Covert problematic anger toward family related to admission to nursing home (continued).	Client will verbalize fears of rejection and abandonment, anger related to dependency on nurses, and sadness about dying.	Provide an environment in which client feels it is "safe" to talk about her fears, anger, and sadness.	Client talks about rejecting family because family rejected her. Client talks about missing her home and being able to visit family rather than having family visit her. Client cries about her situation, loneliness, and having to die.
		Client will share with family her feelings, fear of dying, and loneliness.	Encourage a discussion with family about feelings and fears.	Client discusses her feelings and fears with family. Family members are empathic and share their feelings. Mutual "I love you's" are exchanged.
		Client will cite one problem with nursing home and discuss possible solutions with nurse.	Explore how client could feel more comfortable and less dependent in nursing home.	

SUMMARY

This chapter has explored the factors that interact in the sequence of dying and death. The dying process was considered in terms of the environment, the nurse, the dying person, and the family; and the application of the nursing process to dying persons and their families was examined.

Significant patterns in the environment are the sociocultural mileu of death, including the "death system" of a culture; contexts of awareness of dying (closed, suspected, mutual pretense, and open); and settings in which dying and death take place (emergency rooms and trauma centers, general hospital units, special-care units, clients' own homes, nursing and convalescent homes, and hospices).

Patterns of interaction in the nurse include avoidance, sociocultural aspects, professionalization, attitudes and values, issues of authority and control, identification with dying clients, helplessness and hopelessness, and the "care-cure" conflict.

Patterns of interaction of dying persons include the clinical phases of dying (acute crisis, chronic living-dying phase, and terminal phase), and the responses identified by Kübler-Ross: initial shock and disbelief, denial, anger, bargaining, a sense of loss and depression, and acceptance.

Family patterns of interaction are influenced by the family's degree of awareness and by the nature of family relationships, particularly communication. Two important family patterns are the "emotional shock wave" and "anniversary reactions."

Dysynchronous patterns of interaction can be characterized as dysynchronous denial, anger, and depression; the giving-up–given-up complex; and dysynchronous patterns of pain.

Application of the nursing process to dying clients and their families provides a systematic way of delivering nursing care. *Assessment of the client* needs to address the physical, mental, and spiritual dimensions as they interact with the family and the environment; *assessment of the family* should include the family configuration, the position of the dying person in the family, and the family's overall level of adaptation to life; *assessment of the environment* is essential because the context of care is a major influence on the dying process. *Diagnosis* consists of formulations of problematic patterns that require nursing intervention. Problems of dying clients vary considerably and depend on the phase of the illness, the type of assistance needed, the amount of time involved, and the social context in which care is provided. *Outcome criteria* reflect the purposes of nursing care for dying clients: helping clients to live more comfortably until death, helping families to support dying members, and helping both clients and families to accept death. *Intervention with dying clients* is focused not on "cure" but rather on helping clients to achieve and maintain the maximum quality of life possible. Important aspects of intervention with clients are their "right to know"; the management of pain; clients' feelings and emotions, altered body image, and sexuality; and hope. *Intervention with families* is based on openness and support; nurses need to be available to family members throughout the dying process, to help them ventilate feelings appropriately, and to help them adapt to the changes associated with the client's death. *Evaluation* is based on the outcome criteria. Nurses need to allow clients to live in their own way during the dying process rather than coerce them into a "standard" way of dying.

REFERENCES

1. M. Rogers, *An Introduction to the Theoretical Basis of Nursing*, Davis, Philadelphia, 1970.
2. R. Kastenbaum and R. Aisenberg, *The Psychology of Death*, Springer, New York, 1972.
3. H. M. Tirad, trans., *Book of the Dead*, Oxford University Press, London, 1910.
4. W. Y. Evans-Wentz, trans., *The Tibetan Book of the Dead*, Oxford University Press, New York, 1960.
5. M. G. Netsky, "Dying in a System of 'Good Care': Case Report and Analysis," *Connecticut Medicine*, vol. 41, January 1977, pp. 33–36.
6. J. Howard and A. Strauss, *Humanizing Health Care*, Wiley, New York, 1975, pp. 293–303.
7. B. G. Glaser and A. L. Strauss, *Awareness of Dying*, Aldine, Chicago, 1965.
8. C. A. Garfield and R. O. Clark, "The SHANTI Project: A Community Model of Psychosocial Support for Patients and Families Facing Life-Threatening Illness," in C. A. Garfield, ed., *Psychosocial Care of the Dying Patient*, McGraw-Hill, New York, 1978, pp. 335–364.
9. Elise L. Lev, "An Elective Course in Hospice Nursing," *Oncology Nursing Forum*, vol. 8, Winter 1981, pp. 27–30.
10. Cicely Saunders, "The Management of Terminal Illness," *Hospital Medicine*, 1966, p. 225.
11. Florence S. Wald, Z. Foster, and H. J. Wald, "The Hospice Movement as a Health Care Reform," *Nursing Outlook*, vol. 16, March 1980, pp. 173–178.
12. Elise L. Lev, "Community Support for the Oncology Patient and Family," *Topics in Clinical Nursing*, vol. 7, April 1985, pp. 71–78.
13. "Standards of a Hospice Program of Care," unpublished paper presented to the Board of Directors of the National Hospice Organization, February 23, 1979, Washington, D.C.
14. Interview with Janice Casey, RN, M.S., Administrator, Hospice of Stamford, Connecticut; Director, National Hospice Organization; President, Hospice Council of Connecticut; July 12, 1985.
15. H. Feifel, *The Meaning of Death*, McGraw-Hill, New York, 1959.
16. H. Feifel, "The Function of Attitudes toward Death," *Death and Dying: Attitudes of Patient and Doctor*, Group for the Advancement of Psychiatry, vol. 5., October 1965.
17. J. C. Quint, "Awareness of Death and the Nurse's Composure," *Nursing Research*, vol. 15, Winter 1966, pp. 49–54.
18. M. Bowers et al., *Counseling to the Dying*, Nelson, New York, 1964.
19. B. G. Glaser and A. L. Strauss, "The Social Loss of Dying Patients," *American Journal of Nursing*, vol. 64, June 1964, pp. 119–121.
20. R. Kastenbaum, "Multiple Perspectives on a Geriatic Death Valley," *Community Mental Health Journal*, vol. 3, 1967, pp. 21–29.
21. S. M. Jourard, *The Transparent Self*, Van Nostrand, New York, 1971, pp. 183–188.
22. E. P. Stoller, "Effect of Experience on Nurses' Responses to Dying and Death in the Hospital Setting," *Nursing Research*, vol. 29, January-February 1980, pp. 35–38.

23. C. M. Gow and J. I. Williams, "Nurses' Attitude toward Death and Dying: A Causal Interpretation," *Social Science and Medicine,* vol. 11, 1977, pp. 191–198.
24. J. C. Norman, "The Effects of Death Education on the Value Clarification of Student Nurses and on Their Responses toward the Dying Patient," Ph.D. dissertation, George Peabody College for Teachers, Vanderbilt University, 1982.
25. M. Schrock and E. A. Swanson, "The Effect on Nursing Students of Direct-Care Experience with Death and Dying," *Nursing Forum,* vol. 20, 1981, pp. 213–219.
26. K. Hatano and K. Murata, "Factors Related to Nursing Students' Attitudes and Nursing Behaviors to Terminal Patients," *Kango Kenyu,* vol. 15, Summer 1982, pp. 420–426.
27. S. Rouslin, "Chronic Helpfulness: Maintenance or Intervention?" *Perspectives in Psychiatric Care,* vol. 1, 1963, pp. 25–28.
28. C. A. Garfield, "Elements of Psychosocial Oncology: Doctor-Patient Relationships in Terminal Illness," in C. A. Garfield, ed., *Psychosocial Care of the Dying Patient,* McGraw-Hill, New York, 1978, pp. 102–118.
29. E. M. Pattison, "The Living-Dying Process," in C. A. Garfield, ed., *Psychosocial Care of the Dying Patient,* McGraw-Hill, New York, 1978, pp. 133–168.
30. E. L. Lev, "Developing a Model for Teaching Chemotherapy of Hematologic Disorders," *Journal of the National Intravenous Therapy Association* 4:337–346 (Sept./Oct. 1981).
31. J. Q. Benoliel, "The Realities of Work," in *Humanizing Health Care,* op. cit., pp. 175–183.
32. A. D. Weisman, "Misgivings and Misconceptions in the Psychiatric Care of the Terminal Patient," *Psychiatry* 33:67–81 (1970).
33. Cicely Saunders, "Terminal Care," in C. A. Garfield, ed., *Psychosocial Care of the Dying Patient,* McGraw-Hill, New York, 1978, p. 22.
34. E. Kübler-Ross, *On Death and Dying,* Macmillan, New York, 1969.
35. R. Schultz and D. Aderman, "Clinical Research and the Stages of Dying," *Omega,* vol. 5, 1974, pp. 137–143.
36. A. D. Weisman, *On Dying and Denying,* Behavioral Publications, New York, 1972.
37. S. G. Klagsbrun, "Communications in the Treatment of Cancer," *American Journal of Nursing,* vol. 7, May 1971, pp. 944–948.
38. M. Bluebond-Lagner, *The Private Worlds of Dying Children,* Princeton University Press, Princeton, N.J., 1978.
39. B. Schoenberg, A. C. Carr, D. Peretz, and A. H. Kutscher, eds., *Psychosocial Aspects of Terminal Care,* Columbia University Press, New York, 1972, p. 194.
40. M. Bowen, "Family Reaction to Death," in M. Bowen, ed., *Family Therapy in Clinical Practice,* Aronson, New York, 1978, pp. 321–335.
41. A. R. Albin et al., "Childhood Leukemia," *New England Journal of Medicine,* vol. 280, February 1969, pp. 414–418.
42. Elise L. Lev, "An Activity Therapy Group with Children in an In-Patient Psychiatric Setting," *Psychiatric Quarterly,* vol. 55, 1983, pp. 55–64.
43. J. O. Cavenar, J. G. Spaulding, and E. B. Hammett, "Anniversary Reactions," *Psychosomatics,* vol. 17, 1976, p. 4.
44. G. Caplan, *Principles of Preventive Psychiatry,* Basic Books, New York, 1964.
45. M. McCaffrey, *Nursing Management of the Patient with Pain,* Lippincott, Philadelphia, 1979.
46. G. L. Engel, "A Life Setting Conducive to Illness: The Giving-Up–Given-Up Complex," *Bulletin of the Menninger Clinic,* vol. 32, 1968, pp. 355–365.
47. Cicely Saunders, "The Last Stages of Life," *American Journal of Nursing,* vol. 65, no. 3, 1965, pp. 70–75.
48. R. Melzack, *The Puzzle of Pain,* Basic Books, New York, 1973.
49. Cicely Saunders, "The Moment of Truth: Care of the Dying Person," in L. Pearson, ed., *Death and Dying,* The Press of Case Western Reserve University, Cleveland, 1969, pp. 49–78.
50. R. Abrams, "The Patient with Cancer—His Changing Pattern of Communication," *New England Journal of Medicine,* vol. 274, no. 16, February 1966, pp. 317–322.
51. M. Wasow, "Human Sexuality and Serious Illness," in C. A. Garfield, ed., *Psychosocial Care of the Dying Patient,* McGraw-Hill, New York, 1978, pp. 317–327.
52. M. G. Drellich, "Sex after Hysterectomy," *Medical Aspects of Human Sexuality,* vol. 1, no. 3, 1967, p. 62.
53. R. Amelar and L. Dubin, "Sexual Responses to Disease Processes," *Journal of Sex Research,* vol. 4, no. 4, 1968, pp. 257–264.
54. V. E. Frankl, *Man's Search for Meaning,* Beacon, Boston, 1959.
55. M. C. Kiely, "Bereavement: Royal Victoria Hospital Study Report," cassette 5-70 A, New Horizons, Montreal, September 29, 1983.

PART SEVEN
Community Environment

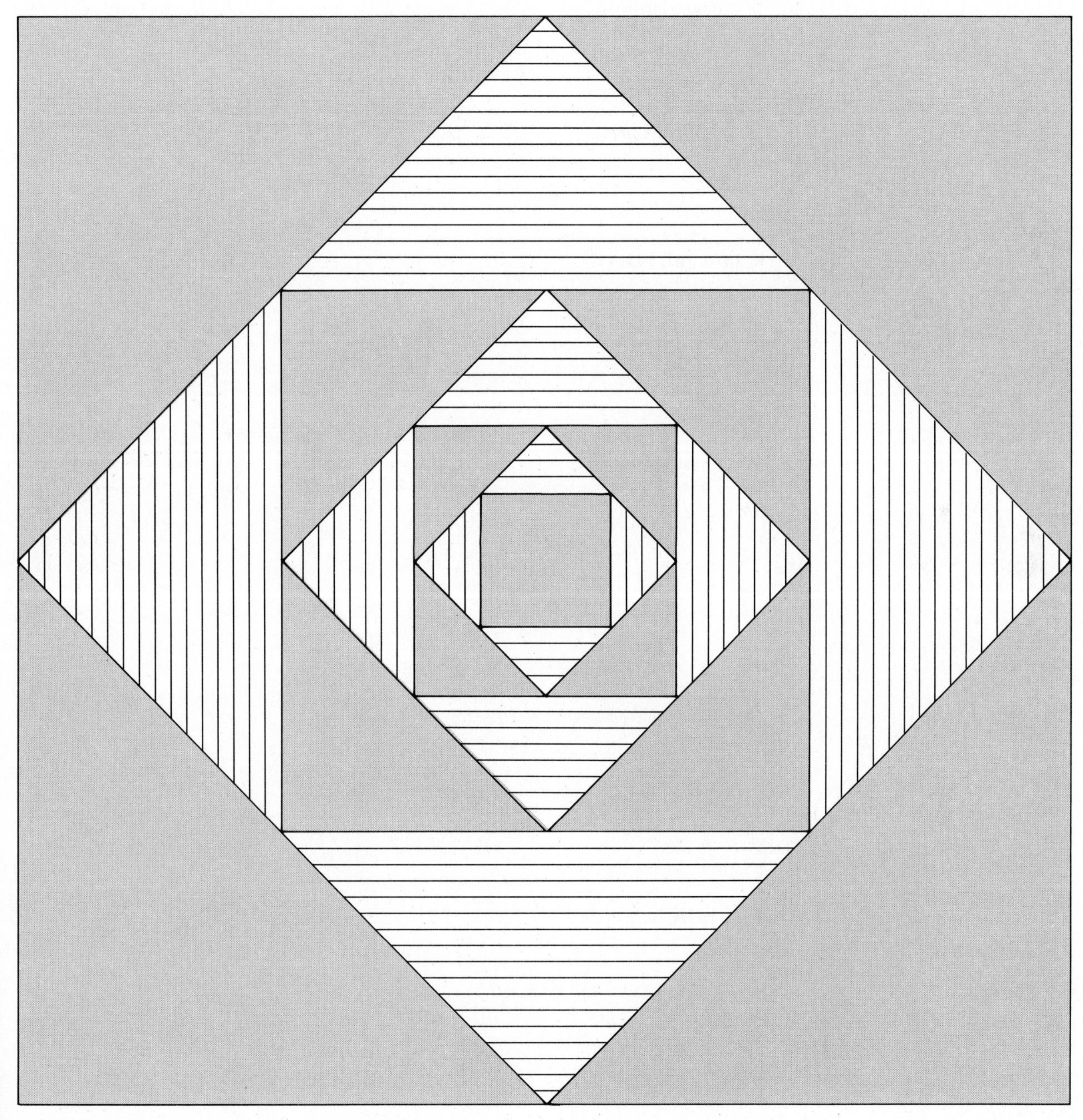

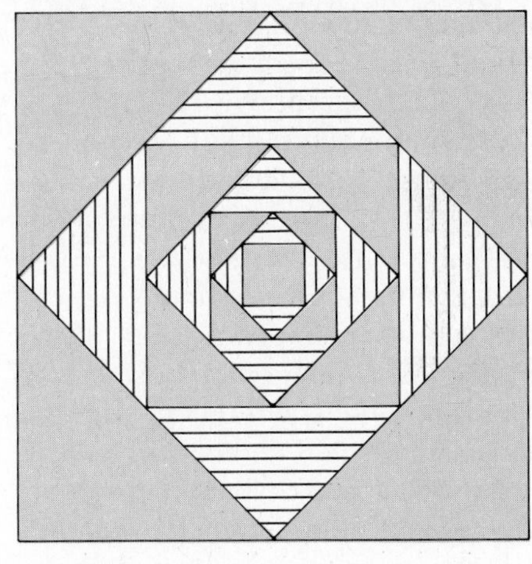

CHAPTER 46
Community

Judith Haber
Pamela Price Hoskins
Anita M. Leach
Barbara Flynn Sideleau

LEARNING OBJECTIVES

After studying this chapter, the student should be able to:

1. Elaborate on the definition of *community*.
2. Recognize the potential of the community as a setting for nursing practice.
3. Analyze interactions among persons and families who are at risk for mental problems in light of the community setting.

From the nursing viewpoint, *community* is both "client" and "setting." In this section, both ideas are developed. Individuals and families at risk may be served directly, or they may be approached by treating the community—changing the environment and thus the level of risk for individuals and families. The purpose of the chapter is to develop the concept of community within the conceptual framework. The definition of *community* will be expanded, and a framework related to community will be provided for Part Seven.

THE CONCEPT OF COMMUNITY

Community is defined as a group of people with common characteristics, location, or interests, living together within a larger society. Expansion of three phrases in this definition will assist students in understanding the meaning of *community.*

Group of People

The mental health professions are concerned with the human community, both as the unique individuals that make it up and as groups which share commonalities. Mental health is most effectively facilitated when each individual is seen in the context of a community. The group context is important; but words such as *conglomeration, assembly,* and *gathering* are not appropriate in the definition of a community. *Group* implies organization, roles, growth, development, and connections among people.

Common Characteristics, Location, or Interests

Connections among people may, conceptually, take three forms: (1) common characteristics, (2) common location, (3) common interests.

Common characteristics are factors that groups share, such as ethnicity, social status, and education. Common characteristics are the "mental dimension" of a community because they are factors which individuals and communities use to develop the concept of self or community.

Location refers to geographic locale; it is the "physical dimension" of a community. Not all communities have a geographic location.

Interests are connections that transcend the physical and mental dimensions; they are the "spiritual dimension" of a community. The spiritual dimension has a cognitive component—a conceptualization of the community—as well as a characteristic ambiance. (The "terrorist community," for instance, conceptualizes itself as people who will change the world, and its ambiance is rage.)

The community is the context within which individuals and families pursue the business of living. The community is the environment with the fewest restrictions on personal choice; however, it does have norms and laws to which individuals and families are expected to adhere. The community (rather than the hospital) is considered the ideal environment for treatment of any health problem as long as the resources needed for treatment are available. Since psychiatric–mental health nurses require very little equipment and few resources to provide services, the community is usually the best setting for mental health care, and this is true whether the client is an individual or a family. (When the client is community, it might be said that the community cannot really be considered the "ideal" or "best" setting but must be thought of as the "only" setting, since there is, of course, no way to hospitalize a community. However, communities sometimes become ghettoized, and that is a form of institutionalization. For a community, therefore, the ideal treatment setting would be the larger society.)

The community offers freedom for nurses to practice and freedom for clients to choose new ways to function; this creates a potential for healing in the community that has only begun to be explored.

Living Together within a Larger Society

The community, which is the environment of individuals and families, is itself part of a larger environment: the society. A community influences and is influenced by society. Growth and development, resources, and attainment of goals are influenced, and to some extent determined, by the larger society. The community interacts as a whole with the society, whether the community is a city, an ideological group, or a group with common characteristics.

RATIONALE FOR THE ORGANIZATION OF PART SEVEN

Part Seven consists of eight chapters dealing with individuals and families who have potential or actual mental health problems and who are treated for those problems in the community setting. The mental health problems dealt with in these chapters have such an intense impact that they are considered community problems.

The chapters may be thought of in terms of promotion, maintenance, restoration, and rehabilitation of health—the goals of nursing. Chapter 47 deals with promotion and maintenance of health in childbearing and child-rearing families. Chapter 48 deals with the characteristics of high-risk families, and Chapter 49 with maintenance and restoration of health of children in high-risk families. Chapter 50 explores the rehabilitative interventions that nurses use with children who have developed severely dysynchronous patterns of interaction with their environments. Chapter 51 and 52 deal with two forms of violence in the community: Chapter 51 with abusive families, and Chapter 52 with rape. Chapter 53 explores the care of the chronically mentally ill in the community. Chapter 54 focuses on the promotion and maintenance of health of the elderly in the community. Taken as a whole, these eight chapters develop a comprehensive nursing approach to individuals and families who are at risk for mental health problems and who are assisted in the community.

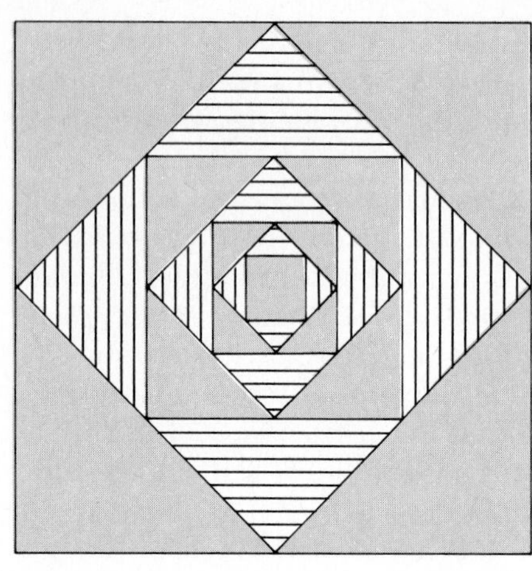

CHAPTER 47
Promotion of Mental Health in Childbearing and Child-Rearing Families

Ann Bello
Alice Marie Obrig

LEARNING OBJECTIVES

After studying this chapter, the student should be able to:

1. Describe the options available to an individual or couple in the childbearing years with regard to parenthood.
2. Describe the common assessment factors for individuals in the childbearing years.
3. Discuss the basis for evaluating nursing intervention with couples who have decided not to become parents.
4. List the emotional tasks confronting the childbearing and child-rearing family.
5. Describe the nursing process in the promotion of mental health in the childbearing and child-rearing cycle.
6. Formulate a plan of nursing intervention to promote mental health in the childbearing and child-rearing cycle.

The nursing profession, regardless of the work setting, is committed to the concepts of *promotion of health* and *primary prevention.* In families, the focus of primary prevention is promotion of health and intervention before dysfunctional behavior develops. Promotion of health and primary prevention begin with the childbearing and child-rearing cycle, and the family provides a natural focus for nurses in a variety of in- and outpatient settings. Nursing intervention is directed toward promoting mental health by expanding the family's knowledge base, exploring feelings, providing anticipatory guidance, and teaching and reinforcing decision-making skills. Such intervention will enhance the family's ability to cope with situational and maturational challenges. The purpose of this chapter is to explore common issues and decisions that are encountered in families during the childbearing and child-rearing years.

ASSESSMENT OF FAMILIES IN THE CHILDBEARING YEARS

Common Factors

The nurse can identify several factors that are common to various situational and maturational crises of the childbearing years:

1. Knowledge base about sex, contraception, conception, and parenting
   a. Information about physiological processes
   b. Information about potential impact of specific procedures
   c. Information about options and resources in specific areas
2. Feelings associated with sex, contraception, conception, and parenting
   a. Role of spiritual beliefs in the life of the couple
   b. Family influences
   c. Emotions associated with sex, contraception, conception, and parenting
3. Factors influencing the decision-making process relating to sex, contraception, conception, and parenting
   a. Reasons for decision
   b. Level of agreement or conflict
   c. Congruence of motivation and commitment
   d. Lifestyle
   e. Availability of extended family, peer, and community support systems
   f. Input from and influence of extended family and peer group
   g. Current communication patterns
   h. Health factors
   i. Division of power, roles, and responsibility
   j. Individual goals, identity, and self-worth
   k. Current practices

Assessment of these factors will enable the nurse to identify the strengths and weaknesses of both individuals and marital units. The nursing diagnosis and nursing intervention will be based on this assessment.

Much nursing intervention in the childbearing family is aimed at primary prevention, that is, anticipating the kinds of problems that are likely to arise and providing the sort of guidance and support that will help the family avoid problems.

Nursing Ethics

A prerequisite for application of the assessment factors is clarity on the part of the nurses about their own strongly held personal ethical or religious beliefs. Lack of such clarity may lead to inaccurate assessment or ineffective intervention.

In addition, the nurse needs to maintain clear boundary definitions that will allow the client to pursue goals which may be unacceptable to the nurse. This is especially important in enhancing the problem-solving abilities of emerging families who are making critical decisions in such controversial areas as contraception, divorce, abortion, artificial insemination, and sterilization. Nurses should develop a referral system for clients whose decisions they cannot support.

In order to achieve clarity, nurses can imagine situations which may occur and think about how they would feel. They may also need to attend value clarification workshops in order to develop a better understanding of their own values.

Before accepting employment, nurses will also want to be aware of the operational beliefs of the setting in which they will work. It is important for the beliefs of the institution and the individual to be compatible. Nurses will want to assess their compatibility with the setting before accepting a job (see Chapter 9).

SYNCHRONOUS AND DYSYNCHRONOUS HEALTH PATTERNS

Deciding Whether or Not to Become a Parent

Having passed through the developmental stages of unattached young adulthood and beginning a marriage, a couple will next face the major decision of whether or not to become parents and, if so, when. Figure 47-1 indicates the choices, or options, available. Before making a decision, the couple must assess their resources, their goals, and the lifestyle they hope to have in the future. Resources include money, support systems, current health status, technologies available to help people become parents, and reasons for wanting a child.

An initial decision *not* to have a child is subject to revision as long as the capacity to reproduce is present or acquiring children through adoption or other sources remains a viable option; changes in family circumstances may alter an initial decision. An initial decision to *have* a child may also be revised—before a child is conceived, of course; and in some cases after conception (see the section below on therapeutic abortion) and even after birth (see the section on placement for adoption). Again, changes in circumstances may make it necessary to reconsider an initial decision.

Common assessment factors relating to the decision to have or not have children are identified in Table 47-1 as they apply to sex, contraception, and sterilization.

Deciding Not to Become a Parent

Postponement of Parenthood

Among reasons for deferring childbearing are the following: fears of pregnancy, labor, and delivery; fears of parental responsibility; and disagreement when one partner wants a child and the other does not. Any one or more of the resources needed for responsible parenthood may simply not be available at the time of the decision. For example, a couple may lack money or housing, may be in school, or may be pursuing challenging careers; they may therefore choose to defer childbearing until they have achieved their current objectives. When couples decide to postpone parenthood, several options are available to them.

CONTRACEPTION. When a couple desire contraception (defined as nonsurgical prevention of conception), the question is where to obtain it. The facility they need may be their physician's office or a hospital clinic. Or they may prefer a freestanding facility such as a family planning clinic.

The role of the nurse in these facilities involves assessing the knowledge and attitudes of the couple, helping them to decide on the best method, helping them to get the knowledge and practice they need to use their chosen method effectively, providing regular checkups, and serving as a resource for answers to questions.

To do this, nurses must be clear about their own feelings. For example, if a nurse believed that contraception was wrong or unhealthy, it would

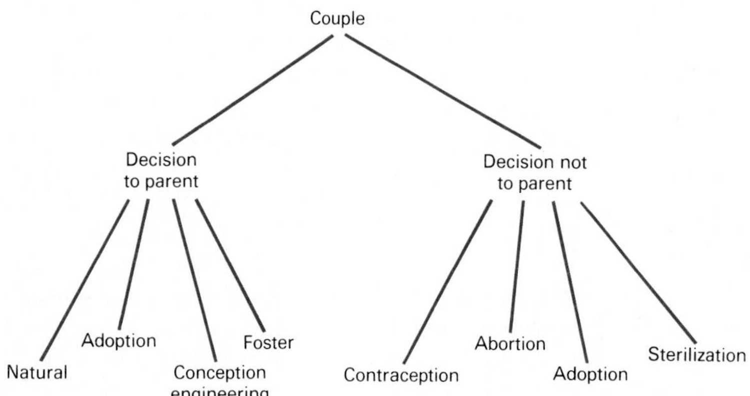

Figure 47-1 Parenting.
Choices regarding parenting available to a couple.

Table 47-1 Sex, Contraception, and Sterilization

Assessment	Assessment Data	Diagnosis	Intervention
		Sex: Knowledge base	
Knowledge about sexual expression: What do you see as the purpose of sex?	1. Wife and husband see sex as pleasurable, a way of having children, a way of feeling close.	1. No problem	
	2. Sex is seen only as a means of procreation, not as pleasurable.	2. Dysfunctional sexual expression related to knowledge gap	Identify gaps in knowledge base about sexuality and sexual activity.
Knowledge about sexual arousal: What sexual arousal techniques for men and women do you each know about? What kinds of positions can people take during intercourse?	3. Both are able to identify and use a wide variety of arousal techniques and positions.	3. No problem	Clarify misconceptions, myths, and stereotypes about sex.
	4. One or both view common arousal techniques as deviant. Couple have divergent views on arousal techniques or on normal positions.	4. Constricted sexual activity related to misconceptions, myths, and unclarified values about sex	Provide factual information about sexual activity and sexuality.
Knowledge about sexual response cycles: What do you both know about the differences between the male and female sexual response cycles?	5. Couple identify and accommodate to differences in their sexual response cycles.	5. No problem	
	6. One or both cannot describe what happens physiologically during sexual activity.	6. Dysfunctional mutuality related to lack of understanding of differences in sexual response cycle	Describe the male and female response cycles. Use a variety of media appropriate to the couple's learning style (for example, films, pamphlets, books, magazines, charts).
		Sex: Feelings about sex	
Spiritual feelings about sex: What has your religion taught each of you about sex?	7. Both partners' religious teachings have facilitated responsible decision making about sex.	7. No problem	
	8. One or both partners' religious teachings have emphasized sin, chastity, and procreation.	8. Inhibited sexual pleasure associated with misconceptions about religious teachings	Identify problematic emotional responses to sexual activity and sexuality. Identify source of problematic feelings.
Feelings about sex—family influence: How did both of your families deal with sex education and your sexuality when you were adolescents?	9. Both partners had open communication with their parents about sex information and clarification of values.	9. No problem	
	10. Sex was never talked about; labeled "dirty." No sex education by parents. Family history of illegitimacy.	10. Impairment of sexual enjoyment related to toxicity of sex as a family issue	Explore reasons for family messages about sexual activity and sexuality.

(Continued.)

Table 47-1 Continued

Assessment	Assessment Data	Diagnosis	Intervention
	Sex: Feelings about sex		
Emotions associated with sexual activity: How do you each feel about having sexual relations?	11. Sex is perceived as enjoyable, exciting, and fun. Couple recognize that both sexual partners have rights and responsibilities.	11. No problem	
	12. Sex is an obligation, dirty, and painful.	12. Distaste for sexual activity related to failure to accept sex as a normal human function	Encourage verbalization about inhibiting emotions and preconceptions, as a way of desensitizing the couple. Facilitate open communication about giving and receiving pleasure. Communicate that fun and playfulness are part of sexual activity. Help couple to clarify their values about the purpose of sexual activity in their relationship. Clarify couple's misconceptions about sexual needs.
	Sex: Decision making		
Decision-making process—division of power roles and responsibility: How do you two decide who initiates sexual activity? How does each of you know when your partner wants to have sex?	13. Either person is free to initiate sexual activity.	13. No problem	
	14. Disagreement about who can initiate sexual activity.	14. Role conflict related to misconceptions about the mutuality of sexual expression	Provide information about the mutuality of sexual expression. Identify whether there is a rigid role structure in relation to sexual activity. Explore values and attitudes that support the role structure around sex.
Level of agreement or conflict: To what extent do you two agree or disagree about innovative approaches to sex? Which of you would be more open about voicing disagreement? How easy is it for each of you to discuss your individual sexual needs with your spouse?	15. Each person feels free to state thoughts and feelings even when they are not congruent with partner's. Couple are willing to discuss sexual needs and innovative approaches.	15. No problem	
	16. Husband and wife are hesitant to voice ideas because of potential conflict. Unable to discuss sexual needs with one another.	16. Impaired communication related to conflicting thoughts and feelings.	Explore both partners' thoughts and feelings about what would happen if they changed their sexual activity pattern. Talk about variations in sexual activity; support couple's desire to try variations.

(Continued.)

Table 47-1 Continued

Assessment	Assessment Data	Diagnosis	Intervention
	Contraception: Knowledge base		
Knowledge about contraception and fertility: What does each of you know about ways to prevent pregnancy?	17. Both understand about the menstrual cycle and fertile periods.	17. No problem	
	18. Couple does not understand about fertile period; for example, one or both believe a woman is fertile only the day she ovulates and that sperm can impregnate only during intercourse.	18. Knowledge gap related to ambivalence about pregnancy	Identify gaps in knowledge base about contraception. Provide factual information about contraception: risks, benefits, and safe use.
Knowledge about contraceptive devices (male and female): How can conception be prevented most effectively?	19. Both identify a variety of reliable contraceptive devices and understand risks and benefits of each.	19. No problem	
	20. Couple do not know about effective contraceptive devices—for example, can identify only one method of contraception, coitus interruptus (which is unreliable).	20. Ignorance about contraceptive methods related to shyness in initiating discussion	Initiate discussion about methods of contraception. Provide hands-on opportunities to examine contraceptive devices. Use media (films, books, pamphlets, and charts) to facilitate learning about selected method. Identify problems of manual dexterity in use of contraceptive device. Give feedback about couple's efforts to use contraceptive methods and about effects on their sexual relationship.
	Contraception: Feelings about contraception		
Spiritual feelings about contraception: What does your religion teach about contraception?	21. Religion has no proscriptions about contraception, therefore, no conflict; or despite religious proscription, couple experience no conflict.	21. No problem	
	22. Conflict of conscience about any method besides natural planning; frustrations caused by use of natural planning method.	22. Decision-making conflict related to frustration about prescribed religious teachings about family planning	Identify problematic religious influences in relation to contraception. Identify the source of problematic feelings—for example, misconceptions about religious teachings and family messages.

(Continued.)

Table 47-1 Continued

Assessment	Assessment Data	Diagnosis	Intervention
	Contraception: Feelings about contraception		
Influences of family of origin: What have your families said about contraception?	23. Both families are open about discussing contraceptive alternatives.	23. No problem	
	24. One or both families do not believe in or use contraception; one or both have many children.	24. Sexual abstinence related to conflict about family messages about the importance of having a large family	Explore reasons for family messages about contraception—for example, family religious beliefs, values about family size, importance of children to the life of the family.
Personal emotions about contraception: How do you feel about using the pill, IUD, diaphragm?	25. Couple have clear preference for one method; are happy with that and have no contraindications.	25. No problem	
	26. One or both fear the pill and IUD and have distaste concerning insertion of diaphragm; or preferred method is contraindicated—for example, woman wants the pill but has a history of cancer.	26. Inhibitions about use of contraceptive methods other than the pill associated with distaste about touching genital area	Facilitate verbalization of feelings about conflicts regarding use of contraception. Explore fears and fantasies about use of various contraceptives. Explore acceptable options for contraception. Recommend use of mirror to view genitalia as a way of facilitating knowlege about body and desensitizing inhibitions related to the use of contraceptive devices.
	Contraception: Decision making		
Decision-making process—reasons for decision to use contraception: Why have you chosen contraception? Do you both clearly understand why you made this decision?	27. Both wife and husband clearly articulate rational reasons for their decision.	27. No problem	
	28. Decision made only on basis of feelings or recommendation of friend. Couple do not use their chosen contraceptive method as indicated, or they use an unreliable method.	28. Misuse of contraceptive method related to misinformation	Identify factors that influence the decision-making process in the relationship.

(Continued.)

Table 47-1 Continued

Assessment	Assessment Data	Diagnosis	Intervention
	Contraception: Decision making		
Level of agreement or conflict: Do you agree about the necessity for use of contraception? Do you agree about using this particular method? Are you using it every time you have sex? How successful do you see yourselves being in terms of long-term commitment to this method?	29. Both partners highly committed.	29. No problem	
	30. One or both partners fail to use the chosen method consistently—for example, wife forgets to take the pill.	30. Unconscious failure to use effective contraception related to unrecognized and uncommunicated desire for pregnancy	Encourage couple to describe how they made a previous decision about sexual activity. Help each to verbalize what he or she sees as a block to joint decision making about the use of contraception.
Division of power, roles, and responsibility: Who is responsible for using the chosen method of contraception? Does your lifestyle (for example, lack of privacy, low income) limit your choice of contraceptives?	31. Mutual agreement about responsibility for current method.	31. No problem	
	32. Wife or husband abdicates responsibility and refuses to talk about responsibility for contraception.	32. Power conflict about responsibility for contraception, related to passive resistance of one partner	Guide couple through a systematic decision-making process about responsibility for contraception and choice of method.
Health factors: Do you have health problems which limit your contraceptive options? Aesthetic problems?	33. Both are in good health and do not place aesthetic limits on contraceptive options.	33. No problem	
	34. Options limited: Varicose veins prevent use of the pill. PID precludes use of IUD. Husband complains that condoms decrease sensitivity. One or both object that diaphragm inhibits spontaneity.	34. Limited contraceptive options related to health and aesthetic problems	If health or aesthetic problems result in a change of contraceptive from original choice, explore repercussions for family.
	Sterilization: Knowledge base		
Knowledge about sterilization: What do you know about methods of sterilization for males and females? What are the risks and benefits?	35. Couple have information about options, procedures, risks, benefits, impact, and irreversibility of sterilization procedures for both male and female.	35. No problem	
	36. Couple lack information that would enable them to make a knowledgeable decision and are unable to formulate questions to acquire needed information.	36. Knowledge deficit about male and female sterilization options related to lack of information	Identify gaps in knowledge about sterilization. Provide needed information in lay language; use teaching materials such as films, charts, and reading materials.

(Continued.)

Table 47-1 Continued

Assessment	Assessment Data	Diagnosis	Intervention
	Sterilization: Knowledge base		
Knowledge about resources for sterilization: Do you know about facilities and services for sterilization? Do you know how to handle the costs involved?	37. Couple know about available services and have health insurance or Medicaid coverage.	37. No problem	
	38. Couple do not know how to locate agencies that provide these services; do not have the needed financial resources.	38. Confusion about where to seek sterilization related to knowledge deficit about services and costs	Provide information about agencies, costs involved, and forms of third-party payment.
	Sterilization: Feelings about sterilization		
Spiritual feelings about sterilization: How do your religious beliefs influence your feelings about sterilization?	39. Couple's beliefs and practices are not in conflict with sterilization.	39. No problem	
	40. Religious teachings of one or both define sterilization as sinful, generating guilt and anxiety or marital conflict.	40. Ambivalence about seeking sterilization related to conflict of conscience	Identify factors that generate feelings of guilt, anxiety, anger, or depression. Encourage verbalization of problematic feelings about sterilization.
Family influence: How do your families feel about sterilization?	41. Families accept sterilization as a safe and pragmatic way to prevent unwanted pregnancies.	41. No problem	
	42. One or both families disapprove of sterilization because they believe it alters sexuality.	42. Reluctance to be sterilized related to family fears about altered sexual desire and performance	Help both partners to clarify their fears and fantasies about the effect of sterilization on sexuality. Acknowledge clients' right to have their own feelings and beliefs about sterilization.
Emotions about sterilization in relation to childbearing potential: What are your feelings about undergoing an irreversible sterilization procedure? How intense are your feelings?	43. Both partners express feelings of relief that potential for unwanted pregnancies will be eliminated.	43. No problem	
	44. One or both have intense ambivalence about termination of childbearing potential.	44. Refusal to be sterilized related to ambivalence about ending childbearing capacity	Encourage verbalization of feelings about sterilization. Identify source of intense feelings.

(Continued.)

Table 47-1 Continued

Assessment	Assessment Data	Diagnosis	Intervention
	Sterilization: Decision making		
Decision-making process—reasons for choosing sterilization: Have you considered options other than sterilization? What circumstances led you to consider sterilization (for example, age, finances, genetics, health)?	45. Couple have weighed pros and cons of sterilization and made a rational decision.	45. No problem	
	46. Anxiety about potential unwanted pregnancy has blocked awareness and consideration of other options.	46. Impaired decision-making ability related to fear of unwanted pregnancy	Identify factors that influence choice of sterilization. Identify factors that block realistic exploration of options. Encourage exploration of factors that block realistic decision making. Encourage use of resource people outside the family, if indicated.
Congruence of agreement: Do you both agree about the decision to undergo sterilization?	47. Open discussion of sterilization between spouses leading to agreement about the benefits of either vasectomy or tubal ligation.	47. No problem	
	48. Disagreement about which partner is to be sterilized, resulting in blocked communication and lack of decision making.	48. Failure to arrive at decision for or against sterilization related to conflict in values	Help each client to identify his or her own position on the decision. Identify health factors that influence the decision.
Family and peer group input and influence: Have your family's or friends' values about sterilization influenced your decision?	49. Family's and peer group's values support decision.	49. No problem	
	50. Family's or peer group's values conflict with decision.	50. Postponement of decision related to conflict of values	Guide clients through a systematic decision-making process.
Current communication patterns: Whom have you both talked to about this decision?	51. Couple have discussed the decision together and come to mutual agreement.	51. No problem	
	52. One or both have discussed the decision with an unsupportive third person.	52. Decision against sterilization related to fears generated by an unsupportive third person	Identify ways of working through intense feelings that the couple have found helpful in the past.
Health factors: Have health factors influenced your decision to undergo sterilization?	53. Both are in excellent health; or one partner's health problem supports need for procedure.	53. No problem	
	54. Health of one partner seen as reason for procedure when no medical indication exists.	54. Guilt feelings in one partner related to factitious health complaints by the other	Recommend postdecision counseling.

be difficult to assist others in a positive way. The nurse might need to refer the couple to other helpers.

Having resolved their own feelings, nurses are then in a position to assess, diagnose, and intervene in the couple's behalf. Assessment factors for decision making in contraception are outlined in Table 47-1.

While nurses will need to look at each assessment factor individually, they also need to look at the total picture to arrive at the final diagnosis. The more agreement there is among the assessment data, the surer the nurse will be in formulating the diagnosis.

STERILIZATION. For the couple who have completed their family, who have decided against children, or who face a high risk of having a genetically damaged child, sterilization (surgical contraception) may be the solution. For families who elect sterilization, the current options are vasectomy, tubal ligation, and hysterectomy. Recent developments in laparoscopy have made tubal ligation easier and the hospital stay shorter; in most cases it may be 12 hours or less. Sterilization is still considered a permanent procedure because only a small percentage of the reversals of vasectomies and tubal ligations result in a viable infant.

Any elective alteration of a person's own body is certain to have a psychological impact. Therefore, sterilization should be discussed by a couple over a period of time in order to be sure that its effects on their relationship will be positive. Possible changes which sterilization and the absence of the option to have children may bring to the family should be assessed. Table 47-1 summarizes the areas which should be considered.

Before beginning to assess the family, nurses need to clarify their own beliefs and be sure their personal knowledge is up to date. Nurses themselves need to go through the same list of assessment factors as the family in order to clarify their feelings.

Problem Pregnancies

A couple faced with an unwanted pregnancy, a pregnancy in which there is a health problem that endangers the life of the mother, or a pregnancy in which the fetus is found to be defective must decide whether to have the child. Modern science and societal changes have given them the options to avoid parenthood at later stages than was possible in past generations. The options—abortion, adoption, or keeping a baby—are often confusing because of the strong feelings and values associated with childbearing and child rearing. The confusion has increased in recent years because of the debates between prolife and prochoice segments of the population. Nurses may find themselves experiencing the same confused feelings as clients. These feelings arise from conflicts between societal values and support, religious values and beliefs, and emotional needs or basic parental instincts.

Table 47-2 summarizes the assessment factors which are involved in the decision after conception has occurred.

Table 47-2 Unwanted Pregnancy

Assessment	Assessment Data	Diagnosis	Intervention
	Knowledge base		
Knowledge about options: Do you know what your options are regarding this pregnancy?	1. Aware of options at given stage of pregnancy.	1. No problem	
1st or early 2d trimester abortion Giving baby up for adoption Keeping baby	2. Lacks knowledge of options. Lacks adequate information about procedure, risks, benefits, and postprocedure physical signs and symptoms.	2. Indecision related to lack of information	Identify gaps in knowledge base about dealing with problem pregnancies. Identify options for dealing with problem pregnancies: adoption, abortion, single parenting. Identify resources for dealing with problem pregnancies.

(Continued.)

Table 47-2 Continued

Assessment	Assessment Data	Diagnosis	Intervention
		Knowledge base	
Knowledge about methods of terminating a pregnancy: What do you know about Methods of terminating pregnancy? Timing of each approach? Risks and benefits of each procedure? Usual postprocedure physical signs and symptoms and potential complications?	3. Aware of options at given stage of pregnancy.	3. No problem	
	4. Lacks realistic information about options available at given stage of pregnancy. Lacks adequate information about procedure, risks, benefits, and postprocedure physical signs and symptoms.	4. Indecision related to lack of information	Identify methods for terminating a problem pregnancy. Clarify misconceptions about abortion procedures. Describe risks and benefits of abortion procedures. Describe the postprocedure physical signs, symptoms, potential complications.
Knowledge about resources: What do you know about community resources for adoption, abortion, or counseling? The costs involved?	5. Has identified services available and has adequate health insurance to cover fees.	5. No problem	
	6. Local services that are available are beyond the financial reach of the person.	6. Indecision about choice of options related to lack of knowledge about services and their cost	Encourage client to ask questions. Provide information about community resources and services. Provide postdecision information on contraception.
		Feelings	
Spiritual feelings about a problem pregnancy: How much do your religious beliefs influence the way you feel about this pregnancy?	7. Religious beliefs do not influence feelings about this pregnancy, nor influence direction of decision making.	7. No problem	
	8. Religious beliefs lead to feelings of guilt about not wanting to continue this pregnancy.	8. Desire to terminate pregnancy, accompanied by guilt related to religious beliefs	Encourage identification of feelings and description of them in a concrete way. Encourage exploration of the source of the feelings. Be nonjudgmental.
Influence of family of origin: How does your family value children? To what extent do your family's views about completing or terminating a pregnancy influence the feelings you are experiencing right now?	9. Family views about children and pregnancy do not pervasively influence feelings about this pregnancy; family supports decision.	9. No problem	
	10. Family values conflict with feelings about this pregnancy and result in a strong feeling of ambivalence; family pressures for continuance or discontinuance of the pregnancy.	10. Ambivalence related to conflict about family values	Explore feelings and values that are interfering with decision making.

(Continued.)

Table 47-2 Continued

Assessment	Assessment Data	Diagnosis	Intervention
		Feelings	
Emotions about this pregnancy: On a scale of 1 to 10 (1 is mild, 10 is very strong), how would you rate your feelings of apprehension about continuing or terminating the pregnancy? What do you think will happen to your feelings after you make a decision?	11. Mild apprehension about making a final decision but no strong feelings about the outcome of the decision.	11. No problem	
	12. Intense anxiety, guilt, or depression because no option is seen as satisfactory.	12. Immobilized decision making related to strong feelings	Teach relaxation exercises. Reinforce importance of postdecision counseling (postabortion or postadoption). Identify ways of working through intense feelings that the client has found helpful in the past.
		Decision making	
Reasons for decision: What reasons do you have for your decision? What options have you considered? What circumstances led you to consider having an abortion? Continuing the pregnancy? Giving the baby up for adoption?	13. Reasons are rational; has weighed most benefits for each available option.	13. No problem	
	14. Reasons are constantly changing, or reason is outside pressure; unable to logically organize and examine pros and cons for each option.	14. Failure to resolve decision-making process related to inability to logically analyze options	Identify factors that influence the choice of options. Guide client through a systematic decision-making process.
Availability of extended family, peer groups, and community support: Whom would you like to participate in this decision? What will happen if you exclude the father of the child, your parents, or both from the decision?	15. Has identified significant others and discussed decision and options with them.	15. No problem	
	16. Lack of emotional support and assistance from significant others; client wants to exclude all others and lacks sufficient resources to carry out decision herself.	16. Anxiety about decision related to lack of extended family emotional support	Encourage use of resource people outside the family if indicated. Identify factors that interfere with the use of significant others as a resource for decision making.
Influence of health factors: Is health or age a factor in the decision to have an abortion or continue the pregnancy?	17. Health is not a factor in the decision to continue the pregnancy or have an abortion.	17. No problem	
	18. Health is a factor, a potential cause for abortion—for example, underlying cardiac problem, cancer, maternal age, amniocentesis findings, renal birth defects, familial hereditary disorders.	18. Resistance to recommended termination of pregnancy related to denial of health problems	Identify health factors which influence the decision to continue or terminate the pregnancy. Refer for genetic counseling as indicated.

THERAPEUTIC ABORTION. When a nurse and a couple have completed the assessment in Table 47-2 and if the couple have decided that abortion is the chosen option, the nurse can begin to work with the client to plan the time, place, and method.

In the past few years community resources for counseling and abortions have increased. Freestanding women's clinics are often available to counsel women and perform first-trimester abortions. Such clinics often have arrangements with local hospitals for the performance of second-trimester abortions. Many hospitals have abortion clinics. In some states, legislation permits physicians to perform first-trimester abortions in their offices, using accepted protocols.

Freestanding clinics may be the least expensive source of abortion for the woman with limited resources. Financial help for the procedure is available from some medical insurance companies. Since the United States Supreme Court decision supporting the Hyde amendment, government financial aid for abortion is determined by the states. In view of this, practitioners will need to keep abreast of current developments in their own states.

In addition to serving as a resource, the nurse also should be involved in promoting the couple's or the woman's mental health. The nurse should encourage the couple to talk about their perceptions of the procedure, answer their questions, and provide needed information about the procedure. Misconceptions about the procedure and its effects on future childbearing and future sexual relations should be cleared up. The nurse should clarify who will go with the client and pick her up after the procedure and who will help her at home. The nurse should also serve as a good listener and provide emotional support, for the couple may need help in expressing their feelings at each stage of the process. These emotions may range from guilt to confusion, anger, and depression. If at all possible, every woman having an abortion should have follow-up counseling including contraceptive counseling and an emotional inventory. This is especially true for women identified as experiencing negative emotions such as guilt. Follow-up studies on women who have undergone elective abortions have shown that if they have had sufficient support for their decisions, there are no measurable emotional sequelae.

However, women whose decision to have an abortion is not consistent with their personal operational value system are at risk of experiencing guilt and associated emotional turmoil. In addition, women who encounter picketers, such as "right to life" groups, at abortion clinics may be thrown into turmoil by having their unresolved ambivalence highlighted at a time of much personal stress and anxiety. Such women may need extensive counseling by the nurse.

A nurse can help a couple prevent further unwanted pregnancies. Repeated unwanted pregnancies are a sign of the need for further professional exploration of the decision not to have children and the available alternatives. In some cases they may be a sign of pathology, and hence referral for psychiatric care may be indicated.

PLACEMENT FOR ADOPTION. Adoption is an alternative not only for young unwed mothers, but also for married couples who have experienced contraceptive failure after completing their family and for young couples who are not ready to begin a family.

When a decision is made that adoption is in the best interests of the child and the couple, help will be needed by the couple or the woman in implementing the decision. Referral to a licensed adoption agency, in order to provide the best placement for the infant, is in order. Homes for unwed mothers are still available, but their number is decreasing. For support during pregnancy, groups such as Birth Right supply counseling and financial aid.

In counseling the couple, the nurse must realize that giving up a baby is experienced as a loss and that the couple, especially the woman (who will carry the child for 9 months), will need to resolve these feelings. This is true not only before the baby is born but also after placement of the baby, before the child is legally given up. The mother or couple will experience all the stages of grief and will need assistance in dealing with the resultant emotions (see Chapter 3).

Additional pressures come from a society which expects every couple to want and keep their children. However, the couple can be helped to ask themselves whether this expectation is congruent with their needs.

Deciding to Become a Parent

Natural Pregnancy

DECISIONS ABOUT CONCEPTION. Couples who have decided to become parents face new decisions—

for example, at what time of year they want the pregnancy and the delivery, and how they should time the pregnancy with respect to their careers. In the future, couples may be faced with deciding whether or not to choose the sex of their child and, if so, which sex to choose. (There is a developing technology for selection of a male.[1]) The increasing number of choices brings a potential for stress and thus a need for support.

DECISIONS ABOUT CARE. Couples who have settled their questions about conception and have succeeded in conceiving a child face decisions related to the pregnancy and the delivery: they need to choose a style of care, a type of institution, and a care provider.

The modality of care that is selected depends on intangibles such as power, ethnic considerations, and knowledge. If the couple feel that all decisions regarding reproduction are the woman's, she will make the decision. Otherwise they can make the necessary decisions together to their mutual satisfaction. In some ethnic groups the grandparents are responsible for the decision. If the nuclear family is isolated, the couple may make a decision based on the advice of friends. When the distant extended family learn of the decision, they may or may not support it. The degree of support received will have an effect on the nuclear family's coping patterns.

Several alternatives exist which have in common a philosophy of family-centered care. This enables the couple to define their roles in the childbearing process, such as having the father present during labor and delivery and allowing both parents to have unlimited access to the infant. It also permits siblings to have access to the mother, father, and new baby during the childbearing process.

Care based on this philosophy is available in different types of settings or institutions. The one which has most recently returned to the urban health care scene is the maternity home or childbearing center. In this setting couples attend classes and finally the wife has a wide-awake delivery assisted by a nurse-midwife. The mother breastfeeds her baby, and they share the same room. Mother and baby leave the center within 12 hours of delivery. The center "operates with rigid rules on the mother's physical condition and with enormous latitude in procedures."[2] Mothers who develop complications make a short trip to the nearest hospital.

Another mode of care which is being popularized because of "consumer satisfaction," and by word of mouth, is home delivery. Home deliveries—when restricted to low-risk clients with adequate transportation to a hospital, made in a safe and prepared environment, and assisted by a physician, a nurse-midwife, or both—have had, in the hands of such groups as the Frontier Nursing Service, very respectable records. However, home deliveries by minimally trained or untrained personnel or by the baby's father are fraught with emotional repercussions should anything happen to the newborn, the mother, or both.

The most widely used mode of care is hospital delivery. For many couples, the reason for choosing a particular hospital is not the excellence of care but rather the warmth and interest conveyed to the family.

Couples who have defined the style of care they want must make a careful search of their area to find the providers who will meet their needs. They may choose an obstetrician or a nurse-midwife. The provider may be located in an individual or group practice or in a public clinic.

In order to find a provider who will meet their expectations, the couple need to decide (1) on a particular style of care, (2) whether they prefer a caretaker of a particular sex or training, (3) on the degree of the participation they want in decision making, (4) on the amount of time they hope the care provider will spend with them, (5) on the amount of money they have to spend, and (6) how far they can travel.

After an initial interview, the couple can change their minds. It is important for both wife and husband to feel that they can trust the provider. For example, it is not uncommon for a husband to find that he is jealous of the depth of his wife's attachment to her male obstetrician.

EMOTIONAL TASKS OF PREGNANCY. In addition to understanding what is involved in a couple's choice of style of care, institution, and provider, the nurse must know the dynamics of the psychological tasks of pregnancy and their normal sequence.[3,4] Table 47-3 provides a summary of assessment questions, assessment data, nursing diagnoses, and interven-

Table 47-3 Application of the Nursing Process: Decision to Become a Parent

Assessment	Assessment Data	Diagnosis	Intervention
	Knowledge base		
Knowledge about conception and fertility: Do you know how to determine when a woman is most fertile? What do you know about the life of a sperm?	1. Can use temperature chart. Can check condition of cervical mucus to identify fertile period. Aware that frequent intercourse and male ejaculations can decrease the sperm count in each ejaculation.	1. No problem	
	2. Lack basic knowledge about fertility.	2. Difficulty in conceiving related to knowledge deficit about fertility	Identify gaps in knowledge base about conception and fertility. Provide factual information about the process of conceiving. Clarify misconceptions, myths, and stereotypes about conception.
Timing of intercourse and positions that facilitate conception: How often do you think you should have intercourse when you are trying to conceive? What do you know about positions that facilitate conception?	3. Have basic knowledge about intercourse.	3. No problem	
	4. Cannot identify fertile period. Have no idea about how long a sperm is viable and can impregnate. Think that intercourse as often as possible during the fertile period will increase the possibility of conception.	4. Difficulty in conceiving related to knowledge deficit about conception	Use a variety of media (pamphlets, charts, films, books, models) appropriate to the couple's learning styles to illustrate the process and timing of conception. Encourage the couple to ask questions.
	Feelings		
Spiritual feelings about conception: What does your religion teach about the purpose of marriage? Family size? Necessity of marriage?	5. Religion teaches responsible parenthood and personal decision making.	5. No problem	
	6. Religious conflicts about purpose of marriage, family size, or necessity of marriage.	6. Depression related to conflict with religious beliefs	Explore conflicts between personal preferences and religious teachings and the related feelings. If needed, clarify feelings about single parenting. Explore family messages about procreation that generate feelings of guilt, anger, or conflict in the relationship.

(Continued.)

Table 47-3 Continued

Assessment	Assessment Data	Diagnosis	Intervention
		Feelings	
Family influence: What would be the reaction of the families of origin to a pregnancy at this time?	7. Both families are happy to become grandparents.	7. No problem	
	8. Both families think pregnancy at this time is inappropriate; or the families differ in their opinions.	8. Conflict about conception associated with disapproval from family of origin	Assist each person in the relationship to identify and label feelings about pregnancy and parenthood.
Personal emotions associated with pregnancy: How would you feel if you found you (or your spouse) were definitely pregnant?	9. Realistic perceptions of pregnancy, labor and delivery.	9. No problem	
How would you feel about the changes in your lifestyle that would occur? How do you feel about your ability to be a parent? How do you feel about the changes in your body (or your wife's body) that will occur during pregnancy? How do you feel about what will happen during labor and delivery? What are your fears and fantasies about pregnancy, labor, and delivery?	10. Irrational fears and fantasies about pregnancy, labor, delivery, becoming a parent; narcissistic overinvestment in body image overriding desire to become a parent.	10. Irrational fears about pregnancy related to folk tales about labor and delivery	Explore irrational fears, fantasies, and misconceptions about pregnancy, labor, delivery and parenting. Provide reality-based information about pregnancy, labor, delivery, and parenthood; use discussions, parent education groups, books, films, pamphlets. Explore the impact of pregnancy and parenthood on the couple's marital relationship, lifestyle, and relationship with extended families and friends. Explore the couple's perceptions about obstacles to being a "good" parent. Communicate that effective parenting can be learned and is not totally dependent on instinct.
		Decision making	
Decision-making process: How do you view having a child? Why do you want a child?	11. Child viewed as an individual.	11. No problem	
	12. Child viewed as a solution to problems—a way to hold marriage together or make one partner grow up.	12. Erroneous reason for desiring a child related to attempt to resolve marital conflict	Explore impact of decision to parent or not to parent on the relationship.
Congruence of motivation and commitment: Have you reached a decision? How did you reach that decision?	13. Decision made after much thought and discussion.	13. No problem	
	14. No decision because couple continue to argue without listening to one another.	14. Conflicted decision about conceiving related to impaired spousal communication	Explore each spouse's perceptions of what it would be like to have a child. Explore peer and extended-family pressures that affect the decision to parent or not to parent.

(Continued.)

Table 47-3 Continued

Assessment	Assessment Data	Diagnosis	Intervention
	Decision making		
Lifestyle: What are your perceptions of the changes in your lifestyle and living arrangements that will occur if you decide to become a parent?	15. Couple have discussed impact of pregnancy.	15. No problem	
	16. Couple do not perceive that parenting will change their lifestyle, or refuse to discuss changes.	16. Misperception regarding impact of parenting associated with failure to project lifestyle changes	Explore the couple's reasons for contemplating, postponing, or ruling out parenthood.
What changes will occur in your financial situation if you have a baby?	17. Couple have adequate financial resources and medical coverage.	17. No problem	
	18. Present debts cannot be managed if one partner stops working or if the couple have to pay for child care out of present salaries.	18. Decision to conceive correlated with failure to recognize financial limitations	Explore financial stresses that would influence the decision to parent or not to parent.
Division of power, roles, and responsibilities: How do you think your marital relationship will change if you have a baby? How will having a baby at this time affect your career plans? Your spouse's career plans?	19. Couple have made a decision to share parenting responsibilities.	19. No problem	
	20. Couple unable to reach joint decision that will prevent parenting responsibilities from interfering with one partner's career plans.	20. Inadequate planning for child care associated with failure to reach joint decision about parenting responsibilities	Assist couple in clarifying their position on parenthood. Explore ways of managing parenting roles and responsibilities.
Availability of extended family, peer group, and community support systems: How geographically available are family and friends? How will your relationship with your extended family change if you have a baby?	21. Families or peer group are available, accessible, and willing to help. Families of origin and extended families celebrate new babies.	21. No problem	Identify potential support systems.
	22. Geographically mobile couple with families physically and emotionally distant; little peer group support. Ethnic and religious issues will generate conflict between families of origin.	22. Lack of support systems related to geographic unavailability of extended family, and ethnic and religious differences	Explore ways that the couple can work with their extended families to facilitate acceptance of their decision. Guide the couple through a systematic decision-making process about whether or not to parent.
Health factors: Are there health factors affecting the decision to become pregnant (medical problem such as diabetes, genetic problem)?	23. No health factors.	23. No problem	
	24. Health problem or family history of Down's syndrome.	24. Ambivalence about conception related to health problem or family history	Refer couple for medical consultation if a problematic health condition is suspected or identified. Refer couple for genetic counseling if a hereditary disease is in question.

tions for use with the couple who are choosing to have a baby.

First trimester. During pregnancy, both the mother and the father are preoccupied with the emotional tasks which compose much of their experience of pregnancy. For the mother, the first trimester is occupied with the psychological process of incorporation of the fetus into her consciousness and self-image. As she begins to care about the fetus as an extension of her body, she turns inward and begins to consider her own needs. This increase in narcissism or concern with self manifests itself in a need to detach herself from previous commitments. This may be upsetting to family, friends, and associates who have come to depend on her. She may also experience increased emotional sensitivity and personality changes. Additionally, changes in sexuality require that the couple communicate their respective interpretations of their shifting emotional states.

Also, in this phase a woman often becomes concerned with the past. She begins to sort out the myths, themes, and scripts that have been passed down over the generations. Now that she is to become a mother herself, she begins to examine the input on mothering from her past and to decide what is necessary and what is not. She begins to see herself as an individual rather than as a daughter. This change in viewpoint may enable her to develop a new adult-to-adult relationship with her mother, but the increasing differentiation may be a problem for the prospective grandmother if she sees herself as someone whose only role as a human being is being a mother who is needed by her children.

The emotional changes in a pregnant woman may be caused by hormonal and metabolic alterations as well as psychogenic factors. She may experience changes such as nausea and mood swings even before she knows she is pregnant. Her increased fatigue in the first trimester decreases her ability to handle stress. Petty annoyances which she might once have overlooked now take on major proportions. If this is not her first child, the other children may become confused by changes in their mother's behavior. The nurse may need to interpret the expectant mother's fatigue to the couple and help them plan rest time for her. If the mother is working, finding a time and place to rest may require ingenuity.

The father is also preoccupied during this period with the realization that his partner is pregnant. It confirms his ability to procreate and is often followed by an unexpected spurt of energy. Another aspect of his role transition is concern about his adequacy as a financial provider. And if he wishes to take an active role in the delivery, he will become involved in choosing the care provider and the site for care. In addition, he may so sympathize with his partner's discomfort that he experiences typical symptoms of the first trimester even when his partner does not have them.[5]

Second trimester. The next recognizable psychological task for the prospective mother generally occurs during the second trimester. It is described as *differentiation,* or the task of recognizing and acknowledging that the fetus—whom she has accepted as present in her body—is not part of her. This begins with the momentous experience of the baby's first movement.

The couple now develop a relationship called *attachment* with this unseen but distinct being. This involvement is very real, so that the loss of the baby from this point on brings not only physical trauma but also psychological grief and mourning.

The father may enter a new crisis situation in the second trimester, in which he struggles with sexual feelings triggered by his partner's expanding size. The psychoanalytic literature discusses revival of oedipal conflicts during pregnancy. Another feature of the father's behavior during this period may be rivalry with his pregnant wife. This may be expressed as increasing unhappiness with his work accompanied by complaints of increasing job politics and competition. Many men express thwarted hopes—for example, "If I were single now, I would . . . ." The father may also feel it difficult to relate to the fetus and may express rivalry with it. Nonetheless, he may become involved in such tasks as picking a name, he may try to guess what sex the baby is, and he may express a preference about the method of feeding the baby.

Meanwhile, the woman often develops an increased concern about and interest in her husband. She wants and needs to know that she can depend on him. His sharing in the experience clearly is important. "Feel the baby move" is a familiar demand directed at him.

The baby's movement is the first concrete proof the husband may receive that the baby is real. This may awaken in him fears about his adequacy as a provider and fears for the safety of his wife and the infant. He is going through his own emotional adjustment to fatherhood. This includes incorporating or rejecting much of what he has previously known about fathering. In the process, he is beginning to view his wife as a mother, and this may reawaken his early feelings about his own mother. At the same time, the expectant wife is continuing to resolve her feelings about her relationship with her mother. Both are striving to shake off the last vestiges of adolescent dependence on their parents and to stand on their own. The extent to which they accomplish this task of achieving independence will influence their new roles as parents (see Chapter 5).

During this second trimester, the couple may have to make sexual adjustments. Frequently, the wife feels an increase in sexual desire, but as the trimester progresses, her expanding abdomen may interfere. This requires adjustment by both partners. They need to discuss their feelings about sexual relations and to adjust their position so that the sex act will be satisfying to both. Adjustments in position can bring up issues of dominance and social and ethnic role orientations. For example, how does a wife who is oriented to a passive sexual role adapt to the superior position?

As the third trimester approaches, the couple's view of the fetus or fear of hurting it may cause difficulty in their sex life. The woman may desire relations more or less often than before, and her changing sexual desires may confuse her husband.

Third trimester. The third trimester usually coincides with the couple's third task: *separation.* Here the mother prepares for delivery, and her main interest is the baby. Dreams, fantasies, and everyday conversations are likely to include the baby. If the couple are able and willing to name the baby, this says much about their anticipation of the birth of a separate and distinct individual to whom they are becoming attached. Thus the first stage of becoming a parent is well under way.

Frequently, the father feels the need to increase the family's living space, and the couple move in the last trimester. Another of his concerns is getting his partner to the hospital on time. He may fear for his wife's and child's safety during labor and delivery. This fear can be reduced by participation in classes and a hospital tour. Campbell and Worthington advocate a class in coaching led by a father who has coached his wife.[6] Such a class would be designed to help fathers deal with discouragement, conflict, or panic during labor. It is also at this period that a man's memories of his father are most likely to emerge.

Couples tend to have very definite expectations about their infant's appearance, age, and future skills. These expectations are often related to the couple's own unfulfilled wishes. They visualize the baby as being at a specific age and having a distinctive personality. They become attached to this view, and if the infant does not fulfill their expectations, they may go through a period of mourning for the fantasized infant before they become willing to accept the real one.

The couple's perception of the fetus may be an indication of how the parent-child relationship will develop. If the couple view the fetus as a problem which interferes with their life, they may continue to view the child as a problem. If their feelings toward the fetus are positive, their initial reaction to the infant is usually positive.

Couples may also see in the infant a chance to fulfill their unrealized dreams. They may invest the fetus with the talents and abilities needed to fulfill these dreams. As long as these expectations are adjusted to reality, this can be a healthy process.

Problems can develop when the fetus is considered to be in danger of dying. The parents may not form a mental image of the baby. This lack of attachment in pregnancy may pose problems if the child is born and lives.

Last but not least, the third trimester is accompanied by an inescapable anxiety about the coming labor and delivery. No matter how slight the impulse to worry, the coming event looms large as the completion of the process of pregnancy nears. Couples use many coping mechanisms in attempts to channel their anxiety about the approaching labor.

Constructive coping mechanisms will enable the couple to develop the skills necessary to manage labor, delivery, and parenting. Among these coping activities are the following: (1) caring for other infants, (2) attending parent-education classes, (3) attending classes preparing for labor and delivery, (4) gathering infant-care items, (5) preparing and freezing meals for after delivery, (6) housecleaning, (7) maintaining open communications, (8) attending self-help meetings for prospective parents sponsored by groups such as La Leche, and (9) other activities the couple can share. Without such activities, couples who are having difficulty in dealing with anxiety may become aimless and may arrive at labor and delivery without preparation.

As the due date approaches, constructive coping activities fade into insignificance; at this point the desire to have the pregnancy over becomes dominant. The woman begins to tire of carrying the extra weight and of having people say, "Are you still around?" "Haven't you had the baby *yet*?"

During the third trimester, *physical changes* and *body image* become significant. Extra body weight is the most striking of the developmental changes in body image, which are especially prominent at this time. The changes bring highs and lows. Buying (or letting out the seams of) maternity clothes can bring deep emotional satisfaction if the baby is a planned and wanted one. But it can also be the cause of feelings of ugliness and clumsiness, especially if the woman is ambivalent about the pregnancy or is receiving little or no emotional support from her husband, friends, or relatives. Other clues to the mother's feelings about her body image are her comments about negotiating her enlarged body through familiar spaces which seem to have shrunk. One example is passing through the supermarket checkout counter, where most women are surprised that they do not fit as easily as before. If the woman is really unhappy about her pregnancy, this discovery can be an upsetting event. Whether happy or sad, the woman wonders whether she will ever get her figure back.

Other physical changes which occur during pregnancy may be either delightful or burdensome, depending on the couple's stability and desire for this child. Chloasma, or the mask of pregnancy, can be seen either as imparting a healthy suntanned appearance or as a disfiguring brown skin rash. Striae, or stretch marks, appear on the abdomen and breasts. If the couple especially prize physical appearance and "youth," striae, which are very visible in a bikini, are highly undesirable. This is especially true because these marks, unlike chloasma, do not disappear completely.

Another concern of the couple during the third trimester is *preparation of the siblings* for the coming of the new baby and the mother's absence from home for a few days. The extent of the preparation will vary with the age of the children, but all questions about the childbearing process should be answered honestly and simply. Correct terminology should be used to avoid future confusion. Reading age-appropriate books can help to focus discussion with the children. The emotional and physical changes which the mother undergoes have a marked effect on her husband and children. In other words, her responses set up responses in the family. This *resonance phenomenon* in the family leads to the term *pregnant family*.

LABOR AND DELIVERY. After 9 months of anticipation, the couple arrive at the childbearing center full of apprehension. During a first pregnancy, there is a particular fear of the unknown. The couple have probably heard many stories about labor and delivery and do not know which ones to believe. Here at last is the culminating event for which they have been exercising, studying, and preparing. For a couple approaching labor and delivery, the experience can be overwhelming as they feel a loss of control over what is occurring. The deep emotional significance of the appearance of new life in itself makes labor and delivery momentous. This is especially true for a couple who have had past disappointments; the event is anticipated as a confirmation of their ability to have children.

The onset of labor also makes the couple more fully aware of their changing roles. There is no turning back; they are about to become parents. This thought may increase the feeling of apprehension.

It is only natural that such a momentous event will be more meaningful if the woman is able to share it with a husband who cares deeply and who will be able in the future to recreate the scene because he was there. This is far different from trying to describe the delivery later. The classes and exercises have set the scene for this sharing; continuing it through labor and delivery is a logical sequel. If the classes have helped to establish between the couple an agreement about the father's role, this should lower his anxiety and facilitate sharing.[7] When the woman wakes up in the middle of the night wondering whether she is experiencing false labor or the real thing, she will find it helpful to receive reassurance from someone who remembers what the instructor said in class. Later, after being admitted to the center, she may be comforted by having a familiar person at hand to coach her in breathing.

Despite a general paucity of research about fathers' participation, we do know that the "coach" (usually the father) requires support by the nurse in order to support the mother. To do this, assessment of the knowledge, skills, and needs of the coach is important. On the basis of this assessment, the nurse can choose strategies such as teaching, reinforcement, encouragement, and praise.[8]

As labor advances, a woman is very dependent on others for her physical needs as well as for emotional support. She is apprehensive and uncomfortable, unable to do anything for herself. She becomes aware that "this is it." The contractions continue unabated despite her momentary, frightened wish to withdraw. She may well feel "caught," somewhat as soldiers do when, under fire, they feel an urge to run away.

Having mastered the most painful phase of labor—the transition phase during which the cervix dilates to 8 to 10 centimeters—the couple may derive real satisfaction from delivery. The satisfaction of having delivered without anesthesia (except perhaps for a local) and the joy of holding the newborn are universal. The prepared couple who have shared this experience are likely to feel well prepared for events to follow. However, those who have not lived up to their mental image of what the well-prepared couple should do may experience feelings of failure and dismay after delivery. Their self-images as competent individuals may be shaken. There are several ways in which their expectations may be disappointed. For example, they may be disturbed by the failure of labor to progress, by the physician's need to use forceps or a vacuum extractor, or by a need to have the baby delivered by cesarean section.

In addition, couples experiencing difficulties in labor are also more likely to encounter fetal monitoring equipment than those not experiencing problems. The strangeness of being attached to a machine increases the sense of helplessness and loss of control. It may also increase tension and anxiety, thus playing a role in increasing pain. The monitor limits freedom of movement and frequently usurps the staff's attention.

The increasing use of fetal monitoring and cesarean births has been coupled with a trend toward preparation for the possibility of monitoring and an explanation of cesarean births in classes preparing couples for childbearing. Such preparation has in many places led to a trend to allow fathers to participate in not only elective cesarean births but also primary cesarean births.

A woman with insufficient knowledge may come to labor and delivery having heard many stories about the pain and dangers of childbirth. She has few facts with which to counter her fears. Since she is unprepared, she is not likely to have anyone with her to share her labor and delivery experience. A woman may prefer to have her sister or another female relative present rather than her marital partner, but she may be unaware that this is possible. Her anxiety level may be so high that she is unable to comprehend what is being said to her. One method of coping is to regard this crisis as the initiation into womanhood. Survival is the requirement, and culturally accepted modes of behavior in childbirth, such as screaming or moaning, provide reassurance that she is one with the women who have gone before her. A father who has had no preparation for labor and delivery may withdraw psychologically by reading a magazine or going to sleep. He is doubly likely to "live suspended somewhere among the roles of husband, lover, partner, protector and father, not knowing which way to turn."[9]

Nursing intervention during labor and delivery depends on continually assessing the reactions of all present. Each stage is characterized by expected physical changes accompanied by more or less predictable emotional reactions in the mother which affect all those present.

If, in addition to the father, the couple's older children are present during labor and delivery, the nursing role also includes responsibility for seeing that their needs for knowledge, support, and encouragement are met. If a support person for the children is present, the nurse should assess whether that person is able to fulfill his or her role.[10]

POSTPARTUM PERIOD. Following the delivery of the infant, the family undergoes profound physical and emotional changes. The infant adjusts to extrauterine life and performs its own vital life functions. The mother's body begins to adjust to not being pregnant and completes the physical changes necessary for breast-feeding. But the major processes at this time are the *psychological tasks of the postpartum period*—the family's attachment to the new baby and adjustment to the changes in family members' roles.

Attachment. The process of being uniquely and totally involved with this particular infant is called *attachment, engrossment,* or *bonding.* It is known to be a unique relationship as well as a two-way developmental process influenced by both infant and parents. The concept or process of attachment includes mutuality. The family claims the baby and expands its identity to include this child. This is illustrated by comments such as, "She has long feet like her father, but her nose is definitely mine."

Ideally the process of attachment begins with planning for pregnancy, progresses through recognition of fetal life and imagining the baby during pregnancy, and culminates in the following behaviors:

1. Mother seeks *eye-to-eye contact* with the baby. This is facilitated by the baby's fixed gaze during the first hour.
2. Looking is accompanied by progressive *touching and stroking,* first with fingertips, then with the whole hand. The mother then embraces the baby and holds it close to her body.
3. The parents talk to the baby in high-pitched voices, and the baby responds by turning toward the sounds.
4. The parents take care of the baby; by feeding and changing diapers, they learn to identify their own child's odor, just as babies can identify their own parents with their eyes closed.[4]

Klaus and Kennell[11] pointed out in their studies that prolonged separation of mothers from high-risk infants resulted in decreased attachment and, therefore, by definition, decreased maternal involvement in the infant. The corollary derived from this is the current belief that attachment is facilitated by initial and continual contact between mother and infant.

However, parents who cannot have early contact with their infants need to be made aware that there is no conclusive evidence that such contact is essential for ideal parent-child relationships. Parents' familiarity with the literature on attachment can lead to undue anxiety when ideal conditions cannot be achieved.

Another potential source of parental anxiety can be the failure to feel immediate love for the baby. This is especially true of mothers who have learned the myth of automatic mother love. Caplan believes that many mothers experience a delay in feeling "mother love," and he regards this delay as normal.[12]

Fathers also have needs to relate to their children. Greenberg and Morris coined the term *engrossment* to describe the father's attachment to his baby. Fathers' responses include those we have already discussed.[13] Other researchers have documented that differences between mothers and fathers lie not in competent care giving or attachment but in distinctive styles of play, the mothers being more verbal and the fathers more physical. This difference provides the child with a wider range of experiences.[14]

If the mother, in her preoccupation with the newborn, excludes the father, as a person, from her field of active concerns, thus leaving him feeling abandoned while he may be additionally burdened by financial concerns, she may establish a pattern which diminishes the quality of his relationship both with her and with the baby. Anticipatory guidance during the postpartum stay in the hospital can be quite helpful in avoiding this situation. Other areas in which such guidance can be helpful include the timing of resumption of normal activities including sexual relations. Both partners often fear pain for the mother. They may have unrealistic fears of ripping episiotomy stitches; such fears can be lessened by an understanding of the rapidity with which the well-vascularized perineum heals, so that normal sexual relations can often be resumed within 3 to 4 weeks.

Rubin has described three psychological tasks of great importance in maternal postpartum adjustment, which she calls *taking in, taking hold,* and *letting go.*[15]

The first stage in the postpartum period is *taking in.* This period lasts 2 to 3 days; during it, the mother's primary concern is with her own needs. She reacts passively and initiates little activity. Adequate sleep and rest are major needs in this period.

So that the mother may have sufficient energy to meet the needs of the infant, the nursing staff must mobilize the environment to meet the mother's individual needs. She requires periods during which she does not have to care for anyone else. She has been through a period of biological stress, and within a few days she will be putting out large amounts of energy in caring for her newborn at home.

In addition to needing rest, the mother needs to have opportunities to talk about and relive her labor and delivery experience. This includes clarifying the events which took place and should lead to the feeling that she has met the challenge successfully.

If the dependency needs of the taking-in phase are well met, the mother will be ready to progress to the next stage, *taking hold.* The taking-hold period lasts about 10 days. During this time, the mother is concerned with her need to resume control of her life in all its phases. She wants to be viewed as competent. It is important to her that everything function well, her own body as well as that of the infant. She seems ready to organize herself and her life. As a mother, she now wants to be in command of her situation. But when problems occur, they are likely to reduce the mother to tears. This sudden emotional frailty may bewilder her husband. He is at a loss to explain what has happened to his confident wife, who seems to have lost her common sense. The wife, in turn, may see the nurse as the perfect mother. The nurse is the one who can get the infant to burp in a few seconds after the mother has spent 10 minutes trying. When the nurse puts a diaper on the baby, it says on; when the mother does so, it falls off. She feels that she is being judged and must measure up in everyone's sight, especially in that of her mother and her mother-in-law. To maintain her self-esteem, she must be as good a mother as they are.

During this phase, the mother needs praise and encouragement for her efforts. The "helping others" should provide support for *her* efforts rather than doing the tasks themselves. They must understand her need for adequate rest in this phase as well. Exhaustion in the pursuit of perfection can be damaging to mental as well as to physical health. This is a danger with first babies as well as when the mother has no help in coping with her other children.

At this time not only the mother but also the rest of the family may want to be with the infant as much as possible. If the concept of family-centered rooming-in (see Table 47-4) and its advantages to the development of the parent-infant attachment have been explained before delivery, mothers will often be eager to have the infant with them. On the other hand, if the infant is suddenly brought to the room to spend the day and the mother is unprepared, she may view the infant's arrival as an indication that the nursing staff does not want to care for the infant. To meet the needs of the family, rooming-in needs to be flexible. The mother needs sufficient exposure to the infant to develop care-giving skills and attachment but not so much as to interfere with the meeting of her own basic needs.

Table 47-4 Family-Centered Rooming-In

Advantages	Disadvantages
Facilitates attachment	Decreases mother's rest
Increases care-giving skills of mother and father, such as bathing, diapering, handling	May be culturally unacceptable to client or her husband
Increases family's knowledge of infant's rhythmic patterns of sleeping, eating, etc.	
Increases siblings' exposure to infant before homecoming	

The final phase, *letting go,* is initiated in the postpartum period and continues throughout life. The mother should begin to see the infant as an individual rather than as an extension of herself. Mothers who are making satisfactory progress in the task of letting go will recognize the child's need for increased independence at various stages of growth and development.

A woman experiences many inner conflicts during this phase. First, she must balance her dependency needs against those of the infant. This may prove a problem if the mother has not previously mastered her own developmental task of resolving the issue of dependence versus independence. If a mother has not developed independence in some spheres of her own life, it will be difficult for her to allow independence to develop in the child.

Second, such a woman may think of the perfect mother as one who always loves her infant and whose infant wakes, eats, and sleeps but never cries. She may need to balance her wish to be the perfect mother against the real situation, in which an infant may cry from time to time for no apparent reason. In addition, the mother may be amazed at how much she resents the infant when it interferes with her needs. The baby may cry when the mother wants to sleep or fuss when the couple are about to eat dinner. The feeling of resentment may be particularly strong if the mother has had no contact with infants and does not realize that such behavior is normal and will subside.

A third internal conflict which may materialize is that between the roles of mother and wife. The woman may accumulate guilt over her inability to be both the perfect wife and the perfect mother. Or in her concentration on the role of motherhood, the role of wife may become lost. Such concentration on the infant may cause the husband to feel he has been abandoned. This makes him withdraw, leading to a breakdown in communications. A nurse can help the couple to reset priorities and reopen communications. The couple will need to arrange time for themselves. The use of household help and baby-sitters to accomplish this should be explored.

A fourth potential source of conflict exists when the postpartum mother has a tubal ligation for which she is not totally ready, either intellectually or emotionally, or for which she does not receive substantial support and acceptance from husband and relatives. If the mother has not made a positive, internally integrated decision for sterilization, she may handle her conflict by spoiling her last child and retarding its movement into independence.

Because of her inner conflicts, the reality of caring for a new infant, and the hormonal changes in her body, the woman may experience a period of emotional readjustment following the birth of the infant. The mother may frequently feel very tired or find herself crying for no apparent reason. The rest of the family may be puzzled; they expect her to be happy with the infant. This period of postpartum blues usually lasts only a few days. The others in the environment can be most helpful if they try to meet the woman's dependency needs so that she will have the energy to meet those of the infant. Extra rest is frequently helpful. Depression which is not relieved by simple measures may require psychiatric referral.

Family readjustment. While the adjustments of mother and infant are occurring, the couple must also adjust to new relationships. The family has now formed a triad (see Chapter 19). Relationships between the husband and wife have to evolve to include the new member. A similar process of change occurs after each subsequent child.

The period of readjustment may be difficult for the couple. The husband may feel jealous of the new infant and all the attention it is receiving. If the relationship throughout pregnancy, labor, and delivery has not been a shared one, he may feel abandoned by his wife. If she has had an episiotomy, she will be too uncomfortable for the first 3 or 4 weeks to have sexual relations, and the unprepared husband may find this, too, difficult to accept. If the couple are geographically isolated from the extended family or for other reasons have not developed a strong kin network, the husband may have to help his wife with the household chores after he has worked all day at his job. The increased responsibility without any immediate, tangible rewards may strain the relationship.

Older children may also be experiencing the strain of a new relationship. Increasing numbers of maternity units are permitting siblings to visit their new brother or sister. This may facilitate a smoother adjustment to having another child in the family. It may also help to prevent older children from feeling that they have been displaced in the mother's affections, thus reducing sibling rivalry and regressive behavior.

Problems in Becoming a Parent

Having made the decision to become parents, some people experience difficulties in achieving their goals. These crises may take the form of infertility, a high-risk pregnancy or infant, or the impairment or death of the desired child.

INFERTILITY. The couple who have decided to have a child but are unable to conceive will feel frustrated. A major component of this frustration is a perceived loss of control over their lives. Their self-concepts will be altered; this will affect not only their feelings about themselves as sexual beings but also their lifestyles, relationships, and life goals. The task of coming to terms with changes in self-concept will, most probably, go along with an extensive infertility workup of both partners. This workup may or may not uncover the reason for the couple's inability to conceive. Most obstetricians will not do an infertility workup without the active participation of both partners, but sometimes the husband is reluctant to participate. He may find the possibility that he is the cause of the problem more of a threat to his masculine pride than he can face.

During the period of the workup the couple need support, and they need to be able to express their feelings and frustrations. Nursing strategies during this period should stress the positive aspects of giving up some control and should also provide support and education.[16] The couple may be referred to Resolve, a peer support group of infertile couples.

If the workup finds no cause or a cause that is not amenable to treatment, the couple need help in (1) grieving for their loss; (2) assessing the importance of parenthood to them; (3) dealing with their feelings of lack of control; (4) exploring their alternatives—remaining childless or acquiring a child by other means such as conception engineering (see below) or adoption. Several authors note that coming to terms with negative feelings is a crucial precondition for becoming effective and happy adoptive parents.[17]

"Conception engineering." Although tubal causes of infertility account for only 20 to 30 percent of all female infertility problems, many of the new technologies have concentrated on this area.[18] One of these technologies, in vitro fertilization and embryo transfer, unites an ovum surgically removed from the mother with sperm from the father in a laboratory culture dish. Two days after fertilization takes place, the embryo is transplanted into the mother's uterus. Since this procedure represents the couple's best and perhaps last chance to achieve pregnancy, the nurse needs to provide support, counseling, and education.[19]

An older method of conception engineering is artificial insemination either with homologous sperm (AIH) or by donor (AID). Unfortunately, AIH is usable by fewer couples than the more controversial AID. A newer and even more controversial variation of artificial insemination is popularly called *surrogate motherhood.* Primarily used when the mother is not able to carry a pregnancy, this arrangement allows another woman ("surrogate") to be artificially inseminated with the husband's sperm or to have an embryo conceived in a culture dish implanted, to carry the pregnancy to term, and to deliver the baby and turn it over to the father and his infertile wife. The legal contract by which the surrogate is paid for the baby is still being tested in courts.

The legal rights of children conceived by the various methods of artificial insemination (except AIH, which causes no legal controversy) are still being decided in the courts. Legal inheritance for children conceived through AID is not established in all states. Some states require that the couple adopt the child.

Assessment of a couple considering AID or surrogate motherhood should particularly emphasize (1) physical examination for infertility, (2) the couple's reasons for wanting the procedure, (3) their feelings about it, (4) their knowledge of the legal implications, (5) other common assessment factors as indicated (see the discussion earlier in this chapter under the heading "Assessment of Families in the Childbearing Years" and Table 47-1).

After diagnosis and goals have been established, the interventions needed will become clear. Counseling sessions may be numerous, and each partner may need to be seen alone. After conception, counseling is continued to enable the couple to work through their feelings. This helps them to sort out the normal feelings of pregnancy from any remaining misgivings about AID. Nurses working with these couples will need to keep abreast of the results of current research regarding the emotional needs of these clients.

Resources from which artificial insemination can be obtained are infertility clinics and private physicians.

Adoption and foster parenting. Adoption and foster parenting are alternative methods of activating the decision to become a parent. Each has potential risks and specific interventions which will be discussed in Chapter 48.

HIGH-RISK INFANTS. If a couple are able to conceive but the infant is high-risk instead of a healthy, full-term baby, then the couple and the nurse encounter other problems. This is particularly true in the case of an older couple whose baby faces a higher risk of Down's syndrome because of the age of the mother. The tension inherent in the decision to have or not to have an amniocentesis, and in waiting either for the test results or for the birth of the baby, highlights the need for use of therapeutic communication techniques. (See Chapter 12.) Even when the couple are expecting an infant with Down's syndrome, they have no way of knowing how mildly or severely the child will be affected. Thus, nursing interventions are directed toward helping the parents to establish realistic expectations for themselves and the child, as well as helping them to set priorities. Such a couple need to receive genetic counseling before they plan future pregnancies.

Perhaps the most common reason for high risk in infancy is preterm birth. (A baby is considered to be preterm if birth takes place less than 38 weeks after conception or birth weight is less than 2500 grams.) In addition to the obvious risks of preterm birth, these infants are at higher risk of abuse and neglect.[20] Normally, women become psychologically and physically prepared for labor during the last few weeks of pregnancy; clearly, preterm delivery cuts this time short. Moreover, preterm labor differs from full-term labor in many respects: (1) it occurs early; (2) there is an atmosphere of emergency; (3) the husband may be excluded; (4) increased use of fetal monitors and tests creates a feeling of danger; (5) there are more people watching the monitor and not the client.

The rapid removal of the high-risk infant to a special nursery can retard the normal attachment process by (1) making the mother feel that she may lose her infant, so that the mother begins to withdraw from the relationship she has established with the fetus; (2) making it more difficult for her to see, touch, and care for the infant—a difficulty that is increased by the special equipment. And in addition to having disturbances in attachment, the mother is often left to deal with her feelings alone.

If the baby is small, the mother may experience feelings of failure and depression. This may be manifested by tearful sadness or by anger. If the baby has medical problems, the mother may blame them on the care she has received. Often she searches her own actions to find a cause. Another common feeling is loneliness, which may occur partly because the mother cannot take care of her baby, whereas she sees other mothers caring for theirs, and also partly because she may have to go home without the infant. Staff members may inadvertently exacerbate the problem by tending to avoid her because they are unsure of what to say. They are accustomed to focusing on the relationships in a happy family.

During this period, the father is also experiencing deep feelings. He is concerned about his wife and infant. If he has been excluded from the delivery room, his concern is first for his wife and then for the infant. As the first parent to see the infant, he may be startled by its small size and by the complexity of the equipment used. He needs support and explanation of each procedure. It is to him that many of the initial decisions concerning medical care will fall. Because he is often asked to make the decisions without consulting his wife, communication between them may be disrupted. While in most cultures the mother is allowed to express her feelings, the father is expected to be stoical and to support her. In order to accomplish this, he needs the support of the nurse. However, at the same time he needs permission to express the myriad of feelings he may be experiencing; the nurse who encourages ventilation on the part of the husband will often find him only too relieved to unburden himself to a nonjudgmental listener. The husband is also faced with the task of explaining what has happened to the other siblings, the family, and friends. The nurse can help him by providing suggestions about how to impart the information to others.

The emotions of both parents may take several forms. They may express general anger with the situation, blaming each other or the caretakers. They may make insistent bids for reassurance and attention. They may feel unable to communicate and may thus withdraw from one another.

The parents' methods of coping with emotions evoked by the infant's problems will generate feelings in the nursing staff. Outbursts of anger or accusations may cause the staff to withdraw at the time when the parents most need support. Staff members need to look at their actions in light of the parents' needs.

Some interventions which may help to meet the family's needs are as follows: (1) change rules in high-risk nurseries to allow parents into the nursery; (2) change rules to allow parents to touch, handle, and possibly feed or diaper the baby; (3) encourage the couple to room in for several days before discharge (this is called *nesting*);[20] make necessary referrals for nursing support at home. These interventions are aimed at facilitating bonding by allowing as much contact as possible between parents and child. The most important long-term goal here is to encourage development of a healthy parent-child relationship.

DEATH OR IMPAIRMENT. If the situation is more extreme and the parents experience a fetal or perinatal death or have a defective child, they will go through the mourning process (see Chapters 3 and 48). They need the nursing staff to support them and listen to them. When a defective child dies, the parents mourn not only the child they have actually lost but also the perfect child they had visualized.

Parenting

NURSES AND PARENTING. The quality of parenting that people receive is probably the most influential factor in their biopsychosocial development and well-being. Effective parenting is a skill that can be learned and is not a set of instinctive behaviors. The abundance of lay literature about parenting is an indication of the widespread interest in the topic. Parents are constantly seeking new knowledge about parenting as well as advice and reassurance about the quality of their parenting skills. By addressing parenting issues, nurses who work with families can help to promote development of effective ways of dealing with the inevitable changes that occur during a child's growth and development, and to prevent the emergence of dysfunctional patterns during maturational crises.

The parent-child relationship is an interactive process. The nurse must understand both the child and the parent in order to identify ways to help them evolve a mutually satisfying and growth-promotive relationship.

Nurses work with families in a variety of settings. Obstetricians' and pediatricians' offices, well-child clinics, health maintenance organizations (HMOs), schools, and public health departments are all settings in which nurses can work with children and families on parent-child issues. Nurses' roles as counselors, advocates, care givers, and teachers permit them to engage in primary prevention.

FACTORS WHICH INFLUENCE CHANGES IN PARENTAL ROLES. Social forces in recent years, specifically the women's movement and variations in family configuration, have led to reevaluation of traditional male and female roles. As men and women examine themselves and explore their values and beliefs about masculinity and femininity, their perceptions of their roles as parents and their expectations of their children are inevitably affected.

In the traditional nuclear family structure, each parent has had a specific role. The father has filled the *instrumental role* of providing financial resources, making and implementing significant decisions, and acting as the major authority figure in the family. The mother has filled the *expressive role* of nurturing the child. The role of wife has traditionally been perceived as subordinate to that of the husband. The exercise of *overt power* through instrumental-role activities has been limited for women. However, in some families, the woman has, over the years, exercised a great deal of *covert power*, particularly with regard to decisions about day-to-day family life such as child rearing, household changes, and other family matters.

Today, many couples are reevaluating traditional parenting roles. Couples are deciding in favor of more flexible parenting roles. They are finding that the instrumental and expressive parenting roles can be shared and negotiated. Fathers are participating more in the nurturing of children, and mothers are participating more in financial support and decision-making and authority issues. This increased flexibility has led to a more effective division of labor and greater freedom for both parents. The possibilities for exploring and developing other interests are expanded for both parents.

Variations in family configuration (see Chapter 19) are another significant factor in modification of traditional roles. For example, an increasing number of single parents find themselves having to fulfill both the instrumental and the expressive roles.

SOURCES OF INFORMATION ON PARENTAL ROLES. People's ideas about parenting roles are derived from a matrix of factors. These factors include the family of origin, the way each person was raised, family myths and scripts about parenting, socioeconomic status, cultural practices, current marital relationship, parents' level of differentiation, and knowledge about child development.

The increase in geographic mobility and the decline of the traditional family structure have deprived new parents of a valuable source of information: the extended family. In former years, parenting skills were learned from observation and practice within the family. In most families, children observed what their parents did, how they behaved, and what was included in the roles of mother and father. Little brothers, sisters, and cousins were frequently available for practice of parenting skills. Following marriage and parenthood, the extended family was usually still available to provide assistance, guidance, and role modeling.

Today, in a highly mobile society, few new parents have the extended family available for those kinds of services. In the absence of the extended family, parents turn to each other and to friends, acquaintances, mass media, and books for advice and support. Information obtained from such sources, as well as from the extended family, is often conflicting and sometimes stereotyped and unreliable.

New parents frequently seek information and advice from health care professionals individually or in parenting classes. Such sources of information are likely to be more reliable. Professionals who constantly interact and intervene with families have multiple opportunities to supply helpful and accurate information about parenting.

NURSING PROCESS

Assessment

Assessment of Parents

Intervention during the childbearing–child-rearing cycle commonly involves primary prevention. In order to provide effective intervention in this area and to determine the need for intervention in other areas, the nurse should first assess the parents' current and potential functioning in their parental roles. The initial assessment can be done at the time the decision to conceive is being considered, during the prenatal period, or at any point during the child-rearing cycle. The common assessment factors identified at the beginning of the chapter are used as a framework for the parenting assessment in Table 47-5. This assessment guide will need

Table 47-5 Application of the Nursing Process to Parenting

Assessment	Assessment Data	Diagnosis	Intervention
	Knowledge base about self as a parent		
Self: What significant problems do you have now that relate to your present stage of life? What do you anticipate will be your problems in the next stage? Do you see how many problems that you are currently having might affect your parenting ability now or in the future?	1. Spouses are clear about how a baby's dependency needs will diminish the ease with which their own needs will be met; each can identify resources for obtaining personal emotional "supplies" and "strokes."	1. No problem	
	2. Spouses are concerned about their lack of time for each other since birth of baby. Colicky baby with irregular sleep pattern.	2. Unmet dependency needs related to role strain	Review or teach stages of adult growth and development. Assess with parents their stages of growth and development. Explore positive ways to meet needs of their developmental stages. If parents' developmental stages are not adequate to meet demands of parenting, refer them for further evaluation and counseling. Use role playing to help parents view themselves accurately.

(Continued.)

Table 47-5 Continued

Assessment	Assessment Data	Diagnosis	Intervention
	Knowledge base about self as a parent		
Characteristic emotional response patterns: How do you respond when you are forced to change your plans to meet the needs of others? What do you think you will do when your child breaks something valuable?	3. Usual reaction to frustration is rational and within control. Expectations of growth and development are accurate; couple have had some exposure to children.	3. No problem	
	Knowledge about children		
Growth and development: How much time have you spent with infants and young children? What do you expect your child to be like? Describe what you think the typical newborn or 1-year-old is like.	4. Usual reaction to frustration is uncontrolled anger or rage. Expectations too high or too low; unable to describe what child will be like; little or no exposure to children.	4. Potential for child abuse related to unrealistic expectations of child	Explore characteristic emotional response patterns. Explore source of reactions; for example, was this reaction a pattern in the family of origin? Use role playing to model new or alternative ways of dealing with negative emotions. Refer for counseling those whose habitual reactions may endanger the child. Reassess parents' knowledge at each stage of growth and development. Explore basis of unrealistic expectations.
Individual differences among children: How does your child's development compare with that of other children of the same age? Do you see your child as fast, average, or slow? Give an example. Have you ever compared your child's development with that described in books on this topic, such as those by Dr. Benjamin Spock? Do you expect your child to react as other children do? What were you like growing up? Were you similar to or different from your child? Are your child's reactions to situations similar to or different from yours? How does your child adjust to changes in schedule or routine, such as sleeping in a strange crib and eating at different times?	5. Parents understand differences in development and temperament; can adapt to child's reaction to new situations; understand how their own personal temperament could contribute to fit or lack of fit with the child's temperament. 6. Parents believe all children develop at the same rate and react alike; they have difficulty in adjusting to child's reactions to situations. For example, they consider the first baby an easy child, the second a difficult child.	5. No problem 6. Impatience with new baby related to failure to recognize individual differences between children	Provide anticipatory guidance as indicated. Arrange for observation of groups of appropriate-age children, as in play groups or on movies or videotapes.

(Continued.)

Table 47-5 Continued

Assessment	Assessment Data	Diagnosis	Intervention
	Knowledge about parenting		
Knowledge about age-appropriate parenting activities:			
What kinds of play activities stimulate physical, social, and cognitive development at your child's age?	7. Couple are able to identify age-appropriate toys, games, and parent-child activities.	7. No problem	
What kind of limit setting and enforcement is appropriate at your child's age?	8. Parents realistically identify limit-setting strategies and enforcement.	8. Inappropriate selection of playthings and activities related to lack of knowledge about the role of play in stimulating age-related learning	Provide information about toys and activities that stimulate age-related learning.
	9. Parents have a realistic view of age-appropriate toys, games, and parent-child activities that may interfere with child's safety needs.	9. No problem	
	10. No limit setting and enforcement, or inappropriate attempts.	10. Abdication of limit setting related to failure to consider child's developmental age	Encourage couple to join and attend parenting groups.
	Feelings about parenting		
Spiritual feelings about parenting:			
What has your religion taught you about the role of parents and children?	11. Religion has taught a positive, flexible view of roles for both parents and children.	11. No problem	
	12. Religion has taught a rigid, negative view.	12. Punitive enforcement of limit setting associated with rigid views about right and wrong	Clarify values about right and wrong. Help parents consider gray areas where there is no clear solution. Explore basis for feelings.
Family influence:			
How do you feel about the influence your parents have on your children? The advice your parents give you about your child-raising practices?	13. Couple feel influence is positive; are able to evaluate advice and use what is helpful.	13. No problem	
How did your family of origin handle Discipline? Money, especially in relation to clothing and allowances? Freedom for the individual child? Were there differences for boys and girls? Do you feel you must follow the practices of your family of origin?	14. Couple feel parents have a negative influence; feel compelled to follow advice even when in conflict with their own desires; or disregard advice because it came from parents.	14. Inconsistent parenting related to periodic extended family influence	Explore behavior learned in families of origin. Explore degree to which couple feel they must follow behaviors learned from or advice given by families, peers, and others. Explore differences in feelings between parents in families of origin. Role-play situations to enable couple to better articulate feelings about religious and family influences.

(Continued.)

Table 47-5 Continued

Assessment	Assessment Data	Diagnosis	Intervention
	Feelings about parenting		
Personal emotions: How do you feel about Being a parent? Staying home with a sick child? The changes having a child has brought in your lifestyle? The progress your child is making? Dealing with a child at this stage of growth and development?	15. Feelings are realistic; couple can articulate both positive and negative feelings; the parents' feelings are in general agreement with one another's.	15. No problem	
	16. Parents relate only negative feelings, or have negative feelings which do not seem appropriate to situation; are in wide disagreement; or express only positive feelings.	16. Critical parenting associated with regrets about decision to be a parent	Explore couple's perception of their own parents' satisfaction in the child-rearing role. Identify couple's unmet needs. Explore their feelings about the satisfaction of their personal needs. Encourage open communication about feelings.
	Decision making about parenting		
Level of agreement: Do you two have difficulty in agreeing on rules for the child? Does your child first ask one parent's permission and then (if he or she does not like the answer) ask the other parent and get a different answer?	17. Parents agree on rules.	17. No problem	
	18. Parents disagree on rules; child plays one parent against the other.	18. Lack of unified parental coalition related to blurred generational boundaries between parents and children	Support open communication about differences and similarities. Explore effect of differences on current functioning. Facilitate definition of generational behavior.
Communication: Whom do you talk to about parenting decisions? What advice do these people give? Do you two spend time privately discussing parenting decisions on a regular basis or only when a major decision is needed?	19. Parents have others with whom they can discuss parenting issues, who discuss options but leave final decision to parents; parents discuss issues with each other on an ongoing basis.	19. No problem	
	20. Parents have no one with whom to talk; others they talk with do not explore options but give only one answer; parents have discussion only when there is a crisis. Couple believe that parents ought to know how to raise their children.	20. Failure to seek resources for parenting decisions related to belief that parenting is instinctive	Give feedback about parents' efforts to increase level of agreement.

(Continued.)

Table 47-5 Continued

Assessment	Assessment Data	Diagnosis	Intervention
	Decision making about parenting		
Availability of support systems: Do you have any support from family? From friends? Whom do you turn to when you need help in child-rearing activities?	21. Support is readily available from friends and is used by parents; family of origin is available on short notice.	21. No problem	
	22. Support is available from family and friends but not used. Or support is not readily available.	22. Intensification of family feelings related to emotional cutoff from extended family and friends	Explore emotional cutoff. Encourage parents to explore all possible alternatives. Explore sources of support for decisions and child-rearing activities. Discuss community support available. Encourage use of support systems.
Division of power, roles, and responsibilities: Who is responsible for Doing household chores? Making major financial decisions? Deciding on rules for the child or children?	23. Division is based on individual interests and abilities; tasks are shared, roles are flexible; parents are satisfied with division.	23. No problem	
	24. Division is based on stereotypical ideas, and one or both parents are unhappy with division.	24. Unsatisfactory balance of power in child system related to parental helplessness	Reexamine allocation of resources. Explore role of family of origin. Examine models with respect to similarities and differences. Explore realistic modifications of power, roles, and responsibilities.

to be updated as children pass through the various developmental stages of child rearing.

The genogram (described in Chapter 19) is also a tool for family assessment. It can assist with the identification of parent-child issues, problems, and patterns as well as personal, family, and community resources. This information highlights parenting issues and the ways in which stresses in other generations might influence parenting patterns in the current generation. For example:

> Ellen G.'s mother developed metastatic cancer of the breast when Ellen was 5 years old. She was in and out of hospitals many times, was often heavily sedated because of pain, and was largely unavailable both emotionally and physically to Ellen and her older sister, Deborah. The girls were cared for by a series of housekeepers while the father spent many hours working. It was as if he was able to avoid his grief by working all the time. They had no extended family nearby. The mother died when Ellen was 11 and Deborah was 15. Ellen remembered sitting on her front steps on the day of her mother's death, vowing that she would not be the kind of mother her mother was. She would be there for her children to help them, guide them, and support them. After graduating from college, Ellen married a man who had a good job but was not overly involved in his work. He was very happy spending a lot of time with Ellen. Within a few years they had a daughter, Suzanne, whom Ellen was with constantly. She tried to divide her time and

energy between her husband and her daughter but found that Suzanne always seemed to come first. Initially, Ellen did not want to have another child because she felt that she would never be able to give two children the kind of attention each deserved. Finally, when her daughter was 5, she had another child, a boy, Peter. Ellen ran herself ragged trying to be the perfect mother and wife. When Peter was 4 months old, she became run-down from getting up at night with him. Peter had an irritable temperament which she found difficult to tolerate or change. Ellen caught a cold that quickly turned into pneumonia. When Ellen was asked how it had happened, she shrugged. Her husband angrily proclaimed that if she had not been trying so hard to be the perfect mother that her mother had not been, she might be in better shape. He said, "I've had it! I'm not playing second fiddle to any kids, or anybody else from here on in."

In this situation, parenting patterns experienced in Ellen's family of origin had a profound effect on her notion of mothering, on her expectations of herself as as parent, on her marriage, and perhaps eventually on her children. A nurse would find it difficult to understand Ellen's total preoccupation with her children unless she had this genogram information.

Assessment of Children

Children also need to be assessed in order to determine their progress through the developmental stages (Chapter 5) and their perceptions of events. Nurses can assess children's developmental progress by using such tools as Brazelton's Personality Inventory of the Newborn or the Denver Developmental Screening Test. Sharing the results of the assessment can form the basis for providing anticipatory guidance to the parents (Table 47-6).

A child's perception of family events can be assessed through storytelling, structured play ses-

Table 47-6 Age-Related Anticipatory Guidance

Age of Child	Information to be Reviewed with Parents	Age of Child	Information to be Reviewed with parents
Newborn	Bathing, feeding, diapering, and other physical care as indicated Irregularity of habits in feeding, sleeping, and elimination Normalcy of fussy periods (Describe variations in temperament.) Need for exposure to variety of sounds—importance of talking to infant Need for visual stimulation Importance of having needs met consistently	9 months	Feeding: three meals with bottle before bed, not in bed; introduction of finger foods Play: choosing toys, use of household articles as toys Safety precautions: poisons, stairs, sharp objects
		12 months	Visual stimulation: name objects and ask child to point Choosing toys Changing appetite Weaning Need for parents to have time to themselves
6 weeks	Above as indicated Signs and symptoms of illness Use of sitter to allow parents time together Need for immunizations	18 months	Safety Need for exploratory behavior Prevention of negative behavior (Give one instruction at a time, praise positive behavior but still expect some negative behavior.) Discipline practices
3 months	Infant becoming more regular Need for visual, oral, and aural stimulation		
6 months	Introduction of solid foods Need for safe environment as infant becomes more mobile Care of emerging teeth Discussion of developing fear of strangers	24 months	First 18 months as indicated Toilet training Advent of food fads Play groups Care of teeth

(Continued.)

Table 47-6 Continued

Age of Child	Information to be Reviewed with Parents	Age of Child	Information to be Reviewed with parents
24 months (continued)	Fears Pros and cons of nursery school Choosing a nursery school	6–10 years	Increasing competence in all phases of activity Importance of friends Changing needs for sleep and rest
3 years	First dental visit Discipline practices Sex education (Answer questions as they occur in language the child understands.)	Pre-adolescence	Preparation for changes taking place: wide variations among children of the same age Prevention of drug addiction and alcoholism Need for changing disciplinary measures Importance of peer groups
4–5 years	School readiness Safety precautions Changing fears		
6–10 years	Safety precautions Allowances if family budget permits Need for wide range of experiences Assignment of age-appropriate household tasks	Adolescence	Prevention of drug addiction and alcoholism Continuing need for sex education Need for increasing independence balanced by need for parental guidance

sions, observation of behavior, and the child's statements concerning important events. Questions such as the following provide broad openings that allow children to express their concerns:

> "What is the most important thing that has happened to you in the last week (or month or some other suitable period)?
>
> What is the best thing that has happened to you?
>
> What is the worst thing that has happened to you?

Assessment of Parent-Child Fit

Parent-child fit refers to the degree of congruence or incongruence between the temperament of the parent and the temperament of the child. Chess, Thomas, and Birch[21] describe individual patterns of response and temperament that seem to be present in each infant at birth. Long before their research had identified temperamental styles, however parents commented on differences between children:

> She always had a mind of her own; it's wonderful that she was so assertive at such a young age.
>
> He was so placid; he would adjust to anything. It was such a pleasure to have him around.

These comments reflect two very different temperamental styles. However, in each case the parent-child fit is congruent. The same styles might be described negatively if the parent-child fit was not congruent:

> That child drove me crazy; she never sat still or listened for one minute.
>
> He was so floppy, like a rag doll; whatever you did with him was OK; he wasn't very responsive.

Parent-child fit is an interactive process; both the parent and the child contribute to and mutually reinforce their temperamental interaction. The temperament of the parent may or may not mesh with the temperament of the child. For example, a very placid, easygoing mother who has an irritable, headstrong, very active child may have difficulty viewing this behavior as "normal" and devising ways to deal with it successfully. She may become upset because she cannot seem to quiet or set limits on the child. She may feel incompetent as a mother and resent the child for making her feel that way. The cycle of parent-child fit is depicted in Figure 47-2. Parent-child fit can change with the child's developmental stage. A parent who competently and happily meets an infant's total dependency needs may have difficulty dealing with

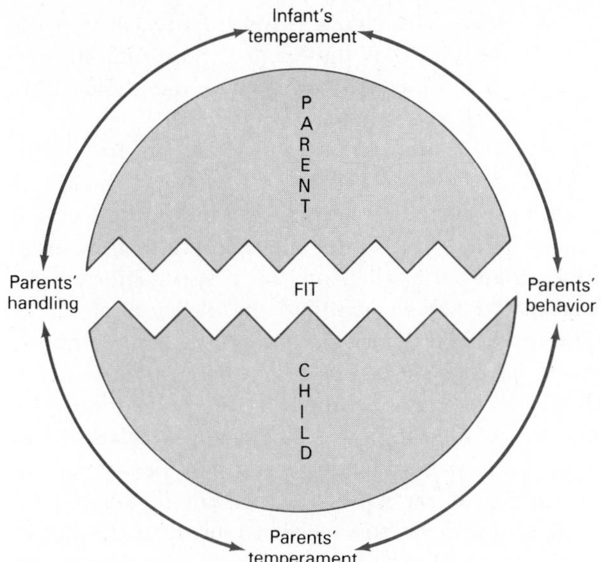

Figure 47-2 Cycle of parent-child fit.

the same child's emerging needs for autonomy and separation at age 2 (see Chapter 49). Parents who have unresolved developmental conflicts may find that these conflicts are reawakened when a child enters the stage at which the developmental conflict originated.

In order to assess the parent-child fit, nurses can ask parents the following questions.

How would you describe your child's level of activity, alertness, and irritability?

How does the child respond to changes in routine, schedule, environment, or care givers?

Is your child's reaction similar to or different from yours?

If there are differences in temperament, are you concerned about them?

Are the differences in temperament creating problems in the interaction between you and your child?

What strategies have you already used to improve the parent-child fit?

What worked? What did not work? How can you explain the success or failure of different strategies?

Strategies for intervention in the area of parent-child fit include providing information about temperament, parent-child fit, and techniques for improving the congruence of parent-child fit so that the interactive process does not become a negatively reinforced spiral. (See Chapter 49 for more information on temperament and parent-child fit.)

Diagnosis and Goals

After completing the assessment with its concurrent identification of areas with and without problems, the nurse can work with the family to develop a nursing diagnosis and goals. A diagnosis such as "potential for growth" will have as its goal the continued promotion of family growth, while a diagnosis such as "parenting, potential alteration in" will have as its goal the prevention of parenting problems.[22]

Intervention

The nursing interventions chosen will be directed toward diminishing problems and reinforcing positive areas. The type of intervention required can vary widely, from providing anticipatory guidance for specific age groups (as indicated in Table 47-6) to referral for family therapy to deal with the more extensive factors that inhibit effective parenting. Some of the interventions which can be used with parents are outlined in Table 47-5; other interventions include special education for parenthood in family health curriculums in schools, as well as prenatal classes, new parents' groups, and parenting classes.

Education for Parenthood

Regardless of the setting, education for parenthood needs to include information about physical, cognitive, and psychosocial growth and development; exploration of basic parenting skills; and an opportunity for the participants to sort out their own feelings.

The first step in an educational process is to assess the needs of the learner. Practitioners can use the parenting assessment in Table 47-5 as an assessment tool to evaluate the learning needs of the group or couple. After an assessment of the learning needs, various techniques can be used to convey the information. Values clarification, role playing, role modeling, audiovisual techniques, group discussion, and hands-on experience are all possible. The method or methods chosen will depend on both the learning styles of the participants and the ability and experience of the nurse.

Preventive Parenting Strategies

Any group of parents or potential parents can be helped to develop general techniques of parenting,[23] including the following:

1. Scheduling a daily period when the parents spend time with the children, concentrating on listening to and paying attention to each child. Consistency is most important here.
2. Knowing the children's friends; encouraging the children to invite their friends home.
3. Planning and carrying out a clear-cut, mutually agreed upon system of rewards and punishments.
4. Planning experiences to share together.
5. Trying to listen when the child talks, using communication techniques such as eye-to-eye contact and reflection and restatement.
6. Assigning age-appropriate tasks to promote independence.
7. Explaining family situations and changes in language the child can understand. What the child imagines is almost always worse than the reality.
8. Giving anticipatory guidance to the child as indicated.

Dual-Career Parents

SPECIAL NEEDS OF DUAL-CAREER FAMILIES. Dual-career parents are under special stress. One part of society supports their efforts, while another condemns them. With larger numbers of these families in the society, whether through choice or economic necessity, specific interventions need to be developed for them. They need to be aware of the changes in the child-development literature. During the 1950s and 1960s the child-development literature suggested that a large quantity of continuous mothering by the mother was necessary for the normal development of the child. More recently, however, evidence has been found that it is the quality rather than the quantity of parenting that is important.

Hoffman and Nye[24] feel that the mother's emotional state is the key factor. If she works willingly or stays home willingly, there is little or no negative effect on the child. The child who suffers is the one whose mother is doing what she does not want to do. Chess, Thomas, and Birch[21] suggest that the only child who may have difficulty in adjusting to a working mother is the child who has difficulty in adjusting to any change.

DIVISION OF LABOR. When an infant is born, its parents need to agree on their working patterns. If both partners continue to work full time, they must renegotiate the division of responsibilities for household tasks, negotiate the division of child-care tasks, and decide on child-care arrangements. If one partner shoulders a larger share of the work, that partner may become too tired to maintain the marital relationship and to develop a relationship with the new family member. In families which do not arrive at an equitable division of labor, it is most likely to be the woman who gets the larger share of the tasks, leading to the "supermom" syndrome. It is she who will have to get up earlier to dress herself and the child, prepare lunches, pack extra clothes, and deliver the child to the day care provider before going to work. After work, she will pick up the child and rush home to prepare dinner and perform some household tasks before falling into bed exhausted—only to arise the next morning and repeat the sequence.

The couple also need to plan ahead for times when the sitter is unavailable or the child is too ill to go out. Who will stay home or be late to work? Will it always be the mother? The father? Or will they handle each occasion on the basis of current needs? Each needs to be aware of the parenting policies of the other's employer.

FINDING CHILD CARE. Perhaps the most difficult task facing the couple is to find reliable, competent child care. They will need to explore the child-care options available near where they live as well as near where both parents work. A small number of companies are beginning to provide day care in or near the workplace, but most couples still need to provide independent care for their children.

In initially choosing a day care arrangement the couple will need to weigh the advantages and disadvantages of each of the options open to them. As the child grows older, the couple may need to reevaluate their choice in light of the child's changing needs.

A sitter who comes to the home is convenient and may give the child more individual attention, but competent sitters are difficult to find and expensive. In addition, if the sitter is unable to come, the couple will have to find a substitute. Taking the child to a sitter's home may be less expensive and easier to arrange, and may also give the child a peer group to interact with. However, such a sitter may provide very limited activities—possibly just a television set—and again, the parents will still on occasion have to find a substitute on short notice. Day care centers provide a peer group, a variety of adult care givers, and a wide range of activities. However, they may be expensive, may have an inconvenient location or hours, and may not provide individual attention.

In choosing a sitter to come to their home, the couple should carefully interview the person, check references, and observe the person with the child. In evaluating options outside the home, the couple should consider:

1. Is the center or sitter licensed? If not, why not?
2. Does the environment seem safe?
3. Are the care givers knowledgeable? What is their educational background?
4. Is the ratio of adults to children satisfactory?
5. What provisions are made for children who become ill or are injured?
6. What are the meal arrangements? If meals are provided by the sitter or day care center, are they nutritious and appealing?
7. Do the children seem happy? Are they involved in activities?
8. What is the center's philosophy of education?
9. What allowances are made for children's individual differences?
10. Is a variety of activities offered?
11. Are the location and hours convenient?
12. Are the fees affordable?[25]

ROLE OF THE NURSE. The main nursing task with working parents is to provide anticipatory guidance and to help them sort out their feelings about the fact that they are both working and the effect of their working on the child. The couple need to be encouraged both to spend time with their child and to spend time alone as a couple. They may also need help in assessing the adequacy of their child-care arrangements.

Nurses may have to help establish adequate child-care facilities in the community to meet the needs of all ages and income levels. They may also be involved in the assessment of children at such centers. In making such assessments, it is important to explore a variety of possible causes for any problems a child may be having. Remember that the parents' dual careers are only one factor affecting the complex development of the child.

SUMMARY

Nurses who work with childbearing and child-rearing families need to be constantly aware of the changing societal pressures which influence families. Each family is unique and needs individual assessment and planning. The family must be involved in developing its own plan of care. A carefully constructed and well-implemented plan can lead to satisfactory development and happiness for the entire family.

REFERENCES

1. Ferdinand Beernink and Ronald Ericsson, "Male Sex Preselection through Sperm Isolation," *Fertility and Sterility*, vol. 38, no. 4, October 1982, pp. 493–495.
2. Nadine Brozan, "New Childbirth Centers: Baby Born in Morning Was Home by Evening," *The New York Times*, March 27, 1976, p. 30.
3. Arthur Colman and Libby Colman, *Pregnancy: The Psychological Experience*, Herder and Herder, New York, 1971.
4. Reva Rubin, *Maternal Identity and the Maternal Experience*, Springer, New York, 1984.
5. Margaret Jensen and Irene Bobak, *Maternity Care: The Nurse and the Family*, 3d ed., Mosby, St. Louis, Mo., 1985.
6. Anne Campbell and Everett Worthington, "Teaching Expectant Fathers How to Be Better Childbirth Coaches," *Journal of Maternal-Child Nursing*, vol. 7, no. 1, January-February 1982, pp. 28–32.
7. Katharyn A. May, "The Father as Observer," *Journal of Maternal-Child Nursing*, vol. 7, No. 5, September-October 1982, pp. 319–322.
8. Charen Elsherif et al., "Coaching the Coach," *Journal of Obstetrical and Gynecological Nursing*, vol. 8, no. 2, March-April 1979, pp. 87–89.
9. Philip Taubman, "Doubts in the Delivery Room," *The New York Times*, October 21, 1984, p. 72.
10. Pauline Perez, "Nurturing the Child Who Attends the Birth of a Sibling," *Journal of Maternal-Child Nursing*, vol. 4, no. 4, July-August 1979, pp. 215–217.

11. Marshall H. Klaus and John H. Kennell, *Maternal-Infant Bonding,* Mosby, St. Louis, Mo., 1976.
12. Gerald Caplan, *Concepts of Mental Health and Consultation,* Children's Bureau, U.S. Department of Health, Education and Welfare, 1959.
13. Morris Greenberg and N. Morris, "Engrossment, the Newborn's Impact on the Father," *Nursing Digest,* January-February 1976, p. 19.
14. Michael Lamb, ed., *The Role of the Father in Child Development,* 2d ed., Wiley, New York, 1981.
15. Reva Rubin, "Puerperal Change," *Nursing Outlook,* vol. 9, no. 12, December 1961, pp. 753–755.
16. Terry McCormick, "Out of Control: One Aspect of Infertility," *Journal of Obstetrical and Gynecological Nursing,* vol. 9, no. 4, July-August 1980, pp. 205–206.
17. Adrienne Kraft et al., "The Psychological Dimensions of Infertility," *American Journal of Orthopsychiatry,* vol. 50, no. 4, October 1980, pp. 618–628.
18. Barbara Macy Friedman, "Infertility Workup," *American Journal of Nursing,* vol. 81, no. 11, November 1981, pp. 2040–2046.
19. Catherine Garner, "In Vitro Fertilization and Embryo Transfer," *Journal of Obstetrical and Gynecological Nursing,* vol. 12, no. 2, March-April 1983, pp. 75–78.
20. Kristine Siefert et al., "Perinatal Stress: A Study of Factors Linked to the Rise of Parenting Problems," *Health and Social Work,* 1983, pp. 107–121.
21. Stella Chess, Alexander Thomas, and Herbert Birch, *Your Child Is a Person,* Viking, New York, 1965.
22. Marjory Gordon, *Manual of Nursing Diagnosis,* McGraw-Hill, New York, 1982.
23. Paul Ackerman and Murray Kappelman, *Signals: What Your Child Is Really Telling You,* Dial, New York, 1978.
24. Louis Hoffman and Ivan F. Nye, *Working Mothers: An Evaluative Review of the Consequences for Wife, Husband and Child,* Jossey-Bass, San Francisco, 1974.
25. Stevanne Auerbach, *Choosing Child Care,* Dutton, New York, 1981.

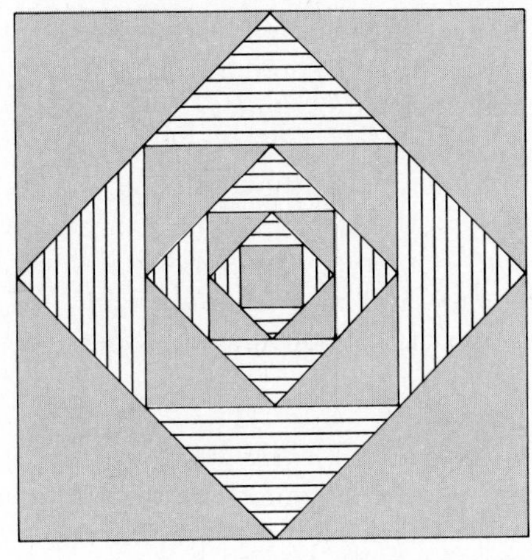

CHAPTER 48
High-Risk Families

Barbara Flynn Sideleau

LEARNING OBJECTIVES

After studying this chapter, the student should be able to:

1. Discuss the impact of a parent's or sibling's death on a surviving child and the family system.
2. Discuss the impact of divorce on children, parents, and the family system.
3. Discuss the factors that contribute to a decision to divorce.
4. Discuss the changes that occur following divorce.
5. Discuss the problems of single parents and their impact on children.
6. Discuss adoption as it relates to adoptive parents, adoptees, and surrendering parents.
7. Discuss the foster placement process as it relates to foster parents and children.
8. Discuss the epidemiological facts related to high-risk families.
9. Discuss individuals' patterns of interaction (attachment, identity formation, and grief) as they relate to high-risk families.
10. Discuss family patterns of interaction (loyalty and impaired gender and generational boundaries) as they relate to high-risk families.
11. Discuss environmental patterns of interaction that influence high-risk families.
12. Apply the nursing process to high-risk families.

Changes inevitably generate losses and are inherently stressful. They dysynchronize mind, body, spirit, and interactions with the environment. If situational supports are unavailable, or if a person, because of immaturity, is unable to adjust to changes and work through losses, then biopsychosocial dysfunction occurs. Children experience greater difficulty than adults in resolving serious losses and managing the resulting changes in their lives, because of the limitations imposed by their developmental capacities.

Death, divorce, single parents, stepparents, adoption, and foster placement all involve the loss of a significant other (or others) and changes in lifestyle. Each of these situations reflects disruption of the family system. Since the family is a primary source of nurturing, security, and refuge, its disruption results in the loss of a major source of support. Without this support the risk of development of a crisis increases.

The purpose of this chapter is to examine the impact of death, divorce, single parents, stepparents, adoption, and foster placement on the family system and its members. Children, because of their immaturity, are the most vulnerable family members. For this reason, greater emphasis is placed on their perspective and problems and on ways to lessen the negative impact on their growth and development. The nursing process is applied to the problems generated by disruptions of family integrity.

DYSYNCHRONOUS HEALTH PATTERNS

Family patterns that increase the risk of problems and crises, particularly for children, include death of a family member, divorce, single parents, stepparents, adoption, and foster placement.

Death

The death of a parent, sibling, or spouse is a major life stress that elicits the grieving process. The disruption of the family system creates an emotional shock wave that extends with a rippling effect horizontally to affect the peer-level generation and vertically to affect the older generation and future generations. The impact on individual members is reflected by the physical and emotional dysfunction that follows the loss. Unfulfilled obligations and expectations that result from premature death continue to influence the family and generations yet to be born.

Children are vulnerable to the loss of significant people in their lives. The loss of a sibling or parent during childhood influences the surviving child's perception of death and may interfere with personality development, schoolwork, and personal relationships.[1,2]

Death of a Sibling

Death of a sibling is an uncommon but devastating event. Immediately following the death, the surviving sibling experiences shock, confusion, depression, anger, numbness, and fear. Difficulty sleeping and eating are common complaints. These youngsters report thinking about the lost sibling frequently. Some also experience hallucinatory phenomena in which they believe they hear or see the dead sibling. Suicidal ideation also occurs among many of these surviving siblings.[1]

When a child dies, the family is left with a sense that a great injustice has been done, since death has occurred before life has been fully lived. This feeling of injustice and its impact on loyalty balancing in the family have serious ramifications for the surviving siblings. Survivors' guilt, which has been described in relation to the survivors of concentration camps and disasters, can be found among children when a sibling has died unexpectedly or after a terminal illness. It is characterized by an attitude of "Why not me?" that may, or may not, be directly expressed. Since idealization of a lost person is a part of the grieving process, it is not surprising that when one measures the living self with its human frailties against an idealized image of the dead person, in this case a sibling, the "perfect" child seems to have died and the "imperfect" child to be living on. Survivors' guilt is a logical response to the situation.

Idealization of a dead sibling sets up an image impossible for surviving children to match. Failure is inevitable because surviving children are real, living people, not idealized images. Some children spend their lives trying to live up to this image in order to attain parental approval and acceptance and to justify their existence. They try to "make up" to their saddened parents for the cruel loss they experienced. In the process, attention to their own needs and grief may be overlooked by them and their parents. Their attempts, which negate their own needs, only further imbalance the family system. Such efforts are doomed to fail because they can never fully undo the injustice.

Some children caught in this survivors' guilt appear to define themselves as the direct opposite of the "perfect" dead child. Their self-destructive acting out seems only to further emphasize the sharp dichotomy between the "perfection" of the dead child and their own "imperfection." Their antisocial behavior is often not recognized as self-punishment to resolve the guilt of surviving.

Regardless of whether a child dies of a sudden, preventable or unpreventable accident or after a long illness, parents often blame themselves. They search their memories and often become preoccupied with such thoughts as "If I only . . . " or "I should have . . . ." The loss of the child is, in a sense, seen as the result of their failure as parents. This belief that they are failures as parents affects surviving siblings.

Children need their parents to be strong, good, and competent. To recognize the parents' perception of themselves as failures is anxiety-producing, and thus children avoid it. Some respond by becoming higher achievers and "good" children in an unconscious attempt to bolster the parents' low self-image. Others, through antisocial, destructive behavior that requires the parents to rescue them, are unconsciously attempting to help the parents recognize what good people they are to try to save such an "imperfect" child.

The surviving sibling, who may now be an only child, is faced with a particularly difficult problem trying to manage the "imperfect" self in light of the idealized "perfect" image of the dead child. When there are several children in a family, they can become a mutually supportive subsystem at times when the parents are unavailable because of their grief. An only surviving child does not have this peer support system and is therefore caught in the intensity of the parent system. Grandparents and other people in the extended family may be helpful to these children in relation to deintensifying the nuclear family's emotional tension.

Parents may become so caught in their own grief, self-blame, or blame of one another that they are relatively unavailable as a support system for the surviving children. These children are acutely aware of their parents' distress. Older children and adolescents are better able to understand what is happening; however, they are also struggling with their sense of loss and self-blame for not being "better siblings" to the dead child. Young children may not fully grasp what is happening because of the developmental immaturity of their concept of death. However, they are aware of, and respond to, the distress surrounding them. They may feel that in some way they are personally responsible for what is happening and are "bad" for causing so much pain. When this happens, they may incorporate this self-perception into their self-concept.

When the dead child was ill for an extended period of time, the child's care and treatment have been a primary, time-consuming concern of the parents. Attention to the other siblings may have been minimal. An older sibling may have been delegated as the "psychological parent" for the younger siblings. This responsibility "parentifies" this child and results in loyalty imbalances that will require retribution. Deprived of parental attention, the other children also are owed unmet parental obligations that will require retribution at some point. Following the death of the sibling, this situation may not be readily resolved and further imbalancing will occur.

Subtle social learning may occur among the siblings when the parents give total attention to the care of the dying child. The lesson learned is that if you are physically ill, you will have your parents' undivided love and attention. When this learning occurs, surviving siblings may unconsciously use physical symptoms and health problems to elicit the parental attention and nurturing they crave.

The stresses imposed on a family during and following the death of a child may be beyond the coping capacity of the siblings as well as the parents. Following the death, it is not uncommon for vulnerable family members to develop physical illnesses such as colitis, asthma, and dermatitis. The development of symptoms, particularly if they are similar to those exhibited by the dead child, may frighten both the child and the parents. If the lost child's disease was first discovered when the child was being treated for a common ailment such as a sore throat or swollen glands, all family members may panic when a surviving child manifests similar symptoms.

Following the death of a sibling, a child who is acutely aware of the mother's distress and sense of loneliness may develop morning stomachaches and headaches. The symptoms prevent the child from going to school and leaving the mother home alone—they legitimize staying home to keep her company. The seeds of school phobia may be sown if this situation is not resolved.

Parents may respond in various ways to an only surviving child and to each other following the death. Stress, blame, and inability to be mutually supportive may lead to divorce for some couples. The surviving child then loses both sibling and family. Other couples become totally and mutually engrossed in their grief. The parental subsystem becomes closed and focused inwardly, excluding the surviving child. Some couples manage their grief and feelings about being "failures" as parents to the lost child by becoming overprotective "superparents" to a single surviving child. This response ensures emotional support for the child but may have a smothering effect that interferes with and impedes normal separation if other children are not born to the family.

It is not uncommon to hear professionals, family members, and friends advise a couple who have lost a child to have another child immediately. In reality, however, the lost child can never be replaced. The couple need to work through the loss of the child before having another child. A "replacement child" is born with the burden of the lost child's identity as an ever-present ghost between him or her and the parents. A child conceived to replace the lost child is often blocked or impeded in developing his or her own identity. If a couple allow themselves to fully experience and mourn the lost child before conceiving another child, there is a greater possibility that the second child will be allowed to be unique, separate, and worthwhile as a person in his or her own right.

Death of a Parent

Death of a parent is an acutely distressing experience. When the death is sudden and traumatic, if the youngster has had problems or if the family environment has been troubled, a stress response syndrome may result.[3,4] Children with a history of poor impulse control, emotional instability, and a tendency to react with explosive rage to frustrating situations are more vulnerable to prolonged emotional difficulties following the death of a parent. If the youngster has experienced a prolonged separation from the parent before the death, there is an increased risk of pathological bereavement.[4]

The loss of the "mothering parent," the one who was the warm nurturing parent, is also likely to generate problems and unresolved mourning. When youngsters engage in self-blaming and have a sense of responsibility for the parent's death, they are especially vulnerable to a prolonged stress response. Both depression and schizophrenia have been associated with early loss of a parent.[4,5] The availability of a substitute surrogate parent to fill the role of the dead parent and the ego strength of the surviving parent seem to foster adjustment and facilitate the mourning process.[4]

Divorce

Divorce does not usually occur without warning. Even when the decision is precipitate, the legal processes take time. Thus, the family experiences a predivorce period that is characterized by conflict, disruption, and stress. This period of family upheaval distresses both spouses and children. Stress during this period may be manifested through physical or emotional dysfunction. Children are particularly vulnerable to such family stresses and strains. In one study, half the children reported somatic symptoms during the predivorce period (vomiting, facial twitches, hair falling out, weight loss or gain, and ulcers). Generally, these symptoms had no adaptive value, since they did not necessarily elicit parental attention.[6]

Precipitating Factors

Factors that may contribute to the decision to divorce include mental illness, unfaithfulness, family crises, a low level of differentiation, pursuer-distancer interactions, and the multigenerational transmission process.

MENTAL ILLNESS. When one spouse has a psychiatric illness, the divorce process may be more difficult. The other, unhappy spouse may make a rational, purposeful, and deliberate decision to divorce his or her mentally ill partner but experience painful psychological conflicts.[7]

On the other hand, a spouse who is experiencing severe psychosocial dysfunction may impulsively seek a divorce. The increase in symptomatic behavior is often punctuated by filing for divorce, despite the fact that the marital relationship has not been conflictual or particularly unhappy. Unfortunately these people lose family support at a crucial time. Their decompensation, which may include bizarre behavior, frightens the children, and the suddenness of the divorce further upsets them. Often the psychiatric symptoms have not been previously recognized. The turbulence in the house increases, and other family members may not understand why the dysfunctional parent is behaving so differently.[7]

UNFAITHFULNESS. Divorce proceedings are sometimes initiated in an attempt to punish or win back an unfaithful spouse. The decision to divorce is usually impulsive. This strategy often fails, and the separation process is characterized by bitterness. The aggrieved partner may continue to rage for years.[7]

In some instances the impulsive divorce is precipitated by a partner who announces his or her intention to seek a divorce and marry a lover when there has been no explicit recognition of marital difficulty. The aggrieved spouse may become enraged or bitter, may threaten suicide, and may become violent. These spouses try to influence the children to join them against the abandoning parent, to enlist them in the battle as allies and confidants.[7]

FAMILY CRISES. Divorces sometimes occur following an internal crisis such as the death of a significant person or a crisis that occurs outside the family. The emotional shock wave felt in families following the loss of a significant person partially explains divorce even when the marriage has not been previously characterized by unhappiness, dissatisfaction, or conflict. The death of a child, parent, or sibling is acutely stressful. In some instances, the birth of a defective child or a tragic accident that leaves a child or parent seriously impaired may be a disorganizing rather than a mobilizing force within the family. Spouses who are under acute stress because of these circumstances may use divorce to flee the situation and protect themselves from overwhelming anxiety or depression.

LOW LEVEL OF DIFFERENTIATION. One of the basic assumptions of family systems theory (see Chapter 19) is that all people seek closeness. However, as people move closer to one another, the level of emotionality increases. The closeness is a threat to boundary maintenance. Some people find it difficult to manage closeness in ways that preserve the integrity of the self as a separate person with unique needs, thoughts, and feelings. Some people have a tendency to fuse. When fusion occurs, personal boundaries and the separateness and uniqueness of the other person are negated. The boundaries overlap and blend. The self may merge or fuse with the other person's self. One person may speak, make decisions, or act for the other. When this happens, one self becomes lost, incorporated by the other. The loss of self generates uncomfortable feelings and the need to distance, in order to find the self again. When people have a low level of differentiation, they are at greater risk of divorce. Their pervasive emotionality interferes with their ability to use cognitive processes and a problem-solving approach to marital problems. They are also less able to tolerate the closeness of the marital relationship because they have a greater fear of losing the self in the relationship.[8]

PURSUERS AND DISTANCERS. Some people persistently and characteristically pursue their spouses. They seek and expect the spouses to gratify all their needs for love, belonging, self-esteem, and recognition. They are inevitably disappointed. They expect their spouses to resolve their inner emptiness and loneliness, feelings that have their roots in early life experiences. They fail to recognize that their pursuit of their spouses is for this reason. They fail to recognize their own loneliness and emptiness, or to act in their own behalf.[9]

Pursuers, those who continually seek interaction and gratification of their needs by others to the point of becoming totally intrusive, often select mates who are more inclined to distance others. The pursuers pursue and the distancers distance. The pursuers periodically become discouraged when their efforts fail to result in the desired closeness or to relieve their sense of emptiness and loneliness. At these times their frustration contributes to the development of either open conflict with their spouses or reactive distancing—when they "crawl into a corner"; "lick their wounds"; and feel hurt, angry, or depressed. In some instances, overwhelmed by their loneliness and emptiness, they may view divorce as a possible solution and act on this perception.[9]

Distancers also experience loneliness and emptiness in the relationship, but because of personality style and past learning, they are unable to seek satisfaction and closeness in the marital relationship. Their style is one of avoiding closeness and conflict and defending against intrusion. Consequently, they become overinvolved in activities outside the family. They invest in these activities to avoid dealing with marital conflict, but the avoidance aggravates the conflict and divorce becomes the solution.

THE MULTIGENERATIONAL TRANSMISSION PROCESS. Divorce seems to run in some families. The "multigenerational transmission process" hypothesis predicts that marital dissolution in preceding generations is a contributing cause of marital dissolution in succeeding generations.[10] This phenomenon has long-range implications, given the present dramatically increasing divorce rates. On the basis of this hypothesis, it can be predicted that rates of marital dissolution will be even greater in future generations. Loyalty balancing, which will be discussed later in this chapter, has been identified as a significant dimension of this multigenerational transmission process.

Role theory has also been used to explain transgenerational influences on family divorce patterns. Those who propose the use of role theory to explain the intergenerational transmission of divorce assume that to become a successful marriage partner, a child must learn culturally appropriate sex roles and marital roles. They propose that this is done best when two loving and competent parents are available to teach these role behaviors and serve as role models. The risk that children of divorce will repeat the pattern increases when their divorced parents do not successfully socialize them with respect to appropriate sex and marital roles.[11]

Parents ideally role-model a deliberate, thoughtful approach to life and its problems. But parents who are impulsive and are unable to delay gratification role-model this behavior for their children. They often fail to foster thought-provoking discussions of problems. Young people who have such role models are at greater risk of early marriages and appear to be at high risk of divorce.

Impact of Divorce on the Child

THE PREDIVORCE PERIOD. Children in conflict-ridden homes may feel insecure and anxious; they may feel torn because loyalty to one parent entails the risk of disloyalty to the other. A complex balance of psychological forces governs the relationship between parents and children in a failing marriage. Marital stress and conflict do not always spill over into the parent-child relationship. In some instances parenting may remain relatively conflict-free. The parents may disagree strongly with each other on a great many issues but be able to communicate effectively and cooperate in the care of the children.[7]

However, Wallerstein and Kelly found that over 40 percent of the children in their study had relationships with their fathers which were exceedingly poor, rejecting, and marked by gross psychopathology or neglect. These men were physically or sexually abusive and corrosive of their child's self-esteem. At least 25 percent of the mother-child relationships were also very poor, marked by serious neglect and abuse or threatened abuse.[7]

When spousal violence occurred, children not only witnessed it but, when it was habitual, came to find it an expectable part of life. This was true for 25 percent of the children in Wallerstein and Kelly's project. Another 25 percent of the children in the study witnessed occasional violence. Regardless of whether the violence between their parents occurred habitually or occasionally, it made a vivid impression on the children and was a source of acute anxiety.

Two paradoxical phenomena seem to be associated with the parent-child relationship during the predivorce period: the negative impact of the marital tension and unhappiness affects the parent-child relationship; and at the same time there are positive gains in closeness and intimacy with the parents because of the unhappiness and frustration in the marital relationship.

The parents' perceptions of the child's response to their decision to divorce seem to reflect which parent was the initiator. The parent who disapproves of the divorce is more apt to see the children as traumatized, suffering, and in crisis. The parent who opted for the divorce tends to see the children as relatively well and adjusting to the situation.[7]

The nature and circumstances of the decision to divorce become factors in the child's capacity to cope before and after the divorce. The child's success in mastering the situation depends in part on the ability to "make good sense" of the sequence of disruptive events within the family. Seeing the divorce as a serious and carefully considered remedy for an important problem and a purposeful, rationally implemented decision—not an impulsive one—helps the child "make sense" out of what is happening to the family. The child is burdened and under stress when the divorce is unplanned, impulsive, pursued in anger or guilt, and characterized by blaming.[7]

In general, parents have difficulty telling children and adolescents about a divorce. They tend to be unsure about when and where to tell, how to tell, and how much to tell their children. Because the parents themselves are distressed, they tend to be overly concerned about their children's responses. In an effort to protect themselves, parents are often reluctant to go beyond a simple pronouncement. Feeling depleted, they are anxious and unconsciously defensive about the children's ventilation of their feelings, particularly their anger or grief. Consequently, when the announcement is finally made, it is brief, awkward, and unaccompanied by any explanation of how family life will be affected. Four-fifths of the youngest children in one study were not provided with either an adequate explanation or any assurance of continued care. Most youngsters do not know why the divorce occurred.[12] Parents, however, perceive their pronouncements as "telling."[7]

CHILDREN'S RESPONSES DURING AND AFTER THE DIVORCE. For children and adolescents, the divorce and its aftermath are a period of shock, distress, and grieving. Few children and adolescents are relieved by their parents' decision to divorce, even if they were often exposed to physical violence during the marriage. Children and adolescents most often must deal with their feelings and problems during, and in the critical months following, the divorce with little help from their parents. The parents, preoccupied with their own feelings and problems and the demands of their new life, have limited physical and psychological energy and time to be sensitive or attendant to their children's needs.

Younger children are more likely to act out than older children, who are more at risk of overt depression.[13] The psychological development of the child may be impaired, particularly if multiple environmental changes occur. In a study of children from intact and divorced families, those from disrupted families exhibited higher levels of inappropriate interpersonal behavior patterns.[14]

Children and adolescents experience heightened vulnerability when the family is disrupted by divorce. They all seek reunion of the parents and restoration of the family—if not consciously, then unconsciously. The exceptions are children who have themselves been physically abused or who have witnessed physical harm to the custodial parent or a sibling.[7]

Children who are young when a divorce occurs usually have few memories of the predivorce and divorce periods but may have recurring dreams about events that occurred during this time. In a longitudinal study of children of divorce, some youngsters were curious about why the divorce occurred but were reluctant to ask their parents. This inhibition may be based on a need to avoid generating anger or upset in the parents. For a significant number of these youngsters, the divorce was still a central, painful issue in their lives that evoked tears, sadness, and a sense of loneliness and deprivation. Over half the children interviewed continued to entertain reconciliation fantasies, in which the parents remarried and the lost family was restored. Regardless of the noncustodial parent's visiting pattern, this parent remained a significant psychological presence in the lives of these children.[15] There was evidence that these youngsters were aware of the tentative nature of the relationship with the noncustodial parent, and took steps to avoid conflict or distress in interactions with this parent.

Adolescents are particularly distressed by a parent who develops a social life that parallels theirs and, in so doing, violates generational boundaries. Their response to this parental behavior is often extreme and problematic. The divorce may exacerbate preexisting problems. These youngsters may experience school problems, emotional instability, withdrawal, acting out (such as sexual promiscuity), severe depression, runaway behavior, delinquency, substance abuse, and impulsive behavior. Those who have no history of problems and whose families have been relatively stable before the divorce may be shocked by the divorce and tend to experience a temporary regression.[16]

Children's and adolescents' perceptions of the divorce and the way they cope with their emotional response to the divorce reflect their age and stage of development. Children's responses to divorce are presented in Table 48-1 (see the following pages, 1054–1055).

Table 48-1 Children's Responses to Divorce

Response	Preschool Children	Young School-Age Children	Older School-Age Children	Adolescents
Fear and anxiety	Difficulty sorting out fantasies and dreams from reality. Diffuse and pervasive feelings. Worry about who will take care of them. Worry about whether they will be fed. Fear of abandonment. Vulnerability to disorganization and regression. Seeing themselves as replaceable if parent remarries.	Fear of abandonment. Fear of loss of independence. Development of physical symptoms.	Feeling the world is turned upside down. Feelings of rejection. Fear of loneliness. Development of physical symptoms such as headaches and stomachaches. Aggravation of preexisting health problems.	Concern with the survival of relationships. Concern with awakening sexual and aggressive impulses. Anxiety produced by seeing parents as sexual people. Concern about their own competence as sexual and marital partners. Worry about how changes in the family finances will affect them.
Anger and aggression	Irritability. Temper tantrums. Frustration focused on younger siblings. Increasing problems with peers. May massively inhibit aggressiveness and deny anger; may become overly compliant. May project aggressive impulses onto others and become fearful that others will do them harm.	Little or no anger toward father. Feelings expressed toward peers. Boys' anger expressed toward mother. Girls blame mother for the divorce.	Expressions of intense anger. Moral indignation and outrage at the parents' irresponsibility in dissolving the family.	Outbursts of anger about the divorce. Use of anger as a defense against sadness and feelings of vulnerability. Resentment about the divorce and its impact on their lifestyle.

(Continued.)

Children who make a better adjustment to the divorce develop more realistic perceptions about money matters than their peers and strategically withdraw to pursue their own interests while maintaining connectedness with both parents. Grandparents, aunts, uncles, siblings, and close or special friends are useful resources. Empathic listening helps these youngsters sort out what is happening. Some of these youngsters avoid heart-to-heart talks that elicit grief and pain but seek out supportive people and use their homes as a "port in a storm." Social activities, hobbies, and sports that may be shared with these supportive people are useful distractions which can also enhance self-esteem.[11]

When youngsters are developmentally able to analyze and interpret what is happening to them, they are better able to set, and to maintain, boundaries between themselves and their parents, and to maintain some control over their lives. Recognizing their separateness from their parents allows them to become more aware of their own needs and wishes, as separate and distinct from those of each parent. It also helps them to relate to each parent as a separate and distinct person.

Table 48-1 Continued

Response	Preschool Children	Young School-Age Children	Older School-Age Children	Adolescents
Guilt feelings	Vulnerability to guilt feelings. Belief that something they did or failed to do was the reason for the divorce.	Not usually experienced.	Not usually experienced.	Not usually experienced.
Grief	Bewilderment about the divorce. Pervasive sadness. Crying and sobbing. Intense feelings of loss influencing all dimensions of their lives.	Response similar to that of preschool child.	Defends against the loss by aligning with one parent against the other. Use of academic and recreational activities to avoid feeling grief.	Experience of profound loss. Suffering from psychobiological symptoms of grief. May act out in dissocial ways.
Functional regression	Regression: thumb-sucking, need for security blanket, lapses in toilet training. Infantile play. Macabre fantasies. Fantasies about parental reunion which help them to master the grief.	Understanding of the meaning of divorce and its impact on them. Anticipation and worry about the inevitable changes in their life. Fantasies focus on their deprivations. May eat compulsively. May hoard or demand new possessons. Idealization of the noncustodial parent.	Interests may be pursued without interruption by painful feelings. Use of social and school activities as defensive strategies to overcome feelings of helplessness and powerlessness. Shame about the divorce. Lying and covering up; may not even tell close friends. Working toward parental reconciliation.	Parents' self-absorption may force a premature separation and independence from the family, accelerating development processes. Worry about right and wrong because of lack of parental support and guidance. If parents are sexually active, adolescents may sexually act out; premarital pregnancy. May withdraw from dating. "Bury" themselves in sports, hobbies, school. Antisocial acting out.

Postdivorce Changes

Following divorce, potential stressors include issues of custody, financial changes, feelings, alterations in physical health, socializing, and sexuality.

CUSTODY. Children cannot survive and maximize their potential without the protection and nurturing provided by adults with whom they have a psychological bond. Society has evolved legislative and judicial mechanisms to protect children and ensure their well-being.[17]

Custody is a legal term used to designate the care and control aspects of a relationship between a child and his or her care givers. It implies watching, security, responsibility, and protection, but not absolute control or ownership. Custody decisions in a divorce can be resolved in either of two ways. One parent may be awarded custody of the children, or the two parents may have a joint custody arrangement.

When one parent has custody, this parent assumes responsibility for the day-to-day care of the children, and the noncustodial parent is awarded the right to visitation. This arrangement often leads to decreased contact with the noncustodial parent. A custodial parent who places little value on the noncustodial parent's relationship with the children may negatively influence the children's perception of the noncustodial parent.[18] This negative influence may generate guilt or sympathy toward the noncustodial parent or may bring about an alliance with the custodial parent and rejection of the noncustodial parent.

Custodial parents often feel humiliated, angry, depressed, and overburdened. Consequently, they have difficulty in coping with the daily demands of the children, much less their acute distress precipitated by the divorce. The children, sensitive to the custodial parent's distress, also tend to become more anxious and depressed. Because of the custodial parent's distress, and the need to protect the custodial parent, the children are unable to share what is happening to them or to seek comfort from this parent.[7]

Noncustodial parents tend to be less available and more worrisome to the offspring. The noncustodial parent is often deeply involved in locating and establishing a residence and beginning a new life. Therefore, during and immediately after the divorce he or she usually has less contact with the children. A noncustodial parent who becomes severely depressed worries the children.[7]

The day-to-day responsibility for child rearing without the participation and support of the other parent can be a burden for the custodial parent. When divorce occurs, both the custodial parent and the noncustodial parent have responsibilities and problems related to parenting. The custodial parent often becomes the one who must set and enforce limits and take responsibility for socializing the children. The noncustodial parent with weekend visiting arrangements may become the "good-time" parent, permissive and overindulgent.

Research findings indicate that both the custodial parent's misuse of power and the noncustodial parent's dependence on the custodial parent's goodwill to maintain a relationship with the children affect the quality of the children's relationships with both parents.

Custodial parents may resent the time children spend with noncustodial parents. Custodial parents may perceive their time with the children as all work and no fun. Consequently, they may demand that noncustodial parents use visitation time to solve disciplinary problems.

Visits with the children may generate ambivalent feelings. If old spousal conflicts are renewed at such times, the noncustodial parent may dread these encounters and wish to avoid the whole scene, in which case the visits may be few and far between.[19] If visiting is restricted to weekends and summer vacations, having the children at these times may interfere with the noncustodial parent's dating or courting. If the attachment to the children is poor, the noncustodial parent may drift away from the children and see very little of them.

Some parents, immediately following the divorce, attempt to include their dates when the children are visiting, or to take the children to their dates' homes. Children may have difficulty accepting a parent's date, but—more important—they may feel rejected by the parent and in "second place" compared with the date.

The custodial parent has greater opportunity to align with, and influence, the children. If the parent is bitter and resentful, he or she may either overtly or covertly influence the children to reject the noncustodial parent. Consequently, the children may choose not to visit with the parent, or they may plan a conflicting activity that prevents visiting. In some instances the children may become openly hostile and angry toward the noncustodial parent.

Research has found that when this relationship is disrupted, the children experience impaired cognitive development. The noncustodial parent who had an affectionate relationship with the children experiences acute loneliness, a sense of loss, and depression following the divorce. The pain associated with intermittent visiting tends to result in diminished visiting.[19]

The more desirable arrangement is joint custody or coparenting. In this situation both parents are involved in child rearing. The children lose neither parent. Both parents are able to maintain a close relationship with the children. If, however, conflict between the parents is acute, the children's adjustment may be impaired.[20] For a couple to continue acting jointly as parents, their relationship must be based on trust and respect. The couple also need to be able to communicate effectively. The logistics of this custody arrangement require joint orchestration.[21]

If the parents maintain residences in the same community and school district and in proximate neighborhoods, the movement from one parent's home to the other's is comparatively easy for the children. Some couples arrange the joint custody so that the child spends alternating weeks at each parent's home. Others use an alternating 3-day, 4-day pattern.

Scheduling toys, clothes, money, and moves between households requires careful planning and attention to detail. When children sense this essential degree of parental cooperation and mutual concern for them, the divorce is less of a threat to their security and less anxiety-provoking.[21]

Since the logistics of residing in two households are complicated and designed in part to meet the child's needs, it is important that the children also participate in planning the schedule, the permanent location of possessions, and what items go back and forth with them.

The joint custody arrangement allows each parent free time to pursue social, work, educational, and recreational activities. Neither has the total burden of rearing the children, and the children do not feel abandoned by the noncustodial parent, as may be the case in other custody agreements.

However, coparenting is not a miracle cure for the problems encountered by parents and children following divorce. Children still become jealous of parents' dates, and parents may feel lonely, experience low self-esteem, and become angry and resentful toward one another. Coparenting does, however, provide opportunities for the children to continue to share love, warmth, and closeness with both parents on an ongoing basis. Furthermore, it helps them to cope effectively with the dissolution of the marriage, the development of self-concept, and eventually their own marital situation.[21]

If parents continue to be bitter, resentful, angry, or in conflict, coparenting can be a disaster. Decisions about the children's education, health care, or privileges may become a parental battleground. Rather than stabilizing the child's world, joint custody may become a threat to the child's physical, emotional, and social well-being. Children need to know that there is an adult responsible for them.[17] If the children become the focus of the parents' continuing conflict, the children will experience guilt and anxiety. They may see themselves as the cause of their parents' problems; and this may impair their self-image if they also see themselves as "bad" for causing the dissolution of the family.[22]

FINANCIAL CHANGES. In most instances, divorce produces changes in the family's economic base that become a focus of concern. The need to support two homes tends to cause a notable decline in the living standard. In one study three-fifths of the men and three-quarters of the women experienced financial problems.[7] The sudden reduction of income may be inconvenient but not serious, or it may be so drastic as to cause one person (usually the woman) to sink to the poverty level of subsistence.[23]

Some degree of bitterness appears to be almost inevitable in relation to the financial agreement no matter what its nature is. The aggrieved spouse's ability to take half the family property may be perceived as the final insult. Initially the person who chooses to terminate the marriage is likely to ask for less or to be generous in the settlement. Later this spouse is apt to become angry about the lopsided arrangement.[7]

Despite the legal requirements in some states that community property accumulated during the marriage be equally divided, women still tend to be affected by severe economic changes more substantially, and more permanently, than men. This is particularly true among middle- and lower-class families.[7] In many instances identification with a particular social class, which had been the core of the woman's self-esteem, had been largely determined by the husband's education, occupation, position in the community, and income. The divorce means a loss of this identification and self-esteem. Men may also be devastated by the divorce and lose self-esteem. However, they do not usually experience the additional stress of a major change in status which disrupts their base of social operations.[7]

FEELINGS. Predivorce feelings of anger, bitterness, anxiety, and depression do not magically disappear when the divorce is final. They must be worked through gradually. Since many of these feelings are part of the grieving process, the first year following the divorce is a significant period. Letting go of the past, living in the present, and anticipating a hopeful future are not easy tasks, but they are necessary. Problematic feelings are not resolved, despite the legal papers that declare the end of the marriage.

Money is the most frequent focus of anger; visiting is the next most frequent.[7]

Some couples become enmeshed in an ongoing, bitter battle in which hatred and vindictiveness may serve as a defense against a more devastating depression. Anger seems to enhance their capacity to maintain a semblance of psychological inner order. These embittered, chaotic people seem to make no effort to shield the children from their raw hostility or the resulting chaos; in many instances, they involve the children in the battle. Custody battles, kidnapping of the children from the parent awarded custody, and interference with the noncustodial parent's visits are often reflections of this bitterness. The children may be told that if they visit the estranged parent, they can leave; or that if the other parent really loved them, he or she would not have abandoned them.[7]

On the other hand, a battling couple, unable to communicate calmly or rationally on any other topic, may present a united front, collaborate, and be mutually supportive when a child develops physical symptoms. Unfortunately, if the couple join together to help the child and this unity is visible to the child, the child may unconsciously use physical symptoms as a way of reuniting the family.

Following the upheaval created by the divorce, the irritations, frustrations, and problems of daily living may be magnified and experienced as overwhelming. For example, burned toast or the breakdown of an appliance may generate intense anger or depression. The grief related to the losses incurred by the divorce and loneliness are the source of these intensified feelings. Some custodial and noncustodial parents withdraw physically and psychologically while they are grieving.

In spite of the anger, the depression, and the sometimes massive changes in lifestyle, some people view divorce as an opportunity for change for the better and for personal growth. For some, the final decree brings a feeling of relief. They are happy to be free of the conflicts and problems—and sometimes the violence—they experienced in the marriage. They happily anticipate a new lifestyle and possibly remarriage.

PHYSICAL HEALTH. Marital conflict and disruption are inherently stressful. Low income has been found to generate high levels of stress and is related to health problems among the divorced.[24–27] The changes and stress caused by divorce may contribute to development of physical and emotional dysfunction among family members.[24,25] Weiss[26] found that loss of a spouse uniformly produces intense distress. The disruption of attachment is a major source of this distress. When the separation is accompanied or followed by basic changes in social role and relationships, the stress is even greater.[26]

Health problems encountered by the divorced people include an increased risk of automobile accidents; psychiatric problems; and medical illnesses such as lung cancer, diabetes mellitus, and arteriosclerotic heart disease. The risk of these health problems appears to be greatest at the time of the separation and when the divorce becomes final.[19]

SOCIALIZING. Loneliness during the postdivorce period may be acute. The tendency is to allow past social relationships to deteriorate. Women especially have a tendency to allow the collapse of these social relationships. They may feel shame or believe that they are unwanted—"the fifth wheel"—at social gatherings. They may also believe, and sometimes rightly so, that their married friends feel threatened by the "contagious" nature of divorce. Friends of the couple often feel unsure, uncomfortable, and inadequate in relating to those who are newly divorced. Because of this discomfort, they may exclude the divorced person from some activities, particularly those that are couple-oriented.[7]

In some instances a geographical move following the divorce interrupts social relationships. Limited financial resources may be an obstacle to entertaining or joining others in many recreational activities. If the children are young, custodial parents may be hampered from developing a social life because of parenting responsibilities and because they cannot afford baby-sitters.

The noncustodial parent, often the man, may have both greater opportunity and adequate finances to develop a social life as a single person. Men usually find it easier to develop a new circle of friends or continue socializing with old friends, particularly when the social activities center on spectator sports or recreational sports such as golf, hunting, or soccer. Men also usually have fewer problems than women in relation to dating.[7]

SEXUALITY. Sexuality after divorce is a significant issue. Because of sexual deprivation and a lack of affection before the breakup, some people look forward to a renewed sexual life, closeness, and affection from new partners.

It is often difficult for both men and women to seek out and become comfortable with new sexual partners if they have been faithful to their spouses during marriage. Following the divorce, some people attempt to deal with their loneliness and exclusion by their married friends by having many superficial sexual encounters.

Men and women who have been rejected by their spouse in favor of a new partner experience a threat to their self-concept and sexual identity. It may be difficult for these people to take the risk of seeking out new partners. Others, who have experienced problems with their sexuality and the sexual relationship in the marriage, may feel a degree of relief to be free of the pressure to have sex. However, these people may be acutely distressed by the loneliness and lack of affection in their lives following the divorce.

Single-Parent Families

The single-parent family structure may result from abandonment or death of a parent, or divorce; or by choice: a woman may bear a child as a single person, and either a man or a woman may become a single adoptive parent. Most single-parent families are headed by women who are in the lower socioeconomic strata of society.[28]

The problems encountered by these families reflect physical, emotional, and socioeconomic stress. These parents tend to feel lonely, guilty, depressed, and at times overwhelmed. Many custodial parents often feel frightened and insecure when they first find themselves with the sole responsibility for rearing their children on a day-to-day basis. When these parents must depend on welfare, child support, and other stigmatizing or unstable sources of income, they feel unable to plan for their lives.[29] The inability to plan for tomorrow or the more distant future contributes to family disorganization. Financial constraints imposed by death or by abandonment by the partner, divorce, or the struggle to support the family with one paycheck may be a continual problem. Unexpected problems having to do with health, the home, or even the family car may cause crises.

Children are upset by the dissolution of the family or death of a parent and may present problems. Custodial or surviving parents may have difficulty recognizing or resolving these problems because they are depressed or have neither time nor energy after working and managing homemaking chores. They may cope by denying the children's problems.

A custodial mother may become heavily invested in succeeding at a new career or educational pursuits outside the home. The transition from the homemaker role and identity to that of career woman or student is often difficult. A custodial father may try to be both mother and father. If he lacks homemaking skills, he may focus on the physical needs of the children and lack sensitivity to their emotional needs.

Surviving and custodial parents who live with or near their parents have the advantage of their support. But they or their children may find this arrangement problematic if the grandparents "take over" and the custodial parent becomes one of the "children." The grandparents may undermine the custodial parent's authority and also interfere with the children's relationship with the other grandparents.

Single parents who have financial resources and a sound support system may manage the new family structure effectively despite the inherent stress, change, and conflict. A study comparing children from single-parent and reconstituted families with children from intact families found that on the whole there is no significant difference in self-concept and functioning between these groups of children. However, children who perceive greater conflict in their families, regardless of whether both parents are present, have significantly lower self-concepts.[30]

Stepfamilies

A stepfamily is a family system in which at least one of the adults is a stepparent. Children of one or both of the adults, who may or may not be married, live in the household or visit regularly.

The words *stepchild* and *stepmother* historically have had a negative connotation. Children's stories, such as "Cinderella" and "Hansel and Gretel,"

Table 48-2 Stepfamilies

Reasons for Self-Imposed Invisibility
1. Feelings about having failed in marriage once and reluctance to admit to problems with the second marriage
2. Unpreparedness for the roles in a reconstituted family
3. Failure to recognize that many of the problems encountered are not unique
4. Tendency of stepparents to have unrealistic expectations of themselves which are inevitably not met and therefore generate guilt or anger
5. Lack of self-confidence in the stepfamily's ability to fulfill their own and others' expectations
6. Inherent competition between the dual sets of parents
7. Stepchildren's reluctance to surrender their wishful fantasy for reunion of their families of origin
8. Sensitivity to the overall discomfort in relation to stepparenting

emphasize the plight of the stepchild and the wickedness of stepmothers.

Stepfamilies tend to maintain a low profile. The reasons for this partially self-imposed invisibility are presented in Table 48-2.

Structure of Stepfamilies

The structure of a stepfamily differs significantly from that of an intact family by virtue of its complexity and the varied legal and genetic relationships among members. The roles of mother, father, and child may be filled by several people, some of whom have neither legal ties nor blood ties. The children are often, to varying degrees, members of more than one household. Stepparents have no legal relationship to a stepchild. The social or parental relationship may last only as long as the marriage.

The original nuclear family is split by death or a divorce. Remarriages may result in four new stepfamilies families, each directly or indirectly influencing the children: "yours," "mine," "ours," and "theirs." The genogram in Figure 48-1 illustrates the complexity of these families. The number and complexity of the roles, relationships, and loyalty ties may interfere with the children's identification and attachment processes and with the development of their self-concept.

Functioning of Stepfamilies

Remarriage and the addition of a new parental figure create loyalty conflicts for children. Feelings of loss may escalate. Rivalries, jealousies, and feelings of alienation and isolation affect children and adults. Young or adult children accept a stepparent more readily than adolescents do.[31] Bonds between one parent and the children who are part of the "remarriage package" predate the couple's relationship. The nonbiological parent may feel left out.

Figure 48-1 Three-generational genogram for stepfamilies.
(SOURCE: Symbols from E. G. Pendergast and C. O. Sherman, "A Guide to the Genogram," *The Family,* vol. 5, no. 1, 1977, pp. 101–112.)

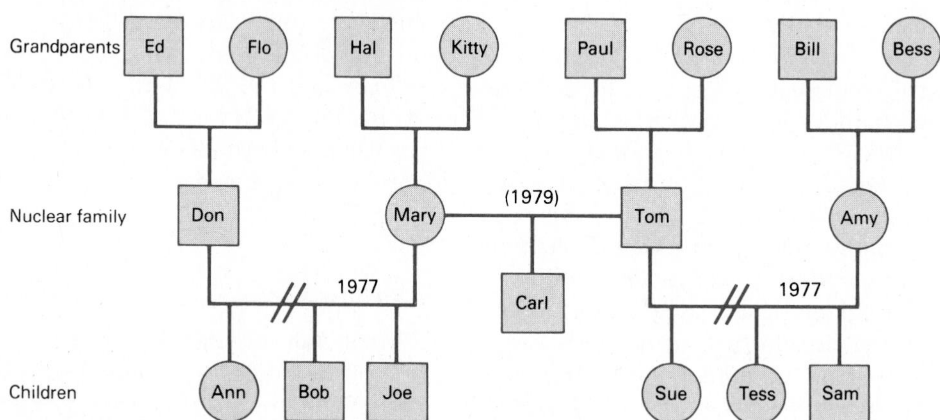

Divorced couples: Don and Mary; Tom and Amy
Stepfamily: Mary and Tom (parents); Ann, Bob, Joe, Carl (children)
Single-parent family: Amy (parent); Sue, Tess, Sam (children)
Stepgrandparents: Paul and Rose

Children may also feel displaced if the remarried couple's relationship excludes them. Stepchildren tend to perceive both their stepfathers and their natural fathers more negatively than children from intact families perceive their fathers.[32] Biological parents often feel very protective of their children. Further, children in stepfamilies have already lived through the turmoil of their parents' divorce and more than likely are still trying to resolve the losses and changes in their lives. Family boundaries are blurred and ambiguous. The blurring and permeability of boundaries may interfere with a child's sense of belonging.

Problems of Stepfamilies

Stepfamilies must deal with the usual problems of sibling rivalry, spousal and parent-child conflict, setting limits, attempts by members to align, and, at one time or another, members' being left out or made scapegoats. The complexity of the stepfamily structure, the leftover feelings from the disruption of the nuclear family or families, and the inherent loyalty conflicts complicate these problems and introduce additional difficulties. Problems unique to stepfamilies are presented in Table 48-3 and discussed in the following sections.

BIOLOGICAL PARENT VERSUS STEPPARENT. The biological parent outside the household may have a considerable impact on the stepfamily, regardless of whether the parent is alive or dead. If the biological parent has died, the children often idealize the lost parent. The stepparent, who is human and real, can never replace or live up to the perfection of the idealized image. Acceptance of the stepparent may also seem to be inherent disloyalty to the dead parent. The deceased parent's picture may be prominently placed in the home and serve as a constant reminder of the preceding marital relationship and family unity.

Remarriage places the ex-spouse in an outside position. Fears of losing the children and competition for their affection and loyalty may produce behaviors that disrupt the newly formed stepfamily. Struggles often emerge around visiting, gifts, and setting limits.

Table 48-3 Stepfamilies

Special Problems
1. There is a biological parent outside the household.
2. Children are members of two households.
3. Two families—with different backgrounds, values, and ways of interacting (and sometimes with at least one member who has a history of marital failure)—are attempting to blend. This creates problems of integration, particularly with regard to making and enforcing rules.
4. There may be one or more "extra" sets of grandparents.
5. Allocation of money within the household may be complicated, and there may also be financial arrangements involving two or more households.
6. Choosing a residence may become an issue.
7. Stepparents' roles are ill defined.
8. The relationships are new and untested.

CHILDREN BETWEEN TWO HOUSEHOLDS. Moving back and forth between two households can be stressful for children. Rules, expectations, and limits may be drastically different, requiring a continual shifting of behavior and ways of relating.

Biological children visiting in a household where stepchildren live are in a no-win position. The children are not members of the visited household, but a biological parent lives there. The biological parent's relationship with the stepchildren living in the home generate jealousies and loyalty conflicts. The visited parent has obligations to the natural visiting children. However, the overall relationship time, availability, and accessibility of that parent are greater for the stepchildren living in the household than for the natural visiting children.

There may also be a sharp discrepancy between the social status and affluence of the remarried and the custodial parents' households. Visiting natural children who reside with their custodial mother may live in far less affluence and may have even lost their original home because of the divorce. The visiting children may feel deprived and rejected, and may feel like second-class citizens, when they visit their more affluent remarried parent. Inner turmoil may be expressed in unpredictable, disruptive ways when they visit.

The stepparent is in a bind. These are not his or her children, and thus attempts to manage the disruption or problematic behavior may be met with hostility from the biological parent and his or her children. If the stepparent is obviously distressed, his or her children may align with the parent. Such alignments split the stepfamily and interfere with the development of cohesiveness and the establishment of family boundaries.[32]

STEPFAMILY INTEGRATION: MAKING AND ENFORCING RULES. Integration of the stepfamily is a function of the passage of time; the definition of roles, relationships, responsibilities, and norms; and the development of a feeling of belonging, cohesiveness, and attraction to the family. Setting and enforcing limits are an area of intrafamily interaction and a basic social process which influences integration or disintegration.

Who makes rules and who is allowed to enforce them are a significant part of the integration process. Rules for making and enforcing rules have a major influence on the development of roles and relationships. Stern[33] found that early in the family's development, the natural mother plays go-between for her children and the stepfather. The same probably happens between a natural father and his children, since he also knows both his children and the stepmother best. If this process becomes entrenched, the natural parent's go-between role interferes with integration.

Stern[33] describes five ways that stepfamilies deal with making and enforcing rules which influence family integration. The structural patterns that interfere with family integration are presented in Table 48-4. The rule-making and rule-enforcing pattern most supportive of integration is characteristically democratic, with no one left out. Setting limits is a part of the total socialization process. The stepparent does not attempt to replace the absent or lost biological parent. Instead, the stepparent makes a friend of the child before assuming a comanagement role with the biological parent. To become a friend, the stepparent demonstrates that he or she is on the child's side. The stepparent is available as an empathic listener and someone who helps to create pleasurable moments. Championing the child's course aligns the stepparent against the biological parent, who may initially resent this new power bloc. When the interference is in the child's best interest, the biological parent eventually recognizes this reality and the child develops a positive perception of the stepparent. This integrative undermining helps the family move toward integration.[33]

Table 48-4 Problematic Stepfamilies

Making and Enforcing Rules
"Not my kid"—Stepparent left out
Biological parent fails to share rule making and enforcing, sabotages the stepparent.
Stepparent distances the children.
Everyone left out
Stepparent moves too quickly in making and enforcing rules.
Biological parent disapproves and sabotages the stepparent by directly confronting the stepparent's authority and right to make and enforce rules or indirectly by ignoring or countermanding the rules.
Children recognize the split and the power they derive from it.
Chaos develops because everyone makes rules and there is no consistent enforcement.
"Anything you say, dear"—Stepparent left out
Biological parent leaves the rule-making and rule-enforcing role to the stepparent.
Because the biological parent has been burdened and overwhelmed by parenting responsibilities before the remarriage, the stepparent's assumption of the responsibility is welcomed.
Stepparent makes a rule; biological parent is expected to enforce it.
Biological parent may not abdicate responsibility for rule making entirely.
Biological parent enforces rules which receive his or her approval.
Biological parent sabotages rules which receive his or her disapproval by ignoring or forgetting them, or violations of the rules become a secret between the biological parent and the children.
Children left out
Biological parent says "take over" to the stepparent and means it.
Stepparent moves in as directed, establishes firm rules, and strictly enforces them.
Children become resentful of this stranger and fight back.
Stepparent counters with harsher rules and punishments.
Children develop severe behavior problems or physically or psychologically withdraw.
Biological parent and stepparent align and children are left out.

SOURCE: P. N. Stern, "Stepfather Families: Integration around Child Discipline," *Issues in Mental Health Nursing*, vol. 1, Summer 1978, pp. 49–56.

GRANDPARENTS AND STEPGRANDPARENTS. Grandparents can be a positive resource for children when a parent dies, during their parents' divorce, and during the remarriage of one parent and the formation of the stepfamily. When a parent remarries, the children may acquire stepgrandparents. These older adults are expected to incorporate the children into their lives. This may be very difficult, particularly if they disapprove of the divorce and the remarriage. Children are sensitive to the significant adults in the family circle. Even if stepgrandparents do not express overt rejection, the step-grandchildren may pick up on subtle messages that reflect an unwillingness to accept them as members of the family.

In some instances grandparents and grandchildren may form a tight unity excluding all others. The disapproval and rejection of the remarriage of a parent become a bonding force for this coalition. This alignment can be destructive to the stepfamily. Supported by the grandparents, the children resist the parent's and stepparent's efforts to integrate the family.[32]

ALLOCATION OF MONEY. Money is a common problem for intact families, divorced families, and stepfamilies. In stepfamilies money and its allocation are an emotional issue. Paying alimony and child support may contribute to a scarcity of money in a stepfamily. One spouse may be responsible for such payments as well as for supporting the stepfamily, including stepchildren. In most families the income available for these allocations is limited. Basic needs and wishes may be affected, and the new stepfamily may be burdened by financial worries. The resulting tensions may influence other areas of family life and may thus impede family integration.

Alimony and child support payments tie ex-spouses together and become a source of continued conflict. The payments reflect the permeability of the stepfamily's boundaries and are a threat to the formation and integrity of these boundaries.[32]

CHOOSING A RESIDENCE. People are by nature territorial. The process of selecting a residence and deciding on whether to settle in his, her, or new "turf" significantly influences and reflects relationships and power balancing within the family. Discussions between the couple about where to live generally conclude with a decision that addresses the needs of either the biological parent, the stepparent, or the children. The decision reflects a designation of the family focus and who holds the pivotal power position in the family. Available space and its allocation can become a source of conflict. Few stepfamilies resolve the allocation of space and resources as logically and agreeably as families in television shows.[32]

The advantages and disadvantages of each option are presented in Table 48-5.

Table 48-5 Choosing a Residence

Residence	Advantages	Disadvantages
New home	Neutral turf for everyone. No member has prior claim to ownership. No one is a guest in the house.	Children are uprooted. Friends are left behind. Adjustment to new neighborhood. Adjustment to new school. Exposure to multiple changes within a short period of time.
Stepparent's home	Stepparent on own turf.	Children are uprooted. Friends are left behind. Adjustment to new neighborhood. Adjustment to new school. Strange turf—children feel like guests in stepparent's home. Stepparent's children feel their turf has been invaded and they have lost territory.
Biological parent's home	Minimizes impact on the biological children. Biological children in their own home. Biological children and parent have a shared history in the home and a sense of ownership.	Maximum impact on stepparent and his or her children. Stepparent and his or her children feel like guests. Stepparent may be outnumbered. Stepparent must live with another person's belongings; attempts to redecorate are met with hostility from stepchildren.

SOURCE: E. B. Visher and J. S. Visher, *Stepfamilies*, Brunner/Mazel, New York, 1979.

DEFINING STEPPARENTS' ROLES. The role of stepparent is poorly defined. The stepparents, the children involved, and society do not know what to expect of stepparents. Their involvement with the education and health care systems of their stepchildren is poorly defined and tends to be confusing to the authorities and the family.[32]

The stepparent needs to negotiate his or her role with the biological parent and the stepchildren and in relation to the school system and the health care of the children. Keeping in mind the importance of the stepparent's defining himself or herself as being on the child's side, it would seem that the role relationship with the school and health care needs are initially seen by the children as helpful and caring. Since neither of these social systems has a very clear notion of how a stepparent fits in, the stepparent may need to assertively define his or her role for these systems. If the stepchildren perceive the stepparent's efforts as championing their cause and looking out for their interests, the stepparent-child relationship will be enhanced.

Stepfathers tend to achieve better relations with stepchildren than stepmothers do. This may be related to their more limited presence and day-to-day involvement in child rearing. Stepmothers fare better in their relationships with stepchildren under age 13 than with teenagers. Stepmothers have been found to be more ambivalent about their stepchildren, to experience jealousy of them, and to be at risk of feelings of anxiety, depression, and anger related to family relations. Their role as stepparent is made more difficult by the lack of a clearly defined status in society.[32]

Stepparents seem to take less personal responsibility for their stepchildren's problems than natural parents, and to blame factors other than themselves for the stepchildren's problems.[34] Stepparents run into problems when they have unrealistic expectations of themselves. When the stepchildren have experienced a traumatic divorce, abandonment, or the death of a parent, the stepparent may attempt to "make up" to the children for the pain and disruption in their lives. It is not possible to "take away" or "make up" for past pain; efforts to do so are doomed to fail. The most a stepparent can do is to provide a positive, warm, empathic relationship that allows the children to work through the losses and find acceptance and affection in the child-stepparent relationship.

When stepparents attempt to recreate the nuclear family as a close-knit, happy stepfamily, they face an impossible task. The hopes and expectations for cohesiveness and emotional closeness are idealistic in nature. The expectation of instant love ends in disappointment. The inevitable conflicts and expressions of anger may be viewed as shattering rather than a part of the evolving family life. The stepfamily can never become the original nuclear family. The stepparent can never replace the lost parent; attempts to do so will create problems for the stepparent and the stepchildren. To replace the lost parent would represent disloyalty.[32]

On the whole, stepchildren, once integrated, consider themselves as happy as children from intact families, and they achieve as much. The consensus is that there is not much long-range detrimental effect on children reared in stepfamilies. Thus, despite the difficulties encountered by these families, the children fare well. However, children from lower-class families find the remarriage more stressful than those from families with higher socioeconomic status. This difference may reflect the effect of deprivations imposed by limited financial resources. The difference may also lie in the reasons for remarriage. People in lower socioeconomic groups tend to remarry to fill the role of the absent parent, particularly the breadwinner. People in higher socioeconomic groups often remarry in an attempt to achieve a satisfying relationship.[32]

Adoption

Throughout the ages societies have used the adoption process as a way of legally providing care for children whose biological parents are unwilling or unable to meet their minimal needs. All cultures have found adoption to be an effective form of substitute care for children deprived of their natural parents.

Parenting, even under the most ideal conditions, is a complex and difficult task. The legal process which transfers parental rights and responsibilities from biological parents to people who volunteer to serve as the child's parents may seem clear-cut, but there are problems inherent in a parent-child relationship that is socially constructed.[35,36]

Unwanted Children

Every child has the right to be wanted. However, in spite of liberalized abortion laws, the availability of contraception, and supposedly adequate supportive welfare programs, many children are born to people unwilling or unable to assume responsibility for their care.

Children become available for adoption by nonrelatives as a consequence of abandonment by or death of their parents, because of illegitimacy, or because their parents decide to relinquish a child they perceive as an economic or psychological burden they do not want or are unable to assume.

Since a considerable percentage of adoptees are illegitimate, the availability and accessibility of prenatal care for the unwed pregnant woman have an impact on adopted children. Research on the relationship between the psychological state of the mother and the condition of the newborn infant suggests that stress during pregnancy has negative consequences.[35]

Decision to Adopt

Historically the childless couple who have adopted a child have been infertile and have been expected by the adoption agency to submit proof of being unable to bear children. In recent times, however, with increasing societal concern about overpopulation, some couples are choosing not to procreate and instead to adopt children. Couples who adopt often subscribe to the American ideology that a family without a child is incomplete and less satisfying.

Many people seeking to adopt a child are older. They are couples who have finally accepted their infertility and seek a "fantasy child" who will enhance the quality of their lives as they grow old. Unfortunately, the well-ordered lives of such couples and their rigid personalities are bombarded by the lively, noisy, ungrateful, growing child they adopt. Relinquishing the fantasized, cheerful, companionable, well-mannered child may be a painful and destructive process for all concerned. When older couples adopt, they may develop a grandparent-grandchild relationship which is either too distant, too permissive, or too incorporative, making adjustment difficult for the child. Similarly, when a young couple adopt an older child, the relationship that develops may resemble sibling-sibling rather than parent-child, thus impairing the necessary generational boundary.

Some couples apply for a baby in the belief that a child will help a foundering marital relationship develop into a satisfying and happy family. Clothier also reports situations in which a couple have been advised that the responsibility of caring for a baby would be the best treatment for the wife's "nervousness."

People also adopt children for a variety of unconscious reasons similar to those of couples who bear children: to be loved, to cope with loneliness in the marital relationship, to be like one's social group and therefore accepted, to meet the expectations of their parents, and as an excuse to leave an unsatisfying career. Both the couple and the child may have problems if these reasons and the accompanying fantasies prevent a realistic appraisal of parenting and its impact on the couple's lifestyle.

Family Structure

The obvious structure of the adoptive family resembles the natural family unit: mother, father, child, and extended kin. What is often forgotten in identifying the subsystems of the adoptive family is the biological parents, because they are not visible. These "hereditary ghosts," even though they may be in reality unknown to the adoptive parents and the adoptee, influence the adoptive family processes by their existence and their biological link to the child, and because of the perceptions of them held by the significant family members in the adoptive family. Thus a genogram of an adoptive family would be modified to include both the adoptive and the natural parents and their extended kin, as illustrated in Figure 48-2 (page 1066).

Parents Who Surrender Their Children

The decision to surrender a child for adoption is not an easy one. A variety of factors have an influence, including financial constraints, lack of situational support, unpreparedness for the parenting role, either family opposition to adoption or pressure to surrender the child, shame, and uncompleted education.[37] Many parents who give up their children are young and unmarried.

There are long-term consequences to the decision to surrender a child for adoption. Having made the decision does not close the issue. One study

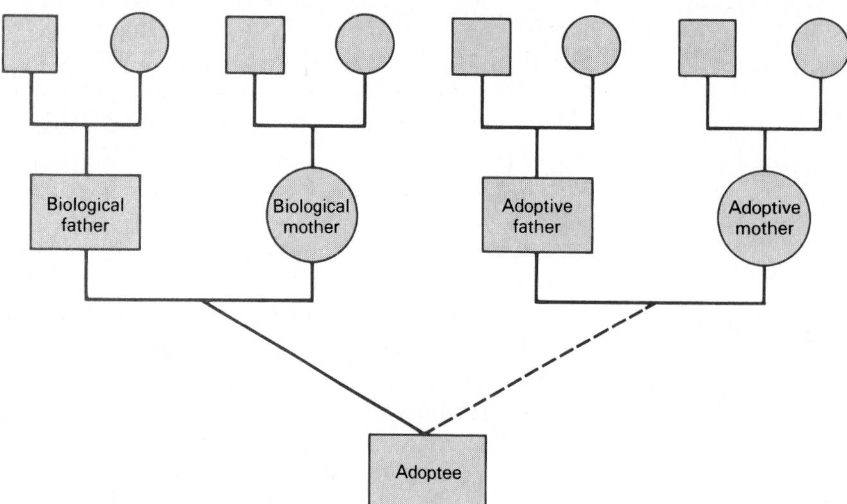

Figure 48-2 Three-generational genogram for an adoptive family.

found that 96 percent of biological mothers consider searching for their child years after the adoption, and 65 percent actually initiate a search. These women also reported that the adoption had had a negative influence on their subsequent marriages, and some reported that it had influenced their reproductivity. Of those studied, 14 percent were unable to become pregnant and 17 percent chose to remain childless. Among those who did bear subsequent children, almost all reported that they tended to be overprotective, compulsive, worried parents, particularly with regard to their children's health and their own difficulty in accepting their growing children's independence.[37]

Foster Care

Foster placement of children disrupts family relationships. The child is removed from the home shared with one or both parents, and in some instances with siblings, and is resettled in the home of the extended family or of strangers, in an institution, or in a group home. Of the children known to be in foster placement, because some social agency was involved in the placement, approximately half are placed for longer than 2 years and one-third are placed for 4 or more years. One-half of these children live in more than one foster home and have as many as four caseworkers. The exact number of children who are in foster homes is unknown, since many arrangements are made among family members and therefore are not reported by the courts or social service agencies.[38]

Placement Process

The child's placement may be effected by one or both parents; by the extended family, whose members believe the child is not being adequately cared for; or by authorities who have determined that the child has been abandoned, dangerously abused, or neglected, or that the parents are dead or imprisoned. Table 48-6 lists, in order of frequency, the reasons for foster placement. Currently, children who require placement away from their own families tend to come largely from families in which the parents' social disorganization or personality disorders are so severe as to affect their ability to provide adequate care.[39]

Legal intervention occurs primarily when the family has had contact with the police, a health care agency, or a social service agency. The parents

Table 48-6 Foster Care

Reasons for Placement
Mental illness of parent
Neglect or abuse
Behavior of the child
Physical illness of parent
Abandonment or desertion by parent
Parent unwilling or unable to provide care
Death of one or both parents
Imprisonment of parent
Parental retardation
Parental alcoholism or addiction
Unavailability of extended family

may be in prison, may have sexually or physically abused the child, or may have psychiatric problems that require long-term hospitalization; or the severity of their physical or emotional problems may impair their ability to function adequately as parents. Parents have been known to simply abandon their children, leaving them without economic support or supervision. In chaotic, disorganized families there may be no relative able or willing to care for the child, and placement in a foster home, institution, or group home is effected through legal procedures. A social agency implements the court's decision.

In many instances, several children in a family must be placed. One study revealed that these families tend to have three or more children in foster homes, and only half the time are siblings placed together.

Some parents, particularly of adolescents, threaten their youngsters with placement out of the family. These parents often use either a psychiatric hospitalization of the adolescent or the youngster's involvement with the judicial system to implement the threat and exclude the child from the family. Four major factors contribute to this action: (1) parents' frustration about their inability to control the child's behavior; (2) marginal family socioeconomic and emotional resources; (3) ambivalence about parenthood; and (4) unresolved feelings on the part of a single parent toward an ex-spouse. Adolescent delinquency, violence, or both may interact with unrealistic parental expectations. The youngster's physical appearance, sex, or personality may be a reminder of a hated person and may thus lead to rejection. Many of these parents have low self-esteem and feel unable to cope with the youngster's increasing needs for autonomy, affection, and guidance. Often the parents themselves experienced foster placement as children. Parents who experienced deprivation during childhood lack the personal resources needed to nurture and guide their children. If the parent is single and lacks support from a spouse and extended family, child rearing may become overwhelming and intolerable when the youngster becomes an adolescent.[40]

These youngsters, regardless of their ages, are confronted with fears of loneliness and abandonment. They are depressed and anxious. Rejected youngsters may cling to their parents in a frantic attempt to stay in the family; or adolescents may defend themselves from the sense of hopelessness and the role of victim by becoming angry and protesting against the rejection. Many blame themselves for their predicament. Whatever the outcome, their sense of trust is impaired. Consequently, their ability to establish and maintain meaningful relationships is jeopardized.[40]

If the family has had contact with the police, a health care agency, or a social service agency, the law may intervene. When children are abandoned or there is no relative available to care for them, a court decides that placement is appropriate, and a social agency carries out the decision.

A child who is placed with relatives has a greater chance of remaining in that home until maturity or until the family of origin is reconstituted. Children placed in homes of nonrelatives have a greater chance of temporary, multiple foster placements. Statistics show that approximately 5 years is the average length of time spent in foster placement and that approximately 83 percent of foster children are never returned to their biological parents.[39] Seventy percent of the parents of these children, who for all intents are permanently placed, retain their parental rights without demonstrating significant interest.[39] These uninvolved parents are often ambivalent toward the children and thus unwilling to relinquish them for adoption.

Foster children are often upset about the dissolution of their families, the separations and losses they have sustained, and the need to adjust to a new living situation and new "parent" figures. Consequently, they may exhibit behavior problems that disrupt the foster home. Difficult children are usually considered undesirable; at the request of the foster parents, they are removed. They are then placed in another foster home or in congregate housing. For some children, whose parents are unable or unwilling to care for them and who refuse to allow their adoption, there is a succession of foster homes. Placement itself is a disruptive experience. Multiple placement is a disorganizing and alienating experience. These children become "nobody's children," and their only stable relationship may be with the social worker who supervises and arranges for the placements. If there is a series of social workers, even this form of stability is unavailable.

Age, race, and sex influence the placement process. The younger the child, the more easily he or she may be integrated into the foster family. Adolescents are more difficult to place and have a more difficult time with integration. Adolescents who have a history of aggressive behavior, drug abuse, or antisocial behavior such as vandalism or stealing are particularly difficult to place in foster homes.[36] Some of these young people may be temporarily placed in a psychiatric treatment setting in hopes of resolving their behavior problems. Eventually these youngsters may be placed in group homes until they are old enough to live on their own.

More than 77 percent of the children in urban foster care are minority children. Proportionately more black children than those of other racial groups are in foster care. This is particularly true in areas where blacks constitute a small proportion of the population. Ethnic differences have been found in relation to length of time in placement. The median time in foster placement is shortest for Asian children, approximately the same for Hispanic as for American Indian children, and longest for black children. White children are placed for longer periods of time than Asian children but for significantly shorter periods of time than black children.[41]

Children's Perception of Foster Placement

The child's stage of development is a significant factor in relation to how he or she perceives the placement and manages the separation from the family of origin.

Infants and very young children who remain with the same foster parents for an extended period of time in a consistent environment perceive the foster parents as their psychological parents. The attachment process can develop, and if there is a subsequent separation from the foster parents, it is traumatic. When there has been maternal deprivation before placement, these very young children have lower cognitive functioning. However, if the "mothering" is adequate in the foster home, the effects of earlier deprivation are reversed.[38]

Children who are older at the time of placement experience the separation from their parent or parents as an acute loss. Placement is experienced as rejection and abandonment. It is difficult for these children to conceive of strangers caring for them if their own parents do not want them. If other siblings remain with the family or other children are born into the family and not placed, the placed child may feel that he or she is "bad" or "worthless." This self-perception is incorporated into the self-concept. Self-esteem is diminished and interacts with the real loss and separation to generate depression.[38]

If a child experiences multiple placements, attachment to parenting figures is impaired. A sense of trust may fail to develop, and needs for love and belonging are never adequately satisfied. Each new set of foster parents are strangers who eventually reject and abandon, or appear to do so when the child is moved to another household.[38]

A young child may regress at the time of placement. The anxiety may be so great that it is severely disorganizing. The child may develop enuresis (bedwetting), encopresis (involuntary defecation), eating disturbances, or acute nightmares. If depression is the primary mood, the child may withdraw psychologically and physically. Increasing isolation may result in a compliant child, but the suppression and repression of feelings and the overall lack of interaction with others suggest a poor prognosis in the long run.[42]

An adolescent may deal with the loss and change through aggressive, angry, antisocial behavior. This expression of feelings often interferes with placement.

Hazards of Foster Placement

Problems of children in foster care reflect the disruption that has occurred in their lives. These problems are presented in Table 48-7. Among the foster children who have been studied, those who developed severe symptomatic behavior had experienced multiple placements, rather than extended time in placement, and had parents who were markedly ambivalent about them. In all studies of foster children, approximately 40 percent have either been returned to their biological parents or remained in one foster home, and 60 percent have received more than one placement, with some experiencing four or more placements.[38,42]

Foster children often tend to be relatively inarticulate and to express feelings through actions rather than words. It would seem that these children may have given up, or have never learned how to verbalize their needs or feelings. Having been rejected once, by the most important people in their lives, they expect rejection from others. They may reject their foster parents and peers and thus exert some degree of control over apparently uncontrollable foster placements. Some foster children

Table 48-7 Foster Placement

Hazards
Identity confusion
Difficulties in interpersonal relationships
Poor school achievement: perform below age-appropriate grade level, particularly during first 2 years
Multiple placements related to symptomatic behavior: stealing, deviant sexual behavior, enuresis, encopresis
Here-and-now orientation; the future is unpredictable because the past has been unpredictable
Poor orientation to time, place, and person: vague about birth dates, addresses, and family relationships: not remembering may be a defense against feelings of loss
Loss of contact with biological family
Interpersonal limbo; confusion related to attachment
Feelings of alienation
Feelings of "being different"
Teasing by peers which generates anger and aggressiveness
Being made scapegoats
Feelings of despair, futility, and helplessness
Feeling that they have been abandoned and that they are responsible and guilty
Feeling that their behavior is to blame for the loss of their family

SOURCE: H. S. Mass and R. E. Engler, *Children in Need of Parents,* Columbia, New York, 1959, pp. 353–354.

"love" everyone and exhibit exaggerated compliance toward adult authority figures. In their own way these children also are attempting to find some degree of security and to manage the anxiety generated by the loss of their family. Their ability to trust others is impaired.[39,40] They approach foster parents, peers, and teachers with belligerence that induces the very antagonism they fear. In some cases the child's preplacement home life had been chaotic, and little parental effort was expended in socializing the child. One or both parents may be emotionally disturbed or massively antisocial, or the family may have been overwhelmed by a parent's debilitating terminal illness. The child may have been severely neglected. Eating, toilet habits, hygiene, ability to relate to others, and sleeping habits may be seriously disturbed before and after placement. These children may exhibit rocking, head banging, or accident-proneness, or they may daydream excessively.

Patterns of Visiting

Patterns of family-of-origin visits to foster children vary greatly and have varying influences on the children's perception of the placement as well as on their growth, development, and ability to cope. Visiting is a significant problem. Studies seem to concur that fewer than 30 percent of children in foster placements are visited by their parents. Furthermore, two-thirds of the children remaining in foster care 5 or more years lose contact with their parents completely. The younger the children at the time of placement, the more likely that they will remain in foster care and have little or no contact with their parents. Older children tend to be visited more, and appear to have a greater claim on parental loyalty.[39,43–46] Patterns of visiting and their impact on the child are presented in Table 48-8.

Coping with Foster Placement

Among the children who do well in foster placement are those who have regular contact with their parents and siblings. They are developmentally and

Table 48-8 Patterns of Visiting

No Visiting
Parents have no specific plans or have unrealistic plans that they make no attempt to implement.
Children have been involuntarily removed from home of biological parents.
Children's lack of contact with parents is experienced as rejection and abandonment.
Parents are apt to obstruct freeing the child for adoption.
Parents may feel guilty and ashamed of the placement; avoid visiting to prevent these feelings.
Parents may believe their not visiting helps the child adjust to foster home more easily.
Parents may be too disorganized or dysfunctional to visit or to release the child for adoption.
Of these children, 5 percent are adopted; but most experience multiple placements.
Parents view placement as a long-term arrangement.
Visiting
Parents usually relinquished children because of a crisis; death of one parent, economic hardship.
Children are visited regularly and consequently show a better sense of well-being.
Parents intend to reestablish the family and view placement as temporary; but some are unable to mobilize resources that would support this goal.
Parents reinforce notion that placement is temporary.
Child's hope of returning to biological family interferes with attachment to foster family; such hope is problematic if return is not probable.

psychologically able to distinguish between their roles and relationships in the foster and the biological family and therefore have less identity confusion. They have a social conscience and are able to relate well to others; this probably reflects their self-esteem. Those who do well are able to follow rules, accept the placement, and realistically recognize the strengths and weaknesses of both their foster parents and their biological parents.[44]

Foster Parents

Foster parents are difficult to find and retain. The demand for foster homes is greater than the supply. Consequently, those that do exist are overcrowded. To further complicate the problem, financial support tends to be inadequate, matches between children and foster homes tend to be inappropriate, and support services tend to be lacking. Many foster families are not adequately compensated and must therefore use their personal income to support the child. This is particularly difficult, since these foster parents tend to be middle-income people already affected by inflation. One study revealed that 93 percent of foster parents used their own financial resources to support the foster child.[47] Because support services are inadequate, many foster parents are not prepared to manage the problems they encounter. However, state groups and National Foster Placement Associations are emerging and helping to address the problems of foster parents.

The average age of foster parents is 46 years. Thus in many instances they have the advantage of child-rearing experience, but at the same time they may be considerably older than the parents of the child's peers.[47]

Adjustment in Foster Families

The foster parents and the child must make adjustments and accommodations in the process of becoming a family. The foster family's capacity to understand the impact on the child and to respond empathically is important to this process. The usual pattern is presented in Table 48-9.

Removal of a child at the foster parents' request tends to occur during the first few months after placement. Reasons for requesting the removal tend to be discouragement, failure to attach, conflict with the foster family's biological child, or the foster father's dissatisfaction with the arrangement. If the child has been given labels that indicate a problem at the time of placement, he or she is at greater risk of rejection by foster parents.[47]

Table 48-9 Adjustment in Foster Families

Patterns in Adjustment Process
First 3 months
Tension in foster family is high.
Foster parents are optimistic.
Child is anxious, fearful, and sad.
Children and foster family are getting to know one another.
More comfortable relationship evolves during this period.
Foster parents have a positive attitude about the placement.
Second 6 months
Foster parents less optimistic about the child's adjustment.
Foster parents tend to feel discouraged.
Foster parents have an increased understanding of the seriousness of the child's problems and the difficulty in effecting change.
Foster parents recognize the need for biological parents to visit but have difficulty accepting the visits.
Foster parents become more emotionally involved with the child.
Foster child begins to feel as if he or she "belongs."
Foster parents believe their role is close to that of a biological parent.
First anniversary
Foster parents are more satisfied and settled in role.
Foster parents' satisfaction is tied to child's improvement, which is recognized through a review of the year.
Child continues to miss biological family but is better able to depend on the foster parents and to seek them out for help.

SOURCE: P. W. Cautley, *New Foster Parents,* Human Science Press, New York, 1980.

DSM III

The problems generated by disruption of family integrity may be correlated with a number of categories in the *Diagnostic and Statistical Manual of Mental Disorders* (DSM III) used with children and adults. The V codes for *conditions not attributable to mental disorder* such as *phase-of-life problem* and *other life circumstance problem* are also used.

Epidemiology

Divorce is endemic in American society. Increases in divorce rates have been dramatic in the last two decades. For example, more than 1 million divorces were granted in the United States in 1980. The dissolution of a marriage affects not only the divorcing spouses but the children as well. Thus, several million people each year are confronted with the stress inherent in the separation and loss incurred by divorce.[19] It is estimated that 1 white child in 3 will experience family disruption before age 16, and the ratio will be even higher for minority children.[12] More than 12 million children live with only one biological parent.[40] It is estimated that another 10 million children live in a household with one natural parent and a stepparent and that these children constitute 1 out of every 8 children living in two-parent families.

Approximately 80 percent of stepfamilies today result from remarriage following divorce, and 60 percent of remarriages involve an adult with custody of one or more children. It has been estimated that well over 15 million children are living with a remarried parent. Since 40 percent of second marriages end in divorce, many children must cope with the dissolution of their family twice or more.[32]

Thirteen percent of all children in the United States are being reared in a remarried family.[31] More than 2 million children are not living with a parent.[40]

As many as 142,000 adoptions occur each year in the United States. Approximately 30,000 of this number are adoptions by stepparents or blood relatives.

PATTERNS OF INTERACTION: PERSON

Patterns of interaction that are core issues in coping with death, divorce, single parenthood, stepfamilies, foster placement, and adoption are the *attachment process, identity formation,* and *grief.*

Attachment Process

Attachment is a primary psychological task of becoming a parent. Affectional and loyalty ties between parent and child result from this process. Bonding is necessary for the development of closeness and the satisfaction of the human need for love and belonging. The importance of the attachment process in biological parenting has been described and documented. A parallel process is necessary when a child is adopted or placed in a foster home. The attachment process in biological parenting is presented, with the counterpart process in adoptive and foster parenting, in Table 48-10.

Table 48-10 Attachment Process

Biological Parents	Adoptive or Foster Parents
Begins with the confirmation of the pregnancy.	Begins with confirmation by the adoption or placement agency that the couple are eligible for a child.
First trimester	
Biological mother is involved with the psychological process of incorporation of the fetus into the concept of her own body.	Adoptive or first-time foster mother may begin to explore and define her identity as a mother, even though she does not experience bodily changes.
Biological mother explores her relationship with her mother.	Adoptive and foster mothers are often older, and their mothers may no longer be alive and may therefore not be available for this work; whether younger adoptive and foster mothers do this needs to be documented.
To the biological father the baby is not yet real; he is concerned about his provider role and money matters.	Same may be true for both adoptive and foster fathers.
Second trimester	
Biological mother engages in the psychological task of differentiation: recognizing and acknowledging that the fetus is not part of her.	Adoptive and foster mothers may wish to deny the child's nonbiological status and the child's shared status.
Biological father feels rivalry toward fetus.	Same may be true of adoptive and foster fathers.
	Older foster parents may need to resolve feelings about the end of their procreative capacities and the temporary nature of the placement.
Young couples work on decreasing the remnants of their adolescent dependence on their parents and increasing their independence.	Adoptive and foster couples are usually older and may have resolved this issue in the past; however, they may be dealing with the introduction of a non-blood-related child into the family.

(Continued.)

Table 48-10 Continued

Biological Parents	Adoptive or Foster Parents
Second trimester	
Termination of the pregnancy of a wanted child precipitates a grief reaction.	Becoming ineligible for an adopted or foster child because of financial reversals, changes in the physical health of one spouse, or some other factor may also precipitate a grief reaction.
Third trimester	**Notification that child will be available within an approximate specified time**
Couple prepare for the birth, set up nursery, purchase baby clothes and equipment.	Couple prepare for child's arrival in same fashion.
Couple have conversations with one another and with others about the baby.	Couple have conversations with one another and with others about the impending arrival of the baby or child and about the adoption or foster placement process.
Couple seriously consider a name for the child.	Adoptive parents discuss whether they will keep the name assigned to the child or change it; if they decide to change it, they need to decide whether they will follow family traditions, such as giving the child one of their names or naming the child after a family member.
	Foster parents do not have the option of renaming the child, which reinforces impermanency of the relationship; child retains given and family names.
Expectant mother and father daydream and fantasize about the child at different ages and rehearse their roles in relation to the child.	Adoptive parents may daydream and fantasize about the child and rehearse their role as parents in the same way as biological parents.
	Foster parents cannot project into the future because of expected transience of the relationship; this may be a barrier to attachment and also a self-protective device to defend against the child's eventual removal from their home.
Beginning of labor.	Adoptive parents experience "psychological labor."
Delivery.	Child's arrival.
Parents inspect, fondle, and care for the baby.	Both adoptive and foster parents behave the same toward the baby as do biological parents.
Characteristic en face position.	Behaviors must be modified if adoptee or foster child is older.
Interaction between infant and mother facilitates attachment process; tactile exchange	
Stroking, fondling, patting, petting, cuddling by the mothering one.	Same by adoptive and foster parents when age-appropriate; verbal counterparts for an older child.
Proximity-maintaining behavior or retrieving behavior	
Mothering parent keeps baby with her or him or in the next room when involved in other tasks.	Same for adoptive and foster parents when age-appropriate; provides time to be with an older child.
Mothering one holds baby for feeding, playing with, and talking to; smiles at and talks to the baby.	Same for adoptive and foster parents when age-appropriate; provides time to talk with an older child.
Couple display affection for the child: kissing, nuzzling.	Same for adoptive and foster parents.
Mothering one responds to infant's crying, smiling, and babbling.	Same for adoptive and foster parents; respond with interest to what older child says or does.
Infant smiles and babbles to attract mothering one.	Same for adoptee and foster infant; older child seeks parents to tell them something or to ask for assistance.
Infant cries when mothering one leaves; protests the departure of mothering one until end of third year and becomes quiet and inactive after mothering one leaves him or her with another person.	Same for adoptee and foster infant and young child.
Infant crawls after mothering one earlier, more consistently, than after other parent.	Same for infant adoptee and foster infant; young child seeks out parent or plays near parent.
Infant clings to mothering one.	Same for adoptee and foster infant; young child plays near or checks with mothering one periodically.
Infant responds joyfully to other parent.	Same for adoptee and foster infants and children.

SOURCES: J. Bowlby, *Attachment*, vol. 1, Basic Books, New York, 1969; M. D. Jensen, R. C. Benson, and I. M. Bobak, *Maternity Care: The Nurse and the Family*, Mosby, St. Louis, 1977, pp. 152–167; B. Sideleau, "Adoption," *Issues in Mental Health Nursing*, Summer 1978, pp. 57–80; M. E. Fairweather, "If a Baby Is To Be Adopted," in I. E. Smith, ed., *Reading in Adoption*, Philosophical Library, New York, 1963, pp. 168–175.

Bowlby[48] states that interpersonal factors, and not simply the provision of quality care for physical needs, are essential to effective attachment. Harmony is a primary ingredient in the facilitative interpersonal process of attachment.

The importance of the first 3 months of life to the growth and development of the child is well documented, and the importance of intrauterine life is thought to be significant. Adequate, consistent, sensitive mothering is critical. A child's early experiences should have a loving, definite rhythm and sameness. Without this nurturing the child will experience impairment. Thus, the emotional and the intellectual development of the child are best promoted by consistency and continuity in the parent-child relationship.[48,49,50]

The attachment process can be impaired by a variety of factors. Those relevant to high-risk families include *dysrhythmic caretaking, failure of "entitlement,"* and *discontinuity in relationships.*

Dysrhythmic Caretaking

The death of a parent before birth or shortly thereafter is a major disorganizing stress for the surviving parent. The capacity to provide sensitive, consistent nurturing may be impaired. The sadness that accompanies the grieving process is likely to be communicated to the infant, who is acutely sensitive to the nonverbal messages a parenting figure sends through the care-giving process. The parent may also need to work, necessitating day care or multiple baby-sitters. Parental anxiety and inconsistent care giving may be upsetting to the baby and interfere with the attachment process.

Research suggests that infant adoptees are potentially vulnerable to disturbances in early object relations. Adopted children who have had transitional institutional or multiple foster home placements may exhibit disturbed object relations because they have been subjected to insensitive, inconsistent handling.[39,51]

Attachment during infancy is a function of maternal sensitivity to and satisfaction of a child's needs and a unique rhythmic pattern to the care giving, which reflects consistency and continuity. If a child has multiple care givers during this critical period, the attachment process and development of feelings of security are interfered with. Placement of the infant in day care and foster arrangements may be potentially problematic if the infant's care is provided by several people. To prevent the negative impact of multiple care givers, it would be in the infant's best interest to have a surrogate mother in either the home or the day care center, who could fill the role needed to facilitate the attachment process.[36]

The absence of a biological tie between the infant and the adoptive mother makes for an inherently labile primary identification. It would seem that this would be as true for the foster mother, if not more so, since the child's presence in the home is only a temporary arrangement. If the attachment process is not carried through in a complete and orderly fashion, the result is unresolved areas which become weak spots that give way under stress.

Anxiety and depression are inevitable consequences of an impaired attachment process. High levels of anxiety interfere with the child's physical, emotional, and intellectual development. The capacity of infants and young children to cope with anxiety is limited by their immaturity. Severe and prolonged anxiety during this stage of life has long-term consequences on the ability to function effectively throughout life.

Failure of "Entitlement"

Jafee and Fanshel[52] have proposed the concept of entitlement as a useful perspective for understanding the dynamics of attachment in adoptive parents. *Entitlement* is the feeling that the adopted child really belongs to them—is their child. These authors state that the successful resolution of the entitlement problem, one can assume, is derived from the parents' ability to master their basic doubts about their worthiness as parents, particularly with respect to the psychological "insult" associated with the problems of infertility.[36,53]

Adoptive and foster parents have no visible physical involvement in preparing for the infant. Adoptive parents may be susceptible to destructive feelings of unworthiness and insecurity because of their infertility. Such feelings may impair the ability of these people to feel comfortable and competent in assuming responsibility for the newly adopted, dependent, and helpless infant, or for someone else's child.

Entitlement remains forever an unresolved issue for foster families. In most cases there is no hope for permanence in the relationship with the child.

Transience characterizes the expectations of the foster parents and of the older foster child.

Discontinuity of Attachment

When a child is not placed directly in an adoptive home after birth but spends time in an institution or foster home, the move to the adoptive home may be traumatic. The period between 9 months and 3 years has been identified as the most critical time for placement of a child in an adoptive or foster home. It is during this stage of development that the child forms and consolidates a discriminating attachment to the parent care givers. Thus removal to the adoptive or foster home implies the loss of parents. At this developmental stage the child cannot use language effectively to communicate the impact of the separation and lacks the intellectual maturity necessary to understand what is happening.[36]

Adoption is not the first family relationship in an older child's life. When older children must break affectional ties with their biological or foster parents, they experience acute grief. These children are absorbed by feelings of sadness and anger, disillusionment, and resentment toward the family that has failed and deserted them. They may experience self-blame for their perceived responsibility for their situation as well as a sense of shame and worthlessness.[36]

To some degree the child's reaction to adoption, removal from family, or placement in another foster home is rooted in the disruption in the continuity of life, the flow and relatedness of memories and tangible associations. It is not the loss of specific individuals that is troublesome as much as it is the gestalt of the loss.

The development of a meaningful parent-child relationship depends on the capacity of each to make adjustments and to accept the other. The child's earlier opportunities and experiences in the primary relationship with the parent will be a significant factor. If early parenting was gratifying, even if there is no conscious memory, the child will have achieved the capacity to establish a meaningful relationship with the adoptive or foster parents.

Older children are more complex. They have lived through and coped with more of life's events, and these experiences can be either assets or liabilities. School-age children can be expected to adjust and become integrated into an adoptive or foster family if they:

1. Have been able to relate to an adult in a meaningful way in the past.
2. Are able to make friends and get along with peers.
3. Accept the fact that they cannot return home to their natural parents or to earlier foster parents.
4. Can say that they want an adoption or will be able to adjust to foster placement.
5. Indicate some ability to measure their own worth and self-respect.
6. Are able to acknowledge realistic fears and anxieties.
7. Can take some responsibility for themselves and recognize that more can be gained by trying to adjust than by resisting.

Whether a child is adopted or placed in a foster home in adolescence or as an infant, the adolescent developmental phase is difficult both for the adoptee or foster child and for the adoptive or foster parents. Adolescence is a maturational crisis for all children, but adoption and foster placement generate special conflicts. The literature on adoption addresses the issues confronting the adopted adolescent, but reference is not made to the special problems inherent in adoption at this age.[36]

Adolescents are difficult to place in adoptive or foster homes. All the problems of the school-age child may be compounded for the adolescent struggling for an identity and independence. This is a period of separation, not attachment, and separation dynamics may interfere with the integration of these young people into the adopted or the foster family. Couples wishing to adopt often look forward to the joys of seeing their child grow and develop and would therefore be hesitant to accept an "almost grown" unrelated child. Some people are willing and able to adopt or accept foster children who are older, handicapped, or of mixed racial heritage, but unfortunately they are few.[36]

Identity Formation

Identity, which is an awareness of being a person separate and distinct from all others, is a dimension of the self-concept. It is a function of identification processes.

Identification

The process of identification has a central role in the development of a child. The parents are the earliest and most influential figures in this process. Other significant people who have attributes that are perceived as necessary or desirable also become identification figures.

When family integrity is disrupted by divorce, foster placement, death, or abandonment by a parent, vulnerability to interference with identification processes and the development of a positive self-concept increases. A parent who is absent is not available as a figure for identification processes or for the realistic feedback that revises early childhood fantasies.

Sexual Identity

During the phallic and genital stages of development, children and adolescents are establishing a sexual identity and developing awareness of the genital area. If these developmental tasks are resolved positively, the person has the capacity to develop satisfactory relationships with the opposite sex. Disruption in these developmental processes may lead to problems related to sexual identity and relationships with the opposite sex and authority figures.

During the phallic stage, male children have an erotic attachment to the mother (Oedipus complex) and female children have a similar attachment to the father (Electra complex). When both parents are present, this attachment is mediated by the same-sex parent and the associated anxiety is maintained at a manageable level. When the same-sex parent is unavailable as a symbol of external control, there is potential for increased anxiety. High levels of anxiety burden the child's and the adolescent's coping capacities. Deterioration may occur in school achievement; relationships with peers, teachers, or both; and sleeping and eating patterns. The adolescent may become impulsive, may become a risk taker, or may act out sexually or with drugs or alcohol.

When divorce takes place and the parent of the opposite sex becomes the custodial parent, the child or adolescent in one sense "wins." Fantasized unconscious wishes associated with the Oedipus or Electra complex to "win" the parent of the opposite sex, which should remain unfulfilled, become a reality. Children and adolescents may find themselves in a similar situation as a result of the death of a parent. When the nuclear family has minimal involvement with extended family or friends, the intensity of the parent-child relationship increases. This intensification of the family relationship increases the child's vulnerability to anxiety related to the Oedipus and Electra complexes. The risk diminishes in a nuclear family in which there are extensive interactions and supportive relations with extended family and friends and in which the same-sex parent or surrogate parent is visible and involved in the parenting.

Adoptive parents who have unresolved feelings about their ability to procreate may have both an impaired sexual identity and an impaired sense of parental entitlement. Consequently they do not serve as stable positive sexual identification models.[52]

A child whose psychosexual development has been frequently interrupted by changes of environment may have limited capacity for identification with love objects. To be comfortable with one's sexual identity depends on learning within the family. If family life is disrupted or dysfunctional, this learning may be incomplete.

Discontinuity and Negative Identification Figures

Divorce, death, and foster placement create situations that increase the risk of impaired identity formation through the break in the continuity of the relationship with one or both parents. This break and the absence of biological parents for the identification processes interfere with the child's identity formation. When a custodial, foster, or surviving parent expresses anger, rejection, and intense dislike toward an absent parent, the child's desire to be like the absent parent means to be like someone who is "bad," "hateful," or "worthless."[54,55]

Foster or adoptive parents may confront a child with the biological parents' failure to care for him or her. Such confrontations may produce anxiety and guilt in the child. Motivation to identify with the noncustodial parents' or the biological parents' qualities and actions decreases or disappears. The child is left with only the custodial parent, or the temporary foster parents, as a model for identification and for development of self-concept.

Since the relationship with the foster parents may be a transient one, and removal from the foster home is perceived as another rejection and abandonment, identification with them has inherent problems. In addition, denial of the link to the positive qualities of the biological parents impairs development of the self-concept, because one can never divest the self of the blood tie.

Adoption or foster placement of an older child in a home that differs racially, ethnically, or socially may interfere with identity formation. Failure to respect the cultural or racial heritage of either the child or the surrogate parent decreases the integration of the child into the family. If the child rejects the surrogate family's cultural or racial identity in a negative or destructive fashion, the family may either isolate the child within the family or expel him or her. If the family denigrates the child's cultural or racial heritage, there is risk of damaging the child's self-concept.

Both failure to identify and identification with the negative image of the lost parent or parents are problems. The child is either deprived of the parent figure needed for an integrated, balanced identity or left with negative attributes such as "worthlessness," "hatefulness," and "badness." Children whose parents die or abandon them are further deprived of the parents' mediation of societal influences and, even more important, lose the feedback that becomes data for development of the self-image.

A rejecting, hostile, or distant parent-child relationship interferes with formation of identity, particularly development of conscience. Such a parent-child relationship results in an impaired conscience and a faulty sense of right and wrong. There is a failure to develop internal restraints that a well-developed conscience would impose. Delinquency and acting-out behavior reflect inadequate parental identification and a failure to incorporate moral and ethical standards.

Children also need to broaden their social circle to gain access to a variety of potential sources of identification. When an overclose relationship develops with a surviving or custodial parent, there may be a constriction of life outside the home, which decreases opportunities for using people outside the family for purposes of identity formation.

Siblings also serve as resources for identification and development of self-concept. Parents' love for and attention to siblings can provide the basis for use of siblings in identity-formation processes. When a sibling dies, the integrity of the family is disrupted, and a resource for identification processes and development of self-concept is lost.

Genealogical Concerns

As adopted and foster-placed children enter adolescence, they become more aware of the biological link of the generations. Their identity formation may be impaired by disruption in their sense of belonging to a genetically related multigenerational family. The increased curiosity about genealogy that occurs normally in adolescence is particularly confusing and threatening to adoptive and long-term foster parents. In order to be helpful to themselves and their child, these parents must recognize the normality of their adolescents' questions about their biological parents, must respect the dignity of their own role, and must accept the reality of the child's adoptive or foster status and of the parenthood they share with the biological parents.

When young adults who have been adopted or placed in a foster home as infants do not know who their biological families are, they often have concerns that they might inadvertently date a sibling or some other close relative. These fears and fantasies may interfere with the developmental tasks of seeking a mate and beginning a family of their own.[36,53]

"Family Romance"

Adoptive and foster children who have no contact with their biological family have a unique problem in terms of identification processes and the development of self-concept.

Freud proposed the "family romance" as a part of normal development. When children are unhappy or dissatisfied with their relationship with their parents, they fantasize an ideal family to whom they "really" belong: a family that is powerful, wealthy, kind, and loving. If they possess a fertile imagination, they may also invent a romanticized scenario to explain the loss of this family and their "adoption" or placement. Freud reported that this fantasy of being adopted occurs before the children are fully aware of the sexual determinants of procreation and that when they become aware of the sexual relationship between their mother and father, the family romance has a "peculiar curtailment."[36,56]

The family romance presents an unusual problem for adopted children, who in reality have two sets of parents. Family romance is not a game for these children; it is a reality. When prolonged, the family romance interferes with the child's identification with the adoptive parents and identity formation. The family romance has potential for supporting the child in splitting the images of the parents—one set of good parents and the other bad.[36]

Family romance may be a transitory fantasy and gain prominence only if the adopted or foster child feels rejected and not integrated into the family. The prolongation of the family romance and its fixation in the adoptive child are a function that the adoptive parents precipitate. When excessive fantasizing or idealization of the biological parents exists, it tends to persist into adult life. The fantasizing provides its own satisfaction for a while, when the child is dissatisfied with family life in the adoptive or foster home. However, eventually it is no longer age-appropriate, and it often serves as motivation to search for the biological parents.[36,53]

Adoptive and foster children who are deprived of information or possess only fragmented data about their biological parents may experience confusion and uncertainty, which can lead to low self-esteem and impair their sense of identity.[36] A lack of knowledge of their real parents and ancestry can be a cause of maladjustment in children. Adoptees and foster children, unable to incorporate known ancestors into their self-concept, are handicapped in the work of identity formation.[36]

Grief

Grief is the psychobiological response to loss of a significant loved object or person. It is resolved through the grieving process, which is the gradual "letting go" of emotionally painful memories of what has been lost and becoming able to invest energy in new relationships. Three aspects of grief are discussed below: (1) mourning, (2) absence of grief, and (3) "quests." (See also Chapter 3.)

Mourning

The losses inherent in divorce, death of a parent or sibling, or foster placement elicit a grief reaction. *Mourning* is a process during which the person *perceives* the loss of a love object and in one way or another *confronts the pain* associated with the loss of gratification desired with the lost person and the impossibility of attaining it. Thus, *perception* of the loss, *emotional pain,* and *confrontation* of the reality are essential components of the mourning process.[55]

Whether a child can engage in the mourning process before adolescence is debated by many theoreticians. Some state that mourning cannot be accomplished until adulthood, or until after detachment from parental figures has taken place. Others find that mourning is possible for children after early latency.[57,58] There is agreement that mourning is not found in very young children.[59,60,61]

Grieving is an affective state of sadness, pain, and desolation in response to loss. The distinction between *grieving* and *mourning* is somewhat arbitrary except that in relation to the child it better explains the extended period of crying and depression associated with the loss without resolution of the loss.

When the mother figure is lost and unavailable because of death, institutionalization, or foster placement during the period between 6 months and 3 to 4 years, a grief reaction occurs and is likely to take a course unfavorable to future development. Bowlby[59] identified the following responses to the loss: thought and behavior are directed toward the lost object; hostility is experienced; appeals for help, despair, withdrawal, regression, and disorganization occur, followed by reorganization of behavior toward a new love object.

Children of elementary school age tend to deal with serious losses with massive denial. Adolescents may recognize loss but also use denial. Both age groups search for substitutes while entertaining fantasies of reunion. Some degree of regression seems inevitable when these young people experience the loss of a significant person. Feelings of protracted grief are avoided. The finality of the loss is denied, fantasies related to the lost person develop, the quest for reunion persists, and rage replaces grief.[55,57] If children become locked into this status, they are unable to seek out, attach to, and derive satisfaction from an available substitute parent. Among 2- to 5-year-olds, there is a tendency to cling to the parent substitute, but they also resist the substitute, who is taking the place of the lost person. When older children accept a substitute parent without conflict, they usually have a conscious reason for rejecting the lost parent.[55,57] Some children adapt to the loss of a parent by identifying with the lost parent, thereby replacing him or her.

Absence of Grief

The "absence of grief" in childhood has consequences in adulthood. The phenomenon of indifference, when a parent has died or has been lost, indicates an absence of grief. This apparent failure to manifest grief may be caused by an intellectual inability to grasp the reality of the death or by inadequate object formation. The ego of the child may not be sufficiently developed to bear the strain of the work of mourning. Primitive defenses are used self-protectively. If the child did not use these defenses, the mourning process might be experienced as overwhelming.[55,60]

When grief is absent, it is displaced in time and emerges at a later point, often when another loss is experienced. When the mourning is incomplete, attachments to the lost object are unresolved. The finality of the loss is denied. Even when children are provided with extensive support and are able to sustain intense affect, the finality of the loss is not fully resolved, and unconscious fantasies continue. Tessman[55] raises the question whether the finality of a loss experienced as a child is recognized even as an adult, or whether there is an external quest for the lost person in disguised forms.

"Quests"

According to Freud, the quest for a wanted but absent person coexists with the mechanism of identification as a means of coping with loss. Reunion wishes and fantasies are inevitable responses to the loss of a significant person.[55]

Quests are secretive. They are often unconscious, because they conflict with what is "known" to be rational and true; they may jeopardize the security of other relationships inasmuch as they are perceived as acts of disloyalty; or they may generate intolerable pain, loneliness, and longing. Magical thinking is a dimension of the quest and reflects the regression that occurs when a significant loss has been incurred. Quests can also be conscious, as in the case of adopted people who seek information about their biological parents.

The quest is a precursor of grief. It helps to defend against the deeper grief that comes with recognizing the finality of the loss of the loved and needed person. The quest may be invested with vitality and creativity or with stagnating rigidity and self-destructiveness.

The diverse expressions of the quest include the following:[55]

1. Searching: acting out or hyperactivity to defend against the emotional pain
2. Remembering: a sense of the lost person's presence
3. Daydreaming
4. Recreating and holding onto painful feelings associated with the loss
5. Magical thinking or gestures meant to recreate the lost relationship
6. Sensing the presence of the lost person
7. Use of transitional objects
8. Suicidal ideation directed toward reunion
9. Denial

SEARCHING. Unconscious searching takes many forms. Restless activity which may seem purposeless is an unconscious quest. In the young child, the search for the lost parent may be a conscious, concrete, room-by-room looking for the person. In the older child, the quest may be expressed unconsciously through stealing or seeking out forbidden experiences. Turning to the external environment for instant gratification may occur among older children and adolescents because dealing with inner feelings is too painful. However, once acquired, the stolen object or forbidden experience fails to produce the reunion, and disillusionment sets in.[55]

Motor restlessness and a frenetic "looking for something to do" combined with an inability to initiate and maintain normal patterns of activity are characteristic of unconscious searching. Once the meaning of such behavior becomes conscious, it tends to lessen or stop, and the person is able to begin dealing with the loss and working it through.[55]

When divorce occurs, all family members incur losses. Each person, depending on his or her level of development, degree of regression, and ego integrity, searches for reunion in some way. The activity and unconscious preoccupation with the search may interfere with family members' capacity to be mutually supportive.

The losses experienced by children at the time of foster placement, after the death of a parent, or upon adoption elicit this phenomenon. Unconscious searching which leads to hyperactivity, restlessness, or stealing can be better understood when related to grief and the quest.

REMEMBERING AND DAYDREAMING. Remembering the lost person is a form of searching. It can occur as the recall of the mental image of the lost person and memories of shared experiences, or as the recreation of bodily sensations. When the loss occurs before the child has developed the capacity to hold on to and recall a mental image of the lost person (object constancy) and the loss is accompanied by severe deprivation, then bodily sensations associated with the loss become the memory. Remembering for these children, even when they are adults, becomes a search to recreate the physical sensations. For example, the associated bodily sensations may be tactile in nature. To remember, the search for the lost object is directed toward experiencing, once again, the tactile sensations.

The developmental capacity to evoke a memory helps adults and children deal constructively with the sense of loss. Daydreams may be the first mental activity directed toward remembering.[55] Effective use of memories is enhanced when these recollections are shared. Sharing experiences with a custodial or surviving parent, in a context in which the lost parent had participated, evokes memories. The remembering can be conveyed by words, feelings, and descriptions of events and examined in a supportive relationship, thus helping to resolve the loss.[55]

RECREATION OF PAINFUL FEELINGS. Painful feelings may also be recreated as a way of searching for the lost person. Painful feelings associated with the loss are used thereafter to get in touch with the lost person. Through the recreation of painful feelings the bereaved person seeks a reunion with the lost person. Children of divorce and those who have lost a parent through death may recreate these painful experiences as a form of quest. These people, as children and adults, choose situations and relationships that evoke painful feelings time and again, unconsciously seeking a reunion with the lost person. Since such a reunion is impossible, the situations and relationships used to accomplish the reunion are disappointing and the feelings of rejection are regenerated. A pattern of recreating the emotional pain associated with the loss may not emerge until young adulthood. At this time the young person seeks a relationship with another for the unconscious purpose of recreating the lost relationship and associated feelings. Since the other person is not the lost person, disappointment and frustration develop, the relationship is broken, and the emotional pain is recreated.

MAGICAL GESTURES AND THOUGHTS. Magical gestures and thoughts are forms of searching that involve the use of an activity that was previously associated with the appearance of the lost person. The use of these gestures and thoughts is based on the belief that they will produce reunion.[20] For example, a father came home every evening while his child was watching a particular television show. After his death the child insists on watching the show every evening because he or she believes on some level that watching the show will cause the father to come home. Again, disappointment is inevitable. The capacity to deal with reality—to accept the finality of the loss—diminishes the perceived power of such gestures and thus decreases the likelihood that they will be repeated. For example, the person who associates playing the piano with the warm, intimate, and secure feelings of a time when the lost person was present plays the piano following the loss to effect reunion.[55]

"PRESENCE." The feeling that a lost person is present or seen in a crowd for a fleeting moment is commonly reported by people, including children and adolescents, who are grieving. This phenomenon occurs more commonly when the lost person is deceased rather than missing as a result of divorce or foster placement. Apparently, long-buried memories are revitalized after the loss and become dreamlike figures that are neither hallucinations nor illusions but projections of memories.[55] For some people this experience is comforting; for others, it is frightening.

TRANSITIONAL OBJECTS. Transitional objects are illusions that form a bridge in a person's relationship with the external world. A magical dependence on the treasured object survives regardless of the person's conscious feelings, behaviors, or intentions toward it. Magical thinking is necessary for attachment to a transitional object to occur.[55]

Magical thinking that occurs in childhood fosters the use of transitional objects. Following the loss of a parent, sibling, or family, the child becomes attached to an object or animal. The family pet or a doll or toy may take on special significance. The presence of this object may be required at all times as a source of comfort and pleasure. When the object is misplaced or out of sight, the child may experience acute anxiety. The phenomenon appears to develop only when the child has experienced satisfying, effective parenting. The transitional object becomes part of the quest for reunion.[55]

SUICIDE. When the quest is self-destructive in nature, the wish for the lost person is balanced against a significant other's devaluation of the lost person. Such an attempt at reunion involves a renunciation of the self and may also require identification with the deadness of the lost person or the internalization of hostility. The drive for reunion is fueled by an unsatisfactory environment and a lack of hope, creating a risk of suicide. An unconscious connection may be made between death and peaceful sleep, both of which are representative of a desire for merging or fusion—the wished-for reunion.[55]

In some instances the self-destructiveness is derived from the wish to be rid of a hated or devalued aspect of the lost person that has been incorporated into the self. An unsupportive environment, identification with a hated aspect of the lost person, or a combination of these two factors increases the risk of suicide. The search for reunion and poorly developed self-boundaries also predispose people to self-destructive thoughts and behaviors.[55] Both children and adolescents may attempt and complete suicide in their search for reunion with the lost person.

DENIAL. Outright denial of the loss occurs more frequently among young children. Older children and adolescents may protect themselves from full recognition of the loss by screening out the memory with stories characterized by wish fulfillment. Adults should recognize that these stories cover up a painful reality and are not being used to avoid punishment.[55]

Children may be accused of lying when they use these stories to alter reality in order to satisfy their wishes. Children in divorced and foster families develop dual truths about their parents. A child who has lost a parent and experienced family disruption may lie to protect the inner self and to handle contradictory knowledge about the lost parent.[7] The lies cover up the truth and appear both to protect the child's inner integrity and to reproach the lost parent for being untruthful in some way.[55]

PATTERNS OF INTERACTION: FAMILY

Patterns of interaction within the family that are significant when people are dealing with death, divorce, single parenthood, stepfamilies, foster placement, and adoption include *loyalty* and *impairment of gender and generational boundaries.*

Loyalty

Family Loyalty

Loyalty is faithfulness and an obligation to defend or support. Loyalty can be defined by the following principles which sustain it: influence of external coercion, conscious recognition of an interest or need to belong, conscious recognition of feelings of obligation, and an unconscious binding obligation to belong. Loyalty commitments are like strong, invisible fibers which bind relationships together.[62]

Family loyalty is based on biological, hereditary kinship. Consanguinity (blood ties) and genetic relatedness, which last a lifetime, are the characteristics that distinguish the family from other multiperson systems.

According to Boszormenyi-Nagy and Spark,[62] the component of ethical obligation in loyalty elicits a sense of duty, fairness, and justice. Failure to comply with obligations leads to guilt feelings. These feelings and the need to avoid them constitute a regulatory force in family systems.

Within loyalty-bound family relationships each person maintains an invisible bookkeeping ledger in which accounts of give-and-take, exploitative use of others, and the exploitation one has experienced are recorded. Family members keep an invisible record of their perception of the balances of past, present, and future give-and-take within the family that affect them.[62] These accounts are balanced through the principle of justice which requires the person to treat others fitly and fairly, giving what is owed or due. Thus, the give-and-take among family members is determined by deserved, merited reward or punishment. Because a family is a multigenerational system of interlocking and interacting relationships, unsettled accounts in one generation influence relationships in subsequent generations. Exploitation of a member in one generation reflects past loyalty imbalances and will be settled in future generations.[62]

A family code guides the various contributions of members to the family system. This code is, in part, a pattern of learned reactions and ways of relating which are based on both genetic relatedness and a shared history. The code determines the equivalence of merits, advantages, obligations, and responsibilities of members that influence members' expectations. To meet the needs for justice and to resolve injustices, members, guided by the family code and their perceptions of justices and injustices, treat each other fitly and fairly. Accounts of justice and injustice in the invisible ledger demand equitable balancing. The rewards and punishments that are meted out reflect what is owed and what is due, and settle the accounts. They may also set up further injustices.[62]

There are vertical and horizontal loyalty commitments in a family. Loyalty commitments which are owed to previous and subsequent generations are vertical commitments; those owed to one's mate, siblings, or peers are horizontal commitments. Table 48-11 presents the pattern of family loyalties. If these patterns are disrupted by a failure to follow through on these loyalty commitments, then injustice occurs and results in a debt in the member's accounts ledger.[62]

Children can never fully repay parents for their lives or for effective and nurturing upbringing. Through reciprocity they can fulfill some obligations and expectations. They can contribute to the partial satisfaction of parental needs for love and belonging through affection for the parents, and they can represent a sense of immortality through their procreation. Children fulfill these obligations by preserving family traditions and values and adhering to the family's religious and ethnic orientation. They also fulfill these obligations by being available and helpful when their parents grow old and need to depend on them. In their turn, they set up an obligation and expectation for their children to treat them in the same way. Adult children who do not procreate or care for their aged parents or who abandon their religion create loyalty imbalances and conflicts. This failure to fulfill their obligations as children demands rebalancing of accounts and will often interfere with fulfillment of the role of spouse or parent.[62]

Table 48-11 Family Loyalties

Patterns
Married couple owe loyalty to each other and a redefined loyalty to their families of origin.
Couple owe loyalty to the children born of their relationship.
Children owe loyalty to their parents and to the older generation.
Siblings owe loyalty to each other.
Blood-related family members owe each other affection and support.
Blood-related family members owe each other respect for the incest taboo.
Parents owe support to their nuclear families.
Parents owe homemaking and child rearing to their nuclear families.
Mothers and fathers owe their children nurturing, a secure environment, the resources to meet basic human needs, and opportunities for personal growth.
Mothers and fathers owe support to their aging or incapacitated parents and relatives.
Family members owe loyalty to their nation, cultural, racial, and religious backgrounds and their values.

Injustices in the family ledger are in some instances related to the loss and exploitation of family members. Balanced reciprocity in a family requires mutuality of both giving and acceptance of giving. Inherent in every relationship is a balance between receiving and being used that is related to justice. Exploitation originates from imbalances characterized by nongiving or nonreciprocal taking. When there is exploitation within the family system, both participants are victims.[62]

Boszormenyi-Nagy and Spark[62] describe intergenerational balancing of what is owed or due members and label the phenomenon the *revolving slate*. Unsettled accounts of injustices between two family members revolve and get between the person who has experienced the injustice and another family member who was not a part of the original injustice but is made a scapegoat to pay the debt. This revolving slate sets up a chain of displaced retribution in families that moves from generation to generation. Because of this revolving slate, exploitative parents may produce exploiting children. The chain reaction of generations of injustices leads to more frustrated and less giving future parents.[62]

Children are loyalty-bound to each parent through these multigenerational patterns, the attachment process, dependency needs, and genuine affection. When the family is intact and functional, loyalty is not a problematic issue.

Disloyalty

DIVORCE AND DISLOYALTY. Divorce reflects family dysfunction. It creates a situation which increases the risk that children will become embroiled in a loyalty conflict in their relationships with their parents.

Rejection of a spouse, marital conflict, and sexual dysfunction, which may lead to divorce, are ways people manage their invisible loyalty conflicts with the family of origin. To rebalance the ledger that was imbalanced by the disloyalty of marrying, people may choose divorce and return to the family of origin.

Injustices are inevitable in divorce. During and immediately following a divorce, the preschool child's dependency needs, inability to understand the ramifications of the marital dissolution, and overall immaturity preclude a companionable or supportive relationship for the parent. The parents usually do not attempt to enlist preschool children in their struggle with each other. For these reasons, young children do not initially experience a loyalty conflict. However, as a child matures and needs the noncustodial parent, loyalty conflicts may emerge, particularly when divorced parents are unable to collaborate on child rearing.[62]

The young school-age child may be actively enlisted by one parent to join him or her against the other parent. These children seem unable to align with one parent against the other. Disloyalty to a parent seems incomprehensible to children in this age group.[62]

The older school-age child may also be actively enlisted by one parent to side with him or her against the other. These youngsters are caught in a bind between their desperate need for parental reconciliation and the reality of the parents' devisive attempts to align with them. Children in this age group can and do become enmeshed in a loyalty conflict. If they align with the noncustodial parent, it is usually for only a brief period of time, perhaps because the alignment lacks daily reinforcement. Alignment with the custodial parent is more likely to occur.

In some cases these children dichotomize their relationships with their parents. One becomes the "good parent" and the other the "bad parent." This dichotomization reflects an immature conscience and perhaps the overt and covert influence of the parent cast in the "good parent" role. Supported by the "good parent's" feedback, these children have a sense of righteousness and unspoken permission to reject, humiliate, or be vengeful toward the other parent. These children are infused with a sense of power and identification with the "winner." There is a lack of awareness on the part of the "good parent" of the destructive effects of this disloyalty on the child's development of self-concept and later relationships with people of the same sex as the "bad parent."[7,62]

"PARENTIFICATION." Adolescents are also vulnerable to loyalty conflicts. Both the adolescent and the older school-age child can, and in many instances do, provide companionship and support to one parent. *Parentification* occurs when the older child or adolescent becomes more the "emotional parent" to the parent than a child in the relationship. Certain needs of both the parent and the child are met through such a relationship, but at the child's expense. The parent's loss of a spouse is an injustice. The parent's account is rebalanced through the parentification of the child, who is exploited by being expected to "parent" his or her parent. The child's "giving" to the parent is excessive and developmentally inappropriate. The child loses the responsible parenting he or she is due. Since parental obligations are not fulfilled, the child's account is imbalanced.[62]

When a parent relates to a child as a generational equal, the child's developmental needs suffer, and the child is exploited. However, the child's sacrificial role is sustained by both the parent and the child. The parent helps to define the child's parentified role and associated expectations to avoid his or her own loneliness. The child wishes to be needed and desires the closeness that comes with "taking care of" the parent. The child also nurtures the parent as insurance against further abandonment by this parent. Children of divorce often fear abandonment by the custodial parent, feeling, "If it could happen once, it can happen again." By being available, affectionate, and compliant, they attempt to defend against this possibility. The child is a willing victim and cooperates by complying with the role expectations.[62]

ABANDONMENT. Parents struggling with divorce, with single parenting, and with establishing their own personal lives as single people and in a new career are often greatly self-absorbed. Time, energy, and emotion are often overcommitted to these pursuits. Awareness of their children's needs and emotional pain may be self-protectively diminished. They may rationalize their unavailablility as fostering their children's independence and self-sufficiency. In reality, these parents may be emotionally abandoning their children. Failure to set limits, provide nurturing, and appropriately delegate care-giving responsibilities for younger siblings parentifies and exploits the children. Not infrequently, these parents were themselves emotionally abandoned by one or both parents. As children they may have lost a parent through abandonment, death, or divorce; or they may have been reared in a home that lacked supportive nurturing and warmth.[62]

The death of a parent or spouse is experienced as abandonment and rejection. When a parent dies, the parental obligation to remain loyal and give affection, support, nurturing, and responsible parenting is not fulfilled. The spousal obligation to give support and affection and to share in the responsibility for child rearing is unfulfilled when the partner dies. These unmet obligations are entered into the ledger as accounts owed.

Rebalancing Injustices

Children who lose a parent, particularly through death, experience an injustice. They may seek retribution and rebalancing of their account by searching for the lost parent through the assumption of a dependent role in their relationships with others. Their neediness is insatiable, and their dependency can be a burden on significant others. Inevitably, other people become exhausted and dissatisfied because their dependency needs are never met within the relationship. In a marital relationship the partner may be cast in the role of "surrogate parent" and thus experience the marriage as one-sided and unsatisfactory. As a result this partner may seek a divorce and, by his or her abandonment, recreate the original rejection and abandonment by the parent who had died.

Some people who have lost a parent during childhood may marry and subsequently seek divorce. Others may never leave the surviving parent. Remaining with the parent for life is the only way the surviving parent's loyalty can be even partially repaid. To leave would be to repay loyalty with disloyalty.

These parents and their children are participating in settling and setting up transgenerational retributive accounts. They are enmeshed in a social context of family obligations, injustices, and exploitations which remain invisible but powerful influential forces, because the family cultivates mystification to perpetuate the status quo. The parents and offspring unconsciously and collusively participate in perpetuating the relationship.[62]

Divorce, death, adoption, and foster placement result in varying degrees of abandonment that reflect and initiate loyalty imbalance. Surviving or custodial parents may evolve a permanent symbiotic relationship with their child. To make up for the losses the child has experienced, to avoid their own loneliness, or for both of these reasons, the surviving or custodial parents are overdevoted and martyrlike in their giving, thus generating guilt-laden feelings in their offspring.

The martyrlike and overdevoted parent sets up an imbalance by overgiving. Such a parent blocks the child's attempt to reciprocate by refusing to take and acts on guilt which is related to feeling responsible for the failure of the marriage. The child experiences guilt because he or she is unable to even partially repay the debt. The scapegoating system becomes circular: guilt against guilt and mutual martyrdom.[62]

Adoption is often characteristically mystified. The process of giving up the child, the adoption agency's policies and procedures, and the adoptive family's self-protective denial of the child's adoptive status all reflect mystification. Adoptive and foster children who have little information about their biological parents develop fantasy images and on some level recognize strong blood ties to their biological parents. Thus, in spite of the physical separation from, and abandonment by, the biological parents, loyalty ties and the ledger continue to exist. Adoption is equivalent to abandonment by the biological parents, and abandonment is an injustice. Parental failure to meet the obligation of responsible parenting demands retribution. Parents who abandon their children by giving them up for adoption or foster placement are disloyal to these children. The injustice is entered in these children's accounts ledger. Foster and adoptive parents, their spouses, and their children may be pulled in through the revolving-slate phenomenon for purposes of retribution. Loyalty commitments to foster or adoptive parents cannot be made, because the original disloyalty of being abandoned by the parents has impaired the children's capacity to make such commitments.

When a person has guilt-laden obligations to a parent, these obligations may also impair the ability to make loyalty commitments. Marriage to an "outsider" would be disloyal. If the person marries despite this inherent disloyalty and the guilt-laden obligations, he or she may not be able to remain in the marriage for any length of time and eventually may seek a divorce or separation, thus loyally returning psychologically, if not physically, to the family of origin.

People who have been adopted or placed in a foster home, or who have lost a parent during childhood through death (abandonment) or divorce have experienced parental disloyalty. Their invisible account ledgers have been imbalanced and will require rebalancing at some future time. The person in the family who is pulled into the revolving-slate phenomenon for purposes of retribution varies. In some instances the care giving "owed" to these people because they were abandoned may be found at the expense of optimal functioning. They become dependent inmates in a psychiatric facility or penal institution, or are forever "children" in their families. They abandon their spouses or children, or parentify their children.

Impairment of Gender and Generational Boundaries

Entry into adolescence is characterized by an emerging sexual identity and an awareness of other family members as sexual beings. Daughters become sexually attractive to their fathers, but the feelings are usually automatically blocked in the father-daughter relationship. Fathers would become highly anxious and frightened if they found this sexual interest in their daughters continuing. To allow themselves to continue to think about their daughters as possible personal sexual partners would be too disturbing. The same is true of the mother-son relationship.

In the relationship between adoptive or foster parents and children, however, there are no automatic sexual barriers, and explicit thoughts may not be blocked out. Without these barriers, the risk of sexual acting out is increased, as is the possibility that the parents may intrude into their children's sexual lives. Prying questions about the adolescent's activities on a date, requests for detailed descriptions, and sexually loaded teasing are ways in which this intrusiveness may be manifested. Intrusiveness is often rationalized as, "I didn't want her to get pregnant the way her mother did," or "All this stuff on television about VD—well, I want to be sure the kid is OK. I don't want him sick or anything." Emotionally mature adoptive parents and foster parents avoid and block out this sexual intrusiveness.[36]

Brothers and sisters in blood-related families interact with each other freely on many sexual levels—teasing, peeking, caressing, fighting. However, there is usually a final, firm barrier against explicit sexual behavior. Blocking and repressing occur, and the incest barrier becomes more firmly entrenched. Adoptive opposite-sex siblings may find it much easier to become intimate and intrusive because there are no blood ties, and consequently less anxiety occurs.[63]

Repression of incestuous feelings by family members may tend to push the parents and adolescents toward emotional emancipation and independence from one another.[63] These repressed feelings serve as a powerful force in moving the adolescent toward maturity and normal adult sexuality. In the adoptive family, when there are impaired sexual barriers and a greater toleration of incestuous feelings, there is risk of closer sexualized interaction and a blurring of gender and generational boundaries. Thus the impetus derived from repressed incestuous feelings is diminished, and emancipation therefore is slowed.[63]

PATTERNS OF INTERACTION: ENVIRONMENT

Disruption of family integrity is becoming commonplace in our society. Divorce, single parents, stepparents, and foster placements are becoming accepted and even commonplace. The social stigma previously associated with such situations is decreasing. Environmental factors that interact with the family and that may influence society's perception of these situations include reform of divorce laws, particularly no-fault divorce; the changing role of women in society; the influence of the media; increasing recognition of the need for group homes for adolescents; and societal attitudes toward adoption.

Reform of Divorce Laws

In recent years over half of the states have incorporated no-fault grounds into their divorce laws. No-fault reform is based on the principle of marital breakdown, which instructs the court to grant a divorce upon proof that the marriage relationship is irretrievable. This represents a liberalization of the divorce laws, since neither spouse need prove fault or innocence to secure a divorce. Liberalization of divorce laws may be contributing to increasing divorce rates.

Women in Society

Women's roles in society are changing. Greater numbers of women are joining the work force. In the past, many women who worked did so to supplement the family income and returned to work after their children had entered school. Most were neither skilled workers nor professionals, and many sought part-time employment.

Greater numbers of women in today's society are preparing for skilled work and professions. Young women are seeking entry into fields that have been male-dominated, and homemakers are returning to school to learn new skills or to update their education before entering the work force. More young women who are presently entering the work force do not view their time in either school or job as an interim before marriage and child rearing. They are seeking careers, financial security, and upward mobility. For many this means delaying childbearing, interrupting their careers briefly to have children, having smaller families, and using day care.

As women make economic gains and achieve upward mobility in the work force, they may acquire as individuals the financial and professional status that would formerly have been derived from their husbands. Furthermore, the social stigma once associated with divorce has been considerably diminished, particularly in urban centers. Thus, the financial and societal forces that were once influential in preventing marital dissolution have been somewhat diminished.

The Media

The communications media (books, movies, television) have a profound influence on society and on individuals and also reflect societal patterns. The way divorce is treated in the media influences people's values, perceptions, and attitudes and, more than likely, their behavior.

Soap operas and evening programs on television, as well as movies, tend to deal with divorce as a common phenomenon. Subtly and persistently the media portray not only divorce but serial marriages and do so in an overall positive frame of reference. Television abounds with single parents who cope good-humoredly and successfully with the trials and tribulations of raising their children alone. Exposure to such presentations desensitizes the viewer to divorce and reinforces its potential and desirability when marital dissatisfaction and conflict occur.

Group Homes

In recent years increasing numbers of adolescents have run away from home, have been ejected from their homes by their families, or have been brought to residential psychiatric treatment settings by their parents, who then refuse to allow them to return home after discharge. Foster home placements for these adolescents are limited in number; foster families prefer young children over adolescents who have histories of acting out, substance abuse, and delinquent behavior. Communities are therefore beginning to recognize that these youngsters need a safe, stable place to live and an opportunity to complete their education. In response to this need there is a trend toward establishing group homes for adolescents. Parents' awareness of this alternative may influence their efforts to exclude the adolescent when they feel overwhelmed or frustrated in their parental roles.

Societal Attitudes toward Adoption

Society tends to view adoption as an adequate, economical, and acceptable way to provide the advantages of family life for children whose natural parents are unable to provide for them. Societal attitudes and values regarding adoption influence adoptive parents, adoptees, and the manner in which relatives, friends, neighbors, and community organizations such as schools relate to the adoptive family and its members.[36]

When people adopt an unrelated child, society views them as kind and generous. On the other hand, the adopted child, who is very likely to be illegitimate or abandoned and only rarely has been orphaned because of the loss of loving parents, is covertly less benevolently viewed by society. There is an unspoken societal expectation that such a child should be "grateful" and respectful because these generous strangers have made sacrifices to rear an "unwanted" member of society.[36] Subtly our society defines the unrelated adoptee as different, as someone who is accepted and loved only because of a stranger's generosity or benevolence. Adoptive parents or their friends may be heard commenting on the child as an "adopted" child, but one does not observe the same need to refer to biological offspring as a "natural" child.[36]

Consequently the adopted child is expected to assume the burden of being a "perfect child." Society, adoption agencies, and couples wishing to adopt children have historically perpetuated this expectation and supported a system which emphasizes the importance of perfection in adopted children. It is interesting to note that when a couple decide to have a baby, the attendant risks are rarely discussed or considered. However, when a couple decide to adopt a child, the risks of physical and emotional defects in the adoptee are given considerable attention. Society expects and accepts the risks inherent in biological parenthood but not those associated with adoptive parenthood.[58]

Society and adoption agencies have also expected "perfect families" for adoptees. In the past, placement agencies have implied, by their extensive and detailed screening and rigid criteria, that perfection is required. These societal expectations for perfection in adoptive couples and adoptees are not only unrealistic but a burden to all involved. They affect adaptation of individual members and integration of the family system.[36]

NURSING PROCESS

Nurses encounter members of families at risk in a variety of health care settings. Promotion of health and prevention of the development of crises are the primary concerns of nursing in relation to these families and their members. Because the family is a social and emotional system characterized by interaction and influence among members, the problems encountered by one person in the family affect other family members and the overall functioning of the family system.

Prevention is the primary goal of nursing. Recognition of the hazards in various life situations guides nurses' assessments of family members to identify potential problems, select nursing interventions designed to prevent their development, or make appropriate referrals. Where problems exist, an understanding of the intra- and interpersonal dynamics that contribute to the problems in these families guides the selection of interventions which will help the families manage the changes and resolve the losses.

When family integrity is disrupted, anger and bitterness do not simply go away. They continue for extended periods of time—sometimes for a lifetime—and continue to be a source of stress.

The delivery of high-quality health care begins when providers and consumers have an ongoing, stable, and consistent collaborative relationship founded in mutual respect and trust and characterized by positive rapport. If nurses personalize their care, children and adults receiving either routine health supervision or treatment for a health problem are known as *people*. The nurse's data base goes beyond the person's physical status, signs, symptoms, and treatment. The nurse makes an effort to learn about the person's neighborhood, living arrangements, work and family life, feelings, concerns, and hopes. The nurse takes time to listen actively and to encourage the client to share personal information about himself or herself. This means that nurses communicate to clients that they have time to listen. They prevent outside interruptions, respond empathically, and ask questions that provide clients with opportunities to talk about their concerns.

Divorce, death of a family member, remarriage, stepparenting, the placement of a child in a foster or adoptive home, and integration of a foster or adopted child are all associated with stress-related health problems. When people experience so much stress that they develop physical or psychosocial dysfunctions, they seek help in clinics, health maintenance organization (HMO) settings, physicians' offices, emergency rooms, and possibly inpatient hospital facilities. Nurses in all these settings have both the opportunity and the need to assemble and record information about each person's problems. A holistic approach will guide nurses to explore with the client factors that may have contributed to the development of symptoms. These nursing activities have a case-finding dimension that helps the nurse identify members of families at risk who need assistance beyond the alleviation of the presenting symptoms.

School health nursing provides exceptional opportunities for early case finding and intervention. Promotion of health and prevention of disabling responses are primary concerns of nurses in these settings.

In many school districts preschool children are screened before admission to kindergarten to identify readiness for school and the need for remedial services. The interview with the parents usually includes information about the child's developmental history. These interviews provide an opportunity for nurses to collect a family health history as well. The information acquired helps the nurse identify children from high-risk families and identify parents' needs in relation to managing problems. Once potential problems have been identified, nurses can monitor children for early signs of distress and refer parents for counseling to prevent or remedy problems (see Chapter 19).

School health nurses need to develop their roles in working with teachers to identify children who are presenting problems in the classroom that may reflect a stress response to problems in the home. Children from distressed families often seek out school nurses on a regular basis because of minor scrapes, bruises, or physical discomforts. Nurses can serve as a liaison between the school and the family in such instances. Since nurses are perceived as "helping people," families usually welcome their interest. Thus, school health nurses have opportunities to find families at risk and to help distressed children directly and indirectly by collaborating with their teachers and families and other providers of health care.

Occupational health nurses develop health educational and screening programs for the employees in their settings. They are perceived and used by the employees in the setting as a source of help for physical complaints. People often have difficulty recognizing that many of their physical discomforts and ills are related to mismanagement of stress. They also know better how to seek help for physical complaints than for personal problems, anxiety, and depression. Nurses can identify families at risk by expanding their interviews with people who seek their help to include data that would reveal marital or parent-child conflicts.

Educational programs that focus on family functioning may also help attendees to prevent and recognize family problems, to identify ways to resolve them, and to seek help for those problems that do not respond to obvious solutions.

Assessment

Children whose family life has been disrupted by abandonment, death, divorce, adoption, or foster placement are at risk of adverse reactions that may impair growth and development. Nurses encounter these children and their families in a variety of settings. Assessment provides the nurse with information that can be used to determine whether health-promotive needs should be addressed, or whether problems exist that require intervention. The process of giving information to the nurse may, in some sense, be an intervention as well. The questions that are asked require the child and parents to reflect on the information contained in the response. This reflection may focus or increase their awareness of important issues they have not considered in the past.

The *genogram* provides a useful tool and guide in collecting both the psychosocial and the overall health history of the family system and its members. It provides a comprehensive data base that reflects a holistic approach to clients better than other tools presently used. It also presents the information in a form that can be quickly scanned and updated.

When genograms are routinely constructed upon admission to a health care setting or school, and periodically updated, families and individuals at risk are identified. Early identification of populations at risk is an important aspect of the responsibility of the nursing profession for promotion of health.

Information that should be included in a genogram in order to help identify families at risk is presented in Table 48-12. The data collected need to be examined to identify significant patterns such as divorce, cause of death, premature death, abandonment of children, mental illness, and interpersonal conflicts. Identification of nodal events or crises may help nurses recognize emotional shock waves, anniversary reactions, and loyalty conflicts that could influence the development of family dysfunction.

The names of family members will reveal whether there is a family tradition of naming children after people in preceding generations and whether expectations are associated with a name that might influence either the family's perception of a child or the child's self-perception. If someone breaks a tradition, this may be a significant issue in the family. For example, if all first-born sons on the father's side are named John, and a couple do not give their first child, an adopted son, the traditional name, are they saying that this child is not a member of the family? Are they also saying that this child can never really be a member of the family? How will this affect the child?

Noting the age of the parents at the time of death can help to identify family members who are vulnerable to unresolved grief, loyalty conflicts, or parentification. Without intervention, these issues may affect the person's ability to parent.

Including the physical locations of family members helps to identify potential support systems and indicates whether there is a pattern of remaining near one another or scattering and settling in geographically distant locations. Geographical distance may preclude or limit visits by a noncustodial parent, for example.

Specific assessment questions which address the problematic issues related to death, divorce, remarriage, stepparenting, and foster placement are presented in Table 48-13.

Table 48-12 Identification of Families at Risk Using the Genogram

Family Structure
1. Identify each member (including stillbirths and abortions) by name, age, sex, date of birth, and date of death (if appropriate).
2. Identify place of birth and present geographical location of each member.
3. Indicate divorces and remarriages.
Family Function
1. Identify close, distant, and conflicted relationships.
2. Specify cause of death for members who are deceased.
3. Identify ethnic, racial, and religious affiliations.
4. Who communicates with whom? How? When and how often? Is one family member a central clearinghouse for information on family members?
5. Where are holidays and vacations spent? With whom?
6. Identify significant family events (nodal points).
7. Who makes which decisions in the family? In previous marriages? In families of origin?
8. How did family members respond to divorce or remarriage? Foster arrangements? Adoption? Stepparenting?
9. Identify children's behavior suggestive of a stress response (see Chapters 49 and 50).
10. Note changes in members' behavior and way of relating after divorce, remarriage, foster placement, and adoption.
11. Who pays child support or alimony and how is it handled?

Nursing Diagnosis

Analysis of the assessment data for potential and existing problems, and conceptualization of the problems, leads to the formulation of nursing diagnoses. Table 48-14 (pages 1090–1095) includes nursing diagnoses relevant to families at risk.

Outcome Criteria

Once nursing diagnoses have been established, outcome criteria need to be formulated and stated in observable, measurable terms so that they can be used in evaluating the effectiveness of nursing interventions. Examples of outcome criteria for families at risk and their members are presented in Table 48-14.

Table 48-13 Assessment Questions for High-Risk Families

Death

1. How was the child told about the death? By whom? When? What explanation was given? Does the child feel responsible in any way for the death?
2. Does the family talk about the lost person? Is the child able to talk to the parent (or parents) about the deceased parent or sibling? Do the children talk among themselves? If there is a taboo on talking, what happens if someone mentions the deceased person's name?
3. What happened to the deceased person's possessions? Does the child have a special memento of the lost parent or sibling?
4. How are the family's feelings about the death expressed?
5. Has blame been attached to anyone for "causing" the death?
6. What is the relationship between the child and the surviving parent (or parents)?

Divorce

1. How was the child told of the divorce? By whom? What was his or her immediate response?
2. Is there evidence that one parent is attempting to align the child against the other parent?
3. Does the child have continued contact with the noncustodial parent's family?
4. What was the extent of the changes in the family following the divorce?
5. What are the visits with the noncustodial parent like?
6. To what extent is money a problem? A source of conflict?
7. If the parents are dating, how does the child perceive and respond to it?
8. What are the child's relationships with the custodial and the noncustodial parent?

Remarriage

1. What is the ex-spouse's response?
2. How will the remarriage affect the child? His or her relationship with the parent?
3. How does the child perceive and feel about the potential stepparent?
4. How does the allocation of resources and space affect family relations and boundaries?
5. Are visiting patterns altered?
6. What was the extended family's response?

Stepparenting

1. Whose turf did the family choose?
2. Who makes and enforces family rules?
3. Whose children live in the household and whose children visit?
4. Who communicates with the school? The physician?
5. Who supervises the purchase of the child's clothes?
6. What is the relationship between the child and steprelatives, particularly the stepgrandparents?

Adoption

Assessment of the adoptive family in the early stages of its development must focus on:

1. How was the decision to adopt made?
2. What are the couple's perceptions, attitudes, and feelings about the child's origins? Extended family?
3. How is the attachment process evolving?
4. What changes have occurred in the marital relationship since the arrival of the child?
5. Is the couple's parenting behavior congruent with the child's needs?
6. What is the child's adaptation to the adoptive family?

At a later point in time, the assessment focuses are:

1. Does the child know of his or her adoptive status?
2. How was the child told? By whom?
3. What is the extended family's response to the adoption? To the child?

(Continued.)

Table 48-13 Continued

Adoption

4. What do the adoptive parents know about the child's background? How do they feel about sharing this information with the child? Have they shared what they know?
5. How do the adoptive parents feel about their inability to procreate?
6. How is the attachment process developing?
7. Is there evidence the child is developing a positive identify and self-concept?

Foster Placement

1. What problems are the foster parents encountering?
2. Are their solutions appropriate?
3. How much experience have they had with child rearing?
4. Is the child visited by the biological parent or parents?
5. Does the child have contact with natural siblings?
6. How likely is it that the natural parents will be able to resume care of the child?
7. How does the child relate to the foster parents? Other children in the home?
8. How is the child progressing in school?
9. What obstacles are there to placing the child for permanent adoption?

Table 48-14 Application of the Nursing Process to High-Risk Families

Loss

1. **Assessment: Impact on young child**
   Child cries excessively; has prolonged periods of crying.
   Child expresses fear of leaving the house.
   Child has night terrors, enuresis, encopresis, somatic symptoms.
   Child exhibits unrealistic fears of common daily activities and common objects.

   Nursing diagnosis: Acute anxiety reaction related to parents' divorce.

   Outcome criteria: Adaptation to noncustodial parent's absence from home, as evidenced by:
   - Use of transitional object to cope with the loss.
   - Talking about loss or use of play to work through loss.
   - Confrontation of feared objects and situations gradually and with support of parent.
   - Increasing periods of time spent comfortably pursuing age-appropriate activities.

   Nursing interventions
   Teach parent how to provide empathtic support and nurturing.
   Help parent identify ways to set limits on avoidance behavior.
   Show parent how to use distraction when child becomes anxious.
   Coach parent on how to help child talk about fears, feelings and fantasies.
   Reassure child during anxiety attack.
2. **Assessment: Death of a sibling**
   Child feels that he or she should have died instead of sibling.
   Child exhibits antisocial or self-destructive behavior.
   Child acts as if deceased sibling were still alive.
   Parent blocks child's expression of grief by crying uncontrollably or refusing to talk about the loss.
   Parents communicate primarily with each other.
   Parents withdraw into their bedroom after supper.
   Parents plan to go on vacation without surviving child shortly after the funeral.
   Survivors feel guilty.
   Denial of sibling's death is developmentally inappropriate.

(Continued.)

Table 48-14 Continued

Loss

2. **Assessment: Death of a sibling** (continued)
   Parents block child's expression of grief.
   Child is psychologically isolated in the family.
   Parents are absorbed with their own grief.

   Nursing diagnosis: Family immobilization associated with child's death.

   Outcome criteria: Working through the loss, as evidenced by:
   - Realistic perception of death.
   - Abandonment of self-destructive or antisocial behavior.
   - Parents' helping child ventilate feelings.
   - Family member's sharing memories of the deceased member.
   - Parents' making efforts to meet specific needs of the child.

   Nursing interventions:
   Provide child with full information about cause of sibling's death.
   Answer child's questions honestly and openly.
   Help child to talk about loss or use play to ventilate feelings.
   Help child reframe past behavior as normal, not as cruelty toward dead sibling.
   Help child to recognize that simply relating to dead sibling (in no special way) was helpful to him or her.
   Encourage parents to involve child in the funeral.
   Help parents to recognize the importance of helping child express his or her feelings.
   Encourage parents to help child select a keepsake memento of sibling.
   Encourage parents to share memories of lost child with surviving children.
   Sensitize parents to child's needs.
   Provide parents with support to increase their capacity to nurture.
   Encourage child's involvement with other supportive adult family members.

3. **Assessment: Loss of same-sex parent**
   Child verbalizes that he or she is "no good" or "not worth" anything.
   Child dresses in clothes of the opposite sex.
   Child exhibits behavior that plays down own gender and exphasizes the opposite sex.

   Nursing diagnosis: Impairment of identity and self-concept related to loss of parent.
   Outcome criteria: Development of a healthy identity, as evidenced by:
   - Selecting and using parent surrogate.
   - Experimenting with gender-appropriate behavior.

   Nursing intervention
   Help parent to recognize child's need for a surrogate parent.
   Help parent to identify a surrogate parent.
   Sensitize custodial parent to child's need to spend time with noncustodial parent and to use the surrogate parent.

4. **Assessment: Impaired gender and generational boundaries**
   Adolescent is sexually promiscuous.
   Parent and adolescent violate each other's right to privacy.
   Parent dates people close to adolescent's age.
   Parent's dating behavior, dress, and socializing is comparable to adolescent's.
   Parent has multiple sexual relationships within the home while adolescent is at home.
   Stepparent initiates sexual activity with stepchild or foster child.

   Nursing diagnosis (see Chapter 39)
   Adolescent's sexual acting out is related to parent's inappropriate behavior.
   Parent's social competitiveness with adolescent is related to recent divorce.
   Parent's sexual behavior is problematic (incestuous or promiscuous); behavior is related to loneliness generated by divorce.
   Blurred generational and gender boundaries in reconstituted or foster family, associated with marital discord.

(Continued.)

Table 48-14 Continued

Loss

4. **Assessment: Impaired gender and generational boundaries** (continued)
Outcome criteria: Establishment of appropriate gender and generational boundaries, as evidenced by:
Parent's discontinuation of blatant sexual promiscuity.
Discontinuation of stepparent's sexual behavior with adolescent.
Enforcement by parents of respect for privacy.
Adolescent's talking about feelings related to parent's behavior.

Nursing intervention
Sensitize parents to the impact of their behavior on their adolescent's behavior.
Facilitate adolescent's exploration of his or her feelings about parent's behavior.
Encourage parents to reinforce adolescent's age-appropriate social or sexual behavior.
Intervene to decrease parent's intrusiveness.
Support respect for privacy.
Help parents to negotiate a sound approach to sex education.
Help family members to communicate with each other regarding feelings.
Provide information about growth and development.

5. **Assessment: Loss of family**
Child expresses anger, bewilderment, or confusion about foster placement.

Nursing diagnosis: Child's failure to understand changes in his or her life is associated with impaired communication with parents.

Outcome criteria: Child will be able to explain what has happened to his or her family and why, in a way that fits his or her developmental level.

Nursing interventions: Counsel parents on telling the child about the foster placement: "how," "when," "who."

6. **Assessment: Overclose parent-child relationship**
Child shares parent's bed after the other parent's death.
Child withdraws from peers and spends time exclusively with the surviving parent.
Child develops a school phobia.

Nursing diagnosis: Overclose relationship with the surviving parent, related to need to comfort him or her.

Outcome criteria: Establishment of appropriate relationship between parent and child, as evidenced by:
Definition and maintenance by parent of boundary between parent and child.
Parent's insistence that child sleep in his or her own bed.
Definition by parent of times and activities that exclude the child.
Insistence by parent that child attend school.
Parent's helping child to find and participate in activities with peers.

Nursing interventions
Help parent make distinction between his or her own perceptions, thoughts, and feelings and the child's.
Help parent recognize how his or her distress affects the child.
Encourage child's participation in activities with peers.
Encourage parent to build a social life that excludes child.
Counsel parent to insist that child sleep the night through in own bed.
Counsel parent to insist that child attend school and to occupy himself or herself outside the home during school hours.

Divorce

Assessment: Conflicts of loyalties
Child overtly expresses anger and hostility toward noncustodial parent.
Child refuses to visit with noncustodial parent; plans activities that interfere with visiting.
Custodial parent bitter and hostile toward noncustodial parent; assumes role of victim.
Custodial parent distant from and cold to child immediately before and after child's visit with noncustodial parent.

(Continued.)

Table 48-14 Continued

Divorce

Assessment: Conflicts of loyalties (continued)

Nursing diagnosis: Child caught in loyalty conflict related to parents' divorce and continued poor relationship.

Outcome criteria: Prevention of loyalty conflicts by parents, as evidenced by:

Collaboration on specific parenting issues.
Honoring of visitation and limit-setting agreements.
Refraining from talking to child about their problems with each other.
Verbally acknowledging one another's strengths.

Nursing intervention

Encourage parents to communicate to child that divorce reflects a marital breakdown to which both partners have contributed.
Sensitize parent to the child's problem: aligning with one parent and disloyalty to the other.
Support parent's collaboration in relation to setting limits, visits, attendance at school functions.
Encourage parents to honor child-rearing agreements.
Sensitize parents to negative impact on child of derogatory comments about the other parent.
Encourage parents to disapprove of child's hostility and vengefulness toward the other parent.
Empathize with parents about how difficult it is to contain anger and bitterness and not enlist child's support and alignment.

Stepfamily

1. **Assessment: Impact on stepchildren**

Continual arguments among stepchildren in reconstituted family.
Physical altercations among stepchildren of both parents in reconstituted family.

Nursing diagnosis: Stepsibling conflict related to territorial conflicts in reconstituted family; impaired parental authority related to sabotage.

Outcome criteria: Prevention by parents of loyalty conflicts, as evidenced by:

Negotiation by parents of allocation of resources with children.
Facilitation by parents of communication among children and with each other.
Enforcement by parents of respect for privacy.

Nursing interventions

Counsel parents to consistently enforce limits on physical conflict.
Counsel parents on cooperative conflict resolution.
Encourage parents to negotiate space allocation democratically.
Counsel parents to enforce mutual respect for privacy among family members.
Counsel parents to encourage children to talk about their problems and feelings rather than act on them.
Counsel parents to discuss setting limits and to support one another.

2. **Assessment: Impact on making and enforcing rules**

Stepparent and parent argue about, undermine, or overrule each other in relation to making and enforcing rules for children.

Nursing diagnosis: Impaired rule making and enforcing related to problems in defining stepparenting role.

Outcome criteria: Making and enforcing reasonable rules, as evidenced by:

Democratic negotiation about rules.
Befriending of stepchildren by stepparents.
Family members' respecting each other's opinions and needs.

Nursing intervention

Counsel stepparent to be stepchild's friend.
Counsel stepparent to use integrative undermining.
Counsel stepparent to avoid attempts to replace child's lost parent.
Counsel family to negotiate stepparent's role in family.

(Continued.)

Adoption

1. **Assessment: Genealogical concerns**
   Adoptive child hostile to adoptive parents.
   Adoptive child perceives biological parents as "good" and adoptive parents as "bad."
   Adoptive parents are critical of child and his or her family of origin.

   Nursing diagnosis: Impaired adoptive parent-child attachment process related to denial of importance of biological parents.

   Outcome criteria: Development by child of balanced perception of biological and adoptive parents, as evidenced by:
   - Realistic perception of both adoptive and biological parents' strengths and weaknesses.
   - Acknowledgment by adoptive parents of their own contribution to child's problematic behavior.
   - Adoptive parents' stopping their criticism of child and biological parents.

   Nursing interventions
   Counsel adoptive parents on helping child to use information about dual parents to see positive and negative qualities in both.
   Help adoptive parents to examine fears, fantasies, and feelings that interfere with attachment.
   Help adoptive parents to explore impact of adoption on their relationship and possible ways to resolve problems.

2. **Assessment: "Telling"**
   Adoptive child knows nothing about biological parents.
   Adoptive child's requests for information about biological parents are discouraged by adoptive parents; this upsets child.
   Child is anxious and upset by fantasy that biological parents were "bad people" and he or she "inherited" their "badness."

   Nursing diagnosis: Child's lack of information about biological parents related to adoptive parents' overprotectiveness.

   Outcome criteria: Establishment by child of a satisfactory "knowledge base" on biological parents, as evidenced by:
   - Support by adoptive parents of child's search for information about biological parents.
   - Adoptive parents' sharing information about biological parents.
   - Adoptive parents' not seeing child's search for information about biological parents as dissatisfaction with them.
   - Acquisition by child of information about biological parents.

   Nursing intervention
   Help adoptive parents to become less sensitive to child's search by talking about their feelings and fantasies.
   Explain to adoptive parents the need for child to acquire more knowledge about biological parents.

Foster Family

1. **Assessment: Impact of placement**
   Foster child's school performance is below grade level.
   Foster child is belligerent and combative toward peers.
   Foster child is involved in stealing.
   Foster child has become enuretic since placement.
   Foster child is argumentative with foster parents and other children in the home.

   Nursing diagnosis
   Child's dysfunction related to foster placement.
   Child fears rejection and copes by rejecting others associated with rejection by biological family.
   Child's regression related to loss of biological family.

   Outcome criteria: Adaptation by child to foster placement, as evidenced by:
   - Decrease in antisocial behavior; then elimination of such behavior.
   - Expression by child of a sense of belonging.
   - Gradual improvement in school performance.
   - Less frequent conflicts with peers and foster family.
   - Cessation of bed-wetting.

   Nursing intervention
   Sensitize foster parents to negative impact of hostile rejection of child's cultural heritage or parents.
   Counsel foster parents to encourage child to talk about feelings rather than act on them.
   Negotiate special help with schoolwork.
   Counsel foster parents to recognize source of child's anger and keep conflicts focused on particular issues.

(Continued.)

Table 48-14 Continued

Foster Family

2. **Assessment: Visiting**
   Biological parents and family members do not visit foster child or make contact by telephone.
   Foster parents were hostile toward biological parents when they visited in the past.

   Nursing diagnosis
   Foster child's abandonment by biological family related to parents' conflict with foster parents.
   Foster parents' interference with visiting by biological parents related to their anger about the child's placement.

   Outcome criteria
   Biological parents visit and telephone child regularly.
   Biological parents make concrete, realistic plans to resume responsibility for the child or agree to give the child up for adoption.
   Child expresses feelings related to parents' failure to visit.
   Child has regular contact with siblings.
   Foster parents facilitate biological parents' contact with child.

   Nursing intervention
   Help child to understand and accept parents' limitations and how these influence their failure to visit.
   Sensitize foster parents to child's need to remain connected with biological family and to facilitate communication when possible and appropriate.
   Help biological parents work toward regaining custody.
   Help biological parents make decision to surrender child for adoption.

3. **Assessment: Foster parenting**
   Foster parents verbalize their sense of helpnesses, inability to cope with child, and wish to give up child.
   Child has temper tantrums and is destructive.

   Nursing diagnosis
   Foster parents' discouragement related to child's acting out and destructiveness.

   Outcome criteria
   Foster parents express satisfaction with their role.
   Foster parents handle day-to-day problems more effectively.

   Nursing intervention
   Help foster parents ventilate their feelings about their role and unmet expectations in relation to child and placement.
   Provide foster parents with information about children's response to foster placement and strategies for helping this child adapt to foster home and loss of parents.
   Refer parents to self-help group of foster parents.
   On the 1-year anniversary, facilitate foster parents' review of placement to identify gains and areas of growth.

Nursing Interventions

Nursing interventions designed to prevent or remedy problems encountered by families at risk are directed toward both family and individual dysfunctions.

Interventions with Adoptive Families

PREADOPTION INTERVENTION. To promote mental health in adoptive children, nursing must begin before risks and vulnerabilities exist. If one subscribes to the belief that every child has the right to be wanted, then conception should be the outcome of a positive act of choice by the parents after they have realistically appraised their ability to provide a loving and nurturing family environment.

An unwanted pregnancy resulting from ignorance is not uncommon among the young, the illiterate, and the poor. Educational programs on reproduction and responsible parenthood aimed at these groups in our society would not eliminate all unwanted pregnancies but would introduce the possibility of choice for many.[36]

Information on contraception and family planning must be made readily available and accessible to women of all ages and socioeconomic levels. Many poor women who are most in need of limiting their families are restricted in foresight, poorly informed about the nature of the help they might seek, and accustomed to seeking health care only on an emergency basis. Thus outreach programs must be developed to educate these women on how to use the health care system and to adopt self-care practices which promote health.[36]

More important, the health care system must go beyond just dispensing information and providing a physical examination. "Telling" clients is not teaching, nor does it facilitate understanding. To use contraceptive devices effectively and to engage in family planning, clients must develop the attitudes and values which support these activities. When care givers take the time to develop a working relationship with clients and use the time to help clients explore their fears, their fantasies, and the perceived obstacles to the prevention of unwanted pregnancies, the clients will be more apt to support a decision not to become parents when socioeconomic factors militate against procreation.[36]

Too often, family planning clinics deliver services on the assumption that provision of information and contraceptive devices is all that is needed, neglecting to assess the clients' ability to assimilate the information and apply it in their unique situations. Cultural, interpersonal, and personal factors affect utilization of information and must therefore be considered in any effort to prevent unwanted pregnancies.[36]

There will also be some who, in spite of their knowledge about reproduction and the availability of contraceptives, will, because of immaturity, unconscious emotional problems, or ambivalent feelings, expose themselves to the possibility of an unintended pregnancy. A sensitive, individualized, educative, and counseling approach may make the difference for some of these clients.[36]

When family planning and contraception fail, unmarried mothers need to confront the psychological pressures of motherhood and to relate them to the realities of their present situation.[47] Society emphasizes parental responsibility and the unnaturalness of giving up one's children. When affected by these attitudes, a decision for placement generates a sense of worthlessness, a feeling of failure, and guilt about rejecting the baby, which may interfere with the ability to make the decision final or may precipitate an impulsive decision based on the mother's need to punish herself or the father who wants the child. Unmarried mothers causing the greatest concern are those who, because of an ambivalent tie to their children, elect long-term foster placement, which is potentially disastrous for these children. If decision making is delayed until the child is older, the insecurity generated by institutional living or multiple placements may cause behavior problems and disturbed object relations. These children often have difficulty establishing a meaningful relationship with their foster parents because their allegiance is divided between their real and foster mothers. In time, they often fall into the "unadoptable" category because of severe behavior problems and are denied the family life to which they have a right.[36]

Some mothers resist exploring adoption as a viable possibility because of their attachment to the father and their hope that the baby will sustain the relationship. Still other unmarried or separated mothers try to ignore the realities of the situation and exhibit more dependent and immature behavior. These mothers choose to keep their babies in spite of insurmountable problems and an inability to provide adequately for them.[36]

Parents who are considering giving their children up for adoption have the right to self-determination and sensitive counseling throughout the decision-making process. Opportunities must be provided to allow them to explore and clarify options, consequences, and related feelings in an accepting climate. Relinquishing one's child is a difficult and painful process. A guided and supported problem-solving approach will help parents arrive at a decision which best meets the needs of all concerned and which helps the parents to feel that they have made the best decision, given their circumstances at that time.[36]

Some children might not become available for adoption if disadvantaged biological families were better supported in maintaining socially and economically stable households. Children have a right, as first choice, to be cared for and reared by their biological parents. The welfare system should be redesigned to preserve the integrity of the family. Rather than being penalized for being intact, the disadvantaged family should be economically rewarded so that financial pressures and a rapidly changing job market will not be destructive to the nuclear family.[36]

ADOPTIVE COUPLES. Couples who seek to adopt a child, even with what appear to be the best intentions, need to realistically examine their feelings and the changes that the child will bring to their life. Many couples romanticize parenthood and fantasize the perfect child. If these distorted perceptions persist, they will interfere with a realistic acceptance of the parenting role.[36] The nurse can facilitate the couple's exploration of their feelings and fantasies and help them begin to think about what they will feel, think, and do when problems emerge.

Prospective adoptive parents cannot reassure themselves about the origins of the child by denying reality. Their feelings about the kind of people who relinquish their children for adoption or have them taken away by the court will affect their acceptance of the child. Likewise, the couple's attitudes and feelings about illegitimacy will influence their perception of the child. At particular points in the child's development, these attitudes can seriously jeopardize the parent-child relationship and the child's ability to deal successfully with the various phases of development.

If the child's origins, particularly illegitimacy, are a sensitive issue for the parents, the nurse can help desensitize it. Helping the couple to talk about and examine how origins influence the child and their perceptions may be useful. Misconceptions about inherited genes that would "cause" the child to be delinquent or promiscuous can be resolved through discussions with the parents and through presentation of facts. Parents need help in recognizing the significant influence of the self-fulfilling prophecy. The nurse can help the family to recognize the important influence of their view of the child and their way of relating to him or her. The nurse can also help the parents develop positive, growth-promotive ways of relating to the child that enhance the child's self-esteem and ability to cope.

Before adoptive parents can realistically perceive the adoptive child as a unique person, they must mourn the loss of the fantasized natural child they never had.[35] This is best accomplished before adoption; otherwise the unresolved feelings and fantasies will interfere with the parenting process. The adoptee may be expected to behave and feel in a way that matches the idealized lost child.

Promotion of mental health for adoptive families who are integrating an infant or toddler addresses not only the attachment process but the transition into the adoptive home. Interventions must be directed at helping the biological parents (or the foster parents) and the adoptive couple focus on the needs of the child and resolve feelings about the adoption process. Issues which are anxiety-provoking and cloaked in secrecy can be demystified by discussing them with a nurse who accepts the fears, fantasies, and feelings and points out that they are normal and manageable. Often these parents need information about growth and development and how to apply it to the day-to-day management of problems.[36]

FACILITATING ATTACHMENT. Adoptive parents often need guidance and support through the attachment process. Reassurance that their fears and feelings of ambivalence, incompetence, and responsibility are normal and comparable with those of biological parents can help these parents develop their role.[36]

Adoptive mothers benefit not only from classes on parenting but from individualized supportive care as well. Most communities are in dire need of programs that help parents accept parenthood and educate them about child and family development. Most people raise their children the way they were raised. People may be able to clearly articulate their perceptions about what their parents did that was good or bad and how they would do it differently. However, when confronted by the stresses and strains of day-to-day living, most people, in a pinch, will revert to acting and sounding just like their parents. To help couples parent more effectively, health professionals need to provide information, an opportunity to share problems with other parents, and supportive recognition of their efforts to manage the parent-child relationship. Most problems encountered by adoptive parents of newborns are transitory in nature if the parents have access to information, support, and realistic reassurance.[36]

"Telling"

One of the most difficult problems facing surviving, adoptive, divorcing, and foster parents is when, where, and how they should tell the child that he or she is adopted, or the circumstances of a divorce, a foster placement, or the death of a parent or sibling. In many respects the manner in which the child learns about these circumstances affects the way the child resolves the other issues in his or her life.

Some families, misguidedly believing that they are protecting the child, or wishing to deny the reality of the situation, opt not to tell the child. Avoidance of "telling" creates more problems than it solves. It is all but impossible to keep such events and circumstances a secret. Inevitably a friend or family member will let it slip. The adoptee may discover a document.[53] The child may accidentally meet the noncustodial parent and his or her "new" family or overhear pieces of conversations about how the parent or sibling died. When the child overhears the information or someone other than a parent tells the child, the sense of trust between the parents and the child, which is essential for relatedness, is jeopardized. Not "telling" also implies that the death, divorce, remarriage, adoption, or placement is shameful, disgraceful, or terrible and that the knowledge of it is potentially destructive; it can also imply that neither the child nor the parents have the capacity to deal with the knowledge.[53]

TELLING CHILDREN ABOUT ADOPTION. Triselotis[53] found that among adoptive families, if "telling" was left until the child was age 10 or older, there was the greatest probability that the child would find out from sources outside the family. Adoptees told by parents when 10 years old or younger were significantly more satisfied than those told later. Triselotis found that there was a close association between "telling" at a later point in time and extreme dissatisfaction. Most of the adoptees who were told initially when they were between the ages of 4 and 8 years expressed the greatest satisfaction even though they did not grasp the real implications of being adopted until adolescence. The same probably holds true for children in other circumstances. Table 48-15 presents positive and negative forms of "telling."[53]

Triselotis[53] also found that when "telling" came as a punitive, hostile, retaliatory exchange, the child felt that having been adopted was something shameful or terrible. If the adoptee did not find out until adolescence or as an adult, the initial reaction was one of shock, followed later by intense anger toward the adoptive parents, particularly the mother.[53] The same outcome, more than likely, holds true for children who need to be told about a parent's divorce, remarriage, or foster placement.

When adoptees are told that their biological parents are dead, but information about the circumstances of their death is avoided, these children often feel guilty and imagine that in some way they were responsible. This is particularly true when the child is told that the biological mother died in childbirth. These adoptees may feel that their birth killed their mother and thus may later face parenthood with undue anxiety and fear that they, too, will either die in childbirth or cause a wife to die while giving birth.[35,36]

Table 48-15 Positive and Negative Forms of "Telling"

Positive Forms	Negative Forms
1. Telling at an early age	1. Waiting until the child is older
2. Making the child feel special or chosen	2. Letting child be told by an outsider
3. Revealing image of natural parents positively, truthfully, openly, and appropriately to the child's age	3. Letting child learn about adoption accidentally, through a document
4. Dealing with the issue sensitively and using an approach analogous to sensible sex education	4. Making the child feel grateful
	5. Making malicious references to illegitimacy or to the mother's morals
	6. Belittling the original background
	7. Responding evasively to questions
	8. Telling in the context of a fabrication which is later disproved

Triselotis points out that "telling" or being able to discuss the adoption easily is not necessarily healthy or a sign of strength. Repeated allusion to the child's adoption or placement can convey that he or she really is a stranger in the family. When adoptive, foster, or stepmothers too readily and unnecessarily volunteer that the child is adopted, a foster child, or a stepchild, it may indicate a tenuous attachment to the child and a failure to integrate the child into the family.[39,53] The nurse can help adoptive parents in relation to "telling" the child about his or her adoptive status. These nursing interventions are presented in Table 48-16.

People have a right to an accurate and complete identification in its broadest meaning.[53] Our identity

Table 48-16 Helping Adoptive Parents with "Telling"

Nursing interventions
Facilitate the parents' expression and examination of their feelings and fantasies about telling the child.
Provide information about "telling" that others have found to be helpful.
Help the parents rehearse what they will say and how.
Provide the parents with feedback and rehearsals.
Help the parents review "telling" after the fact.
Help the parents plan how and when they will provide additional information and reinforce previously shared information.

includes what we know about ourselves and about our origins and also what we have been able to take out of our life experience. Identity is a matrix of multiple family, personal, and sociocultural influences. A person's identity is an accumulation of past experiences in the context of the family, both nuclear and extended, and the environment. These experiences form the core of identity. Thus, successes and failures contribute to a sense of being either a competent, related person or an incompetent, isolated person.[53]

Lineage alone does not create one's identity, but one's heritage is integrated into the self. Young adopted and foster children identify unquestioningly with the adoptive or foster family. However, when they realize that they were born to another tribe and have some qualities or talents which cannot be explained by reference to the adoptive or foster family, they develop an increased need to know about their heritage so as to continue developing their sense of identity. Adoptees who prolong the family romance live in a world of imaginary alternative parents. There is greater possibility of delaying acceptance of the adoptive parents, with their normal human qualities, thus slowing identification with them.

The more that adoptees and foster children know about their heritage, the less they have to use imagination. The background knowledge of the biological family necessary for the construction of the mental and emotional structure (mental picture) includes: (1) quality of the biological parents' interest and involvement that went into the original planning for the child, that is, the extent to which their plan represented a genuine desire to obtain security for him or her; (2) factors which interfered with their ability to care for him or her; (3) what the mother and father looked like, for example, hair and eye color; (4) facts nonadopted people know about their family's health, such as diseases and life span; (5) place of birth, where and when they were adopted, and who made the arrangements; (6) age of biological parents at time of the child's birth; (7) interests and hobbies of biological parents; and (8) existence of brothers and sisters.[36,53]

Triselotis[53] found that the greater the amount of positive genealogical and other similar information made available, the less the adoptees' involvement and preoccupation with the natural parents. He concluded that if this information was shared in a positive way, it helped the adoptees identify with a good image of the natural parents and lessened the likelihood of a search for the biological parents. The concept of self seemed influenced by what they thought the original mother was like. When illegitimacy was revealed, it was not necessarily received as negative, nor did it diminish a positive perception of the biological parents.

TELLING CHILDREN ABOUT DIVORCE. Couples who are contemplating divorce may come into contact with the health care system because of stress-related physical symptoms. When opportunities occur, nurses may be of help to such couples. Referrals for counseling may help these couples either work through their problems or manage their separation and their parenting responsibilities more effectively.

When couples divorce, their children need to be told about what is happening to their family. Children (except for infants) need to be told that a parent is moving out of the household before it happens. The nurse can counsel parents to sit down with the children and share the information presented in Table 48-17.

The age of the children affects the way information is shared. Parents must also be counseled to help the children express their fantasies, feelings, and questions related to what is happening to themselves and their family. Nurses can help couples anticipate both the children's reactions and their own reactions, and plan how they will manage

Table 48-17 Children and Divorce

What to Tell Children
When the parent expects to leave the household
Where the parent will be living
Telephone number where the parent can be contacted
When and how often the parent will visit with them
Whether they also will be moving
Concretely how their life will be changed following the separation and divorce
Whether a parent is planning to remarry after the divorce is finalized
That the conflict between the couple has not changed and will not change the parent's feelings toward the children
That the couple are not happy living together; that they have discussed their disagreements and that these areas of conflict are related only to their relationship as husband and wife
That the children did not cause the parents to decide to divorce

both effectively. Secrets in a family can have a potent negative influence. Thus, parents need to be advised that to tell half-truths or to fail to explain the divorce may contribute to greater problems than if they were open and honest. When a parent moves out of the house and immediately begins to live with or marries another person, the custodial parent may be reluctant to share this information with the children. The reluctance serves the parent's own need to avoid and deny; however, it leaves the children in a vulnerable position. Hearing about a parent's living arrangement or remarriage from someone outside the family may be painful and may jeopardize a trusting parent-child relationship.

The nurse needs to counsel divorced couples about the need for them to work together on how they will cooperate in their parenting responsibilities. Despite their interpersonal conflict, they need to recognize the importance of effectively communicating with one another about their children. The nurse may need to help the couple recognize how they use the children as "go-betweens" when they give the children messages to carry to the other parent or use the children to gather information about the parent and his or her lifestyle.

TELLING CHILDREN ABOUT FOSTER PLACEMENT. Foster children also need information that will help them understand their placement. Questions about their biological parents need to be answered directly and honestly. If the foster parent does not have the information, the nurse needs to encourage the use of available resources to acquire it for the child.

When an older child is to be placed in an adoptive or foster home, the child needs to be told as soon as the decision is made. Biological and foster parents can help the child understand the advantages of the placement and by their approval help the child feel less insecure.[36]

TELLING CHILDREN ABOUT DEATH. The death of a spouse or child causes anguish in the survivors. References to the deceased person or even mention of his or her name may escalate the feelings related to grieving. Surviving parents may wish to protect themselves and the surviving children from emotional pain. Consequently, they may avoid telling the children about the cause of death or the circumstances surrounding it. The nurse needs to help surviving parents recognize the importance of telling the children what they need to know to have a realistic understanding. Most important, children need to know the cause of death, to know that everything possible was done, and to know that the person died peacefully. Religious beliefs can be used to help the child to understand and accept the loss.

The nurse also needs to support these parents in feeling that they will be able to provide the information in a sensitive, supportive, and developmentally appropriate way. Role-playing and rehearsals with the nurse help prepare these parents for the difficult task. Self-help groups can provide them with further direction and support.

Managing Grief and Loss

The nurse can help surviving, adoptive, foster, and divorced parents recognize that each child has his or her own way of handling the feelings generated by loss. Threatening, aggressive, hostile, or impulsive behavior may reflect past problematic living arrangements or mask depression. Antisocial behavior distances the parents, other adults, and peers, thus reinforcing the child's belief that the world is a hostile place and that he or she is unlovable. Withdrawn and compliant children who do not manifest anxiety may create less turmoil in the household. These children may be mislabeled as "making an adjustment" when in reality they, too, are struggling with their feelings and in need of help. These children may fear the expression of negative feelings lest they lose another family member.[36] Nurses can help parents to understand the dimensions of the pain and loss experienced by their child and to reassure the child that these feelings are natural and that it is OK to verbalize sadness and rage.[36]

To some degree children's reaction to death, divorce, foster placement, and adoption is rooted in the disruption in the continuity of life, the flow and relatedness of memories and tangible associations. As was noted earlier, it is not the loss of specific individuals that is difficult to deal with as much as it is the gestalt of the loss.

Very young children are essentially preverbal and may regress following a loss. Parents need to be counseled to use a nonverbal approach to console and to help these children cope with their anxiety and grief. Play is also a way in which parents can help these children express their feelings and give meaning to what has happened.

The foster parents, biological family, or institution can facilitate the transition of a child to the adoptive family or foster family by forwarding detailed descriptions of the child's eating, sleeping, bathing, and playing schedule. Familiar toys and other items such as a favorite blanket should accompany the child, and the adoptive or foster family should be helped to understand the importance of these objects to the child during the period of transition. Often the adoptive or foster parents lavish new toys upon the child and feel confused and hurt when the child rejects them for a soiled and ragged favorite stuffed animal. Adoptive or foster parents need help to understand that their adopted child is no different from a biological child who becomes attached to a doll or stuffed animal which, over time, begins to show the wear and tear of the loving it has received. They also need to know that the child is not rejecting them when the old, familiar toy is preferred; rather, the child is gaining security from the familiar and comforting object.[36]

If at all possible, it is also helpful to implement placement by a gradual transition process. For adoptive parents a series of care-giving sessions in the foster home with the foster parents helps the child associate familiar sensations with the adoptive parents and optimizes maintenance of consistent rhythmic and synchronous care giving. The foster mother who has established a relationship with the infant and recognizes the infant's cues for specific needs can help the adoptive mother "tune in" to the child, thus facilitating the development of synchrony in the mother-child relationship.[36] Factors that contribute to the effectiveness of the transition process are presented in Table 48-18.

In spite of the most carefully planned and implemented transition process, the child will experience anxiety. It is not uncommon for children to initially experience mild somatic reactions such as diarrhea, nausea, vomiting, rashes, or colicky stomach pains when they are relocated to a foster or adoptive home. The parents need to be assured that these symptoms will usually be transitory if the parents are able to effectively manage their own tension and uncertainty.[36]

Nurses need to help adoptive and foster parents understand that children who blame themselves for the loss of their family may feel abandoned and rejected. Children who have a history of multiple placements or who have experienced abuse, neglect, or emotional deprivation will be affected by this past. The parents need to recognize that these children will not trust easily or quickly. Some of the old memories and associated feelings will be accessible for working through, but some will be repressed. The adoptive and foster parents need to understand that consistent, positive experiences over time will lessen the influence of these bad memories.[36]

Table 48-18 Foster Placement

Factors That Can Ease the Transition
Ability of the biological or foster parents to manage their own sense of loss and be genuinely helpful to the adoptive or foster parents
Ability of the foster or biological parents to prepare the child for the move into the adoptive or foster family
Ability of the adoptive or foster parents to lessen the trauma to the child by accepting elements of the previous care-giving style so the child will be less disrupted by the move
Ability of the adoptive or foster parents to understand and accept the child's expression of anxiety and grief

Facilitating Integration

Integration of an adoptive, foster, or stepfamily requires the active participation of all members. Nurses need to help the older children recognize the importance of sharing their feelings with their parents. Nurses can also provide feedback to these children that will help them realize their potential for making appropriate changes in thinking, feeling, and behaving that will enhance positive relationships in the family. They can help the parents facilitate integration of the family by promoting the parenting behaviors listed in Table 48-19 (page 1102).

Adoptive and foster parents are able to credit themselves for their adoptive or foster children's successes, but where failings are concerned, they may have a tendency to blame the child's heritage. In some cases there is even a disowning process when serious problems arise. Nurses may need to empathically, sensitively, and persistently help these parents recognize the child's need for their support.

Table 48-19 Family Integration

How Parents Can Facilitate Integration
Help the child to develop at his or her own pace and in his or her own way
Respect the child's individuality and independence without expecting direct expressions of appreciation
Foster flexibility, humor, and resilience when coping with the inevitable stresses, strains, and crises
Accept the residual scars the child bears as a result of past traumatic experiences by avoiding negative labels
Consistently communicate empathy, patience, love
Recognize the difference that foster placement or adoption makes and that their child is a shared child with biological parents who also have meaning to the child
Recognize the need for reasonable age-appropriate limits, establish them, and enforce them consistently

Time Concept and Placement

Depending on their age, children experience any given time period not according to its actual duration, as measured objectively by calenders and clocks, but according to subjective perception. Their time concept influences their perception of abandonment in instances of divorce and foster placement. Parents' absences from day-to-day activities tax the child's ability to cope when the time concept is not fully developed.

Goldstein and others[17] recommend a guideline, based on the child's sense of time, that would require the courts and state and social agencies to "act with all deliberate speed to maximize each child's opportunity to . . . restore stability to existing relationships or to facilitate the establishment of a new relationship or to replace old ones through adoption."

In adoption, the child should be placed before birth when possible.[36] In divorce, the placement of the child needs to be determined by accelerated proceedings and rapid final decision making. Other issues in the divorce proceedings may be dealt with separately, and these proceedings may continue at their own rate.[41] Nurses are often in a position to help clients recognize the child's needs and to explain how children's time concept influences their perceptions of placement.

Evaluation

Evaluation of nursing care provided to children and adults experiencing disruption in family integrity is a significant dimension of the nursing process. An example of evaluation is presented in Table 48-20.

SUMMARY

Dysynchronous patterns are often associated with death of a parent or sibling, divorce, single-parent families, stepfamilies, adoption, and foster placement. This chapter has identified and discussed such patterns with regard to parents and, especially, children.

Divorce may be precipitated by mental illness, infidelity, family crises, low levels of differentiation, a pattern of "pursuing and distancing," and processes of multigenerational transmission. Its impact on children is significant, before it actually takes place, while it is taking place, and after it is an accomplished fact. Changes after a divorce that affect families include arrangements for custody of children; financial changes; and family members' feelings, physical health, social life, and sexuality.

A single-parent family may be formed as a result of death, divorce, or desertion, or by choice—a woman who is single may decide to bear and keep a child, and single men and women sometimes adopt children. Most single-parent families are poor and headed by women. Problems of single-parent families include physical, emotional, and socioeconomic difficulties and stress.

Stepfamilies have distinctive structures and functions, and also distinctive problems. Problems are particularly likely to arise because there are both biological parents and stepparents, children are members of two households, family integration (especially making and enforcing rules) is difficult, there may be "extra" grandparents, finances are complicated, choosing a residence may be controversial, and stepparents' roles are not well defined.

Adoption can also create problems having to do with unwanted children, making a decision to adopt, structure of adoptive families, and biological parents.

Foster placement disrupts family relationships. Dysfunctional patterns may characterize the placement process itself, children's perceptions of placement, visiting, and family adjustment. In addition, there are specific hazards of foster placement; and foster parents may need support.

Table 48-20 An Example of Evaluation

Assessment	Diagnosis	Outcome Criteria	Intervention	Evaluation
Adopted adolescent daughter knows nothing about biological parents. Adopted adolescent's requests for information about biological parents are discouraged by adoptive parents. Adolescent is anxious and upset by fantasy that the biological parents were "bad" people and that she may have inherited their "badness." Adoptive parents feel hurt and rejected when adolescent asks about biological parents. Adoptive parents know that their adopted daughter's biological mother was an unwed teenager and the biological father was a married man.	Adolescent's lack of information about biological parents related to adoptive parent's overprotectiveness and fear of rejection.	Daughter establishes a satisfactory knowledge base on biological parents, and adoptive parents become less sensitive about daughter's need for this knowledge, as evidenced by: 1. Adoptive parents' supporting daughter's search for information about biological parents 2. Adoptive parents' sharing information they have about the adoption and the biological parents 3. Adoptive parents' verbalizing recognition that their adolescent daughter's search for information is not an indication of her dissatisfaction with them as parents 4. Daughter's acquiring information about biological parents' appearance (hair and eye color, height), ethnic background, health, reason for surrendering her for adoption	Help adoptive parents explore fears and fantasies about why daughter wants information about biological parents and what will happen if she acquires this information. Encourage adoptive parents to help daughter in search for information and to offer the information they have. Help daughter to understand the adoptive parents' fears and her legitimate right to know about her biological parents.	Adoptive parents are able to verbalize their fears and discuss them with their daughter. Adoptive parents provide daughter with information about her origins. Adoptive parents and daughter share the search for information. Adoptive parents and daughter are able to discuss the information they find.

Three important patterns of interaction in the person are (1) the attachment process, (2) identity formation, and (3) grief. Impaired attachment can result from dysrhythmic caretaking, failure of "entitlement," and discontinuity. Several aspects of identity formation are important: identification, sexual identity, discontinuation, "negative identification figures," geneology, and the concept of the "family romance." With regard to grief, significant factors are mourning, absence of grief, and "quests."

Two important patterns of interaction in the family are (1) loyalty and (2) impairment of gender and generational boundaries. The concept of family loyalty includes the concept of disloyalty—which may be considered in terms of divorce, "parentification," and abandonment.

Five important patterns of interaction in the environment are (1) reform of divorce laws, particularly no-fault divorce, (2) the role of women in society, (3) the influence of the media, (4) a growing awareness of the need for group homes for adolescents, and (5) attitudes of society toward adoption.

Nurses encounter high-risk families—families dealing with death, divorce, single parenthood, stepparenting, foster placement, and adoption—in many settings; and the primary goal of nursing is prevention of dysfunction. In nursing assessment, the genogram is especially useful. Nursing interventions may involve helping adoptive families; helping adults tell children about adoption, divorce, foster placement, and death; helping clients manage grief and loss; and relating children's concepts of time to placement.

REFERENCES

1. D. Balk, "Effects of Sibling Death on Teenagers," *Journal of School Health,* vol. 53 no. 1, 1983, pp. 14–18.
2. A. Roy, "Early Parental Death and Adult Depression," *Psychological Medicine,* vol. 13, 1983, pp. 861–865.
3. M. J. Horowitz, D. S. Weiss, N. Kaltreider, et al., "Reactions to the Death of a Parent," *Journal of Nervous and Mental Disease,* vol. 172, no. 7, 1984, pp. 383–392.
4. E. Elizur and M. Kaffman, "Factors Influencing the Severity of Childhood Bereavement Reactions," *American Journal of Orthopsychiatry,* vol. 53, no. 4, 1983, pp. 668–676.
5. "Parental Death and Schizophrenia," *Science News,* vol. 116, no. 5, 1979, p. 85.
6. D. A. Leupnitz, "Which Aspects of Divorce Affect Children?" *Family Coordinator,* January 1979, pp. 79–85.
7. J. S. Wallerstein and J. B. Kelly, *Surviving the Breakup,* Basic Books, New York, 1980.
8. T. Fogarty, "Systems Concepts and the Dimensions of Self," in P. Guerin, ed., *Family Therapy: Theory and Practice,* Gardner, New York, 1976, pp. 144–153.
9. T. F. Fogarty, "Marital Crisis," in P. Guerin ed., *Family Therapy: Theory and Practice,* Gardner, New York, 1976, pp. 325–334.
10. M. Bowen, "Theory in the Practice of Psychotherapy," in P. Guerin ed., *Family Therapy: Theory and Practice,* Gardner, New York, 1976, pp. 42–90.
11. C. W. Mueller and H. Pope, "Marital Instability: A Study of Its Transmission," *Journal of Marriage and the Family,* vol. 39, no. 1, February 1977, pp. 83–92.
12. A. K. Mitchell, "Adolescents' Experiences of Parental Separation and Divorce," *Journal of Adolescence,* vol. 6, no. 2, 1983, pp. 175–187.
13. W. F. Hodges and B. L. Bloom, "Parent's Report of Children's Adjustment to Marital Separation: A Longitudinal Study," *Journal of Divorce,* vol. 8, no. 1, 1984, pp. 33–50.
14. A. L. Stolberg and J. M. Anker, "Cognitive and Behavioral Changes in Children Resulting from Parental Divorce and Consequent Environment Changes," *Journal of Divorce,* vol. 7, no. 2, 1983, pp. 23–41.
15. J. S. Wallerstein, "Children of Divorce: Preliminary Report of a Ten-Year Follow-Up of Young Children," *American Journal of Orthopsychiatry,* vol. 54, no. 3, 1984, pp. 444–458.
16. J. C. Westman, "The Impact of Divorce on Teenagers," *Clinical Pediatrics,* vol. 22, no. 10, 1983, pp. 692–697.
17. J. Goldstein, A. Freud, and A. J. Solnit, *Beyond the Best Interests of the Child,* Free Press, New York, 1973, pp. 21–23, 27, 57.
18. C. R. Ahrons, "Predictors of Paternal Involvement Postdivorce: Mothers' and Fathers' Perceptions," *Journal of Divorce,* vol. 6, no. 3, 1983, pp. 55–69.
19. J. W. Jacobs, "The Effect of Divorce on Fathers," *International Journal of Family Therapy,* vol. 6, no. 3, 1984, pp. 177–191.
20. A. P. Derdeyn and E. Scott, "Joint Custody: A Critical Analysis and Appraisal," *American Journal of Orthopsychiatry,* vol. 54, no. 2, 1984, pp. 199–209.
21. M. Galper, *Coparenting,* Running Press, Philadelphia, 1978.
22. G. Dullea, "Is Joint Custody Good for Children?" *New York Times Magazine,* February 3, 1980, p. 32.
23. T. J. Espenshade, "The Economic Consequences of Divorce," *Journal of Marriage and the Family,* vol. 41, no. 3, August 1979, pp. 615–625.
24. B. S. Dohrenwend and B. Dohrenwend, eds., *Stressful Life Events: Their Nature and Effects,* Wiley, New York, 1974.
25. R. S. Weiss, "The Emotional Impact of Marital Separation," *Journal of Social Issues,* vol. 22, no. 1, 1976, pp. 1135–1145.
26. H. Carter and P. Glick, *Marriage and Divorce: A Social and Economic Study,* 2d ed., Harvard University Press, Cambridge, Mass., 1976.
27. N. D. Colletta, "Stressful Lives: The Situation of Divorced Mothers and Their Children," *Journal of Divorce,* vol. 6, no. 3, 1983, pp. 19–31.
28. J. A. Horowitz and B. J. Perdue, "Single Parent Families," *Nursing Clinics of North America,* vol. 12, no. 3, September 1977, pp. 503–511.
29. S. Bould, "Female-Headed Families: Personal Fate Control and the Provider Role," *Journal of Marriage and the Family,* vol. 39, no. 2, May 1977, pp. 339–349.
30. H. J. Raschke and V. J. Raschke, "Family Conflict and Children's Self-Concepts: A Comparison of Intact and Single-Parent Families," *Journal of Marriage and the Family,* vol. 41, no. 2, May 1979, pp. 367–374.
31. P. K. Knaub, S. L. Hanna, and N. Stinnett, "Strengths of Remarried Families," *Journal of Divorce,* vol. 7, no. 3, 1984, pp. 41–55.
32. S. M. Halperin and T. A. Smith, "Differences in

Stepchildren's Perceptions of Their Stepfathers and Natural Fathers: Implications for Family Therapy," *Journal of Divorce,* vol. 7, no. 1, 1983, pp. 19–30.

33. P. N. Stern, "Stepfather Families: Integration around Child Discipline," *Issues in Mental Health Nursing,* vol. 1, Summer 1978, pp. 49–56.
34. S. G. Willard and E. B. Gasser, "Stepmothers and Natural Mothers: A Study of Maternal Attitudes," *International Journal of Family Therapy,* vol. 4, no. 4, 1982, pp. 242–251.
35. K. W. Watson, "Adoptive and Foster Parents," in L. E. Arnold, ed., *Helping Parents Help Their Children,* Brunner/Mazel, New York, 1978, pp. 315–327.
36. B. Sideleau, "Adoption," *Issues in Mental Health Nursing,* vol. 1, Summer 1978, pp. 57–80.
37. E. Y. Deykin, L. Campbell, and P. Patti, "The Post-adoption Experience of Surrendering Parents," *American Journal of Orthopsychiatry,* vol. 54, no. 2, 1984, pp. 271–280.
38. A. R. Gruber, *Children in Foster Care,* Human Sciences, New York, 1978.
39. D. Fanshel and E. B. Shinn, *Children in Foster Care,* Columbia, New York, 1978.
40. S. Z. Moss, "Threat to Place a Child," *American Journal of Orthopsychiatry,* vol. 54, no. 1, 1984, pp. 168–173.
41. S. Jenkins and B. Diamond, "Ethnicity and Foster Care: Census Data as Predictors of Placement Variables," *American Journal of Orthopsychiatry,* vol. 55, no. 2, 1985, pp. 267–276.
42. H. S. Mass and R. E. Engler, *Children in Need of Parents,* Columbia, New York, 1959, pp. 353–354.
43. M. D. Ainsworth, "Reversible and Irreversible Effects of Maternal Deprivation on Intellectual Development," in *Maternal Deprivation,* Child Welfare League of America, New York, 1962.
44. W. H. Missildine, ed., "Problems of Children in Foster Care," *Feelings,* Ross Laboratories, Columbus, Ohio, 1963.
45. A. R. Gruber, *Foster Home Care in Massachusetts,* Governor's Commission on Adoption and Foster Care, Commonwealth of Massachusetts, Boston, 1973, p. 18.
46. E. V. Mech, *Public Welfare Services for Children and Youth in Arizona,* Joint Interim Committee on Health and Welfare Services, 29th Legislature, Arizona, April 1970, p. 72.
47. P. W. Cautley, *New Foster Parents,* Human Sciences, New York, 1980.
48. J. Bowlby, *Attachment,* vol. 1, Basic Books, New York, 1969.
49. E. S. Wertheim, "Person-Environment Interaction: The Epigenesis of Autonomy and Competence," *British Journal of Medical Psychology,* vol. 48, 1975, pp. 95–111.
50. E. H. Erickson, *Identity, Youth and Crisis,* Norton, New York, 1968.
51. S. Reece and B. Levin, "Psychiatric Disturbances in Adopted Children: A Descriptive Study," *Social Work,* vol. 13, 1968, pp. 101–111.
52. B. Jafee and D. Fanshel, *How They Fared in Adoption: A Follow-up Study,* Columbia, New York, 1970.
53. J. Triselotis, *In Search of Origins,* Routledge, London, 1973.
54. M. Rosenberg, *Conceiving the Self,* Basic Books, New York, 1979, p. 10.
55. L. H. Tessman, *Children of Parting Parents,* Aronson, New York, 1978, pp. 42, 90, 92–94, 103, 108, 116, 133, 135.
56. J. B. Newman et al., "Adoption," *Medical Journal of Australia,* vol. 2, November 1972, pp. 1098–1099.
57. M. Wolfstein, "How is Mourning Possible?" *Psychoanalytic Study of the Child,* vol. 21, 1966, pp. 93–122.
58. H. Nagera, "Children's Reactions to the Death of Important Objects: A Developmental Approach," *Psychoanalytic Study of the Child,* vol. 25, 1970, pp. 360–400.
59. J. Bowlby, "Grief and Mourning in Infancy and Early Childhood," *Psychoanalytic Study of the Child,* vol. 15, 1960, pp. 9–52.
60. H. Deutsch, "A Two-Year-Old Boy's First Love Comes to Grief," *Neuroses and Character Types,* International Universities Press, New York, 1965.
61. A. Freud, "Discussion of Bowlby," *Psychoanalytic Study of the Child,* vol. 15, 1960, pp. 54–94.
62. I. Boszormenyi-Nagy and B. G. Spark, *Invisible Loyalities,* Harper and Row, New York, 1973, pp. xix, 18, 28, 39, 51–53, 111, 152.
63. W. Easson, "Special Sexual Problems of the Adopted Adolescent," *Medical Aspects of Human Sexuality,* July 1973, pp. 92–103.

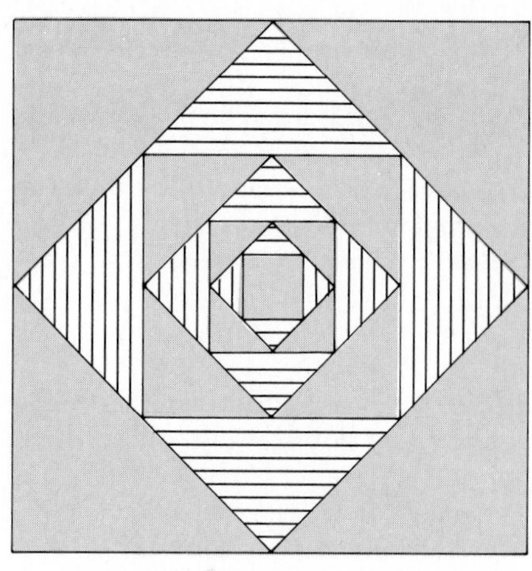

CHAPTER 49
Maintenance and Restoration of Mental Health in Child-Rearing Families

Jane Norbeck
Patricia Pothier

LEARNING OBJECTIVES

After studying this chapter, the student should be able to:

1. Identify physical and behavioral symptoms of distress in children.
2. Discuss patterns of interaction—in persons and families—that contribute to the development of symptoms of distress in children.
3. Discuss environmental patterns of interaction that influence parent-child relationships and mental health care of infants and children.
4. Discuss the problems encountered in delivering mental health services to families with infants and young children.
5. Apply the nursing process to infants and children with symptoms of distress and to their families.

Young children are vulnerable to stress in the family. Patterns of parenting interact with the development of the child's mind, body, and spirit. Effective parent-child patterns of interaction promote growth, development, and overall well-being; dysynchronous patterns interfere with the child's maturation and generate biopsychosocial health problems. The Joint Commission on the Mental Health of Children[1] identified five categories of problems that play a role in the genesis of emotional and mental disorders in infants and children:

1. Faulty training and faulty life experiences
2. Surface conflicts between children and parents which arise during the performance of such adjustment tasks as establishing and maintaining relationships with adults, peers, and siblings; involvement in school; academic performance; and social and sexual development
3. Deeper conflicts which become internalized and create emotional conflicts within the child
4. Difficulties associated with physical handicaps and disorders
5. Difficulties associated with severe mental disorders such as pervasive developmental disorders and severe mental retardation

Stressors for infants and young children fall into two categories: developmental and situational.[2] Common *developmental* stressors are the "rapprochement" period (see Chapter 5), entry into school, and mastery of social and academic skills. *Situational* stressors include family disruption such as a death, divorce, or illness; abuse or neglect; and economic or social disasters.

These stressors interact with the child's ability to cope and with any existing vulnerability found in the child's or the family's functioning. In the child, vulnerability can result from impairments of physiological integrity; low tolerance for frustration; a "difficult child" temperament; impaired ability to pay attention, to sustain attention, or to perceive reality accurately; poorly developed cognitive, problem-solving abilities; and an inability to use resources that are available. In the family, vulnerability can result from an inability to provide a secure, predictable nurturing environment, and cultural or ethnic incongruence with the larger society.

The purpose of this chapter is to examine the risk factors for infants and young children that contribute to the development of mental health problems. The chapter also addresses the application of the nursing process to maintain and restore mental health in child-rearing families.

DYSYNCHRONOUS HEALTH PATTERNS

It is unusual to find crystallized and circumscribed symptom profiles in infants and children indicating early evidence of dysfunction. The symptoms that do appear vary and may include evidence of behavioral or physical disturbance or a combination of both. These symptoms reflect mismanagement of stress and a dysfunctional parent-child relationship. There are early signs of mismanagement of stress and deprivation that indicate mental health problems in infants and young children;[3,4] these are presented in Table 49-1 (page 1108).

DSM III

Several diagnostic categories found in the *Diagnostic and Statistical Manual of Mental Disorders* (DSM III) encompass the early signs of mental health problems in infants and children. These categories include *attention deficit disorder, conduct disorder* (undersocialized, aggressive; undersocialized, nonaggressive; and socialized, nonaggressive), *anxiety disorders* (separation anxiety disorder, avoidant disorder, overanxious disorder), *other disorders of infancy, childhood, or adolescence* (reactive attachment disorder, oppositional disorder), *eating disorders,* and *other disorders with physical manifestations.*[4]

Epidemiology

The Joint Commission on the Mental Health of Children has estimated that 10 to 12 percent of people under 25 years of age (approximately 10 million people) are in need of mental health services. However, only about 5 to 7 percent (approximately 500,000) of the children who need mental health care are being served.[1] In 1978 the President's Commission on Mental Health reaffirmed the extent of these unmet needs for children and young people.[5]

Table 49-1 Early Warning Signs of Mental Health Problems in Infants and Young Children

Physical Symptoms	Behavioral Symptoms
Delayed or disordered growth and development: Poor weight gain; retarded skeletal growth; failure to thrive, which may occur even when food intake is adequate; obesity; weak rooting and grasping responses during feeding	Accident-proneness, excessive clumsiness
Delayed acquisition, loss, or deviant nature of motor skills and activities (walking, self-feeding and dressing, right-left discrimination); control over sphincters; communication (use of speech; idioglossia, or barely comprehensible speech; stuttering or stammering; continued use of baby talk, socially inappropriate gestures, and other nonverbal modes); intellectual processes (illogical or impaired focal attention, that is, inability to attend to a task for an extended period of time; an inability to learn not attributable to physical or organic disabilities)	Excessive running and climbing; act as if "driven by a motor"
Specific organ-system symptoms: Gastrointestinal disturbances (vomiting, poor absorption of food, diarrhea, colitis, constipation, anorexia, peptic ulcers), skin disturbances (rashes, hives, eczemas, warts, angioneurotic edema), respiratory disturbances (rhinorrhea, asthma, wheezing), endocrine disturbances (juvenile diabetes mellitus, thyroid disturbances), circulatory disturbances (headaches)	Habit patterns: Nail biting, tics, hair pulling
Behavioral Symptoms	Impulsive temper tantrums
Sleep disturbances: Nightmares, night terrors, difficulty falling asleep, sleepwalking, excessive sleeping	Shy and withdrawn, apathetic
Disturbances in activity-rest patterns	Restless, fidgety, easily distractible, low achievement in school
Eating disturbances: Too much or too little food intake, disturbance in appetite, avoidance of foods, ingestion of inedible substances (pica), anorexia, bulimia	Aggressive and destructive: Fail to respect the rights of others
Elimination disturbances: Enuresis, encopresis	Excessively ritualistic, perfectionistic tendencies
Disturbed capacity to play: Become upset with messy play; regressed selection and use of play materials; inability to stick to activities for age-appropriate time periods	Asocial behavior: Stealing, lying, setting fires
	Sexually inappropriate behavior: Exhibitionism; seductiveness; excessive or public masturbatory behavior; molesting other children; cross-gender dressing
	Delayed or disturbed relationships with others: Marked isolation; inability to relate to peers and teachers; difficulty separating from mother or father; refusal to attend school (school phobia)
	Do not seem to listen to others
	Not affectionate; lack empathy toward others; not attached to others
	Absence of age-appropriate guilt
	Tendency to blame others
	Excessive distress upon separation or anticipated separation from attachment figure
	Unrealistic worry about losing attachment figure
	Unrealistic worry about anticipated situations
	Mood disturbances: Overreaction to minor stresses; sadness; prolonged anger; anxiousness; fears of familiar and new situations and persistent doubts about capacity to master these situations; pervasive mood of unhappiness; inappropriate feelings under normal conditions

PATTERNS OF INTERACTION: PERSON

Children are considered to be at risk when they are vulnerable in certain ways or when they have been exposed to traumatic situations. There are several types of factors that contribute to putting children at risk. Each is listed here, along with an example or examples:[2]

- Genetic (familial schizophrenia)
- Reproductive (prematurity)
- Constitutional (temperamental type)
- Developmental (medical problems at a given stage)
- Physical (acute or chronic illness)
- Environmental (psychotic parent)
- Traumatic (physical abuse, separation from the mothering parent)

Initially, situational conflicts may not be distinguished easily from deeper, internalized conflicts. The persistence of symptoms, despite the efforts of the child and others to change them, is a cardinal clue to intrapsychic conflicts. Thus, if the first line of intervention (that is, problem-focused intervention) fails to bring about a change in the problem behavior, the possibility is that deeper conflicts are involved. Likewise, with problems in parenting, if problem-focused interventions are not successful, the possibility exists that the parents' practices are sustained by their own pathological needs. It is also possible that problem behavior manifested by an infant or child can be detected early and remedied. When the problem is related to ineffective parenting, it is usually long-standing and requires more intensive, prolonged treatment. In many cases, however, parental anxiety and lack of knowledge about normal child development account for the conflicts that arise between parent and child.

In assessment of problem behavior in a child, another distinction to be made is between the original factors related to the *development* of the maladaptive behavior and ongoing factors related to the *maintenance* of the behavior. For example, a child might have begun to show clinging, dependent behavior at age 3 when displaced by a sibling, but—long after the original situation—the behavior continued because it was rewarded, either positively or negatively. Parents are often unaware that negative reinforcement, such as excessive criticism, can maintain the very behavior it seeks to suppress.

"Difficult Child" Syndrome

Alexander Thomas, Stella Chess, and Herbert G. Birch[6] have identified a type of vulnerable child they labeled the *difficult temperamental type*. Such a child is characterized from early infancy onward by irregularity in bodily functions (for example, unpredictable sleeping and feeding schedules), high intensity of reactions or responses, a tendency to withdraw in the face of new stimuli, slow adaptability to changes in the environment, and negative mood. The constellation of traits of the "difficult" tempermental type is presented in Table 49-2 in comparison with the "easy" and "slow to warm up" temperamental types. Difficult children composed 10 percent of the study sample. Approximately 70 percent of these difficult children developed behavior problems, in contrast to 18 percent of the easy children.[6] However, when parents can maintain consistent approaches based on an objective view of the child's reaction patterns, the child is able to adapt slowly to step-by-step demands for normal socialization.[6] Thus, such a child requires a high degree of consistency and tolerance in his or her upbringing; the parents may need help in defining and understanding the child's special needs as well as support in handling the day-to-day behavior.

Cumulative Stress from Major Life Events

The death of a parent is a major life event that is clearly traumatic for a child. What is less frequently considered is the cumulative stress from a number of life events or changes. Examples of highly stressful life events for preschoolers or children of elementary school age are death, divorce, or marital separation of parents; jail sentence of a parent for

Table 49-2 Temperamental Types

Type of Child	Activity Level (Proportion of active periods to inactive ones)	Rhythmicity (Regularity of hunger, excretion, sleep and wakefulness)	Approach-Withdrawal (Response to a new object or person)	Adaptability (Ease with which a child adapts to changes in the environment)	Intensity of Reaction (Energy of response, regardless of its quality or direction)	Quality of Mood (Amount of friendly, pleasant, joyful behavior as contrasted with unpleasant, unfriendly behavior)
"Easy"	Varies	Very regular	Positive approach	Very adaptable	Low or mild	Positive
"Slow to warm up"	Low to moderate	Varies	Initial withdrawal	Slowly adaptable	Mild	Slightly negative
"Difficult"	Varies	Irregular	Withdrawal	Slowly adaptable	Intense	Negative

NOTE: Temperamental characteristics for traits which differentiate among three temperamental types. In the original research, 65% of the children could be so categorized; 35% displayed a mixture of traits.
SOURCE: Alexander Thomas, Stella Chess, and Herbert G. Birch, "The Origin of Personality," *Scientific American*, vol. 223, no. 2, August 1970, pp. 102–109.

1 year or more; marriage of a parent to a stepparent; death of a brother or sister; serious illness requiring hospitalization of the child; acquisition of a visible deformity; serious illness requiring hospitalization of a parent; birth of a brother or sister; and full-time employment of the mother outside the home.[7]

The frequency or severity of stress from major life events determines the amount of readjustment required by the child. With increased levels of stress from recent life events, more time is required to accomplish readjustment. A few high-stress events or several lower-stress events occurring within a single year may overload the child's capacity to adjust to the changes. In a study of the significance of life events as etiologic factors in the diseases of children, a research team found that, compared with healthy children, 2 to 3 times as many children in each of four client groups (rheumatoid arthritis, general pediatric hospitalization, surgical patients, and psychiatric patients) had an overload of stress from life events before the onset of disease.[8]

Children's responses to change and their ability to readjust are influenced by their strengths, weaknesses, and resources. For example, a child characterized by a difficult temperament would be likely to respond with great intensity and to adjust quite slowly to life events or changes. A child who has emotional support during the period of readjustment to major life events is more likely to have a favorable outcome.

PATTERNS OF INTERACTION: FAMILY

Many of the dysynchronous patterns seen among infants and children are a function of faulty training and socialization, life experiences, and disordered family-child relationships.[4] Faulty training can result from unclear or contradictory expectations, inconsistent or inappropriate discipline, reinforcement of undesirable or developmentally unproductive behavior, or lack of reinforcement for positive or developmentally appropriate behavior.

Faulty or inadequate life experiences can block the child's achievement of developmental tasks because of unmet developmental needs; for example, the lack of a continuous relationship during infancy can interfere with the development of trust and the ability to form normal attachments.

Undifferentiation in the family, the family projection process, the multigenerational transmission process, parentification, and loyalty conflicts are involved in the development of symptoms of distress in infants and children. These dynamics contribute to the way the parents perceive, relate to, and influence the child. They affect the recognition of individual family members' unique idiosyncratic and developmental needs, the separateness and uniqueness of individual members, and the personal boundaries that define the family system.

PATTERNS OF INTERACTION: ENVIRONMENT

The delivery of mental health services to children and families occurs in the context of a larger environment. Both families and care providers are affected by economic, social, and cultural factors.

Economic factors influence the incidence of mental health problems and the availability of services. Studies indicate that with every 1 percent rise in unemployment there is an increase in admission to mental health facilities, related to suicide attempts and child abuse.[9] At the same time the status of the nation's economy affects the funding that is available to lower-income families for support of social, medical, and mental health services.[10] These factors greatly affect the lower-income working families who are not eligible for medical assistance. Many health-insurance plans do not provide adequate coverage for psychiatric services, and there are not enough low-cost programs to meet the needs.

Maternal employment is another major economic factor affecting the mental health of children. The 1980 U.S. Census indicated that 43 percent of mothers with children under 6 years of age were in the labor force and that 50 percent of the children 3 to 5 years old were in some type of day care. Of this group of children, 94 percent were in unregulated family day care arrangements.[11] Many of these children are inadequately cared for while their mothers work, and many child-care arrangements lack the stability that children, particularly those under 3 years of age, need. The younger the child, the more dependent he or she is upon a consistent and continuous relationship with one person. Thus an important area to assess in families with a working mother is the adequacy of the child care that is provided. For an infant it is, of course, important to establish continuity, but the care giver must also be willing to enter into a responsive, nonrejecting, and stimulating relationship with the infant. Recent research indicates that when adequate child care is provided, maternal employment has a beneficial effect on mothers, children, and families.

Social factors that affect the behavior of clients and care providers are changing family patterns, sex roles, and lifestyles. Many recent changes in patterns of family life call for the reinterpretation of assumptions about the nuclear family. The divorce rate in this country has increased. More than 1 million children below the age of 18 are affected by divorce. Not only does divorce require major adjustment and coping by children and parents, but a series of readjustments in the formation of a stepfamily are required when parents remarry. Just as the providers of mental health care cannot assume that the intact nuclear family is necessarily normal or healthy, they cannot assume that the single-parent family is dysfunctional. In either case, an objective assessment of family resources and functioning is needed. Likewise, changing patterns of child care within the family must be evaluated as they relate to children's needs rather than to traditional roles.

Cultural factors influence communication and interaction between clients and care providers in several ways. Cultural differences exist in values regarding behavior, attitudes and practices of child rearing, and patterns of using outside help for problems. Although families and subcultural groups have the right to hold differing child-rearing attitudes and philosophies, some basic principles of effective child rearing transcend these values. For example, whether the family values conformity or creativity, a child still needs clear, unambiguous messages about what kind of behavior is expected. The developmental stage of a child should be considered in determining expected standards or levels of behavior.

Nurses and other providers of health care should be aware of their own values and their feelings about various child-rearing attitudes and practices. When these practices are harmful (for example, excessively punitive or rejecting), professionals must be prepared to intervene; however, where attitudes and practices are merely different from one's own, one should attempt to convey acceptance and understanding so as to facilitate a collaborative relationship with the family. Consultation with a professional from the client's subculture can be used to gain information about cultural patterns and viewpoints as well as insight into the family's needs and behavior.

There are two major limitations in the delivery of mental health services to children. First, existing mental health services are reaching only a small percentage of the identified population of children and young people in need.

Second, the group aged 3 years old and under tends to be neglected. Many children disappear from professional surveillance during the period from birth to entry into school or preschool programs. The various mental health disciplines have not focused training on the assessment and treatment of children who suffer from emotional disorder in the first years of life, and families do not take advantage of existing services. Yet the first 3 years are the most crucial in the life of a child. The foundations of development in all areas—physical, intellectual, linguistic, emotional, social, and spiritual—are laid down at this time; likewise, barriers to normal development can be erected during this period. The effects of early emotional and experiential deprivation can be seen in much later periods. Children under 3 are rarely exposed to responsible adult observation outside the family. Since not all children attend preschool programs, society has no clear responsibility for the child until he or she reaches school age. Consequently many problems of development go unnoticed until the child enters school. By this time the maladjustment patterns may be deeply entrenched and difficult to treat.[1]

NURSING PROCESS

Evidence of dysynchronous biopsychosocial health problems in infants and children calls for nursing care that focuses on maintenance and restoration of health. The goals of restorative nursing care are to reduce the duration of symptoms and to prevent

Table 49-3 **Early Intervention: Developmental Issues, Clients, and Settings**

Developmental Stage	Developmental Issue	Client	Setting
Perinatal	Bonding Attachment	Newborn Mother Father	Maternity unit Nursery Infant intensive-care unit
Infancy	Strengthening of human bonds Development of trust	Infant Family	Home Clinic
Preschool	Mastery Coping Problem solving	Child Family Care-setting personnel	Home Day care Nursery school Pediatric mental health services (outpatient and inpatient)
Primary school	School entrance Adjustment to learning situation	Child Family School personnel	School Pediatric mental health services (outpatient and inpatient)

more severe or complex emotional disorders from developing.[12] The guiding principles in health maintenance are (1) early identification and (2) early intervention. The focus of early intervention is on infants and children who have diagnosed physiological syndromes or defects, and those who are at risk of developing problems. Common health maintenance activities that nurses might be involved in are surveillance, developmental teaching and demonstration, anticipatory guidance, counseling for developmental or situational crises, extending support systems, advocacy, referral and liaison to appropriate services, and consultation. Table 49-3 summarizes the issues for the developmental stages that are of concern to nurses in health maintenance and restoration and lists the clients who are the recipients of nursing care and the settings where nurses encounter these clients.

The early warning signs of stress indicate that the infant or child's adaptive equilibrium is altered; however, the nature of the stress must be determined by further assessment of the child and the family. One must also determine whether the difficulty is transitory, within the range of individual differences, or an early manifestation of maladaptation.

Three factors to be considered in weighing the significance of early warning signs are the *extent*, or severity, of the behavior; the *duration* of the behavior; and the *number* of early warning signs present. If any one sign is manifested to a great extent or has persisted over a long period of time, further assessment of the child and family is indicated. Likewise, if more than one early warning sign is present, further assessment is needed.

ASSESSMENT

Assessment of the child and the family provides information about the significance, and possibly the origins, of the early warning signs of stress or problem behavior exhibited by the child. This information is useful in determining the most effective level in the system for intervention (the parenting, the family situation, or the child's behavior or characteristics).

Assessment of the Child

Assessment of the child for early intervention differs from both screening and a comprehensive psychiatric examination. Deeper in scope than screening, this assessment seeks to determine the developmental level attained by the child and to identify problems that may interfere with the development of sensorimotor, language, or psychosocial skills. Unlike a comprehensive psychiatric examination, assessment does not explore or evaluate intrapsychic levels of functioning. The elements of the assessment include developmental screening, interviewing of parents, and observations of the child in a variety of settings.

DEVELOPMENTAL SCREENING. The current developmental level of an infant or young child is assessed through standardized screening procedures. Several developmental tests exist, each measuring development in four main areas: gross motor abilities (integration of the central nervous system and the musculoskeletal system), communication skills (comprehension, expression, hearing, and speech), fine motor skills (eye-hand coordination), and personal-social behavior (self-care and interaction with others).[13] Developmental tests are insufficiently standardized and lack the sensitivity to provide precise diagnostic data; therefore, the results should be interpreted as a screening only—an indication of whether further evaluation is indicated.

The Denver Developmental Screening Test[14] is the mostly widely known by nurses; it is also familiar to pediatricians, social workers, and psychologists. This test is used for detecting developmental delays during infancy and the preschool years. As with any testing, one must bear in mind that the results can be influenced by the rapport established by the examiner and by factors related to the child's psychosocial environment.

Testing of the school-age child frequently consists of evaluating problems in learning. Emotional problems are usually associated with impaired school achievement, but in the cases in which specific learning disabilities (for example, impaired visual or auditory memory) are found, the emotional problems are secondary. To gain a comprehensive picture of the child's learning difficulties, one selects a battery of tests sensitive to the child's overt problem areas. The testing is usually done by a clinical psychologist or an educational specialist.

INTERVIEW WITH PARENTS. Three main areas are covered in an interview with parents: the parents' perception of the child's current functioning, the child's developmental history, and the child's history of previous episodes of behavioral difficulty or difficult life experiences.

In the interview the parents are encouraged to describe their perceptions of the child's current behavior and adjustment. From this discussion, one can learn whether the parents feel there is a problem; if so, how severe they feel it is; and whether they have sought help or considered seeking help.

To gain a picture of the child's previous progression of development, one should take a brief history. The developmental landmarks that parents can usually report are holding the head up, sitting without support, crawling, saying "dada" or "mama," walking alone, using short sentences, and achieving bowel and bladder control. Although the parents' memory of the actual months of occurrence of these developmental landmarks may not be accurate, one can get an estimate of their occurrence and of the parents' ideas about the appropriateness of the time of occurrence.

In addition to information about sensorimotor and language development, inquiry about interpersonal behavior provides information about the child's psychosocial development. Some of the psychosocial adjustment tasks the parents should be asked about involve separation from mother and father, sibling rivalry, socialization with peers, and adjustment to school.

Possible relationships of current behavioral and adjustment problems to the child's past development and experiences can be discovered by inquiring about previous areas or episodes of troublesome or inadequate behavior or the occurrence of difficult life experiences (for example, hospitalization or major illness, or separation from the mother during infancy or early childhood). Sometimes a current problem behavior first occurred during a difficult life experience, and through secondary gain the behavior persisted as a habit.

OBSERVATIONS OF THE CHILD. Observations of the child at home, at school, in a play situation, and interacting with peers can provide data about the child's relationships with parents, other family members, peers, and teachers; the child's play and exploratory behavior; the child's presentation of self (for example, hostile, aggressive, withdrawn, shy); and the child's characteristic mood. Observations over a period of time are helpful in distinguishing between enduring behavioral characteristics and transitory reactions.

From the testing, interview, and observations one can identify problems related to (1) specific developmental lags or learning disabilities, (2) difficulties in the mastery of psychosocial adjustment tasks,

(3) problem behavior which has become established as a habit, or (4) difficulties in relationships.

Assessment of the Family

Assessment of the current functioning of the family includes obtaining information about current stressors, needs, and problems as well as current resources and strengths. Inquiry into the following areas will provide a picture of the current functioning of the family: the current situation, the family constellation and roles, the history of problem solving and coping with stress in the family, and parenting knowledge and skill.

Assessment of the current situation of the family includes obtaining information related to the economic and living conditions of the family, the health status of each family member, recent or impending stressful events or major life changes, and the family's perception of the current family problem.

Data on the family constellation include the name, age, and sex of all persons in the living unit, persons temporarily out of the living unit, and persons who exert influence on or provide support to the family. Identification of the persons who fill the following roles should be made: economic provider, primary parenting figure, support person for the primary parenting figure, marital-type relationship for each adult, adult emotional support relationship for each child, and peer support relationships among the children. Among the support relationships, the absence of a support person for the primary parenting figure is the most detrimental to effective parenting; and the absence of an emotionally supportive adult for a given child is the most detrimental to the well-being of that child.

The family assessment also includes identification of nodal points in the family life cycle. These significant events may have produced crises that were disruptive of family function. The emotional shock waves that were created may be a contributing factor in the present difficulties of the child and the family. The history of previous problem-solving experiences and ways of coping with stress in the family provides information about family strengths, weaknesses, and stability. Important areas to cover concern the early marital history and the adaptation of the parents to the first child. The health history of each pregnancy, the parents' response to each baby, and the adjustment of siblings to each new baby are factors in the resolution of common maturational crises faced by most families. Other life crises that may have occurred are family illness, parental disharmony, unemployment, disasters, and death in the family. The genogram, described in Chapter 19, provides both a guide to the assessment process and a visualization of the family structure, relationships among members, and the deaths of significant family members that may have produced an emotional shock wave contributing to symptomatology in the target child.

The assessment of parenting knowledge and skill is useful in planning intervention, since treatment frequently consists of imparting and demonstrating healthy and effective child-rearing patterns. Ideally, parents should have basic knowledge of the needs of children as they progress through the developmental cycle. For example, the curiosity drive of an infant or small child leads to exploratory behavior that can be bothersome to parents; yet an absence or curtailing of opportunities for exploration and manipulation of the environment is detrimental to the intellectual development of the child. In addition to understanding the needs of children, parents should be able to tolerate—and, one hopes, enjoy—the child's unfolding behavior in order to perceive needs accurately and to respond positively. Other important elements of successful parenting are age-appropriate child-rearing techniques (for example, setting limits appropriate to the child's developmental gains), general agreement and consistency in child-rearing attitudes and practices, sharing of responsibility, and mutual support. Parents' expectations for their child may not be appropriate for the child's actual behavior, temperament, or potential. Unrealistic or inappropriate expectations interfere with the parents' selection of age-appropriate child-rearing techniques and can contribute to disagreement and inconsistency in the handling of conflict or areas of difficulty.

In summary, the identification of difficulties in parenting includes (1) identification of gaps in the parents' understanding of child development and needs; (2) identification of limitations in the parents' understanding of age-appropriate child-rearing techniques; (3) identification of limitations in the parents' ability to recognize or discriminate among needs, to meet needs or tolerate behavior, or to use specific child-rearing skills effectively; (4) identification of incongruities between parents' expectations and the child's actual characteristics; (5) identification of areas of inconsistent discipline or handling of behavior by parents; and (6) identification of areas of conflicting child-rearing attitudes and practices of parents. Parenting may also be interfered with by situational factors such as unfilled role functions in the family, family crises, marital disharmony, pathological needs of parents, or severely dysfunctional family patterns.

Assessment of the Environment

The interacting environment must be assessed to determine if intervention is needed to foster the child's and family's effective functioning . The following questions can be used to guide this assessment:

1. What is the economic health of the community?
2. What community mental health resources are available to help the child and the family?
3. What social stressors exist within the community?
4. How accessible are day care centers?
5. What is the quality of available day care centers?
6. Is safe, affordable housing of adequate size available?

Diagnosis

Nursing diagnoses for infants and children need to address the interactive nature of the parent-child relationship. Examples of nursing diagnoses are presented in Table 49-4.

Outcome Criteria

Outcome criteria for nursing care need to be expressed in terms of the remission of the child's problems and development of effective parenting. Outcome criteria for maintenance and restoration of health should be expressed in terms of normal development or functioning in light of the child's characteristics and the family situation. Examples of outcome criteria are provided in Table 49-4.

Intervention

The nurse who is relating to children with behavioral manifestations of maladaptation should be sensitive to the children's feelings or concerns about their adequacy, differentness, problems, or special situations. Although infants and very young children may not be aware of their standing in relation to other children, older children are often acutely aware of being singled out. Professionals should avoid talking about children in front of them or their peers. On the other hand, it is appropriate for nurses to point out that they are interested in the children, aware of their special needs, and available for support or help.

In working with the family, the nurse should avoid taking a critical stance but instead attempt to establish a relationship of collaboration in problem solving and intervention. The nurse's capacity for showing acceptance of others is severely limited

Table 49-4 Nursing Diagnoses, Outcome Criteria, and Nursing Interventions

Nursing Diagnosis	Outcome Criteria	Nursing Intervention
Perfectionistic, ritualistic tendencies related to insufficient knowledge of child development and needs	Parents' expectations of child's behavior appropriate to developmental capacity. Evidence: Fewer critical comments by parents when child's performance is not perfect. Less ritualism in child. Less overt anxiety in child when a mistake is made.	Educate parents regarding growth and development. Encourage parents to lower performance standards for child. Help child recognize that mistakes are learning opportunities.
Aggressive, destructive behavior related to parents' deficient child-rearing skills	Parents' setting limits on aggressive, destructive behavior appropriate to child's age. Evidence: Encouraging child to talk about what upsets him or her. Acceptance by child of limits imposed by parents.	Provide parents with general principles for selecting and imposing limits on child's behavior. Demonstrate child-rearing skills. Correct misconceptions about child development and needs. Facilitate parents' collaboration in the employment of parenting skills. Teach child social skills.

(Continued.)

Table 49-4 Continued

Nursing Diagnosis	Outcome Criteria	Nursing Intervention
Child's eating and sleeping problems related to parents' conflicts about child rearing	Identification by parents of their own and each other's child-rearing beliefs, attitudes, and practices, including areas of agreement and conflict. Evidence: Open communication about conflict and concerns of child rearing. Parents' supporting each other in areas of agreement or compromise. In areas of conflict, agreement to try one approach for a specified time, then to reach a compromise or try another approach for a trial period. Identification of clear expectations and rules for child's behavior. Awareness of unclear or contradictory clues about expectations for behavior; sending of clear, unambiguous messages. Following through on establishing expectations and enforcing limits.	Help parents to identify areas of conflict. Explore feelings to resolve conflicts. Help parents to share responsibility for child rearing and to provide mutual support. Explore with parents their child-rearing attitudes, beliefs, and practices.
Child's apathy and delayed motor development related to parents' failure to recognize and appropriately meet child's needs	Recognition by parents of their child's basic needs for food, rest, safety, stimulation, acceptance, and love. Evidence: Providing stimulation (audio and visual) that is age-appropriate. Recognition of the child's need for naps. Protecting the child from household dangers while allowing the child to explore the environment. Discriminating between cries of hunger and pain. Providing child with affectionate interactions.	Provide education for parents regarding child's needs for sensory stimulation, affection, and sensitive interactions. Help parents provide a safe environment for the child's exploratory behavior. Help parents become aware of child's responses to their interventions. Provide referral for evaluation by specialist. Facilitate entry into specific remedial program (for example, infant stimulation) if indicated.
Lack of support for the primary parenting figure related to failure to recognize need for support	A family member is actively involved in providing consistent contact and support to the primary parenting person, or a new source of support has been identified and recruited to provide consistent contact and support.	Help parenting figure recognize the need for support. Reinvolve withdrawn family member to fill the support role. Establish alternative sources of support.
Feelings of dissatisfaction and incompetence in parenting role related to child's "difficult" temperament	Satisfaction and feeling of competency in parents. Evidence: Recognition and accurate assessment of their child's reactions and needs. Ability to apply techniques for successful managing of their child's special needs and behavior. Recognition of their own needs for assistance or respite in day-to-day management of their child.	Help parents to cope with child's irregular eating and sleeping patterns. Help parents to understand the child's reactions and needs. Help parents to follow appropriate principles of managing daily trials and tribulations and to use community resources for support. Suggest books and pamphlets to facilitate learning about children's growth, development, and needs and about parenting. Help parents to become aware of how their feelings can influence their child.
Acute anxiety related to separation from mother	Child tolerates separation from mother without acute anxiety. Child is able to play with peers without mother being present.	Help parents recognize inappropriateness of child's reaction to separation from the mother. Help parents to establish and implement program for gradual mother-child separation. Use goal-directed play sessions with child to explore and implement mother-child separation.

if the nurse operates from an idealistic position or imposes his or her values, beliefs, and expectations on the family. Particularly when working with families with a different cultural background, the nurse must guard against imposing his or her own cultural assumptions about child rearing on the family. Even when the nurse refers the case to another professional, a positive rapport with the family is important to ensure cooperation in following the referral and acceptance of the referral agency by the family.

Nurses' expectations of the helping process may also interfere with their effectiveness in helping parents alter their behavior. Since child-rearing behavior is based on long-standing life experiences—usually the child rearing that the parents experienced as children—simply telling parents what to do or teaching them new approaches is insufficient. Parents also need an opportunity to talk about their reactions to suggestions and to express their feelings and concerns about trying new ideas. Similarly, if the nurse takes over to show the parents how to deal with their child, the parents are likely to feel a diminished sense of competence.

Anticipatory guidance is the major intervention used to accomplish goals related to maintenance and restoration of health. Parents can be prepared for emerging developmental stages in their children, and children can be prepared for impending life events or changes in the family.

Perinatal and Postnatal Interventions

For all infants and parents the successful management of the birth process and care immediately after birth are essential in providing the infant with opportunities for optimal development. For infants at risk, this stage is especially significant. There is documentation that approximately 31 percent of live births in the United States are at risk.[15]

A longitudinal study[16] found that there are both long- and short-term effects of perinatal stress. In this study 660 newborns were evaluated for perinatal complications. A follow-up study of these children was done at 2, 10, and 18 years of age; it was found that perinatal stress was linked with mental health problems and learning disabilities in childhood. Those children who were most affected were from less advantaged homes.

Beyond medical management of mother and infant during the perinatal period, the most crucial issue is the attachment process in the infant-mother relationship.[17] Premature babies and babies of low birth weight, particularly those receiving extensive medical treatment that interferes with the parent-infant relationship, are at risk of an impaired attachment process.[18,19] There is also evidence that infants who have physiological problems or who are temperamentally different from norms or the parents' expectations are vulnerable not only to poor attachment but to physical abuse.[20] Early intervention that provides the mother of an infant who is at risk or disabled with coaching on how to interact effectively with the infant prevents future impaired mother-child interactions.[21]

Intervention in Infancy

One of the major issues in the care of the infant is to provide an environment which continues to strengthen the attachment with the parents and does so in such a way as to instill a sense of basic trust in the developing infant. Providing an environment that has the appropriate level and amount of sensory, motor, social, and emotional stimulation is essential to helping the infant accomplish the developmental tasks of infancy.

For the infant who is at risk but who does not have any symptomatology, surveillance intervention in the home or clinic setting provides the opportunity to institute more intensive intervention if necessary. In some situations where parents are not able to provide basic, safe care (for example, in the case of abusive, retarded, or emotionally ill parents), intervention may include removal of the infant from the home situation. The contacts can also include demonstrations of appropriate stimulation, anticipatory guidance, coaching, and counseling as needed. Nurses may also foster development by helping the parents expand their support network and utilize community services for their special needs.

Intervention with Preschoolers

For infants who have had a secure, trusting relationship with their parents during the first few months of life, the next stage of separation and individuation is more easily accomplished. Preschool children use their freedom as mobile, social, emotional beings to explore their environment and continue to develop mastery of developmental tasks, coping, and problem-solving skills.

The preventive interventions described for infants continue to be appropriate for toddlers and preschool children; however, surveillance and intervention is more likely to occur at home or in settings such as day care centers, developmental centers, nursery schools, and well-baby clinics. Nurses who have access to this age group are in key positions to detect behavioral problems that could lead to poor school adjustment in subsequent years. Nurses with a knowledge of child development can provide consultation to the staff members in day care or nursery school settings that will help them foster coping, problem-solving, and mastery skills in preschoolers.[22]

Nurses have opportunities for preventive intervention with preschool and young school-age children who become ill, sustain injuries in accidents, or for some reason need to be involved with medical or surgical health care services. Anticipatory guidance and crisis counseling for these children and their families provide opportunities for early detection of problems and interventions.[23]

Intervention with Young Schoolchildren

Federal legislation mandates that all youngsters entering school be screened for special health needs and that programs be developed for them where necessary. But children with mild behavior problems or early signs of potential problems are not usually the ones to receive the services provided, because of the minimal funding available to carry out the legislation.

One school district, however, has focused on prevention of mental health problems for over 20 years and provides a model for a program in which nurses could be involved. The Primary Mental Health Project (PMHP)[24] provides systematic early detection and prevention of school-adjustment problems. It focuses on primary grades because a child in this age group is most amenable to constructive help before school-adjustment problems crystallize and the child's self-esteem is seriously compromised. The program starts with early detection through psychological screening, interviews with parents, and behavior rating by teachers. The three groups of adjustment problems that become the targets for preventive interventions are (1) aggressive, disruptive behaviors; (2) shy, withdrawn behaviors; and (3) learning difficulties. After problems have been identified, individual goals are formulated for each child. The direct interventions are then carried out with individual children by trained nonprofessional mental health aides under the supervision of mental health professionals. The major focus of these interventions is on facilitating successful coping and problem-solving skills. Evaluation of this type of intervention indicates that it has been effective in helping children to overcome school-adjustment problems, thereby diverting them from lives of academic and social failure.[25]

As noted previously, the child again enters a routine surveillance system as he or she enters school. Many children entering the school system have not had the benefit of preschool experiences that help them develop coping and problem-solving skills. They enter kindergarten or first grade with low self-esteem and low competence; they are, therefore, unlikely to succeed in the school environment. These children are appropriate targets for preventive interventions, and the school setting is the ideal place for these interventions to occur because (1) children spend more time in school than in any other institution, (2) schools provide convenient access to large numbers of children, and (3) education provides a medium for preventive intervention.

Examples of nursing interventions for infants and young children and their families are presented in Table 49-4. Nurses who identify problems that require more extensive intervention and the services of other health professionals need to refer the children and their families to these services.

Referrals

Referring a family for mental health services is a complex process involving several elements. The agency selected must be appropriate and must match the needs of the family.

Three steps have been identified in the preliminary process of bringing about the parents' cooperation in providing mental health services for children. These steps are (1) acknowledging the reality of their child's emotional disturbance, (2) overcoming their concerns about using mental health services, and (3) dealing with realistic issues in seeking and starting these services. Often a series of interviews is necessary to establish rapport and to work through these steps.

In helping the parents acknowledge the reality of their child's emotional disturbance, the nurse can clarify and support the parents' concerns about their child's behavior and provide information about the seriousness of the problem and the need for prompt intervention. If the parents are unaware of their child's symptoms or if they distort or minimize the significance of the distress signals, they may be using denial to avoid accepting the reality of their child's problem. These parents need help to work through their feelings before they can act on a referral.

Families often have concerns about using mental health services, and they may have distorted ideas about what these services are like. The nurse can encourage family members to express their perceptions and concerns and then correct misconceptions by providing accurate information about the helping agency and the helping process. To help bridge the gap between the known and the unknown, the nurse can compare the preliminary interviews to the kind of help that the agency might provide.

Once the need for help is admitted and conflicts about using mental health services are reduced, the nurse can assist the family with realistic issues in seeking and starting these services. When an appropriate agency has been found, the nurse can facilitate the family's actually going to the agency by acting as a liaison between the family and the agency. A personal telephone call to the referral agency on behalf of the clients, to establish contact with the agency and to arrange for the initial appointment, is an effective referral method. Assistance with other practical problems, such as providing for a bilingual interpreter, will also increase the likelihood of a successful referral.

After the initial appointment has been made and the family has had contact with the referral agency, a follow-up visit is useful to convey continued interest and concern for the family and to deal with any remaining issues or problems that may have arisen around seeking or using help.

Evaluation

In the initial evaluation of the effectiveness of the intervention, data are obtained that relate to the behavioral criteria which were established to indicate a remission of the child's problem behavior or signs of stress. The extent of improvement, lack of improvement, or worsening of the child's problems should be described in all areas of the child's functioning, both at home and at school.

There should be at least one more evaluation a few months later to determine the effectiveness of the intervention over time and its generalization to other potential problem areas which might have arisen.

The evaluation process is illustrated in the following case study and Table 49-5:

A woman who was receiving public health nursing visits for major health problems had also reported problem behavior by her 4-year-old son, Randy. He

Table 49-5 Evaluation: Randy and His Family

Diagnosis	Outcome Criteria	Intervention	Evaluation
Misperception of developmentally appropriate behavior related to inappropriate expectations of child's behavior	Recognition by mother of age-appropriate activity level. Evidence: Acknowledging dysynchrony between her expectations and child's activity level Acknowledging Randy's behavior as normal Making arrangements for Randy to visit playground daily Making arrangements for Randy to attend a nearby low-cost preschool program	Facilitate mother's ventilation of exasperation and failure. Provide relevant developmental information. Discuss the concept of individual differences among children in relation to mother's inappropriate expectations. Help mother identify opportunities for Randy to be active in a safe, appropriate way.	Mother shares feelings generated when her expectations of Randy are not met. Mother listens attentively and asks relevant questions. Mother verbalizes a connection between her expectations of Randy and her perception of a problem. Randy has opportunity to play actively with peers. Mother has relief from parenting while Randy attends preschool program. Randy's behavior at home is no longer a problem. Mother is a more effective parent.

had recently become disobedient, inconsiderate, mean to his younger brother, and frequently angry.

Assessment of the child revealed a normal but active boy who could not comfortably comply with the quiet, sedate standards of behavior expected by his mother and successfully met by his older sister. Assessment of the family indicated that the family was poor and somewhat isolated, but the parents were stable and intelligent. The family lived in a third-floor apartment located on a busy urban street, and the three children spent most of their time indoors.

The parents had not had difficulty with Randy during his infancy or toddler period, but as he moved into the heightened activity level characteristic of 4-year-olds, his boisterous behavior became intolerable to his mother.

SUMMARY

Promotion of mental health and prevention of psychiatric disabilities must address early warning signs of stress among infants and children. Case finding among children during infancy and the preschool years is more difficult because these children are often lost to the health care system.

Physical symptoms and evidence of delayed, regressed, or disordered growth and development are early warning signs of distress in children. Observed and reported disturbances in bodily functions such as sleeping, eating, eliminating, rest and activity patterns, playing, and relating are significant criteria. Asocial behaviors such as lying, stealing, setting fires, and sexually inappropriate behavior are also indicative of problems. Children who are overly aggressive or withdrawn and those with mood disturbances are suffering from stress. The child's temperamental style is a factor in the parent-child relationship and may contribute to the definition of the target child.

Family dynamics associated with disturbances in childhood include undifferentiation, the family projection process, the multigenerational transmission process, parentification, and loyalty conflicts. Faulty training and socialization may reflect a deficit in the parents' knowledge, but in varying degrees underlying pathognomic family dynamics influence the parents' ability to recognize their own and the child's needs; meet needs; maintain the integrity of personal and family boundaries; and acquire, integrate, and use knowledge about effective parenting and growth and development.

Case finding is an important role for nurses. Settings for case finding include well-child clinics, obstetrical-care clinics, private physicians' offices, postpartum units, various community health and screening projects, and camp and school settings.

Application of the nursing process provides a systematic way of addressing problematic parent-child interactions and symptomatology in children. Diagnosis of the most significant problems leads to the formulation of specific outcome criteria that are used to evaluate the effectiveness of intervention. Interventions must be directed toward the child's behavior, the marital relationship, and parenting practices.

When the assessment process or outcomes from the interventions indicate a pervasive developmental disorder, a referral process must be initiated. When disturbances are extreme, hospitalization may be appropriate.

REFERENCES

1. Joint Commission on the Mental Health of Children, *Crisis in Child Mental Health: Challenge for the 1970's*, Harper and Row, New York, 1970, p. 251.
2. E. James Anthony, "A Risk-Vulnerability Intervention Model for Children of Psychotic Parents," in E. James Anthony and Cyrille Koupernik, eds., *The Child in His Family: Children at Psychiatric Risk*, vol. 3, Wiley, New York, 1974, pp. 99–121.
3. C. E. Schafer and H. L. Millman, *Therapies for Children*, Jossey-Bass, San Francisco, 1977.
4. American Psychiatric Association, *Diagnostic and Statistical Manual of Mental Disorders*, 3d ed., APA, Washington, D.C., 1980.
5. The President's Commission on Mental Health, *Task Panel Reports*, vol. 3, app., pp. 612–660, Washington, D.C., 1978.
6. Alexander Thomas, Stella Chess, and Herbert G. Birch, "The Origin of Personality," *Scientific American*, vol. 223, August 1970, pp. 102–109.
7. R. Dean Coddington, "The Significance of Life Events as Etiologic Factors in the Diseases of Children: I. A Survey of Professional Workers," *Journal of Psychosomatic Research*, vol. 16, March 1972, pp. 7–18.
8. J. Stephen Heisel et al., "The Significance of Life Events as Contributing Factors in the Diseases of Children: III. A Study of Pediatric Patients," *Journal of Pediatrics*, vol. 83, July 1973, pp. 119–123.

9. Harvey Brenner, "Mental Health Employment and Unemployment: Research Abstracts," *American Journal of Orthopsychiatry,* 1983, p. 9.
10. Children's Defense Fund, *A White Paper: Children and Federal Health Care Cuts,* CDF, Washington, D.C., 1983.
11. *Social and Economic Characteristics of American Children and Youth, 1980,* ser. P-23, no. 114-450, Washington, D.C., 1980.
12. Caplan, *Prevention of Mental Disorders in Children,* Basic Books, New York, 1961.
13. Mari Siemon, "Mental Health in School Aged Children," *American Journal of Maternal and Child Nursing,* vol. 3, no. 4, 1978.
14. William K. Frankenburg, Arnold D. Goldstein, and Bonnie W. Camp, "The Revised Denver Developmental Screening Test: Its Accuracy as a Screening Instrument," *Journal of Pediatrics,* vol. 79, December 1971, pp. 988–995.
15. T. Mercer, "The Nurse and Maternal Tasks of Early Postpartum," *American Journal of Maternal and Child Nursing,* vol. 6, 1981, pp. 341–345.
16. E. Werner and S. Smith, "An Epidemiological Perspective on Some Antecedents and Consequences of Childhood Mental Health Problems and Learning Disabilities: A Report from the Kauai Longitudinal Study," in Stella Chess and Alexander Thomas, eds., *Annual Progress in Child Psychiatry and Child Development,* Brunner/Mazel, New York, 1980.
17. Susan Blackburn, "A High Risk Environment," *American Journal of Nursing,* 1982, vol. 82, pp. 1709–1712.
18. K. Klaus and John H. Kennel, *Parent-Infant Bonding,* 2d ed.. Mosby, St. Louis, 1982.
19. M. Schaefer, P. Hatcher, and D. Barglow, "Prematurity and Infant Stimulations: A Review of the Research," *Child Psychiatry and Human Development,* vol. 10, no. 4, 1979, pp. 199–209.
20. M. Cooper and D. Schraeder, "Developmental Trends and Behavior Styles in Very Low Birth Weight Infants," *Nursing Research,* vol. 31, 1982, pp. 68–72.
21. Tiffany Field, "Interaction Coaching for High-Risk Infants and Their Parents," in H. A. Moss, Hess, and Swift, eds., *Early Intervention Programs for Infants,* Haworth, New York, 1982.
22. L. Forquer, "Developing Coping Skills in Early Childhood: Theory and Techniques," in Mary Frank, ed., *Primary Prevention for Children and Families,* Haworth, New York, 1982.
23. D. Prugh and K. Jordan, "Physical Illness and Injury: The Hospital as a Source of Emotional Disturbances in Child and Family," in Irvin N. Berlin, *Advocacy for Child Mental Health,* Brunner/Mazel, New York, 1975.
24. L. Cowen, "Primary Prevention: Children and the Schools," in Mary Frank, ed., *Primary Prevention for Children and Families,* Haworth, New York, 1982.
25. P. Weissberg, L. Cowen, and B. S. Lotyczewski, "The Primary Mental Health Project: Seven Consecutive Years of Program Research," *Journal of Consulting Clinical Psychology,* vol. 55, 1983, pp. 100–107.

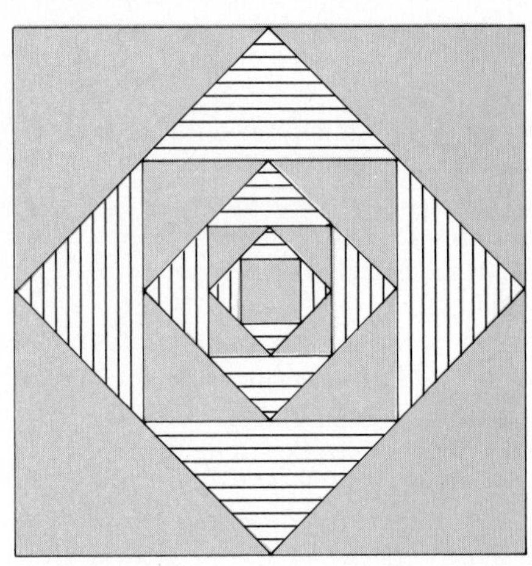

CHAPTER 50

Rehabilitation of Mental Health in Child-Rearing Families

Nada Light

LEARNING OBJECTIVES

After studying this chapter, the student should be able to:

1. Discuss the dysynchronous health patterns associated with pervasive developmental disorders.
2. Discuss the dysynchronous patterns of interaction—in person, family, and environment—associated with pervasive developmental disorders.
3. Apply the nursing process to children with pervasive developmental disorders and to their families.

Pervasive developmental disorders reflect impairment of multiple psychological functions. The dysfunctions that occur interfere with development and interaction with the environment. The dysfunctions occur in the development of social skills, primarily; these skills involve language skills, attention, perception, and orientation to reality.

Profound emotional, psychological, and developmental disorders reflect severe dysynchrony of the mind, body, and spirit. These disorders also involve dysfunctional patterns of interaction between the person and the environment. Profoundly dysfunctional children generate emotional pain in their families and their care givers. The number of children affected by profound emotional, psychological, and developmental disorders is much smaller than the number of those with less severe dysfunction, but the extent of the impairments is significantly greater. Both these children and their families need extensive and often long-term support.

The purpose of this chapter is to examine the theories relevant to the development of pervasive developmental disorders, the manifestation of these disorders, and the related dysynchronous patterns of interaction. The application of the nursing process to children with these profoundly dysynchronous patterns and to their families is also presented.

DYSYNCHRONOUS HEALTH PATTERNS

The profound emotional, psychological, and developmental dysynchronous patterns that are usually first evident in infancy or childhood are characterized by many severe impairments of basic areas of psychological development. Multiple extreme intrapersonal and interpersonal dysfunctions are present. The manifestations of pervasive disorders do not indicate developmental delays. Instead, they indicate abnormal, distorted development.

The dysynchronous health patterns that reflect pervasive developmental disorders include impaired communication, interpersonal relationships, motor skills, visual and perceptual abilities, and affective patterns; and self-mutilation.

Communication Patterns

These children's ability to communicate is impaired. Their nonverbal interactions (eye contact, facial expressions, and gestures) may be socially inappropriate or altogether lacking. If they develop language, it is characterized by persistent immature grammatical structure, echolalia (where the last phrase or word heard is repeated), and an inability to name objects or use abstract words appropriately. Fragmentary speech, confusion over meanings of words, and difficulty in understanding sounds may occur. Speech patterns may be melodic, monotonous, or questionlike.[1,2]

Interpersonal Patterns

Some children fail to develop interpersonal relationships, while others exhibit varying degrees of asocial behavior. Failure in relatedness appears to be in part a function of a lack of responsiveness to people, a lack of interest in people, and an absence of bonds of attachment.

The social smile that appears first as a reflex in the normal child remains a reflex in the autistic child. Other social cues are absent in the growing baby with a severe disorder. For example, there are no anticipatory behaviors from the child when the parent approaches—arms are not extended toward the parent—and there is no molding to the parent's body when the child is held. The infant seems more content to play alone and does not seek the parents during the crawling and earlier toddler stages. Further, if the child cries when hurt, comforting offered by the parents does not console the child. Clinging behavior is mechanical rather than affectional and relational.

These children often show more interest in and attachment to objects. They may have a particular fascination with spinning or shiny objects. Sometimes they become strongly attached to an object, such as a cup, piece of colored ribbon, or toothbrush, which they need to have in hand at all times. These objects usually lack the qualities of a soft blanket or stuffed animal that healthy children become attached to for security or comfort.

Children with profound developmental disorders do not develop peer relationships. They may develop the ability to participate in a peer group activity, but this participation is characterized by passivity, a lack of cooperation, and separateness. As these children grow older, they may develop some connectedness to parents, siblings, peers, or care givers.

Motor Patterns

For some children with these disorders, the milestones of motor development do occur; however, these children have an excessive interest in motions such as rocking, riding, swinging, and spinning. Some flap their arms, jump, and walk on tiptoe to an excessive degree. These children may exhibit peculiar posturing and hand or finger movements. Ritualistic behavior may also develop.[1]

Visual and Perceptual Patterns

By age 2 or 3, these children exhibit distorted visual and perceptual patterns. The ability to separate figure from background develops slowly. Peripheral vision is preferred over more controlled vision; there is a characteristic avoidance of eye contact, involving looking past people and objects. However, moving objects are recognized more easily than stationary ones; thus, the child recognizes a dog on television or a live dog more easily than a picture of a dog in a book. This characteristic is demonstrated further when these children are older. When studying a stationary object, these children do so by moving it up and down or moving their heads from side to side. Very complex visual stimuli, including people, are avoided; this may account for some of the interpersonal avoidance. This response may indicate a defense against a flooding of stimuli.[1] These children also respond abnormally to sounds and smells. They may be unable to comprehend auditory stimuli or attach meanings to sounds.[2]

Affective Patterns

Abnormalities of mood are most apparent by ages 3 and 4. These children appear remote and aloof at these ages. Interestingly, by 5 or 6 years of age, an increase in affection toward familiar people is often observed, but any new person or situation evokes withdrawal. Emotional outbursts of tears, rage, stamping, or kicking occur as a reaction to frustration, fears, changes in the environment, or for no apparent reason. Bursts of giggling and laughter may also occur without provocation.

These children often lack the fear of real dangers such as height and moving cars. However, they exhibit an exaggerated, illogical fear of harmless things and situations such as wearing shoes, looking at a particular piece of furniture, bathing, or brushing their teeth. Some exhibit excessive and sudden anxiety, rage, or catastrophic pain in reaction to apparently neutral events or situations, while others respond in ways that seem constructed, or artificial, and inappropriate.

During childhood, those affected by pervasive developmental disorders may have bizarre thoughts and fantasies. They may also become preoccupied with morbid thoughts or interests or with particular events.

Self-Mutilation

Some of these children engage in self-mutilative behavior. They may bang their heads, bite or hit themselves, or dig at their skin with their fingernails or toys. If scabs or recent injuries are present, these children may pick at these injuries, inflicting further damage.

DSM III

The diagnostic category of *pervasive developmental disorders* in the *Diagnostic and Statistical Manual of Mental Disorders* (DSM III) addresses conditions that are evident in infancy and childhood and that are distinct from mental retardation or schizophrenia. The subcategories include infantile autism and childhood-onset pervasive developmental disorder. Infantile autism is evident before 30 months of age; the symptoms of childhood-onset pervasive developmental disorder occur after 30 months of age and before 12 years of age.[1]

Epidemiology

Of all the children who need mental health services, barely 10 percent suffer from pervasive developmental disorders.[1,2] Infantile autism is very rare (2 to 4 cases per 10,000), as is childhood-onset pervasive developmental disorder.[1,2] Autism is much more common in males than females. A high proportion of parents of autistic children are above average in intelligence and in socioeconomic status.[2]

PATTERNS OF INTERACTION: PERSON

With regard to the *person*, patterns of interaction related to pervasive developmental disorders are organic in nature. They involve basic defects in neurological functioning, genetic predispositions, and infection.

The work of Rimland[3] and Bender[4] suggests that the symptoms seen in severe childhood disturbances are the result of an impairment in the reticular formation of the brain stem. Widespread neurophysiological changes are seen even in the absence of severely faulty parenting. According to Bender severe psychiatric disturbance is a biological disorder in the integration of the central nervous system and in the processes of behavioral maturation. Children with these disturbances exhibit disordered development characterized by embryonic features such as plasticity (capacity to be molded). Bender views parenting difficulties as a result of living with a profoundly disturbed child.[4] It appears that the earlier the severe symptoms are recognized, the greater the probability that the disorder has an organic basis rather than a basis in impaired parenting. A basic defect in perception, particularly in the integration of sensory stimuli, has also been cited as a cause of disturbance.[1]

Genetic factors may also influence the development of infantile autism; siblings of autistic children are at greater risk (50 times as great) of developing this disorder than children whose family is unaffected. Other predisposing factors include maternal rubella, phenylketonuria, encephalitis, viral disease, meningitis, tuberous sclerosis, and immune deficiencies.[1,2]

PATTERNS OF INTERACTION: FAMILY

Family patterns of interaction that are held to be related to the occurrence of pervasive developmental disorders fall into two categories: parent-induced dysynchrony and dysfunctional family interactions.

Parent-Induced Dysynchrony

Several theorists have proposed that pervasive developmental disorders seen in infancy and early childhood are parent-induced. Symbiosis, schizophrenogenic mothering, and "icebox" mothering will be discussed here.

Symbiosis

Mahler[5] defined the term *symbiotic psychosis* as a child's profound affective state of panic and regression that occurs when there is separation from the mother. She used the term to refer to an intrapsychic rather than a behavioral condition. She was referring not to physical clinging but to a primitive cognitive-affective feature of the infant, where differentiation between self and mother has not taken place. Mahler was concerned that the profoundly disturbed young child never felt a wholeness of self and a sense of human identity. She viewed autism and symbiosis as two extremes of disturbances in identity: primary infantile autism as a frozen wall between the child and others, and symbiosis as a fusion, meeting, or lack of differentiation between the mothering figure and the child.

Because of the developmental nature of the first year of life, the clinical symptoms of symbiosis, although grossly distorted, may not be readily apparent until the period of normal symbiosis ends. The child begins to sense impending separation. Retrospectively, the parent describes the child's unusual dependence on the mother. When this real or fantasized threat to the mother-child relationship occurs, the child shows intense separation anxiety; for example, the child may exhibit panic tantrums, clinging, and regressive behaviors often accompanied by the giving up of speech. The last of these may be the symptom which causes most concern and the one that brings the child to a clinical setting. By then, other profoundly disturbed behaviors may have developed, such as emotional aloofness, autistic behaviors, distortions of reality, and autoaggressive behaviors.

Rank's[6] working hypothesis is that the child experiences a highly ambivalent parent during the years antedating the burst of profoundly disturbed behavior. This process may be one of rapidly alternating overgratification and needless frustration coupled with a lack of nurturance and appropriate sensory stimulation. Historically, the infant may be described as fretful, sleepless, tense, and excessively demanding. For a while, these infants continue to demand that basic needs be met, but eventually they give up, feeling helpless and hopeless. Their gradual withdrawal into their own isolated world may be misinterpreted by their parents as calming down, finally being able to play alone, and not needing as much attention. Some of these observations may seem at first to describe the developing autonomous behaviors of a normal preschooler. However, this isolation is premature and may be misunderstood by the parents, who then reinforce the developmentally inappropriate behavior.

Schizophrenogenic Mothering

The concept of the *schizophrenogenic mother* flows from work at the James Jackson Putnam Center in Boston. Rank[6] and her colleagues developed a research project which used as its client population families composed of disturbed parents and a psychotic child. Three broad conclusions can be drawn from their work:

1. The mother-child relationship was disturbed in the first years of life and was characterized by unusually high ambivalence in the mother.
2. The father-child relationship was disturbed.
3. The infants had suffered severe gastrointestinal and respiratory embarrassments in infancy. A current traumatic event centering on separation from the parent precipitated the acute psychotic symptoms.

"Icebox" Mothering

Kanner's[7] work at Johns Hopkins supports the theory that childhood psychosis is parent-induced. In his work on infantile autism, Kanner developed the concept of the *icebox mother.* The mothers of Kanner's autistic clients were cold, detached, and interested in their children only intellectually. These same mothers were often quite different with other children in the same family. The empathic bonding that takes place in the first years of life was absent in these disturbed mother-child relationships, which consequently produced psychosis.

Dysfunctional Family Interactions

Dysfunction in the family system has been related to impairment of the child. Undifferentiation and fusion, the projection process, loyalty conflicts and parentification, abandonment and rejection, and erratic parenting are potentially influential phenomena that may be involved in the occurrence of pervasive developmental disorders. Moreover, a child's organic impairment interacts with family functioning.

Undifferentiation, Fusion, and Projection

When parents lack a sense of self and are dominated by emotionality, their self-system boundaries become blurred. This undifferentiation fosters *fusion,* a loss of separateness between the couple. The lack of distinct boundaries and the diffusion of emotionality interfere with the couple's ability to relate effectively with one another and with their offspring. To maintain their relationship when inevitable conflicts arise, the couple may attempt to diffuse or avoid the resulting tension by forming a triangle[8,9] (see Chapter 19).

Dysfunctional projection patterns that evolve out of parental undifferentiation operate within the mother-father-child triangle. The parental fusion and consequent periods of discomfort are managed by the parents' triangling of the child and their projection of their own disturbances and distorted perceptions onto the child. The emotional investment in the child, maternal anxiety, and paternal support of the projection process cast the special child into a fixed role. This child becomes the target of the projection process. The emotional tensions displaced onto the child help the parents avoid discussing their conflicts by talking about problems in terms of the child.[8,9]

When one parent, usually the mother, develops a high emotional investment in the child, the automatic emotional processes facilitate an overclose relationship. The overclose relationship violates the child's personal boundaries and inhibits self-definition and self-determination.

If, through the projection process, a child is perceived as mentally disordered or as being special, the parental interactions with that child will be distorted and not congruent with the child's real personality or mental status. Over time these distorted interactions will influence the developing child and contribute to a self-fulfilling prophecy. The consistent and repetitive distorted parental projections are integrated by the child and in time influence the child's self-perception and behavior. The child exhibits behavior which is congruent with the parents' projections and expectations.

Loyalty Conflicts and Parentification

Loyalty is a reliable, positive attitude of an individual toward another person or group. It is based on trust, merit, commitment, and action. In families it is a dynamic process derived from consanguinity and genetic relatedness. Loyalty commitments are invisible bonds that influence members' relationships while remaining outside awareness. These commitments and obligations evolve from each member's perception of the give-and-take with other members, particularly in relation to the parent-child relationship. Appropriate balancing of the give-and-take maintains effective multigenerational relationships. When serious imbalances occur, dysfunctional relationships and behavior develop.

In the natural order of parent-child relationships, parents primarily give to children, and children receive from them. Periodically and in temporary situations children may repay parents by their trustworthiness and support, and in the process learn how to be responsible. If, however, the parents and child reverse roles so that the child gives to the parents and is thus exploited, then *parentification* occurs. This parentification is pathological and imbalances the multigenerational family system.[10] When people are parentified as children, they experience deprivation of nurturing. The debt incurred by this deprivation persists into adulthood and may impair the ability to be a nurturing parent. Having been the recipient of inadequate parenting, these people have limited capacity to nurture their own offspring.

Abandonment and Rejection

Some parents physically abandon their children by leaving the home. Others may be imprisoned or confined to psychiatric institutions. Parents may be lost through death or divorce. Loss of parents may be compounded by the consequent loss of home, familiar surroundings, and sometimes even siblings if there is a foster home or institutional placement. Regardless of the reason for the loss of the parents, children tend to perceive it as abandonment and rejection. Without intervention the child's self-esteem is diminished when the conception of self-worth is influenced by the perception of parental rejection.

Erratic Parenting

Erratic, inconsistent parenting creates an unpredictable world for the child. The adults that people the child's world are so undependable that to count on them for consistent satisfaction of basic human needs or predictable interpersonal relationships is inevitably disappointing. The emotional climate and daily living activities in such an environment become precarious and are thus highly stressful. To cope, these children may prefer to relate to inanimate objects or animals that they can control.

Organic Impairment and Family Interactions

A holistic perspective on the occurrence of pervasive developmental disorders focuses on the interaction between the child's organic impairment and the family.

Mahler[5] and Escalona and Bergman[11] in their respective work include an emphasis on constitutional predisposition. Each understood that an infant who was "different" could elicit irrational responses from the parents, especially as the mother and father grew more perplexed, discouraged, and tired of trying to understand the child's needs. Even Kanner, who had viewed these profound disturbances as parent-induced, in his later work acknowledged multiple causation. The intellectual inadequacy seen in disturbed children may be the outcome of organic limitation or cultural deprivation. Affective inadequacy may reflect an organic dysfunction, affective deprivation, faulty parenting, or some combination of these factors.

Goldfarb's[12] position is the clearest endorsement of both the organic and the nonorganic hypotheses. He views the whole area of childhood psychosis on a continuum: at one end, the preponderance of data suggests that the etiology of a particular child's disturbance is organic; at the other end of this continuum is a group of children who by history and assessment have more environmentally induced psychoses. Thus, the children found at midpoint on the continuum contribute evidence *against* either single-causation theory. Examination of clinical data points to multicausation based on inadequate nurturing, environmental deprivation, and an organic predisposition.

Findings support the thesis that a child's vulnerability preexists and the birth into a disturbed family combines with it to produce a child who could potentially become profoundly disturbed. Most severe disorders in childhood appear to be a mixture of organic problems that interact with dysfunctional parenting, which may emerge because of the frustration and bewilderment in relation to the child's behavior or may derive from the parents' own psychiatric disturbance. Research findings of studies designed to identify the influence of genetic, biochemical, neurological, or transactional factors are limited by the extreme rareness of the disorders, which inevitably results in a small sample.[2]

PATTERNS OF INTERACTION: ENVIRONMENT

A number of environmental factors have been associated with pervasive developmental disorders. Psychosocial circumstances within the family and treatment setting are presented in Table 50-1.

Children with disordered affect and thinking are easily distracted and influenced by environmental stimuli. Noise, lights, and demands for interaction with a number of people are potential stressors that can disorganize these children. New people, situations, or changes in daily routines can be upsetting and interfere with treatment approaches. The people who make up these children's social environment can create a climate that is secure and predictable or one that is perceived by the child as threatening and overstimulating. Both the physical environment and the psychosocial environment are important dimensions in relation to the child's ability to cope. The regulation of stimuli and the provision of significant role models are important to the child's functioning and growth.

Table 50-1 Psychosocial Stressors

Circumstances within the Family
Parental drug or alcohol abuse
Parental discord
Parental separation or abandonment
Parental divorce
Death of a parent, sibling, or significant grandparent
Marriage of a single parent
Birth of a sibling
Remarriage of a divorced parent
Acute, severe conflict with a sibling
Intrafamily violence
Incestuous encounters
Disabling physical or psychiatric illness of a significant family member
Geographical move
Catastrophic loss of home (for example, through fire or storm)
Immigration
Foster placement
Dysfunctional parenting
Insufficient social or cognitive stimulation
Dangerous environmental conditions
Crowded, unsafe, substandard housing
Circumstances in the Treatment Setting
Separation from home and family
Tendency of care givers to focus on the child's deviant behavior
Depersonalized care giving
Sociocultural and socioeconomic disparity between client and care givers
Tendency of care givers to negate the child's uniqueness
Inconsistencies in care giving inherent to multiple providers during each 24-hour period
Unfamiliar surroundings
Lack of special educational resources that individualize learning
Unavailability of safe transportation services to day treatment

NURSING PROCESS

Assessment

The setting, the presenting problem, and the nurse's role may modify the assessment process. Regardless of whether the child is in a hospital unit, a residential setting, or the community, an ongoing assessment which includes the child, the family, and any other care givers is required. A child in crisis with distraught parents may require a modified and condensed assessment until a more thorough evaluation is feasible later on. The nurse may function as a primary care giver, a liaison to others directly responsible for care, or a member of the treatment team.

The nursing interview is the major tool in the nurse's assessment of a disturbed child. Ideally, a brief meeting with the parents and the child begins the contact and sets a clear goal of gathering information about the family unit in order to solve or alleviate part or all of the presenting difficulties.

The nurse can observe the interaction between parents and child and hear their respective views. A separate interview with each is needed, for several reasons. For the parents, this is an opportunity to express their special concerns about their child without the inhibiting and shaping influence of the child's presence. Also, marital and family problems and needs may emerge more spontaneously. And last, the parents can provide an understanding of their child's past development.

Assessment of the Child

The child needs a chance to be seen without direct parental influence. The nurse can observe the differences in the child with and without the parents. Some children may not separate easily from a parent; with them, information gathering must be done cautiously and tactfully over a period of several joint interviews until a physical separation is possible. Young children will be unable to tell clearly what is troubling them or their family. However, the nurse can listen with a "third ear" as the child answers unloaded questions about a child's world; the nurse can also observe the way play materials are manipulated. Even a very disturbed child without speech or interactional language may be observed in order to gather primary data.

Bringing the family unit back together at the end of the interview provides the nurse with an opportunity to articulate observations and interventions that may be useful. While a nursing diagnosis or complete understanding of the issue is rarely possible at the end of an initial interview, the family will have observed and experienced a systematic process, and the beginning of a therapeutic relationship will have been established.

In addition to the nursing interview, the data base may include information from other disciplines. For example, a psychiatric examination may identify psychopathology that requires the use of psychotropic drugs. Psychological assessment through intelligence testing and projective techniques can identify strengths and weaknesses in cognitive and personality functioning that may be useful in designing a treatment plan. A general health examination is necessary, especially for a very young child—in whom concurrent problems involving hearing, vision, and kinesthesia may exist. Self-mutilation, toilet problems, seizures, and other abnormalities with a mixed etiology must be clearly identified, and organic bases either ruled out or treated appropriately. Finally, any past records from other treatment facilities or agents may be helpful in gaining the scope that will be needed for effective planning.

The nursing assessment focuses on the child's response to the problems posed by the physical deficits and affective disturbances as well as on the child's ability to interact effectively with the environment and with other people. The data on the child needed for planning can be obtained through the answers to the questions presented in Table 50-2 (page 1130).

Assessment of the Family

Because of the interaction between the child and family, the nurse using a systems framework must collect data about the family system. This information contributes to the planning of care and the selection of interventions.

Considerable information is available through observing parent-child interactions during visiting hours or when the parents leave or pick up their child in day care settings. The interactions and the behavior generated in parents and children reveal the positive and negative dynamics. These data can also be used to provide the parents with feedback that can help them alter pathological ways of relating and enhance their positive interactions with their child.

The parents have thoughts, perceptions, and feelings about their child and their situation that influence the situation and the treatment. For example, there may be other children in the home with whom the parents are having problems or who are experiencing difficulties not recognized by the parents because their attention is continually absorbed by the disturbed child. Therefore, the assessment of the family must also include the siblings and their state of well-being.

The psychosocial stressors identified in Table 50-1 occur in many families and do not predictably cause the degree of disruption seen in families with a profoundly disturbed child. The family's perceptions of these events and their impact on the family are significant. Therefore, each stressor must be carefully explored and evaluated for the following: (1) the actual amount of change experienced by each member, (2) each member's degree of control

Table 50-2 The Child

Assessment
1. Is there evidence of developmental lag?
2. Is there a lack of responsiveness to people, with avoidance of eye contact?
3. Does the child engage in self-stimulating rather than interactive behavior?
4. Does the child exhibit a strong problematic response to new people or situations?
5. Does the child respond with inordinate fear toward neutral, harmless objects but lack fear of real danger?
6. Is there an absence of relief when the child is given comfort and nurturing after a painful or distressing experience?
7. What activities diminish distress when the child is upset?
8. Do incidents of separation elicit excessive anxiety and problematic behavior?
9. Does the child exhibit temper tantrums inappropriate to the developmental age?
10. Is the child's speech appropriate to the developmental age?
11. Do the child's verbal messages or behavior seem out of touch with reality?
12. Is there a paucity of communication with others: care givers, parents, peers?
13. Is the child becoming socially isolated—withdrawing from family and peers?
14. Does the child exhibit ritualistic behaviors or report obsessional thoughts?
15. Does the child make inappropriate facial expressions or lack appropriate disturbances?
16. Are there language disturbances?
17. To what extent are the child's body boundaries intact?
18. Does the child exhibit impulsivity?
19. What is the degree of regression?
20. Does the child engage in self-mutilating behavior?
21. Is there evidence of bizarre behavior?
22. Does the child exhibit outbursts of aggressive or assaultive behavior?
23. Can the child distinguish between reality and fantasy?
24. Are there areas of self-care the child has mastered (feeding, dressing, toileting)?
25. Does the child play with or destroy toys?
26. Which toys does the child choose?
27. How does the child play with the toys?
28. Do the pictures drawn by the child represent reality?
29. Are these drawings appropriate to the child's developmental age?

over the event, and (3) the number of other stressors occurring at the same time.

The data base on family functioning can be obtained through the construction of a genogram (see Chapter 19) and the answers to the questions presented in Table 50-3.

Table 50-3 The Family

Assessment
1. Do the parents exhibit problems or express fears about normal separation from the child?
2. How does each family member perceive or react to the child's behavior?
3. Are the siblings exhibiting behavior suggesting that they are negatively affected by the family situation?
4. How does each spouse describe the marital relationship and the relationship with extended family?
5. What are the parents' expectations of the child and therapy?
6. Which are the close and which are the distant relationships in the family?
7. What was happening in the family when the child with the problem was conceived and born?
8. How does each parent describe the child from birth up to the present?
9. What kinds of stressors have the family members encountered since the birth of the child?
10. Do the parents express a desire to keep the child at home or place the child in an institution?
11. Is there evidence (in the interactions observed) of parent-child role reversal?

Table 50-4 The Environment

Assessment
1. Are there adequate community resources to help the family meet the child's educational, recreational, and other needs?
2. Are there adequate community resources to help the family members meet their needs?
3. Is the household adequate in terms of space, ambient temperature, safety, and comfort?
4. Is there adequate transportation to and from treatment services?
5. Is the residential treatment setting able to provide holistic, individualized care?
6. Is the participation of the family in the care-giving process encouraged by the health care setting or educational system?
7. Do the care givers have access to nurse consultation, inservice education, and continuing education?

Assessment of the Environment

The child also interacts with environments other than the immediate family. The context of care influences the child's and the nurse's behavior. Thus, an assessment of the child's problem needs to include data on the way the child interacts with his or her physical and social environments. The data base on significant environmental influences can be obtained through the answers to the questions presented in Table 50-4.

Diagnosis

The data assembled through the assessment phase contribute to the conceptualization and formulation of the child's and family's problems. The statements that reflect this analysis of data are nursing diagnoses. Examples of nursing diagnoses for the child are presented in Table 50-5. Examples

Table 50-5 The Child: Nursing Diagnoses, Outcome Criteria, and Interventions

Diagnosis	Outcome Criteria	Intervention
Impaired interpersonal responsiveness related to probable organic factors	Child has 15-second periods of eye contact.	Positively reinforce eye contact, no matter how brief, with favorite food or toy. Replace this reinforcement as quickly as possible with a social reward that is comfortable for the child.
Lack of interest in human contact related to visual and perceptual impairment	Child tolerates body contact with another person for 2 to 5 minutes.	Plan gradual, deliberate intrusion into child's solitude to force beginnings of social interaction. Begin by sitting next to the child, touching playfully, turning child's face to force face-eye contact.
Impaired langauge development related to dysfunctional integrative capacities	Child uses sound fragment or word to indicate a message between self and another person.	Mouth back any sounds or word fragments uttered by child. Use sign language as a tool with children who have little or no language.
Inability to sustain attention on a single activity related to restlessness and distractibility	Child can sit in chair for part of a meal or a project for 2 to 5 minutes without leaving chair.	Seek pharmacological evaluation initially. Administer medications as needed. Employ structured exercise tasks to develop neuromuscular efficiency and concentration. Use positive social reinforcement for appropriate behavior.
Panic reaction related to confinement in a room with closed doors and windows	Child tolerates door and window being shut for short intervals of time until complete closing is possible.	Very gradually, use positive reinforcement as child's anxiety decreases and tolerance increases. Have child close doors if anxiety is not overwhelming, or do it with child. Measure and mark extent of opening of door and window to show gradual progress and make the progress visible to child.
Obsessional attachment to blue shoe associated with impaired ability to relate to people	Child tolerates gradual weaning from holding the shoe until shoe is no longer needed.	Plan with parents for a gradual withdrawal from these transitional objects. Begin by encouraging child to release clutched object. Allow child to have object nearby but not hold it. Have child place object in another part of the room, then outside the room, finally leave it at home. Give positive reinforcement through deliberate intrusion into obsession and deliberate coupling of reinforcer.
Ritualistic behavior associated with increased anxiety	Time spent in ritualistic behavior gradually decreases. Child verbally identifies anxiety-provoking situations.	Identify possible anxiety-provoking stimuli (sudden loud noises, certain people, fighting parents, or strangers) and eliminate them. Provide gradual desensitization to noxious stimuli; for example, one cannot eliminate sudden loud noises or new faces, but child and nurse can explore origin of noise or possibly greet and identify stranger.

(Continued.)

Table 50-5 Continued

Diagnosis	Outcome Criteria	Intervention
Autoerotic behaviors (excessive masturbation, rocking) related to impaired relatedness	Autoerotic behavior extinguished when someone attempts to engage child in an interaction. Rocking behavior decreases when child is presented with toys or when on a swing or rocking horse.	Repatterning process: observe (with parents' help) when behaviors occur, remove anxiety-producing stimuli. Intervene prior to these times with alternative motor patterns (motor pattern relieves anxiety and interrupts habitual response); for example, substitute an appropriate rubbing activity for inappropriate one. Use swings, rockers, or walking patterns.
Self-mutilation (banging head, biting and scratching self, and picking sores) related to impaired integration of sensory stimuli	Self-mutilating behavior ceases.	Identify behaviors or stimuli that trigger self-mutilating behavior and interrupt pattern before it begins. Repattern child into more satisfying movements. Provide ongoing protection (wearing head helmet, elbow restraints, bandages over open sores). Develop outer stimuli more satisfying than child's body. Avoid restraining in any way, if possible, since it may cause increased anxiety.

of nursing diagnoses for accompanying family dysfunction are presented in Table 50-6.

Outcome Criteria

Outcome criteria for both the child and the family are needed. These criteria should be congruent with the overall treatment plan and reflect interdisciplinary collaborative efforts and coordination of services. Examples of outcome criteria for the child are presented in Table 50-5; for the family, in Table 50-6.

Intervention

The nurse may function in both psychiatric and nonpsychiatric settings. The latter may include schools, public health nursing agencies, well-child clinics, emergency rooms, and inpatient pediatric units. In these settings, the nurse can apply knowledge of pervasive developmental disorders as a case finder, a supportive professional in the treatment process, or both. Community mental health centers and outpatient child psychiatric clinics are now recognizing the prepared nurse as a primary therapist who can render direct therapy to the child and the family. Partial hospitalization programs have utilized the nurse as a therapeutic role model, supporter of health, and liaison with parents. The nurse in a residential center can also provide a holistic approach to the child, enabling child-care workers to function more effectively. Wherever nurses practice, they can strengthen a working relationship with the parents by listening to the parents describe how they have coped with the disturbed behaviors.

Whatever the setting, the first step is to engage the family in the treatment process. Engagement is significant if the therapeutic process is to proceed. Either initially or periodically families will resist the treatment process. When families miss appointments or fail to visit their hospitalized child, it is important to diagnose the problem. Thus, follow-up telephone calls and home visits are important.

Sometimes families are overwhelmed and need nurses to reach out to them supportively. In other instances they experience an encounter with the staff as a rejection. They may perceive that they are being blamed and therefore defensively withdraw because of angry or guilty feelings.

Interventions must be selected for the child, the family, and the environment. For example, often siblings have experienced stress because of the turmoil created by the disturbed child's behavior.

Table 50-6 The Family: Nursing Diagnoses, Outcome Criteria, and Interventions

Diagnosis	Outcome Criteria	Intervention
Inability of family members to handle feelings and attitudes about having severely disturbed child (for example, they actively deny bizarre behavior, cover up for child's destructiveness, rationalize that child is just immature and will outgrow disturbances) related to the use of denial	Parents use psychiatric language (diagnosis, symptom names, some terminology) in referring to their child. Parents make a contract, and keep it, to talk regularly with mental health personnel about child and family.	Hold family meetings with and without child. Use videotape or audiotape to demonstrate disturbances parents may try to deny. Provide information and resources to cope with behavior; do not agree that there is no problem Provide supportive counseling while family contracts with a psychotherapist; listen empathically, clarify feelings and conflicting values of parents.
Parental conflict related to inability to tolerate child's bizarre behavior	Parents openly disagree about issues. Parents disagree without yelling at each other. Parents able to tolerate the child's bizarre behavior without engaging in a loud verbal altercation.	Point out child's behavioral response to parents' arguing. Help parents learn how to argue and disagree without rageful disruptiveness. Assess family and explore areas in family life that may be helped with education, financial assistance, better decision making; these stresses may be precipitating dysfunctional parenting. Help parents see how they experience conflict and argue when child behaves bizarrely.
Inability to accept child's need for residential treatment related to lack of knowledge and unresolved mourning of the fantasized healthy child	Parents are involved in concrete details of separation process (able to talk about possible placements, perhaps visit if feasible, help plan departure). Parents verbalize grief over child's problems.	Provide a forum for family members to talk about the placement and to discover and discuss their feelings about it. Provide essential details (including information on visiting privileges) to help parents resolve feelings of "losing" their child. Offer supportive counseling and contact after placement occurs to help with feelings of loss, guilt, and mourning.
Excessive guilt, anger, and blaming within family related to inability to accept the child's problem	Decreased use of protective blaming of others as a defense mechanism. Decrease in angry words and expressed feelings at family meetings. Identification of source of guilt for each person in the family.	Hold family meetings to explore and discuss these feelings and attitudes. Identify projection process that is occurring and help each distressed member take responsibility for his or her own feelings of guilt.

The parents may not recognize these problems; or they may initially be too exhausted physically and emotionally to deal with them effectively, even with professional help. To point out the problems of the other children prematurely might overload the parents and the family system. Initially the child ("identified patient"), the parents, and the family system may be best helped by interventions that provide temporary relief from the chaos that has existed. It may be appropriate at this point to help the family select a way of providing opportunities for all involved to be free of the daily stresses and strains of living together. Treatment in a day hospital or brief residential treatment may give this type of relief and provide an opportunity for the family to restabilize and develop more functional dynamics. Throughout this process the nurse needs to be available to each family member and to provide empathic support for the ventilation of feelings and perceptions.

Intervention with the Child

Autistic children may be cared for in residential treatment settings or remain at home and receive day care treatment. These are difficult children to care for. Their behavior is problematic regardless of the setting. Table 50-5 lists selected interventions for the severely disturbed child.

Children with childhood-onset pervasive developmental disorders exhibit disturbed behaviors which reflect their anxiety. Since their behavior may be unmanageable in the home situation, hospitalization may be required until they are better able to cope within the family system. The nursing interventions listed in Table 50-5 can be utilized either in the home, in day care, or in a residential setting.

The boundaries of the severely disturbed child may be fluid—unfixed and undefined. Even though the nurse may have a comfortable way of using touch to achieve closeness with clients, physical contact must be used judiciously with the disturbed child, who may be overwhelmed by closeness but may nevertheless desire some safe contact or connectedness.

A holistic approach is used to help these children. *Drug therapy* is used in conjunction with educational therapy and psychotherapy. The more potent but less sedative of the major tranquilizers are better tolerated by young, severely disturbed children. Barbiturates tend to disorganize the severely disturbed child and may have a negative effect. Principles that guide the use of these drugs with children and that are a concern of nursing include the following:

1. As the child grows, the response to the medication changes, and so the dosage must be changed.
2. Side effects can be severe.
3. Regular laboratory evaluations and physical examinations must be a part of the larger treatment plan.

The nurse may be directly responsible for administering medications. This task potentially contains elements of both positive and negative effects on the child. For example, the more disorganized child may feel relieved to have control facilitated by the medication and to feel less anxious; the child who has hallucinations may experience relief at feeling stronger than, for example, an auditory command. However, other children may be highly anxious about ingesting oral medication, viewing this as an invasion of or intrusion into their bodies. Injections become a difficult procedure for a child who has a limited capacity to comprehend that the nurse wants to be helpful. Nurses can also be particularly useful in transmitting and reinforcing to parents and child care workers essential knowledge about the medications that are used.

Milieu therapy can include both educational therapy and psychotherapy. Emphasis is on the whole experience and environment, and therapy can take the form of half-day, whole-day, or residential care. If the program is educationally oriented, the thrust may be to habilitate and educate the child using the teacher-pupil model. Classroom experiences focus on visual and motor training, language skills, socialization through group projects, and other ways of dealing with learning disabilities. Daily activities become learning situations. Behavior-modification techniques have been useful in shaping more functional behaviors. Nurses play a major role in creating a therapeutic milieu and in supervising the health care of these children in collaboration with other disciplines.

Play therapy is another technique nurses use in working with these children. A precise definition of play therapy is difficult to formulate, since the words *play* and *therapy* have different meanings for different therapists. The notion of using play as a modality for assessing and treating disturbed children is based on the fact that play is the child's natural medium of self-expression. There also seems to be an inner need and motivation among children and adults for self-realization and personal growth. Play provides an opportunity for self-expression. Furthermore, in an accepting, understanding, secure, and predictable climate, the child is allowed to experience autonomy, limits, and self as a unique separate individual. Play therapy is therefore an approach to helping children express feelings and work through problems.[13] Young children experience painful emotions and complex problems. Impaired and regressed language development and limited vocabulary make full expression of thoughts and feelings difficult and limit children's ability to describe their perceptions. Furthermore, young children lack the emotional and intellectual capacity to use a verbal interpersonal process to explore their difficulties and feelings.[13] The way the child selects and uses play materials and the child's activities and dramatizations provide assessment data and help the child release problematic tensions without fear of retaliation.

If the nurse is caring for a severely disturbed child in a *nonpsychiatric* setting—for example, a general pediatric surgical or medical unit—the procedures used in treating the child will require specialized approaches and explanations. Routine hospital care can disorganize a normal youngster and can certainly do the same more readily to a child who depends on routine to manage anxiety. Therefore, special efforts must be made to help the child comprehend the situation and cope with the anxiety it generates. It is helpful to limit the number of persons providing care so that the demands on the child to adjust to strangers are minimized. The presence of familiar objects and favorite toys also helps to reduce the strangeness of the environment. With these children, it is very important that all who are providing care be taught about the management of behavior problems and special personal rituals. These nursing orders will provide greater consistency in care giving and lessen the possibility of provoking anxiety-producing situations which will subject the child to further stress.

Intervention with the Family

Parental support is an imperative part of nursing care. Parents of children with pervasive developmental disorders suffer guilt and ambivalence. Some children do improve with growth; however, the parents usually have experienced an excessively long period in which they have spent sleepless nights and have been in a state of chronic anxiety. They have felt depressed, angry, resentful, and at a loss to understand the nature of their own child. If the parents blame each other, guilt is generated; this is counterproductive as far as helping the child is concerned. Where disturbed parenting exists, it needs to be replaced by more healthy parenting through education of the parents, role modeling, and supportive counseling.

Since a very young child may not be eligible for a day treatment program, home treatment techniques are an area in which the nurse can be helpful. Suggestions may be needed by the family regarding expanded and protected play space, safer and more practical furniture until destructiveness is controlled, methods of feeding, and satisfying other family members' needs. The advantages of home treatment even for an older child include the following:

1. Parents are more relaxed in their own homes.
2. Problems at home require different management from clinic or office problems.
3. Home treatment is cheaper than institutionalization.
4. If a child does experience prolonged hospitalization, there is marked regression when the child is discharged home, thus diminishing valuable gains regarding time and treatment.
5. Greater progress over time has been observed in homes where there has been increased parental involvement.

Sometimes a family cannot move beyond placing blame and feeling guilty about the presence of a disturbed child. These feelings often take the covert form of overprotection or unwillingness to relinquish part of the child's care to outside resources. The nurse can provide supportive counseling during this period of adjustment. The provision of daytime relief through schooling, weekend care, overnight camps, and occasional baby-sitting reduces the family's feeling that they have no options.

While a few children may have a schizophreniform psychotic episode and reconstitute with minimal residual problems, the child who is severely disorganized early in life generally remains chronically disturbed. This burden becomes intolerable for some families as the child grows and hope of major change and improvement disappears. Eventually placement in an institutional setting becomes the only choice when family growth is compromised. Support during this decision and process is essential if the family is to be left feeling that it can continue to function without being burdened by excessive guilt and a sense of failure.

Table 50-6 presents suggested interventions for the care of the family.

Intervention with the Environment

Maintaining a child with pervasive developmental disorders in the community with the family is potentially a difficult undertaking. These families need support to cope with the problems they encounter. The health care system needs to be sensitive to the emotional drain on the family resources. If therapeutic day care facilities are lacking or support groups for parents are nonexistent, nurses need to assume a leadership role in establishing these services.

Families are often ashamed of and embarrassed by their child's bizarre behavior in public. People in the community often feel at a loss or are critical toward the parents of these children. Public education can demystify the problems of children with pervasive developmental disorders and their families. Again, nurses need to take an active leadership role in helping make the environment a supportive resource. This leadership role may be implemented through helping the media, schools, local civic groups, and parent-teacher associations become more knowledgeable about and more sensitive to the problems.

Evaluation

Evaluation is an important dimension in the delivery of effective services. The nurse uses the outcome criteria and nursing diagnoses as guides to measure whether the selected interventions have been effective in lessening or eliminating symptoms of distress in the child and family. They are also used in conjunction with developmental theories to determine whether the child and family are functioning in a more effective, healthy fashion. Of course, in such evaluation, allowances must be made for deficits that cannot be corrected or that can be ameliorated only by normal maturation over time. An example of the evaluation process is presented in Table 50-7.

The nurse's self-evaluation is an important dimension of the evaluation process. Working with these children and their families can become stressful over time. Progress is slow. Total resolution of the symptoms or the dysfunctions is not always possible. Nurses are therefore vulnerable to discouragement. To protect themselves from feelings

Table 50-7 Evaluation

Assessment	Diagnosis	Outcome Criteria	Intervention	Evaluation
Exhibits a panic attack when mother leaves the room. Clings to mother continuously. Refuses to sleep in own bed. Has temper tantrums when mother disengages from child and attempts to move away.	Inability to manage separations related to a lack of awareness of self as separate from others	Demonstrates awareness of self as separate from mother. Evidence: Ability to sit and play on floor next to mother. Sleeps in own bed. Allows mother to leave room for 15 minutes without showing anxiety or rage reaction. Moves from mealtime situation to activity without temper tantrums or throwing dishes. With adequate warning (10 to 15 minutes), leaves project and moves to next activity cooperatively.	Strengthen body boundaries ("me" separate from "you") by: Reinforcing any behavior which differentiates child from environs (for example, self-feeding—inside-outside self—exploring objects and persons). Having mirrors available for child to see self. Encouraging appropriate touching of others to feel difference between self and others. Encouraging eye contact and positively reinforcing it with favorite object and then with social reinforcers (smiles, hugs, kind words). Helping mother reward separation behavior. Anticipatory planning where possible to provide for gradual introduction of change and desensitization to separation. Demonstrate how one leaves table; point to any role models; warn against doing it inappropriately. Interrupt tantrum and throwing. Use body to hold erratic behavior in check, literally lending your ego controls.	Child able to play on floor with mother at the opposite side of the room. Child continues to play when mother leaves the room for brief periods of time. Mother identifies ways to reward child for tolerating separations. Mother is able to tolerate separations without becoming anxious.

of helplessness and purposelessness, nurses may gradually lower their expectations to a point where a subtle sense of apathy develops. Ongoing self-evaluation of thoughts, perceptions, feelings, and interactions related to the care-giving process helps nurses recognize a decrease in hopefulness, creativity, and motivation and to persist when progress is slow.

SUMMARY

Although profoundly disturbed children are a small segment of our population, they generate great concern among health professionals, educators, and their families. The pervasive developmental disorders that affect children's intellect, affect, and behavior and the disruption that occurs in their families are painful to all involved.

Many theories have been postulated regarding the cause of these disturbances. It seems that the earlier the symptoms appear, the more likely it is that an organic basis is the source of the problem. Evidence of symptoms at a later point and regression are more likely to be the product of multiple interacting factors.

The symptoms exhibited by these children are extreme and serious. There is major impairment of the ability to interact effectively with the physical and social environments. Perceptions of reality are distorted. The impairment of reality testing, perception, relatedness, and language development interferes with the ability to communicate and use feedback.

A variety of therapeutic approaches are employed to maximize the child's and family's health potential. The context of care selected for treatment is dependent on many factors, particularly the needs of the child and the family.

The child's and family's interaction with the physical and social environments plays an important role in the resolution of symptoms and the facilitation of growth and development.

Application of the nursing process to the care of these children and their families requires the acquisition of a broad data base, a thoughtful analysis of the findings, and collaboration with the family and other resource people. The interventions selected are directed toward relieving the symptons, resolving the underlying problems, and facilitating growth and development.

REFERENCES

1. American Psychiatric Association, *Diagnostic and Statistical Manual of Mental Disorders,* 3d ed., APA, Washington, D.C., 1980.
2. M. Weissberg, *Dangerous Secrets,* Norton, New York, 1983.
3. B. Rimland, *Infantile Autism,* Appleton-Century-Crofts, New York, 1964.
4. L. Bender, "The Brain and Child Behavior," *Archives of General Psychiatry,* vol. 4, 1961, pp. 531–548.
5. M. S. Mahler, "On Child Psychosis and Schizophrenia: Autistic and Symbiotic Infantile Psychoses," in S. I. Harrison and J. F. McDermott, Jr., eds., *Childhood Psychopathology,* International Universities Press, New York, 1952.
6. B. Rank, "Intensive Study and Treatment of Preschool Children Who Show Marked Personality Deviations or 'Atypical Development' and Their Parents," in S. I. Harrison and J. F. McDermott, Jr., eds., *Childhood Psychopathology,* International Universities Press, New York, 1952.
7. L. Kanner, "To What Extent Is Early Infantile Autism Determined by Constitutional Inadequacies?" *Proceedings of the Association for Research on Nervous and Mental Diseases,* vol. 33, 1954, pp. 378–385.
8. M. Bowen, "Theory in the Practice of Psychotherapy," in P. J. Guerin, ed., *Family Therapy: Theory and Practice,* Gardner, New York, 1976, pp. 76–84.
9. T. F. Fogarty, "System Concepts and the Dimensions of Self," in P. J. Guerin, ed., *Family Therapy: Theory and Practice,* Gardner, New York, 1976, pp. 146–148.
10. J. Boszormenyi-Nagy and G. M. Spark, *Invisible Loyalties,* Harper and Row, New York, 1973, pp. 22, 37, 39.
11. S. Escalona and P. Bergman, "Unusual Sensitivities in Very Young Children," in *Psychoanalytic Study of the Child,* vols. 3 and 4, International Universities Press, New York, 1948.
12. W. Goldfarb, *Childhood Schizophrenia,* Harvard University Press, Cambridge, Mass., 1961.
13. M. S. Miles, "Play Therapy: A Review of Theories and Comparison of Some Techniques," *Issues in Mental Health Nursing,* vol. 3, no. 1, 1980, pp. 63–75.

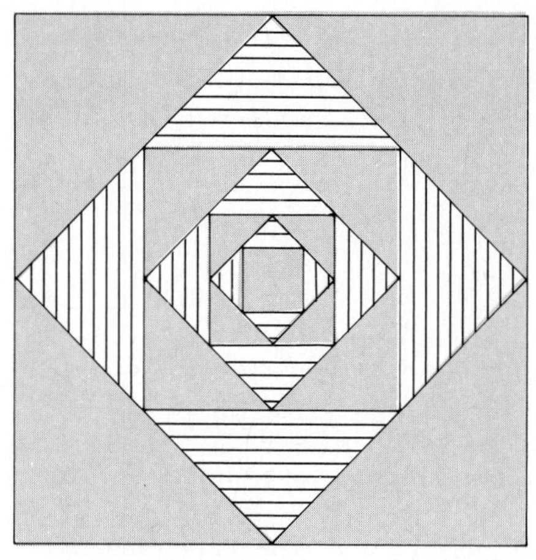

CHAPTER 51
Patterns of Abuse

Barbara Flynn Sideleau

LEARNING OBJECTIVES

After studying this chapter, the student should be able to:

1. Recognize evidence of physical, verbal, and sexual abuse; neglect; and psychological unavailability.
2. Discuss the problems associated with the acquisition of accurate statistics on the extent of abuse within families, abuse of people who are institutionalized, and abuse of children by unrelated adults.
3. Discuss patterns of interaction within the person associated with the neglect and abuse of children, spouses and cohabitants, elderly people, and those who are institutionalized.
4. Discuss family patterns of interaction associated with abuse.
5. Discuss environmental patterns of interaction associated with abuse.
6. Apply the nursing process to cases of abuse.

Violence is as old as humankind. It is pervasive in our society. The abuse of the powerless and helpless is as much a problem in our highly technological and sophisticated society as it was during earlier times. The prevention and resolution of abuse are serious and difficult problems that must be addressed holistically not only by the health care delivery system but by society as well.

From a holistic perspective, abuse is a product of the interaction of victim, victimizer, past generations, the present environment, and other forces which lead to pathological management of stressful situations. The dynamics of violence within the family and within institutions can be viewed in terms of sociocultural, intrapersonal, and interpersonal contexts. The aspects of such violence that are related to the social structure include (1) the power structure of the family or institution, (2) the socializing framework of beliefs and values, and (3) the power and social structures of the larger society. A family and a residential institution consist of a hierarchy of interpersonal relationships, with superordinate and subordinate roles as well as rivalries that often elicit the use of force. Authority relations, milieu climate, hierarchical positions in the structure, values, and beliefs influence the expression of violence in the family and institutional environments.

Abuse demoralizes the mind, body, and spirit of the victim and reflects demoralization of the victimizer. The dysynchronous patterns of interaction that develop indicate a dysfunctional value system, an absence of respect for the rights of others, and a failure to empathize with the needs and plights of others.

The purpose of this chapter is to examine the interactive influences in situations of abuse within families and institutions. It also addresses the application of the nursing process to these situations for the purpose of prevention of abuse and restoration or rehabilitation of synchronous health patterns.

DYSYNCHRONOUS HEALTH PATTERNS

There are five major categories of abuse: (1) physical abuse, (2) neglect, (3) psychological unavailability, (4) verbal abuse (verbal hostility), and (5) sexual abuse. Each type of abuse seems to be associated with a characteristic impact on the person who is the recipient of the abuse.[1]

Physical Abuse

Physical abuse involves nonaccidental injury inflicted by someone whose purpose is to cause physical harm. Examples of this type of abuse are presented in Table 51-1 (page 1140). Physical abuse may be so severe that it results in the death of the victim.[1,2]

Neglect

Neglect is a deliberate failure to provide for the satisfaction of basic human needs (physiological safety, love and belonging, and self-esteem).[3] There is also usually a failure to provide needed preventive, restorative, and rehabilitative health care. The deprivations that result are willfully inflicted, and they are not a function of poverty. Examples of this type of abuse are presented in Table 51-2 (see page 1140).

Psychological Unavailability

Psychological unavailability is a style of parenting that is characterized by (1) failure to recognize the child as a dependent individual with developmental limitations and with needs that can be met only through parental assistance and (2) lack of response to the child's verbal or nonverbal expressions of need.[1] It is also a style of caretaking of retarded, disabled, or elderly adults that lacks warmth, sensitive personalized attention, and sociability. Examples of psychological unavailability are presented in Table 51-3.

Verbal Abuse

Verbal abuse, or verbal hostility, involves the use of words and actions to threaten or terrorize, or to depreciate the person's self-worth. Efforts are directed toward convincing the person that he or she is worthless, stupid, crazy, unwanted, or unloved. Examples of this type of abuse are presented in Table 51-4.

Table 51-1 Physical Abuse

Forms
Slapping, kicking, or punching, particularly giving blows to head, face, and genitals that produce hematomas
Hitting or whipping with blunt instruments such as belts, ropes, sticks, and electrical cords
Pulling hair out at the roots
Inflicting burns with lighted cigarettes or appliances such as stoves or irons
Immersing in scalding water, causing burns—to thighs, perineum, hands, or feet, for example
Throwing person to the floor, down the stairs, against furniture, or out of a window
Choking or tying a gag over the person's mouth
Tying to bed, crib, or chair, using cords, ropes, or chains
Locking in dark closets, cellars, or small and bare rooms for extended periods of time
Attempting to drown or hang

Table 51-2 Neglect

Forms
Failing to provide foods that meet nutritional needs
Failing to provide for hygiene needs: baths, clean clothes, clean diapers as needed, clean sheets and skin care for the elderly or disabled person
Failing to provide a bed to sleep in, or bedding for warmth in cold weather
Failing to provide sensory stimulation, recreational activities, developmentally appropriate learning activities, or growth-promoting activities
Failing to provide health-promotive care (for example, immunization, periodic physical examinations)
Failing to provide health-restorative care (for example, eyeglasses, medications)
Failing to protect against accidental falls (for example, out of beds or chairs, or down the stairs)
Failing to protect against the ingestion of poisons
Failing to provide safe play area or toys for child

Table 51-3 Psychological Unavailability

Forms
Ignoring person (child, elderly or disabled person)
Failing to provide sufficient affection or warmth
Failing to appreciate accomplishments
Failing to appreciate competence
Failing to respect elderly or disabled person's privacy
Failing to recognize need for human contact
Failing to respect preferences and opinions
Failing to interpret and understand needs for nurturing and comfort when a distressful or painful situation has occurred
Failing to share pleasant experiences
Failing to share mealtimes and social events

Table 51-4 Verbal Abuse (Verbal Hostility)

Forms
Using words as weapons: calling the person names; using insulting words such as *dumb, stupid, bad, dirty, slut, whore, worthless, rotten*
Directing obscenities toward the person
Telling the person, "You're crazy"
Telling the person, "You should never have been born"
Telling the person, "You've outlived your usefulness"
Telling the person, "If you were dead, everyone would be better off"
Being extremely critical
Holding the person to unrealistic expectations and then being verbally aggressive when the expectations are unmet
Using verbal and nonverbal behavior to humiliate or shame
Declaring elderly family members incompetent, coercing them or stealing from them to gain access to their financial resources and property (thereby increasing their helplessness and powerlessness)
Provoking fear of violence or isolation
Threatening to have the elderly person put in a nursing home
Threatening to have the elderly person committed to a psychiatric hospital

Sexual Abuse

Sexual abuse includes assaultive and violent traumatic sexual contact and sexual exploitation of a nonviolent type. For the purpose of this discussion, *incest* is a type of sexual abuse which includes any sexual activity or intimate physical contact that is sexually arousing between members of the same family who are not married to each other.

In this chapter, the discussion of sexual abuse focuses on the victimization of people who, because of age or intellectual capacity, are unable to legally consent to the sexual activity initiated by the abuser. These victims include children, elderly people, and people who are institutionalized because of mental or physical disabilities.[4] Examples of sexual abuse are presented in Table 51-5.

Epidemiology

In 1984, 4.1 million incidents of family violence came to the attention of the justice system in the United States.[5] Many more unreported incidents occurred. Statistics on intrafamily abuse reveal only the tip of the iceberg. Abuse of children, elderly

Table 51-5 Sexual Abuse

Forms
Oral-genital contact
Mutual masturbation
Fondling and caressing the genitals
Anal intercourse
Sexual intercourse
Rape and sodomy
Sadistic manipulation of the genitals
Threatening to kill victim or someone else if the sexual activity is reported to anyone
Maiming or killing a small animal to illustrate what will happen if the sexual activity is reported to anyone
"Renting out" child to pedophiles and pornographers
Making the victim participate in sexual activity that emphasizes deviant and erotic activities (such as group sex, sadomasochistic rituals, bestiality)
Exposing the genitals to the victim (exhibitionism)
Masturbating while exposing oneself

people, or spouses is, more often than not, a closely guarded family secret. The abused, the abuser, and other family members who are spectators in the episodes of abuse tend to collude, for various reasons, in keeping the situation a secret. They do not tell people outside the family, and rarely discuss it within the family.

Statistically, abuse *appears* to be more common in families of low socioeconomic status and educational achievement, but such findings are inaccurate. Abuse occurs in families of all socioeconomic statuses and levels of education. The inaccuracy of statistics is related to the reporting of incidents. Lower-class families with low levels of education tend to seek treatment in emergency rooms or clinics. In these settings, because of the discrepancies between the health care providers' and clients' socioeconomic and educational backgrounds, abuse is more easily recognized and more likely to be reported to welfare authorities than it is when treatment is provided by a private physician. Families in the upper classes are more likely to seek treatment from private physicians, who are less likely to doubt the explanations given for the injuries; to recognize that the injuries are the result of abuse; and, therefore, to report the situation to the welfare authorities.[4,6]

The number of identified cases of *child abuse* in the United States is rising. From 1976 to 1981 the number of reported cases doubled. The incidence of reported cases has continued to rise more than 10 percent a year since 1981.[7] More than 2 million cases of child abuse are reported annually. One in five abused children who are identified as abused die as a result of mistreatment. Estimates indicate that more than 200,000 children die each year from abuse or neglect. This figure does not include the many more than 1000 who die annually from suspicious accidents such as falling out of windows.[1] Since the passage of the Mondale bill (Child Abuse and Treatment Act of 1973), all states have enacted legislation to protect children from abuse. The legal requirements for reporting that resulted from the Mondale bill have undoubtedly influenced the increased incidence of reported child abuse. Since 1976, there has been a 200 percent increase in reported cases of sexual child abuse alone.[7,8]

Statistics on the *abuse of spouses* include reported incidents in which serious or repeated injury was inflicted by a person who was a legal spouse or who had a relationship with the victim involving cohabitation and sexual intimacy. Domestic violence resulting in one spouse's murdering another accounts for 15 to 20 percent of all homicides committed in the United States. Wife abuse is reported considerably more frequently than husband abuse. It is estimated that annually nearly 6 million wives are abused by their husbands, and between 2000 and 4000 are beaten to death. Battering is the major cause of injury to women, occurring more frequently than automobile accidents, rapes, or muggings.[9]

Women may become victims more frequently than men because of their status in society and their inferior physical strength. However, the disparity in the numbers of reported incidents of wife abuse compared to husband abuse may not be as great as it appears. More men than reported may be abused by their wives, but they may be reluctant to report their victimization. There is little doubt that abuse of spouses of either sex is underreported.[10]

Abuse of elderly people by family members has only recently been recognized as a societal problem. As with abuse of children and spouses, abuse of elderly people has been and is underreported. It has been estimated that 1 in 10 elderly people living with a family member are abused, and that as many as 2.5 million elderly people are victims of intrafamily abuse.[2] All social classes, in rural, urban, and suburban areas of the country, are affected.[11] As the number of elderly people increases in our society, the potential number of victims also increases. As both health professionals and the public become more aware of the problem and the number of potential victims increases, the number of reported incidents of abuse of elderly people will predictably increase dramatically in the near future.

The extent of *abuse of elderly, retarded, and mentally ill people who are institutionalized* is unknown, but undoubtedly such abuse is underreported. Periodically, instances of extensive abuse of residents in convalescent homes and in institutions that provide long-term care for retarded and mentally ill people are reported in the news media. The publicity tends to generate an immediate outcry for improving conditions in these institutions and for greater protection of the residents from abuse. However, there has been a failure to follow through with efforts directed toward determining the extent of abuse in institutions across the country and how the abuse can be prevented.[12]

Recently, across the country, there has been extensive media coverage of the *sexual abuse of young children* by day care personnel and of older children by teachers, physicians, and adult leaders of church and social youth groups. This type of sexual abuse of children is not a new phenomenon. In the past, however, there was little publicity, and the few formal, verifiable complaints were treated as isolated incidents; in addition, a child's complaint of sexual abuse was often dismissed as a lie or a product of imagination. Findings of one study suggest that 19 percent of all women and 9 percent of all men have been sexually victimized as children.[4] Arrest records and confessions found 73 victims for each heterosexual child molester and 30 victims for each homosexual child molester. Statistics also indicate that more female children than male children are molested. There is evidence, however, that sexual assault of male children occurs more frequently than is reported.[13]

The increased media coverage of sexual abuse and exploitation of children has increased public awareness of the problem. One agency reported that the number of such cases investigated increased by 38 percent from 1982–1983 to 1983–1984.[13] The rash of media reports in 1984 about the sexual abuse of young children in day care and about the prosecution of day care operators suggests that reporting of incidents by victims has increased. Future statistics will undoubtedly reveal a sharp increase in the sexual abuse of children.

The incidence of *rape-murder* of children is very low. A rapist of children is most likely to be reported and arrested if the offender is a stranger. However, the offender is rarely a stranger, and, therefore, child rape is often not reported.[14] Estimates are that only 1 in 10 incidents is reported to the police, and only 1 in 10 of those reported ever goes to court.

Incest, a form of sexual abuse, has existed in most civilizations throughout the ages.[15] Despite legal and religious prohibition, incestuous relationships have continued to be widespread. Recently the FBI reported that more than 10 percent of all American families may be affected by incest and that, contrary to popular belief, incest occurs most commonly in middle-class families.[13] Meaningful statistics on the incidence of incest are lacking, however. The sociocultural taboo against incest reinforces the conspiracy of silence. Family members collude to keep the incestuous relationship a secret. The strong emotional reaction associated with violation of the taboo further contributes to the tendency of health care professionals to defend themselves through denial, avoidance, and distancing.[6,15]

A study of women who were victims of incest as children revealed that the average age of onset of the incestuous relationship was 9.4 years of age and that the average duration of the relationship was 3.3 years.[16] Another study found that the average age of onset was 7 years of age.[17] These studies indicate that vulnerability to incest is great in childhood and dispels the myth that adolescence is the stage when the risk of involvement in an incestuous relationship is greatest. Study findings also indicate that victims of incest tend to come from large families.[16,18]

PATTERNS OF INTERACTION: PERSON

Victims

The victims of abuse are today, as always, those who have least power in society. Children, adolescents, women, people who are institutionalized, and aged people have little capacity to defend themselves against physical assault and emotional abuse or neglect. These victims often possess special characteristics or fill special roles which engender intense feelings in the abusers. Not only do they lack the physical power to adequately defend themselves, but also they tend to experience their situation as hopeless and themselves as helpless.

Children

The phrase *battered child syndrome* was coined by C. Henry Kempe[19] in 1962 to describe the physical injuries found among infants and children who had been physically abused by their parents. Kempe's work initiated further investigation into the problem of child abuse.

Infants and young children are particularly vulnerable to inadequate parenting and emotional and physical neglect. The consequence of deprivation by parents is failure to thrive. An infant or child whose nutritional, sensory, oral, and dependency needs are met satisfactorily will direct energy toward growth and development. When these basic needs are not met, the process is disturbed. In time, the child's physical growth will be slowed or stopped, the development of motor skills will be delayed, and social and emotional withdrawal will occur. Such infants are more susceptible to infection and impaired physiological functioning, which may even result in death. A study of premature and ill newborns revealed an increased risk of abuse in these special infants.[20] These children as well as apparently healthy infants and toddlers cannot protect themselves from the shaking and slapping inflicted by immature, frustrated parents.

Children most likely to be physically battered by their parents are infants and preschoolers because they are defenseless, demanding, and nonverbal. Children from birth to 3 or 4 years of age have been identified as particularly vulnerable. Two-thirds of physically abused children are under 3 years of age. Infants who cry persistently because of colic pains and active, curious toddlers who say, "No," to all requests frustrate parents.

School-age children do not necessarily escape physical abuse, however, despite these statistics. Underreporting may be a function of the children's actively preventing detection of the abuse by teachers and school health nurses. Some fear reprisals if they tell, some remain silent because they are ashamed, and others have come to believe that they are bad and deserve the abuse. There are still others who, because of the family's religious orientation, believe that the abuse is punishment for their sins, and that if they did not receive the punishment, they would become the "devil's helpers" and "be cast into hell forever" when they died.

Abused adolescents usually have a history of parental abuse. Reciprocal violence may occur as the adolescent becomes more physically mature. Often these young people become runaways. An adolescent may become involved in marital conflict through an attempt to protect the mother from abuse by the father or boyfriend (surrogate father). When this happens, the husband may vent his abuse on the adolescent, any other children, or both.[10] Because a woman in this situation tends to be dependent on and fused with her spouse, she is likely to remain in the relationship, and the rescuing adolescent is likely to leave the household and be further victimized.

The characteristics of the child which generate hostility in the abusing parent are often unique to the relationship. But a child's developmental stage and the behavioral characteristics of the phase may also trigger specific conflicts in the parents. Also, control is more of an issue in certain developmental phases. The impulsive drive to experience the environment and the innate messiness of toddlers are disruptive to compulsive parents who place a high value on neatness and obedience. Another critical point in the parent-child relationship is adolescence, when the child is striving ambivalently for independence.

Children who exhibit age-appropriate sexual behavior may be in conflict with their parents. Toddlers who explore or manipulate their genitals may be perceived as abnormal by their parents. This behavior evokes the parents' anxiety about their own unacceptable impulses, which lie buried in their subconscious. These impulses are ascribed to the child by denial of their ownership and projection into the child. Parents may administer prophylactic punishment to prevent an older child from becoming delinquent or pregnant out of wedlock.

A child's sex, physical appearance, or personality may have the potential for triggering a conflict the parent experienced in the past. The parent reenacts the conflict with the child (who becomes the victim). If the parent is separated, divorced, or abandoned by a mate, the child may be seen as the cause and, therefore, may become the focus of the parent's anger and abuse.

Negative attention is better than no attention in a child's world. Although being beaten is not a healthy way of making contact with the parent, it has the elements of interaction and sensory input desired by the child. Thus, to receive attention from the adults in the environment, the child may learn to be provocative and invite abuse. This pattern becomes very evident when these children are placed in foster homes and continue to exhibit provocative behavior with the foster parents. Extinguishing such behavior requires time, patience, and understanding on the part of the surrogate parents or care givers.

As was noted above, victims often possess unique or special characteristics that engender intense feelings in their abusers. For example:

> Tom, a lively 3-year-old with curly red hair and blue eyes, clearly resembled his father. His mother also saw him as having a personality similar to that of his father, who abandoned the family shortly after Tom's birth. Tom was frequently and severely beaten by his mother, while his two older sisters, who resembled the mother's family, were never the targets of abuse. Tom's physical appearance, probably the fact he was male, and the perceived similarity of his personality to his father's triggered the mother's anger and resentment of her husband, which she displaced onto her son.

Race can be a significant variable which places the child in a special position within the family. For example:

> Jamie was a 7-year-old from his white mother's common-law marriage to a black laborer. His mother had been abandoned and subsequently married a white shopkeeper. This marriage produced two children, a boy and girl who were fair-skinned and blond like their father. Jamie's skin was light brown and his hair dark brown and very curly. This child represented a very difficult and unhappy period in the mother's life, and his mixed racial appearance was a sharp reminder of her earlier liaison. The present marriage and family life seemed stable and relatively happy except for Jamie's role in the family. He was frequently and severely beaten by his mother. Once, when he was admitted to an emergency room, the back of his body—from shoulders to ankles—was severely lacerated from a beating with a belt, and his shoulder was broken. In this family, Jamie had become the scapegoat for the denied family stresses and the mother's bad self-image.

Sometimes, a child in a violent family kills either the abusive parent or a sibling. In most cases, the child who kills in this situation is acting as the unwitting lethal agent of an adult, usually a parent, who unconsciously prompts the child to kill so that the adult can enjoy vicariously the benefits of the act. A history of parental brutality is a significant factor in the homicidal adolescent's attack on a parent. Young children can also be provoked to and are capable of homicidal rage when there is a perceived threat to their position in the family system, but more often they are the recipients of covert messages from their adult environment to kill.

Daughters in incestuous relationships with their fathers usually have poor relationships with their mothers, who may be physically as well as psychologically unavailable. These girls may develop a seductive posture to gain attention from their fathers. Failure to identify with the mother may contribute to a fixation on the father and the desire to possess him; this is called the *Electra complex*. Sons in a comparable situation are said to be suffering from an *Oedipus complex*. These daughters and sons may believe that they are in pivotal family roles and responsible for keeping their families together and taking care of the parents of the opposite sex.[21] This belief is reinforced and supported by both parents.

Incest is always a devastating and emotionally disturbing experience for the victim. The psychological impact extends well beyond the immediate episode and lasts long after the relationship is terminated.[22,23] There is a high rate of emotional disturbance among adults who experienced incestuous relationships as children.[24] Even as adults, many feel inadequate and inferior, have low self-esteem, and tend to be socially isolated.[15] They invest considerable energy in keeping their secret and dealing with their guilt. When these victimized children become adolescents, they tend to become sexually promiscuous. They describe themselves as "witches" or "bitches." They date and marry at an earlier age than their peers, probably as a means of escaping from their incestuous relationships. Frequently, they become substance abusers to deaden the feelings generated by the incest.[16]

Some children cope with repeated sexual abuse that extends over years by developing multiple personalities. Their psychopathology often goes unrecognized and untreated until adulthood.[6] Adolescents often run away from home to escape the situation. Their premature separation from their families and their dysfunctional parent-child relationships contribute to their involvement in delinquent activities, substance abuse, and prostitution.[6,24]

One study found that 17 out of 22 children who were victims of incest had abnormal electroencephalograms (EEGs) and 6 suffered from seizures. Of the 22, 18 reported depersonalization experiences. The EEG abnormalities that were found have been associated with cerebral mechanisms in the temporal and limbic regions of the brain which mediate identity formation and a sense of personal boundaries. This neurospsychiatric handicap may influence the child's need for closeness and perception of personal boundaries. Children in families in which gender and generation boundaries are poorly developed or impaired may be more vulnerable to the breakdown of the incest taboo.[25]

When the perpetrator is a loved relative, the incest relationship causes ambivalence, anxiety, and depression. Children are frightened by the experience. In one study, half of the victims reported feeling disgusted, shocked, and confused. They did not know how to react or what to do.[26] Very young children are uncertain, uncomfortable, and easily intimidated. Since the mothers are usually psychologically unavailable, these children do not know who they can tell, who would believe them, or even how to describe their experiences. Their ambivalence toward the perpetrator may inhibit them from telling anyone, and fear may inhibit them from seeking help. Usually disclosure by the child is spontaneous and accidental. An older child or adolescent is more likely to disclose what has occurred intentionally and sometimes angrily.[15] When a victimized child or adolescent tells the nonabusive parent about the incestuous relationship, the response may or may not be supportive. Very young children as well as adolescents experience guilt and fear of retaliation when they tell.[15] When an adolescent discloses the incestuous relationship to the nonabusive parent, only to find this parent aligning with the abuser and providing no protection, the risk of a suicide attempt is high.[6] A supportive parental response involves listening to the child, accepting the description as fact, seeking help (police, protective services, physician), and requiring the perpetrator to leave the household. Unfortunately, a supportive response was found to occur in only one-fourth of the families in one study of children in treatment for symptoms caused by incestuous relationships. If the incest becomes publicly known, these children are blamed by their peers as well as adults for being seductive and provocative or for letting it happen. This reinforces the children's sense of guilt.[17]

Many people go through life never sharing the secret. Some after years of psychotherapy are able to confront the perpetrator and share what occurred with siblings. Some become distressed after they have left home and recognize that a younger sibling has been recruited, and only then do they reluctantly return to confront the perpetrator and protect the sibling.

As adults these victimized children continue to suffer from guilt. They often have flashbacks of their experiences which are acutely distressing.[6,17] Many seek out relationships that repeat the abusive situation. As victims again, and lacking an understanding of how and why they were victims in the past, they become psychologically paralyzed and remain passive.[26] Others deal with their sexuality and sexual feelings through promiscuity, which provides a barrier to intimacy; homosexuality; or asexuality. In a study of prostitutes, 99 percent reported immediate emotional harm resulting from sexual abuse they experienced as children, and 70 percent indicated that the sexual exploitation they experienced influenced their decision to become prostitutes.[27]

Spouses or Cohabitants

A *spouse* is a partner in a legally constituted marriage. The term is also used in relation to a partner in a *common-law marriage,* which is the relationship of a heterosexual couple who share the same household and represent themselves as married. A *cohabitant* is a partner in a couple who are emotionally and sexually intimate and share the same household without being legally or religiously married. The terms *wife* and *husband* that appear in the literature on abuse refer to either a married or a cohabiting couple. The couple may share living quarters, be separated and living apart, or be divorced. When the couple are not living in the same household, the abusive spouse returns to the home to perpetrate the abuse.

The most common victims of family violence are women attacked by their husbands or ex-husbands.[5] Not all this spousal abuse involves physical violence. Psychological battering—verbal and nonverbal threats of violence—creates an environment that is humiliating, degrading, and terrifying. Unpredictable, rageful destruction of property, household objects, and pets can terrify the abused spouse.[10] Hopefulness and a period of calmness follow episodes, but this is temporary. Tension once again increases, and the cycle is repeated.[9]

Battered wives do not differ from nonabused women in terms of social class, religious affiliation, educational level, or racial background.[28] The abuse usually begins early in the marriage. Sometimes the first episode occurs with the confirmation that the wife is pregnant, or shortly thereafter. Usually there were warnings of potential abuse before the marriage that were rationalized or ignored.[10,28] However, women who have been reared in families that believed in physical punishment, or in which abuse of children and spouse was accepted, often initially viewed their husbands as "diamonds in the rough." These women believe that hitting a spouse is normal,[28] and they accept it as a part of life.[29] For some women the physical or psychological abuse was unexpected because the abusers had carefully controlled their temper during the courtship period. If these women do not have a family history of domestic violence or neglect, then they are not likely to tolerate the abuse. They perceive the beatings as coercive, hostile, and intended to cause injury, and they are more likely to leave the relationships than are women reared in abusive homes.[29,30] Regardless, ambivalent feelings about the situation are not uncommon. Loyalty ties and affection sustain the hope that things will change. Between episodes these women often act as if they have forgotten what has happened. Many feel that they are responsible for the outbursts and their husbands' actions—that they somehow provoked the violent episodes. They seek ways to please their husbands and behave so as not to provoke additional outbursts.

Not all of these women are masochistic. To say that they are and to explain their remaining in abusive relationships in this way is only a form of blaming the victim.[9] Women remain in abusive situations for various reasons. A woman who is pregnant or who has young children may believe that her children need a father; she may rationalize that her life is not as bad as it could be and that tomorrow will be better. A woman who rationalizes her predicament seeks refuge only after incurring severe injuries. She may remain in a shelter for only a brief period of time and then return to her husband.[29] Sometimes a woman believes that she has nowhere to go and could not survive alone without a husband. A woman who is emotionally and financially dependent on the abuser and who lacks job skills may be reluctant to leave the relationship, particularly if she has dependent children. A woman may remain in the abusive situation out of fear for her life and the lives of her children and other members of the family. The more aggressive and assaultive the husband becomes, the more fearful the wife becomes and the more she feels trapped and powerless.

Because these women have low self-esteem, are socially isolated, and accept unilateral responsibility for their marriages, they fear the failure of their marriages and they feel ashamed and embarrassed about their situation. They may feel guilty for provoking their husbands' attacks even when reality does not support this perception. Some women continue to believe in their husbands' omnipotence and their own powerlessness. Learned helplessness and a sense of powerlessness sustain a willingness to comply with an abusive husband's demands and to remain in the relationship. Such a woman may view leaving the home as impossible.[31] Instead, she may hide for hours, waiting for the husband to vent his feelings in the destruction of household objects and calm down.[10] In 1984 the New Jersey Supreme Court accepted expert testimony on the behavior of women subjected to sustained abuse by their spouses and acknowledged the battered wife syndrome as an explanation for not leaving the abusive situation.[32]

Husband abuse is very probably underreported for a variety of reasons. Some wife-beating incidents that are reported begin with the wife's physical assault on the husband. Research has revealed that 20 out of every 100 wives studied assaulted their husbands under highly stressful situations, but only 14 out of every 100 husbands assaulted their wives in similarly highly stressful situations. In the absence of high stress, wives are less violent toward their husbands. Under ordinary stressful situations, the rate of wife beating is generally about twice that of husband beating.[33]

Elderly People

Abuse of elderly people has always existed. In this society it is rapidly becoming a major mental health problem as greater numbers of people are living long after they have stopped being economically productive.[12] Medical advances that extend life into very old age often do so at the expense of the elderly person's physical, social, and economic independence.

The abuse of elderly people who are not institutionalized usually occurs when they reside with adult children or other relatives and are no longer able, for physical or economic reasons, to maintain their own homes. Research describes those who are the most vulnerable to abuse as widowed, white, middle-class females who are severely impaired (major mental or physical health problems). Because of their impairments, most are dependent on family members for nutrition, administration of medications, cleanliness, and ambulation.[2]

Elderly people may contribute to conflicts with their abusers. For some elderly people, the loss of independence caused by physical impairments generates frustration and anger, which are expressed through excessively demanding, belligerent, and aggressive behavior. This style of coping engenders frustration and anger in the caretaking relatives, which may lead to abuse or neglect. Some elderly people cope by surrendering to their disabilities. Their posture and mode of interacting is one of helplessness and hopelessness. They generalize their disabilities and thereby increase their dependence. Their failure to attempt to maintain their independence where possible further burdens caretaking relatives, who may withdraw, neglect, or aggressively abuse as ways of dealing with the consequent frustration and anger.[2]

Abused elderly people fail to seek help for many reasons. Some who are physically able are ashamed to tell anyone that their adult children have physically or sexually abused them. If an adult child has, through misrepresentation or coercion, taken an elderly person's money and assets, the latter may believe that he or she has no alternative but to stay in the abusive situation. This sense of helplessness may be compounded by threats to have the elderly person committed to a psychiatric facility or placed in a home. Fear of reprisals may further inhibit seeking help. Some abused elderly people are unable physically or mentally to contact someone who could rescue them. They are kept isolated, deprived of the use of a telephone, and closely watched when interacting with anyone outside their families.[12,34]

Institutionalized People

Elderly people in nursing homes and mentally and physically disabled people who are institutionalized are dependent on their care givers for meeting their needs for basic survival as well as growth. The physical and mental incapacitation of these people, their dependency on their care givers, and in some instances their impaired ability to communicate their needs and wishes effectively contribute to their powerlessness and their victimization.

Children in Day Care

The trend of women continuing in the work force after the birth of children has increased the use of day care facilities for preschool children. Recently there have been numerous nationwide reports citing the sexual abuse of children in day care centers. In some instances the children were sexually abused by the staff, while in other instances the children were "rented out" to pedophiles and pornographers. In many cases the sexual abuse continued for an extended period of time before it was discovered.

The delay in discovering the sexual abuse is related to several factors. Many young children who are abused have little or no understanding of what they are experiencing and lack the vocabulary to describe it; they are therefore hampered in explaining what is happening to them. They tend instead to manifest their distress somatically or behaviorally. Since young children are unable to describe their experiences clearly, their parents do not understand what has happened. Moreover, sexual abuse of young children is so abhorrent that many parents may have difficulty comprehending and accepting the fact that such abuse is occurring in a day care facility they believed to be reputable. Finally, many children are afraid to tell anyone of their experiences because of threats made by the staff. Some children have been told that they or members of their families would die if they told. To reinforce this threat, they were made to watch a staff member torture or kill a small animal and warned that this is what would happen to them if they told.

Children who experience sexual abuse in these situations are confused, frightened, and even terrorized. Since the experience is usually not a single isolated incident but involves multiple encounters with abusers, the impact is overwhelming. Even after the abuse has been stopped and the child is no longer at risk, the fears continue. The child's sense of trust, safety, and security has been destroyed. Reestablishing trust in adults and a feeling of being safe and secure is a difficult process, and it can be distressing to these young children. They have suffered psychological and sometimes physical harm. The extent of the psychological harm will not be known for years.

Victimizers

The abuser is usually physically stronger and in one way or another more powerful than the victim. In the spousal or cohabitation relationship, the husband or male friend is usually the offender. However, the woman may be the abuser, and the man the passive recipient. Parents, older siblings, baby-sitters, or related adults may be the abusers, physically, psychologically, or sexually abusing and neglecting children. Adult children and their spouses and children may abuse and neglect elderly people at home. In residential situations and day care centers, providers of care may abuse or neglect children and mentally incompetent or aged people under their supervision.

Parents

Morris[35] has identified four types of parents who physically abuse their children: (1) parents who are distressed and guilty about their relationship with and treatment of their child; (2) undercontrolled, impulse-ridden parents who are angry about their relationship with their child and who blame the child for the family problems; (3) overcontrolled parents who feel that they are "correct" in punishing their child, even if the punishment results in injury; and (4) parents who respond to an inner psychotic world rather than to the real world and the child.

Abusers tend to have many hypochondriacal complaints and frequently undergo elective surgery. They exhibit a flight from parenthood through illness and work. They seem to live in fear of their own parents' opinion of them and see their parents as threatening and destructive influences in their lives. In their marital relationships, the men are frequently sexually demanding and the women compliant but lacking interest. There is a marked absence of satisfaction or enjoyment in their sexual acts.[36]

When speaking of their child, abusive parents reveal their ambivalent attitudes, and these are a corollary to the ambivalence with which they view themselves. They describe the child as both lovable and hateful; they exhibit extreme and intense emotions as they describe incidents that illustrate the child's offensive behavior. These descriptions often sound as if the conflict had occurred between adults, reflecting the parents' unrealistic expectations and inability to view the child as a child.[36]

MOTHERS AS ABUSERS. Asch[37] describes a postpartum syndrome in which the mother experiences an emotional response which may range from a "blue feeling," to a deeper depression, to a massive psychotic reaction. Some hostile impulses and thoughts both toward the fetus before birth and toward the newborn infant are not unusual and well within the normal range of maternal ambivalence. They tend to evoke guilt and shame, which the woman supresses. These reactions derive from experiences involving the person's mental representations of pregnancy, parturition, and motherhood; they are not confined to biological mothers, since this phenomenon has been observed in adoptive mothers as well.

If the attachment proceeds along a healthy course, these feelings are effectively suppressed, and warm, nurturing feelings emerge and predominate. Where the attachment process is weak or absent, the mother may experience obsessive infanticidal thoughts that may be manifested by the reaction formation of obsessive concern for the baby's care and health. If postpartum psychosis occurs, the woman experiences marked negative feelings toward the baby. Disordered thought processes may impel the woman to rid herself of her "bad part," and suicide may be attempted. She may also displace these suicidal drives onto the infant; that is, the distinction between the self and the infant may be blurred. Her depression is experienced in reaction to the sense of loss after delivery, and her psychological development may be so distorted that infanticide looks to her like the only way of alleviating her pain.[37]

Although the first act of physical abuse is reported, in the majority of instances, when the child is about 1 year old, it seems reasonable to suppose that the first reported instance will have been preceded by earlier incidents and that the battering may very well have begun during the postpartum period. According to Asch,[37] this behavior derives from a reawakening of the mother's childhood conflicts. It is renewal of an older conflict between the new mother and her mother, the infant's grandmother, which is acted out with the baby. She identifies with the original aggressor in the abusing relationship, but now she is not the victim but the aggressor.

The mother may have wanted someone to love and someone to love her in return. She expects the child to gratify her needs for dependency, self-esteem, love, and belonging. These needs are intensified as the child demands nurturing. An infant does not give or return love; rather, it makes demands on the care giver, who in this instance is emotionally impoverished and has little to give. If the infant also suffers from colic or is premature or irritable, there is even less satisfaction in mothering, and such a situation may increase the mother's feelings of inadequacy. The mother's unconscious desire for a role reversal cannot be fulfilled. As the mother reenacts with the child her own abused and rejected childhood, she feels anxiety and guilt. The loss of self-esteem threatens the mother's fragile, narcissistic equilibrium. She projects her "bad" self-image and unacceptable feelings onto the child and attacks the child, who now symbolizes her inadequacies. This identification with the agressor in her past allows her to actively master the traumatic rejection she had passively experienced as a child.[38]

Not all abusive mothers physically abuse their children. In some instances they neglect the child and are psychologically unavailable because of impaired capacity to nurture; often, this impaired capacity is a multigenerational phenomenon. Neither the child's mother nor her extended family is able to provide the physical care or the social interactions needed by the child. If the family has the capacity to provide adequate child care, the impairment of the mother is remedied by the father or relatives. When neglect and psychological unavailability prevail, a low level of differentiation is present among family members. All potential "mothering" adults are experiencing acute deprivation and are therefore unable to give to the infant and young child. Nurturing is not necessarily an instinctive activity. One must have experienced a warm, sensitive, and caring relationship in order to know how to behave in this way toward another.

In mother-son incest, the mother may directly initiate sex or invite and accept the sexual advances made by the son. In these instances, the son is assigned to the role of a spouse.[21]

FATHERS AND MALE FRIENDS AS ABUSERS. In situations where the mother is not abusive but has allowed a husband or male friend to batter her child, there is a variation to the psychodynamics. In this case, the interaction between mother and child is similar. However, Green[38] points out that the bad self-image is partly retained and partly projected onto the child. The internalized "bad mother" image is projected onto the abusive mate. Consequently, the mother identifies with the child victim. In most instances where the mate is abusing the child, he is also abusing the mother. The mother tolerates this cruelty as a masochistic repetition of her childhood experience. Her extreme emotional dependency and linking with her mate and the extent of her feelings of worthlessness serve to bind her into this pathological relationship. However, if the mother is abandoned by the abusing mate, it is not uncommon to find such a woman assuming the role of aggressor and abusing her children.

Abusive behavior exhibited by a father or a male friend toward a newborn may be based on envy of the woman's pregnancy. Old feelings of sibling rivalry for attention which have resurfaced along with revived feelings and fears may be associated with the oedipal conflict. If the resolution of this conflict was defective or if the ability to tolerate competition with authority has been inadequate, such a revival of feelings may precipitate neurotic or even psychotic behavior. Manifestations of this intensified conflict include transient mood changes, sudden and compulsive extramarital affairs, the breakthrough into consciousness of homosexual impulses, or severe affective or psychotic difficulties. Overwhelmed with these fears and fantasies, the father may assault his child.[36]

A father may justify his physical abuse by redefining his loss of control and infliction of harm as simply disciplining his offspring. Usually such a father was subjected to physical abuse as a child and therefore sees no problem in meting out the same to his children.

A man who has an incestuous relationship with his daughter continues to remain emotionally tied to his mother or a fantasy mother. The daughter is cast into the role of the "good mother" and is expected to care for the father.

The patriarchal father's authoritarianism and overinvested family orientation is used to socially isolate family members. This type of father establishes and fosters an expectation that all needs must be met within the family. In some instances the father operates as a benign, overly protective, smothering parent. In other instances he is a tyrannical child who batters the mother and children, but usually excludes the sexually exploited daughter from the battering if she is cooperative.[16,22] The marital relationship deteriorates before the incestuous relationship with the daughter begins.[16]

Profiles of fathers in father-daughter incest are presented in Table 51-6. Stepfathers or surrogate fathers are 5 times more likely than biological fathers to engage in such incest, and girls with stepfathers or surrogate fathers are also 5 times more likely to be abused by a friend of the family.[21]

The mother may be ill, disabled, absent from the home much of the time, and generally overwhelmed by family responsibilities. As she withdraws from her roles as wife and mother, she exchanges these roles with the eldest daughter. This exchange helps the mother address her own unmet dependency needs and distance her husband. The daughter becomes the homemaker; surrogate mother to younger siblings; and father's friend, confidante, and lover.[22] The mother participates in the father-daughter incest by ignoring or denying the obvious.[16]

The mother may find sex with her spouse unsatisfactory, and the daughter's involvement with the father frees her from this aspect of the marital relationship. By keeping herself tired and worn out, working long hours outside the home, and delegating the care of the home and younger children to the daughter, she supports the incest. Because she tends to be weak and passive and feels emotionally and economically dependent on the spouse, she may refuse to believe that the problem exists even after she has been confronted with it, and she will choose husband over daughter. In some instances the mother may be indifferent or promiscuous—a poor role model for sexual behavior. A profile of the mother in families where father-daughter incest exists is presented in Table 51-7.

Table 51-6 Profiles of Fathers Engaging in Father-Daughter Incest

Type	Description
Symbiotic type	Uses child to meet strong unmet needs for love, warmth, closeness, intimacy. May be a depressed, lonely, isolated introvert rejected by wife; uses persuasion or sympathy to engage daughter.
Substance abuser	Abuses drugs or alcohol. Claims loss of control precipitated incident. Incestuous activity claimed to have occurred during blackout. May bully, physically abuse, or force child. Tyrannical; uses sex with child to feel dominant, superior, or powerful.
Rationalizer	Sees nothing wrong with incestuous behavior. Sees self as helpful to daughter. Sex is goal. Rationalizes behavior as a way of teaching daughter about sex or protecting her from "predatory" peers because he "loves" her; or views his bloodline as elite and wants sex with his own child to produce "pure" offspring.
Psychopath	Sexually promiscuous; pansexual. Impulsive and regressive. Does not experience guilt. May be persuasive and disarming or brutal and physically abusive toward child. Sex is goal. Uses child to gain a sense of power and control.

Table 51-7 The Mother in Families Where Father-Daughter Incest Exists

Profile
Usually not sexually or emotionally involved with husband
Acts helpless
Fails to protect self against involuntary childbearing
History of being sexually abused as child
Exchanges wife and mother roles with daughter
Fearful of questioning father's authority
Absents herself from home during the evenings to work or visit others; or is ill or disabled

If the perpetrator is a loved and trusted parent or stepparent and the need for parental love and attention is great, the abuser manipulates, bribes, and coerces the child. The parent may imply to the child that it is her duty to cooperate and the parent's right to have sex with her. Fathers and adult male relatives tend to use some kind of force (physical force, emotional coercion, threats, or promises) or a combination of forces. In one study more than half of the victims of incest reported being physically held down.[17,26]

A single incident of incest is rare.[26] The relationship is generally maintained for years (3 to 7 years).[17] Adolescents often terminate the relationship by running away, and the perpetrator transfers attention to a younger sibling and involves that child in an incestuous relationship.

When the parents are unsupportive, they do nothing to protect the child. They may ostracize the child and support the abuser's denial. They may tell the child that he or she is lying, that the subject will not be discussed with the abuser, and that the child is forbidden to tell anyone. When a parent responds in this manner, there is a great deal of investment in maintaining current family roles and equilibrium even if the child must be sacrificed to this end.

Siblings

Younger children in a family may become the victims of physical and sexual abuse at the hands of their older siblings. Ongoing sibling incest occurs more frequently when parents are passive, preoccupied, or overtly sexually promiscuous. Conditions within the home may be chaotic. There is usually no strong parental figure to exert leadership or enforce limits.

Physical and sexual abuse by a sibling may occur as a single violent, destructive incident, perhaps related to drug or alcohol abuse. However, this is rare; more often, a pattern develops and is sustained until either the victim or the victimizer leaves home.

Spouses

The husband who abuses his wife tends to have been abused as a child and to have observed wife beating in his family of origin. He feels insecure in the marital relationship and in his roles outside the home. To cope with these insecurities, he pretends to be supertough and independent by projecting a macho image. His male self-image is fragile and he often has morbid fears about his sexual potency. He may hold a rigid set of beliefs about how he and his wife should behave and interact with each other and with outsiders. Any deviation in behavior that conflicts with these beliefs triggers a violent outburst.[10] He may be chronically suspicious of his wife's fidelity, and his jealousy may reach delusional proportions. When he perceives a threat to his self-image, he explodes into a violent rage in an attempt to protect himself.[4] Perceived threats to the self-image may occur outside the household, but the abusive husband typically is inhibited in confronting the source. Instead he returns home and vents his frustrations by abusing his wife (and sometimes children as well). Some of these men describe an experience of sudden blind rage. They are usually unable to connect a previous event with their rage reaction. They also seem unaware of the long-term consequences of their explosive episodes.[10]

The abusive husband has a tendency to blame his wife for his violent outbursts, claiming that either her verbal aggressiveness or her failure to meet his demands satisfactorily was provocative. He may experience remorse but will justify his behavior by blaming his wife. He tends to be immature, self-centered, impulsive, and chronically aggressive and hostile. His rigid and compulsive personality, low self-esteem, and lack of warmth interfere with his ability to sustain relationships. As a consequence, he tends to feel lonely. The cyclical conflicts with his wife may in a distorted way provide moments of closeness.

Battering men hold many irrational beliefs that contribute to their explosive rage reactions and abuse of others. They tend to believe that they must be in control of all situations at all times.[10] Since this is an impossible expectation, their daily interactions with others are constantly generating events that could trigger a rage reaction. These men also believe that they have little or no control over their feelings. If a situation elicits a feeling, they believe its expression is uncontrollable and necessary, despite the consequence. They have little or no insight into their participation in the generation of aggressive and hostile feelings or the impact of the ventilation of these feelings on others. From their perspective, other people and events are the source of their misery, anger, and aggression and, therefore, are blamed for any violent outburst.[10] Since their wives or children are the safest and most vulnerable target for the ventilation of aggressive feelings and frustrations, they choose to abuse them physically or psychologically. Following abusive episodes these men tend to blame their wives for provoking them, thus justifying their behavior. If confronted with their participation and the consequences of their actions, they tend to distort and minimize what has occurred.[10] They perceive beating as a positive act, intended to facilitate communication or end arguments.[30] These men wish to be close to their wives, and to control them and their behavior, but they fail to recognize that their violent behavior drives their wives away from them.[9]

Family Members Who Abuse Elderly People

The primary abuser of the elderly person is usually the adult child with whom the person resides. This abuser is most likely a daughter in her forties or fifties.[2] One study found that daughters were the perpetrators twice as often as any other relatives, followed by sons, granddaughters, husbands, and siblings (usually sisters).[39]

Even if there are several adult children available to care for the elderly parent, usually only one is elected and chooses to take the responsibility. The inclusion of the elderly parent into the household is disruptive of family routines and may restrict the freedom of not only the caretaker but other family members as well. Conflicts develop over lifestyle and allocation of space, money, and time. The caretaker and spouse may have completed child rearing and be looking forward to enjoying their new freedom. Resentments, a lack of gratification, and frustration may develop and contribute to abuse. External stresses, such as a loss of a job, health problems, or children's problems, may interact with this situation. These additional stresses may compound intrafamily stress and contribute to the abusive situation.[2]

Care Givers in Institutions

Care givers single out the clients they abuse for reasons unique to the relationship. Those who provide care to physically and mentally impaired people who are institutionalized are at risk of developing an identification with clients that produces negative transference. Unresolved conflicts are revived, and these are reenacted in relationships with clients. Because care givers who abuse clients tend to be immature, impulsive, aggressive, and dissatisfied with their jobs or status in society, the demands made by the confused, incontinent, or hostile client tax their ability to provide sensitive, therapeutic care. They focus their anger and frustration on the vulnerable client, who then becomes the victim of abuse.

In instances of abuse, emotional linking is an important factor. Intimate relationships involve characteristic emotional ties that can generate strong feelings. The intimacy of long-term care, the dependency of the client, and the inadequacy of emotional support in both the work setting and the home situation all heighten the negative feelings of care givers toward their clients. The abuser's inadequate coping mechanisms and limited impulse control increase the risk of abusive outbursts.

Other factors that increase the risk of neglect and abuse in institutions that provide long-term care include dissatisfaction with chances for advancement and a lack of a sense of accomplishment when the client either makes no progress or deteriorates. Many abusive care givers experienced extreme physical discipline as children and therefore are likely to view physical punishment as normal behavior. Care givers who are unable to use others for support when they are distressed are also likely to vent their frustration on the vulnerable clients. Research also indicates that abusive care givers consume a greater quantity of alcohol than those who are not abusive.[39,40]

Abusers in Day Care Centers

Owners of day care centers and staff members involved in the sexual abuse of children have differing motives. Those who rent out children to pedophiles and pornographers appear to be motivated to do so primarily for monetary gain. However, they may also be consumers of child pornography. In renting out the children, they not only have access to the pornographic media they desire, but may request what they want to have portrayed. Some of the people who sexually molest children in their care are pedophiles.[13,36] Profiles of these offenders are presented in Table 51-8.

PATTERNS OF INTERACTION: FAMILY

Abuse within the family and in care-giving relationships has its basis in preceding generations. The behavior is transmitted from one generation to the next and brought to the fore when various stressors

Table 51-8 Pedophiles

Profile
Fixated offenders
Claim to be in love with children.
Are shy and introverted; loners.
Were frequently sexually abused as children.
Confine sexual activity to just girls or just boys.
Are usually single.
Engage in sex play and exhibitionism.
Tend to wallow in self-pity.
Live in fantasy world and find reality distasteful.
Have no outstanding successes; are underachievers.
Regressed offenders
May have led normal married lives in the past.
Sexual activity with children is triggered by sudden crisis (rejection by mate; midlife crisis).
Are generally successful within limits of abilities and education.
Sexual preferences vary between boys and girls.

interact and deplete the abuser's ability to cope. Violent multigenerational patterns may be a product of imitation. If family violence, neglect, or psychological unavailability were normal behavioral patterns in the family of origin, then it is likely that the patterns will be repeated.[2,33] Loyalty conflicts and the "revolving slate" (see Chapter 48) may also contribute to this multigenerational phenomenon. Steinmetz[41] found that 1 in 400 children reared in a nonviolent family abused an elderly parent, while 1 out of every 2 who were reared in a violent family abused an elderly parent. The low level of differentiation found in abusive families may also support multigenerational influences. The characteristic dominance of emotionality and minimal use of cognitive processes may contribute to family members' reactivity and impulsivity when stress occurs.

Abusive families tend to experience considerable social stress and to manage it ineffectively. Scores on tests that measure the number of life changes have been found to be higher in a group of abusive family members than in a matched control group. The episodes of abuse or escalations of abuse are often preceded by the death of a significant family member, physical or mental illness of a parent, turmoil associated with the developmental changes of adolescence or midadolescence, loss of a job, or geographical moves. These families tend to experience sex difficulties, changes in financial status, trouble with in-laws, and changes in living conditions.

Impaired ability to approach problems thoughtfully and emotional reactivity interfere with appropriate fulfillment of needs. Lack of self-awareness combined with emotional and impulsive reactions, can lead to either blaming the victim for the problems and the consequent neglect or abuse or using the victim as an object for sexual satisfaction. Aggressiveness toward spouse, children, elderly parent, or clients and the sexual use of these victims are employed to meet needs for love and belonging, for recognition, and for a sense of power that will enhance low self-esteem.

Abusive families also tend to be socially isolated and distrustful of others. To further complicate the family situation in our society, there has been a movement from the kinship structure of extended families to the nuclear family. Abusive families often live in isolation. When alienation from the extended family exists, there is often a concomitant isolation from friends and community. When family members are unable to share problems and solutions or to give and receive support from significant others, tension within the family builds and avenues for release tend to become focused within the family.

Among those families who are not socially isolated but who abuse their children are members of some fundamentalist religious groups. These people believe that God expects them to punish their children vigorously in order to raise them correctly. Families on military bases are also vulnerable to using physical abuse as a way of disciplining their children.[19]

Alcohol abuse is a significant factor contributing to the abusive situation. Rage—along with impulsive, assaultive, and sexually aggressive behavior—is more easily triggered when inhibitions are diminished by excessive consumption of alcohol.

In some families, one member may manipulate another into the role of abuser and establish the expectation that physical punishment must be inflicted to maintain control of the situation.

Incestuous families often differ in appearance from those that physically batter or neglect their offspring. On the surface, they appear to be harmonious, close, stable, and strongly patriarchal, middle- or upper-middle-class families, usually with more than three children. Once the facade is cracked, dysfunctional family patterns are evident. Gender and generational boundaries are violated, and role confusion exists.[15,20,22] When incest occurs, multi-generational patterns exist.[20]

Spousal abuse tends to occur in cycles. The time frame for these cycles varies among couples. Since the need for closeness and intimacy is great, but the ability to tolerate it is impaired for both spouses, the daily sharing of space and interpersonal interactions generate tension. Lacking effective coping skills, these people allow tension to build up. In some instances there is awareness of this, but often only one or neither spouse recognizes what is occurring and neither is able to defuse it. The tension peaks, and a violent outburst occurs. Once the episode is over, a period of remorse and apologies occurs.

Some theorists have proposed that abuse of elderly people may occur when the adult children have failed to resolve the stage of adolescent rebellion toward their parents. Consequently, old conflicts reemerge when the adult child must care for the elderly parent and escalate when the caretaking is burdensome and frustrating.[41] The inevitable stress in the life cycle of the family is compounded by the responsibility of caring for an elderly, dependent parent. The physical and emotional demands and the role reversal with a parent may be overwhelming to the caretaker. One study found that two-thirds of the care givers were exhausted and anxious and believed that their own health had deteriorated.[2]

PATTERNS OF INTERACTION: ENVIRONMENT

Society's attitudes toward the use of force as a legitimate means of attaining ends (especially in imbalanced interpersonal relations such as male-female, care giver–client, adult-child, and adult–elderly person) and the tendency in our society to resort to force to deal with conflicts contribute to the rate of abuse. Abuser-abused relations are intimately linked to prevailing social attitudes and the common concept of human beings and their rights. The use of force toward women, children, and aged and incompetent people is also related to the way in which these people are seen by society and how their rights are defined.

In our society, those who are socially unacceptable and those who are unable to care for themselves are relegated to institutions out of the mainstream of life. The rights of this population are not always adequately protected. The problems of neglect and abuse these people face are often not brought to public attention except when they become political or media issues.

Alienation from work may be an influential societal factor in abuse.[40] A work environment with a hierarchical and authoritarian structure which is competitive and exploitative creates psychological stress and in some instances causes deviance in the employees. The place most frequently perceived as safe for releasing tension generated in the workplace is the nuclear family, where the spouse or children become the victims of anger. In residential care settings, the care givers may vent similar feelings on the clients.[42]

Beliefs and values derived from the sociocultural context may foster violence. Cultural norms concerning the child's right to protection are, in practice, vague and perhaps deliberately so. Children "belong" to parents and are considered to have only limited rights. The expansion of children's legal rights is often seen by society in general and by parents especially as an infringement of parental authority. Our cultural norms of child rearing allow the use of a certain amount of physical force toward children by their adult care givers. Children in our society are not protected by the law against bodily attack in the same way as adults are. There are still some school districts in the United States where children are the recipients of physical punishment at the hands of school authorities for purposes of discipline. Laws regarding incest tend to be outdated and fail to address adequately the sexual misuse of children. The issue that needs to be considered is the child's right to healthy development. Incest and physical abuse are always violations of the child's rights.[20]

For years schools and local police have implemented programs to educate children on how to protect themselves from strangers who are potential child molesters. Until recently, however, no efforts were made to help children deal with the more pervasive problem of incest. Children have been unsupported in coping with sexual molestation in the home. This situation reflects a societal attitude toward incest that is characterized by denial.

The divorce rate in recent years has produced large numbers of single-parent and blended families. Many of these families are under stress, emotionally and financially. Geographical mobility has scattered nuclear families, leaving many without the support of an extended family. Consequently, nuclear-family relationships are intensified, increasing the risk of conflict and abuse.

A cultural pattern of denial operates to prevent the recognition that men beat, torture, and kill the women they live with. Many women live desperately in a world of almost incredible violence. Their stories are commonplace to lawyers, doctors, psychiatrists, the clergy, and court officials. These wives delay, often for years, reporting the harrowing experiences of their married lives, even to friends and relatives, out of shame, fear, and hopelessness.[43]

Both the police and the legal system have tended to view domestic violence differently from violence between unrelated people. Consequently, there has been a failure to perceive and to deal with offenders as criminals. The tendency of both these societal systems to assume a mediating stance has contributed to a failure to protect the victim.

Elderly people are not respected in this youth-oriented culture. Their needs and problems are not adequately recognized or addressed. This devaluation of elderly people increases their risk of mistreatment.

Social welfare services are inadequately funded and understaffed. Early case finding and prevention are often beyond the scope of available resources. Caseloads of staff members are formidable and permit only superficial assessments, referrals, or brief intervention. Follow-up of even serious cases of abuse of children, spouses, and elderly people is often cursory. Society has been unwilling to invest in social welfare services, and the victims of abuse who need these services are not powerful enough to influence the political system. Regulation and supervision of day care facilities and residential institutions need to be increased.

The prevention of abuse requires fundamental changes in the philosophy and values underlying our social institutions and human relationships. It requires a reconceptualization of childhood and the status of "noncontributing" dependent people in society, a reconsideration of their rights, and a recognition of their needs. It calls for a rejection of the use of force as a means for achieving social ends. Poverty must be eliminated, along with alienating conditions in work and housing environments. The social processes that trigger abuse must be changed.

NURSING PROCESS

The nursing process provides a systematic way of holistically identifying and resolving problems of abuse. Abuse within the family is to a large extent a hidden problem with multigenerational ramifications. There are large numbers of institutionalized people of all ages and children in day care at risk of abuse by care givers; children at risk of parental abuse; spouses vulnerable to physical attack from their partners; and elderly people at risk of mistreatment by their adult children. These people have the right to lives free from neglect and abuse.

Assessment

A broad data base that includes information about the people involved directly and indirectly in the situation, and the environment in which the abuse occurs, is necessary for effective planning and intervention. Promotion of health, prevention of abuse, and remediation of chronic abuse require recognition of the abuse and the need for intervention. Careful and thorough assessment provides the information used in determining the need for care and in planning the care. The assessment process is directed toward identifying problems from both the nurse's and the client's perspective. It also focuses on the identification of a client's or family's strengths and resources and community resources.

Potential victims of physical abuse, neglect, psychological unavailability, verbal abuse, and sexual abuse are encountered by nurses in a variety of settings. Since abuse is often a silent crime, protected from discovery by the abused, the abuser, the family, and the institution, it often goes unrecognized. When nurses are aware of the pattern of physical, behavioral, and interpersonal signs and symptoms of abuse, they are better prepared to recognize the problem.

When abuse is suspected, nurses and other professionals are generally uneasy pursuing the assessment process. Their anger, anxiety, and disgust and their own wish to deny the situation interfere with the interview process. The attitudes conveyed by the nurse during the assessment interview have a profound influence on both the victim's and the offender's ability to disclose important information and on their later participation in treatment.

The initial assessment interview sets the tone of the relationship between the family and the nurse. Care givers must communicate care, concern, and a desire to understand the victim's and offender's predicament. They must define their role as one of giving support and assistance. Confrontation will only increase the offender's need to be defensive. An interview technique must be employed which allows victim and offender to maintain ego and family integrity. The helping process begins when family members can talk about their frustrations, anxieties, and problems. Thus, a sound, trusting relationship must be developed before the members will be able to work with the nurse and expose their fears, feelings, and problems. Once a level of trust is established, the offender and victim will test the sincerity and commitment of the nurse. There will be times when these clients become closed and withdrawn, avoiding contact with the nurse. If the nurse remains available, concerned, caring, and accepting, they may venture to trust again. Both victim and offender fear rejection; they have low self-esteem and little self-acceptance. Consequently, it is difficult to get close to them and to develop a trusting relationship.[30]

The nurse's self-awareness is essential to an effective assessment interview and the development of a holistic care plan. To understand the totality of the abusive incident, nurses must recognize their own biases, values, conflicts, and reactions and must understand that these have an impact on the clients. The nurses must be "tuned in" to their perceptions and how they are influencing their emotions. Self-awareness contributes to a more sensitive and effective relationship with both the victim and the offender and to a more accurate data-collecting process.

It is the pattern of findings from an assessment of a suspected victim that either supports or refutes a diagnosis of neglect. A physical assessment provides data on whether there are new or old injuries, whether the location and type of injury are suspicious, and whether the explanation about how the injury occurred fits the type and location of injury. Examples of injuries associated with abuse and neglect are presented in Table 51-9.

Table 51-9 Physical Signs of Abuse and Neglect

Appearance or Characteristics of the Victim
Bruises in the form of a hand on face or body
Evidence of multiple previous injuries (scars or bruises) in various stages of resolution
Bruises of thumb and fingers on neck
Striped bruises or lacerations on back, buttocks, back of legs, or chest
Rectangular, linear, or round bruises on back, arms, buttocks, or legs
Circumferential bruises or marks caused by chafing on ankles or wrists that suggest the person has been tied up
Bruises at corners of mouth from gags
Human bite marks
Burns at various stages of resolution, particularly of the type inflicted by cigarettes
Injuries on feet, hands, buttocks, or perineum that suggest scalding
Black eyes; deviated septum; fractured jaw; split lip; or loose, missing, or chipped teeth
Bruises and lacerations of lips and ears
Shortness of breath and loud crying when lifted or moved, which suggest fractured ribs
Bald spots with bruising of scalp
Torsion fractures
Dislocated shoulder
X-ray reports indicating healed fractures without explanations that adequately fit the extent and type of injuries present
Retarded growth or development of the child with no history of pathology
Clothing inappropriate to weather conditions
Evidence of poor hygiene; bedsores
No immunizations appropriate to the child's age
Evidence that prescribed medications have not been given as directed

During the physical assessment, during the treatment of the injuries, and after the treatment, data are also collected on how the victim behaves. This behavioral assessment encompasses the victim's reaction to the injury, interactions with care givers, interactions with family members, and interactions with care givers from the referring agency. Examples of behavioral signs associated with physical abuse and neglect are presented in Table 51-10.

Observations of the behavior exhibited by family members or care givers from the referring agency also provide information that can be used in the diagnosis of an abusive situation. Often the person who accompanies the victim is either the abuser or someone who is colluding in keeping the abuse a secret. Examples of behaviors of people other than the victim that suggest abuse are presented in Table 51-11.

Table 51-10 Behavioral Signs of Abuse and Neglect

Behaviors of the Victim
Child is wary of adults or care givers from the referring facility and of physical contact.
Child adapts to hospital unit quickly and without protest.
Child does not seek out or cling to parents for comfort or affection.
Child does not cry when parents leave.
"Grabbing reaction" or "lap hunger" is exhibited by the young child.
Child shows provocative behavior that generates anger in others.
Abnormal eating or drinking habits (for example, drinking from toilet).
Cries excessively, or not at all, when treated in the emergency room for injuries or when receiving injections.
Exhibits either extreme fear or no fear of authority figures.
Behavior is extremely aggressive or very withdrawn and compliant.
Sudden movements by new care givers cause child to flinch.
Disturbed sleeping patterns observed or reported.
Reluctant to talk about injuries, particularly if parent, spouse, adult caretaking child, or care giver from the referring agency is present.
Checks with parent, spouse, adult child, or care giver from referring agency before answering questions.
Allows parent, spouse, adult child, or care giver from referring agency to do all the talking while watching and listening; neither verbally nor nonverbally agreeing, disagreeing, or contributing information.
Becomes evasive when specific questions about the injury are asked.
Avoids eye contact with new care giver.
Asks no questions and makes no requests for information.
Vacant or frozen stare during treatment in the emergency room or during examination in the clinic or home.
Adolescent reveals, or it is reported by others, that he or she has run away or engaged in delinquent activity.
Adolescent reveals, or it is reported by others, that he or she is chronically truant from or late for school and remains very late after school.
Adolescent or child always wears long sleeves and high-necked clothing to hide bruises or self-mutilation scars.
Adolescent or young child noncommittal about relationship with parents.
No social interaction with whoever brought victim in for treatment.
Adult victim appears apologetic and anxious about seeking treatment.
Adult victim does not protest when a family member refuses permission for a diagnostic test such as x-ray.

Table 51-11 Behavioral Signs of Physical Abuse

Behaviors of Family Members and Care Givers from Referring Agency
Parents . . .
Quickly leave child with new care givers and retreat to waiting room or leave setting
Refuse to permit diagnostic tests
Try to silence rather than comfort crying child
Fail to offer comfort or nurturing when victim cries or otherwise shows distress
Parents and care givers . . .
Fail to question treatment, extent of injury, or prognosis
Volunteer little or no information about victim or injury
Generally noncommunicative with the staff members
Appear irritated when questioned about victim or injury
Are critical, angry, impatient, or unsympathetic toward victim
Become evasive or contradict themselves if confronted with questions about the circumstances of the injury
Appear to monitor what the victim says
Insist on remaining in treatment area and maintain constant eye contact with victim
Use nonverbal or verbal silencing strategies if victim volunteers information or expands on an answer to a new care giver's question

When abuse is suspected, the victim must be examined carefully, and all injuries must be documented on the chart. The victim's or, in the case of a child, the parents' explanation of how the injury occurred and the care giver's observations are also documented. The victim's behavior may also be significant, and in such instances it, too, must be documented.

Typical, well-nurtured children cling to their parents in an emergency room; they refuse or are reluctant to go to nurses; they turn to their parents for comfort, assurance, and affection; they protest having to be in the hospital and want to go home. If admitted to an inpatient unit, well-nurtured children protest loudly and tearfully when their parents depart. The behavior of abused children differs markedly. Both in an emergency room and in an inpatient unit, they do not seek out their parents and may seem wary of making contact with them. When admitted to an inpatient unit, they settle into the unit routine quickly and usually continue to size up the situation. At some point they often state that they do not want to go home but would rather stay with the nurses. It is not uncommon to find that these children are hyperactive or have impaired motor activity suggestive of organic brain damage. Younger children, once oriented to the unit, may exhibit a "grabbing reaction." They will bite or grab the care giver and shout for attention. Such behavior stems from a desire to become involved in a "belonging" relationship—a desire of such intensity as to cause these children to grab at care givers and their property. Once an object (or person) is grabbed by a child, it appears to lose the attribute of "property" and thus loses its value for the child, who discards it to seek something else. This behavior is a derivative of "lap hunger," which is an excessive need to be held by care givers.[35]

When a child or adult exhibits injuries that do not fit the description of the reported accident, and abuse is strongly suspected, the current incident may not have been the first to occur. A person who physically abuses his or her child, spouse, or elderly parent frequently "shops" for hospitals. The central registry for the area must be contacted to determine whether the victim has been treated by or is receiving services from another agency because of a previous abusive incident. The data obtained may help to confirm suspicions of abuse, prevent duplication of services, and coordinate services in the follow-up care.

Not all victims of abuse are identified through emergency room treatment for injuries. Nurses employed in schools, well-child clinics, and occupational settings have opportunities for identifying victims, and even abusers in some cases. Adolescents or school-age children may become frequent visitors to the nurse's office. Their complaints may be minor, but in their own way they may be reaching out for help with a much more serious problem of physical or sexual abuse. The assessment of sexual abuse may be guided by the physical and behavioral signs of sexual abuse listed in Table 51-12.

Table 51-12 Physical and Behavioral Signs of Sexual Abuse

Victim's Appearance and Behaviors
Vaginal discharge in infant or child.
Bloody underpants or diapers.
Genital redness, pain, itching, or bruising.
Difficulty walking or sitting.
Urinary tract infections.
Venereal disease.
Somatic complaints: chronic headaches, stomachaches.
Sleeping problems: nightmares, fear at bedtime and nap time, waking up frequently during the night.
Onset of bed-wetting.
Changes in eating habits.
Abrupt change in behavior (becoming withdrawn or hyperactive).
Onset of problems getting along with peers.
Unwillingness to go to a day care center or stay alone with a particular family member or babysitter.
Fear of strangers, particularly men.
New or excessive sexual curiosity or play.
Constant masturbation.
Curling into fetal position.
Excessively seductive behavior by young child.
Hysterical seizures.
Phobias about particular places, people, or things.
Adolescent runs away from home, exhibits delinquent behavior, is promiscuous, is a substance abuser, attempts suicide, or mutilates self.
Child or adolescent has major household responsibilities because mother is ill or out of home for long periods of time.
Child or adolescent acts like wife and mother.
Youngster's school performance and attendance changes abruptly.
Youngster seems withdrawn and less involved with peers.

Nurses who work in nursing homes and other residential care institutions have a responsibility to supervise the care delivered by nursing assistants. This responsibility includes the assessment of clients for evidence of neglect and physical abuse. Failure to provide adequate hygiene for clients who are unable to care for themselves or who are incontinent constitutes neglect. Clients who are unable to feed themselves and who need assistance in maintaining adequate nutrition are vulnerable to neglectful and abusive care givers. Progressive weight loss in the absence of an organic problem may indicate that the client is not being helped sufficiently at mealtime. Bedridden clients and those confined to chairs who exhibit bruises or lacerations that are not the result of a fall may be the victims of aggressive care givers.

Since abuse and neglect are interpersonal phenomena, an assessment of the suspected abuser is needed. This person is as much a client as the victim. Observations of and interactions with this person provide a data base that contributes to the pattern of findings indicating whether an abusive situation exists. A list of behaviors associated with the abuser is presented in Table 51-13.

Table 51-13 The Abuser

Profile
Evidence of dysfunctional attachment to infant in new mother.
Ignores, is critical of, or withdraws from victim.
Fails to nurture or comfort distressed victim.
Verbalizes fears that he or she will hurt the client.
Has history of being abused during childhood.
Evidences psychotic thinking and behavior.
Abuses alcohol or drugs.
Exhibits low self-esteem and low self-acceptance.
Is hostile and depressed.
Is socially isolated and cut off from extended family and peers.
Is impulsive.
Lacks knowledge about child's developmental capacities.
Justifies need to inflict physical punishment by describing the victim's "badness" or lack of cooperation.
Has multiple hypochondriacal complaints and history of several minor surgical interventions.
Explains need for physical punishment to raise "God-fearing" children who know "right" from "wrong."
Has unrealistic expectations of child given developmental age or of elderly person given impairments.
Asks few questions of care givers while victim is being treated.
Refuses to allow child or elderly person to be hospitalized.
Monitors victim's interactions with care givers.
Is belligerent, uncooperative, and resistant during admission of victim to the emergency room for treatment of injuries or when referral to the emergency room is made during a home visit.
Behaves in an aloof manner toward crying or injured child; is not comforting or affectionate.
Describes victim as "difficult" or "hateful."
Father appears to be overprotective of child, limiting relationships with peers.

Diagnosis

The data collected on the abused person, abuser, episodes of abuse, family dynamics, and environment are analyzed and conceptualized. Table 51-14 presents examples of assessment data, nursing diagnoses related to physical and sexual abuse, and the theoretical bases for their formulation.

Outcome Criteria

Once the nursing diagnoses have been formulated, the nurse, in collaboration with the client, establishes a prioritized list of changes in perceptions, attitudes, thinking, and behavior that would resolve the identified problems. These goals serve as outcome criteria for evaluating the effectiveness of the interventions selected by the nurse to facilitate needed changes. In Table 51-15, previously identified nursing diagnoses are presented with related outcome criteria.

The following are examples of outcome criteria for interventions with abusive care givers:

Care giver experiments with new ways to minimize the resistant behavior of clients.

Care giver uses nurse as a resource when problems with a client's cooperation with care are encountered.

Care giver collaborates with nurse in formulating realistic, attainable outcome criteria for clients.

Care giver evaluates client's care and progress with the nurse, using the outcome criteria.

Table 51-14 Nursing Diagnoses

Assessment Data	Theoretical Base	Nursing Diagnosis
Husband-wife sexual relationship is unsatisfying. Mutual masturbation and oral-genital contact by father and daughter. Father rejected by wife. Father abuses alcohol.	Need theory	Sexual abuse of daughter associated with father's low self-esteem and need for love and affection
Oldest preteen daughter given major responsibility for the care of younger siblings and household management. Mother has history of having similar responsibilities as a child and adolescent. Mother sexually abused as child. Mother works full-time in evenings.	Family theory: parentification	Mother-daughter role reversal related to mother's loyalty conflict with her family of origin

(Continued.)

Table 51-14 Continued

Assessment Data	Theoretical Base	Nursing Diagnosis
Male child sleeps with mother. Father is absent from home. Child has overclose relationship with mother. Child exhibits seductive behavior. Child has excessive curiosity about sexual matters.	Systems theory: dysfunctional boundary management	Sexual overstimulation of child associated with impaired generation and gender boundaries
Father was beaten by parents as child. Father punches and beats son with a leather strap. Son has ruptured spleen and multiple bruises and lacerations on back.	Family theory: multigenerational transmission process	Child battering related to intergenerational family pattern of child abuse
Mother ties 2-year-old to potty chair after child wets her pants. Keeps child tied for entire day. Child has bruises and lacerations of wrists and ankles caused by rope used to tie her to potty chair. Mother is 17 years old, unwed, living alone in welfare hotel. Child is dirty and unkempt, has head lice.	Development theory	Physical abuse and neglect of child associated with lack of knowledge about growth and development, immaturity, and lack of support

Table 51-15 Outcome Criteria

Nursing Diagnosis	Outcome Criteria
Sexual abuse of daughter associated with father's need for love and affection Mother-daughter role reversal related to mother's loyalty conflict with her family of origin	Cessation of sexual abuse accompanied by effective family functioning, as evidenced by: Ending of incestuous relationship Active participation in therapy sessions Keeping all appointments for therapy Mother changing from evening to daytime working hours and resuming management of the household Daughter becoming involved in after-school activities Daughter no longer caring for younger siblings Father acknowledging responsibility for incestuous relationship Daughter verbalizing guilt about the relationship Daughter verbalizing anger toward father and mother Couple requesting marital counseling Fewer conflicts between mother and daughter Father acknowledging alcohol problem and seeking help Father participating regularly in AA meetings
Sexual overstimulation of child associated with impaired gender and generation boundaries	Establishment and maintenance of gender and generation boundaries, as evidenced by: Child sleeping in bed in own room Father limiting overnight business trips Mother joining bowling group and leaving son with sitter one evening a week Parents making arrangements for son to be enrolled in nursery school Couple actively participating in counseling Mother developing strategies for managing her feelings when son protests and cries when she leaves him Parents socializing with other couples with children (organizing picnics and entertaining other families) Mother considering part-time employment while son is in nursery school

(Continued.)

Table 51-15 Continued

Nursing Diagnosis	Outcome Criteria
Child battering related to intergenerational family pattern of child abuse	Cessation of multigenerational patterns of abuse, as evidenced by: Cessation of physical abuse of child Active participation of couple in group for abusive parents Father seeking individual therapy Both parents reading literature on child growth and development provided by nurse Parents discussing setting limits with nurse and how to handle them with their son Child ventilating anger toward father and fear of father Child decreasing avoidance of father Child less frequently attempting to provoke father's anger Father discussing feelings about his own abuse Father setting realistic limits with mother and enforcing them without physical punishment
Physical abuse of child associated with lack of knowledge about growth and development, immaturity, and lack of support	More effective parenting by mother, as evidenced by: Cessation of physical abuse of child Participating in YWCA mother-child groups Suspending attempt to toilet train child for 2 months Asking questions about what she has read in booklet provided by nurse on children ages 2 and 3 Investigating cooperative nursery Discussing advantages and disadvantages of getting high school diploma through home-study program and of going to work Tolerating child's exploratory behavior while talking with the nurse Discussing toilet training (strategies and expectations) with nurse Initiating and following through on application for apartment in new subsidized apartment house Contacting family members Beginning toilet training with an expectation that it may take several months Joining cooperative nursery Using nurse as a resource when feeling under stress Calling nurse and requesting visit because she feels depressed and anxious and child is "getting on her nerves" Improvement in child's condition, as evidenced by: Seeking comfort from mother (for example, when finger is pinched by toy) and receiving cuddling, soothing, and affection Being clean and properly dressed Gaining weight and exhibiting new motor-coordination skill in manipulating toys

Intervention

The theoretical formulation of the nursing diagnoses and outcome criteria contributes to the process of selecting nursing interventions. Table 51-16 presents the application of the nursing process to selected problems related to abuse.

If father-daughter incest has been uncovered and charges are being pressed, the father may be convicted and sent to jail. When this occurs, the underlying issues are never resolved. The family is often destitute. The child victim is often blamed for the disruption of the family and left to feel guilty and worthless. If treatment opportunities are not provided for all the members of the family system, the problem may recur when the father returns, and in future generations. If the victim is separated from the family because of either foster placement or running away, the long-term consequences for this child may be devastating. If at all possible,

Table 51-16 Nursing Intervention

Problem	Intervention	Nursing Order
Emotionally deprived child (seeking human relationships by grabbing and exhibiting lap hunger).	Satisfy child's needs for nurturance.	Hold, cuddle, and rock child for a few minutes every hour. Give child what is asked for. Encourage play with toys; start with child on lap and gradually make transition to play which is out of physical contact of care giver. Communicate with child while feeding and giving care. Praise child for interacting and playing appropriately with toys.
Guilty, abusive, hostile parents withdraw from child during visiting hours.	Therapeutic use of self. Involve parents in child's care. Enhance parents' self-esteem.	Initiate contact with family members and inform them of child's progress. Involve parents in the care of child; have them help feed and bathe child; encourage them to play with child. Remain with parents and work with them, giving positive feedback for nurturing behavior. Express concern about how they are managing and the turmoil in the household caused by child's hospitalization.
Impaired decision making associated with immature, isolated, impulsive parents.	Foster thoughtful decision making. Teach parents problem-solving process. Encourage them to socialize.	Guide parents in solving immediate problems that they see as important, using a systematic approach; point out alternatives and explore their consequences. Help parents explore ways to find friends and become involved in the community. Model discussion and analysis of problems, expressions of feelings, and acceptance of differing opinions.
Rigid, dependent parents lack knowledge of normal growth and development and have unrealistic expectations of child.	Provide education on parenting. Explore areas of potential flexibility and reasonableness.	Explore parents' expectations of child. Describe expected behavior for a child this age. Identify the relevant areas of parent-child conflict. Explore alternatives for resolving conflicts with child.
Battered wife.	Facilitate wife's taking responsibility for her own safety.	Refer wife to community shelter for abused women. Determine the capacity and willingness of couple to participate in family therapy. Make referral if both desire to participate in counseling. If husband is resistant to intervention, help wife explore alternatives and her feelings about herself, her husband, and her present situation. Discuss with husband and wife, together or individually, the impact of intrafamily violence on wife and children.
Aides are abusive to confused elderly clients: feed them forcibly; handle them roughly.	Assist aides in revising perceptions, values, and attitudes toward dependent and resistant clients.	Provide information about the needs of elderly people. Explain how elderly clients' behavior is a form of communication. Provide information about how an organic mental disorder can affect a client's behavior. Explain importance of a sense of autonomy to client's well-being. Encourage aides to explore what clients' resistant behavior may mean. Encourage aides to explore their feelings about these clients. Provide positive feedback when aides are patient with clients. Work with aides to identify ways to help clients maintain autonomy and collaborate in their own care. Collaborate with aides in establishing and implementing a reality-orientation program for clients.

keeping the family intact, monitoring the child's safety, and involving the family in therapy is the most desirable course of action.

When a child has been physically abused, seriously neglected, or sexually molested, and requires hospitalization for an extended period of time, the vulnerability of the child and the pain caused by the abuse may lead the nurses to project their own emotional needs onto the child and to entertain rescue fantasies. If these dynamics develop, the parents are excluded and the child is placed in an even more untenable position. The nurse cannot fulfill the rescue "contract," and the child is further isolated from the family. For example:

> Mike, a 3-year-old hospitalized after being abused by his mother, became the favorite of Ms. D., a member of the nursing staff. This nurse stayed overtime to feed him, bought him toys, and spent as much time as possible during the working day playing with him. When Mike's mother visited, Ms. D. excluded her from her son's care and spoke to her in a curt, hostile manner. In time, the mother visited less frequently and interacted minimally with her son and the staff. When it was time for discharge, social services decided to return Mike to his home with follow-up counseling. The day Mike was discharged, he resisted being dressed by his mother and cried for Ms. D. The mother was visibly angry and reluctantly allowed the nurse to dress him. Ms. D. disagreed with the discharge plans but was unable to intervene. Mike could not remain in the hospital; no space was available in the community child-care facility; no foster home was available; and the mother had agreed to accept counseling. Ms. D. could not actualize her rescue fantasy, and the child was returned to his mother. Because of the nurse's overinvolvement, the mother was rejected by her child. The mother learned nothing about her own or her child's needs and how they could be met. Since it was highly probable that she would not follow through with counseling, the risk of another abusive incident remained.

In this case, the nurse participated in the development of a situation that left the mother in an outside position. A more effective nursing approach would be to involve the mother in the child's care to the greatest extent possible; periodically and briefly model effective mothering behaviors; empathize with the mother's situation; help her work through her feelings; and be available as a helpful resource.

Evaluation

The nursing care plan is designed to change the interaction of those who are significantly involved in an abusive or neglectful situation. Outcome criteria, which interact with the nursing diagnoses and the interventions, are used to evaluate the effectiveness of the actions taken to resolve the problem. If the outcome criteria are discrete and observable, they provide feedback to both client and care giver on progress and issues that require further intervention. The use of outcome criteria in the evaluation process is illustrated by the case study given below; the nursing care plan for the abuser in the case (Mrs. C.) is presented in Table 51-17, and the nursing care plan for the victim (Mrs. K.) in Table 51-18:

> Mrs. K. is an 80-year-old woman with severe arthritis, periodic impaired bladder control, and recent rapid development of cataracts. She refuses to wear any type of pad to absorb urine. She needs assistance to move from bed to chair. She refuses to use a walker. An avid reader, she is now deprived of this activity because of cataracts. Up until a year ago, she resided in her own home, was independent, and was even able to drive a car. One year ago, she fell and fractured her hip. During her convalescence, her arthritis progressed and her hip did not heal as expected. At the time of discharge from the hospital, she had limited mobility and was judged not capable of living independently. She moved into her daughter's home and has since resided there.
>
> Mrs. C., age 50, has full responsibility for the care of her mother. Her younger siblings, at the time of the mother's discharge from the hospital, refused to have Mrs. K. in their homes. All were working full time and had no room for their mother. Mrs. C.'s last child had left home. She and her husband agreed to the mother's moving in with them. The first 6 months were uneventful, according to Mrs. C. Her mother participated in her own care. She was able to be left alone for periods of time during the day and evenings. Recently, however, she refuses to help herself in any way. If she is left alone for any length of time, she purposefully slips out of her chair. She is belligerent and hostile. Increasingly, Mrs. C. has been feeling overwhelmed, physically exhausted, and angry about the situation. Her marital relationship has deteriorated.
>
> Last weekend Mrs. C. had planned to attend a party with her husband. Mrs. K. adamantly refused to go to bed and threw objects at a hired sitter and her daughter. The sitter left, refusing to stay. The husband went to the party without Mrs. C. Mrs. C. physically

Table 51-17 Evaluation: The Abuser (Mrs. C.)

Diagnosis	Outcome Criteria	Intervention	Evaluation
Physical abuse associated with caretaker daughter's burnout	More effective management of care of elderly parent, as evidenced by: Selecting option that provides periodic relief from responsibility.	Provide feedback on extent of burden and need for relief. Explore caretaking options (nursing home, home health aide, involvement of siblings). Ascertain financial capability for options. Encourage active decision making.	Client selects live-in housekeeper and part-time home health aide to assume responsibility for care.
	Ventilating feelings of guilt about abuse.	Facilitate expressions and resolution of feelings.	Verbalizes feelings about abuse in context of caretaking burden.
	Ventilating anger toward siblings for not being supportive.	Explore feelings about options.	Verbalizes anger and resentment toward siblings.
	Recognizing personal decision making that led to the assumption of responsibility.	Encourage active decision making.	Vacillates between feeling that she chose the burden and feeling that it was dumped on her.
	Recognizing reluctance to confront siblings or ask for help.		Admits reluctance in asking for support and acknowledges that she expected siblings to volunteer.
	Confronting siblings and enlisting their financial support.		Enlists financial contribution from all siblings.
Substance abuse associated with mismanagement of stress in caretaking role	Reduces or stops alcohol consumption.	Confront client on excessive alcohol consumption.	Drinks only on social occasions and never to excess.
Marital conflict associated with overinvestment in care of mother	Recognizes her sense of powerlessness when mother is demanding.	Explore options for personal lifestyle.	
	Recognizes when mother is manipulating her.		Continues to allow "guilt tripping" to occur in relation to mother.
	Chooses not to let mother interfere with planned activities with husband.		Agrees to take a long weekend vacation with husband.
	Participates in work or social activities outside home.		Continues to remain at home to supervise housekeeper and home health aide.

dragged her mother to a bed and hit her several times, causing a black eye and a fractured wrist. Mrs. C. admits to a recent problem with alcohol abuse. The community health nurse contacted the family after a referral.

SUMMARY

Abuse within families and institutions, including physical abuse, neglect, verbal abuse, psychological unavailability, and sexual abuse, is widespread; but it is often unrecognized by health professionals and largely unreported.

The abuse of the powerless in our society has roots in the past. Violence is a part of our culture, and it is not likely to be eradicated easily in the near future. It is learned and passed on from generation to generation.

Prevention, case finding, and treatment are challenges that nurses in all health care settings must accept. Each member of society has the right to have his or her basic needs met and deserves the

Table 51-18 Evaluation: The Victim (Mrs. K.)

Diagnosis	Outcome Criteria	Intervention	Evaluation
Belligerent and oppositional behavior associated with increased dependence and physical disabilities	Refusal to participate in abusive situation, as evidenced by:		
	Abstention from throwing objects.	Confront client on throwing and slipping out of chair.	Client has thrown no objects at anyone for 3 weeks.
	Cessation of slipping deliberately out of chair.	Explore other ways of getting attention or help.	Stays in chair but yells and bangs on table for attention rather than using bell provided.
	Talking about frustration of being dependent, and unable to read. Talking about sadness related to losing home.	Encourage verbalization of feelings about situation.	Verbalizes feelings to nurse. Talks once in a while with daughter about frustration and sadness.
	Participating in self-care.	Insist on participation in self-care within physical limitations.	Sporadically makes attempts to wash and dress herself.
	Using walker.	Teach client how to use her walker. Collaborate on developing daily routine.	Uses walker with assistance.
	Agreeing to see eye doctor.	Explore remediation of cataract problem. Meanwhile, provide large-print reading material from library and "talking books."	Is unwilling to go to physician for evaluation of cataracts. Uses resources. Complains about what is available.
	Agreeing to use pads for urinary incontinence.	Explain advantages of pads for urinary incontinence.	Uses pads willingly except when daughter provides care.
Vengeful attitude toward daughter associated with abusive incident	Recognizes how own management of feelings is expressed and the impact of this expression on daughter.	Explore the mutual participation of client and daughter.	Client acknowledges some participation but counters with unrealistic expectations of duties of a daughter.
	Berates daughter less for her failings; praises the siblings (who refused to take her into their homes) less.	Discuss and provide feedback on daughter's attempts to support and care for mother and daughter's feelings when mother criticizes her and praises siblings (who visit mother only for a short period of time every other month).	Is less critical of caretaking daughter. Occasionally still confronts daughter about abusive incident. Uses telephone to berate other siblings for abandoning her.

opportunity to strive to fulfill growth-promoting needs. Nurses are in strategic positions in a variety of health care settings to help both victims and offenders.

The application of the nursing process to abusive situations provides a systematic way of helping victims and offenders alter their destructive patterns of interaction and develop more effective patterns that promote growth and are mutually satisfying.

REFERENCES

1. J. E. Brody, "Emotional Deprivation Seen as Devastating Form of Child Abuse." *The New York Times*, December 20, 1983.
2. N. H. Giordano and J. A. Giordano, "Elder Abuse: A Review of the Literature," *Social Work*, May-June 1984, pp. 232–236.
3. J. H. Daniel, R. L. Hampton, and E. H. Newberger, "Child Abuse and Accidents in Black Families: A

Controlled Comparative Study," *American Journal of Orthopsychiatry*, vol. 43, no. 4, 1983, pp. 645–653.
4. B. J. Justice and R. Justice, *The Abusing Family*, Human Sciences Press, New York, 1976.
5. "Brawl in the Family," *Science News*, May 5, 1985, p. 287.
6. J. Herman, "Recognition and Treatment of Incestuous Families," *International Journal of Family Therapy*, vol. 5, no. 2, 1983, pp. 81–91.
7. E. Magnuson, M. Grant, and J. Wilde, "Child Abuse: The Ultimate Betrayal," *Time*, September 5, 1983, p. 20.
8. R. S. Kempe and C. Kempe, *The Common Secret: Sexual Abuse of Children and Adolescents*, Freeman, New York, 1984.
9. J. O'Reilly, B. Dolan, D. Taylor, and E. Taylor, "Wife Beating: The Silent Crime," *Time*, September 5, 1983.
10. J. L. Edleson, "Working with Men Who Batter," *Social Work*, May-June 1984, pp. 237–242.
11. L. Burder, "Ward Orders More Arrests in Domestic Violence," *The New York Times*, April 3, 1984.
12. D. Robinson, "How Can We Protect Our Elderly?" *Parade Magazine*, February 17, 1983, pp. 4–7.
13. "A Hidden Epidemic," *Newsweek*, May 14, 1984, pp. 30–36.
14. "Most Victims Acquainted with Child Sexual Abuser," *Bridgeport Post*, May 9, 1984.
15. A. C. Serrano and D. W. Gunzuburger, "An Historical Perspective of Incest," *Family Therapy*, vol. 5, no. 2, 1984, pp. 70–80.
16. L. Ledray, "Victims of Incest," *American Journal of Nursing*, August 1984, pp. 1010–1014.
17. J. Herman and L. Hirschman, "Families at Risk for Father-Daughter Incest," *American Journal of Psychiatry*, vol. 138, July 1981, pp. 967–970.
18. C. Adams-Tucker, "Proximate Effects of Sexual Abuse in Childhood: A Report on 28 Children," *American Journal of Psychiatry*, vol. 139, no. 10, 1982, pp. 1252–1256.
19. C. Henry Kempe et al., "The Battered Child Syndrome," *Journal of the American Medical Association*, vol. 181, July 1962, pp. 17–24.
20. R. S. Hunter et al., "Antecedents of Child Abuse and Neglect in Premature Infants," *Pediatric Currents*, vol. 27, no. 7, 1978, p. 55.
21. B. Justice and R. Justice, *The Broken Taboo*, Human Sciences Press, New York, 1979.
22. R. Summit and J. Kryso, "Sexual Abuse of Children: A Clinical Spectrum," *American Journal of Orthopsychiatry*, vol. 48, 1978, pp. 237–251.
23. M. de Young, "Incest Victims and Offenders: Myths and Realities," *Journal of Psychosocial Nursing and Mental Health Services*, vol. 19, no. 10, 1985, pp. 37–39.
24. B. DeMott, "The Pro-Incest Lobby," *Psychology Today*, vol. 3, 1980, pp. 11–12 and 15–16.
25. A. Silber, "Childhood Seduction, Parental Pathology and Hysterical Symptomatology: The Genesis of an Altered State of Consciousness," *International Journal of Psychoanalysis*, vol. 60, no. 1, 1979, pp. 109–116.
26. "Incest and Vulnerable Children," *Science News*, October 15, 1979.
27. M. H. Silbert and A. M. Pines, "Early Sexual Exploitation as an Influence in Prostitution," *Social Work*, vol. 20, 1983, pp. 285–289.
28. V. R. Lichtenstein, "The Battered Woman: Guidelines for Effective Nursing Intervention," *Issues in Mental Health Nursing*, vol. 3, no. 3, July-September 1981, pp. 237–250.
29. U. Dibble and M. A. Straus, "Some Social Structure Determinants of Inconsistency between Attitudes and Behavior: The Case of Family Violence," *Journal of Marriage and the Family*, February 1980, pp. 71–80.
30. D. K. Snyder and L. Fruchtman, "Differential Patterns of Wife Abuse: A Data-Based Typology," *Journal of Consulting and Clinical Psychology*, vol. 49, no. 6, 1981, pp. 878–885.
31. "Battered Wives . . . and Coeds," *Science News*, September 17, 1983, p. 187.
32. D. Margolnick, "Use of Experts on Battering Is Upheld in Women's Trials," *The New York Times*, July 25, 1984.
33. "The Era of Family Violence," *Science News*, November 3, 1979.
34. P. Eastman, "Elders under Siege," *Psychology Today*, January 1984, p. 30.
35. M. G. Morris et al., "Toward Prevention of Child Abuse," *Children Today*, vol. 4, no. 2, 1974.
36. R. Gladston, "Preventing the Abuse of Little Children," *American Journal of Orthopsychiatry*, vol. 45, no. 3, 1975, pp. 372–380.
37. S. Asch et al., "Postpartum Reactions: Some Unrecognized Variations," *American Journal of Psychiatry*, vol. 131, 1974, pp. 870–874.
38. A. Green et al., "Child Abuse: Pathological Syndrome of Family Interaction," *American Journal of Psychiatry*, vol. 131, August 1974, pp. 882–886.
39. E. Lau and J. Kosberg, "Abuse of the Elderly by Informal Care Providers: Practice and Research Issues," paper presented at the 31st Annual Meeting of the Gerontological Society, Dallas, Tex., November 20, 1978.
40. M. D. Haddock and W. M. McQueen, "Assessing Employee Potentials for Abuse," *Journal of Clinical Psychology*, vol. 39, no. 6, 1983, pp. 1021–1029.
41. S. Steinmetz, "Battered Parents," *Society*, vol. 15, 1978, pp. 54–55.
42. M. R. Block and J. D. Sinnott, *The Battered Elder Syndrome: An Exploratory Study*, University of Maryland Center on Aging, 1979.
43. M. Van Stolk, "Beaten Women, Battered Children," *Children Today*, vol. 5, no. 2, 1976, pp. 8–12.

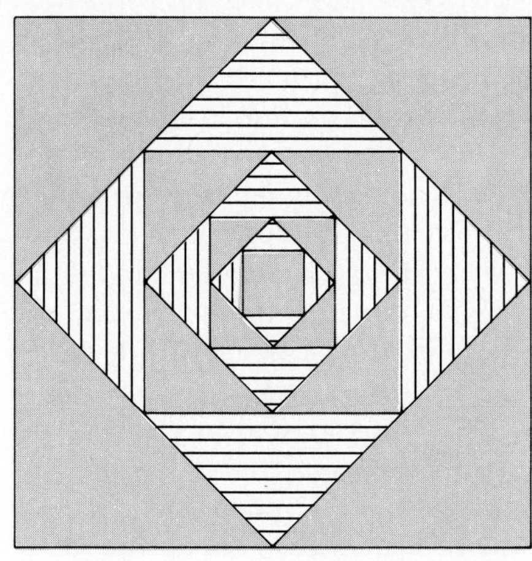

CHAPTER 52
Rape

Anita M. Leach

LEARNING OBJECTIVES

After studying this chapter, the student will be able to:

1. Define *rape.*
2. Describe motivations of rapists.
3. Describe acute rape syndrome.
4. List behaviors expected of clients and their families in the follow-up phase of a rape crisis.
5. Apply the nursing process in the care of rape victims.
6. Evaluate the nursing care of rape victims.
7. Discuss individual and community efforts aimed at preventing rape.

Rape, a form of abuse, is legally defined as an act of sexual intercourse, such as penile-vaginal contact, that is forced upon an unwilling victim.[1] It is considered a violent crime and an act of aggression against a person that degrades, dehumanizes, and violates the victim's sense of self.[2] The impact of a rape is felt in every part of the self. The painful physical assault and the emotional and spiritual trauma have serious implications not only for the victim but for the legal and health care system, and for the social, cultural, economic, and political environment of both victim and rapist.

Nurses need to know about rape, its victims, and its perpetrators because they intervene with victims and rapists in all areas of their practice. An emergency room nurse is generally the first health care professional to whom a victim relates after an assault. A psychiatric nurse or a community health nurse may intervene on a crisis hot line during the follow-up phase of treatment. When the physical injuries resulting from a rape are serious, the victim is admitted for inpatient care by medical-surgical and gynecological nurses. Nurses who work in prisons treat not only rapists but also victims of homosexual rape that occurs within the prison system. Finally, rape occurs in communities and has a profound impact on their resources.

The purpose of this chapter is to acquaint students with the dynamics of male-female rape and rape trauma syndrome (RTS), and with the nursing care of rape victims.

DYSYNCHRONOUS HEALTH PATTERNS

Rape Trauma Syndrome

Rape trauma syndrome is a crisis that occurs in two stages, disorganization and reorganization. Physical, emotional, and behavioral stress reactions occur in both stages and may be acute or persist over a long period of time.[3]

Types of Rape

Rape is the sexual invasion of a victim's body by force. It is a violation not only of the physical being but also of the victim's mental and spiritual wholeness. For the purposes of discussion and study, rape may be classified in various ways.

Burgess and Holmstrom[4] outlined three types of rape on the basis of the degree to which the victim withholds *consent.* The first type of rape is *sex without consent;* the victim is simply taken unaware and raped. The second type is *statutory rape;* the victim is not able to consent to the sexual act because of either chronological age or developmental age. Children, the mentally disabled, and the elderly may be victims of statutory rape. The third type is rape in a *"sex-stress" situation;* the victim initially consents, or implies consent, but later withdraws consent because something goes drastically wrong in the relationship. For example, a married woman may refuse to have sex with her husband because he is drunk and violent. If he uses force to have intercourse, that would be considered rape.

A second way to analyze or classify rape is to examine its *causes.* Such an analysis (unlike analysis on the basis of consent) is in terms of the rapist rather than the victim. A number of research studies have attempted to find the causes of rape; the findings indicate that alcohol abuse is frequently a factor in rape and that rape is more likely to be committed by people who lack social or personal control.[3] Social control may be absent during wars or among people in prison, for example. When personal control is absent, the rapist has no moral reason to refrain from rape.

A third way to analyze rape is in terms of *styles;* here again the focus is on the rapist. Burgess and Holmstrom reported two main styles used in rapes. A *blitz rape* occurs when the rapist and the victim have had no previous interaction; the victim is taken unaware. An *impulsive rape* occurs during another crime; the presence of a victim is exploited for rape as well as the original crime.[4]

Rape has also been analyzed in a fourth way, in terms of the rapist's *motivation. Sexual-gratification rape,* as the term implies, has sexual gratification as its goal; force is the means for achieving the goal. *Power rape* occurs when the rapist is motivated to some extent by a need for sexual gratification but has a simultaneous need to demonstrate power and control over the victim. It is the need to demonstrate power and control that is primary. In this type of rape, then, force is both the means and the end. *Anger rape* has as its goal violence and the degradation and humiliation of the victim. In this type of rape, sexual gratification is the means for achieving the goal. About 35 percent of convicted rapists are "anger rapists." The anger rapist is most likely to injure a victim fatally; it is this kind of rapist who is most often portrayed by the media.

A fifth way to consider rape is in terms of *circumstances*. For example, when there has been some interaction between rapist and victim before the assault and deceit or betrayal is used to obtain access to the victim, the rape is called a *confidence rape*.[4] A woman who is hitchhiking and is picked up by a man who drives her to a deserted area and rapes her is a victim of a confidence rape. *Group rape* is the victimization of a person by more than one assailant. It is characterized by "sexual performance behavior" on the part of the rapists and is motivated by anger or the need for sexual gratification or power and control. Some researchers see group rape as a form of extreme acting-out behavior.[4] Some group rapes of women by men involve the participation of women other than the victim who either entrap the victim or willingly participate in intercourse with the men.

The classifications of rape described above apply primarily (although not exclusively) to male-female rape. There are, however, other kinds of rape. Male-male rape is an increasingly common phenomenon; it occurs most frequently in same-sex institutions such as prisons and has all the characteristics of male-female rape. Some male-male rapes may be motivated by the need for sexual gratification, but such rape more often represents a need for power and dominance on the part of the rapist.[3] The nursing process discussed in this chapter may be modified when nurses care for rape victims who are male.

DSM III

There is no specific diagnostic category for rape trauma syndrome in the *Diagnostic and Statistical Manual of Mental Disorders* (DSM III), although *posttraumatic stress syndrome* has been applied as an appropriate medical diagnosis. Unresolved rape trauma may leave the victim with one or several of the anxiety disorders, including phobia, panic disorder, or a generalized anxiety disorder.

Epidemiology

Rape is one of the fastest-growing forms of abuse in the United States. The Uniform Crime Reports of 1980 showed 82,088 reported cases of rape compared with 37,000 cases reported in 1970.[1] Despite this tremendous increase, the prevalance of rape as a health care problem is probably considerably larger than the reported statistics indicate. It is estimated that only one-third of all rapes are reported in victimization surveys.[2] Fear of retaliation, shame, or a false sense of guilt may influence a considerable number of rape victims to fail to report the crime. The victims who most frequently fail to report forced sexual intercourse as rape are married women sexually victimized by their husbands, children raped by family members, and college-age women.[2]

Statistics indicate that rape by a stranger occurs most frequently in urban areas, during the summer months, in public places such as parks and playgrounds, and near the victim's home. Black women are victims twice as often as white women, and weapons are used about 45 percent of the time. Rape victims range in age from 4 to 80, although the largest number of female victims are between the ages of 16 and 24. In addition to painful penetration, 92 percent of rapes involve other injuries such as cuts, bruises, black eyes, and scratches. About 10 percent of victims of rape by a stranger also receive internal injuries, broken bones or teeth, and gunshot or knife wounds.[2]

PATTERNS OF INTERACTION: PERSON

The victim's emotional response to rape is known as *rape trauma syndrome* (RTS). The most common reactions observed in clients immediately after rape include fear of injury, mutilation, and death; feelings of humiliation, degradation, shame, and guilt; embarrassment; self-blame; anger; and wish for revenge. The typical guilt reaction, for example, is expressed in questions like "Why me?" and "What did I do to provoke this?" According to Burgess, rape trauma syndrome occurs in two stages: *disorganization* and *reorganization*. In the immediate and acute phase, the victim's life is completely disrupted or disorganized by the crisis. This is followed by a long-term process during which the victims reorganize their lifestyle. Physical, emotional, and behavioral stress reactions resulting from the life-threatening rape occur in both stages.[5]

Behaviors in the acute stage of RTS include many physical symptoms as well as a wide range of emotional reactions, including those described above. In the long-term or reorganization phase, the victim's behaviors may include changing residence, seeking support from a social network, and dealing with nightmares and transitory phobias. In response to discussion of rape, some victims willingly express feelings of anxiety, fear, or anger by talking, shaking, crying, smiling, muscle tenseness, and restlessness. Burgess and Holmstrom labeled this an *expressed* emotional style. Other women respond in a *controlled* emotional style, masking their feelings with a subdued, calm, or composed affect. A *compounded reaction* to rape occurs when the victim has a previous history of psychiatric, physical, or social difficulties.[5]

Because a significant number of women do not report rape, nurses should be alert to *silent rape syndrome,* a reaction that occurs in a victim who has not told anyone she has been raped.[5] Silent rape syndrome is characterized by long periods of silence during an interview, blocking of associations, stuttering, and minor physical distress that are manifestations of anxiety and emotional discomfort. Reports by the client of sudden marked irritability, avoidance of relationships with men, or a marked change in sexual behavior are signs of unresolved emotional reactions to rape. The sudden onset of phobic reactions to being alone, going outside, or being inside are all indications to the nurse that intervention is necessary. Some rape victims also experience a loss of self-confidence and self-esteem. Others develop an attitude of self-blame; find themselves feeling paranoid; or experience nightmarish, violent dreams.[5]

PATTERNS OF INTERACTION: FAMILY

When a woman is the victim of rape, the significant man in her life (spouse, father, brother, boyfriend) will also react emotionally. Not infrequently, significant relationships deteriorate as a result of the crisis of rape. Reactions of fathers, husbands, brothers, and boyfriends range from indignation to denial. Overprotectiveness, revengefulness, helplessness, and withdrawal are also responses of significant others.[6]

Real feelings are sometimes denied by the family, and the feelings that are expressed may be just the opposite of what they are experiencing. Family members may "rally around" during the crisis, providing emotional support, but "move out" after the acute reactions have subsided. One victim tearfully described her parents' distrust of her story about her rape, stating that they chose instead to believe that she had in some way provoked the assault. Another woman described the pain she had felt when her brothers had accused her of not resisting the attack and had implied that she could have prevented the rape.

Typically, the frequency of sexual activity with one's usual partner sharply decreases following a rape incident. In one study, only 19 percent of women reported no change in sexual activity. Among the women in this study, 50 percent reported changes in their responses to their usual sexual partners, including worry about their partner's reaction, aversion to certain activities, and discomfort and pain during intercourse.[7]

Integration and resolution of feelings after a rape take varying lengths of time but are positively facilitated for the victim when family and significant others are supportive. When the family and the significant male partner are supportive, the rape victim is likely to adjust outwardly within a short time after the rape.

PATTERNS OF INTERACTION: ENVIRONMENT

Rape is a societal problem unrelated to the victim's age, social class, culture, or race. It involves not only health care professionals but the criminal justice system and the entire community. Police officers gather evidence, file reports, make arrests, and assist the victim in identification of suspects. Victims may need lawyers to help them with the process of filing charges and testifying at a trial. Health care professionals provide crisis, supportive, and preventive services.

Ideally, nurses or professionals in rape crisis centers form a network of advocates for the rape victim. Advocates arrange for needed services during the acute phase as well as follow-up services such as long-term counseling and legal assistance.

When there is a well-planned and comprehensive community program of education, prevention, and intervention, victims usually receive the necessary support. On the other hand, when police officers, medical helpers, or the legal system are unsupportive or judgmental, nurses need to assume a strong advocacy role to protect the victim.

NURSING PROCESS

Before nurses can work successfully in programs for prevention of rape, and before they can intervene skillfully in dealing with rape victims, they must be aware of their own responses to rape, as well as to societal biases and myths. Self-awareness is a prerequisite. If the nurse is a woman, she may have feelings of generalized anger about the violence and may identify with the helplessness of the victim. Some nurses, whether male or female, may have personal values or preconceptions about rape that cloud what they hear of victims' stories. Still other nurses may themselves have been rape victims; their feelings, if unresolved, may affect their ability to intervene successfully.

Because a nurse is frequently the first person with whom the victim feels "safe," the nurse may become the object of the victim's rage. In such circumstances, nurses must remain calm and therapeutic. Table 52-1 suggests questions that will facilitate self-assessment of a nurse's reactions to rape victims and their families. Being aware of one's reactions to rape and taking measures to correct inappropriate responses will facilitate therapeutic interaction with the victim.

Table 52-1 Rape

Nurse's Self-Assessment
How am I reacting to the rape victim?
What are my feelings about the rape victim?
Are my feelings interfering with my care of the client?
Have I been able to maintain a "neutral" position with the rape victim and her family?
Am I identifying with the rape victim? With her spouse?
What are my biases about rape?
Do I have preconceptions that cloud the accuracy of my perceptions of the rape victim's story?
What are my feelings about the client's family? About her spouse?
Am I sufficiently involved in community efforts to prevent rape?
Do I use self-protective measures as a means of preventing rape?

Assessment

The Victim

When applying the nursing process to victims of rape, nurses must consider both the short-term crisis and the follow-up phase of care. Rape victims are to be considered normal people who were capable of managing their lives before the crisis. The nurse uses the same assessment guidelines for assessing any crisis. The victim's perceptions of the event and the presence or absence of supportive significant others are additional components of the assessment process. Another crucial component is the physical examination of the victim.

HISTORY OF THE RAPE. The following questions will elicit the necessary information about the rape itself:

1. When and where did the rape take place?
2. Did you know your assailant? If so, what was your relationship to him?
3. What was the nature of the sexual act?
4. How long ago did the rape occur?
5. Did you struggle with the assailant?
6. What conversation, if any, occurred between you and your assailant? What did he say? What did you say?
7. Did you struggle before, during, or after the rape?
8. Did your assailant threaten you physically or verbally?
9. Was this a first sexual experience?
10. What were your feelings about sex before the rape?
11. How have your feelings about sex changed?
12. Have you been raped or attacked before?

SILENT RAPE SYNDROME. If silent rape syndrome is a possibility, the following questions are appropriate:

1. Have you been avoiding relationships with men? If so, since when?
2. Has there been a sudden onset of excessive fear?

3. Does the client's spouse complain of marked changes in sexual behavior?
4. Is the client afraid to be alone?

PHYSICAL ASSESSMENT. Following are guidelines for the physical assessment:

1. What is the client's general appearance?
2. Ask the client: Have you bathed, douched, showered, urinated or defecated, changed clothes, inserted or removed a tampon, or treated a wound since you were assaulted?
3. What are the vital signs?
4. Are there any signs of physical trauma such as bruises, scratches, swellings, teeth marks, or abrasions? Where are they located?
5. How long are scratches, what size are bruises, etc.?
6. Does the gynecological examination show signs of penetration?
7. Have vaginal specimens been collected, in order to test for the presence of semen and venereal disease?
8. Have the specimens been accurately labeled?
9. In the case of sodomy, has the mouth, throat, or anus been swabbed?
10. If the victim scratched the assailant, have fingernail scrapings been taken?

EMOTIONAL AND MENTAL ASSESSMENT. Following are guidelines for the emotional and mental assessment:

1. Is the victim reacting in an expressed or a controlled emotional style?
2. How is the client behaving (crying, sobbing, silent, pacing, shouting, hyperventilating, etc.)?
3. What is the client's mental status?
4. Are the client's behaviors consistent with or different from usual patterns of coping? How?
5. Ask the client: What were you feeling at the time of the rape?
6. Ask the client: How are you feeling now?
7. Ask the client: What is most painful or difficult for you to remember?
8. How does the victim describe the attack? (Quote the victim's exact words in the record.)

SPIRITUAL ASSESSMENT. Following are guidelines for the spiritual assessment:

1. What are the client's values and attitudes about her body?
2. How will those attitudes influence her reaction to rape?
3. What strengths does the client have that will help in resolving the rape crisis?
4. What religious beliefs of the victim will help in resolving the crisis?
5. What beliefs of the client will hinder resolution of the crisis?
6. How has the victim transcended difficult situations in the past?
7. How will the victim's philosophy of life help or hinder recovery from the rape attack?
8. Does the client have a supportive relationship with a therapist, counselor, or minister?
9. Is the client angry with God because of the rape?

THE LEGAL RECORD. A complete assessment of a rape victim for legal purposes includes physical findings as well as data about the emotional, mental, and spiritual state of the client. Nurses have crucial roles in the legal proceedings that follow a rape. They are frequently called as witnesses when a suspect is apprehended and a trial is held. Prosecution often depends on the care with which the physical examination was performed and documented. The victim's medical record will be a major source of evidence in a trial; it should be complete and accurate, and should include exact details. Since the court assumes that the medical record is correct, it should contain as many of the victim's words as possible.

A complete history of a rape includes the time lapse between the rape and the examination, as well as whether or not the victim bathed, douched, showered, urinated, defecated, treated her wounds, or changed clothes before the medical examination. It should also include a complete physical assessment. The presence and location of abrasions, bruises, swellings, lacerations, or teeth marks should be noted. The gynecological record should indicate whether penetration took place, whether or not genital injury occurred, and the results of screening tests for venereal disease and pregnancy. If the victim gives permission, photographs should be taken of injuries both before and after clothing is removed. Clothing should be checked for blood stains and the presence of semen. Clothing should then be carefully removed from the victim and given to the police. The record should also note what other material evidence was collected and to whom it was given.

A brief, concise, and complete description of the incident should also be entered in the medical record. In addition to the physical findings, described above, the signs of mental, spiritual, and emotional trauma should be noted. Tears, trembling, sobbing, hyperventilation, and withdrawal should be recorded. Negative as well as positive findings should be noted and may assist in protecting everyone involved in the incident and its investigation.

The Family

The family and social support system of the victim, as well as the effect of the rape on the significant man in the victim's life, need to be assessed by the nurse. The following questions will supply the nurse with a data base about the victim's family and social support system:

1. Does the victim have friends?
2. Who are they?
3. How will they respond to the event?
4. Who is the significant man in the victim's life (husband, father, boyfriend, brother)?
5. How is he coping?
6. Is the victim able to talk with significant others about the rape?
7. Can the victim rely on others? Or does she feel she will be rejected?
8. Do the family and friends want to talk to a counselor?
9. Are the family responding with caring or with blaming?
10. Who will accompany the victim home after the initial examination?
11. What does the victim do for entertainment?
12. Does she have hobbies?
13. How soon does the victim return to social and leisure-time activities?

The Community

Following are guidelines for use in assessing the community:

1. Have the police been notified?
2. How supportive is the involvement of personnel from the criminal justice system?
3. What network is already established for assisting the rape victim?
4. What community groups has the victim been involved with recently?
5. Can any community groups be relied on to support the client during the acute and follow-up phases of intervention?

Diagnosis

Nursing diagnoses of the rape victim will be related to the phase of the crisis and the specific requests for assistance made by the client. Clients may be seeking medical or police intervention or may want only counseling to restore their emotional well-being. Burgess and Holmstrom[5] noted that most rape victims look for concern and empathy and a person to whom they can ventilate their feelings about the rape. Others seek clarification of their feelings or advice about physical, social, legal, emotional, or spiritual problems associated with the rape.

Table 52-2 outlines selected nursing diagnoses appropriate in the acute and follow-up phases of a rape crisis.

Table 52-2 Nursing Diagnoses: Rape Crisis

Acute Phase
Evidence of sexual penetration associated with violent rape
Crying, skeletal muscle tension, anger, fear, hyperventilation, self-blame, stomach upset related to rape trauma
Uncertainty about wanting to involve police related to embarrassment and self-blame
Multiple bruises, lacerations, and abrasions
Verbalization of need for physical, mental, and spiritual care related to rape trauma
Marked changes in sexual relationship with husband or boyfriend related to silent rape syndrome
Follow-Up Phase
Insensitivity by family members correlated with lack of accurate information about rape
Decreased sexual activity for past 4 months related to rape trauma
Nightmares associated with rape that occurred 4 months ago
Precipitous change of job related to silent rape trauma
Verbalization of feelings about rapist associated with resolution of rape crisis

Outcome Criteria

Outcome criteria established by nurses caring for rape victims depend on the client's request. The victim may request medical, police, or psychological intervention; may be uncertain about her needs; or may ask for help with a general inability to verbalize needs and wants.[5] The planning of health care professionals aims at restoring the victim's previous functioning, self-respect, and dignity. The ultimate goal is restoration of the client's emotional control so that feelings related to the rape do not reactively determine actions and judgments. Specific outcome criteria appropriate when nursing the rape victim include the following:

1. The victim and the family will verbalize the need for intervention and cooperate with interventions that are offered.
2. The victim and the family will be referred to a supportive network of services.
3. The victim and the family will verbalize the ability to return for additional help if delayed symptoms occur.

Intervention

Intervention with the Client

Short-term, issue-oriented intervention begins immediately in order to facilitate the victim's recovery from the physical, sexual, emotional, social, and spiritual trauma caused by the rape. In the initial, acute stage of intervention, focus is on the present rape situation, and not on previous difficulties; the nurse assumes that before the rape, the victim had been managing life adequately. Table 52-3 suggests several interventions that are appropriate in the acute phase of rape trauma syndrome. Interventions are grouped as responses to specific requests of clients. In most rape intervention situations, all the interventions listed in Table 52-3 may be appropriate.

Nurses may also become involved with rape victims in the follow-up phase of intervention. Follow-up intervention with the rape victim is initiated by the counselor and is done by a telephone call or home visit rather than an office appointment. During this follow-up contact, the nurse needs to be alert for signs of controlled reactions to rape.

Table 52-3 Interventions: Rape Trauma Victims

Acute Phase
Client requests police assistance
Notify police. Note time, date, and name of officer notified.
Encourage the victim to prosecute the rapist.
Explain legal procedures to victim.
In the presence of a witness, collect evidence for use during court trial: (1) Photographs of clothing and physical condition. (2) Clothing. Note tears, stains, presence of blood or semen. (3) Fingernail scrapings. (4) Swabs and smears of vagina, etc. Label all evidence carefully.
Carefully document findings in the medical record.
Client requests medical assistance
Observe client's general physical appearance.
Obtain medical history.
Obtain history of the rape.
Perform pelvic examination and note signs of trauma, redness, lacerations, or bruises.
Determine and note condition of anus and rectum.
Observe for signs of vaginal or anal bleeding.
Obtain vaginal swabs and smears to determine the presence of semen or VD.
Inform client that a follow-up examination for VD should be performed in 6 weeks.
Carefully note all bruises, lacerations, abrasions, swelling, redness, and scratches.
Measure size and note location of injuries.
Evaluate vital signs.
Carefully note findings in the medical record.
Rape trauma syndrome is present
Initiate crisis intervention according to an established crisis format.
Adopt an empathic, understanding approach.
Allow and encourage victim to talk about the rape.
Note client's coping style (expressive or controlled).
Clarify happenings for client.
Help client to focus on immediate feelings.
Offer referrals for ongoing counseling.
Facilitate moral and spiritual peace.
Client requests control
Provide client with a safe and private environment.
Explicitly discuss the physical, social, legal, and psychological issues associated with rape.
Allow client time and space to think through the crisis.
Client is uncertain about needs
Explore whether victim is present in emergency room because of free choice or because of pressure from family, legal system, or other source.
Discuss appropriate action with the client.
Discuss client's options about physical care.
Encourage client to ventilate concerns.
Explain legal process in detail.
Explore client's ambivalence.
Suggest follow-up counseling.
Clarify and give advice about specific issues.
Offer victim a selection of referrals.

When a victim is experiencing difficulty adjusting to work, social, or family routines, the following interventions are appropriate:

- Initiate family counseling.
- Suggest social networking (women's groups, church groups, self-defense classes, etc.).
- Structure activities of daily living.
- Explore client's anxieties and fears.
- Encourage resumption of normal lifestyle.

When the client shows evidence that resolution of the crisis has begun, the following interventions are important:

- Remain available to the client.
- Initiate contact by telephone calls, visits, etc.
- Facilitate further ventilation by encouraging the victim to reflect back on feelings and thoughts.
- Explore the client's feelings about the rapist.
- Explore the client's current feelings about herself.
- Channel the client's energies and efforts to prevent rape into taking a self-defense course or working in a rape crisis center.

Intervention with the Family

The support network of the rape victim is a major factor in successful resolution of a rape crisis. Female victims whose significant male family members are supportive and nonjudgmental make the most rapid, strongest recovery. Counseling and education for families are essential in the process of restoration of health. If victims work or go to school, they should also be encouraged to share the fact of the rape with significant people in these environments.

Anticipatory guidance in the form of suggesting to the family what emotional responses they can expect from the victim is another helpful approach. The victim should be encouraged to resume active involvement with the extended family and the previous social network. Ongoing assessment of the victim's sexual relationship will indicate the degree of sexual counseling and education that is necessary. If the husband views the victim as "damaged," this puts a serious strain on the marital relationship; marital counseling by an accredited therapist is essential.

Intervention with the Environment

Because it is a crime, rape is a broad social issue and not just the private concern of individual victims. Primary prevention of rape requires a broad-based community focus aimed at educating police officers, emergency room personnel, the clergy, teachers and other educators, physicians, lawyers, and social workers about rape. Increasing public awareness and providing for public safety are other aims of programs.

Community agencies such as rape crisis centers and hot lines need to be established. Courses in self-defense and workshops on rape crisis and security issues need to be offered.

Some self-protective strategies for preventing rape which have direct environmental implications are suggested in Table 52-4. Nurses can be influ-

Table 52-4 Self-Protection: Preventing Rape

Suggestions	Suggestions
Environmental protection	**Psychological protection**
Provide adequate light at entrances.	Keep a clear head.
Have visitors identify themselves.	Know the route home.
List only first initial and last name in telephone directory.	Rehearse in your head the action you would take if attacked.
Have key *ready* before getting out of car.	
Give your home a lived-in look.	**Be knowledgeable of high-risk areas**
Physical protection	Avoid dark alleys, streets, etc.
Carry a "weapon."	Be wary of suspicious-looking men.
Wear a whistle.	If followed, walk or run to a house or apartment with lights on and ring the doorbell.
Wear nonrestrictive clothing, so that you will be able to run.	
Avoid carrying a purse.	
Walk in the middle of the sidewalk.	

(Continued.)

Table 52-4 Continued

Suggestions	Suggestions
Self-protection if attack is imminent If you suspect you are being followed, turn and check. Head for a well-lighted or well-inhabited area. Begin to run suddenly, and start shouting. Act in a bizarre manner. Stay calm, and think as clearly as possible. Size up the assailant. You may be able to talk your way out of the situation. If the assailant wears glasses, rip them off. Yell *fire, help,* or *rape.* Step on your assailant's foot. If in a house or apartment, make noise to attract neighbors. **Self-defense** Take a course in self-defense. Remember that the eyes and throat are the most vulnerable parts of the body to strike. Use a "karate chop" to the neck.	**Protection while traveling** Lock doors and keep windows partly rolled up when traveling in a car. Sit near the driver or conductor on public transportation. Avoid hitchhiking. **Protection against being powerless** Observe assailant for identifying features such as height, weight, or hairstyle and color. Memorize assailant's license plate number, style, and color of car. If driven to another location, note distance, direction, speeds, landmarks, odors, and time in transit. **Collective action** Organize community anticrime groups. Organize groups to educate others about rape. Pressure community officials and landlords to provide safety measures.

ential in seeing that rape prevention strategies are discussed and implemented in the communities and health care agencies in which they live and work.

Evaluation

Ongoing contact with rape victims should occur at regular intervals, usually quarterly. Nurses should assess the physical, emotional, social, spiritual, and sexual functioning of the victims. Although definitive research on the long-term effects of rape has not been performed, the assumption is that effective crisis intervention and ongoing counseling will enable victims to return to their previous levels of functioning.

Table 52-5 illustrates the use of the nursing process and the evaluation of one problem associated with the acute phase of rape trauma syndrome, in the following case:

> Jane T. is a 23-year-old white single female seen at a rape crisis clinic after being assaulted and raped while walking in a park near her home. She is hyperventilating and crying, and her clothes are soiled and torn. After calming Jane and obtaining the necessary physical and legal evidence, the nurse can evaluate the client further.

Table 52-5 Rape: Case Study (Jane T.)

Evaluation
Assessment Ask the client: How are you feeling now? What were you feeling at the time of the rape? What is most painful or difficult for you to remember about the rape? Are you able to stop crying? How have you dealt with previous upsets in your life?
Diagnosis Hyperventilation and crying related to rape trauma syndrome
Outcome criteria Jane will cease crying and verbalize her emotional state.
Intervention Adopt an empathic, soothing approach. Encourage Jane to ventilate her feelings about the rape. Allow time and space for the client to think through the crisis. Explore her coping style. Clarify happenings for the client. Include physical and legal proceedings. Help Jane to focus on her immediate feelings.
Evaluation Jane has stopped crying and her hyperventilating has stopped. She is able to talk about the rape with appropriate affect. A follow-up appointment will be made with the rape trauma clinic for 1 week from today.

SUMMARY

Rape is a physical and psychological act of aggression against a person that degrades, dehumanizes, and violates the victim's sense of self. It is one of the fastest-growing forms of abuse in the United States. Rape may be motivated by a need for sexual gratification, by anger, or by a need for control or power.

The common behaviors observed in rape victims include fear of injury, mutilation, and death; feelings of humiliation, degradation, shame, and guilt; embarrassment; self-blame; anger; and revenge.

Victims respond to rape in predictable but individualized ways. Victims who have not told others that they were raped may experience silent rape syndrome. A family's responsiveness to a rape victim may be supportive or blaming. To be effective in counseling rape victims, nurses need to be aware of their own feelings and biases.

Assessing a rape crisis involves obtaining a history of the rape, doing a physical examination, and determining the emotional and spiritual reactions of victims. Gathering and documenting evidence that will be legally helpful is a primary task of health care professionals during the immediate rape crisis period. Victims of rape may request police or medical assistance, psychological support, or help in restoring a sense of control; or they may be uncertain of their needs. Intervention involves crisis management and follow-up counseling with victims and their families. Community education helps to prevent rape.

REFERENCES

1. Uniform Crime Reports for the United States Federal Bureau of Investigation, U.S. Department of Justice, Washington, D.C., 1980.
2. J. McDermott, *Rape Victimization in 26 American Cities*, U.S. Department of Justice, Law Enforcement and Assistance Administration, Washington, D.C., 1979.
3. E. R. Mohoney, *Human Sexuality*, McGraw-Hill, New York, 1983, pp. 423–455.
4. L. L. Holmstrom, and A. W. Burgess, "Sexual Behavior of Assailants during Reported Rapes," *Archives of Sexual Behavior*, vol. 9, 1980, pp. 427–439.
5. A. W. Burgess and L. L. Holmstrom, *Rape: Victims of Crisis*, Brady, Bowie, Md., 1974.
6. D. Sredl, C. Klenke, and M. Rojkind, "Offering the Rape Victim Real Help," *Nursing '79*, July 1979, pp. 38–43.
7. A. W. Burgess, and L. L. Holmstrom, "Rape: Sexual Disruption and Recovery," *American Journal of Orthopsychiatry*, vol. 49, no. 6, June 1979, pp. 648–657.

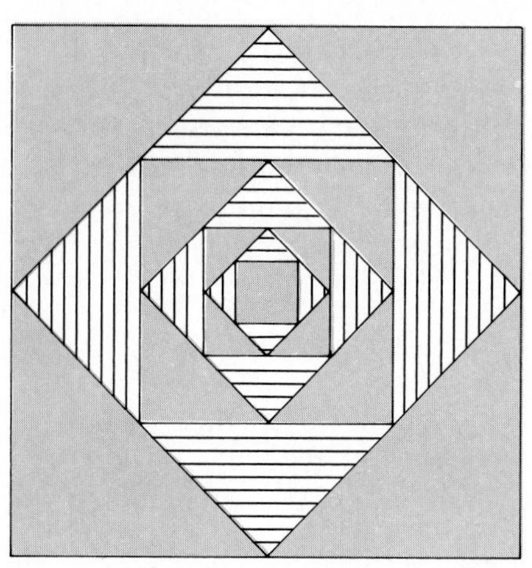

CHAPTER 53
The Chronically Mentally Ill in the Community

Pamela Price Hoskins

LEARNING OBJECTIVES

After studying this chapter, the student should be able to:

1. Describe the two populations of chronically mentally ill psychiatric clients.
2. Analyze the effects of deinstitutionalization of chronically mentally ill people on the community.
3. List the dysfunctional patterns of the chronically ill population.
4. Discuss theories of chronic mental illness.
5. Plan nursing care for a chronically ill client in the community.
6. Identify and build on strengths of a chronically ill client.
7. Work with a chronically ill client to set appropriate short- and long-term goals.
8. Evaluate the appropriateness of living arrangements for chronically ill clients.
9. Delineate the services offered by community nurses to the chronically ill psychiatric population.

Treatment of the chronically ill psychiatric population is emerging as one of the most important issues of the 1990s. The United States has made a commitment to treat the chronically ill in the least restrictive environment possible, which for most is the community. However, the nation has not allocated the financial resources necessary to follow through on that commitment.

The purpose of this chapter is to help the student understand the role of nursing in rational, appropriate health care for the chronically ill psychiatric population living in the community. The history and trends of the community movement, the identification of the chronically ill population, the impact of the chronically ill on the family and the community, and the contribution of the nursing profession to treatment of chronically ill psychiatric clients will be explored.

HISTORICAL PERSPECTIVE

Until the 1950s, severely disturbed psychiatric clients were admitted to psychiatric hospitals, where they lived for years. Mostly untrained personnel were expected to offer humane custodial care. Because there were few effective treatments, few clients were discharged. Admission to a psychiatric hospital implied chronic illness with long-term hospitalization as the treatment of choice.

With the advent of phenothiazine drugs in the 1950s, an upheaval took place in the treatment of the mentally ill. The most bizarre psychiatric symptoms were ameliorated, and discharge from psychiatric hospitals became possible for many clients. As discharge placements were made, several difficulties became apparent, among them the following:

1. Many clients had no family who could provide a home, necessitating other community arrangements.
2. Many clients exhibited symptoms in close relationships that, while not bizarre, were difficult to live with.
3. Many clients had become "institutionalized," an iatrogenic condition created by the institutional setting. The institutionalization syndrome was perceived to be as devastating to health and personality as the original psychiatric illness had been. People who had been institutionalized were able to live in the community only if placed in another institution, a nursing home, or an adult home.

The need for treatment resources in the community became apparent as institutionalized clients were prepared for discharge, and as the institutionalization phenomenon became known. The public as well as mental health professionals began to ask why people had to be admitted to hospitals, especially if the institutional setting itself compounded the client's problems. Nurses were instrumental in envisioning treatment programs in the community; the community setting was a familiar one in which nurses had offered therapeutic health services for clients with many kinds of problems.

The community mental health ideology is best summarized in the following statement made by the Joint Commission on Mental Illness and Health in 1961:

> The objective of modern treatment of persons with mental illness is to enable the patient to maintain himself in the community in a normal manner. To do so, it is necessary (1) to save the patient from debilitating effects of institutionalization, (2) to return him to home and community life as soon as possible, and (3) thereafter, to maintain him in the community as long as possible. Therefore, aftercare and rehabilitation are essential parts of all service to mental patients, and the various methods of achieving rehabilitation should be integrated in all forms of services, among them day hospitals, night hospitals, aftercare clinics, public health nursing services, foster family care, convalescent nursing homes, rehabilitation centers, work services, and expatient groups.[1]

The community mental health movement began when funding for community mental health centers was appropriated by the federal government in 1963. Once community services had begun to be developed, institutionalized clients were discharged into the community in large numbers. Only those who were simply unable to live in the most protected community environment were allowed to remain in hospitals.

Communities were not prepared for the onslaught of chronically ill psychiatric clients. Financial support for and commitment to the concept, an accepting community attitude, and facilities for housing and treating large numbers of clients had not yet been developed. Many communities began to see themselves as "dumping grounds," and clients found no place where they belonged. The "revolving-door syndrome" developed; the same clients were repeatedly admitted and then discharged. In addition, discharge plans were difficult to make because so few resources were available.

Today, there is still inadequate development of community resources, little financial support for disabled clients, little financial commitment to development of more effective treatment modalities, and little commitment to maintaining the resources available in the institutional setting.

On the positive side, psychiatric personnel are better prepared to deal with chronicity and many community resources have been developed for the chronically mentally ill. Repeated admission is seen as a necessary adjunct to the ongoing community treatment a client receives.

DYSYNCHRONOUS HEALTH PATTERNS

Since the community mental health movement began, statisticians have had difficulty determining the number of people who are chronically mentally ill (CMI). Part of the difficulty was deciding on a definition for chronic mental illness (also abbreviated CMI). Originally, *chronic mental illness* was defined by the number of hospitalizations and length of stay; however, since deinstitutionalization began, a chronically ill client may have been hospitalized once or twice for only a few days. Members of the older CMI population are readily identified, but the young CMI constitute "a transitional generation which is not *de*institutionalized but *un*institutionalized."[2] Hence, though number of hospitalizations and length of stay contribute useful information, the current distinguishing characteristics of CMI are severe and prolonged functional disability, and a need for mental health services lasting 2 years or more.

Epidemiology

While it is difficult to determine the number of CMI, several studies have found that there are approximately 7 million people who have been treated for mental health problems. Approximately 3 million of these fall into the CMI category; 1.7 million have been hospitalized for prolonged periods. Approximately 900,000 of these remain institutionalized, and 700,000 are severely disabled but have not been hospitalized for prolonged periods. About 600,000 have received a diagnosis of severe mental disorder and have the potential to develop chronicity.[3]

Only those who are thought to be harmful to self or others and those who are unable to function are admitted to hospitals. Length of stay may be as short as 1 day and as long as a lifetime. However, 80 percent of all clients admitted to state and county mental hospitals, and 100 percent of all clients admitted to private mental hospitals and general psychiatric units, are discharged within 90 days.[2] Studies of readmission have estimated that 30 to 40 percent of clients return within 6 months, 40 to 50 percent within 1 year, and 65 to 75 percent within 3 to 5 years.

The CMI live in a variety of settings. Figure 53-1 indicates the living arrangements in 1977. In the last 10 years, further development of community housing, such as group homes and room-and-board facilities, has occurred. However, many of the older

Figure 53-1 Care of chronically mentally ill clients.

Location of the chronically mentally ill in the United States as of 1977. (SOURCE: Steering Committee on the Chronically Mentally Ill, *Toward a National Plan for the Chronically Ill*, DHHS Publication No. ADM 81-1077, 1981, Department of Health and Human Services, Washington, D. C., December 1980.)

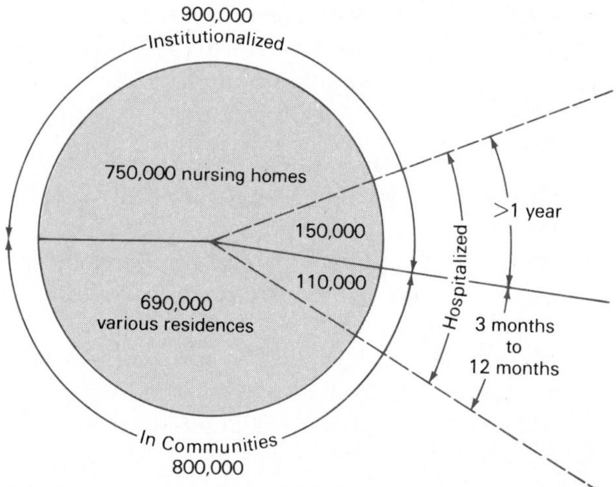

CMI continue to live in nursing homes, especially as their own families age and are no longer able to care for them. Nursing homes tend to give custodial care to CMI clients; therefore, nursing homes may be the "back wards" in the community.[2]

DSM III

There are basically two populations of CMI in the community: the older deinstitutionalized population, and the young chronic population between 18 and 30 years old. Organic mental disorders, schizophrenic disorders, major affective disorders, paranoid disorders, and other psychotic disorders predominate in the older population. As a group, these people are system-dependent.

The young adult population tend to have multiple diagnoses and a high incidence of substance abuse and suicide attempts. In addition, disruptive social behavior and rejection or inappropriate use of mental health services are characteristic of this group. Both populations depend partially or totally on public assistance, family, or both for financial support.[4] There are three hypothesized subgroups of the young CMI: the low-energy, low-demand (system-dependent) subgroup; the high-energy, high-demand subgroup; and the high-functioning subgroup. Table 53-1 shows the differences among the subgroups. Each subgroup differs from the others in terms of self-perception, functional levels, and attitude toward mental health services.[5]

PATTERNS OF INTERACTION: PERSON

How does a person with mental health problems come to be chronically mentally ill? Theories of chronicity and symptoms of chronicity combine to provide some understanding of this question.

Theories of Chronicity

There are seven theoretical approaches to chronicity in mental illness: (1) medical, (2) epidemiological, (3) sociological, (4) intrapsychic, (5) integrated, (6) comprehensive, and (7) myth. Each approach has a different focus and interventions. Table 53-2 (page 1182) presents a summary of the approaches.

The *medical* approach to chronic mental illness is organic. Research is geared to biological explanations and physically oriented treatment modalities.

The *epidemiological*, or statistical, approach has provided a data base and some notions of causality. This approach does not dictate interventions but provides information for decision making and ways to test the effectiveness of interventions in the population.

The *sociological* approach focuses on society rather than individuals, and treats chronicity as learned social behavior reinforced by social structure. Interventions are geared to the structure and function of society's institutions of socialization.

Table 53-1 Hypothesized Typology of Young Adult Chronic Patients

Low-Energy, Low-Demand Group	High-Energy, High-Demand Group	High-Functioning Group
Well-ensconced in role of patient	Able to shop around from agency to agency to get what they want	Generally higher socioeconomic status and better appearance
Unable to do well, even in remission	Fluctuating functional abilities and interests	New to mental health system
Concretely attached to programs and program places	"Give me what I want or stay out of my life" attitude toward mental health services	Resist involvement in mental health programs on basis of convictions
Passive, poorly motivated	Low tolerance for frustration. Frequent acting out, encounters with the law	May enter mental health system because of alcohol or drug abuse
Accepting of mental health services	Frequently evicted, mobile	Want to understand their disorders and to learn ways of preventing relapses
Appear burned out at an early age	Includes revolving-door patients and street people	Want to blend into general population without being identified as mental patients

SOURCE: J. L. Sheets et al., "Young Adult Chronic Patients: Three Hypothesized Subgroups," *Hospital and Community Psychiatry*, vol. 33, March 1982, p. 201. Used with permission.

Table 53-2 Current Theoretical Perspectives on Chronic Mental Illness

Model	Focus	Interventions
Medical-technical (science)	Ills of the body	Physical treatments Research
Epidemiological (science)	Ills of the body and the group	Research Planning and prevention
Sociological (social science)	Ills of the group	Social engineering Change in institutional structures
Intrapsychic (social science)	Ills of the mind	Psychotherapy Alterations in interpersonal environment
Integrated (social science)	Ills of the individual in relationship with the family or group and community	Individual therapy Family or group therapy Social values clarification and realignment
Comprehensive (social science)	Analysis of the needs of individuals with chronic medical illness, including mental illness	Prevention and management of medical crises Control of symptoms Regimens for carrying out treatments Prevention of social isolation Adjustment to changes in the course of the disease Normalizing lifestyles and interactions with others Funding
Myth (ethics)	Ills of the spirit	Tolerance of deviance Client advocacy Political and legal reform

SOURCE: Adapted from J. B. Krauss and A. T. Slavinsky, *The Chronically Ill Psychiatric Patient and the Community*, Blackwell Scientific Publications, Boston, 1982, p. 13. Used with permission.

The *intrapsychic* approach focuses on the individual human mind rather than on social structure. Interventions are geared to intrapersonal and interpersonal change.

The *integrated* approach combines the medical, epidemiological, sociological, and intrapsychic approaches to form a holistic approach. Chronic mental illness is considered present when an illness is severe, permanent, stigmatized, and contagious.[6] The integrated approach suggests interventions that are broad in nature, focusing on intrapersonal, familial, social, and functional factors, as well as biological factors.

The *comprehensive* approach does not attempt to explain chronic mental illness but rather is treatment-oriented.[7] Seven aspects of intervention based on this approach are listed in Table 53-2.

The *myth* approach dismisses the configurations of behavior called "mental illness" as a figment of the cultural imagination. This does not imply intervention in the usual sense but instead focuses on values clarification; that is, it questions the right of a society to incarcerate people for relatively harmless behavior, and to strip them of their constitutional rights.

Each of these seven approaches has made significant contributions to the understanding of the causes of, effects of, and approaches to chronic mental illness. Research and theory development using each approach will provide more ways to prevent, treat, and cure mental illness. The integrated approach is most congruent with the conceptual framework used in this text.

Symptoms of Chronicity

There are seven symptoms of chronic mental illness: (1) dependence, (2) social incompetence, (3) stigma, (4) the sick role, (5) long-term relationships with institutions, (6) symptomatic behavior, and (7) a low level of functioning. Each symptom is explored below in light of physical, mental, and spiritual dimensions of the person.

Dependence

Dependence is defined as reliance on others to meet basic needs for love, affection, nurturing, shelter, protection, security, food, and warmth. People have an inborn need for relationships with others; and many people have a need for a relationship with a higher being. Clients who are CMI tend to develop one of two extremes: they either need nobody and nothing, or they sense no inner resources and need everybody and everything. Developmentally, they may function at an infantile level, depending on others to meet all their needs; or they may function at the autonomy level of, say, a 3-year-old: "I can do it myself." The client does not assess self, family, and community strengths and weaknesses and make sound judgments about appropriate interdependence. It is appropriate for the CMI to be dependent, and they should be encouraged to be appropriately dependent. However, extremes of dependency are not acceptable in this society and therefore make functioning in society very difficult. For instance:

> A man who looked about 30 years old got on the subway. He was dressed in jeans and a black wool, mud-splotched overcoat. He smelled very strongly of body odor, urine, and feces. He crawled onto a seat and assumed a fetal position. He began sucking his completely ulcerated thumb, apparently wounded from almost constant exposure to saliva over a very long period of time. At that point, almost everyone else on the crowded subway car left and went to other cars.

At the other extreme, the totally independent person refuses to be integrated into society. For instance:

> A 65-year-old man dug a hole in the ground, fixed up a semblance of a home, including a place for food storage, and crawled in. At the last report, he had been living there for 9 years. He comes out in the spring and summer to find food to store for the winter; he never comes out in the winter, because the heat that has accumulated in the hole would escape and he would freeze. Twice a year his sister goes out to see if he is still alive. He has stated that he never wants to deal with people for any reason again.

The relationship of dependence to the meeting of physical needs is illustrated in both examples. One person was not meeting the most basic cleanliness and hygiene needs; the other foraged for food and sometimes went hungry rather than dealing with people to meet a basic need. Relationships with others deviate significantly from the norm for both men, and indicate very different meanings and purposes for life.

Social Incompetence

Social incompetence is inability to navigate the norms expected for functioning and interpersonal relationships. People who are CMI are almost totally devoid of interpersonal skills. While there is a need for relationships with others, the CMI cannot meet that need through intimate relationships; closeness is intolerable. Those who suffer from schizophrenia disorders have the most difficulty with intimacy. When too much is expected in the way of participation and interaction, deterioration in social functioning is the outcome.[2] For example:

> After discharge from a psychiatric unit, John lived in a garage apartment and got a job cleaning a clothing store in the evenings. He refused to speak to the manager on the street one day, certain that she had followed him to see if he was taking drugs. When a therapist confronted him with the irrationality of this idea, he said, "You don't understand; you can be nice to people because you know how. I don't have a choice." John has continued to live in seclusion, having no friends and only distant relationships with his family, and to work at menial jobs where he doesn't have to interact with people. Any suggestion of a change in level of relationship creates extreme anxiety which incapacitates him for days.

Stigma

Stigma is defined as a sign of disgrace. In ancient times, a stigma was a mark burned into the skin of a slave or criminal, a sign of infamy, disgrace, or reproach. While the mentally ill today do not have physical scars to communicate their illness, mental illness does carry a social stigma. The mentally ill are treated in this society as if they earned and deserved their disease, and as if the illness itself were a disgrace and a reproach. Even people who seem to feel compassion for a mentally ill person may not want that person to be a friend, coworker, or neighbor. The desire for distance from the mentally ill is based on a societal norm of reproach for mental illness. When this societal attitude is operational, neighborhoods don't want group homes or halfway houses located in their vicinity; employers don't want to hire people who have been or are being treated for mental illness; and former friends no longer call.

Those afflicted with mental illness are socialized to the same norms as the rest of society; consequently, they feel the same reproach as their neighbors but direct the feelings toward themselves. Feelings of infamy, disgrace, and shame, and a desire to be "away from themselves," are characteristic of the mentally ill.

The mentally ill live with the stigma, the mark. As their condition becomes chronic, the mental illness is seen as their most important characteristic. The disorder is compounded by the stigma, and the person may be more entrapped by the stigma and the resulting rejection than by the disorder itself. The continuing low level of functioning is the mark, worn by the person and recognized by society, that reinforces the attitudes of reproach and shame. The resulting destructive interaction between the person and society deprives the community of the resources that could be contributed by the CMI and deprives the mentally ill person of the support and sense of belonging needed for healthy functioning.

Sick Role

Parsons defined the *sick role* as a set of institutional and societal expectations that people who are ill must meet. The expectations are: forfeiting decision making to professionals who know how to care for the sick person; tolerating any treatment without complaint, no matter how personal, invasive, or dehumanizing; and abandoning the sick role as soon as possible.[8] The CMI are caught in the paradoxical expectations—unable to abandon the role and consequently stigmatized. Their attempts to abandon the role lead to exacerbation of symptoms and rehospitalization. The influence of chronic mental illness on the enactment of the sick role is outlined in Table 53-3.

Young CMI clients reject the expectations of the sick role outlined in Table 53-3 and are difficult to find; planning and implementing adequate assistance is also difficult. Older CMI clients, particularly those with histories of prolonged hospitalization, are difficult to resocialize to a new role, more appropriate for community living.

Relationships with Institutions

The CMI, by definition, have prolonged relationships with mental health services. At one time,

Table 53-3 Expectations and Characteristics of the Sick Role and the Influence of Chronic Mental Illness

Expectations	Characteristics	Influences of Mental Illness
Sick person forfeits decision making to health care professionals.	Passivity, dependency	Person needs assistance with activities of daily living, making the most minor decisions. Needs sheltered living environment.
Sick person tolerates any treatment without complaint, no matter how personal, invasive, or dehumanizing.	Feelings of loss, fear, anxiety, and depersonalization Altered self-concept and body image	Chronic sense of loss and grieving. Loss of sense of self as capable, worthy of dignity and respect. Feelings of entrapment in body, with self that will never change. Loss of sense of self.
Sick person cooperates with treatment, works toward getting well, and gives up sick role as soon as possible.	Cyclic attempts to become independent; sometimes seen as rebellion Cyclic attempts to begin making own decisions	Vacillation between total removal of self from support systems and total dependency requiring hospitalization. Poor judgments. Loss of social skills; loss of ability to perceive reality accurately. Sick role becomes the permanent, and sometimes the sole, role the person enacts.

mental health professionals perceived rehospitalization of psychiatric clients as failure of the treatment process. A client who has suffered acute illness, has been treated, and does not need extended community treatment is considered cured. The chronically mentally ill, however, need treatment for at least 2 years. Like any other chronic illness, mental illness requires follow-up care, monitoring, adjustment of medication, and assistance in developing a healthy lifestyle while living with a chronic condition. As with any other chronic illness, periodic hospitalization may be part of the ongoing treatment process, and may be used to establish new, more productive patterns of living.

Symptomatic Behavior

Classic behaviors, such as hallucinations and posturing, are symptomatic of chronic mental illness. The CMI population as a whole exhibit symptoms that create discomfort for others. The symptoms signal chronicity, and chronicity reinforces symptomatology. Symptoms include difficult interpersonal relationships, side effects of medications, and inappropriate behavior.

Difficulty with intimacy keeps interpersonal relationships off balance and difficult to maintain. The extrapyramidal symptoms exhibited as side effects of prolonged phenothiazine medication are disquieting and sometimes embarrassing. Some CMI clients have never been socialized to appropriate behavior, and they exhibit behavior similar to that of a 3-year-old. For instance:

> Pat, 42 years old, can be seen at the shopping center on Saturday mornings with her mother. Pat blows her nose and wipes it on her sleeve; she eats with her hands, burps loudly, and chews with her mouth open. Pat is of average intelligence, but attempts to teach her to behave appropriately in public precipitate anxiety attacks.

Some CMI clients in the community exhibit classic signs of psychosis. They can be seen hallucinating in public places such as bus stations and fast-food restaurants, even to the point of having loud verbal battles with imaginary companions. The police and FBI take multiple calls from CMI clients who report that imagined thefts, attempts at murder, and other criminal activity are aimed at them.

Such symptoms are disturbing, both to the client and to the community. Some clients may be helped to reduce their unsocialized or symptomatic behavior. Others, who may always exhibit bizarre behavior, will always need the same long-term tolerance and compassion that should be given to all chronically ill people in the community.

Level of Functioning

Another diagnostic criterion for chronic mental illness is prolonged impaired functioning in the following areas:

- Activities of daily living, including hygiene and comfort
- Independent living
- Ability to support oneself financially

The CMI may have difficulty in one, two, or all three areas. Some clients may work and hold a job but are not able to live independently. Some clients may take care of their hygiene and comfort needs well but are unable to live independently or to work. Clients who are so incapacitated that they are unable to meet their own basic needs are usually hospitalized until they have gained or regained this level of functioning.

Some CMI may function at high levels in all three areas, but then experience exacerbations that immobilize them. Brief, intense treatment helps them to regain their former levels of functioning, and they return to home and job.

There are several patterns of functioning with the CMI, from profound adverse effects to minor, inconvenient influences. Determining the kinds of supports and resources needed to maintain the highest level of functioning is a major focus of clinical research. Such research holds out the hope that, once appropriate resources are placed at their disposal, the CMI population may become functioning, contributing members of society.

PATTERNS OF INTERACTION: FAMILY

Approximately 65 percent of clients are discharged to their homes (*home* means living with parents or spouse), and about 25 percent of those are CMI.[2] Two major patterns of interaction are important when nurses are considering the family with regard to chronic mental illness: patterns that influence the client's functioning, and patterns that influence the family's functioning. One factor has changed over the past 10 years: the family used to be seen as the culprit in mental illness but is now seen as an "active partner" in a "rational treatment approach" to mental illness.[2] Chronic mental illness has a severe impact on the family regardless of where the CMI person lives.

The family of a CMI person has a different lifestyle from the ordinary family and copes with a different reality. Five aspects of reality influence the lifestyle of such families: (1) grieving, (2) search for meaning and purpose, (3) the burden of illness, (4) feelings of guilt, and (5) the family's perceived needs. The following paragraphs discuss each of these.

First, a family goes through the *grieving* process as it comes to terms with the fact that a loved one is CMI. The cyclic nature of the illness creates a grieving cycle that never ends. (This is much like the experience of a family with a developmentally challenged child.)

Second, the family *searches for meaning and purpose* in the face of chronic mental illness. These families must deal with the questions "Why?" and "Why us?" This is not an attempt to assign blame, but an attempt to understand why there can be such tragedy in a world that is expected to make sense. Nurses assisting families are effective when they deal with this question as a universal, existential issue. A referral to a rabbi, priest, or minister may be useful if the nurse is uncomfortable dealing with spiritual matters.

Third, CMI places a tremendous *burden* on a family—physically, mentally, emotionally, spiritually, financially, and socially. It is a great challenge for such a family to create a loving, supportive, accepting climate that encourages the highest level of functioning. The CMI member often becomes the center of activity and concern in the family, and a disproportionate amount of family resources may be expended on that member. Consequently, the needs of other members and of the family as a whole may not be adequately met, and psychiatric symptoms may begin to emerge in other members. Family members report a keen sense of loss of time and energy for leisure activities and interpersonal relationships[9]—in other words, for normal family life. The financial strain is also great and may affect a family's lifestyle and financial security.

A fourth aspect of reality for a family faced with CMI is feelings of *guilt*. These guilt feelings will be exacerbated by mental health workers who believe that the family is to blame for mental illness. As long as nurses focus on deficiencies in families, families will feel that they are being accused or blamed. On the other hand, when families and mental health workers have similar perceptions of the family's situation, there is empathy, cooperation, and satisfaction with service.[2]

A fifth aspect of reality is the family's *perceived needs*. Hatfield found that families identified their three most important needs as knowledge and understanding of the CMI person's symptoms, specific assistance with coping with CMI behaviors, and opportunity to talk with other people who have CMI family members.[10] In a study of 138 families, 21 needs were ranked;[11] it is significant to note that baccalaureate nurses are able to meet 12 of them. (See Table 53-4.)

Table 53-4 Family Needs that Baccalaureate Nurses Can Meet

Need	Frequency, N	Chosen, %
Reduction of anxiety about patient	96	70
Learning to motivate patient to do more	89	64
Understanding appropriate expectations	89	64
Help for care giver in accepting the illness	78	57
Locating community resources	76	55
Understanding medications and their use	76	55
Learning potential side effects of medication	74	54
Learning appropriate responses to symptoms such as hallucinations, talking to self, paranoia	62	45
Help in gaining order and control over household	61	44
Achieving compliance with medication regime	54	39
Getting patient to practice better hygiene habits	47	34
Finding time for personal life	47	34

SOURCE: Adapted from A. B. Hatfield, "What Families Want of Family Therapy," in W. R. MacFarlane, ed., *Family Therapy in Schizophrenia*, Guilford, New York, 1983, pp. 41–63.

PATTERNS OF INTERACTION: ENVIRONMENT*

Individuals and families depend on communities for social, leisure, living, and work activities. Normalizing activities and relationships must happen in the community. The CMI population not only depend on but also have difficulty in achieving access to these resources in the community. Client, family, and community must make an effort in order to overcome these difficulties. Patterns of interaction between communities and the CMI range on a continuum from "totally integrated" to "totally segregated or isolated." The degree of community integration varies from community to community, and one community may change its degree of integration over time. An important variable influencing the degree of integration is community acceptance of CMI people. A high degree of community acceptance makes possible the needed opportunities for normalizing experiences and relationships.

One factor influencing community acceptance is the number of CMI a given community is expected to absorb. For instance:[12]

> Asbury Park, New Jersey, was expected to integrate between 1000 and 1500 persons into the community, a figure representing 10 percent of its population. This number exceeded the community's level of acceptance, and the response was opposition to deinstitutionalization. The community ultimately addressed its problem through community involvement in planning for its CMI population.

This example demonstrates that with adequate planning, a community can integrate a CMI population.

The experience at the other end of the continuum, isolation and segregation, is a common community phenomenon. Communities may simply have no room for people who deviate from the community norm, even if these people are not mentally ill. For example, a small, rural, northern community recently brought such strong social pressure to bear on a homosexual couple that the couple felt forced to move out of town.

* For additional discussion of the community, see Chapter 18, "Outpatient Contexts of Care."

Living Arrangements

Basic necessities include a place to live. CMI people may live at home or in alternative settings, but a community attitude of acceptance is necessary if the arrangements are to be successful. In well-integrated communities, families can, for example, take a CMI member to a neighborhood picnic; there is a basic assumption that people will be tolerant of one another's idiosyncracies. In a closed community, by contrast, mentally ill family members are treated shabbily and the family may be ostracized. Neighbor children may throw stones and taunt the ill person, and their parents may tolerate their behavior.

For CMI people who do not live at home, the situation in a closed community is exacerbated. The CMI may live on the streets and are sometimes imprisoned. The housing provided in a particular community, such as single-room-occupancy hotels, room-and-board homes, and nursing homes, may be woefully inadequate for the needs of the CMI.

Social Activities

The social activities of well-integrated communities are open to the public. Community education programs and public facilities such as swimming pools and libraries are available for all citizens. Community events are usually listed in local newspapers, accompanied by a description of the event, location, and fee. These are excellent opportunities for CMI people, since they can use the facilities without having much expected of them in the way of participation. In communities that have a high level of integration, several people who look and act a little different are usually seen in community social settings. In closed communities, however, the CMI are systematically excluded from social activities.

Leisure Activities

Businesses that provide leisure activities, such as swimming and bowling, are concerned about their reputations and are an excellent reflection of the degree of community acceptance. If a community has a high level of integration, a bowling league of former mental patients may compete in the local bowling tournament along with other groups. In a closed community, by contrast, such a group may have to make special arrangements, come at an unusual time, and bowl in a special place.

Opportunities for Work

Competition for work opportunities is heavy. Business, government, industry, and service organizations are looking for the best-qualified workers for the least amount of money. Mental illness, or even the possibility that a person may have had emotional problems, is usually considered a negative aspect of an application. The stigma of mental illness is especially pronounced in the work arena, and consequently, the mentally ill ordinarily do not reveal their medical histories. For instance:

> Amanda, 49 years old, began having problems with mood swings some years ago and was admitted twice with a medical diagnosis of bipolar disorder, manic phase, with psychotic features. She has maintained herself in the community for the past year but has been unable to salvage her business. She was offered an excellent position in another state and has even been staying in her new employer's home while looking for a place to live. She has not told her new boss about her history of mental illness because, as supportive as her employer is, Amanda does not believe she would have been hired had her medical history been disclosed.

The problems of CMI people are even greater than the problems of people who, like Amanda, have had one or two episodes of mental illness. Ordinarily their work histories show patterns of unreliability, interpersonal difficulties, and problems with authority and responsibility. Their personal habits and appearance may indicate to interviewers that they suffer from chronic mental illness.

Campaigns have been successfully launched to hire the mentally retarded and the physically challenged; a similar campaign is needed for the chronically mentally ill. While chronically mentally ill people have some severe limitations, they also have many strengths. Matching community need with this untapped resource would positively influence the health of the community as well as the individual. In this society, people are socialized to value themselves in accordance with what they are able to produce. When the CMI are not allowed to produce by doing constructive work, the result is lower valuation of themselves. Their low self-valuation is reinforced by the community.

Volunteer work is an excellent starting point for a CMI person in the process of rehabilitation. Other opportunities include sheltered workshops and rehabilitation programs. Such opportunities may be readily available in communities with a high level of integration, whereas there are fewer opportunities in closed communities.

Social life, living arrangements, leisure activities, and work are needed by everyone in a community but may represent special problems for the CMI population. Degree of *integration* in a community is a reflection of degree of *access.*

NURSING PROCESS

The nursing process is as important for CMI clients as for any other recipients of nursing services. A failure to provide adequate nursing services can, in part, be blamed on inadequate planning for discharge and inadequate adaptation of the nursing care plan.

Assessment

Assessment of the CMI client in the community deals with the person, the family, and the community.

The Person

Assessment of an individual CMI client includes, in addition to the usual assessment of the person, an evaluation of specific problems afflicting the chronically mentally ill:

- Dependence
- Social competence
- Stigma
- Sick role
- Level of functioning
- Relationships with institutions
- Symptomatic behavior

Table 53-5 provides some assessment questions for each of these areas. The CMI client may have difficulty answering the questions, and sometimes the client and significant others give different an-

Table 53-5 Assessment of the Chronically Mentally Ill Client

Dependence

Direct questions

Tell me about the people who depend on you.

Upon whom do you depend? How does that person help you?

What is your living situation?

What is the source of your income?

Observation

Degree of ability to make adequate decisions about daily living without assistance.

Degree of ability to independently provide structure for daily activities.

Degree of dependence developed in the nurse-client relationship.

Social Competence

Direct questions

How do you spend your time every day?

What do you do to relax?

Who is your best friend? Tell me about that relationship.

How comfortable are you when you meet new people?

Observation

How comfortable is the client in the nurse-client relationship? With social communication? With therapeutic communication?

Degree to which client prefers isolation.

Degree to which community members leave client alone.

Nature of casual interactions.

Degree to which client exhibits social graces.

Degree to which client fits in with community.

Opinion of others concerning client's ability to fit in.

Stigma

Direct questions

To what extent do you feel different because of your illness?

Do people treat you differently than they treat others? If so, to what do you attribute this?

Have you had difficulty being served in restaurants, getting work, or making friends because of your illness? If so, to what specific factors do you attribute this?

Observation

Verbalizations that indicate self-reproach for mental illness.

Verbal and nonverbal behavior by family and significant others that indicates stigma.

Degree to which people in the community shun the client or family.

Sick Role

Direct questions

What is the best thing about your illness? The worst thing?

What do you think your life will be like 5 years from now because of your illness?

In what ways do you change your lifestyle because of your illness?

Sick Role

Observations

Degree of ambivalence concerning sick role.

Degree of appropriate enactment of sick-role expectations.

Extent to which the role itself is assisting and hurting the client.

Level of Functioning

Direct questions

What daily activities do you perform for yourself?

How "together" do you feel?

How "together" do you act? What activities show how "together" you are?

How much time do you spend alone?

Who takes care of your living quarters? Where do you live? With whom? What are your duties at home? How well do you do those duties?

Do you work? What does your job entail? Do you meet deadlines? How do you get along with your boss? Your peers?

What arrangements have you made to take care of your money?

Observations

Degree of ability to take care of basic hygiene, carry out activities of daily living.

Strengths and weaknesses in handling stressful situations.

Tolerance for stressful situations.

Degree of flexibility in working with people.

Level of motivation, energy, purposeful activity.

Ability to set realistic goals for self.

Relationships with Institutions

Direct questions

Have you been hospitalized for psychiatric reasons? How many times? For what problems?

Have you received outpatient therapy? What kind? Reasons for termination?

Have you taken medications for your illness? What were they? How often per day? Reasons for discontinuation?

Observations

Get permission from the client to review records from agencies that have provided services.

Get history of relationships with institutions from relative or friend.

Symptomatic Behavior

Direct questions

Have you ever thought that someone might try to harm you in any way? Do you have these thoughts now?

Do you see or hear things that others don't see or hear?

Do you find that you have no choice but to do certain things? What are those things?

Observations

Relative amounts of client's socially inappropriate and socially appropriate behavior.

Control of bodily functions.

Amount of ritualistic behavior.

Presence of hallucinations, delusions.

swers to the same questions. It is important to collect data from a variety of sources.

The Family

Assessment of the family includes the client's relationships with family members and significant others, as well as the extent of the family's burden. The following specific areas need to be assessed:

- Grieving
- Search for meaning and purpose
- Physical, mental, spiritual, emotional, social, and financial burden
- Guilt feelings
- Perceived needs (see Table 53-4)

The Community

Assessment of the client's community focuses both on the client's degree of connectedness and on the community's acceptance of the CMI.[13] Questions for use in assessing community acceptance are given in Table 53-6. Assessment of the client's links to the community is important and should include:

- Informal links, such as friends, social activities, leisure activities, and use of community facilities
- Formal links, such as job, ongoing therapy and self-help activities, and use of a family health care provider

Table 53-6 Community Acceptance of CMI

Assessment Questions to Ask Community Members
1. Do you believe that ex-patients of mental hospitals can function well in this community?
2. Would you object if a club you belonged to accepted as a new member someone who had previously been mentally ill?
3. Would you object if someone who had previously been mentally ill moved in next door to you?
4. Can you imagine yourself becoming a close friend with someone who is now mentally ill?
5. Would you object if a halfway house for mentally ill people were located in your neighborhood?
6. If a mentally ill person asked for your help in getting a job where you work, would you be willing to help?
7. Would you object if a halfway house for mentally ill people were located next door to you?
8. Would you regularly participate in programs in your neighborhood which helped mentally ill people?

SOURCE: Peter Johnson and Joseph Beditz, "Community Support Systems: Scaling Community Acceptance," *Community Mental Health Journal*, vol. 17, Summer 1981, p. 153–160. Used with permission.

Table 53-7 Nursing Diagnoses for CMI Clients

Examples
Systematic, structured approach to work related to successful management of anxiety level
Low self-esteem associated with poor hygiene habits
Preference for repetitive tasks associated with memory lapses and short attention span
Financial distress related to lack of money management skills
Intimacy-isolation struggle associated with history of poor judgment about people's trustworthiness
Tolerance for long periods of isolation related to discomfort in interpersonal relationships
Emotions of depression and defeat associated with unrealistic expectations for the self
Difficulty getting a job related to lack of job skills
Fear of leaving home related to physical and psychological harassment by neighbors
Tolerance of considerable stress associated with supportive family

Diagnosis

Nursing diagnoses should include strengths as well as problems in clients' interaction with family and community. During assessment, many of a client's strengths become apparent. By giving feedback on these strengths, the nurse can provide a basis for building new skills, and can help the client to recognize that his or her situation has positive aspects. Clients' strengths may include:

- Education
- Job skills
- Hobbies or nonvocational skills
- Special aptitudes or resources
- Intellectual abilities
- Organizational skills
- Aesthetic sensitivity
- Ability to form and maintain relationships

Some diagnoses that reflect both problems and strengths are found in Table 53-7.

Outcome Criteria

When working with a CMI client, long- and short-term goals and accompanying outcomes need to be set. The outcomes should be realistic and should reflect low expectations. Unhealthy patterns of interaction between the client and the environment were created over time, and multiple physical, mental, spiritual, and social factors were involved.

Even minor changes are major gains for a CMI client; the nurse who can appreciate the personal pain and risk required to take the smallest step is able to work well with the CMI.

Outcomes need to be set with the participation of the client. Often, CMI clients have no personal goals. Helping them to think about the future, to develop hope, and to consider their circumstances are major accomplishments. The process of setting goals is itself a therapeutic activity and may be a worthy outcome criterion.

With chronic mental illnesses, even so-called short-term goals may involve a longer time than would ordinarily be considered appropriate. Thus a short-term goal for an acutely ill or recovered person, such as joining a self-help group, may be a long-term goal for a CMI person; and achieving several other short-term goals may be required before the CMI client can actually join the group. The other short-term goals may consist of learning the art of social conversation, controlling spontaneous jerking of limbs, choosing a group, finding out what the membership qualifications are, arranging transportation, role-playing anxiety-producing situations, and identifying and overcoming barriers the client personally feels would hinder the outcome.

It is important to set realistic, practical goals. For instance, if a client has been unemployed for 5 years because of mental illness, circling three want ads in the newspaper every day for 7 days would not be a practical goal. A more realistic goal might be choosing what to wear on a job interview, with the nurse's encouragement and with a week's notice.

CMI clients have experienced multiple failures; setting unrealistic goals, or setting realistic goals without appropriate anticipation of the associated problems, does the client a disservice. For instance:

> Nancy A. (a nurse) worked with Tom B. (a client) on applying for a job similar to one he had held for many years. Though he had not been employed for 4 years, Tom felt that he still had the job skills because he had continued to receive his trade journals and had kept up his reading. Nancy had worked with Tom on interview skills, completion of applications, dealing with his history of mental illness, and several other important issues. Tom got to the door of the personnel office, had an anxiety attack, and was taken to the emergency room.

Change involves the risk of failure. Nurses must be ready with contingency plans when working with the CMI population. In the situation described above, Tom had several options; for example, he could have managed the anxiety attack and followed through with the interview, or he could have cancelled the interview at the last minute. The nurse can help the client to anticipate several possible outcomes and options so that falling back on symptomatic behavior, as Tom did, will not be necessary. The creativity of both nurse and client can be used to develop plans which will enhance the client's self-esteem and functional ability.

Intervention

Interventions for CMI clients and their families are described below. In addition, approaches to community planning and change are suggested, in an effort to address some of the needs of both the CMI population and the community.

Intervention with the Person

The four major arenas of the client's life in the community are living arrangements, social life, leisure activities, and work. Each must be dealt with by the nurse and the client together, in order for the client to survive in the community.

LIVING ARRANGEMENTS.* The chronically ill client's survival and rehabilitation depend on appropriately supportive and structured living arrangements. Living arrangements in the community are a major concern when plans for discharge are formulated. Some clients are able to live independently in an apartment or home or with their families. When family support is available in the form of warmth and acceptable levels of emotional involvement, clients tend to have fewer readmissions to the hospital.[14] However, some clients have no appropriate family support, have no family, or have a family in which dysfunctional patterns of interaction are reinforced. In such cases, alternative living arrangements must be made. Several possibilities are described below.

Clients may be candidates for a *halfway house* which provides a bridge between the hospital and

* Portions of this section from Lynn R. Bernstein, "Helplessness," in the second edition of this book.

gradual assumption of an independent lifestyle. The goals of the halfway house are enhancement of socialization skills and vocational rehabilitation.

Other clients may be placed in a *group home* on a temporary or permanent basis. A group home provides supervision, focusing on stabilization of chronicity and social recovery in a protected environment. *Satellite housing* is a type of group home in which there is professional supervision but no live-in staff; apartments in which four clients live together work out well. It is in keeping with the goal of community integration to locate only a few group homes in a given neighborhood.

Some clients are discharged to a state-approved *boarding home* in which they occupy a single or double room. They receive three meals a day, minimal staff supervision, and, in some states, supervision of medications.

Severely disabled clients may be placed in a *locked skilled-nursing facility.* These facilities house people who can survive outside state hospitals only if their living facilities are sufficiently structured to compensate for their lack of internal controls.[15]

Still other clients may be placed in a *foster home,* in which five or fewer clients live with a family. If clients are matched properly with the home milieu, their social functioning may improve. A study of schizophrenic clients found that much home activity and close supervision were associated with deterioration of clients.[16] Too much nurturing and closeness and too little opportunity to withdraw from social stimulation are thought to hinder the adjustment of these clients.[2]

Another possible "living arrangement" for mentally ill clients is *jail.* Because the present rate of discharge from hospitals is high and inpatients' stays are shorter, clients may not become stabilized on medications before discharge and thus may experience psychotic episodes that involve misdemeanors or felonies. Sometimes their behavior is so bizarre that the police cannot leave them on the street. Community health nurses must be aware of this problem, because clients whose medications have not been stabilized need close monitoring after discharge to prevent these episodes. Police departments report that they would take clients to emergency rooms rather than to jail if this did not entail hours of waiting and the possibility of no admission after the wait.[2] Close cooperation between community health nurses and local police departments may help to prevent inappropriate housing of the CMI in jails.

MAINTAINING BASIC NEEDS. Krauss states that nursing services for the CMI client must include:

- Provision of basic necessities of life
- Help in finding meaningful ways to use time
- Access to medication
- Support for family members
- Integrated medical, nursing, and social services[17]

As nurses plan for and provide care for the CMI, these services must be kept in mind. Nurses who work with clients in community settings play an important role in assessing basic functioning, monitoring health care practices and medication compliance, providing support to families, and coordinating services. Table 53-8 describes nursing interventions for clients living in unstructured home settings. The goal of such interventions is not only the stabilization of the client in the community but movement toward higher levels of functioning. The psychiatric nurse is uniquely suited to coordinate the activities of professional services with family and community helping networks.[6]

Nurses who work with clients in structured settings such as halfway houses or group homes may provide supervision or consultation to resident counselors in these settings, teaching them how to intervene to help clients meet basic needs and move toward higher levels of functioning. Another function unique to these transitional settings is preparing clients to cope with an independent lifestyle once they leave the halfway house or group home.

REHABILITATION PROGRAMS. Wherever discharged CMI clients live, aftercare is a necessity. Studies show that appropriate aftercare increases the length of time a client stays in the community. Increasing the variety and intensity of rehabilitation-oriented services has more positive influence than services consisting simply of chemotherapy, counseling, and case management.[18]

The various rehabilitation programs that have been established to deal with aftercare are described below. Many of them are alternatives to complete hospitalization. Each such program offers a specific service, has a different amount of structure, and works toward a different goal.

Table 53-8 Nursing Intervention for Clients Living in Unstructured Home Settings

Intervention	Example
Assess basic functioning.	1. Assess adequacy of physical surroundings and of living arrangements. 2. Assess adequacy of public transportation. 3. Assess adequacy of client's financial resources to meet basic needs. 4. Assess client's ability to shop for groceries, buy clothing, and pay bills. 5. Assess client's ability to meet basic health needs, such as proper hygiene and grooming, independently. 6. Assess client's ability to solve problems and make independent decisions. 7. Assess client's social and vocational skills.
Monitor degree to which client is meeting basic needs.	1. Monitor degree to which client is: a. Bathing b. Wearing clean clothes c. Shopping for groceries d. Preparing and eating nutritious meals e. Keeping the living quarters clean f. Paying bills 2. Monitor appropriateness of client's decisions. 3. Monitor client's level of social relatedness or isolation. 4. Monitor consistency with which client goes to work and attends the aftercare program.
Monitor client's medication compliance.	1. Monitor client's medication compliance: a. Does client have an adequate supply of medication? b. Is he or she taking prescribed medication in the proper amount and at the appropriate time? c. Does client understand the side effects of the medication? d. Does client understand the medication regimen? e. Is client attending a medication clinic? 2. Are there factors such as motivation or lack of information that inhibit compliance?
Teach skills that enhance client's ability to meet basic needs.	1. Help client plan a daily schedule for taking care of basic needs. 2. Teach client how to make a shopping list. 3. Teach client how to plan a balanced meal. 4. Teach client how to use public transportation. 5. Teach client how to shop for groceries. 6. Teach client how to cash a check and pay bills. 7. Teach client how to use a laundromat. 8. Teach client how to make up a medication schedule. 9. Teach client about medication side effects. 10. Teach client how to contact medication clinic for appointments and problems.
Provide support for family members.	1. Explore and validate appropriate concerns. 2. Help family members divide responsibility for supervising and caring for client. 3. Help them find free time for themselves. 4. Teach them how to set limits on problematic behaviors. 5. Help them find ways to let client be a contributing family member. 6. Involve them in community support groups with which they can share common problems.
Coordinate services.	1. Provide a dependable person whom client can contact on a 24-hour basis. 2. Act as liaison between client and community agencies such as welfare, day care center, vocational rehabilitation center, and clinic, as well as community support groups. 3. Initiate coordination of mental health services into an effective treatment plan by collaborating with members of the health team. 4. Initiate referral of client to community support groups such as social groups, AA, and church groups. 5. Inform client about available community resources. 6. Initiate rehospitalization process if client's level of functioning threatens well-being of self or others.

SOURCE: From Lynn R. Bernstein, "Helplessness," in the second edition of this book.

Partial hospitalization. One kind of rehabilitation program is partial hospitalization. The three most common types of partial hospitalization are the day hospital, day treatment, and day care. A *day hospital* serves the same population and provides the same services as an inpatient unit; it exists to prevent hospitalization. *Day treatment* provides therapeutic experiences for 2 to 3 months to clients who are making the transition from hospital to community. *Day care* provides long-term care for patients who are not expected to show improvement or progress beyond the day care setting; it keeps clients from deteriorating to the point where hospitalization would be necessary. While these programs are theoretically separate and distinct, in reality they may overlap considerably.[19]

In partial hospitalization programs, a variety of therapeutic activities are provided, including structured activities such as dance, art, and hobbies as well as discussion groups which facilitate reality orientation, socialization, problem solving, task mastery, and increasing self-direction. The day hospital population is regarded as a community to which all members are responsible in different ways. Clients are expected to contribute to the effective functioning of this community. Additional services such as medication clinics, therapy sessions, and coordination with vocational rehabilitation services are often part of the program. Nurses, as members of the day care team, participate in evaluation of new clients and care planning, lead groups, provide one-to-one therapy, work in medication clinics, and help to coordinate other services.

Mental health clinics. A second kind of rehabilitation available in the community is the mental health clinic. Mental health clinics offer a variety of services, commonly including evaluation, individual therapy, group and family therapy, medication follow-up, and community outreach programs. The clinic often becomes a client's ongoing link to mental health services, and clients are able to utilize the services provided by the clinic on an open-ended basis. A nurse may be involved as primary therapist for a client. In this role the nurse not only deals with therapeutic issues in an individual or group milieu but inevitably also acts as liaison between the client and other community agencies. Table 53-9 provides examples of group activities that may be initiated by mental health clinics.

Vocational rehabilitation. A third kind of rehabilitation available in the community is vocational rehabilitation. Vocational rehabilitation programs are another dimension of the coordinated care plan. Clients are helped to return to former areas of vocational expertise or to develop new areas of skill. Some clients lack job skills, others have never held a job, and still others may have worked only for brief periods of time. Vocational counseling helps such clients identify areas in which they have interests and abilities. Specific training programs help them acquire the credentials and skills to meet job requirements. Efforts are made to coordinate clients' vocational interests and skills with job placements.

Not all clients are able to cope with the stress of a full-time job that involves considerable responsibility; they may be more successful in full- or part-time jobs in low-stress environments. For those who are unable even to cope with such comparatively low levels of stress, volunteer work or employment in a sheltered workshop is often possible.

In general, a client's involvement in a work program should take place in a series of progressive steps that make the likelihood of success at each step probable. If successful, the work program provides a vehicle for meaningful productivity, enhancement of self-esteem, socialization, and independence. Nurses generally act as liaisons between vocational rehabilitation programs, the mental health center, and the client.

Crisis intervention. A fourth kind of rehabilitation available in the community is crisis intervention. CMI clients are easily upset and need a crisis intervention service. This service is often provided by the professional, often a nurse, responsible for the client's ongoing case management. However, because many CMI clients (perhaps, according to some estimates, as many as 60 percent) do not maintain ongoing therapeutic relationships, additional crisis intervention services must be provided by the community. Aggressive, appropriately timed crisis intervention may help clients to remain in the community. CMI clients are even more dependent than the usual client in crisis, and the therapist must be prepared for and accommodate the high level of dependence. Crisis intervention theory and application are explored in Chapter 22.

Self-help groups. A fifth kind of rehabilitation available in the community is the self-help group.

Table 53-9 Client Groups Sponsored by Mental Health Clinics

Type of Group	Goal	Examples
Activities of daily living	Help clients to acquire or reestablish self-care behaviors.	A reentry group for outpatients which begins before discharge and which clients continue to attend after discharge. It teaches clients how to meet hygiene needs, cook a meal, clean an apartment, budget money, shop for groceries, and use public transportation.
Activity	Involve clients in activities in which they can succeed. Develop recreational and leisure interests. Encourage resocialization.	Photography, ceramics, dance, and current events groups provide a topical or activity focus which is goal-directed and can be participated in on many levels.
Social	Decrease isolation. Increase socialization skills. Decrease feelings of being threatened by relatedness. Expand clients' support systems and social networks.	Social groups sponsored by clinics may organize an activity—perhaps bingo, a dance, or a party with food and conversation. A speaker may be the focus of the meeting or the activity may just be an informal get-together.
Community education	Increase awareness and knowledge of issues and problems common to families coping with psychiatric illness. Increase family coping skills. Increase community awareness. Develop community resources.	A community series on chronic psychiatric problems discussing what they are, whom they affect, and what community members can do to help. A series of talks and discussions for families on how to manage behavioral problems common to people with chronic psychiatric conditions.

SOURCE: J. B. Krauss, "The Chronic Psychiatric Patient in the Community—A Model of Care," *Nursing Outlook*, vol. 28, 1980, pp. 308–314.

Self-help groups have been shown to provide social support, to prevent illness and death, and to reduce the need for hospitalization.[20] Nurses need to assess the availability of self-help groups in the local community; if such groups are needed, nurses may initiate and work with them.

Intervention with the Family

In order to intervene effectively with the family of a CMI person, the nurse adopts the position that the client is a member of the family rather than either a victim or the center of the family and the most important person in it. It is also important to remember that:

- The family is in the most strategic position to offer consistent long-term support to the client.
- The other family members must have support so that they will be able to provide the resources needed by the client.

Goldman synthesized from the literature four solutions to the problem of the family's burden.[9] The first of these is *family-oriented rehabilitation and treatment services*. The purpose of this solution is to foster the view that the client is a member of the family, to shore up the family's natural support system, and to recognize the stress in the family's situation.

The second solution is *home visiting*. The purpose of home visiting is to "reinforce the client's natural support system." Goldman refers to home visiting as both effective and time-consuming. Among the advantages of home visiting are these: family members are in familiar surroundings and behave naturally; family strengths are more apparent and more easily reinforced in the home; interventions are more effective when specifically designed for the family's unique physical and psychological environment; and the ambience of the home is accessible only to those who visit there.

Relatives' groups are the third solution. Their purpose is to address the family's burdens of stigma and guilt feelings through a broad-based, inexpensive approach. These groups are now also addressing consumer issues such as civil rights, improvements in services, and benefits for people who are disabled permanently or for a long time.

Community support systems are the fourth solution. The purpose of community support systems is to bolster the natural supports, including families, of chronically disabled people living outside institutions. A community support system is a comprehensive network of health, mental health, and social welfare services and benefits. Community services should include respite care to give families a vacation from the responsibility of home care for brief periods.

Intervention with the Community

The community is amenable to change and will have to respond to the needs of diverse groups of community members needing special services. Some of these groups are the elderly, minorities, people from other countries, and the chronically mentally ill. Two directions can help in effecting change in communities: community organization approaches and planning for community services.

COMMUNITY ORGANIZATION APPROACHES. Rothman suggests three models of community organization that help professionals to understand how they can participate in community change.[21] The first model, the *community-development* approach, is designed to create conditions of economic and social progress for the whole community. President Reagan's approach to economic recovery is an example of the community-development approach.

The second model, the *social-planning* approach, emphasizes a technical process of solving problems surrounding specific major issues. The plan, cited earlier, for integration of CMI people into the community of Asbury Park, New Jersey, is an example of the social-planning approach.

The third model, the *social-action* approach, is used on behalf of a specific disadvantaged segment of the population. The deinstitutionalization movement that began in the 1960s is a social-action approach.

PLANNING FOR COMMUNITY SERVICES. In offering principles for planning community services, Bachrach[22] suggests that planning services for the CMI population is more difficult than the usual planning of services for several reasons:

- The needs of the CMI endure.
- The needs are comprehensive and intense.
- Paradoxically, communities do not want to treat the people who are most severely disabled.
- There is a stigma attached to CMI.
- Efforts are often uncoordinated.[22]

Bachrach's planning principles include the following:

1. State precise goals, and give objective rather than idealistic or global directions.
2. Set priorities specifically for the CMI population.
3. Reassess available mental health services to find an appropriate place for institutions among the services offered.
4. Use a range of service interventions to provide a flexible network of interrelated programs, including screening and referral, crisis stabilization, residential alternatives, a range of treatment settings and services, transportation, information, and evaluation.
5. Set up cooperation and linkages between agencies to reduce duplication and increase communication.
6. Match clients with programs on an individual basis to increase effectiveness of treatment and appropriate utilization of services.
7. Make sure the services to be provided are culturally relevant to the local setting and local clients. (Note that this principle precludes imitation of a successful program from another region.)
8. Provide a format flexible enough to respond to the ever-changing needs of individual clients as they grow and change.
9. Use caution and restraint. Apply adequate thought, study, and funding to the situation before developing the services.[22]

Local and state professional nursing organizations, as well as individual nurses, have opportunities to address the needs of the CMI population. The nursing profession can work effectively with the community in solving some difficult issues related to provision of services for the CMI population.

Evaluation

Evaluation of the success of the nursing care plan for a CMI client relates to the outcomes established with that client. The goal is to promote, maintain, or restore the client's maximum possible level of functioning. An adaptation of Albee's formula[23] for level of functioning is as follows:

$$\text{Level of functioning} = \frac{\text{mental and spiritual stress} + \text{physical vulnerability}}{\text{social supports} + \text{coping skills} + \text{competence}}$$

Working with each aspect of this formula should have a positive effect upon the client's level of functioning.

A case study will illustrate the process of evaluation:

> J. R., 26 years old, has a 10-year history of psychotic episodes. He has lived at home throughout this period, except for one hospitalization of 21 days. He has been maintained on medications, crisis intervention during psychotic episodes, and case management, in which he is seen every 2 months. J. R. finished high school but has not been able to sustain employment. His family consists of his mother, father, and two sisters, both younger than J. R. The family have provided J. R. with an accepting environment and have managed to weather his psychotic episodes at home with comparative calm. The family contacted the nurse case manager, who wrote and implemented the care plan.

The care plan in Table 53-10 illustrates assessment data adequate to support the nursing diagnosis. The outcome criteria reflect agreement by the client, the family, and the nurse about the goals they think will resolve the crisis. The interventions are designed to address the second part of the nursing diagnosis (the weakening of the family support system). The evaluation documents both the outcome criteria and the usefulness of the nursing process.

Table 53-10 Nursing Process to Illustrate Evaluation of Care for a CMI Client (J. R.)

Assessment

Currently, J. R.'s 20-year-old sister is dating a young man very seriously and has become embarrassed because J. R. is behaving obnoxiously. He is also behaving seductively with his 16-year-old sister's girlfriends. The 16-year-old is angry and rebellious, accusing the parents of catering to J. R.; she is staying out all night and refusing to accept restrictions placed on her for unacceptable behavior. The parents are having difficulty knowing how to handle these new problems and are having more serious disagreements more often, which are followed by periods of silence. In the past week, J. R. cornered one of the 16-year-old's friends and frightened her with vulgar language and attempts to fondle her. He has become loud and demanding during his usually quiet times. He is unable to concentrate on his stamp and butterfly collections, which he can usually spend hours on. He is refusing to cooperate with home routines. In the past he maintained his medication regimen without supervision, but he is now requiring monitoring by his father to do so.

Diagnosis

Impending exacerbation of psychotic symptoms related to weakening of family support system

Outcome Criteria

J. R. will maintain intact ego within 4 weeks as evidenced by:

1. Use of current coping skills
2. Development of one new support system
3. Ability to handle a new daytime environment
4. Maintenance of medication regimen
5. Control of sexual and demanding acting out

Interventions

1. Interventions addressed to J. R.:
   a. Enroll J. R. in day care program for CMI, 8 A.M. to 5 A.M., Monday to Friday.
   b. Arrange for weekend care for J. R. every other weekend for 3 months at the Respite Care Center.
   c. Refer J. R. to physician for increased dose of antipsychotic medication.
2. Interventions addressed to the family:
   a. Provide family crisis intervention aimed at: reestablishing order, routine; dealing with launching phase of family development when the eldest is not launched; increasing the family's problem-solving skills.
   b. Decrease family burden by: encouraging acceptance of long-term day care for J. R.; assisting in weekly plans for individual, spouse, and family leisure activities; referring family to a support group for families of the CMI; assisting parents in development of a system of rewards for appropriate behavior by J. R. and sisters; encouraging realignment of responsibilities among family members.

Evaluation

Evaluation completed 4 weeks from date of emergency telephone call.

Evaluation of outcome criteria

J. R. has experienced no psychotic symptoms in the past month.

1. He is concentrating on his collections for an hour at a time each evening.
2. He has made two new friends and they have gone for pizza and a movie twice in the past 2 weeks.

(Continued.)

Table 53-10 Continued

Evaluation	Evaluation
Evaluation of outcome criteria (continued) 3. He has adjusted well to day care setting. 4. Physician increased medication dosage, which initially helped; dosage now needs to be reevaluated because J. R. is drowsy in the late morning and early evening. Father is no longer monitoring medication, and J. R. reports comfort in monitoring his own medication again. 5. J. R.'s sisters report no sexual or obnoxious behavior; however, their friends have been coming over much less often, which makes this behavior difficult to measure. The day care center reports no unacceptable sexual behavior on J. R.'s past. **Evaluation of nursing interventions** 1a. The day care center worked well short-term, but the environment may not be stimulating enough long-term. 1b. The family appreciated the respite care, though they voice some guilt. They all express missing each other, but J. R. announced he wanted to go to the Respite Care Center "forever." He enjoyed the activities and was not forced to interact with a lot of people. 1c. Increased medication was effective.	**Evaluation of nursing interventions** (continued) 2a. Parents continue to show lack of insight into family dynamics; daughters see no connection between their developmental needs and J. R.'s acting out. J. R. continues to express the family's unacceptable impulses. The parents did make some "hard and fast" rules for all three children that has placed the parents back in control of their home. 2b. The family's burden has been relieved by having J. R. out of the home all day, every other weekend, and two evenings. His hobbies remove him from the family another hour each day. Leisure activities continue to be a problem; the 16-year-old's activities continue to cause anxiety to the parents, though her staying out and rebelliousness have declined considerably. Parents feel they can't enjoy themselves because they must be alert for the 16-year-old and J. R. Parents "planned to go to support group twice but something came up." Daughters and J. R. showed interest in discussing privileges as rewards for appropriate behavior, and parents came through somewhat for 16-year-old. Parents "see no need" for rewards for J. R., who "can't help himself," or for the 20-year-old, who "is no problem and never has been." All family members are comfortable with their responsibilities; though there is a lot of complaining, no one is interested in trading jobs. 2c. Am unsure that the way they established the rules increased their problem-solving skills.

SUMMARY

Historically, the chronically mentally ill population were given custodial care in state hospitals and were not expected to return to the community. With the advent of antipsychotic medications and funding for community mental health centers in the 1960s, many people were discharged from state hospitals, and fewer clients were admitted. The result was deinstitutionalization of the mentally ill, with the result that most of the CMI began to live in the community. Community resources are being developed to respond to the needs of the CMI, but the low level of financial resources available is a serious problem.

Since the community mental health movement began, statisticians have had difficulty determining the number of CMI in the United States. There are thought to be about 3 million CMI, out of a total of 7 million people who have been treated for emotional or mental problems. There are basically two populations of CMI: the older, deinstitutionalized population and the younger, never institutionalized population. The groups differ in symptoms, medical diagnoses, treatment patterns, and interaction with the community. Both groups require financial assistance from family, government, or both because of severe, prolonged disability. There are seven theoretical perspectives of chronicity: medical, epidemiological, sociological, intrapsychic, integrated, comprehensive, and myth. The symptoms of chronicity are dependence, social incompetence, stigma, the sick role, ongoing relationships with institutions, symptomatic behavior, and a low level of functioning.

Whether a client lives at home or elsewhere, the family carries a heavy responsibility. To prevent this responsibility from becoming a burden that threatens the family's ability to provide the necessary support for the client, assistance for the family may be offered in the form of family-oriented rehabilitation and treatment, home visiting, relatives' groups, and community support systems.

The community offers opportunities for living, social activities, leisure pursuits, and work; but the chronically mentally ill often have difficulty in taking advantage of these opportunities. Communities find the CMI a burden and respond in a variety of ways. The goal of integration is accomplished through working toward community acceptance of the CMI and through community participation in planning and funding resources. Community development models provide ways to work with the community toward integration of the CMI population.

The nursing process is the same for the CMI client as for any other. Particular attention to outcome criteria is necessary, however, since long- and short-term goals are different for the CMI population. Goal setting for these clients is a challenge for the CMI as well as for the nurse. Establishing a time frame for goals is difficult as well. The most effective nurses are those who appreciate the personal pain and risk encountered by the CMI client in attempting to accomplish even the most minor goal.

The care of the CMI population is expected to be one of the primary health care issues of the 1990s. This is an area in which nursing can make a major contribution to the well-being of individuals, families, and communities.

REFERENCES

1. Joint Commission on Mental Illness and Health, *Action for Mental Health,* Basic Books, New York, 1961.
2. John A. Talbott, ed., *The Chronic Mental Patient: Five Years Later,* Grune and Stratton, New York, 1984.
3. *National Plan for the Chronically Mentally Ill,* final draft report to the Secretary of Health and Human Services, Washington, 1980.
4. J. R. Woy, I. D. Goldstrom, and R. W. Manderscheid, *The Young Chronic Mental Patient: Report of a National Survey,* NIMH-OP-79-0031, National Institute of Mental Health, Washington, 1982.
5. J. L. Sheets et al., "Young Adult Chronic Patients: Three Hypothesized Subgroups," *Hospital and Community Psychiatry,* vol. 33, 1982, pp. 197–203.
6. J. B. Krauss and A. T. Slavinsky, *The Chronically Ill Psychiatric Patient and the Community,* Blackwell Scientific Publications, Boston, 1982.
7. A. Strauss, *Chronic Illness and the Quality of Life,* Mosby, St. Louis, Mo., 1975.
8. T. Parsons, *The Social System,* Free Press, New York, 1951.
9. H. H. Goldman, "Mental Illness and Family Burden: A Public Health Perspective," *Hospital and Community Psychiatry,* vol. 33, July 1982, pp. 557–560.
10. A. B. Hatfield, "Help-Seeking Behavior in Families of Schizophrenics," *American Journal of Community Psychology,* vol. 7, July 1979, pp. 563–569.
11. A. B. Hatfield, "What Families Want of Family Therapy," in W. R. MacFarlane, ed., *Family Therapy in Schizophrenia,* Guilford, New York, 1983, pp. 41–63.
12. Peter Breyer and Donald Malafronte, "Promoting Community Involvement in Deinstitutionalization Planning: The Experience in One Community," *Hospital and Community Psychiatry,* vol. 33, August 1982, pp. 654–657.
13. Peter Johnson and Joseph Beditz, "Community Support Systems: Scaling Community Acceptance," *Community Mental Health Journal,* vol. 17, Summer 1981, pp. 153–160.
14. C. E. Vaughn and J. P. Leff, "The Influence of Family and Social Factors in the Course of Psychiatric Illness," *British Journal of Psychiatry,* vol. 139, 1981, pp. 102–104.
15. H. R. Lamb, "Structure: The Neglected Ingredient of Community Treatment," *Archives of General Psychiatry,* vol. 37, 1980, pp. 1224–1228.
16. M. W. Linn et al., "Foster Home Characteristics and Psychiatric Patient Outcome," *Archives of General Psychiatry,* vol. 37, 1980, pp. 129–132.
17. J. B. Krauss, "The Chronic Psychiatric Patient in the Community—A Model of Care," *Nursing Outlook,* vol. 28, 1980, pp. 308–314.
18. P. Solomon et al., "Discharged State Hospital Patients' Characteristics and Use of Aftercare: Effect on Community Tenure," *American Journal of Psychiatry,* vol. 141, 1984, pp. 1566–1570.
19. M. S. Edwards, "Psychiatric Day Programs: A Descriptive Analysis," *Journal of Psychosocial Nursing,* vol. 20, September 1982, pp. 17–21.
20. A. J. Gartner and Frank Riessman, "Self-Help and Mental Health," *Hospital and Community Psychiatry,* vol. 33, 1982, pp. 631–635.
21. J. Rothman, "Three Models of Community Organization Practice, Their Mixing and Phasing," in F. M. Cox et al., eds., *Strategies of Community Organization: A Book of Readings,* Peacock, Itasca, Ill., 1979, pp. 25–45.
22. L. Bachrach, "Principles of Planning for Chronic Psychiatric Patients: A Synthesis," in J. A. Talbott, ed., *The Chronic Mental Patient: Five Years Later,* Grune and Stratton, New York, 1984, pp. 165–182.
23. George Albee, "An Ounce of Prevention: Reorienting Mental Health Priorities," *Self-Help Reporter,* vol. 5, 1981, pp. 1–2.

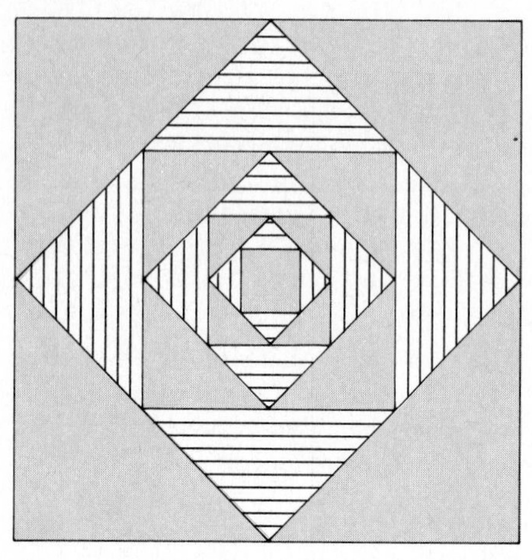

CHAPTER 54

Mental Health Issues of the Elderly

Anita M. Leach

LEARNING OBJECTIVES

After studying this chapter, the student should be able to:

1. Describe the aging process.
2. Identify emotional responses and mental health problems common among older people.
3. Discuss patterns of interaction—person, family, and environment—among older people.
4. Identify stages of transition to the role of widowhood among older people.
5. Describe the levels of housing for the aged, and give examples of each.
6. Discuss the adult child's position in relationship to aging parents.
7. List the phases of retirement.
8. Apply the nursing process in the care of the elderly.
9. Utilize a variety of frameworks to assess older clients' needs.
10. Formulate multifaceted nursing diagnoses.
11. Evaluate intervention strategies.
12. Construct a holistic nursing care plan for an elderly client.

Old age, the time after age 65, is a dynamic stage in the overall life-span continuum. Aging is accompanied by physical, emotional, cognitive, and spiritual changes that compound a person's preexisting strengths and weaknesses.

Aging can be a comfortable and happy time of life for people who are in reasonably good physical health, maintain strong family and environmental bonds, have adequate finances, and enjoy ease and warmth in interpersonal relationships.

Despite many years of involvement in the care of the elderly, the nursing profession has only recently been recognized for its contribution to geriatric care. Not until 1967 did the Division of Geriatric Nursing Practice of the American Nurses Association begin developing standards of practice for geriatric nursing. In 1976, the association adopted the term *gerontological nursing* to differentiate holistic nursing care of the elderly from a more medical geriatric approach:

> Gerontologic Nursing is concerned with assessment of the health needs of older adults, planning and implementing health care to meet these needs, and evaluating the effectiveness of such care. Emphasis is placed on maximizing independence in the activities of everyday living and promoting, maintaining and restoring health.[1]

Geropsychiatric nursing, a subspecialty of psychiatric nursing, is a relatively new field for nurses.[2] The purpose of this chapter is to acquaint nursing students with the principles of geropsychiatric nursing. The chapter will examine the physical, mental, and spiritual dimensions of elderly persons, the common family and environmental issues of the older adult, and some mental health problems of the aged. The nursing process will be used to demonstrate the way in which nurses interact with older clients. Because this chapter deals with a population rather than individuals, it begins with patterns of interaction (person, family, and environment) and then takes up dysynchronous health patterns and the nursing process.

PATTERNS OF INTERACTION: PERSON

People grow old in different ways. *Aging,* the process of growing old, is not a rigid or fixed process but is influenced by social, emotional, ethnic, physical, racial, religious, and economic factors. The way in which people grow old is influenced by the environment, and society in turn influences both structures and functions of the elderly. Butler and Lewis[3] define the major developmental task of the elderly as clarifying, deepening, and finding use for what has already been attained through a lifetime of learning and adapting. They state that older people must teach themselves to conserve their strength and resources and to adjust to those changes and losses that occur as part of aging.

Several factors have been identified as positively influencing older people's place in society:

- Ownership of property
- A sense of control over their destiny
- Strong religious and cultural traditions
- Strong kinship, social network, and extended family bonds
- The ability to use and contribute to community resources
- A sense of independence and autonomy[3]

Psychosocial, cognitive, and personality theories about aging focus on a person's emotional or intellectual response to the aging process. Mental health involves emotional and cognitive dimensions as well as self-esteem. Older people's self-esteem is maintained when their achievements are recognized, they receive positive feedback, they are treated with respect and courtesy, they maintain decision-making power and control of their destiny, they have satisfying interpersonal relationships, and they meet the basic needs of everyday living. Mentally healthy older adults are able to fulfill appropriate roles, accept new challenges, negotiate age-related changes, accept losses, remain flexible, and interact with their environment in gratifying ways.

Erikson states that the developmental issue of older adulthood is *ego integrity versus despair.* Ego integrity allows a person to view life as meaningful, with both positive and negative characteristics, to accept this reality, and not to be threatened by it. Integrity provides a person with the basis for approaching the end of life with a feeling of having lived completely.[3] Despair is the result of rejecting oneself and one's past. It arises when a person rejects the decisions made in the process of living and simultaneously realizes that there is not enough time left to alter this self-assessment. Despairing older adults are prone to depression and are afraid of dying.[3] Neugarten suggested that peoples' personalities and emotional makeup do not change with aging but that their behavior becomes more predictable. Her *continuity theory* states that people's patterns, habits, commitments, preferences, and methods of adaptation serve as the basis for predicting their mental and emotional state as they grow older.[4]

Physical Patterns

Many theories about the physiological processes of normal aging have been proposed. These may be summarized by stating simply that aging is a universal, progressive, intrinsic, and selective slowing down of physiological and biological processes.

Several physical explanations for the aging process have been proposed. Aging may result from some or all of the following factors:

- Hereditary, genetic programs that set limits on growth, aging, and longevity
- Slowed molecular functioning
- Lowered efficiency of the immune system
- Increased autoimmune reactions in which antibodies are produced that destroy normal cells
- Decreased efficiency of endocrine control of various vital functions
- Age-related decline in the capacity of the nervous system to speedily and efficiently maintain body integrity and prevent body deterioration[5]

The elderly, like other segments of the population, are affected by many acute and chronic physical conditions. Certain illnesses commonly associated with the elderly include arthritis, congestive heart failure, glaucoma, cataracts, deafness, blindness, hypertension, and osteoporosis. Although these physical conditions are accompanied by emotional and spiritual dimensions, a detailed discussion of physically based syndromes is beyond the scope of this chapter. Several comprehensive texts on aging provide in-depth discussions of the specific biological and physiological changes that occur in the elderly person. Impairments in psychomotor and sensory processes, common among older adults, are discussed in this chapter because they have implications for mental health.

Psychomotor Processes

The psychomotor responses of older people are generally slower than those of younger people. Reaction time increases with age, causing people to take longer to respond to environmental stimuli. Speed and accuracy of movement decline as people grow older, and complex tasks take longer periods of time to complete. The implications for nursing care are obvious.

Some diseases of old age, such as arthritis and osteoporosis, affect an older person's psychomotor ability and may cause severe pain. People who have limited mobility, severe pain, or both may respond with withdrawal, isolation, loneliness, and depression.

Sensory Processes

The senses are the means by which people experience the world outside themselves as well as their internal functions. *Vision* allows experience of color, intensity, distance, and field angle. As a person ages, many changes occur in the eye. Older people take longer to accommodate to darkness and need higher levels of illumination and more intense color for satisfaction. Twenty-five percent of people over 70 have cataracts (a *cataract* is a clouding of the lens that causes impairment of vision). Although only a small percentage of older Americans are blind, it is interesting to note that the majority of blind people in the United States are older.[6] *Impaired hearing* is common among older people, who generally have more difficulty in hearing both high-pitched sounds and sounds of low intensity. *Elevated taste thresholds,* that is, a need for a more intense stimulus in order to taste things, may also occur. On the other hand, there seems to be no change in an older person's sense of *smell.* Sensitivity to *touch* increases with age, but older people appear less sensitive to pain.[5]

Loss of vision, hearing, or any other sense can be partly compensated for by increased use of another sense, but when several senses decline simultaneously, as happens with many older people, adaptation to the environment becomes a serious problem. Such people often become increasingly isolated, lonely, and depressed because of the decrease in sensory input.

Mental Patterns

Cognitive processes do not decline simply because of the aging process. There are apparent cognitive changes in older people, but these are generally caused by malfunction of the circulatory or neurological systems rather than by the aging process itself. *Intelligence, learning, memory, thinking,* and *creativity* are the mental processes of greatest concern to mental health practitioners.

Intelligence

The intelligence of the elderly as a group has been difficult to study, primarily because of the many variables in this age group. However, Jacewicz and Hartley[7] found that when younger individuals were matched with older individuals in terms of life experience and other variables, there were no significant differences in spatial relationships, verbal skills, or psychomotor skills (all these are components of intelligence). The elderly are sometimes deficient or slower during learning, need more time to store and retain new information, and have overall slower retrieval time for stored information,[4] but they do not experience any significant change in intelligence.[5]

Learning

For most older people, learning capacity continues well into the eighties. The elderly may be either impeded or helped by earlier learning, and it is known that they need longer time frames in which to learn new tasks. Practice, particularly of new tasks, greatly improves performance. When the material to be learned is meaningful, and when they can control the pace and rate of learning, the elderly learn as well as their younger counterparts of equal intelligence.[5]

Memory

Memory is linked to learning in the elderly. Many older people complain that they have difficulties with their memory. They are generally referring to *short-term memory,* the ability to remember the recent past. Misplaced keys, dentures, and eyeglasses are frequently the concerns voiced to the nurse. Forming a habit of always putting these items away in the same place usually solves the problem. Many older people have excellent *long-term memory,* the ability to recall the distant past. They may be very adept at reminiscing about their childhood and young adulthood. Reminiscing can be a useful therapeutic tool in intervention with elderly clients.

Memory deficits among the elderly may occur when tasks are meaningless or are paced too quickly. When many changes are required in the performance of a task or when the task requires high levels of visual rather than auditory acuity, the older person is likely to have difficulty. *Memory interference* is the inability to remember because of some previously stored memory.[2] For example, when there is anxiety attached to some event of the past, the older adult will "forget" the event.

When organic processes are dysfunctional, an older person's intelligence, memory, and ability to learn are generally impeded. Chapters 33 and 44 discuss substance abuse and organic mental disorders, respectively. Both of these problems impair cognitive functioning.

Thinking

Thinking is defined as the process of developing new ideas.[5] Thinking helps put order into multiple data by differentiating and categorizing the data into concepts. Studies show that, as age increases, a person's ability to form concepts declines. However, observation indicates that older people may remain adept at concept formation but simply become "set in their ways" because of personality or environmental factors.[5]

Creativity

Creativity is problem solving that is unique, original, and inventive.[5] The ability to be creative does not come to an abrupt halt when a person becomes older; rather, there is a gradual decline in creative effort. A crucial issue in the creativity of older people is the presence or absence of social supports for creative efforts. In order for the elderly to continue being creative, encouragement is needed from others in their environment. Frequently, increased leisure time facilitates a person's discovery of some previously unknown creative talent.

Spiritual Patterns

A holistic approach to older people requires consideration of the spiritual self. Self-actualized people consider alternative ways of viewing themselves and the universe, and many believe in forms of life and energy beyond present reality and knowledge. As death approaches, people are called upon to transcend the ordinary events of life and to perceive commonplace happenings in entirely new ways. Finding meaning in the later years and accepting death are major developmental tasks of the elderly.

Personal meaning and *self-fulfillment* have as many varied expressions as there are people. Some people transcend themselves through mystical or religious experiences, while others leave artistic legacies or express themselves through objects, deeds, crafts, progeny, or autobiographical statements. Some people view life as having at its end only death. For these people, trancendent expression of self includes developing and enhancing the virtues of hope, wisdom, courage, humor, faith, and idealism. A sense of duty, prestige, secularism, and pragmatism are more practical expressions of life's meaningfulness.

Religious practices, dreams, symbols, fantasies, daydreams, and visions are all expressions of the spiritual dimension of self. *Religious practice* has been found to be positively correlated with feelings of happiness, usefulness, and personal adjustment and to be a support system for those in failing health. In a study by Devine, marital status, health problems, and availability of transportation were factors that affected the religious attitudes and activities of the older people studied.[8]

Jung stated that one of the major goals of the last half of life was the reconciliation of a person's various repressions by the use of *dreams, myths,* and *symbols.* The process of individuation and transcendence requires embracing not only conscious reality but the hidden self as well. For all people, including the elderly, dreams serve to reveal the unconscious, to compensate for or modify self-deficits, to help resolve conflicts, to warn of danger, to share in and touch the collective unconscious of all humanity.[9]

Fantasies are waking dreams or mental images conjured in the imagination that fill reverie states and carry the person into situations that are otherwise inaccessible. Older people tend to fantasize and daydream less than the young, but to engage instead in memory images. *Memory images* are visualized experiences accompanied by affective changes. Present needs are uncovered through past memories. The technique of reminiscing makes use of memory images.

Visualizations are mental images that tap the subconscious and facilitate the revelation of hidden parts of the self. Guided affective imagery and directed daydreams are ways in which visualization helps the elderly transcend such realities as pain, dying, and depression.[10]

Older people leave many legacies. In a *living legacy* a person donates his or her body or body parts to science for transplants. *Spatial legacies* involve written or verbal autobiographical accounts of a person's environment. *Physical legacies* may include property, assets, and personal possessions. Grandchildren and other descendants may also be part of an elderly person's legacy. People who have found meaning for their lives by facing the inevitability of death as the beginning of an afterlife specify their legacies in very concrete and vibrant ways. They have in a sense discovered the secret of immortality.

PATTERNS OF INTERACTION: FAMILY

Only 5 percent of the elderly in the United States live in institutions. The remaining live in family households in the community.[11] Bonds of interdependence, intimacy, and belonging are basic needs of elderly family members which often find their fulfillment within the structure of the family. The dynamics created in the family with an older member are not unlike those discussed in Chapter 19. These elderly people contribute to family life in their unique roles as spouses, parents, grandparents, great-grandparents, siblings, and family sages. However, some older people do not live in the context of family. The never-married, the widowed, and the divorced are those most likely to be cut off from close family bonds.[5]

Couples

About half the older population in the United States are married and live with a spouse in an independent household. Seventy percent of older men and 36 percent of older women are married.[11] In addition to married couples, there are unmarried heterosexual and homosexual couples over age 65 who live as mates. Late marriages, that is, marriages in old age, are increasing, probably in part because of an increased awareness of gerontic sexuality.

The couple relationship becomes a focal point for many older people because of the increased amount of contact between the spouses and the corresponding decreased contact with fellow workers or grown children. Older couples are characterized by a high degree of interdependence and caring. Marital satisfaction is a central factor in overall life satisfaction for the elderly. Happily married older couples share many activities, have few unfulfilled expectations, are satisfied with their roles as wife and husband, and exhibit considerable equality between partners. Only about 15,000 couples over the age of 65 are granted divorces each year.

Couplehood has several functions, including emotional and sexual intimacy, a sense of belonging, and interdependence. Intimacy involves mutual affection, regard, and trust as well as sexual intimacy.

The *sexual intimacy* of older people reflects their physical capacity; their emotional needs; and cultural, social, and religious norms. It is usually physically possible for sexual intimacy to continue into the later years provided the couple have established a pattern of sexual intimacy in their middle years. Several major factors have been found to reduce the possibility of sexual intimacy in the elderly:

- Boredom with one's partner
- Mental and physical fatigue
- Overindulgence in food or drink
- Physical or emotional infirmities
- Fear of poor performance or fear that one's partner is uninterested
- Previous low performance or lack of interest

One study found that 80 percent of older people are sexually active[7] and are more sexually satisfied than they were earlier in their marriages. They stated that leisure time, lack of fears about pregnancy, and the privacy to be spontaneous are major factors in their increased satisfaction.[12]

The empty nest and retirement increase a couple's *sense of belonging* to each other. Frequent opportunities for companionship tend to decrease the potential for conflict.

Interdependence involves sharing housework as well as income and other resources. It has been found that interdependence increases in importance for the elderly. Major difficulties occur, however, when care giving is no longer mutual and shifts from interdependence to dependence. The physical disability of one spouse, a common occurrence in old age, is a major cause of such a shift. The consequent resentment causes a reduction in the quality of the relationship and simultaneously reduces intimacy between spouses, resulting in further conflict.

Single People

The single older population includes people who have never married, people who are widowed, and people who are divorced. In 1981, only 5 percent of older people in the United States had never married.[11] Older single people who had never married had developed autonomy and self-reliance to a higher degree than their married counterparts.[13] Single people who have tended to be lifelong isolates state that they are not particularly lonely in old age. Older women who are single tend to maintain more contact with their family of origin than do older men.

Divorced People

In 1981, 6 percent of the older population were found to be divorced. The sequelae to divorce among the elderly are not unlike those experienced by younger couples. They are, however, compounded by scarcer financial resources and by decreased family and environmental supports. Older women are particularly vulnerable following a divorce in later life. Many are without career skills and have never lived alone.

Widowhood

Women and men who are single because of the death of a spouse are called *widows* and *widowers*, respectively. Widowhood is felt throughout the entire family system. Personality disorganization for the bereaved spouse, changed economic resources, and increased contact with adult children are among the more obvious shifts. Burnside[2] discussed stages of transition to the role of widow or widower. These are outlined in Table 54-1 (page 1206) with predicted time frames and common behaviors.

Adult Children

About 80 percent of the older American population have living children, and about 10 percent of older

Table 54-1 Stages of Transition to the Role of Widow or Widower

Stage	Time Span	Behaviors
1. Reaction	First few weeks	Disbelief, anger, indecision, and detachment Inability to communicate in a logical sustained manner Searching for the mate Visions, hallucinations, depersonalization.
2. Withdrawal	First few months	Depression, apathy, physiological vulnerability, slowed movements, slowed cognition, insomnia, waves of grief, anorexia
3. Recuperation	Second 6 months	Feelings of depression, alternating with capabilities approaching those before the death of the spouse Return of feelings of having life under control
4. Exploration	Second year	Beginning new projects Testing new roles Anniversary reactions
5. Integration	Fifth year	If grief is resolved, full integration into role of widow or widower

SOURCE: Adapted from I. Burnside, *Nursing Care of the Aged*, McGraw-Hill, New York, 1981.

adults have adult children who are over 65. As aging parents live longer, adult children are assuming significant roles in their care. The growing trend toward early discharge from hospitals and the emerging phenomenon of the four-generation family have together been responsible for the assumption by adult children, many of whom are themselves in their middle and late years, of care-giving roles with their aging parents. When older people recognize adult children as individuals with their own rights, needs, limitations, and unique life histories, and when the adult children are mature and secure, satisfactory relationships usually develop.

For adult children, a number of stressors are associated with caring for aging parents: financial problems; competing responsibilities for family, spouse, and work; unresolved parent-child conflicts; changes in family roles; and uncertainty about the future. Even for people who ordinarily have effective coping skills, the intensity of family relationships caused by an ill elderly parent may lead to guilt, depression, loneliness, avoidance, withdrawal, loss of identity, role uncertainty, anger, and loss of power or control.[14]

Grandparents' Roles

Seventy-five percent of older people are grandparents, and about 5 percent of all households headed by older people include grandchildren. For most people, grandparenthood offers symbolic satisfaction but is not so meaningful in terms of actual relationships with grandchildren. The most satisfying period of grandparenting usually takes place when the grandchildren are small; however, one study found that young adults rated their relationships with grandparents as very significant and that most see their grandparents three to four times a year.[15] The role of valued grandparent is achieved rather than automatically ascribed and is based on the personal qualities of the older adult.

Contributions of grandparents to families include roles as surrogate parents, providers of income, homemakers, baby-sitters, support persons in times of crisis, teachers, and confidants. Neugarten and Weinstein described grandparenting styles that included the formal grandparent, the fun seeker, the parent surrogate, the reservoir of family wisdom, and the distancer.[16]

Siblings and Other Relatives

Eighty percent of persons over 65 have living brothers and sisters. As people grow older, they tend to renew family relationships and to make efforts to visit siblings, even those living far away. Except when there has been a long-standing gulf, siblings are a logical source of primary relationships for the elderly. Many older people form households with siblings following the death of their spouses. Death of siblings, like that of spouses and other people, reminds people of their own mortality, and death takes on immediacy.

Relationships with other extended family members are usually activated on special occasions such as weddings, funerals, holidays, and reunions. Older people may have favorite nieces or nephews, but this is based on individual characteristics rather than on any trend toward closeness of relationship.

PATTERNS OF INTERACTION: ENVIRONMENT

The environment of older people includes their personally significant space and territory as well as the larger geographic environment. The concept of personal space has to do with the need for privacy, solitude, and anonymity. Research has also indicated that the elderly need more light, less noise, and warm, bright colors in their physical environment.[2] Elements in the environment that have special significance for the elderly include *territoriality, housing, isolation and loneliness,* the impact of *retirement, transportation and mobility, victimization, deviance and crime,* and use of *leisure time.*

Territoriality

The term *territory* refers to a person's designated personal space, sometimes also called *body* or *interactional territory.* The *individual* territory is the place a person calls "home," and the *public* territory is his or her life space. Older people, like people of any age, may maintain a sense of personal space by cluttering, by gathering environmental props, which are usually significant personal items, and by behaving in a possessive manner.[2] A need for personal territory accounts for such behavior as the hoarding of string, newspapers, or greeting cards, as well as being rigid about a particular seat at the table or in a group, having favorite furniture, and being possessive about personal items such as pictures or religious articles. Possessive traits tend to escalate in direct proportion to a person's loss of control over environmental circumstances.[2]

Housing

An elderly person's residence may be a symbol of independence, may serve as a focal point for family gatherings, may involve many memories, and may be a link with neighborhood and community. Ninety-five percent of the elderly live in the community either alone, with a spouse, with their married or single children, or with their middle-aged or elderly siblings. The remaining 5 percent are institutionalized. Table 54-2 (page 1208) looks at the independent and group housing needs of the elderly on a continuum according to levels of independence, and gives criteria and examples for each level.[17]

Housing needs are at the root of many of the psychosocial problems of the aged. A lack of finances with which to maintain their home of many years, or an unwanted move to smaller, more convenient housing following the death of a spouse is often at the root of elderly people's depression. Adult children may visit less frequently after the home in which they grew up has been sold, contributing further to the family's collective sense of loss. Even couples who plan and look forward to a move to a retirement community are faced with a translocation crisis. Some elderly people who have lived their middle years in relatively safe urban areas find themselves in deteriorating and unsafe neighborhoods, which may precipitate fear, loneliness, and isolation. Still other older people are unable to find suitable, safe, and affordable housing. Severe grief reactions and depression follow or accompany a translocation crisis or concerns about a place to live.

Loneliness and Isolation

Feelings of isolation, loneliness, and hopelessness are thought to be among the major emotional problems faced by older people in the United States. If *loneliness* is defined as a reactive response to separation from persons and things in which people have invested themselves, then it is likely that all older people will experience some degree of loneliness. Some causative factors in the loneliness and environmental isolation of the elderly include:

- Death of a spouse
- Loss of functions
- Loss of sensory acuity
- Death, relocation, or physical illness of a sibling, neighbor, or roommate
- Loss of a pet
- Geographic move
- Language barriers
- Lowered energy levels

Table 54-2 Levels of Housing for the Elderly

Type of Housing	Significant Criteria	Examples
Fully independent	Independent household.	Private home.
	Self-contained.	Condominium or cooperative in retirement community.
	Self-sufficient.	Self-contained apartment in adult child's home.
Semi-independent	Self-contained but not entirely self-sufficient household.	Independent household augmented by community services such as Meals on Wheels or homemaker services.
	Occupants require assistance with household chores or cooking.	Adult foster care.
		Self-contained apartment in adult child's home. Meals and household chores taken care of by adult child.
Congregate housing	Self-contained housing but less self-sufficient.	Share a Home Program.
		Independent household shared by elderly siblings.
	Cooking and household chores shared by occupants.	Independent housing units with common dining room, medical, and recreation facilities.
Personal care home	Neither self-contained nor self-sufficient.	Adult home.
	Supervised residential unit.	Single-room occupancy (SRO) hotel.
	Help is given with personal care, grooming, transportation, and health care needs.	Health-related facility (HRF) within nursing home.
Nursing home	Neither self-contained nor self-sufficient. Total care including health, personal, and household functions is provided by health care personnel.	Skilled-nursing facility (SNF).
		Rehabilitation center.

SOURCE: Adapted from K. J. Reichstein and L. Bergofsky, "Domiciliary Care Facilities for Adults: An Analysis of State Regulations," *Research on Aging*, vol. 5, no. 1, 1983, pp. 25–44.

- Immobilizing pain
- Changes in body image
- Economic changes
- Organic problems
- Eccentricity
- Structural barriers

Loneliness is often difficult to diagnose, since many elderly people will not admit that they feel lonely. For others, the lonely feelings occur only at certain times (usually at night) and are not readily observed by care givers. Still others, because of their personalities or because of a need to project an image of the "picture of health," fail to recognize their loneliness and isolation; they unconsciously disguise or overcompensate for their symptoms. For example:

> Mr. G., an elderly man with a long-standing medical diagnosis of osteoporosis, has felt very isolated and lonely since the death of his wife. He overcompensates for his feelings and disguises them by being the "perfect widower." He states that his arthritis is keeping him from "getting out." His family and friends may perceive his behavior as appropriate expression of grief, not being aware that Mr. G. is unnecessarily isolating himself from his environmental support system.

Retirement

Retirement is a process that involves withdrawing from a job and taking on the role of retired person. A *retired person* has been operationally defined as anyone who is not gainfully employed, or who is receiving retirement pension benefits. Retirement is a complex process that affects a person's finances, family, and life course.

Retirement may be an event or a role. The retirement *event* is a rite of passage in which a person begins to deal with the opportunities and obligations of the retirement *role*. As a role, retirement offers people free time and geographic freedom; it requires them to have physical, social, and financial independence and to be certain about their personal life goals.

Phases of retirement have been identified in a series of empirical studies by Atchley, Cottrell, and others.[18] These phases are outlined in Table 54-3, and anticipated behaviors in each phase are noted.

Table 54-3 Phases of Retirement

Phase	Characteristics
Remote preretirement	When planned during middle age, retirement is seen as a vague possibility for the future.
Near preretirement	People begin to orient themselves to their own specific retirement dates.
"Honeymoon"	The time immediately following retirement is a period of euphoria during which the newly retired plan and do many things they "always wanted to do." This period is usually characterized by a hectic and fast-paced lifestyle.
Retirement routine	A daily, weekly, and monthly rhythm is established. Activities are chosen and time is set aside to enjoy them.
Rest and relaxation	A period of low activity, in marked contrast to the "honeymoon" stage; "taking it easy." After sufficient rest and relaxation, restlessness occurs.
Disenchantment	A period of letdown and depression. Disenchantment may result from failure of preretirement plans or because of illness or death of a spouse.
Reorientation	People who are depressed or disenchanted "take stock" and pull themselves together. They begin to view retirement realistically.
Routine	The individual retirement style is well developed; life proceeds in a reasonably comfortable, predictable fashion. Retirees are self-sufficient adults managing their own affairs.
Termination	Role is canceled by return to work, by illness, or by disability. Loss of independence or loss of health may necessitate the change.

Source: Adapted from R. C. Atchley, "Issues in Retirement Research," *The Gerontologist*, vol. 19, no. 1, January 1979, pp. 44–54.

The decision to retire involves several elements: how the person makes the decision to retire, the factors that influence the person to consider retirement, and the timing of retirement. Pressure to retire comes from employers, peers, the person's own desire, changes in health status, and compulsary retirement laws.[18] Adjustment to retirement is influenced by:

- Personality
- Attitude toward retirement
- Attitudes of significant others
- Strength of the work ethic
- Perception of how retirement will affect prestige
- Wages or salary before retirement
- Pension and other financial resources after retirement
- Level of job satisfaction
- Meaning the job has for the person
- Perceived or real physical and mental demands of the job
- Physical status
- Overall morale and satisfaction with life

The interaction of these and other factors determines the person's adjustment to the retirement. Some people make healthy, productive use of their retirement years, while others become socially isolated from the community or depressed. However, mild feelings of loss and boredom are to be expected in the early weeks of retirement. Some older people move to retirement communities. Studies of the impact of retirement on the marital dyad found that husbands adjusted more readily to their own retirement than did their wives.[18] The level of happiness of a retired couple was directly correlated with their overall level of happiness before retirement.

Transportation and Mobility

Transportation needs and resources change radically as people grow older. Some researchers have said that the aged experience a crisis of mobility.[19] The factors that make transportation a crisis for the aged include:

- Declining eyesight which impairs ability to drive an automobile
- Limited access to public transportation
- Declining physical health

Table 54-4 Transportation Services for the Elderly

Examples
Dial-A-Ride
Informal, volunteer drives
Demand-response transit vehicles
Minibuses and "senior jitneys"
Barrier-free buses
Specially constructed vehicles for the handicapped
Charter buses
Reduced-rate taxi services

- Geographic location that limits accessibility to public transportation
- Limited economic resources

Transportation services for the elderly are available in many communities but are often sporadic and limited. Generally, less public transportation is available in rural than in urban areas. The ideal transportation plan to service the elderly includes:

- Fare reductions or discounts on public transportation
- Adequate scheduling and routing of existing transportation
- Discounted taxi fares for the disabled and infirm
- Specially purchased and equipped vehicles to transport the elderly in rural areas and in other areas where public transportation is nonexistent or inadequate

Table 54-4 lists transportation services that are available in some communities.

Victimization

The most common forms of criminal victimization of the elderly are medical swindles and quackery. Economic exploitation through misleading claims and the sale of worthless devices are also common forms of fraud against the elderly. Older people fear violent crime but are statistically less likely than the general public to be victimized. However, when they are victims, they experience more physical, emotional, and spiritual damage as a group then younger people do. Abuse and neglect are common crimes against older adults and range in seriousness from *passive neglect* (leaving the elderly alone and isolated or forgotten) to actual *physical abuse* (hitting or slapping). In *verbal and emotional abuse* the elderly are frightened, insulted, humiliated, treated like children, or treated in a demeaning or overprotective way. *Active neglect* consists of forced confinement, isolation, or withholding of food or medication. Restraining the elderly is another form of physical abuse.[20]

The most common family problem leading to abuse and neglect of the elderly is a poor initial relationship among family members, combined with severe dependency needs on the part of the older person. Chapter 51 discusses abusive family patterns in detail.

Deviance and Crime

Deviants are people who follow a life course that is considered different in our society. Shopping-bag women, tramps, and occupants of single-room-occupancy hotels are sometimes considered deviants. Most of these people are elderly. Formerly institutionalized mentally ill persons also are often considered deviant, and large numbers of older people are included in this population. Chapters 18 and 53 discuss the problems of this chronic population.

Contrary to a commonly held idea, the elderly as a group are no more moralistic or conforming than the general population. They are less likely than younger people to be involved in serious crime. The elderly do, however, commit violent crimes, such as assault and manslaughter, and crimes that involve property, such as shoplifting, stealing, and real estate fraud. Alcohol-related crimes, including driving while intoxicated, are common among older people.

Leisure

Leisure activities are relatively self-determined, psychologically pleasant tasks that provide opportunities for recreation, personal growth, and service to others. Older, retired people have more leisure or unstructured time than the young and the middle-aged. For older people, leisure may be a celebration of life and an end in itself; it may also be therapeutic and serve as an instrument of control and healing.

Leisure activities may be stimulating or restful, expressive or appreciative, and active or passive. The elderly may engage in solitary pursuits such as gardening or crocheting, or they may become involved in sociable activities such as group card games, political activism, and work in community organizations. Some older people remain active through participation in sports, religious organizations, hobby or craft groups, or volunteer work. Watching television, reading and "just plain resting and relaxing" are other leisure activities common among older people.

DYSYNCHRONOUS HEALTH PATTERNS

The emotional responses of the elderly are not unlike those of the general population; people who were labeled *mentally ill* in their younger years will continue, though in less acute ways, to be clients of the mental health care system.[6] Among the dysynchronous emotional responses of older adults are grief, hypochondriacal preoccupations, depression, loneliness, anxiety, guilt, and despair.

People whose functional mental disorders begin in later life have usually become depressed by social or physical losses. Many common events of life—including relocation, retirement, death of a spouse or friends, loss of health, and loss of ability to function independently—are stressors for the elderly.

Problematic Patterns

Cognitive Impairment

Many older people and many health professionals mistakenly believe that mental deterioration is concomitant with old age. Some organic disorders do affect cognitive function and mimic the symptoms of mental illness, but cognitive impairment is not an expected component of the aging process. Physiological distress, sensory and perceptual disorders, overwhelming cumulative stresses, and functional psychiatric impairment may, however, produce what is known as *pseudodementia*. True organic mental disorders are characterized by true dementia, an irreversible mental state that involves changes in intellect, personality, judgment, and affect.

Reversible acute organic mental disorders caused by toxic states, malnutrition, acute infections, and abrupt translocation or loss are common among the elderly. Alzheimer's disease, cerebrovascular accidents, Wernicke-Korsakoff psychosis, Parkinson's disease, and Huntington's chorea are chronic and irreversible organic mental disorders common among the elderly.[6] A complete discussion of organic mental disorders is given in Chapter 44.

Depression

Depression is one of the most common dysynchronous health patterns of the elderly. The history of an older person with onset of depression in the later years usually reveals relatively well-adjusted patterns of emotional, social, and psychosexual behavior earlier in life. Depression in the elderly usually begins soon after some traumatic event such as bereavement, the moving away of children, retirement, physical illness, or illness of a spouse. Depressive disorders in adults of all ages are usually the result of a combination of biological, psychosocial, and cultural factors.

Depression in the elderly is often masked and consequently goes unnoticed. Apathy, preoccupation and "staring into space," reduced eye contact, overreactivity and extreme annoyance with others, sleep disturbances, confusion, fatigue, constipation, slowing of movements and speech, emptiness, withdrawal, and irritability are symptoms of depression that may be overlooked and attributed to the aging process.[3]

Depression may also be associated with the physical ailments common in elderly persons, especially those that cause incapacitation or pain. Some drugs, particularly antihypertensives and tranquilizers, also cause depression in older people. Nursing care for people with depression is discussed in Chapter 34.

Suicide

The highest rate of suicide occurs in white men in their eighties; a severe loss of status is believed to be the major causative factor. The wish to control the circumstances, timing, and method of one's own death is another motivation, particularly among the terminally ill. Suicide pacts between spouses and rational or philosophical decision making also contribute to suicide among older adults. Suicide may also be related to depression. People over age 65 who attempt suicide are likely to succeed in killing themselves. Chapter 36 discusses the dynamics of suicide and the care of suicidal clients.[3]

Alcoholism

Studies indicate that the overall incidence of alcoholism among the elderly is lower than among their younger counterparts. Even so, alcoholism is often a hidden problem for older people. Elderly widowers have the highest rate of alcoholism of all age groups. Some diagnostic clues that an older person is drinking too much are symptoms of insomnia, impotence, uncontrolled gout, multiple unexplained bruises, rapid onset of confused states, uncontrollable hypertension, and unexplained falls.[5]

Alcohol more severely impairs older people than younger ones. Over time the elderly alcoholic will experience slower reaction times, memory gaps, and impaired physiological tolerance to alcohol. Older people also recover more slowly from intoxication. Chapter 33 discusses the nursing care of alcoholics.

Hypochondriasis

Hypochondriasis, a somatoform disorder, is overconcern with one's physical and emotional health, accompanied by various bodily complaints for which there is no physical basis.[3] For older people, hypochondriacal complaints stem from their sense of defectiveness and deterioration. Somatic complaints may become a pattern of interaction and, as such, may be a means of overcoming loneliness. The somatic complaint provides the older person with something to talk about, guaranteeing communication with family members, other elderly people, and health care professionals. Older people who have multiple psychosomatic complaints may also be identifying with deceased family members and friends or displacing anxiety about other concerns. Chapters 42 and 43 provide information about patterns of behavior and the nursing care of clients with symptoms of hypochondriasis.

Drug Abuse

Intentional or accidental drug abuse and drug dependence are major ways in which the elderly cope with stress and depression. Patterns of misuse and abuse include *overuse, underuse,* and *erratic use.* The prescription drugs most often subject to use and misuse are psychotherapeutic; they include Valium, Librium, and Compazine. Over-the-counter drugs such as aspirin, laxatives, and antacids are widely misused. Prescribed drugs for hypertension, diabetes, and arthritis are erratically used by many older people. The most common pattern of erratic use is taking the prescribed medication only when severe or acute symptoms occur, rather than on a regular basis as prescribed.

The problem of drug abuse among the elderly is complicated by a high rate of prescribing by physicians, pressures from the media and pharmaceutical advertising, use of multiple physicians and pharmacists by the elderly, and the unknowing mixing of incompatible drugs.[10] Chapter 33 discusses the nursing care of clients who abuse drugs.

DSM III

The accuracy of classification and diagnosis of the mental disorders of older adults improved with the publication of the *Diagnostic and Statistical Manual of Mental Disorders* (DSM III). The new multiaxial approach takes into consideration physical diseases, current stresses in a client's life, recent changes in functioning, degrees of functional impairment, and the course of the disorder. These are of particular importance in diagnosis of the elderly.

Mental illness statistically increases in old age, a factor that is explained by the rising occurrence of depression and organic mental disorders (OMD).[2] While the acute onset of schizophrenia is rarely seen in the elderly, many people who have developed specific types of schizophrenia in earlier years carry the symptoms into old age.[3] Paranoid behavior in older people is common but needs careful assessment to distinguish it from valid reactions to real events in a person's environment.

Affective disorders, particularly depression, are the most common emotional illnesses of older people. Neurotic disorders common among the elderly include anxiety, phobias, and hypochondriasis. Dissociative disorders sometimes occur, in which an older person's consciousness, identity, or motor behavior is suddenly and temporarily altered, resulting in vague states, stupor, amnesia, and confusion.

Epidemiology

One of the fastest-growing segments of the American population is the elderly. In 1980, 11.3 percent of the population was over age 65, and it is projected that by the year 2030, about one-fifth of the total population will be in this age group.[11]

The elderly population has generally been getting older and is expected to continue doing so for the next several decades. Contributing factors include longer life spans and improved quality and availability of health care. If present trends continue, the future elderly will be better educated and will continue to work in higher-salaried occupations, factors which also contribute to longevity.

Ninety-five percent of the elderly are community-based. The remaining 5 percent, or approximately 1 million, are in nursing homes or related facilities.[11] A significant portion of the institutionalized elderly are in psychiatric or mental health care facilities. The elderly are therefore identified as a special target population in need of comprehensive mental health services that include crisis intervention and emergency programs, specially designed nursing home facilities, outpatient group and family therapy, specialized housing, and preventive educational and counseling services. While there is an identified need and a growing population, relatively few elderly clients receive mental health services beyond the custodial physical level. Even fewer seek out therapy directed toward conflict resolution and personality growth even when it is offered. Contributing factors include the lack of interested and specially prepared professionals, the limitations of funding, the complexity of emotional disorders of aging, and the negative attitudes and distrust of the aged toward mental health services.

NURSING PROCESS

One of the greatest challenges to the nursing profession today is the care of elderly clients. No other group of clients requires so holistic an approach to individuals, nor so greatly taxes the research, assessment, diagnostic, and planning skills of the nurse. Nurses who care for the aged need to practice not only researched, scientific skills, but also the art of nursing.

Assessment

A holistic assessment of an older person is a multifaceted process. It involves gathering a data base about the physical, mental, and spiritual dimensions of the older person, the family, and the larger environmental context in which the person lives. Several of the assessment frameworks[4,21,22,23] that have been developed for use with the elderly are listed in Table 54-5 (pages 1214–1215). Review of the table shows that comprehensive assessment is crucial to correct diagnosis of and appropriate intervention with the elderly. In addition to the data base suggested in Chapter 11, the major components of a basic nursing assessment of an elderly person include several unique considerations.

The first consideration in the assessment process is establishing rapport with the older person. This requires that the nurse, often considerably younger than the client, be aware of his or her own feelings about aging. It involves accepting the older person, being knowledgeable about the aging process, and treating the person as an intelligent and feeling adult.

Second, the assessment process takes more time with older people. Interviews, examinations, and testing should be unhurried and relaxed. The complete assessment should be divided into short sessions and should take place at a time of day when the older person is most alert. Some clients experience *sundown syndrome;* their cognitive ability diminishes in late afternoon and evening, and they may even feel disoriented, confused, and apathetic. *Sunrise syndrome* is early morning confusion that may be caused by insomnia or by the effects of sedatives or hypnotics.

Hearing impairment is a third consideration, since a client's impaired hearing may present a problem during assessment. Minimizing background noise, being sensitive to and acknowledging the problem, sitting close, observing and using nonverbal communication, and speaking distinctly and clearly while maintaining a constant voice volume are all ways to facilitate the assessment process with clients who are hard of hearing.

Fourth, older people who have had a stroke also need special consideration during assessment. The nurse should approach these clients on the unaffected side; should be patient with their struggles to speak, if they have aphasia; should supply words only when absolutely necessary; should, if need be, use an audiovisual aid such as a writing pad, blackboard, or typewriter for asking questions and receiving answers; and should always treat the clients as intelligent and worthwhile people.

Table 54-5 Assessment Frameworks for Use with the Elderly

Model	Theoretical Framework	Areas Assessed
FANCAPES (A mnemonic device used to recall areas of assessment)	An assessment tool based on a survival needs framework with emphasis on function. Assesses ability, basic needs, and the extent to which assistance is necessary.	Fluids Aeration Nutrition Communication Activity Pain Elimination Social skills
OARS (Older Americans Resources and Services)	Specifically designed to evaluate abilities and disabilities of older people. Assesses level of function.	Social resources Economic resources Physical health Mental health Capacity for activities of daily living
Self-assessment health history	An assessment tool to be completed by clients. A comprehensive questionnaire about an individual's self-perception of health.	Personal data Family background Economic and social data Insurance information Mental status History of health and illness
Life review	Based on reminiscing techniques. Both an assessment tool and a therapeutic technique. Comprehensive review of all aspects of life intended to prepare older people to plan for the remainder of their life. Reminiscence is guided by the nurse and is usually characterized by feelings of nostalgia, regret, or pleasure. Extreme emotional pain, despair, depression, guilt, obsessive rumination and panic may complicate the process. The expected outcomes of the life review are atonement, serenity, constructive reorganization, and creativity.	**Background information** Personal data; religion; ethnic, racial, and cultural background. Family status, family history. Education, work history, retirement, economic status. Residence, transportation, and mobility. Interests and pleasures; active community involvements; friendship patterns. Predjuices directed against older adults. **Medical information** History. Accidents, surgery. Circulatory disorders, heart problems, arthritis, lung conditions, diabetes, cancer, thyroid problems, anemia, gastrointestinal problems, bladder problems, menopause or prostate problems, allergies, foot problems. Physical limitations; loss of hearing, vision, or memory; dentures, prosthetic devices. Speech problems. **Daily living habits** Overeating, drinking history, caffeine consumption, smoking history, exercise, sleep patterns. **Drug use** Prescription and over-the-counter drugs. **Sexual activity and concerns** **Psychiatric information** Presenting problem, observed behaviors, previous treatments, home remedies, goals of therapy. **Attitudes toward aging and death; self-view** Appearance, personality, strengths and liabilities; review of happy and sad times.

(Continued.)

Table 54-5 Continued

Model	Theoretical Framework	Areas Assessed
Social Adjustment Rating Scale	Based on stress theory. Evaluates the impact of various life events on a person. It provides a rating with corresponding criteria for adjustment to stress.	Life events, each rated according to amount of stress involved. Solicits information about events such as marriages, deaths, retirement, and geographic relocation.
Self-drawings and use of mirrors	Projective techniques designed to elicit rich, spontaneous responses from older people. Provides cues for collaborative self-exploration. The older client is an active participant.	"Reality factors" about appearance Personality factors that are lifelong or related to the aging process Organic factors Communication patterns
Mental Status Questionnaire (MSQ) or Short Portable Mental Status Questionnaire (SPMSQ)	Standarized questionnaire designed to measure mental status of older people. The degree of cognitive impairment is an important assessment criteria in diagnosis.	The MSQ is a gross measurement of mental status (cognitive functioning). The SPMSQ yields a score that indicates a person's level of disability.

SOURCES: "FANCAPES"—P. Ebersole and P. Hess, *Toward Healthy Aging*, Mosby, St. Louis, 1981. "OARS," "MSQ," and "SPMSQ"—E. Pfeiffer, *Multidimensional Functional Assessment: The OARS Methodology*, Durham, N. C., Center for the Study of Aging and Human Development, Duke University Press, 1975. "Life review"—R. N. Butler and N. Lewis, *Aging and Mental Health: Positive Psychosocial and Biomedical Approaches*, 3d ed., Mosby, St. Louis, 1982. "Social Adjustment Rating Scale"—T. H. Holmes and R. H. Raye, "The Social Readjustment Rating Scale," *Research*, vol. 11, 1967, pp. 213ff. "Self-drawings"—B. L. Neugarten, *Personality in Middle and Late Life*, Atherton, New York, 1964.

Fifth, with elderly clients the nurse assesses not only basic health but also changes in health status that have evolved over the person's life span. The *physical* changes include a series of declines that begin in middle age. Alterations in physical appearance and a decrease in the functioning of organ systems are expected, but the different meanings these have for each person need to be assessed. Nutritional status, hearing, vision, and taste, and pace of and capacity for physical work also require assessment.[24] The nurse also solicits information about whether or not use of prescribed medication or over-the-counter drugs may be the cause of physical symptoms or changed behavior.

The *psychological* changes that need to be assessed include level of independence, ability to cope with loss and with declines in all levels of functioning, and ability to relinquish power. Affective changes may also be occurring. Self-perception and responses to the aging process are essential components of psychological assessment.

Assessing *spiritual* changes includes asking about the person's philosophical perspective on life, and observing whether the "life review" process has begun. The role of religious practice in the older person's life and the person's preparations for death are also important basic data.

The *sociocultural factors* and *environmental factors* that need careful scrutiny include reaction to retirement, geographic moves, changes in family structure, limited mobility, and use of leisure time.

Additional questions that will help in gathering data about the elderly are to be found in clinical sections throughout this book. Of particular concern in work with the elderly are questions which assess level of anxiety (see Chapter 30), alcoholism and drug abuse (see Chapter 33), depression (see Chapter 34), and organic mental disorders (see Chapter 44).

Diagnosis

Formulating definitive diagnoses of the elderly is a complex process often carried out by making a series of "working" or "trial" statements. Diagnosis of elderly people is usually multifaceted because of their many health care problems. Any number of nursing diagnoses may be related to the aging

Table 54-6 Nursing Diagnosis of the Elderly

Person
Physical patterns
Disturbances in sleep patterns associated with environmental changes
Nocturia associated with alteration in bladder tone
Guarding behavior associated with pain in lower limbs
Inability to bathe associated with decreased strength
Perceptual distortions related to hearing loss
Mental patterns
Depressed affect associated with sociocultural isolation
Suicidal thoughts related to decreased sensory acuity
Excessive alcohol intake associated with loneliness
Social isolation correlated with suspiciousness
Disorientation to time related to misuse of over-the-counter drugs
Spiritual patterns
Grief reaction correlated with death of spouse
Expressed concern about meaning of old age
Anger toward God correlated with meaningless personal suffering
Spiritual distress related to inability to practice religion
Family
Passive neglect correlated with geographic distance of caring family
Rejection by grandchildren associated with rigid personality structure
Physical abuse associated with unresolved parent-child relationships
Family immobility related to inability to make decisions about nursing home placement
Family stress related to lack of financial resources
Environment
Diminished social contacts related to limited access to transportation
Decrease in nutritional intake related to translocation crisis
Loneliness and isolation associated with retirement
Potential for injury related to motor and sensory deficits
Deficit in leisure activity related to immobility

process, and a comprehensive list of them would be beyond the scope of this chapter. Table 54-6, however, presents a selection of diagnoses for consideration by psychiatric nurses.

Outcome Criteria

Outcome criteria are statements about expected results or goals of nursing interventions. These results should be measurable, specific in content and time, and attainable by the client. Outcomes in the care of older people need to be realistic and to reflect the interrelationship among the physical, emotional, and spiritual aspects of the client. Goals often need to be adjusted downward for the elderly—and this runs contrary to a "cure" mentality.[2] For example, one outcome criterion for a young adult who is depressed may be independent maintenance of self as evidenced by improved grooming and clean clothes. For the older person, the analogous outcome criterion may be to accept interdependence as evidenced by cooperation with a health care aide who performs certain grooming functions.

Interventions with the elderly are aimed at the ultimate goal of maintaining quality of life rather than at restoration of health. Outcome criteria should consider the strengths and weaknesses of the client, the environmental limitations, and available family and community resources.[25] Table 54-7 lists several examples that are applicable to elderly clients.

Table 54-7 Outcome Criteria

Examples
Client will walk unassisted to the dining room for meals.
Client is able to identify the side effects of medication and report them to the nurse.
Client will discuss his plans for retirement with his wife and children.
Client will utilize hearing aid when conversing with others.
Client will discuss spiritual distress with the chaplain twice weekly.
Client will ask to visit the nursing home in which she will be placed while recuperating from a fractured hip.
Client will not develop the preventable complications of an indwelling Foley catheter.
Client will walk to the mailbox each morning using four-legged cane.
Client will be accompanied by nursing staff until he verbalizes relief from suicidal ideation.

Intervention

Intervention with older adults is a holistic process that begins with attempts to relieve the client's presenting problem. For example, a client who seeks help because of loneliness is referred to

Table 54-8 Specific Nursing Interventions for the Elderly

Intervention	Definition
Person	
Life-review therapy	Positive psychotherapeutic function which provides opportunities for older people to reflect on their lives, to heal, and to reorganize and reintegrate their concerns and problems.
Reminiscing groups	Perceptions, historical life events, and generational attributes are reviewed in the context of a group. The group provides opportunities for therapeutic holding on to and letting go of the past.
Reality-orientation techniques	Behavioral therapeutic approaches that aim to increase awareness of time, place, and person.
Health intervention groups	Professionally led groups that provide clients with preventive instruction about health care needs such as diet, medication, and exercise.
Family	
Groups for adult children	Professionally led groups that support family members who care for their aging parents. One such group, Children of Aging Parents (COAP), allows members to ventilate feelings and share problem-solving approaches in a rational, systematic manner.
Foster grandparents	Provides opportunities for older people and children to share, meet needs, and experience gratification across generations.
Environment	
Gray Panthers	An advocacy group founded by Margaret Kuhn to lobby for change and social justice.
Senior citizens' centers	Comprehensive local groups organized to meet the health, nutritional, social, and legislative needs of the elderly.

SOURCE: R. N. Butler and M. Lewis, *Aging and Mental Health: Positive Psychosocial and Biomedical Approaches,* 3d ed., Mosby, St. Louis, 1982. L. Casandra, *Interview with Founder COAP,* Children of Aging Parents, Suffolk County Department of Mental Health, New York, 1985. M. Stanhope and J. Lancaster, *Community Health Nursing,* Mosby, St. Louis, 1984.

appropriate social resources. The source of the loneliness is then explored, and other appropriate services are networked for the client. In the process, a complete physical and mental assessment is performed, the family is contacted, and the environment is explored.

Discussion of physical interventions is beyond the scope of this book. Specific mental and spiritual interventions are similar to those discussed in earlier chapters and differ only in the approach nurses take to aging clients.

Some specific intervention techniques and approaches that have been found helpful in working with older people are listed in Table 54-8. Much of the care of older people involves getting to know the specific agencies in the community that service their needs and working these agencies into the care plan.

Evaluation

Evaluation of the nursing process and whether goals and outcomes were achieved is an essential component of the care of the elderly. Satisfactory evaluation ensures reimbursement of Medicare, Medicaid, and third-party payers for services provided to clients. Evaluation begins with nurses themselves. *Formative evaluations,* or process scrutinies of self and client, occur while care is taking place. Nurses look at whether clients are improving or achieving the outcomes planned. Plans are updated and revised if necessary. *Summative evaluations,* or outcome audits, are conducted by individual nurses, the agency, and survey visitors, usually after the client is discharged. Summative evaluations are based on what is recorded in the client's record.[26,27] Table 54-9 (page 1218) shows a nursing care program for an elderly client (Virginia K.) and how it is evaluated:

> Virginia K. is an 89-year-old woman who was recently widowed. She was admitted to the nursing home 4 months ago. She cries frequently and is moody and apathetic. The night nurse says that Virginia has nightmares. Virginia has been overheard saying to other residents, "Life has no meaning for me any more," "Why do I have to suffer like this?" and "Why is God allowing this to happen to me?" She has refused to talk to the chaplain, although her family reports that she went to daily mass while living in her own home before her husband's death.

Table 54-9 Case Study (Virginia K.)

Nursing Care Program for an Elderly Client
Assessment
Will you tell me what you are feeling?
Is your crying related to the death of your husband?
Do you miss your home? Your church?
Have you always been so sad?
What would help you feel better?
Are you able to say any of your prayers here?
How could we help you practice your religion while you are living here?
Diagnosis
Spiritual distress related to inability to participate in usual religious practices.
Healthy grieving related to loss of husband.
Anger toward God related to recent losses and placement in nursing home.
Outcome criteria
Virginia will verbalize her anger at God to her parish priest.
Virginia will stop frequent crying behavior within 2 months after beginning therapy sessions with nurse.
Virginia will attend daily mass in neighboring parish.
Virginia will attend bereavement groups twice a week.
Nightmares will decrease in frequency.
Intervention
Arrange to have pastor of Virginia's former home parish come and visit.
Meet with Virginia's former pastor, the nursing home chaplain, the neighboring parish priest, and Virginia to discuss attendance at mass.
Encourage Virginia to talk about her losses and grief.
Be supportive of Virginia's tears and crying behavior.
Reminisce with Virginia about happier times in her life and her unfulfilled dreams.
Encourage Virginia to ventilate anger about nursing home placement and death of husband.
Give permission for her to express anger appropriately.
Encourage Virginia to join widows' bereavement group.
Suggest that Virginia's family participate in multifamily group therapy for children of aging parents.
Arrange for community volunteers to drive Virginia to daily mass in a neighboring parish.
Evaluation
Virginia verbalized anger and distress to parish priest.
Virginia attends mass weekly at present. More volunteers are needed before frequency can be increased.
Virginia attends bereavement group, but does not participate. Encourage her to verbalize her feelings in group at least once every 2 weeks.
Crying has decreased in frequency.
Nightmares have decreased in frequency.

SUMMARY

Old age, defined as the time after age 65, is a dynamic stage in the overall life-span continuum and not a static, isolated stage of development. Aging involves a universal, progressive, intrinsic, and selective slowing down of physiological and biological processes. Aging is accompanied by physical, emotional, cognitive, and spiritual changes that compound preexisting strengths and weaknesses. The major developmental task of the elderly is acquiring the ability to clarify, deepen, and find use for what has already been attained during a lifetime of learning and adapting.

The mental health of older people involves emotional, cognitive, and spiritual dimensions as well as an innate sense of self-esteem. The self-esteem of the elderly is maintained when their achievements are recognized, they receive positive feedback, they are treated with respect and courtesy, they maintain decision-making power and control of their destiny, they have satisfying interpersonal relationships, and their basic needs of everyday living are adequately met.

Cognitive processes in older people change and are generally caused by malfunction of the circulatory or neurological systems rather than by the aging process itself. A holistic approach to older people requires consideration of their spiritual well-being. Self-actualized people consider alternative ways of viewing themselves and the universe, and many believe in forms of life and energy beyond present reality and knowledge. Some older people find transcendence through mystical or religious experiences; others leave artistic legacies or express themselves through objects, deeds, crafts, progeny, or autobiographical statements. Religious practices, dreams, symbols, fantasies, daydreams, and visions are expressions of the spiritual dimension.

The elderly contribute to family life in their unique roles as spouses, parents, grandparents, great-grandparents, siblings, and family sages. As aging parents live longer, adult children, many of whom are themselves over 65, are assuming new roles in the care of their parents. The intensity of family relationships caused by illness of elderly parents can lead to emotional responses such as guilt, depression, loneliness, avoidance, withdrawal, loss of identity, uncertainty about roles, anger, and feelings of loss of power or control.

The environment of old people includes their

personally significant space and territory as well as the larger geographic environment. Factors to be considered in the environment of old people include housing; loneliness; social isolation; the process, stages, and influences of retirement; transportation and mobility needs; victimization; deviance; and crime.

The nursing process involves a multifaceted holistic assessment of old people, their families, and their larger environmental context. Assessment frameworks include FANCAPES, OARS, life review, mental status, questionnaires, self-assessment, health histories, social adjustment rating scales, and self-drawings. Special considerations in assessment of the elderly include establishment of rapport; time needed for assessment; hearing impairments; effects of stroke; and the gathering of information about physical, psychological, sociocultural, and environmental changes. Nursing diagnoses and outcome criteria are formulated for the multidimensional problems of the aged. Specific interventions include "life review" therapy, reminiscence groups, reality-orientation techniques, groups for adult children, foster grandparents' groups, and community organizations such as senior citizen centers and the Gray Panthers.

REFERENCES

1. American Nurses Association, *Standards of Gerontological Nursing Practice*, ANA, Kansas City, Mo., 1976.
2. I. Burnside, *Nursing Care of the Aged*, McGraw-Hill, New York, 1981.
3. R. N. Butler and M. Lewis, *Aging and Mental Health: Positive Psychosocial and Biomedical Approaches*, 3d ed., Mosby, St. Louis, 1982.
4. B. L. Neugarten, *Personality in Middle and Late Life*, Atherton, New York, 1964.
5. R. C. Atchley, *Social Forces and Aging*, Wadsworth, California, 1985.
6. R. Andres, E. L. Bierman, and W. R. Hazzard, *Principles of Geriatric Medicine*, McGraw-Hill, New York, 1985.
7. M. Jacewicz and A. Hartley, "Rotation of Mental Images by Young and Old College Students: The Effects of Familiarity," *Journal of Gerontology*, vol. 34, 1979, p. 396.
8. B. A. Devine, "Attitudes of the Elderly toward Religion," *Journal of Gerontological Nursing*, vol. 6, 1980, p. 679.
9. A. Storr, ed., *The Essential Jung*, Princeton University Press, Princeton, N. J., 1983.
10. M. Caroselli-Karinja, "Drug Abuse and the Elderly," *Journal of Psychosocial Nursing and Mental Health Services*, vol. 23, no. 6, June 1985, pp. 25–30.
11. Office of Human Development Services, *Need for Long Term Care: Information and Issues*, Washington, D.C., 1981.
12. B. D. Starr and M. B. Weiner, *Sex and Sexuality in the Mature Years*, McGraw-Hill, New York, 1981.
13. R. C. Atchley, L. Pignatiello, and E. Shaw, "Interactions with Family and Friends: Marital Status and Occupational Differences among Older Women," *Research on Aging*, vol. 11, no. 2, February 1979, pp. 83–94.
14. P. Mulvaney, V. K. Gray, and K. Carrol, "An Exercise in Understanding: A Way of Improving Communication between Aging Parents and Their Adult Children," *Human Development*, vol. 3, no. 4, Winter 1982, pp. 23–27.
15. T. A. Hartshorne and G. J. Manaster, "The Relationship with Grandparents: Contact, Importance, Role Conception," *International Journal of Aging and Human Development*, vol. 15, no. 7, 1981, pp. 233–245.
16. B. Neugarten and K. Weinstein, "The Changing American Grandparent," *Journal of Marriage and Family*, May 1964, p. 201.
17. K. J. Reichstein and L. Bergofsky, "Domiciliary Care Facilities for Adults: An Analysis of State Regulations," *Research on Aging*, vol. 15, no. 5, May 1983, pp. 25–44.
18. R. C. Atchley, "Issues in Retirement Research," *The Gerontologist*, vol. 19, no. 1, January 1979, pp. 44–54.
19. C. F. Longino, K. A. McClelland, and W. A. Peterson, "The Aged Subculture Hypothesis," *Journal of Gerontology*, vol. 35, no. 10, October 1980, pp. 758–767.
20. T. Hickey and R. L. Douglas, "Neglect and Abuse of Older Family Members: Professionals' Perspectives and Case Experiences," *The Gerontologist*, vol. 21, no. 1, January 1981, pp. 171–176.
21. P. Ebersole and P. Hess, *Toward Healthy Aging*, Mosby, St. Louis, 1981.
22. E. Pfeiffer, *Multidimensional Functional Assessment: The OARS Methodology*, Center for the Study of Aging and Human Development, Duke University Press, Durham, N.C., 1975.
23. T. H. Holmes and R. H. Raye, "The Social Readjustment Rating Scale," *Research*, vol. 11, 1967, p. 213.
24. M. D. Mesey, L. H. Rauckhorst, and S. A. Stokes, *Health Assessment of the Older Individual*, Springer, New York, 1980.
25. L. J. Carpenito, *Nursing Diagnosis Application to Clinical Practice*, Lippincott, Philadelphia, 1983.
26. L. Casandra, *Interview with Founder COAP*, Children of Aging Parents, Suffolk County Department of Mental Health, New York, 1985.
27. M. Stanhope and J. Lancaster, *Community Health Nursing*, Mosby, St. Louis, 1984.

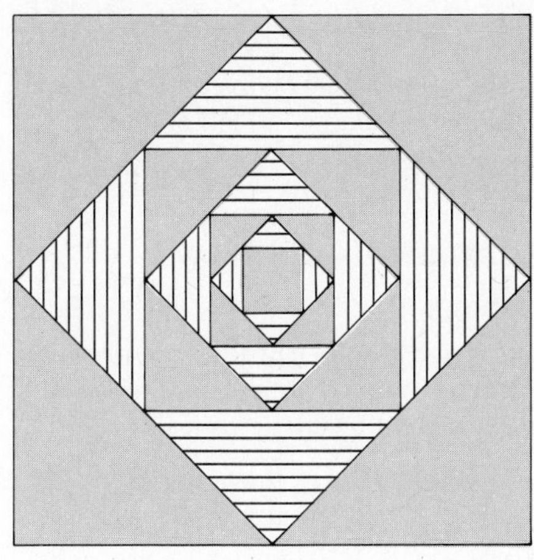

APPENDIX 1

Standards of Psychiatric and Mental Health Nursing Practice

American Nurses Association
Division of Psychiatric and Mental Health Nursing Practice

Standard I. Theory

The nurse applies appropriate theory that is scientifically sound as a basis for decisions regarding nursing practice.

Standard II. Data Collection

The nurse continuously collects data that are comprehensive, accurate, and systematic.

Standard III. Diagnosis

The nurse utilizes nursing diagnoses and/or standard classification of mental disorders to express conclusions supported by recorded assessment data and current scientific premises.

Standard IV. Planning

The nurse develops a nursing care plan with specific goals and interventions delineating nursing actions unique to each client's needs.

Reprinted with the permission of the American Nurses Association (ANA).

Standard V. Intervention

The nurse intervenes as guided by the nursing care plan to implement nursing actions that promote, maintain, or restore physical and mental health, prevent illness, and effect rehabilitation.

Standard V-A Intervention: Psychotherapeutic Interventions

The nurse uses psychotherapeutic interventions to assist clients in regaining or improving their previous coping abilities and to prevent further disability.

Standard V-B. Intervention: Health Teaching

The nurse assists clients, families, and groups to achieve satisfying and productive patterns of living through health teaching.

Standard V-C. Intervention: Activities of Daily Living

The nurse uses the activities of daily living in a goal-directed way to foster adequate self-care and physical and mental well-being of clients.

Standard V-D. Intervention: Somatic Therapies

The nurse uses knowledge of somatic therapies and applies related clinical skills in working with clients.

Standard V-E. Intervention: Therapeutic Environment

The nurse provides, structures, and maintains a therapeutic environment in collaboration with the client and other health care providers.

Standard V-F. Intervention: Psychotherapy

The nurse utilizes advanced clinical expertise in individual, group, and family psychotherapy; child psychotherapy; and other treatment modalities to function as a psychotherapist, and recognizes professional accountability for nursing practice.

Standard VI. Evaluation

The nurse evaluates client responses to nursing actions in order to revise the data base, nursing diagnoses, and nursing care plans.

Standard VII. Peer Review

The nurse participates in peer review and other means of evaluation to assure quality of nursing care provided for clients.

Standard VIII. Continuing Education

The nurse assumes responsibility for continuing education and professional development and contributes to the professional growth of others.

Standard IX. Interdisciplinary Collaboration

The nurse collaborates with other health care providers in assessing, planning, implementing, and evaluating programs and other mental health activities.

Standard X. Utilization of Community Health Systems

The nurse participates with other members of the community in assessing, planning, implementing, and evaluating mental health services and community systems that include the promotion of the broad continuum of primary, secondary, and tertiary prevention of mental illness.

Standard XI. Research

The nurse contributes to nursing and the mental health field through innovations in theory and practice and participation in research.

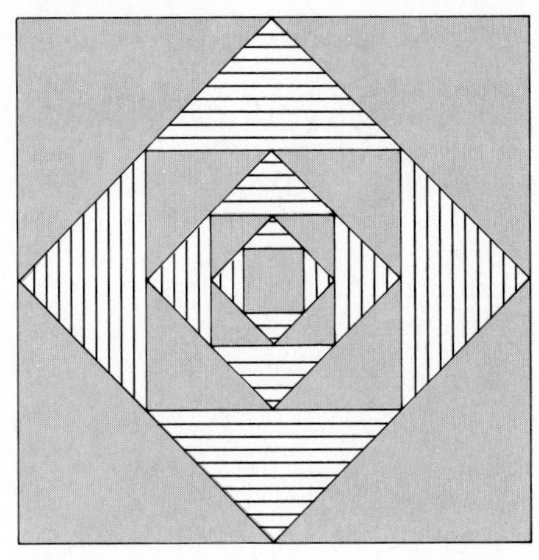

APPENDIX 2
DSM III Classification: Axes I and II, Categories and Codes

American Psychiatric Association

All official DSM III codes and terms are included in ICD-9-CM. However, in order to differentiate those DSM III categories that use the same ICD-9-CM codes, unofficial non-ICD-9-CM codes are provided in parentheses for use when greater specificity is necessary. The long dashes indicate the need for a fifth-digit subtype or other qualifying term.

DISORDERS USUALLY FIRST EVIDENT IN INFANCY, CHILDHOOD, OR ADOLESCENCE

Mental Retardation

Code in fifth digit: 1 = with other behavioral symptoms (requiring attention or treatment and that are not part of another disorder), 0 = without other behavioral symptoms.

317.0(x) Mild mental retardation, ______
318.0(x) Moderate mental retardation, ______
318.1(x) Severe mental retardation, ______
318.2(x) Profound mental retardation, ______
319.0(x) Unspecified mental retardation, ______

From *Diagnostic and Statistical Manual of Mental Disorders*, 3d ed., American Psychiatric Association, Washington, D.C., 1980. Used with permission.

Attention Deficit Disorder

314.01 with hyperactivity
314.00 without hyperactivity
314.80 residual type

Conduct Disorder

312.00 undersocialized, aggressive
312.10 undersocialized, nonaggressive
312.23 socialized, aggressive
312.21 socialized, nonaggressive
312.90 atypical

Anxiety Disorders of Childhood or Adolescence

309.21 Separation anxiety disorder
313.21 Avoidant disorder of childhood or adolescence
313.00 Overanxious disorder

Other Disorders of Infancy, Childhood, or Adolescence

313.89 Reactive attachment disorder of infancy
313.22 Schizoid disorder of childhood or adolescence
313.23 Elective mutism
313.81 Oppositional disorder
313.82 Identity disorder

Eating Disorders

307.10	Anorexia nervosa
307.51	Bulimia
307.52	Pica
307.53	Rumination disorder of infancy
307.50	Atypical eating disorder

Stereotyped Movement Disorders

307.21	Transient tic disorder
307.22	Chronic motor tic disorder
307.23	Tourette's disorder
307.20	Atypical tic disorder
307.30	Atypical stereotyped movement disorder

Other Disorders with Physical Manifestations

307.00	Stuttering
307.60	Functional enuresis
307.70	Functional encopresis
307.46	Sleepwalking disorder
307.46	Sleep terror disorder (307.49)

Pervasive Developmental Disorders

Code in fifth digit: 0 = full syndrome present, 1 = residual state.

299.0x	Infantile autism, ______
299.9x	Childhood onset pervasive developmental disorder, ______
299.8x	Ayptical, ______

Specific Developmental Disorders

NOTE. These are coded on Axis II.

315.00	Developmental reading disorder
315.10	Developmental arithmetic disorder
315.31	Developmental language disorder
315.39	Developmental articulation disorder
315.50	Mixed specific developmental disorder
315.90	Atypical specific developmental disorder

ORGANIC MENTAL DISORDERS

SECTION 1. Organic mental disorders whose etiology or pathophysiological process is listed below (taken from the mental disorders section of ICD-9-CM).

Dementias Arising in the Senium and Presenium

Primary Degenerative Dementia, Senile Onset

290.30	with delirium
290.20	with delusions
290.21	with depression
290.00	uncomplicated

Code in fifth digit: 1 = with delirium, 2 = with delusions, 3 = with depression, 0 = uncomplicated.

290.1x	Primary degenerative dementia, presenile onset, ______
290.4x	Multi-infarct dementia, ______

Substance-Induced Disorders

Alcohol

303.00	intoxication
291.40	idiosyncratic intoxication
291.80	withdrawal
291.00	withdrawal delirium
291.30	hallucinosis
291.10	amnestic disorder

Code severity of dementia in fifth digit: 1 = mild, 2 = moderate, 3 = severe, 0 = unspecified.

291.2x	Dementia associated with alcoholism, ______

Barbiturate or Similarly Acting Sedative or Hypnotic

305.40	intoxication (327.00)
292.00	withdrawal (327.01)
292.00	withdrawal delirium (327.02)
292.83	amnestic disorder (327.04)

Opioid

305.50	intoxication (327.10)
292.00	withdrawal (327.11)

Cocaine

305.60	intoxication (327.20)

Amphetamine or Similarly Acting Sympathomimetic

305.70 intoxication (327.30)
292.81 delirium (327.32)
292.11 delusional disorder (327.35)
292.00 withdrawal (327.31)

Phencyclidine (PCP) or Similarly Acting Arylcyclohexylamine

305.90 intoxication (327.40)
292.81 delirium (327.42)
292.90 mixed organic mental disorder (327.49)

Hallucinogen

305.30 hallucinosis (327.56)
292.11 delusional disorder (327.55)
292.84 affective disorder (327.57)

Cannabis

305.20 intoxication (327.60)
292.11 delusional disorder (327.65)

Tobacco

292.00 withdrawal (327.71)

Caffeine

305.90 intoxication (327.80)

Other or Unspecified Substance

305.90 intoxication (327.90)
292.00 withdrawal (327.91)
292.81 delirium (327.92)
292.82 dementia (327.93)
292.83 amnestic disorder (327.94)
292.11 delusional disorder (327.95)
292.12 hallucinosis (327.96)
292.84 affective disorder (327.97)
292.89 personality disorder (327.98)
292.90 atypical or mixed organic mental disorder (327.99)

SECTION 2. Organic brain syndromes whose etiology or pathophysiological process either is noted as an additional diagnosis from outside the mental disorders section of ICD-9-CM or is unknown.

293.00 Delirium
294.10 Dementia
294.00 Amnestic syndrome
293.81 Organic delusional syndrome
293.82 Organic hallucinosis
293.83 Organic affective syndrome
310.10 Organic personality syndrome
294.80 Atypical or mixed organic brain syndrome

SUBSTANCE USE DISORDERS

Code in fifth digit: 1 = continuous, 2 = episodic, 3 = in remission, 0 = unspecified.

305.0x Alcohol abuse, ______
303.9x Alcohol dependence (Alcoholism), ______
305.4x Barbiturate or similarly acting sedative or hypnotic abuse, ______
304.1x Barbiturate or similarly acting sedative or hypnotic dependence, ______
305.5x Opioid abuse, ______
304.0x Opioid dependence, ______
305.6x Cocaine abuse, ______
305.7x Amphetamine or similarly acting sympathomimetic abuse, ______
304.4x Amphetamine or similarly acting sympathomimetic dependence, ______
305.9x Phencyclidine (PCP) or similarly acting arylcyclohexylamine abuse, ______(328.4x)
305.3x Hallucinogen abuse, ______
305.2x Cannabis abuse, ______
304.3x Cannabis dependence, ______
305.1x Tobacco dependence, ______
305.9x Other, mixed or unspecified substance abuse, ______
304.6x Other specified substance dependence, ______
304.9x Unspecified substance dependence, ______
304.7x Dependence on combination of opioid and other nonalcoholic substance, ______
304.8x Dependence on combination of substances, excluding opioids and alcohol, ______

SCHIZOPHRENIC DISORDERS

Code in fifth digit: 1 = subchronic, 2 = chronic, 3 = subchronic with acute exacerbation, 4 = chronic with acute exacerbation, 5 = in remission, 0 = unspecified.

Schizophrenia

295.1x disorganized, ______
295.2x catatonic, ______
295.3x paranoid, ______
295.9x undifferentiated, ______
295.6x residual, ______

PARANOID DISORDERS

297.10 Paranoia
297.30 Shared paranoid disorder
298.30 Acute paranoid disorder
297.90 Atypical paranoid disorder

PSYCHOTIC DISORDERS NOT ELSEWHERE CLASSIFIED

295.40 Schizophreniform disorder
298.80 Brief reactive psychosis
295.70 Schizoaffective disorder
298.90 Atypical psychosis

NEUROTIC DISORDERS

NOTE. These are included in Affective, Anxiety, Somatoform, Dissociative, and Psychosexual Disorders. In order to facilitate the identification of the categories that in DSM II were grouped together in the class of Neuroses, the DSM II terms are included separately in parentheses after the corresponding categories. These DSM II terms are included in ICD-9-CM and therefore are acceptable as alternatives to the recommended DSM III terms that precede them.

AFFECTIVE DISORDERS

Major Affective Disorders

Code major depressive episode in fifth digit: 6 = in remission, 4 = with psychotic features (the unofficial non-ICD-9-CM fifth digit 7 may be used instead to indicate that the psychotic features are mood-incongruent), 3 = with melancholia, 2 = without melancholia, 0 = unspecified.

Code manic episode in fifth digit: 6 = in remission, 4 = with psychotic features (the unofficial non-ICD-9-CM fifth digit 7 may be used instead to indicate that the psychotic features are mood-incongruent), 2 = without psychotic features, 0 = unspecified.

Bipolar Disorder

296.6x mixed, ______
296.4x manic, ______
296.5x depressed, ______

Major Depression

296.2x single episode, ______
296.3x recurrent, ______

Other Specific Affective Disorders

301.13 Cyclothymic disorder
300.40 Dysthymic disorder (or Depressive neurosis)

Atypical Affective Disorders

296.70 Atypical bipolar disorder
296.82 Atypical depression

ANXIETY DISORDERS

Phobic Disorders (or Phobic Neuroses)

300.21 Agoraphobia with panic attacks
300.22 Agoraphobia without panic attacks
300.23 Social phobia
300.29 Simple phobia

Anxiety States (or Anxiety Neuroses)

300.01 Panic disorder
300.02 Generalized anxiety disorder
300.30 Obsessive compulsive disorder (or Obsessive compulsive neurosis)

Post-Traumatic Stress Disorder

308.30 acute
309.81 chronic or delayed
300.00 Atypical anxiety disorder

SOMATOFORM DISORDERS

300.81 Somatization disorder
300.11 Conversion disorder (or Hysterical neurosis, conversion type)
307.80 Psychogenic pain disorder
300.70 Hypochondriasis (or Hypochondriacal neurosis)
300.70 Atypical somatoform disorder (300.71)

DISSOCIATIVE DISORDERS (OR HYSTERICAL NEUROSES, DISSOCIATIVE TYPE)

300.12 Psychogenic amnesia
300.13 Psychogenic fugue
300.14 Multiple personality
300.60 Depersonalization disorder (or Depersonalization neurosis)
300.15 Atypical dissociative disorder

PSYCHOSEXUAL DISORDERS

Gender Identity Disorders

Indicate sexual history in the fifth digit of Transsexualism code: 1 = asexual, 2 = homosexual, 3 = heterosexual, 0 = unspecified.

302.5x Transsexualism, ______
302.60 Gender identity disorder of childhood
302.85 Atypical gender identity disorder

Paraphilias

302.81 Fetishism
302.30 Transvestism
302.10 Zoophilia
302.20 Pedophilia
302.40 Exhibitionism
302.82 Voyeurism
302.83 Sexual masochism
302.84 Sexual sadism
302.90 Atypical paraphilia

Psychosexual Dysfunctions

302.71 Inhibited sexual desire
302.72 Inhibited sexual excitement
302.73 Inhibited female orgasm
302.74 Inhibited male orgasm
302.75 Premature ejaculation
302.76 Functional dyspareunia
306.51 Functional vaginismus
302.70 Atypical psychosexual dysfunction

Other Psychosexual Disorders

302.00 Ego-dystonic homosexuality
302.89 Psychosexual disorder not elsewhere classified

FACTITIOUS DISORDERS

300.16 Factitious disorder with psychological symptoms
301.51 Chronic factitious disorder with physical symptoms
300.19 Atypical factitious disorder with physical symptoms

DISORDERS OF IMPULSE CONTROL NOT ELSEWHERE CLASSIFIED

312.31 Pathological gambling
312.32 Kleptomania
312.33 Pyromania
312.34 Intermittent explosive disorder
312.35 Isolated explosive disorder
312.39 Atypical impulse control disorder

ADJUSTMENT DISORDER

390.00 with depressed mood
309.24 with anxious mood
309.28 with mixed emotional features
309.30 with disturbance of conduct
309.40 with mixed disbturbance of emotions and conduct
309.23 with work (or academic) inhibition
309.83 with withdrawal
309.90 with atypical features

PSYCHOLOGICAL FACTORS AFFECTING PHYSICAL CONDITION

Specify physical condition on Axis III.

316.00 Psychological factors affecting physical condition

PERSONALITY DISORDERS

NOTE. These are coded on Axis II.

301.00 Paranoid
301.20 Schizoid
301.22 Schizotypal
301.50 Histrionic
301.81 Narcissistic
301.70 Antisocial
301.83 Borderline
301.82 Avoidant
301.60 Dependent
301.40 Compulsive
301.84 Passive-aggressive
301.89 Atypical, mixed, or other personality disorder

V CODES FOR CONDITIONS NOT ATTRIBUTABLE TO A MENTAL DISORDER THAT ARE A FOCUS OF ATTENTION OR TREATMENT

V65.20	Malingering
V62.89	Borderline intellectual functioning (V62.88)
V71.01	Adult antisocial behavior
V71.02	Childhood or adolescent antisocial behavior
V62.30	Academic problem
V62.20	Occupational problem
V62.82	Uncomplicated bereavement
V15.81	Noncompliance with medical treatment
V62.89	Phase of life problem or other life circumstance problem
V61.10	Marital problem
V61.20	Parent-child problem
V61.80	Other specified family circumstances
V62.81	Other interpersonal problem

ADDITIONAL CODES

300.90	Unspecified mental disorder (nonpsychotic)
V71.09	No diagnosis or condition on Axis I
799.90	Diagnosis or condition deferred on Axis I
V71.09	No diagnosis on Axis II
799.90	Diagnosis deferred on Axis II

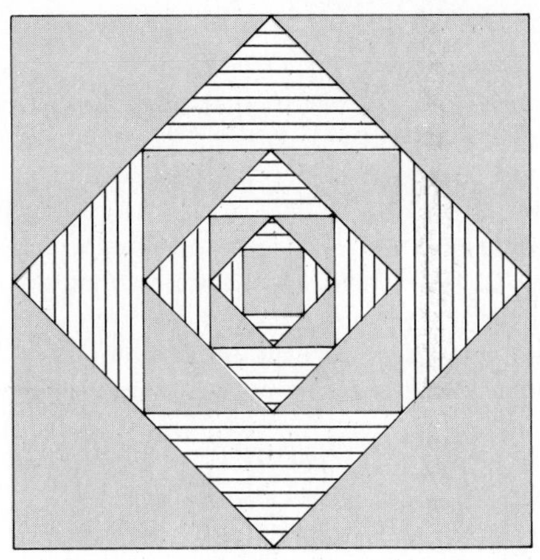

Glossary

Abandon. To withdraw protection, support, or help from another; to break a close association with another person and show complete lack of interest in him or her.

Abandonment depression. A complex of six constituent feelings—depression, rage, fear, guilt, passivity, and emptiness—that arises when attempts at separation from the mother are met with her withdrawal of emotional availability.

Abasement. A state of feeling humiliated or degraded.

Abreaction. The expression of emotions associated with distressing, anxiety-provoking, and repressed ideas. This often occurs when such ideas are brought up during therapy.

Abuse. Willful, nonaccidental injury inflicted with an attitude and purpose of causing physical harm. Four kinds of abuse are hostile verbal abuse, sexual abuse, battering, and psychological unavailability.

Acceptance. A favorable reception of another human being.

Accountability. The process of answering to another for one's actions.

Acculturation. The degree to which members of a culture other than the dominant one have internalized the dominant culture's values and norms.

ACTH (adrenocorticotropic hormone). Substance produced by the pituitary which stimulates the adrenal cortex.

Acting out. A highly compelling and often habitual response to internal signals of distress through some kind of action other than words; a means of discharging feelings to avoid having to experience them.

"Activities of daily living" (ADL) groups. Educative therapy groups focused on helping clients learn to cope with the requirements of day-to-day living.

Activity therapy. Therapy which focuses on the acting out of impulses, conflicts, and deviant behavior in a group setting.

Adaptational energy. The body's capacity to cope with stressors.

Adaptation phase. The final phase of group therapy, characterized by openness and acceptance among group members.

Addiction. Compulsive use of chemical substances, involving physical and psychological dependence.

Addison's disease. A condition characterized by a deficiency in the secretion of adrenocortical hormones.

Adjustment. A person's adaptive relation to society and to the inner self.

Adolescence. Period of growth and development from puberty to maturity.

Adoption. Legal transfer of rights and responsibilities from biological parents to people who volunteer to serve as a child's parents.

Adultery. Voluntary coitus on the part of a married person with someone other than his or her spouse.

Adulthood. Stage of growth and development that follows adolescence.

Affect. Emotional feeling tone attached to an object, idea, or thought; includes inner feelings and their external manifestations.

Affective psychosis. A psychotic reaction in which the predominant feature is a disturbance in emotional feeling tone, usually depression or elation.

Aggression. Physical or verbal behavior that is self-assertive, forceful, or hostile.

Agitation. State of anxiety associated with severe motor restlessness.

Agoraphobia. Fear of the outdoors or going out, especially alone. It is the most common phobia.

Akathisia. Continuous uncontrolled muscular movements and restlessness.

Akinesia. Muscular weakness in which a person has fatiguelike symptoms; sometimes referred to as *rubber legs.*

Alcoholism. Any use of alcoholic beverages that causes damage to an individual, to society, or to both. The following clinical features are evident: chronicity as a disease or disorder of behavior; undue preoccupation with intake of ethyl alcohol; loss of control over the drinking pattern; use of alcohol in a way that is damaging to the drinker's physical health, interpersonal relations, or economic functions; use of alcohol as a universal solution to problems.

Alienation. The feeling of being detached from oneself or society; the avoidance of emotional experiences; generalized estrangement.

Aloneness. A state of social isolation; physical apartness from others in the sense of being an only, sole, or single person, or without company.

Ambivalence. The simultaneous presence of strong, often overwhelming, but contradictory attitudes, ideas, feelings, and drives toward an object, person, goal, or situation.

Amenorrhea. Absence of menstruation.

Amnesia. A dissociative experience in which a person's recollection is lost or split off from conscious recall. The cause of amnesia may be organic or functional.

Amniocentesis. Procedure whereby a sample of amniotic fluid is obtained from the uterus during pregnancy.

Anal stage. In Freud's framework, the stage of growth and development lasting from 18 months to 3 years.

Analogic communication. Nonverbal communication.

Androgyny. A state in which there is a blending of and freedom from traditional sex role behaviors.

Anergia. A state of inactivity and sluggishness.

Anger. A burst of energy in reaction to an insult to one's sense of self, including one's values.

Angina. A paroxysmal severe pain radiating from the heart to the shoulder and sometimes down the left arm.

Anilingus. Oral stimulation of the anal area.

Anniversary reactions. Time-specific psychological or physiological events that occur or recur in response to a traumatic event in a person's past or in the past of another person with whom that person closely identifies.

Annoyance. A physiological and psychological response to stimuli that are unwanted and disturbing to a person.

Anorexia nervosa. An eating disorder characterized by a phobic fear of being fat, resulting in a serious weight loss due to failure to ingest sufficient nutrients.

Anovulation. Absence of ovulation.

Anticipatory grief. Grief occurring before the actual loss with which it is associated.

Anticipatory guidance. A process that aims to help people cope with a crisis by discussing the details of the impending difficulty and problem solving before the event occurs.

Anxiety. Apprehension cued by threats to values which people hold essential to their existence as personalities; continuum of discomfort ranging from mild to panic level; unpleasurable affect consisting of psychophysiological changes in response to an intrapsychic conflict.

Apathy. Lack of feeling or affect; lack of interest or emotional involvement in one's surroundings.

Aphasia. Disturbance or loss of ability to comprehend, elaborate, or express speech concepts; inability to speak, comprehend, name an object, or arrange words in proper sequence.

Appearance. The way in which a person uses clothing and other personal objects to convey a personal image.

Arthritis. A systemic disorder characterized by inflammatory changes in the articular and associated structures.

Artificial insemination. Process of medically instilling into a woman's cervix sperm from a donor who may or may not be her husband.

"As if" behavior. Superficially acceptable behavior that is adopted in a defensive effort to conceal one's unacceptable feelings and aims and to ignore one's underlying feelings of powerlessness in interpersonal situations.

Assaultiveness. Violent behavior involving a physical or verbal attack on another.

Assertive behavior. An expression of emotion that is appropriate to the existing situation, as opposed to the expression of subjective anxiety (anxiety unrelated to the facts of the existing situation).

Assessment. A systematic collection of health-related data about a client's internal and external environment.

Assistance. Help given to clients, and the presence of the care giver.

Ataxia. Incoordination or involuntary movement.

Attachment phase. Bonding of mother and infant.

Attending. The use of the body in a physical and psychological way which communicates to another person that one is listening and paying attention to what is being said.

Attention deficit disorder. A neurological condition that produces "soft" neurological signs, motor-perceptual dysfunction, and problematic behavior characterized by developmentally inappropriate inattention and impulsivity.

Atypical developmental psychosis. Psychotic process in early childhood characterized by autistic behavior, symbiotic behavior, or both.

Audit. A method used to document the extent to which structure and process achieve specific outcomes.

Aura. A sensation—such as fear or olfactory, auditory, or visual hallucinations—experienced by a person just before a grand mal seizure; a peculiar epigastric sensation or a welling up in the throat.

Authority. The right of designated people to make decisions and issue commands.

Autistic thinking. A form of thinking that attempts to gratify unfulfilled needs and desires in a way which is not reality-oriented. Objective facts are distorted, obscured, or excluded to varying degrees, and personal and private meanings are applied to situations and words.

Autoaggression. Aggression directed against the self.

Autoeroticism. Sexual self-arousal without the participation of another person. The term *autoeroticism* is sometimes used interchangeably with *masturbation.*

Autonomy. A condition characterized by independence or self-governance.

Avoidance. A person's escape, through physical and emotional distancing maneuvers, from relatedness to others; withdrawal.

"Awareness of dying" context. A schema for describing the conscious knowledge and interactions of dying people; interactions are "closed," "suspected," "mutual pretense," and "open."

Balance theory. A theory which refers to equilibrium between inducements for a person to join an organization and contributions the person will make to that organization.

Basic assumption. That aspect of group life which is essentially unconscious; it operates through the expression of dependency, fight-flight responses, and pairing.

Battered-child syndrome. A term used to describe the physical injuries found among infants and children who have been physically abused by their parents or surrogate parents.

Behavior modification. A method of reeducation based on the principles of Pavlovian conditioning. Some of the methods are response prevention, modeling, desensitization, shaping, flooding, and implosion.

Bisexuality. Enjoyment of sexual contacts with members of both sexes.

Bitterness. "Gall of the spirit" that pollutes and destroys everything it touches.

Bizarre behavior. Eccentric behavior, or actions which do not conform to social expectations in a situation.

Blocking. Involuntary cessation of thought processes or speech because of unconscious emotional factors; also known as *thought deprivation.*

Blunting of affect. A disturbance of affect manifested by dullness of externalized feeling tone.

Body boundary. A mental idea related to how definitely or indefinitely one experiences the "line of separation" between one's body and the rest of the world.

Body image. A mental representation of one's body derived from internal sensations, emotions, fantasies, posture, and experience of and with outside objects and people.

Borderline personality disorder. A personality disorder in which a client may exhibit either neurotic or psychotic symptoms; it is characterized by fluctuations in mood, behavior, and self-image.

Bulimia. An eating disorder characterized by episodic, uncontrolled, rapid ingestion of large quantities of food over a short period of time (bingeing) followed by attempts to avoid weight gain through self-induced vomiting and laxative abuse (purging).

Bureaucracy. A systematized and centralized governmental structure.

Case management. A method of assigning responsibility for systems coordination to one person who works with a given client in accessing necessary services.

Castration. Surgical removal of testes in males and ovaries in females.

Catatonic state (catatonia). A state characterized by immobility, with muscular rigidity or inflexibility. The catatonic state may also be manifested by excitability.

Cathexis. A conscious or unconscious investment of psychic energy in an idea, concept, or object.

Change agent. An outside force or person acting for another in a deliberate effort to improve a situation.

Childhood psychosis. A basic disorder of personality manifested by disturbances in thinking, affect, perception, motility, speech, reality testing, and object relations.

Centrifugal dynamics. Forces within the family that diminish the integrity of the family system's boundaries and foster the premature separation of offspring.

Centripetal dynamics. Forces within the family that interfere with the permeability of the family system's external boundary, preventing the developmentally appropriate separation of offspring.

Chronic disease. An illness which is not curable, may be progressive, and usually involves some ongoing treatment and permanent disability.

Circumstantiality. A disturbance in associative thought processes in which a person digresses into unnecessary details and inappropriate thoughts before communicating a central idea.

Clarification. An attempt by a nurse to clearly understand the communication of a client when it is vague, confusing, or unclear.

Client. A recipient of nursing services; may be a person, family, group, or community.

Clinging. A style of interpersonal behavior marked by excessive demandingness, neediness, and dependency.

Coercive power. Power based on the others' belief that someone has the ability to punish and that punishment will be unpleasant and frustrate a need.

Cognition. The mental process of knowing or becoming aware.

Cohabitants. Two people who are emotionally and sexually intimate and share the same household without being legally married.

Cohesiveness. A group phenomenon; the resultant of all forces acting on members to remain in the group; a sense of group belongingness; also called *cohesion.*

Coitus. The sex act; copulation; intercourse; penetration of penis into vagina.

Commitment. The act of hospitalizing persons for psychiatric treatment through legal means.

Communication. An ongoing interaction through which people relate to one another; a process of discovering and conveying meaning, of moving toward one's life purpose.

Community. An identifiable group of people living in the same locality under similar conditions and having common interests.

Community development. An approach to community organization that is designed to create conditions of economic and social progress for the whole community.

Community meeting. A large group meeting held at regularly scheduled intervals; a prime characteristic of a therapeutic community.

Community mental health. The synchronous interaction between and among individual members of a community and within the community as a whole; it is reflected primarily in mental indicators such as acceptable norms, open atmosphere, socialization that fosters pursuit of life purposes, healthy relationships with one another, and freedom to pursue a personal relationship with God or another spiritual being. Community mental health is influenced by and reflects the mental health of people within it.

Community milieu. The spiritual aspect of a community; may be therapeutic or nontherapeutic.

Community support systems. Resources that are mobilized to bolster the natural support systems (including the family) of chronically disabled people living outside of institutions.

Competition. Rivalry between and among individuals in a group.

Complementarity. A term referring to the two-sidedness of relationships, where both parties provide both stimuli and responses. All interaction involves complementarity.

Compromise. Conflict resolution whereby the solution is acceptable to everyone even though participants give up something.

Compulsion. An irrational urge to act which cannot be resisted without extreme difficulty.

Concept. An abstract idea having its origins or reference points in the real world.

Conceptual framework. The relationships among concepts.

Concreteness. The clear, direct expression of personally relevant perceptions, values, and feelings as they exist in the present relationship.

Conditioning. A process which involves associating a certain stimulus (or stimuli) with a predictable behavioral response or response pattern.

Confabulation. Compensating for memory gaps with imaginary stories which the teller believes to be true.

Confirmation. True positive or negative information relevant to the current situation; validation.

Conflict. Active striving for one's own preferred outcome—which, if attained, precludes the attainment by others of their preferred outcomes. Hostility is a product of conflict.

Confrontation. Communications that call attention to significant discrepancies in another's experience; verbal messages which are intended to help another to recognize information which is not consistent with the other's self-image.

Confusion. A state of mental perplexity or bewilderment resulting from disorientation.

Conscious. A term describing all the elements of thought and feeling that come to mind readily.

Consensual validation. The verification of reality with someone else.

Consumer. A client, or a person accepting health services; the public.

Content message. Information which is conveyed verbally.

Contingency theory. A theory which states that the structure necessary for the work outcome of an organization is supported by and depends upon environmental variables.

Conversion. A process whereby repressed instinctive tendencies are expressed through (or "converted" into) sensory or motor manifestations, such as paralysis of a limb or blindness, which have no organic bases.

Coparenting. Parenting by divorced or separated parents in which both parents have joint legal custody of a child and are equally involved in child rearing.

Coping. Action-oriented efforts directed toward managing stressors in one's internal and external environments; involves mastering, tolerating, reducing, or eliminating changes and conflicts.

Counterfeit role. A role that is not covertly but overtly accepted in order to protect the self from a penalty.

Counterphobia. A state of actual preference on the part of the phobic person for the very situation of which he or she is afraid.

Countertransference. A conscious or unconscious emotional response of a therapist to a client; through countertransference, the therapist transfers onto the client feelings, wishes, and conflicts which originated in the therapist's own relationships with significant others.

Covert. Hidden or disguised.

Creuzfeldt-Jakob disease. A rare, sporadic, and familial transmissable dementia.

Crime. Conduct that is in violation of the law.

Crisis. A turning point in a person's life; a conflict or problem of basic importance perceived as hazardous which cannot readily be solved by using the usual coping mechanisms; a state of psychological disequilibrium.

Crisis groups. Groups made up of clients undergoing a crisis (for example, recent victims of rape).

Crisis intervention. An intervention process aimed at reestablishing a level of functioning equal to or better than the precrisis level.

Crohn's disease. An inflammatory disease of the small bowel and sometimes the colon.

Cult. A contemporary religious sect considered by society as promoting a deviant religion.

Cultural relativism. The idea that judgments are based on experience and that experience is interpreted by people in terms of their unique culture.

Culture. The learned patterns of values, beliefs, attitudes, customs, and behaviors that are shared by a group in a particular social environment.

Cunnilingus. Oral stimulation of the female genitalia.

Cushing's syndrome. A complex of symptoms resulting from hypersecretion of the adrenal cortex.

Custody. A legal term used to designate the care and control aspects of a relationship between a child and his or her care givers.

Day care. Long-term care provided for clients who are not expected to show improvement or progress; keeps clients from deteriorating to the point that hospitalization is necessary. (*Also:* Supervision of and facilities for preschool children during the day.)

Daydreams. Fleeting fantasies or distracting images that intrude suddenly into waking thoughts.

Day hospital. A structured and protected environment that provides treatment on a per diem basis for clients, generally the chronically ill or those in transition back to their community. Clients return to their family or another shelter for the night. It is partial hospitalization existing to prevent full hospitalization.

Day treatment. Therapeutic experiences provided for 2 to 3 months to clients who are making the transition from hospital to community.

Defense mechanism. An operation outside of awareness which the person calls into play to protect against anxiety; a coping mechanism, a security operation, a mental mechanism.

Delegating dynamics. Forces within the family that influence adolescent members to act as emissaries or proxies for their parents at the expense of their own growth and development.

Delegation. The process of assigning part or all of one's responsibility to another person or persons.

Delirium. A disturbance in the state of consciousness that stems from an acute organic reaction.

Delirium tremens. Delirium associated with prolonged, excessive use of alcohol, usually thought to be induced by abrupt cessation of alcohol intake; a part of alcohol withdrawal syndrome (AWS).

Delusion. A false, fixed idea that arises within a person without appropriate external stimulation; an idea that is inconsistent with a person's knowledge and experience. (The following five entries are examples of delusions.)

Delusion of control or influence. A false belief that one is being controlled by others.

Delusion of grandeur or importance. A false belief in which one's own importance is greatly exaggerated.

Delusion of infidelity. A false belief that one's lover or spouse is unfaithful.

Delusion of persecution. A false belief that one is being harassed by others.

Delusion, somatic. A false belief about one's body or organ systems wherein the focus is on one's physical condition.

Dementia. A loss of intellectual abilities of sufficient severity to interfere with social or occupational functioning.

Denial. An unconscious mental mechanism whereby one refuses to acknowledge or attempts to deny some anxiety-provoking aspect of self or external reality.

Dependency. A person's reliance on others to meet basic needs for love, affection, nurturing, shelter, protection, security, food, and warmth.

Depersonalization. An affective disturbance in which a person experiences feelings of unreality or strangeness concerning either the environment, the self, or both.

Depression. A feeling of profound sadness, low self-esteem, and hopelessness about one's life. A change in mood and responsiveness that ranges from mild and transitory to severe, intense, pervasive, and persistent.

Desensitization. The gradual systematic exposure of a client to feared situations under controlled conditions.

Desirable hope. Belief that if a set of expectations were to be realized it would be nice but that those expectations will not be realized.

Detachment. The condition of being separated or apart.

Detumescence. Return of the penis to its flaccid state following erection and ejaculation.

Devaluation. Attributing of exaggerated "badness" or negative qualities to a person or object.

Developmental crisis. A maturational event during a transition from one developmental period to another in which a person experiences severe stress requiring psychological intervention.

Developmental lag. Physical or emotional development which is less than that expected for a child's chronological age.

Deviance. Behavior that diverges or is different from norms established by a group.

Differentiation. The degree of separateness or fusion between the intellectual system and the emotional system; the degree to which a person defines the self as separate from others.

Digital communication. Verbal communication.

Direct client services. Personal relationships between a nurse and clients—individuals, families, or communities.

Disability. A chronic condition which makes a person unable to perform in a usual manner.

Disconfirmation. A transpersonal defense mechanism whereby a person denies the truth and confirms false images held by another.

Discontinuity. A loss of a sense of continuity between past, present, and future.

Discrimination. The ability to notice similarities and differences in like situations.

Disordered thinking. Cognitive ideational or informational experiences characterized by lapses from logical thinking, use of neologisms, circumstantiality, primary-process thought, and blocking.

Disorientation. A loss of one's bearings or position with respect to time, place, or person.

Displacement. Unconscious defense mechanism; the discharge of emotions, feelings, or ideas upon a subject other than the one that elicited the feelings.

Dissociality. Sociopathic behavior patterns evident in criminals and others who ignore societal restrictions; lack of awareness of right and wrong.

Dissociation. The unwitting splitting off from conscious awareness of those aspects of experience that are intensely anxiety-provoking; such experience comprises the "not me" component of the self-system.

Distance. Movement in a family system that pertains to the amount of physical and emotional space a person puts between self and other family members.

Distancing. An interpersonal style marked by avoidance of closeness, intimacy, and emotional contact with others.

Double-bind communication. A message in which a person is commanded both to do and not to do something, so that no adequate response is possible.

Double standard. A set of rules regarding sexuality that differs for males and females.

Dream. A sequence of pictures or images that embodies the ideas or conceptions of the dreamer.

Dream analysis. A technique used in helping unconscious material to become conscious; the interpretation of symbolism contained in a reported dream.

Drive. Motivation; can be either biological or learned.

Drug addiction. Compulsive drug use which involves craving, psychological dependence, physical dependence; tolerance for increasing doses; and the appearance of withdrawal symptoms.

Drug dependence. A psychological or physical dependence on a drug that is taken periodically or on a regular basis.

Drug habituation. Repeated use of a drug to the point where psychological dependence develops.

Dynamics. Emotional forces that work to produce behavior patterns or symptoms in persons, groups, families, and organizations.

Dysattention. A failure to focus attention on those elements of the environment that are most relevant to the tasks at hand, ranging from distractibility to complete inattention to, or loss of contact with, the environment.

Dysmenesia. Impairment in the ability to retain and recall information.

Echolalia. Automatic repetition by one person of what is said by another.

Echopraxia. Meaningless imitation of motions made by others.

Ecomap. A diagrammatic summary of a nuclear family system within the context of the larger world of neighborhood and community; shows the relationship of family members to society and systems outside the structural boundaries of the nuclear household.

Educative group therapy. A kind of group therapy in which the leader presents didactic information in the form of lectures or written material which is then discussed by the clients.

Ego. The aspect of personality that appraises the environment, assesses reality, stays in touch with bodily and environmental changes, directs the motor activity of the body, and governs defensive operations, self-identity, and sense of reality.

Ego-dystonic. Characterized by incongruence between one's values and one's thoughts, feelings, and behavior.

Ego-dystonic homosexuality. Incongruence between the desire for a heterosexual relationship and the reality of an overt homosexual relationship and arousal.

This conflict is an unwanted and persistent source of distress.

Ego ideal. Part of the developing ego, which eventually fuses with the superego.

Ego pathology. A deviation from normal defensive functioning, self-identity, and sense of reality.

Ego strength. The relative ability of the ego to maintain a sense of reality, to keep unconscious material buried, and to deal effectively with the forces of id and superego.

Ego-syntonic. Characterized by congruence between one's conscious values and how one thinks, feels, and behaves.

Ejaculation. In the male, the transport of semen out of the body.

Electroconvulsive therapy (ECT). Therapeutic use of an electric current to produce a convulsive seizure and unconsciousness.

Electroencephalogram (EEG). A tracing to record electrical discharges in the brain.

Elope. To leave a treatment setting without the awareness of the caretakers or permission from them.

Emotional cutoff. The physical or emotional separation from, isolation from, or denial of the importance of one's family of origin.

Emotional lability. An affective disturbance characterized by excessive and inappropriate emotional responses.

Emotional pain of dying. The psychic pain caused by the perception of an inability to control one's fate during the dying process.

Emotional shock wave. Physical, psychological, and social symptoms generated by "underground aftershocks" in the nuclear and extended family system that occur in the months or years following a serious emotional event in the family.

Emotions. Attitudes toward a social environment which have a definite beginning and run a characteristic course; defined, affective inner experiences and attitudes toward people and social situations.

Empathic understanding. The temporary experiencing of another's feelings; expressions which convey recognition of the feelings, motives, and meanings underlying another person's communications.

Empathy. An objective and insightful awareness of the meaning and significance of the feelings, emotions, and behavior of another person; to be distinguished from *sympathy,* which is usually more subjective.

Empirical-rational change strategy. A strategy for change in which one rationally explains the benefits of change.

Enculturation. A process by which culture is passed from one generation to another.

Endogenous rhythms. Internal, regularly recurring biological phenomena such as fluctuations in various biochemical processes, steroid and electrolyte levels, body temperature, heart rate, and respirations.

Environment. The relevant systems and processes external to and in interaction with the client.

Environmental supports. Those material objects in the environment that the client depends on in time of stress. Examples include financial supports, adequate housing, and employment.

Epidemiology. A science and a specialized field of public health that concerns itself with the health of whole populations. Specifically, epidemiology is concerned with factors related to the distribution and control of disease and promotion of health in identified populations at risk for the development of disease.

Ethic. A standard of valued behavior, or beliefs adhered to by individuals or a group; describes what ought to be, rather than what is.

Ethical decision. A freely made personal choice which originates from inside the self and is based on belief in and adherence to principles.

Ethical dilemma. A conflict that occurs when there are two or more alternatives to choose from in making an ethical decision; also called a *moral conflict.*

Ethical norm. A standard of behavior.

Ethics. A system of objectively given moral norms which determines moral truth in a concrete, present way.

Ethnic group. A group of people who consider themselves, and are regarded by others, as alike by virtue of a common ancestry.

Ethnocentrism. The idea that the way that things are done in one's own culture is the correct way.

Euphoria. An exaggerated feeling of physical and emotional well-being that is not congruent with objective stimuli or events. It may have a psychogenic origin or be due to an organic brain syndrome.

Evaluation. A judgment concerning the relevance, effectiveness, and efficiency of the client outcomes achieved as well as the nursing interventions provided.

Exogenous Regularly recurring phenomena that are external to the person.

Expectational hope. A composite of beliefs and a set of expectations that have some possibility of fulfillment.

Experimental extinction. A process by which undesired behavior is evoked but not rewarded and therefore becomes progressively weaker.

Expert power. Influence that is based on the perception that a person has expertise which is useful.

Extended family. The nuclear family and others related by descent, marriage, or adoption.

External boundaries. Limits delineating a group's identity, position, and function.

Extinction. Lack of reinforcement of behavior patterns, designed to decrease the rate of response.

Factitious disorders. Conditions characterized by repeated simulations of a physical or mental disorder for no apparent purpose other than obtaining immediate treatment and attention.

Faith. Assurance of things that are hoped for but have not yet become reality.

Family. A small social system made up of people held together by strong reciprocal affections and loyalties; sometimes, a permanent household that persists over years.

Family boundary. A real or imagined barrier or limit that encircles a family unit or an individual family member.

Family development. The process of progressive structural differentiation and transformation during a family's history.

Family functioning. The processes by which a family operates.

Family processes. Metaphysical, intangible methods used by people to determine how the family evolves its structure, makes decisions, and maintains itself as a unit.

Family romance. Fantasy experienced in childhood of being adopted by and belonging to another, ideal family.

Family structure. The configuration of family members.

Family therapy. Treatment which involves the total family or specific family members who meet to explore relationships and process; focus is more on the resolution of current reactions to one another than on the problems of individual members.

Fantasy. Waking dreams or mental images conjured in the imagination that fill reverie states and bring a person into situations that are otherwise inaccessible.

Fear. Respect for the power of another. Healthy fear allows constructive interaction with the powerful one; unhealthy fear compromises clear thinking, intelligent action, and assertive interaction.

Feedback. A phase in the communication process in which the receiver of information conveys a negative or positive message back to the sender.

Feelings. The background emotional "coloring" or "tone" of pleasantness or unpleasantness that one experiences in relation to something in the environment; a person's transitory responses to sensations and perceptions.

Fellatio. Oral stimulation of the male genitalia.

Fetishism. The association of sexual pleasure with inanimate objects.

Fiedler's contingency model. A model which measures effectiveness of leadership according to a group's productivity.

Fixation. The concentration of psychic energy at the stage or stages of psychosexual development where one's needs have been over- or undergratified.

Flat affect. A form of mood change in which there is a loss of feeling tone, so that a person often feels "blah," inert, and incapable of any emotional display.

Flight of ideas. A sudden, rapid shift from one idea to another before the preceding one has been concluded.

Flooding. The use of real or imaginery situations to evoke strong anxiety responses.

Focusing. Efforts to keep the flow of communication goal-directed, specific, and concrete.

Formal role. A role that is ascribed.

Fornication. Voluntary coitus between a man and a woman who are not married to each other.

Foster care. Placement of a person with a family for the purpose of encouraging skills in cooperative living. (*Also:* Temporary placement of a child with a caretaking family other than the parents.)

Free association. A technique used in encouraging unconscious material to become conscious; unselected verbalization by the client of whatever comes to mind.

Frigidity. Inability of the female to achieve orgasm.

Frustration. A buildup of energy that was to have been used to pursue a purpose or objective but which has been blocked.

Fugue state. A dissociative state characterized by amnesia and actual physical flight from an intolerable situation.

Gentleness. Touch without invasion; approach to another that respects boundaries while making one's presence known.

"Great man" theory. The theory that some persons are born to lead while others are born to follow.

Guilt. A sense of sin or wrongdoing against oneself or another.

Handicap. A negative response to a disadvantage which makes achievement in some area of functioning difficult.

Helplessness. Inability to act effectively under compelling circumstances.

Identity. Gestalt of self-awareness made up of experiences, memories, perceptions, emotions, and sensory input; awareness of being a person separate and distinct from all others.

Impulsiveness. A tendency to act suddenly, without conscious thought.

Inappropriate affect. A display of emotion that is out of harmony with reality. The mood shown and experienced is incongruous with the situation or the accompanying thought content.

Inauthentic emotions. Affective reactions which are acted out in an exaggerated fashion and serve as a reaction formation to actual feelings, which are experienced only superficially.

Incest. A type of sexual abuse which involves any sexual activity or intimate physical contact that is sexually arousing between members of a family who are too closely related to be married.

Indirect client services. Services which involve administration, research, public relations, procurement and allocation of resources, and formation and implementation of policy.

Indirect self-destructive behavior (ISDB). Any activity that is detrimental to one's physical well-being and might lead to death, such as smoking.

Individuation. The process by which the child differentiates between self and others, and by which one's unfolding individuality emerges.

Infantile autism. In a young child, a neurological, perceptual, and physiological dysfunction characterized by a psychotic state.

Informal groups. Groups in which members provide such satisfactions as affiliation, identification, emotional support, and protection; most commonly seen among people who work together.

Insight. A perception of the connection between conscious behavior and previously unrecognized feelings, wishes, and conflicts.

Integrity. The state in which a person is functioning as a whole being.

Intentional suicide. Endangering one's own life for the purpose of terminating it.

Interactional theory. A theory which states that leadership style is determined by the interaction between a situation and the personality of the leader.

Interest. A feeling of genuine curiosity; a desire to know another person or situation.

Internal boundary. An individual's identity separate from a group.

Interventions. Activities planned by a nurse with a client to achieve established outcomes.

Intimacy. Interaction characterized by knowledge of, availability for, and respect for one another's needs. A closeness which is developed and shared.

Intrapsychic. Within the mind.

Introjection. An unconscious defense mechanism; a symbolic taking in or incorporation of a loved or hated object or person into a person's own ego structure.

Intuition. The act or faculty of knowing without the use of rational processes.

Isolation. An unconscious defense mechanism; the exclusion from awareness of the feelings connected with a thought, memory, or experience. The person remembers the experience or thought but does not reexperience the emotion that originally accompanied it.

Joy. Fullness of heart that strengthens and energizes.

Judgment. A function of the ego involving the capacity to anticipate consequences of one's behavior.

Kinesics. The study of body movement as a form of nonverbal communication.

Kinesthesia. The sense by which one is aware of the position and movement of the various body parts.

Kin network. Groups of related nuclear families living close enough to exchange goods and services.

Labeling. A sociological concept that refers to assigning a particular impression or diagnostic specification to a client on the basis of culturally determined norms.

Lability. Emotional instability; rapidly changing emotions.

Latency. In the Freudian framework, the stage of growth and development lasting from age 6 to age 12.

Leadership. A set of actions or processes that influences members of a group to set and attain goals.

Legitimate power. Influence based on the follower's belief that the leader has a legitimate right to influence and that the follower is bound to accept.

Lesbian. A female homosexual.

Libidinal supplies. The resources made available to children by a mother that support and sustain their physical and emotional well-being; such resources include nurturance, warmth, interest, approval, support, care, attention, and emotional investment.

Libido. Psychic energy; sexual motivation; urge or desire for sexual activity.

Line. The hierarchy of personnel that extends from leaders at the top of an organizational structure to workers at the bottom. Line workers are responsible for performing or supervising the primary functions of the organization.

Living legacy. Donation of bodies or body parts for scientific research or for transplants. Spatial legacies involve written or verbal autobiographical accounts of a person's environment. Physical legacies include property, assets, or personal possessions.

Locked skilled-nursing facilities. Housing for severely disabled people who can survive outside state hospitals only if they have a sufficiently structured facility in the community to compensate for their lack of internal controls.

Loneliness. A restless search for ultimate connectedness with one's "center"; lies at the hub of life and is a state that cannot be avoided in the process of becoming a whole person. The inevitable human search for the meaning of one's life, by necessity, leads a person to the existential, creative, and spiritual experience of loneliness.

Lonesomeness. The conscious recognition of one's aloneness and a simultaneous desire to be with others.

Long-term memory. The ability to recall the distant past.

Looseness of association. A type of disordered thought process in which a person expresses successive ideas which appear to be unrelated or only slightly related to one another. The person does not indicate an intention to change the subject or explain transitions as they are communicated.

Love. Giving oneself to another unconditionally, without demanding anything in return.

Loyalty. A reliable, positive attitude of one person toward another that is based on trust, merit, commitment, and action.

Loyalty commitments. Invisible bonds that influence family members' relationships while remaining out of awareness.

Loyalty conflict. A forced choice to be loyal to one person at the expense of disloyalty to another.

Lust dynamism. A term used by Sullivan to describe clearly stated sexual desires and abilities.

Magical thinking. A type of primitive thought process in which a person attaches personal meaning or power of unrealistic proportions to objective events or neutral situations. To the person involved, the thought may be the same as the act.

Maintenance of health. Continuity or preservation of a client's current health status through nursing activities.

Malevolence. A combination of spite, hate, and malice.

Management by objectives. A process by which a leader and subordinate worker jointly identify the worker's goals and designate his or her areas of responsibility.

Managerial theory. A theory which states that the leader influences group behavior through the processes of planning, organizing, directing, and controlling.

Mania. A mood of extreme euphoria and excitement with loss of reality testing. Can be one of the phases of manic-depressive psychosis.

Manic-depressive psychosis. A major emotional illness marked by severe mood swings between elation and depression.

Manipulation. The process of influencing another to meet or comply with one's own needs and wishes, regardless of the needs and wishes of the other.

Masochism. Sexual pleasure or gratification obtained by experiencing physical or mental pain and humiliation.

Masturbation. The sexual arousal of oneself or another through manual, oral, or mechanical stimulation of sexual organs.

Maternal deprivation. Inadequate physical and emotional care of an infant or young child by a consistent caretaker.

Maturational crisis. Developmental crisis; a predictable life event or turning point which occurs for most people.

McGregor's X and Y theories. Theories which utilize assumptions about motivation. Theory X states that people dislike and avoid work. Theory Y states that people are self-directed and will engage in goal-directed behavior by choice.

Medication education groups. Therapy groups which focus on teaching clients about the medications they are taking.

Melancholia. Severe depression.

Memory interference. The inability to remember because of the existence of previously stored memory.

Mental dimension. The aspect of people relating to their ability to think and feel.

Mental health. The ability to cope effectively with the life process.

Mental illness. Maladaptation to the life process.

Mental status examination. Examination in which the following mental processes are reviewed: appearance and behavior, thought content, sensorium and intellect, thought processes, emotional tone, and insight.

Metacommunication. Communication about communication.

Migraine. An intensely painful episodic headache.

Milieu therapy. Treatment that emphasizes appropriate socioenvironmental manipulation for the benefit of a client. The term *milieu* refers to those social and cultural aspects of a treatment setting which can be influential in reducing the behavioral disturbances of clients.

Mind guard. A role performed by some members of groups characterized by "groupthink," in which they appoint themselves to protect the leader and other members from adverse information that may undermine the confidence of the group.

Minimal brain dysfunction (MBD). A syndrome characterized by deviations in cerebral function such as impairment of perception, conceptualization, language comprehension, control of attention, impulse control, and motor function.

Monopolizer. A person who talks constantly, preventing others from talking.

Moral image. The perception and feeling of what one should be.

Mother measures. Those actions taken by the "mothering" figure which nurture the child and fulfill the child's needs.

Mourning. A process during which a person perceives the loss of a love object and in one way or another confronts the pain associated with the loss of desired gratification and the impossibility of attaining it, and thus resolves the loss by letting go of the love object (person or ability).

Multigenerational transmission process. The process by which family interaction patterns are passed along from generation to generation.

Multi-infarct dementia. An abrupt, rapid, "patchy" stepwise deterioration in intellectual functioning in the presence of focal neurological signs and symptoms and evidence of cerebrovascular disease.

Multiple personality. The existence within a person of two or more distinct personalities, one of which is dominant at any particular time.

Mystification. A transpersonal process which consists of misdefining issues.

Narcissism. A psychoanalytic term meaning "self-love" or "self-interest," which is normal in childhood but pathological when seen in a similar degree in adulthood.

Negative feedback. Any communication that maintains the status quo in the relationship.

Negativism. Strong resistance to suggestions or advice.

Neologism. A made-up word or condensation of several words that has special meaning for the person using it and lacks consensual validation.

Neurosis. A mental disorder characterized by anxiety which may be experienced and expressed directly or through an unconscious psychic process; the anxiety may be converted, displaced, or somatized.

Night hospital. A hospital that provides clients with supervision and treatment at the end of a day which has been spent either at a job or at a rehabilitation center in the community.

Noise. Unwanted and undesirable sound.

Nonverbal communication. Communication using symbols other than words. It is conveyed by body language, gestures, eye movements, facial expressions, personal appearance, and dress.

Normative-reeducative change strategy. A process by which a change agent directly intervenes in the learning and relearning process.

Norms. Unspoken rules of conduct or standards of expected behavior for group members; ideal cultural patterns that specify what people should and should not do in given circumstances.

Nuclear family. The basic unit in society; a group of people united by kinship or adoption which consists of legally married parents and their children.

Nuclear family's emotional system. The patterns of emotional functioning in a family in a single generation.

Nursing. A goal-directed process that promotes synchronous patterns of interactions between the client and environment.

Nursing diagnosis. A statement reflecting judgment and decision about the pattern of interaction between the client and the environment, from which outcomes and interventions are logically derived. A nursing diagnosis may include strengths as well as actual or potential health problems.

Nursing homes. Permanent living arrangements in which residents have no responsibility for tasks associated with home life; some residents, however, may have an opportunity to participate in tasks as part of their treatment program.

Nursing interventions. Activities planned by the nurse, with the client's input, that are designed to achieve client outcomes.

Nursing process. A scientific method used by nurses to systematically assess and diagnose clients' health status, formulate client outcomes, determine interventions to be used with them, and evaluate the quality and outcomes of care planned for them and in conjunction with them.

Obesity. An abnormal amount of body fat, related to an imbalance between food eaten and energy expended.

Object constancy. The capacity to evoke a stable, consistent mental image of the mother, whether she is there or not.

Object image. The mental representation of people in the external environment. The earliest object image formed is of a mother or a mother substitute.

Object relations. A function of the ego involving the capacity for emotional attachment to others.

Obsession. A repetitive thought which a person is unable to control.

Occupational therapy. A form of therapy in which clients are encouraged to perform useful tasks and develop interests which may either reestablish old skills and knowledge or initiate new ones.

Oculogyric crisis. A side effect of a drug, characterized by sudden onset of uncontrolled rolling back of the eyes.

Oligospermia. Deficiency of sperm in the semen.

Oral phase. In psychoanalytic theory, that phase of an infant's psychosexual development characterized by a concentration of psychic energies in the oral zone and strong dependency needs for oral gratification.

Organic brain syndrome. A term used to refer to a constellation of psychological or behavioral signs and symptoms without reference to etiology.

Organic mental disorder. An organic brain syndrome in which the etiology is known or presumed.

Organigram. A visual representation of an organizational structure; an organizational chart.

Organizational structure. A systemic and goal-directed arrangement of the work of an organization.

Orgasm. Highly pleasurable sexual peak response; feeling of physiological and psychological release from maximum levels of sexual excitement.

Orientation. The phase of a therapeutic relationship in which the nature and purpose of the relationship are explained.

Outcome criteria. Measurable statements of a client's goals that are expected to result from nursing interventions. Client outcomes relate directly to, and are determined by, the nursing diagnosis.

Overaggressive phase. The second phase of group therapy, characterized by aggressive behavior among group members.

Palilia. A pathological repetitious use of words and phrases.

Panic. An attack of acute, intense, and overwhelming anxiety accompanied by a considerable degree of personality disorganization.

Paradoxical injunction. A technique in family therapy prescribing the symptom or reversal; the therapist instructs family members to do consciously what they have been doing unconsciously.

Paralanguage. A type of communication involving tone of voice, inflection, spacing of words, emphasis, and pauses.

Parallel process. Duplication of behavior at different levels in a hierarchy.

Paranoid behavior. Behavior characterized by grandiose delusions, suspicion, and mistrust of others. Paranoia also involves persecutory delusions, hostility, and hallucinations.

Paranoid disorder. A psychotic disorder characterized by delusions of reference, persecution, and grandiosity.

Paraphaia. A misuse of spoken words or word combinations.

Paraphilia. Sometimes referred to as *sexual deviation;* involves sexual arousal in response to sexual imagery, objects, or acts that are not part of the normative arousal-activity patterns of society. The paraphilias include fetishism, transvestism, zoophilia, pedophilia, exhibitionism, voyeurism, sexual masochism, and sadism.

Paraprofessional. A mental health worker who does not hold a professional degree; also called a *psychiatric aide* or a *psychiatric technician.*

Parataxic mode. The mode of perception in which the undifferentiated whole is broken into parts that are momentary, illogical, and disconnected.

Parental coalition. Union of parents for the common purpose of rearing children so as to best meet the latter's needs.

Parentification. A process by which an older child becomes the "emotional parent" to his or her parent and assumes parental responsibilities for younger siblings; the parent relates to the child as a generational equal.

Partly compensatory interventions. Activities used in situations in which both the client and the nurse perform care measures; use varies with the client's limitations, knowledge, and skill, and with his or her readiness to perform or to learn needed care measures.

Part object image. An unintegrated mental representation of a person as being "all good" or "all bad."

Passive-aggressive behavior. Behavior such as lateness, obtuseness, forgetting, or making "mistakes" that is seemingly passive but is motivated by unconscious anger; it elicits anger and frustration in others.

Path-goal theory. A theory explaining the effect of a leader's behavior on a group; the conditions in which the leader's behavior affects members' satisfaction are specified.

Pathological loneliness. Social alienation and the unnoticed inability to do anything while alone.

Patience. Giving oneself and others the time, space, and nurturance needed for growth.

Peace. Prevailing calm that continues in spite of difficult circumstances.

Pedophile. An adult who engages in sexual activities with children.

Perception. Mental processes by which data—intellectual, sensory, and emotional—are organized meaningfully.

Permission. Consent or authorization to behave in new ways.

Person. A living being with physical, mental, and spiritual dimensions, who functions in identifiable patterns with the environment to achieve a chosen life purpose.

Personal distance. The normal spacing that is maintained between members of a species.

Personality disorder. A mental disorder that originates within the character structure of a person.

Personification. A symbolic conception of the other and of self as "good" or "bad."

Pervasive developmental disorders. Severe disturbances in the following areas of functioning: intellectual, behavioral, emotional, physical, and developmental.

Phallic stage. In Freud's framework, the stage of growth and development lasting from ages 3 to 6.

Phantom pain. Perception of pain in a body part which has been surgically or accidentally separated from the body.

Phantom phenomenon. The continued experiencing of a lost body part as if it were still present.

Phase-specific splitting. The period in object-relations development when splitting is used as an adaptive mechanism of the ego owing to its immaturity.

Phobia. An irrational fear of an object or an environmental situation.

Physical dimension. The body; the anatomy and physiology of a person.

Pica. An eating disorder characterized by the ingestion of nonnutritive substances such as starch, dirt, and paper.

Plasticity. Quality of being capable of being molded or changed.

Play therapy. A type of therapy used with children which employs toys and games to reveal their problems, fears, and underlying conflicts.

Populations at risk. All members of a specific population who might, under particular conditions, be vulnerable to a particular disease.

Positive feedback. Any communication that leads to change in a relationship.

Posttraumatic stress disorder. Anxiety and stress symptoms that occur after a massive traumatic event; such symptoms might include feeling as if the event were reoccurring.

Power. The moral and physical force that maintains the right to authority; any force that results in behavioral change.

Power-coercive change strategy. The use of power to force compliance with change.

Powerlessness. A state in which a person perceives a lack of personal control over certain events or situations; it is manifested by feelings of apathy, anger, and depression.

Precocity. Unusually early development of mental or physical traits.

Preconscious. A term describing elements that are difficult to remember but can be recalled with help.

Prejudice. A negative stereotype which is emotionally charged and not easily changed by new information.

Premature grieving. Early withdrawal of emotional investment from a relationship with a dying person.

Prescription of the symptom. A therapeutic technique in which the therapist suggests that the client increase or in some way manipulate the manifestation of symptomatic behavior; therapeutic technique used by Watzlawick.

Prevalence. The number of established or diagnosed cases of an illness in a given population at a particular time.

Primary degenerative dementia. A progressive multifaceted loss of intellectual abilities and other higher cortical functions; changes in personality and behavior for which there is no specific cause.

Primary gain. The reduction of tension or conflict through neurotic illness.

Primary prevention. Actions taken to reduce the incidence of disease in populations at risk. Primary prevention emphasizes promotion of healthy personality development, healthy families, and healthy communities through the reduction of factors considered harmful to these systems.

Primary-process thinking. Illogical thinking with a tendency toward concreteness, condensation of separate psychological items into one item, and displacement of feelings from one item to another.

Principle. A basic truth, law, or assumption.

Privacy. The quality or state of being apart from company or observation.

Processes. Organized patterns or operations that are purposeful.

Projection. A psychological defense mechanism in which feelings, thoughts, impulses, or desires which originate from within the self are disavowed as arising from the self but are perceived as originating from objects in the external world; used excessively in a wide variety of normal situations by clients with paranoid thought patterns.

Projection process. A way in which fusion in a family is handled. Anxiety that occurs in the family is projected onto a child.

Promiscuity. A pattern of engaging in indiscriminate or multiple casual sexual encounters.

Promotion of health. Nursing activities that facilitate clients' patterns of interaction with the environment which contribute to more synchronous patterns of interaction.

Prophylactic activities. Activities designed to prevent disease or harmful events.

Protection. Ensuring safety.

Prototaxic mode. The mode of perception in which the self and the universe form an undifferentiated whole.

Proxemics. The study of space relationships during personal interactions.

Pseudodementia. A syndrome of cognitive and memory impairments that appear in the course of a functional psychiatric disorder such as depression; such impairments lead a diagnostician to believe that they are related to a neurologic disease.

Psychoanalysis. A treatment modality based on Freudian constructs; the analysis of the relationship that the client develops with the psychoanalyst.

Psychodrama. A structured, directed, and dramatized acting out of a client's personal, emotional, and interactional problems.

Psychodynamics. The theoretical assumption that present behavior is influenced by past experiences; the science of the mind, mental processes, and affective components that influence human behavior.

Psychogenic. Originating in the mind.

Psychological unavailability. A style of interacting with a significant other (such as a child or a dependent elderly person) in which the actor fails to recognize the other person as a dependent person with developmental or physical limitations; responsivity to verbal and nonverbal expressions of need is lacking, as is emotional warmth, sensitive personalized attention, and sociability.

Psychopathology. Morbidity of the mind; mental illness.

Psychosexual development. The maturation and development of the psychic phase of sexuality from birth to adult life.

Psychosis. A state in which a person's mental capacity to recognize reality, communicate, and relate to others is impaired, thus interfering with the person's capacity to deal with the demands of life.

Psychotic depression. A state of depression of great intensity, in which reality testing is impaired and physiological disturbances are pronounced.

Race. Biologically inherited characteristics that are observable as physical traits.

Rage. An engulfing experience of destroying and being destroyed.

Rallying around. Supportive family behavior manifested by frequent visiting, supplying of resources, and show of concern.

Rank. The position of a member relative to the evaluation of other members of the group.

Rape. An act of sexual intercourse (especially penile-vaginal contact) forced upon an unwilling victim.

Rationalization. An unconscious defense mechanism that is universally employed; an attempt to make one's behavior appear to be the result of logical thinking rather than of unconscious impulses or desires; utilized when a person has a sense of guilt or uncertainty about something that has been done; a face-saving device that may or may not deal with the truth. Rationalization relieves anxiety temporarily.

Reaction formation. An unconscious defense mechanism; it occurs when a person expresses an attitude that is directly opposite to unconscious feelings and wishes.

Reactive depression. A state of depression for which the precipitating stress or loss can be identified and seen to be of some magnitude.

Reality testing. A function of the ego involving distinguishing stimuli that are internally based (subjective) from those that are externally based (objective), and making objective evaluations of and judgments about the external environment.

Reconstructive group therapy. Group therapy based on exploration and analysis of both individual intrapsychic structures and group processes; the goal of such exploration is for permanent change to occur.

Referent power. Power based on the desire of the follower to identify with a charismatic leader.

Regression. A defense mechanism in which the ego returns to an earlier stage of development in thought, feeling, or behavior. Regression is a normal component of the developmental sequence and appears temporarily during times of stress, when it is utilized as a retreat from anxiety and conflict.

Regressive phase. The third phase of group therapy, characterized by regressive behavior of group members.

Rehabilitation of health. Nursing activities that interfere with a client's well-established patterns of dysfunction to facilitate the establishment of more functional patterns.

Reinforcement. A reward for a response.

Rejection. Refusal to acknowledge, accept, or consider a person or idea.

Relationship message. A message that conveys information about the relationship between the people sending messages; it occurs nonverbally.

Relatives' groups. Support system for relatives of mentally ill clients in which family burdens of stigma and guilt are addressed through a broad-based, inexpensive approach.

Representative power. Power that is delegated upward to a leader by a group; the group agrees to follow as long as the leader consults the followers and leads in the direction they want to go.

Repression. A widely used unconscious defense mechanism. Through repression, painful experiences, disagreeable memories, and unacceptable thoughts and impulses are barred from consciousness. Selfish, hostile, and sexual impulses are also usually repressed. A constant expenditure of energy is required to keep repressed material out of awareness; consequently, less energy is available for constructive activity.

Repressive-inspirational group therapy. Therapy that uses clients' present ego strengths and inspiration in order to help them repress problems more successfully than they have done in the past.

Rescue fantasy. An unrealistic belief in one's ability to help a client with his or her problem, save the client, or resolve the client's conflict.

Resentment. A feeling of indignation which is an outgrowth of unexpressed or unresolved anger at having been, in one's own perception, injured or unfairly treated.

Resistance. Active opposition to the uncovering of unconscious material.

Resolution. A phase in the development of a relationship during which the events that have occurred in the relationship are summarized.

Resonance phenomena. Mechanisms that perpetuate characteristic behavior in a family.

Respect. Communication of acceptance of another's ideas, feelings, and experiences. Recognition of another person's potential for self-actualization.

Responsibility. The obligation people have to perform an assigned or delegated task.

Restoration of health. Return of health status to previously experienced levels, through nursing activities.

Retirement. A complex process that involves withdrawing from a job and taking on the role of a nonworking person. The process affects the economy, the family, and individual people. Retirement may be an *event,* a rite of passage in which a person begins to deal with the opportunities and obligations of the retirement role; or a *role,* an obligation in which a person should use freedom of time and space and have physical, social, and financial independence and certainty about personal life goals.

"Revolving door" syndrome. A pattern whereby clients are repeatedly admitted to a health-care facility and discharged back to the community.

Revolving slate. An intergenerational balancing of what is owed or due to members of a family.

Reward power. Influence based on the perception that the leader has the power to reward followers in a satisfying manner.

Rhythms. Patterns of regularly recurring phenomena occurring within and between the person and the environment. There are exogenous and endogenous rhythms.

Right. A claim by an individual or group, made to another individual or group, that calls for the application of ethical principles or enlightened conscience and not necessarily legal rulings.

Ritual. An automatic activity of psychogenic or cultural origin.

Role. A culturally defined set of behavioral performances and expectations, with accompanying status.

Role blurring. The lack of clarity and consensus on role expectations and associated performance behaviors and qualities.

Role conflict. Incompatibility between two or more roles that a person is expected to perform in a given situation.

Role expectations. Those behaviors defined as appropriate, anticipated, and desired by self, others, and society.

Role internalization. The adoption of roles by people; the roles become a part of their self-concept.

Role model. A person who provides an example or standard for others to use in role performance.

Role-playing. A technique in family or group therapy in which members act out the parts of other members.

Role reversal. Exchange of assigned patterns of behavior and responsibility between two related people.

Role strain. Difficulty or stress in fulfilling the demands of required roles.

Rumination. Persistent thinking about and discussion of a particular subject.

Runaway. A child or adolescent who stays out of the home for at least 24 hours without the parents' consent or knowledge about whereabouts.

Sadism. Sexual pleasure and erotic gratification derived from the infliction of pain.

Satellite housing. A method of providing group homes with professional supervision.

Scalar chain. Vertical growth of an organization consisting of a number of levels of a hierarchy.

Scapegoat. A family or group member who acts out unconscious family issues and is perceived as "bad" or "sick" by the others.

Schizophrenic disorders. A group of psychotic disorders characterized by regression, thought disturbances (including delusions and hallucinations), bizarre dress and behavior, poverty of speech, abnormal motor behavior, ritualistic behavior, and withdrawal.

School phobia. A young child's sudden fear of attending school and refusal to go to school.

Sculpting. A technique in family therapy; family members arrange others as they perceive them relationally.

Secondary gain. The "fringe benefit" people derive from the environment as a result of their physical or emotional illness.

Secondary prevention. A form of prevention which aims to reduce the prevalence of disease through early case finding and effective treatment; secondary prevention places emphasis on referrals and appropriate health services, accessibility of services for clients, and rapid initiation of active treatment.

Security operation. A term used in interpersonal theory to denote those behaviors which are used to avoid or lessen anxiety; analogous to the terms *coping mechanism* and *defense mechanism.*

Selective inattention. A phenomenon in which, owing to heightened anxiety, a person is not aware of what is going on in situations peripheral to his or her immediate focus of attention.

Self. The body, body image, and nonbodily parts; a concept of one's own person as distinguished from other people or objects in the environment; the separate, whole person.

Self-actualization. Process of becoming everything one is capable of becoming.

Self-awareness. The recognition of one's own existence

and uniqueness and of the evaluations of others toward the self.

Self-concept. A perception of oneself that is a synthesis of perceptions, feelings, and beliefs. It includes characteristics, personality traits, and an evaluation of the worth of these traits. Achieving a self-concept is a developmental process and consists of self-system, personification, self-feelings, and self-awareness.

Self-determination. A person's control of decisions that influence his or her life.

Self-esteem. The degree to which one feels valued, worthwhile, or competent; the internal image of oneself formed by the interaction of one's bodily experiences with influential factors in the environment at a particular stage in one's life span.

Self-harm. Willful, painful injury to self without the intent of terminating life.

Self-image. What and who one thinks one is; the mental representation of self.

Self-mutilation. Destructive, disfiguring actions toward one's own body.

Self-system. An organization of experiences that exists to defend against anxiety and to secure necessary satisfaction. The total organization and integration of the self, comprising the interrelationships of organic, emotional, and social components.

Semidirect client services. Activities which facilitate the work of providers of direct client services. Nurses who work in semidirect service roles must themselves be expert care givers, since much of their job is to help providers of direct care in their work with challenging clients and to serve as role models.

Senile plaque. A patch of tissue on the wall of a cerebral blood vessel that has a central core of a degenerated neuron or its fibers; adhering to this core is an amyloid substance.

Sensorium. Consciousness; awareness of the environment.

Sensory deprivation. Lack of meaningful stimuli.

Sensory overload. Sensory input beyond the limits with which a person can adequately cope.

Sex therapy. The active treatment of sexual dysfunctions by a qualified therapist.

Sexual abuse. Assaultive and violent sexual contact and sexual exploitation.

Sexual dysfunction. A psychosomatic disorder which makes it impossible for a person to have or enjoy coitus; impotence and ejaculatory problems in the male; vaginismus, frigidity, or orgasmic dysfunction in the female.

Sexual intercourse. Oral-genital, anal-genital, and genital-genital stimulation. *Coitus* is the term used for vaginal-penile intercourse.

Sexuality. The culmination and coming together within a person of biological, psychological, spiritual, and cultural influences that result in a unique expression of the sexual aspect of self.

Short-term memory. Remembering of the recent past.

Sibling position. The place and role one learns and assumes in a family that is established by one's birth order, position, and sex.

Sibling rivalry. Competition among brothers and sisters.

Sick role. A set of institutional and societal expectations that people must meet when they are sick. The expectations are forfeiting decision making to professionals who know how to care for a sick person; tolerating any treatment without complaint, no matter how personal, invasive, or dehumanizing it may be; and abandoning the sick role as soon as possible.

Signal anxiety. Anxiety brought on by the anticipation of danger, by the feeling of being threatened.

Single-room-occupancy (SRO) dwellings. Room and bath facilities provided for clients. Clients are usually expected to vacate their rooms during the day.

Situational crises. Unanticipated or sudden external events in people's lives which threaten their biological, social, or psychosocial integrity.

Situational theory. A theory which states that the leader is in a position to institute change when a situation demands change or is ready for a change.

Social action. Measures taken by people using a community organization approach to address the needs of a specific disadvantaged segment of the population.

Social distance. The situationally defined distance beyond a personal "bubble" in which contact with others is allowed.

Social identity. The integrated self, developed by social labeling processes which classify the person within a societal context.

Social incompetence. The inability to live up to the norms expected for functioning and interpersonal relationships.

Social loss. Loss of all the valued social characteristics embodied in a dying patient.

Social pain of dying. The psychic pain caused by isolation of a dying person.

Social planning. A technical process used to solve problems related to specific major issues in a community; such a process is a community organization approach.

Societal regression. Emotional problems in society that are similar to the emotional problems in families.

Sociopathic personality. A client who engages in chronic antisocial behavior, fails to keep jobs, and often abuses drugs; also called *antisocial personality* or *psychopathic personality*.

Sodomy. Any sex act other than face-to-face coitus between a man and a woman; the legal meaning varies from state to state.

Somatic therapy. Treatment of an emotionally ill or incapacitated client by physiological means.

Somnambulism. Sleepwalking or motor activity during sleep, commonly seen in children.

Space. An invisible distance extending without limit in all directions within which all material things are contained.

Span of control. The number of people a manager can effectively supervise.

Spiritual assessment. A determination of a person's sense of meaning and purpose in life, sense of relatedness or belongingness, and status of giving and receiving forgiveness.

Spiritual dimension. The aspect of a person involving his or her ability to dream, to be aware of mortality, and to articulate and commit himself or herself to God or some power beyond the self.

Spiritual pain of dying. The psychic pain during the dying process caused by an inability to conceptualize the meaning of life within the dying person's belief system.

Splitting. A primitive psychological defense mechanism in which affects of opposite qualities are separated from each other. Its function is to prevent the "all good" object from being contaminated with the aggressive affect linked with the "all bad" object (or self); both states remain in consciousness, but they do not influence each other.

Staff. People who function to support those in the line organization. Staff personnel are usually not involved in decision making and do not command authority.

Stalls in communication. Blocks that are encountered by clients and nurses in their work together.

State anxiety. Anxiety brought on by a situation which is perceived as stressful and conflictual and over which a person feels the absence of control.

Status. The prestige attributed to particular people in a group; a collection of rights and duties is conferred upon those people which is specific for the status involved.

Stereotype. A simplistic picture of a cultural group.

Stereotyped behavior. Persistent mechanical repetition of speech or motor activity, commonly seen in schizophrenia. Examples include echolalia and echopraxia. Also called *stereotypy.*

Stigma. Feelings and thoughts associated with negative societal stereotypes concerning people with mental illness; a sign of disgrace.

Stress. A state of imbalance within an organism that is elicited by an actual or perceived disparity between environmental demands (stressors) and the organism's capacity to cope with these demands.

Stressor. A factor capable of eliciting a stress reaction in the body.

Structural organization. Family relationship patterns common to all families which are modified by the idiosyncrasies of each family according to its traditions, culture, and socioeconomic situation; such patterns are also adapted to meet the family's functional requirements.

Structuring. A term used to describe activities aimed at establishing a working partnership with a client.

"Styles of leadership" theory. A theory which states that forces within a group's leader, within group members, and within a situation in which the group is involved determine the amount of control a leader utilizes. Subcategories of leadership style include autocratic, paternalistic, collaborative, democratic, collegial, permissive, liberal, and laissez-faire.

Subculture. An entire group of people within a society who share values, beliefs, and behaviors that differ from those of the dominant culture.

Subgrouping. The formation of small cliques in which members find more satisfaction in the interaction among themselves than they find in the interaction with the group as a whole. Also called *clique formation.*

Sublimation. Transformation of psychic energy associated with unwanted sexual or aggressive drives into conscious, constructive activities. The activity or its object is changed, but the energy is nevertheless discharged.

Substitution. An unconscious defense mechanism involving the replacement of a highly valued, unacceptable object with a less valued object that is acceptable.

Subsystem boundaries. Limits which define people who can participate in subsystem functions and how they can accomplish the functions.

Suicide. Self-inflicted harm or endangerment which results in death.

Sundown syndrome. The diminishing of cognitive ability in late afternoon and evening that sometimes causes disorientation, confusion, and apathy.

Sunrise syndrome. Early-morning confusion that may be due to sleeplessness, insomnia, or the effects of sedatives or hypnotics.

Superego. The aspect of the personality that contains the rigid, absolute rules directing the person's thoughts, feelings, and actions. The superego is that part of the personality which is associated with internalized parental and societal controls (that is, standards, morals, and self-criticism).

Support groups. Groups of relatively healthy people who meet regularly to discuss specific problems that are common to all of them.

Supportive-educative interventions. Activities used in situations in which a client is able to or should learn to perform self-care but needs assistance such as support, guidance, provision of a developmental environment, or teaching.

Symbiosis. The close interdependence of two people to

the point where the psychic differentiation between them is blurred. Symbiosis is normal between infant and mother.

Symbiotic psychosis. A child's profound affective state of panic, regression, and delusion that occurs when there is separation from the mother.

Symbol. Anything that takes the place of, stands for, or refers to something or someone, created by arbitrary agreement or social custom.

Symptom. An objective or subjective manifestation of pathology.

Synchronous patterns of interaction. A term synonymous with *health* or *high-level wellness.*

Syntaxic mode. The mode of perception that forms whole, logical, coherent pictures of reality which can be validated by others.

Synthetic object image. Artificially created mental representation consisting of parts of objects that have coalesced into an image and are perceived as a whole object.

System. A complex of components in interaction; a group of people, issues, and feelings in interaction with one another; organized structures that influence and are influenced by the client.

Systems theory. A theory which stresses the interrelatedness and interdependency among elements of a specific whole.

Tardive dyskinesia. A side effect of drugs, characterized by bizarre facial and tongue movements, a stiff neck, and difficulty in swallowing.

Tavistock group. A form of group psychotherapy based upon the theory of Wilfred Bion; members examine unconscious group themes and particular ways in which members deal with group tension.

Team. A forum for psychiatrists, social workers, psychologists, nurses, and others to democratically share expertise and develop a comprehensive therapeutic plan of action for clients. A client may be considered a member of a team.

Temperance. Disciplined balance of all aspects of one's person and lifestyle.

Territoriality. A state characterized by possessiveness, control, and authority over an area of physical space.

Tertiary prevention. A form of prevention which aims to reduce, through rehabilitation, the disability associated with disease. Emphasis is placed on preparing clients and families for clients' discharge from institutions and return to communities.

Theoretical framework. Organization in which relationships among concepts are made very specific in theoretical statements, and in which relationships among those statements are also made specific.

Theory. The most advanced conceptualization of knowledge; a fully developed theoretical framework.

Therapeutic communication. The art and process of "touching" a person with messages designed to facilitate health.

Therapeutic community. A complex system which provides an effective environment for behavioral changes in clients through emphasis on their interpersonal functioning. The therapeutic community views illness as an interpersonal and social phenomenon.

Therapeutic nursing relationship. A goal-directed process that promotes synchronous patterns of interaction between the client and the environment.

Thyrotoxicosis. A condition characterized by hyperactivity of the thyroid gland.

Time. A conceptual experience; a way of perceiving the order of things. Time is sensed rather than defined both as motion (passing of time) and as duration (length of time).

Tolerance. The phenomenon occurring in drug or alcohol addiction where increasing amounts of the substance must be used in order to achieve the desired effects.

Trait anxiety. The overall amount of anxiety that a person characteristically experiences.

Trait theory. A theory which supports the notion that characteristics needed by a successful leader can be identified by studying the personality traits of established leaders.

Transaction. A communication sequence between two people consisting of a stimulus and a response.

Transactional analysis. A treatment modality developed by Eric Berne; it involves the analysis of communications between two people.

Transference. Unconscious phenomena in which the feelings, attitudes, and wishes originally linked with significant figures in one's early life are projected onto others who have come to represent these people in current life.

Triangle. An emotional configuration consisting of two people and a third person, an object, a group, or an issue. The triangle is a way of describing relational patterns among people.

Tumescence. The erectile process in the male.

Uncertainty phase. The first phase of group therapy, lasting up to 20 sessions, which is characterized by high anxiety.

Unconscious. Unremembered thoughts, feelings, actions, dreams, and experiences. It is very difficult to become conscious of this material.

Undoing. An unconscious defense mechanism whereby a person negates an act by behaving in a manner opposite to that which was done before.

Unintentional suicide. Self-induced termination of life in which the terminator fails to recognize the risk involved or does not mean to terminate life.

Vaginismus. Irregular and involuntary contraction of the muscles of the vagina whenever there is an attempt at coitus.

Validation. Interpersonal acknowledgement of another's experience; confirmation.

Value. A perspective or view of something or a way of looking at it. An action-oriented, productive, personal belief about the truth, beauty, or worth of a thought, object, or behavior.

Values. Measures of worth; system of individualized rules by which people live. Values govern and influence the way people behave.

Values clarification. An evolutionary process that fosters the making of choices and facilitates decision making about conflicting values by making one's own thoughts and priorities clear.

Value system. A set of priorities.

Vigilance. A state of watchfulness.

Violence. A physical or moral force; unjust strength or power applied to any purpose. Violent acts may be perpetrated deliberately, as in premeditated homicide, or they may occur because a person loses control over aggressive impulses.

Waxy flexibility *(cerea flexibilitas)*. A condition (found in catatonic schizophrenia) in which the extremities have a waxlike rigidity and will remain for long periods of time in any placed position, no matter how uncomfortable it may be.

Whole object image. An integrated mental representation of a person as having both "good" and "bad" aspects.

Wholly compensatory interventions. Activities used in situations in which a client has no active role; the nurse performs all required care measures, including activities of daily living. Such interventions compensate for the client's inability to engage in self-care and support the client in the recipient role.

Withdrawal. A person's pattern of facilitating escape from relatedness through physical and emotional distancing maneuvers.

Women's awareness groups. Therapy groups focused on teaching clients about issues of women's health.

Word salad. A form of speech in which words and phrases have no apparent meaning or logical connection.

Work group. A group that focuses on a task using rational, scientific methods of problem solving.

Zaleznik's executive-functions theory. A theory which states that executive functions are homeostatic, mediative, and proactive. *Homeostatic functions* are those which maintain the status quo. *Mediative functions* include conscious efforts to alter behavior and attitudes in response to environmental forces. *Proactive functions* are those which induce change by creatively employing resources.

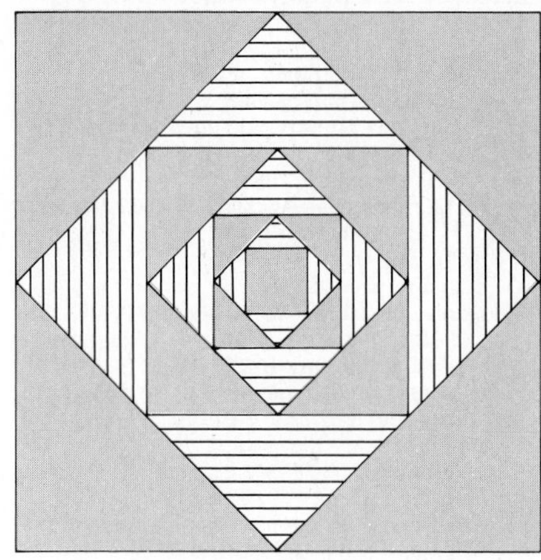

Index

Page numbers in *italic* indicate illustrations or tables.